The new ShopIngenix.com redesigned by an expert in the industry…

YOU.

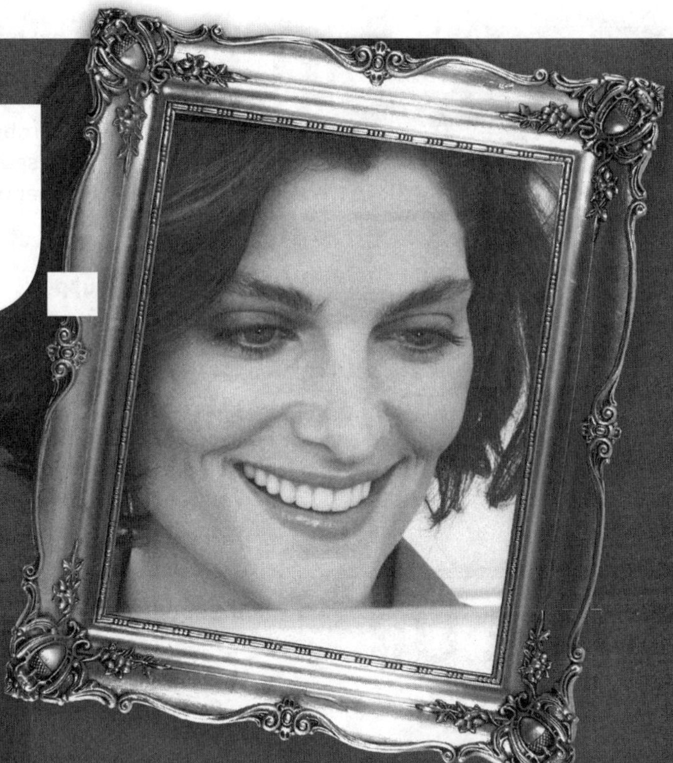

You asked.

We've answered.

Check out the new ShopIngenix.com

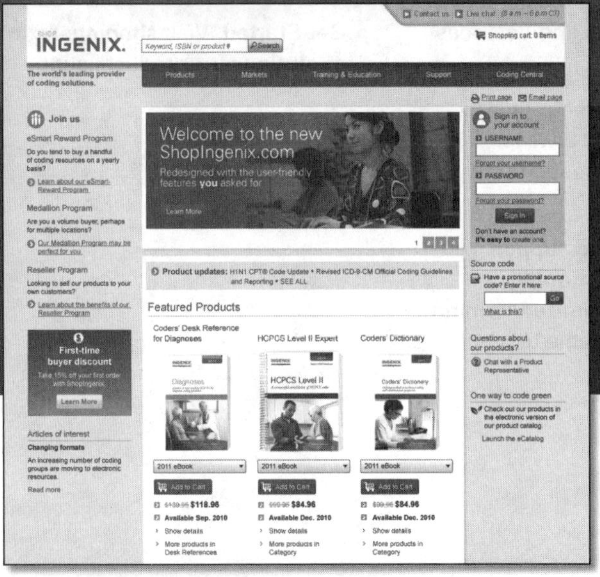

Redesigned with the user-friendly features **you** asked for, the new ShopIngenix.com is ready to make your online shopping a snap.

Log in for a fully customized web experience that includes your order history, shipment status and tracking, and invoice and payment history. You can pay outstanding invoices online, manage your address book, and get product recommendations based on your order history. But that's just the beginning. **Use source code FB11M to get 20% off your next ShopIngenix.com order.**

SHOP INGENIX®

www.shopingenix.com

www.shopingenix.com

INGENIX® *e*solutions

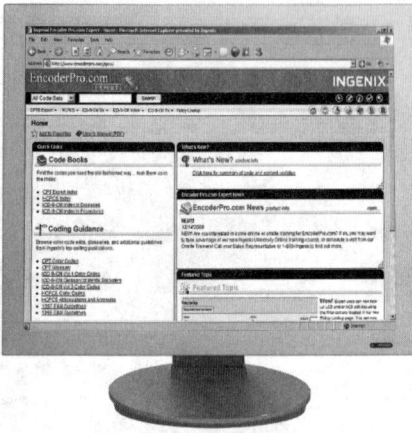

Electronic coding, billing and reimbursement products.

Ingenix provides a robust suite of eSolutions to solve a wide variety of coding, billing and reimbursement issues. As the industry moves to electronic products, you can rely on Ingenix to help support you through the transition.

← Web-based applications for all markets

← Dedicated support

← Environmentally responsible

Key Features and Benefits

Using eSolutions is a step in the right direction when it comes to streamlining your coding, billing and reimbursement practices. Ingenix eSolutions can help you save time and increase your efficiency with accurate and on-time content.

- **Simplify ICD-10 transition.** ICD-10 mapping tools provide crosswalks between ICD-9-CM and ICD-10 codes quickly and easily

- **Save time and money.** Ingenix eSolutions combine the content of over 37 code books and data files

- **Increase accuracy.** Electronic solutions are updated regularly so you know you're always working with the most current content available

- **Get the training and support you need.** Convenient, monthly webinars and customized training programs are available to meet your specific needs

- **Rely on a leader in health care.** Ingenix has been producing quality coding products for over 26 years. All of the expert content that goes into our books goes into our electronic resources

- **Get Started.** Visit **shopingenix.com/eSolutions** for product listing

SAVE UP TO 20%
with source code FB11B

 Visit **www.shopingenix.com** and enter the source code to save 20%.

 Call toll-free **1.800.INGENIX** (464.3649), option 1 and save 15%.

Ingenix | Information is the Lifeblood of Health Care | Call toll-free 1.800.INGENIX (464.3649), option 1.

100% Money Back Guarantee If our merchandise ever fails to meet your expectations, please contact our Customer Service Department toll-free at 1.800.INGENIX (464.3649), option 1, for an immediate response. Software: Credit will be granted for unopened packages only.

Also available from your medical bookstore or distributor.

| www.shopingenix.com |

INGENIX
2011 Essential Coding Resources

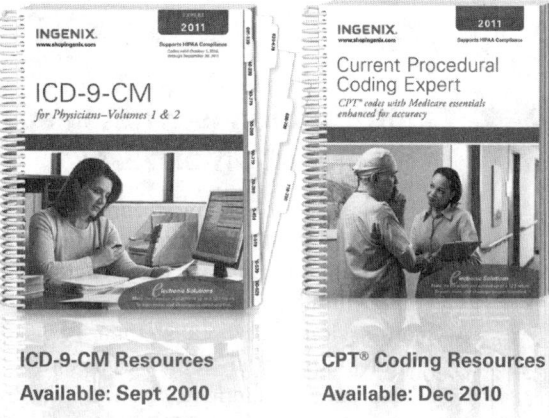

ICD-9-CM Resources
Available: Sept 2010

CPT® Coding Resources
Available: Dec 2010

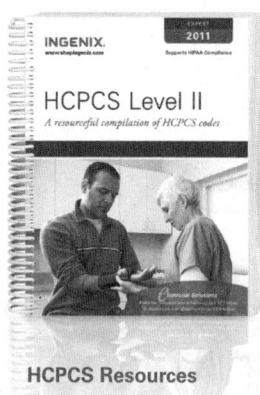

HCPCS Resources
Available: Dec 2010

SAVE UP TO 20%
with source code FB11D

 Visit **www.shopingenix.com** and enter the source code to save 20%.

 Call toll-free **1.800.INGENIX** (464.3649), option 1 and save 15%.

2011 Essential Coding Resources

Looks can be deceiving. Competitors attempt to imitate Ingenix code books because interpreting coding and reimbursement rules correctly and understanding the professional workflow is what we've helped coding professionals do successfully for over 25 years. Count on Ingenix to deliver accurate information, familiar features, industry-leading content, and innovative additions that help you improve coding practices, comply with HIPAA code set regulations, and realize proper reimbursement.

← A professional team's expertise
← Trusted and proven ICD-9-CM, CPT® and HCPCS coding resources
← Industry-leading content
← More value, competitive prices

Key Features and Benefits

Select from a range of formats for your ICD-9-CM, CPT,® and HCPCS coding resources to fit your individual preferences, skill level, business needs, and budget—you can trust your resource to be accurate and complimentary to your daily work when it's under an Ingenix cover.

2011 ICD-9-CM
Physician, Hospital, Home Health, and Skilled Nursing (with Inpatient Rehabilitation and Hospices) editions available

- New Look! Modified font and more vibrant colors increase readability
- New! Highlighted coding informational notes
- New! Snap-in tab dividers (*Expert* spiral editions only)
- More official coding tips and ICD-10 Spotlight codes
- Hallmark additional digit required symbols, intuitive color-coded symbols and alerts, QuickFlip™ color bleed tabs, dictionary headers, and symbol keys

2011 Current Procedural Coding Expert
- Code "Resequencing" identification
- Interventional radiology guidance section
- Reimbursement and mid-year changes information not found in the American Medical Association's CPT® code books
- Easy-to-navigate design
- Comprehensive and up-to-date listings with an extensive, user-friendly index
- PQRI icons and appendix

2011 HCPCS Level II Expert
- Comprehensive code updates for accurate reporting of supplies and services in physician, hospital outpatient, and ASC settings
- User-friendly format and expanded index to ease code look-up
- Important coding indicators and icons, PQRI icons, detailed illustrations, glossary of terms, and special MUEs

Ingenix | Information is the Lifeblood of Health Care | Call toll-free 1.800.INGENIX (464.3649), option 1.

100% Money Back Guarantee If our merchandise ever fails to meet your expectations, please contact our Customer Service Department toll-free at 1.800.INGENIX (464.3649), option 1, for an immediate response. Software: Credit will be granted for unopened packages only.

Also available from your medical bookstore or distributor. CPT is a registered trademark of the American Medical Association.   FB11D

www.shopingenix.com

INGENIX®
Coder Education

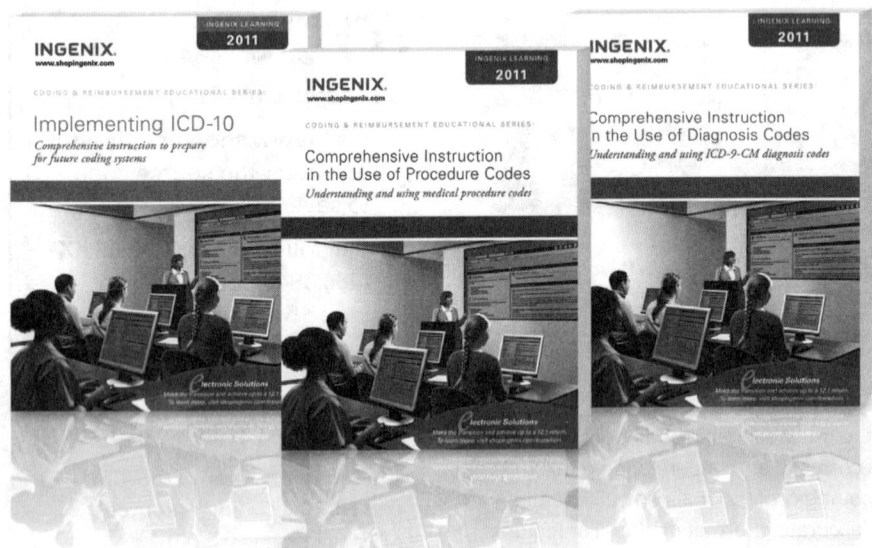

Information is what keeps an expert an expert.

Ingenix Coder Education Series provides comprehensive education and training programs that provide opportunities for health care professionals to increase their knowledge, enhance their skills and keep pace with industry trends. The result is a more capable workforce that enables health care organizations to continually improve their services.

← Convenient and self-paced

← Deep and diverse industry expertise

← Comprehensive coding curriculum

SAVE UP TO 20%
with source code FB11A

 Visit **www.shopingenix.com** and enter the source code to save 20%.

 Call toll-free **1.800.INGENIX (464.3649)**, option 1 and save 15%.

Key Features and Benefits

Ingenix Coder Education Series provides a robust curriculum with a variety of courses that focus on urgent coding and claims review training needs.

- **Satisfy your coding needs by creating your own coder.** Customized curriculum to meet your individual practice needs

- **Keep up-to-date with coding and regulatory changes.** Ingenix experts develop new content based on current guidelines and rules so you and your staff are always up-to-date and prepared in case of an audit

- **Streamline your revenue cycle with knowledgeable coding professionals.** Quickly reap the benefits of knowledgeable coding professionals: fewer denied claims, faster reimbursements and increased revenue

- **Save time and money.** Reduce overall training costs by eliminating travel expenses and reducing costs associated with instructor time and salary

For our full curriculum, visit Training and Education on www.shopingenix.com.

Ingenix | Information is the Lifeblood of Health Care | Call toll-free 1.800.INGENIX (464.3649), option 1.

100% Money Back Guarantee If our merchandise ever fails to meet your expectations, please contact our Customer Service Department toll-free at 1.800.INGENIX (464.3649), option 1, for an immediate response. Software: Credit will be granted for unopened packages only.

Also available from your medical bookstore or distributor.

FB11A

Are You Ready to Make a Successful Transition to ICD-10?

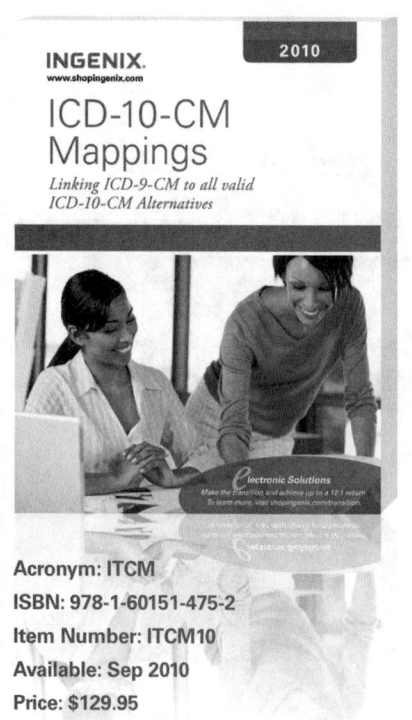

Acronym: ITCM
ISBN: 978-1-60151-475-2
Item Number: ITCM10
Available: Sep 2010
Price: $129.95

SAVE UP TO 20%
with source code FB11L

 Visit **www.shopingenix.com** and enter the source code to save 20%.

 Call toll-free **1.800.INGENIX** (464.3649), option 1 and save 15%.

2010 ICD-10-CM Mappings

It's not too early to start improving documentation habits now in preparation for increased documentation requirements under ICD-10. This new tool will help you focus your ICD-10 training without learning the entire code set. By mapping the most frequently used ICD-9-CM codes for your practice or facility to their corresponding ICD-10-CM codes, you can identify areas needing increased documentation and evaluate how additional specificity may impact your revenue.

← **Simplify your transition**

← **Get ready for future documentation and coding needs**

← **Verify code choices in the new code system**

Key Features and Benefits

Jump-start your implementation plan. Start improving documentation habits now in preparation for increased documentation requirements under ICD-10.

- Perform impact analysis to identify and focus on high priority coding issues. Using the ICD-9-CM codes you already know as your guide, you'll be able to quickly identify the ICD-10-CM codes that are pertinent to your office or facility and zero-in on codes to focus on for training and system transition

- Easily identify documentation issues

- Update super bills, forms, reports, and EHRs/PHRs that meet your specific clinical and coding criteria

- Verify software accuracy, evaluate new software, and assist in conversion planning

- Easy-to-use table format lists ICD-9-CM codes with titles and the corresponding ICD-10-CM codes with titles

Also available....
New ICD-10 Draft Code Set Resources

Ease into the new classification system with the most current and complete drafts of the official ICD-10 code sets. Redesigned with the familiar look and feel of an Ingenix ICD-9-CM code book with hallmark color and additional character required symbols.

ICD-10-CM & ICD-10-PCS versions available as printed code books or CD eBooks.

NEW Hallmark color coding and symbols

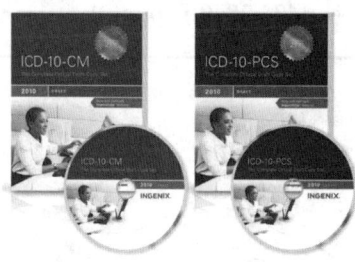

ICD-10-CM
Book
Item# ITEN10
Price: $99.95

eBook
Item# 1780
Price: $119.95

ICD-10-PCS
Book
Item# ITPC10
Price: $99.95

eBook
Item# 1781
Price: $119.95

Used by the AAPC for ICD-10 training

Ensure You're ICD-10 Prepared
For more information, updates on the final rule, and resources available from Ingenix to help guide your transition, visit the new *Coder's Corner* section on www.icd10prepared.com.

Also available from your medical bookstore or distributor.

www.shopingenix.com

INGENIX®

Create Your Own Package

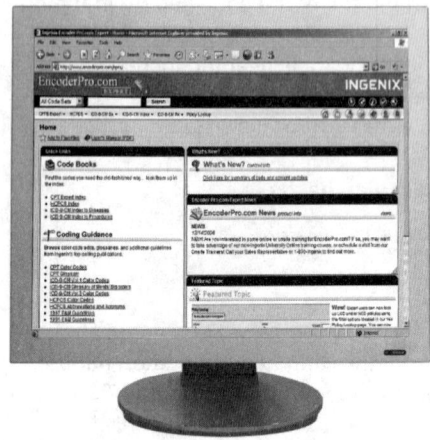

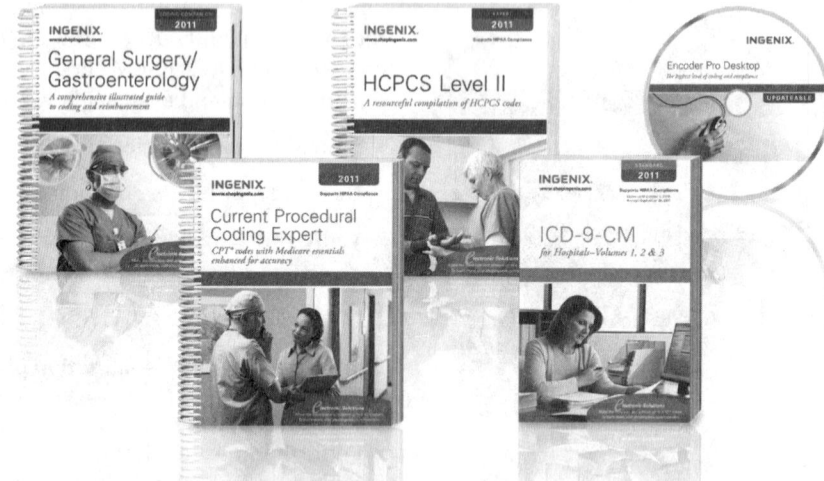

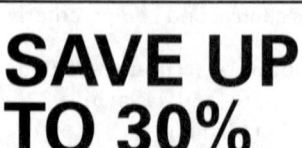

SAVE UP TO 30%

with source code **FB11E**

 Visit **www.shopingenix.com** and enter the source code to save up to 30%.

 Call toll-free **1.800.INGENIX** (464.3649), option 1.

Build your own coding library with the resources you need.

Ingenix resources are tailored to meet your specific needs. Now, you can combine the resources you want—nothing more, nothing less.

← Buy 2–3 items – save 20%

← Buy 4–5 items – save 25%

← Buy 6 or more – save 30%

Key Features and Benefits

Imagine how much time you could save if you could get to the code information you needed, faster. Our resources are designed to shave time off the coding process so you can work smarter, not harder. In addition, we have a dedicated team of experts who research changes in codes and regulations so our resources are updated with the most current information to help you stay compliant.

Buy more and save on the following product categories:

- 2011 Essential Code Books
- 2011 Specialty Reference
- 2011 Desk References
- Coding, Billing and Payment
- Training
- Electronic Resources

Visit **www.shopingenix.com/packages2** to determine what products apply.

Ingenix | Information is the Lifeblood of Health Care | Call toll-free 1.800.INGENIX (464.3649), option 1.

100% Money Back Guarantee If our merchandise ever fails to meet your expectations, please contact our Customer Service Department toll-free at 1.800.INGENIX (464.3649), option 1, for an immediate response. Software: Credit will be granted for unopened packages only.

Also available from your medical bookstore or distributor.

INGENIX®

Coding Companion for Orthopaedics—Upper: Spine & Above

A comprehensive illustrated guide to coding and reimbursement

2011

Publisher's Notice

Coding Companion for Orthopaedics —Upper: Spine & Above is designed to be an authoritative source of information about coding and reimbursement issues affecting orthopaedic procedures. Every effort has been made to verify accuracy and all information is believed reliable at the time of publication. Absolute accuracy cannot be guaranteed, however. This publication is made available with the understanding that the publisher is not engaged in rendering legal or other services that require a professional license. If you identify a correction or wish to share information, please email the Ingenix customer service department at customerservice@ingenix.com or fax us at 801.982.4033.

American Medical Association Notice

CPT codes, descriptions, and other material only copyright 2010 American Medical Association. All rights reserved.

Fee schedules, relative value units, conversion factors and/or related components are not assigned by the AMA, are not part of CPT, and the AMA is not recommending their use. The AMA does not directly or indirectly practice medicine or dispense medical services. The AMA assumes no liability for data contained or not contained herein.

CPT is a registered trademark of the American Medical Association.

The responsibility for the content of any "National Correct Coding Policy" included in this product is with the Centers for Medicare and Medicaid Services and no endorsement by the AMA is intended or should be implied. The AMA disclaims responsibility for any consequences or liability attributable to or related to any use, nonuse or interpretation of information contained in this product.

Copyright

Copyright 2010 Ingenix

All rights reserved. No part of this publication may be reproduced or transmitted in any form or by any means electronic or mechanical, including photocopy, recording, or storage in a database or retrieval system, without the prior written permission of the publisher.

Made in the USA

ISBN 978-1-60151-445-5

Acknowledgments

Kelly Armstrong, *Product Manager*
Karen Schmidt, BSN, *Technical Director*
Stacy Perry, *Manager, Desktop Publishing*
Lisa Singley, *Project Manager*
Jillian Harrington, MHA, CPC, CCS-P, *Clinical/Technical Editor*
Kelly V. Canter, BA, RHIT, CCS, *Clinical/Technical Editor*
Tracy Betzler, *Desktop Publishing Specialist*
Hope M. Dunn, *Desktop Publishing Specialist*
Toni Stewart, *Desktop Publishing Specialist*
Kimberli Turner, *Editor*

Our Commitment to Accuracy

Ingenix is committed to producing accurate and reliable materials.

To report corrections, please visit www.shopingenix.com/accuracy or email accuracy@ingenix.com. You can also reach customer service by calling 1.800.INGENIX (464.3649), option 1.

Technical Editors

Jillian Harrington, MHA, CPC, CPC-P, CPC-I, CCS-P, MHP

Ms. Harrington has more than 16 years of experience in the health care profession. She recently served as President and CEO of ComplyCode, a health care compliance consulting firm based in Binghamton, NY. She is the former Chief Compliance Officer and Chief Privacy Official of a large academic medical center, and also has extensive background in both the professional and technical components of CPT®/HCPCS and ICD-9-CM coding. She teaches CPT® coding and is an approved instructor of the Professional Medical Coding Curriculum, awarded by the American Academy of Professional Coders (AAPC). She has spoken frequently on health care compliance and health information management issues at regional and national professional conferences. She holds a Bachelor of Science degree in Health Care Administration from Empire State College and a Master of Science degree in Health Systems Administration from the Rochester Institute of Technology. She is a member of the American Academy of Professional Coders (AAPC) and a former member of their National Advisory Board, a member of the American Health Information Management Association (AHIMA) and the Health Care Compliance Association (HCCA), and is an associate of the American College of Healthcare Executives (ACHE).

Kelly V. Canter, BA, RHIT, CCS

Ms. Canter is a clinical/technical editor for Ingenix with expertise in hospital inpatient and outpatient coding and reimbursement; ambulatory surgery coding; and ICD-9-CM, CPT, and HCPCS coding. Ms. Canters' experience includes conducting coding audits and coding staff education, revenue cycle management, and concurrent review. Most recently she was responsible for auditing and compliance of a health information management services company. She is an active member of the American Health Information Management Association (AHIMA).

Contents

Getting Started with Coding Companion i
Integumentary..1
Nails..9
Repair..18
Destruction...53
General Musculoskeletal 55
Neck/Thorax...100
Spine...121
Shoulder...159
Humerus/Elbow..222
Forearm/Wrist..302
Hand/Fingers..409
Casts and Strapping 517
Endoscopy..530
Hemic..554
Spinal Nerves 557
Extracranial Nerves 597
Appendix..632
CCI Edits 669
Evaluation and Management 671
Index...691

Getting Started with Coding Companion

Coding Companion for Orthopaedics—Upper: Spine & Above is designed to be a guide to the specialty procedures classified in the CPT book. It is structured to help coders understand procedures and translate physician narrative into correct CPT codes by combining many clinical resources into one, easy-to-use source book.

The book also allows coders to validate the intended code selection by providing an easy-to-understand explanation of the procedure and associated conditions or indications for performing the various procedures. As a result, data quality and reimbursement will be improved by providing code-specific clinical information and helpful tips regarding the coding of procedures.

For ease of use, *Coding Companion* lists the CPT codes in ascending numeric order. Included in the code set are all surgery, radiology, laboratory, medicine, and evaluation and management (E/M) codes pertinent to the specialty. Each CPT code is followed by its official CPT code description.

Resequencing of CPT Codes

The American Medical Association (AMA) employed a resequenced numbering methodology beginning with *CPT 2010*. According to the AMA, there are instances where a new code is needed within an existing grouping of codes, but an unused code number is not available to keep the range sequential. In the instance where the existing codes were not changed or had only minimal changes, the AMA assigned a code out of numeric sequence with the other related codes being grouped together. The resequenced codes and their descriptions have been placed with their related codes, out of numeric sequence.

CPT codes within the Ingenix *Coding Companion* series display in their resequenced order. Resequenced codes are enclosed in brackets for easy identification.

Surgery Codes

A full page is dedicated to each surgical procedure or to a series of similar procedures. Following the specific CPT code and its narrative, you will find a combination of the following features. A sample is shown on page iv. The black boxes with numbers in them correspond to the information on the following page of the sample.

Supplies

Some payers may allow physicians to separately report drugs and other supplies when reporting the place of service as office or other nonfacility setting. Drugs and supplies are to be reported by the facility only when performed in a facility setting.

Appendix

Some CPT codes are presented in a less comprehensive format in the appendix.

Category II and III Codes and Descriptions

Category II codes, which are published January 1 and July 1 of each year, are supplemental tracking codes used for performance measurement only. They describe components usually included in an evaluation and management service or test results that are part of a laboratory test. Use of these codes is voluntary. However, they are not to be used in lieu of Category I codes. Category II codes will not be published in this book. Refer to your CPT book for code description.

In this section, we provide each Category III code appropriate to the specialty, with the official CPT code descriptions. The codes are presented in numeric order, and each code is followed by an easy-to-understand description of the Category III procedure.

These codes are temporary tracking codes to identify new and emerging technologies. This allows health care professionals to indicate emerging technologies, services, and procedures for clinical efficacy, utilization, and outcomes.

Radiology Codes and Descriptions

In this section, we provide each CPT radiology code appropriate to the specialty, with the official CPT code description. The codes are presented in numeric order, and each code is followed by an easy-to-understand lay description of the radiological procedure.

Remember that radiology codes have a technical and a professional component. When physicians do not own their own radiology equipment and send their patients to outside testing facilities, they should append modifier 26 to the radiology procedural code to indicate they performed only the professional component.

Pathology and Laboratory Codes and Descriptions

In this section, we provide each CPT pathology and laboratory code appropriate to the specialty, with the official CPT code description. The codes are presented in numeric order, and each code is followed by an easy-to-understand lay description of the pathology or laboratory procedure.

Medicine Codes and Descriptions

Some medicine codes are expanded into full-page formats, similar to the surgical codes. Only the codes that are directly related to the specialty will be included in this format; general codes that apply across many specialties might be in an appendix in the back of the book. In the appendix section, we provide additional CPT medicine codes appropriate to the specialty, with the official CPT code description. The codes are presented in numeric order, and each code is followed by an easy-to-understand lay description of the medicine service or procedure.

ICD-9-CM Coding System

This section provides a list of codes commonly reported by orthopedics.

CCI Edit Updates

The *Coding Companion* series includes the most up-to-date ICD-9-CM, CPT, and HCPCS codes available at print time. The codes in the Correct Coding Initiative (CCI) section are from version 16.3, the most current version available at press time. Ingenix maintains a website to accompany the *Coding Companions* series and posts updated CCI edits on this website so that current information is available before the next edition. The website address is www.shopingenix.com/NonProd/3709/.

Evaluation and Management

This resource provides documentation guidelines and tables showing evaluation and management (E/M) codes for different levels of care. The components that should be considered when selecting an E/M code are also indicated.

Index

A comprehensive index is provided so you can easily access the codes you seek. The index entries have several axes. You can look up a code by its procedural name, or by the diagnoses commonly associated with it. Codes are also indexed anatomically. For example:

23190   Ostectomy of scapula, partial (eg, superior medial angle)

could be found in the index under the following main terms:

Ostectomy
Scapula, 23190

Excision
Scapula
Ostectomy, 23190

Resequenced CPT Codes 2011

The following CPT codes are not found in numerical order in CPT or in the *Coding Companion* series. The full definition is given and the code that precedes the resequenced code is given to help you find the correct placement.

Code	Full Description	Follows Code
11045	Debridement, subcutaneous tissue (includes epidermis and dermis, if performed); each additional 20 sq cm, or part thereof (List separately in addition to code for primary procedure)	11042
11046	Debridement, muscle and/or fascia (includes epidermis, dermis, and subcutaneous tissue, if performed); each additional 20 sq cm, or part thereof (List separately in addition to code for primary procedure)	11043
11047	Debridement, bone (includes epidermis, dermis, subcutaneous tissue, muscle and/or fascia, if performed); each additional 20 sq cm, or part thereof (List separately in addition to code for primary procedure)	11044
21552	Excision, tumor, soft tissue of neck or anterior thorax, subcutaneous; 3 cm or greater	21555
21554	Excision, tumor, soft tissue of neck or anterior thorax, subfascial (eg, intramuscular); 5 cm or greater	21556
23071	Excision, tumor, soft tissue of shoulder area, subcutaneous; 3 cm or greater	23075
23073	Excision, tumor, soft tissue of shoulder area, subfascial (eg, intramuscular); 5 cm or greater	23076
24071	Excision, tumor, soft tissue of upper arm or elbow area, subcutaneous; 3 cm or greater	24075
24073	Excision, tumor, soft tissue of upper arm or elbow area, subfascial (eg, intramuscular); 5 cm or greater	24076
25071	Excision, tumor, soft tissue of forearm and/or wrist area, subcutaneous; 3 cm or greater	25075
25073	Excision, tumor, soft tissue of forearm and/or wrist area, subfascial (eg, intramuscular); 3 cm or greater	25076
26111	Excision, tumor or vascular malformation, soft tissue of hand or finger, subcutaneous; 1.5 cm or greater	26115
26113	Excision, tumor, soft tissue, or vascular malformation, of hand or finger, subfascial (eg, intramuscular); 1.5 cm or greater	26116
27043	Excision, tumor, soft tissue of pelvis and hip area, subcutaneous; 3 cm or greater	27047
27045	Excision, tumor, soft tissue of pelvis and hip area, subfascial (eg, intramuscular); 5 cm or greater	27048
27059	Radical resection of tumor (eg, malignant neoplasm), soft tissue of pelvis and hip area; 5 cm or greater	27049
27329	Radical resection of tumor (eg, malignant neoplasm), soft tissue of thigh or knee area; less than 5 cm	27360
27337	Excision, tumor, soft tissue of thigh or knee area, subcutaneous; 3 cm or greater	27327
27339	Excision, tumor, soft tissue of thigh or knee area, subfascial (eg, intramuscular); 5 cm or greater	27328
27632	Excision, tumor, soft tissue of leg or ankle area, subcutaneous; 3 cm or greater	27618
27634	Excision, tumor, soft tissue of leg or ankle area, subfascial (eg, intramuscular); 5 cm or greater	27619
28039	Excision, tumor, soft tissue of foot or toe, subcutaneous; 1.5 cm or greater	28043
28041	Excision, tumor, soft tissue of foot or toe, subfascial (eg, intramuscular); 1.5 cm or greater	28045
29914	Arthroscopy, hip, surgical; with femoroplasty (ie, treatment of cam lesion)	29863
29915	Arthroscopy, hip, surgical; with acetabuloplasty (ie, treatment of pincer lesion)	22914

Code	Full Description	Follows Code
29916	Arthroscopy, hip, surgical; with labral repair	22915
46220	Excision of single external papilla or tag, anus	46946
46320	Excision of thrombosed hemorrhoid, external	46230
46945	Hemorrhoidectomy, internal, by ligation other than rubber band; single hemorrhoid column/group	46221
46946	Hemorrhoidectomy, internal, by ligation other than rubber band; 2 or more hemorrhoid columns/groups	46945
46947	Hemorrhoidopexy (eg, for prolapsing internal hemorrhoids) by stapling	46762
51797	Voiding pressure studies, intra-abdominal (ie, rectal, gastric, intraperitoneal) (List separately in addition to code for primary procedure)	51729
80104	Drug screen, qualitative; multiple drug classes other than chromatographic method, each procedure	80101
82652	Vitamin D; 1, 25 dihydroxy, includes fraction(s), if performed	82306
87906	Infectious agent genotype analysis by nucleic acid (DNA or RNA); HIV-1, other region (eg, integrase, fusion)	87901
88177	Cytopathology, evaluation of fine needle aspirate; immediate cytohistologic study to determine adequacy for diagnosis, each separate additional evaluation episode, same site (List separately in addition to code for primary procedure)	88173
90665	Lyme disease vaccine, adult dosage, for intramuscular use	90668
95800	Sleep study, unattended, simultaneous recording; heart rate, oxygen saturation, respiratory analysis (eg, by airflow or peripheral arterial tone), and sleep time	95806
95801	Sleep study, unattended, simultaneous recording; minimum of heart rate, oxygen saturation, and respiratory analysis (eg, by airflow or peripheral arterial tone)	95800
99224	Subsequent observation care, per day, for the evaluation and management of a patient, which requires at least 2 of these 3 key components: Problem focused interval history; Problem focused examination; Medical decision making that is straightforward or of low complexity. Counseling and/or coordination of care with other providers or agencies are provided consistent with the nature of the problem(s) and the patient's and/or family's needs. Usually, the patient is stable, recovering, or improving. Physicians typically spend 15 minutes at the bedside and on the patient's hospital floor or unit	99220
99225	Subsequent observation care, per day, for the evaluation and management of a patient, which requires at least 2 of these 3 key components: An expanded problem focused interval history; An expanded problem focused examination; Medical decision making of moderate complexity. Counseling and/or coordination of care with other providers or agencies are provided consistent with the nature of the problem(s) and the patient's and/or family's needs. Usually, the patient is responding inadequately to therapy or has developed a minor complication. Physicians typically spend 25 minutes at the bedside and on the patient's hospital floor or unit	99224
99226	Subsequent observation care, per day, for the evaluation and management of a patient, which requires at least 2 of these 3 key components: A detailed interval history; A detailed examination; Medical decision making of high complexity. Counseling and/or coordination of care with other providers or agencies are provided consistent with the nature of the problem(s) and the patient's and/or family's needs. Usually, the patient is unstable or has developed a significant complication or a significant new problem. Physicians typically spend 35 minutes at the bedside and on the patient's hospital floor or unit	99225
0253T	Insertion of anterior segment aqueous drainage device, without extraocular reservoir; internal approach, into the suprachoroidal space	0191T

20680

20680 Removal of implant; deep (eg, buried wire, pin, screw, metal band, nail, rod or plate)

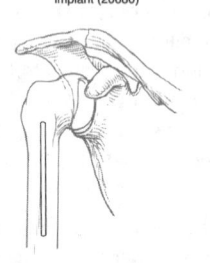

Example of a deep implant (20680)

Explanation

The physician makes an incision overlying the site of the implant. Deep dissection is carried down to visualize the implant, which is usually below the muscle level and within bone. The physician uses instruments to remove the implant from the bone. The incision is repaired in multiple layers using sutures, staples, and/or Steri-strips.

Coding Tips

This is a unilateral procedure. If performed bilaterally, some payers require that the service be reported twice with modifier 50 appended to the second code, while others require identification of the service only once with modifier 50 appended. Check with individual payers. Modifier 50 identifies a procedure performed identically on the opposite side of the body (mirror image). When 20680 is performed with another separately identifiable procedure, the highest dollar value code is listed as the primary procedure and subsequent procedures are appended with modifier 51. If two separate, unrelated incisions are performed to remove different implants, report 20680 twice and append modifier 59 to the second procedure. For removal of an implant, superficial, see 20670. Surgical trays, A4550, are not separately reimbursed by Medicare; however, other third-party payers may cover them. Check with the specific payer to determine coverage.

ICD-9-CM Procedural

- 78.60 Removal of implanted device, unspecified site
- 78.61 Removal of implanted device from scapula, clavicle, and thorax (ribs and sternum)
- 78.62 Removal of implanted device from humerus
- 78.63 Removal of implanted device from radius and ulna
- 78.64 Removal of implanted device from carpals and metacarpals
- 78.69 Removal of implanted device from other bone
- 80.02 Arthrotomy for removal of prosthesis without replacement, elbow
- 84.57 Removal of (cement) spacer

Anesthesia

20680 00600, 00620, 00630, 01120, 01170, 01630, 01740, 01830

ICD-9-CM Diagnostic

- 996.40 Unspecified mechanical complication of internal orthopedic device, implant, and graft — (Use additional code to identify prosthetic joint with mechanical complication, V43.60-V43.69)
- 996.49 Other mechanical complication of other internal orthopedic device, implant, and graft — (Use additional code to identify prosthetic joint with mechanical complication, V43.60-V43.69)
- 996.67 Infection and inflammatory reaction due to other internal orthopedic device, implant, and graft — (Use additional code to identify specified infections)
- 996.78 Other complications due to other internal orthopedic device, implant, and graft — (Use additional code to identify complication: 338.18-338.19, 338.28-338.29)
- V54.01 Encounter for removal of internal fixation device
- V54.10 Aftercare for healing traumatic fracture of arm, unspecified
- V54.11 Aftercare for healing traumatic fracture of upper arm
- V54.12 Aftercare for healing traumatic fracture of lower arm
- V54.19 Aftercare for healing traumatic fracture of other bone
- V54.20 Aftercare for healing pathologic fracture of arm, unspecified
- V54.21 Aftercare for healing pathologic fracture of upper arm
- V54.22 Aftercare for healing pathologic fracture of lower arm
- V54.29 Aftercare for healing pathologic fracture of other bone
- V54.81 Aftercare following joint replacement — (Use additional code to identify joint replacement site: V43.60-V43.69)
- V54.89 Other orthopedic aftercare
- V67.4 Treatment of healed fracture follow-up examination

Terms To Know

dissection. Separating by cutting tissue or body structures apart.

implant. Material or device inserted or placed within the body for therapeutic, reconstructive, or diagnostic purposes.

prosthesis. Man-made substitute for a missing body part.

CCI Version 16.3

0213T, 0216T, 0228T, 0230T, 11000, 11010✦, 11040-11044, 12001-12007, 12011-12057, 13100-13101, 13120-13121, 13131-13132, 13150-13152, 20526-20553, 24300, 25259, 26340, 27704✦, 29075, 29105-29125, 29345, 29405-29425, 29515, 29847✦, 36000, 36400-36410, 36420-36430, 36440, 36600, 36640, 37202, 43752, 51701-51703, 62310-62319, 64400-64435, 64445-64450, 64479, 64483, 64490, 64493, 64505-64530, 64708, 64714, 64718, 64722, 69990, 76000-76001, 93000-93010, 93040-93042, 93318, 94002, 94200, 94250, 94680-94690, 94770, 95812-95816, 95819, 95822, 95829, 95955, 96360, 96365, 96372, 96374-96376, 99148-99149, 99150, J0670, J2001

Note: These CCI edits are used for Medicare. Other payers may reimburse on codes listed above.

Medicare Edits

	Fac RVU	Non-Fac RVU	FUD	Assist
20680	11.03	15.41	90	80

Medicare References: 100-2,15,260; 100-4,12,30; 100-4,12,90.3; 100-4,14,10

1. CPT Codes and Descriptions
This edition of *Coding Companion* is updated with CPT codes for year 2011.

2. Illustrations
The illustrations that accompany the *Coding Companion* series provide coders a better understanding of the medical procedures referenced by the codes and data. The graphics offer coders a visual link between the technical language of the operative report and the cryptic descriptions accompanying the codes.

3. Explanation
Every CPT code or series of similar codes is presented with its official CPT code description. However, sometimes these descriptions do not provide the coder with sufficient information to make a proper code selection. In *Coding Companion,* you will find a step-by-step clinical description of the procedure, in simple terms. Technical language that might be used by the physician is included and defined. *Coding Companion* describes the most common method of performing each procedure.

4. Coding and Reimbursement Tips
Coding and reimbursement tips provide information on how the code should be used, provides related CPT codes, and offers help concerning common billing errors, modifier usage, and anesthesia. This information comes from consultants and technical editors at Ingenix and from the coding guidelines provided in the CPT book.

5. ICD-9-CM Procedural Codes
Volume 3 of ICD-9-CM lists procedural codes hospitals use in reporting charges to the government. In this field, we cross-referenced the CPT code to its corresponding ICD-9-CM Volume 3 code or codes.

6. Anesthesia Codes
The appropriate CPT anesthesia code(s) for the procedure being referenced is listed in this field. There are procedures, however, for which specific codes cannot be indicated, or anesthesia is already included in the surgery code. In these instances, the following abbreviated indicator appears in this field:

Not Applicable (N/A): Some procedures are performed without any type of anesthesia or are performed with a local anesthetic that, by CPT guideline definition of the global surgical package, is included with the surgery.

7. ICD-9-CM Diagnostic Codes
ICD-9-CM diagnostic codes listed are common diagnoses or reasons the procedure may be necessary. This list in most cases is inclusive to the specialty. In some cases, not every possible code is listed and the ICD-9-CM book should be referenced for other valid codes.

8. Terms to Know
Some codes are accompanied by general information pertinent to the procedure, labeled "Terms to Know." This information is not critical to code selection, but is a useful supplement to coders hoping to expand their knowledge of the specialty.

9. Correct Coding Initiative (CCI)
This section includes a list of codes from the official Centers for Medicare and Medicaid Services' National Correct Coding Policy Manual for Part B Medicare Contractors that are considered to be an integral part of the comprehensive code or mutually exclusive of it and should not be reported separately. Mutually exclusive codes are identified with an icon (❖).

To conserve space, we have listed codes in ranges whenever possible. The two codes listed and any codes that fall into the numeric sequence between the two codes listed, are considered part of the National CCI unbundle edit.

The *Coding Companion* includes the most up-to-date ICD-9-CM, CPT, and HCPCS codes. The codes in the CCI are from version 16.3 (10-1 through 12-31-10), the most current version available at press time. Ingenix maintains a website to accompany the *Coding Companions.* Ingenix posts updated CCI edits on this website so that current information is available before the next book update. The website address is www.shopingenix.com/NonProd/3709/

10. Medicare Information
Medicare edits are provided for most codes. These Medicare edits were current in November 2010.

Relative Value Units
In a resource based relative value scale (RBRVS), services are ranked based on the relative costs of the resources required to provide those services as opposed to the average fee for the service, or average prevailing Medicare charge. The Medicare RBRVS defines three distinct components affecting the value of each service or procedure:

- Physician work component, reflecting the physician's time and skill
- Practice expense (PE) component, reflecting the physician's rent, staff, supplies, equipment, and other overhead
- Malpractice insurance component, reflecting the relative risk or liability associated with the service

There are two RVUs listed for each CPT code. The first RVU is for nonfacilities (Non-fac Total), which includes services provided in physician offices, patients' homes, or other nonhospital settings. The second RVU is for facilities (Fac Total), which represents services provided in hospitals, ambulatory surgical centers, or skilled nursing facilities.

Medicare Follow-Up Days (FUD)
Information on the Medicare global period is provided here. The global period is the time following a surgery during which routine care by the physician is considered postoperative and included in the surgical fee. Office visits or other routine care related to the original surgery cannot be separately reported if they occur during the global period.

Medicare Assist at Surgery
Procedures with an N/A in this field are not allowed an assist at surgery. Procedures with a 80 in this field are allowed an assist at surgery without providing documentation to justify the assist. Procedures with a 80 in this field are allowed an assist at surgery with documentation. Payment for the assistant is equal to 16 percent of the global surgical procedure's allowable amount.

Medicare Official Regulatory Information

Medicare Official Regulatory Information provides official regulatory guidelines. Also known as the CMS Online Manual System, the Internet-only Manuals (IOM) contain official CMS information pertaining to program issuances, instructions, policies, and procedures based on statutes, regulations, guidelines, models, and directives. Ingenix has provided the reference for the surgery codes. The full text of guidelines can be found online at http://www.cms.gov/manuals.

11010-11012

11010 Debridement including removal of foreign material at the site of an open fracture and/or an open dislocation (eg, excisional debridement); skin and subcutaneous tissues
11011 skin, subcutaneous tissue, muscle fascia, and muscle
11012 skin, subcutaneous tissue, muscle fascia, muscle, and bone

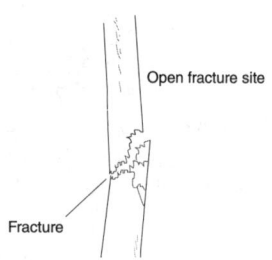

Explanation
The physician surgically removes foreign matter and contaminated or devitalized skin and other tissue in and around the site of an open fracture or open dislocation. Debridement reported with this service includes prolonged cleansing of the wound; removal of all foreign or dead tissue or material using forceps, scissors, scalpel, or other instruments; exploration of all injured soft tissue, including tendons, ligaments, and nerves; and irrigation of all tissue layers. Contamination of a wound by foreign matter is typically associated with open fractures; this excisional debridement is done in preparation for treating the fracture, to reduce swelling and bleeding, and to leave behind viable tissue. Report 11010 for debridement of skin and subcutaneous tissue; 11011 for debridement of skin, subcutaneous tissue, muscle fascia, and muscle; and 11012 for debridement of skin, subcutaneous tissue, muscle fascia, muscle, and bone.

Coding Tips
These codes have been revised for 2011 in the official CPT description. Debridement associated with open fractures and/or dislocations may be reported separately when gross contamination requires prolonged cleansing and removal of appreciable amounts of devitalized or contaminated tissue. When debridement is performed with another separately identifiable procedure, the highest dollar value code is listed as the primary procedure and subsequent procedures are appended with modifier 51. For debridement of skin, subcutaneous tissue, muscle, and bone not associated with an open fracture/dislocation, see 11042–11047. Surgical trays, A4550, are not separately reimbursed by Medicare; however, other third-party payers may cover them. Check with the specific payer to determine coverage.

ICD-9-CM Procedural
- 79.60 Debridement of open fracture, unspecified site
- 79.61 Debridement of open fracture of humerus
- 79.62 Debridement of open fracture of radius and ulna
- 79.63 Debridement of open fracture of carpals and metacarpals
- 79.64 Debridement of open fracture of phalanges of hand
- 79.69 Debridement of open fracture of other specified bone, except facial bones

Anesthesia
11010 00300, 00400
11011 00300, 00400, 01170, 01610, 01710, 01810
11012 00300, 00400, 00450, 00470, 01120, 01170, 01630, 01740, 01830

ICD-9-CM Diagnostic
- 810.11 Open fracture of sternal end of clavicle
- 810.12 Open fracture of shaft of clavicle
- 810.13 Open fracture of acromial end of clavicle
- 811.11 Open fracture of acromial process of scapula
- 811.12 Open fracture of coracoid process
- 811.13 Open fracture of glenoid cavity and neck of scapula
- 812.11 Open fracture of surgical neck of humerus
- 812.12 Open fracture of anatomical neck of humerus
- 812.13 Open fracture of greater tuberosity of humerus
- 812.19 Other open fracture of upper end of humerus
- 812.31 Open fracture of shaft of humerus
- 812.51 Open fracture of supracondylar humerus
- 812.52 Open fracture of lateral condyle of humerus
- 812.53 Open fracture of medial condyle of humerus
- 813.11 Open fracture of olecranon process of ulna
- 813.12 Open fracture of coronoid process of ulna
- 813.13 Open Monteggia's fracture
- 813.15 Open fracture of head of radius
- 813.18 Open fracture of radius with ulna, upper end (any part)
- 813.31 Open fracture of shaft of radius (alone)
- 813.32 Open fracture of shaft of ulna (alone)
- 813.33 Open fracture of shaft of radius with ulna
- 813.51 Open Colles' fracture
- 813.53 Open fracture of distal end of ulna (alone)
- 813.54 Open fracture of lower end of radius with ulna
- 815.11 Open fracture of base of thumb (first) metacarpal bone(s)
- 815.13 Open fracture of shaft of metacarpal bone(s)
- 815.14 Open fracture of neck of metacarpal bone(s)
- 816.11 Open fracture of middle or proximal phalanx or phalanges of hand
- 816.12 Open fracture of distal phalanx or phalanges of hand

Terms To Know
debridement. Removal of dead or contaminated tissue and foreign matter from a wound.

subcutaneous. Below the skin.

CCI
Due to the excessive number of CCI edits associated with this code range, a complete listing may be found in the CCI Edits section at the back of this book.

Medicare Edits

	Fac RVU	Non-Fac RVU	FUD	Assist
11010	8.23	13.89	10	N/A
11011	8.84	15.25	0	N/A
11012	12.63	20.45	0	N/A

Medicare References: 100-2,15,260; 100-4,12,30; 100-4,12,90.3; 100-4,14,10

11042 (11045)

11042 Debridement, subcutaneous tissue (includes epidermis and dermis, if performed); first 20 sq cm or less

11045 each additional 20 sq cm, or part thereof (List separately in addition to code for primary procedure)

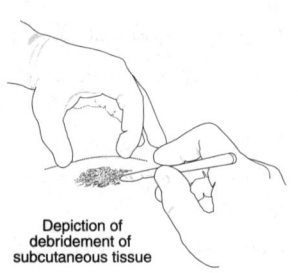

Depiction of debridement of subcutaneous tissue

Explanation

The physician surgically removes foreign matter and contaminated or devitalized subcutaneous tissue (including epidermis and dermis, if performed) caused by injury, infection, wounds (excluding burn wounds), or chronic ulcers. Using a scalpel or dermatome, the physician excises the affected subcutaneous tissue until viable, bleeding tissue is encountered. A topical antibiotic is placed on the wound. A gauze dressing or an occlusive dressing may be placed over the surgical site. Report 11042 for the first 20 sq cm or less and 11045 for each additional 20 sq cm or part thereof.

Coding Tips

Code 11042 has been revised for 2011 in the official CPT description. Code 11045 is new for 2011. It is a resequenced code and will not display in numeric order. As an "add-on" code, 11045 is not subject to multiple procedure rules. No reimbursement reduction or modifier 51 is applied. Add-on codes describe additional intra-service work associated with the primary procedure. They are performed by the same physician on the same date of service as the primary service/procedure, and must never be reported as a stand-alone code. Report 11045 in conjunction with 11042. When reporting debridement of a single wound, the deepest level of tissue removed determines the correct code. The debridement of multiple wounds at the same tissue level may be added together to determine the appropriate code. Different tissue depths should not be added together for code selection. According to the AMA, the debridement of skin (epidermis/dermis) is reported with the codes describing active wound care management (97597 or 97598). Surgical trays, A4550, are not separately reimbursed by Medicare; however, other third-party payers may cover them. Check with the specific payer to determine coverage.

ICD-9-CM Procedural

83.39 Excision of lesion of other soft tissue
86.22 Excisional debridement of wound, infection, or burn

Anesthesia

11042 00300, 00400
11045 N/A

ICD-9-CM Diagnostic

The application of this code is too broad to adequately present ICD-9-CM diagnostic code links here. Refer to your ICD-9-CM book.

Terms To Know

debridement. Removal of dead or contaminated tissue and foreign matter from a wound.

dermis. Skin layer found under the epidermis that contains a papillary upper layer and the deep reticular layer of collagen, vascular bed, and nerves.

devitalized. Deprivation of vital necessities or of life itself.

dressing. Material applied to a wound or surgical site for protection, absorption, or drainage of the area.

epidermis. Outermost, nonvascular layer of skin that contains four to five differentiated layers depending on its body location: stratum corneum, lucidum, granulosum, spinosum, and basale.

excision. Surgical removal of an organ or tissue.

subcutaneous. Below the skin.

ulcer. Open sore or excavating lesion of skin or the tissue on the surface of an organ from the sloughing of chronically inflamed and necrosing tissue.

CCI Version 16.3

0183T, 0213T, 0216T, 0228T, 0230T, 10060-10061, 11000, 11010-11012❖, 11100, 11719-11721, 15852, 17250, 20551-20553, 24300, 25001❖, 28289❖, 29086, 29125, 29445, 29515, 29540-29581, 35761, 36000, 36400-36410, 36420-36430, 36440, 36600, 36640, 37202, 43752, 49000, 51701-51703, 62310-62319, 64400-64435, 64445-64450, 64479, 64483, 64490, 64493, 64505-64530, 69990, 75710, 76000-76001, 93000-93010, 93040-93042, 93318, 94002, 94200, 94250, 94680-94690, 94770, 95812-95816, 95819, 95822, 95829, 95955, 96360, 96365, 96372, 96374-96376, 97597-97598, 97602, 99148-99149, 99150, G0168, J2001

Also not with 11042: 10060, 11010-11011❖, 11040-11041, 20526, 25259, 26340, 29131, 29280, 29365-29425, 29700, 29730, 64505-64553, 64565, 72295, 97022

Note: These CCI edits are used for Medicare. Other payers may reimburse on codes listed above.

Medicare Edits

	Fac RVU	Non-Fac RVU	FUD	Assist
11042	1.4	2.56	0	N/A
11045	0.53	0.91	N/A	80

Medicare References: 100-2,15,260; 100-4,12,30; 100-4,12,90.3; 100-4,14,10

11043 (11046)

11043 Debridement, muscle and/or fascia (includes epidermis, dermis, and subcutaneous tissue, if performed); first 20 sq cm or less

11046 each additional 20 sq cm, or part thereof (List separately in addition to code for primary procedure)

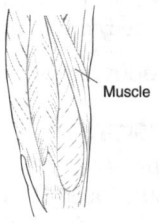

A debridement into the muscle

Explanation
The physician surgically removes necrotic muscle and/or fascia, including epidermis, dermis, and subcutaneous tissue, if performed. The physician uses a scalpel to excise the affected tissue into the muscle layer. The dissection is continued until viable, bleeding tissue is encountered. Depending on wound size, closure may be immediate or delayed. The wound may be packed open with gauze and require immediate or delayed reconstruction. Report 11043 for the first 20 sq cm or less and 11046 for each additional 20 sq cm or part thereof.

Coding Tips
Code 11043 has been revised for 2011 in the official CPT description. Code 11046 is new for 2011. It is a resequenced code and will not display in numeric order. As an "add-on" code, 11046 is not subject to multiple procedure rules. No reimbursement reduction or modifier 51 is applied. Add-on codes describe additional intra-service work associated with the primary procedure. They are performed by the same physician on the same date of service as the primary service/procedure, and must never be reported as a stand-alone code. Report 11046 in conjunction with 11043. When reporting debridement of a single wound, the deepest level of tissue removed determines the correct code. The debridement of multiple wounds at the same tissue level may be added together to determine the appropriate code. Different tissue depths should not be added together for code selection. According to the AMA, the debridement of skin (epidermis/dermis) is reported with the codes describing active wound care management (97597 or 97598). Surgical trays, A4550, are not separately reimbursed by Medicare; however, other third-party payers may cover them. Check with the specific payer to determine coverage.

ICD-9-CM Procedural
- 82.36 Other myectomy of hand
- 83.39 Excision of lesion of other soft tissue
- 83.45 Other myectomy
- 86.22 Excisional debridement of wound, infection, or burn

Anesthesia
11043 00300, 00400, 01610, 01710, 01810
11046 N/A

ICD-9-CM Diagnostic
The application of this code is too broad to adequately present ICD-9-CM diagnostic code links here. Refer to your ICD-9-CM book.

Terms To Know
debridement. Removal of dead or contaminated tissue and foreign matter from a wound.

dermis. Skin layer found under the epidermis that contains a papillary upper layer and the deep reticular layer of collagen, vascular bed, and nerves.

dressing. Material applied to a wound or surgical site for protection, absorption, or drainage of the area.

epidermis. Outermost, nonvascular layer of skin that contains four to five differentiated layers depending on its body location: stratum corneum, lucidum, granulosum, spinosum, and basale.

excision. Surgical removal of an organ or tissue.

fascia. Fibrous sheet or band of tissue that envelops organs, muscles, and groupings of muscles.

muscle tissue. Network of specialized cells for performing contraction to produce voluntary or involuntary movement of body parts, and skeletal, cardiac, or visceral muscles.

necrotic. Pathological condition of death occurring in a group of cells or tissues within a living part or organism.

reconstruction. Recreating, restoring, or rebuilding a body part or organ.

CCI Version 16.3
0183T, 0213T, 0216T, 0228T, 0230T, 10060-10061, 11000, 11010-11012❖, 11100, 11719-11721, 15852, 17250, 20551-20553, 24300, 25001❖, 28289❖, 29086, 29125, 29445, 29515, 36000, 36400-36410, 36420-36430, 36440, 36600, 36640, 37202, 43752, 51701-51703, 62310-62319, 64400-64435, 64445-64450, 64479, 64483, 64490, 64493, 64505-64530, 69990, 75710, 93000-93010, 93040-93042, 93318, 94002, 94200, 94250, 94680-94690, 94770, 95812-95816, 95819, 95822, 95829, 95955, 96360, 96365, 96372, 96374-96376, 97597-97598, 97602, 99148-99149, 99150, G0168, J2001

Also not with 11043: 11040-11042, 12002, 12011, 29405-29425, 29540-29581, 35741-35761, 49000, 64712, 75820, 76000-76001, G0127

Note: These CCI edits are used for Medicare. Other payers may reimburse on codes listed above.

Medicare Edits

	Fac RVU	Non-Fac RVU	FUD	Assist
11043	3.61	5.63	0	N/A
11046	1.13	1.59	N/A	80

Medicare References: 100-2,15,260; 100-4,12,30; 100-4,12,90.3; 100-4,14,10

11044 (11047)

11044 Debridement, bone (includes epidermis, dermis, subcutaneous tissue, muscle and/or fascia, if performed); first 20 sq cm or less

11047 each additional 20 sq cm, or part thereof (List separately in addition to code for primary procedure)

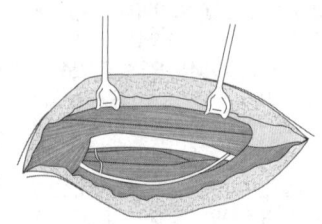
Debridement into the bone

Explanation
The physician surgically removes foreign matter and contaminated or devitalized bone (including epidermis, dermis, subcutaneous tissue, muscle, and/or fascia, if performed) caused by injury, infection, wounds (excluding burn wounds), or chronic ulcers. The physician uses a scalpel to excise the affected tissues into the bone. Depending on wound size, closure may be immediate or delayed. The wound may be packed open with gauze and require immediate or delayed reconstruction. Report 11044 for the first 20 sq cm or less and 11047 for each additional 20 sq cm or part thereof.

Coding Tips
Code 11044 has been revised for 2011 in the official CPT description. Code 11047 is new for 2011. It is a resequenced code and will not display in numeric order. As an "add-on" code, 11047 is not subject to multiple procedure rules. No reimbursement reduction or modifier 51 is applied. Add-on codes describe additional intra-service work associated with the primary procedure. They are performed by the same physician on the same date of service as the primary service/procedure, and must never be reported as a stand-alone code. Report 11047 in conjunction with 11044. When reporting debridement of a single wound, the deepest level of tissue removed determines the correct code. The debridement of multiple wounds at the same tissue level may be added together to determine the appropriate code. Different tissue depths should not be added together for code selection. According to the AMA, the debridement of skin (epidermis/dermis) is reported with the codes describing active wound care management (97597 or 97598). Surgical trays, A4550, are not separately reimbursed by Medicare; however, other third-party payers may cover them. Check with the specific payer to determine coverage.

ICD-9-CM Procedural
- 77.60 Local excision of lesion or tissue of bone, unspecified site
- 77.61 Local excision of lesion or tissue of scapula, clavicle, and thorax (ribs and sternum)
- 77.62 Local excision of lesion or tissue of humerus
- 77.63 Local excision of lesion or tissue of radius and ulna
- 77.64 Local excision of lesion or tissue of carpals and metacarpals
- 77.69 Local excision of lesion or tissue of other bone, except facial bones
- 82.36 Other myectomy of hand
- 83.39 Excision of lesion of other soft tissue
- 83.45 Other myectomy
- 86.22 Excisional debridement of wound, infection, or burn

Anesthesia
11044 00450, 00470, 01120, 01170, 01630, 01740, 01742, 01830
11047 N/A

ICD-9-CM Diagnostic
The application of this code is too broad to adequately present ICD-9-CM diagnostic code links here. Refer to your ICD-9-CM book.

Terms To Know
closure. Repairing an incision or wound by suture or other means.

debridement. Removal of dead or contaminated tissue and foreign matter from a wound.

dermis. Skin layer found under the epidermis that contains a papillary upper layer and the deep reticular layer of collagen, vascular bed, and nerves.

epidermis. Outermost, nonvascular layer of skin that contains four to five differentiated layers depending on its body location: stratum corneum, lucidum, granulosum, spinosum, and basale.

fascia. Fibrous sheet or band of tissue that envelops organs, muscles, and groupings of muscles.

infection. Presence of microorganisms in body tissues that may result in cellular damage.

muscle tissue. Network of specialized cells for performing contraction to produce voluntary or involuntary movement of body parts, and skeletal, cardiac, or visceral muscles.

reconstruction. Recreating, restoring, or rebuilding a body part or organ.

subcutaneous. Below the skin.

CCI Version 16.3
Also not with 11044: 0183T, 0213T, 0216T, 0228T, 0230T, 10060-10061, 11000, 11010-11012❖, 11040-11043, 11100, 11719-11721, 12001-12005, 12013, 12021-12032, 12042, 12052, 15852, 17250, 20551-20553, 24300, 25001❖, 28289❖, 29086, 29125, 29130, 29445, 29515, 29580-29581, 35761, 36000, 36400-36410, 36420-36430, 36440, 36600, 36640, 37202, 43752, 51701-51703, 62310-62319, 64400-64435, 64445-64450, 64479, 64483, 64490, 64493, 64505-64530, 64718, 69990, 75710, 75716, 93000-93010, 93040-93042, 93318, 94002, 94200, 94250, 94680-94690, 94770, 95812-95816, 95819, 95822, 95829, 95955, 96360, 96365, 96372, 96374-96376, 97597-97598, 97602, 99148-99149, 99150, G0168, J2001

Note: These CCI edits are used for Medicare. Other payers may reimburse on codes listed above.

Medicare Edits

	Fac RVU	Non-Fac RVU	FUD	Assist
11044	6.25	8.56	0	N/A
11047	1.96	2.61	N/A	80

Medicare References: 100-2,15,260; 100-4,12,30; 100-4,12,90.3; 100-4,14,10

11400-11406

11400 Excision, benign lesion including margins, except skin tag (unless listed elsewhere), trunk, arms or legs; excised diameter 0.5 cm or less
11401 excised diameter 0.6 to 1.0 cm
11402 excised diameter 1.1 to 2.0 cm
11403 excised diameter 2.1 to 3.0 cm
11404 excised diameter 3.1 to 4.0 cm
11406 excised diameter over 4.0 cm

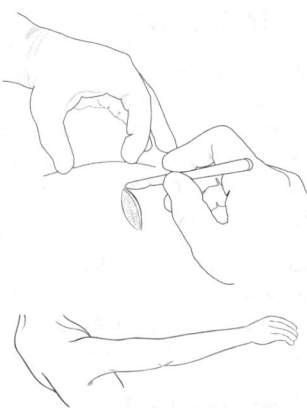

Codes 11400 through 11406 report excisions of benign lesions that occur on the arms (and elsewhere) and are reported according to the diameter of the excision. Report 11400 for excisions 0.5 cm or less; 11401 for excisions 0.6 to 1.0 cm; 11402 for excisions 1.1 to 2.0 cm; 11403 for excisions 2.1 to 3.0 cm; 11404 for excisions 3.1 to 4.0 cm; and 11406 for excisions greater than 4.0 cm in diameter

Explanation

The physician excises a benign (noncancerous) lesion, including the margins, except a skin tag, on the trunk, or arms. After administering a local anesthetic, the physician makes a full-thickness incision through the dermis with a scalpel, usually in an elliptical shape around and under the lesion, and removes it. The physician may suture the wound simply. Complex or layered closure is reported separately, if required. Report 11400 for an excised diameter 0.5 cm or less; 11401 for 0.6 cm to 1 cm; 11402 for 1.1 cm to 2 cm; 11403 for 2.1 cm to 3 cm; 11404 for 3.1 cm to 4 cm; and 11406 if the excised diameter is greater than 4 cm.

Coding Tips

Prior to local infiltration, clinical lesion diameter is determined by measurement at the greatest diameter of the lesion plus the narrowest margins required for adequate removal of the entire lesion. Excision of a benign lesion requires a full-thickness incision and removal of the lesion. Local anesthesia is included in the service. It includes simple (non-layered) repair of the skin and/or subcutaneous tissues. If intermediate repair involving layered closure of deeper subcutaneous or non-muscle fascia is required, it is reported separately. For excision of a malignant lesion, see 11600–11606. Surgical trays, A4550, are not separately reimbursed by Medicare; however, other third-party payers may cover them. Check with the specific payer to determine coverage.

ICD-9-CM Procedural

86.3 Other local excision or destruction of lesion or tissue of skin and subcutaneous tissue

Anesthesia
00300, 00400

ICD-9-CM Diagnostic

214.1 Lipoma of other skin and subcutaneous tissue
216.5 Benign neoplasm of skin of trunk, except scrotum
216.6 Benign neoplasm of skin of upper limb, including shoulder
228.01 Hemangioma of skin and subcutaneous tissue
238.2 Neoplasm of uncertain behavior of skin
239.2 Neoplasms of unspecified nature of bone, soft tissue, and skin
448.1 Nevus, non-neoplastic
686.1 Pyogenic granuloma of skin and subcutaneous tissue — (Use additional code to identify any infectious organism: 041.0-041.8)
701.1 Acquired keratoderma
701.3 Striae atrophicae
701.4 Keloid scar
701.5 Other abnormal granulation tissue
702.11 Inflamed seborrheic keratosis
702.19 Other seborrheic keratosis
706.2 Sebaceous cyst
709.01 Vitiligo
709.09 Other dyschromia
709.1 Vascular disorder of skin
709.2 Scar condition and fibrosis of skin
709.4 Foreign body granuloma of skin and subcutaneous tissue — (Use additional code to identify foreign body (V90.01-V90.9))
757.32 Congenital vascular hamartomas

Terms To Know

benign. Mild or nonmalignant in nature.

excision. Surgical removal of an organ or tissue.

hemangioma. Benign neoplasm arising from vascular tissue or malformations of vascular structures. It is most commonly seen in children and infants as a tumor of newly formed blood vessels due to malformed fetal angioblastic tissues.

lipoma. Benign tumor containing fat cells and the most common of soft tissue lesions, which are usually painless and asymptomatic, with the exception of an angiolipoma.

pyogenic granuloma. Small, erythematous papule on the skin and oral or gingival mucosa that increases in size and may become pendulum-like, infected, and/or ulcerated.

CCI Version 16.3

00400, 0213T, 0216T, 0228T, 0230T, 11100, 11900-11901, 12001-12007, 12011-12018, 17250, 36000, 36400-36410, 36420-36430, 36440, 36600, 36640, 37202, 43752, 51701-51703, 62310-62319, 64400-64435, 64445-64450, 64479, 64483, 64490, 64493, 64505-64530, 69990, 93000-93010, 93040-93042, 93318, 94002, 94200, 94250, 94680-94690, 94770, 95812-95816, 95819, 95822, 95829, 95955, 96360, 96365, 96372, 96374-96376, 96405-96406, 99148-99149, 99150, G0168, J0670, J2001

Also not with 11400: 10060-10061❖, 12031-12057, 13100-13153

Also not with 11401: 10061❖, 19120❖

Also not with 11402: 10061❖, 19120❖

Also not with 11403: 10061❖, 19120❖

Also not with 11404: 10061❖, 19120❖

Also not with 11406: 19120❖

Note: These CCI edits are used for Medicare. Other payers may reimburse on codes listed above.

Medicare Edits

	Fac RVU	Non-Fac RVU	FUD	Assist
11400	2.25	3.45	10	N/A
11401	2.98	4.22	10	N/A
11402	3.28	4.7	10	N/A
11403	4.19	5.4	10	N/A
11404	4.64	6.14	10	N/A
11406	7.0	8.76	10	N/A

Medicare References: 100-2,15,260; 100-4,12,30; 100-4,12,40.2; 100-4,12,90.3; 100-4,14,10

11420-11426

11420	Excision, benign lesion including margins, except skin tag (unless listed elsewhere), scalp, neck, hands, feet, genitalia; excised diameter 0.5 cm or less
11421	excised diameter 0.6 to 1.0 cm
11422	excised diameter 1.1 to 2.0 cm
11423	excised diameter 2.1 to 3.0 cm
11424	excised diameter 3.1 to 4.0 cm
11426	excised diameter over 4.0 cm

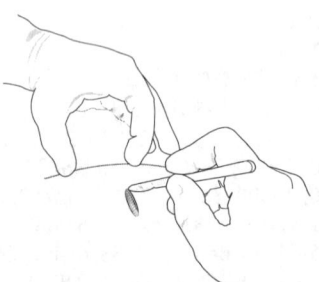

Codes 11420 through 11426 report excisions of benign lesions that occur on the hands (and elsewhere) and are reported according to the diameter of the excision. Report 11420 for excisions 0.5 cm or less; 11421 for excisions 0.6 to 1.0 cm; 11422 for excisions 1.1 to 2.0 cm; 11423 for excisions 2.1 to 3.0 cm; 11424 for excisions 3.1 to 4.0 cm; and 11426 for excisions greater than 4.0 cm in diameter

Explanation

The physician excises a benign (noncancerous) lesion, including the margins, except a skin tag, on the scalp, neck, hands, or genitalia. After administering a local anesthetic, the physician makes a full-thickness incision through the dermis with a scalpel, usually in an elliptical shape around and under the lesion, and removes it. The physician may suture the wound simply. Complex or layered closure is reported separately, if required. Report 11420 for an excised diameter 0.5 cm or less; 11421 for 0.6 cm to 1 cm; 11422 for 1.1 cm to 2 cm; 11423 for 2.1 cm to 3 cm; 11424 for 3.1 cm to 4 cm; and 11426 if the excised diameter is greater than 4 cm.

Coding Tips

Prior to local infiltration, clinical lesion diameter is determined by measurement at the greatest diameter of the lesion plus the narrowest margins required for adequate removal of the entire lesion. Excision of a benign lesion requires a full-thickness incision and removal of the lesion. Local anesthesia is included in the service. It includes simple (non-layered) repair of the skin and/or subcutaneous tissues. If intermediate repair involving layered closure of deeper subcutaneous or non-muscle fascia is required, it is reported separately. For excision of a malignant lesion, see 11600–11606. Surgical trays, A4550, are not separately reimbursed by Medicare; however, other third-party payers may cover them. Check with the specific payer to determine coverage.

ICD-9-CM Procedural

86.3	Other local excision or destruction of lesion or tissue of skin and subcutaneous tissue

Anesthesia
00300, 00400

ICD-9-CM Diagnostic

214.1	Lipoma of other skin and subcutaneous tissue
216.6	Benign neoplasm of skin of upper limb, including shoulder
216.8	Benign neoplasm of other specified sites of skin
228.01	Hemangioma of skin and subcutaneous tissue
238.2	Neoplasm of uncertain behavior of skin
239.2	Neoplasms of unspecified nature of bone, soft tissue, and skin
448.1	Nevus, non-neoplastic
686.1	Pyogenic granuloma of skin and subcutaneous tissue — (Use additional code to identify any infectious organism: 041.0-041.8)
686.9	Unspecified local infection of skin and subcutaneous tissue — (Use additional code to identify any infectious organism: 041.0-041.8)
700	Corns and callosities
701.1	Acquired keratoderma
701.4	Keloid scar
701.5	Other abnormal granulation tissue
701.8	Other specified hypertrophic and atrophic condition of skin
702.0	Actinic keratosis
702.11	Inflamed seborrheic keratosis
702.19	Other seborrheic keratosis
702.8	Other specified dermatoses
706.2	Sebaceous cyst
709.00	Dyschromia, unspecified
709.01	Vitiligo
709.09	Other dyschromia
709.1	Vascular disorder of skin
709.2	Scar condition and fibrosis of skin
709.4	Foreign body granuloma of skin and subcutaneous tissue — (Use additional code to identify foreign body (V90.01-V90.9))
709.9	Unspecified disorder of skin and subcutaneous tissue
757.32	Congenital vascular hamartomas
757.33	Congenital pigmentary anomaly of skin
757.39	Other specified congenital anomaly of skin
782.2	Localized superficial swelling, mass, or lump

Terms To Know

hemangioma. Benign neoplasm arising from vascular tissue or malformations of vascular structures. It is most commonly seen in children and infants as a tumor of newly formed blood vessels due to malformed fetal angioblastic tissues.

lipoma. Benign tumor containing fat cells and the most common of soft tissue lesions, which are usually painless and asymptomatic, with the exception of an angiolipoma.

CCI Version 16.3

00400, 0213T, 0216T, 0228T, 0230T, 11100, 11900-11901, 12001-12007, 12011-12018, 17250, 36000, 36400-36410, 36420-36430, 36440, 36600, 36640, 37202, 43752, 51701-51703, 62310-62319, 64400-64435, 64445-64450, 64479, 64483, 64490, 64493, 64505-64530, 69990, 93000-93010, 93040-93042, 93318, 94002, 94200, 94250, 94680-94690, 94770, 95812-95816, 95819, 95822, 95829, 95955, 96360, 96365, 96372, 96374-96376, 96405-96406, 99148-99149, 99150, G0168, J0670, J2001

Also not with 11420: 10060-10061✤, 11719, 12031-12057, 13100-13153

Also not with 11421: 10061✤, 11719

Also not with 11422: 10061✤

Also not with 11423: 10061✤

Note: These CCI edits are used for Medicare. Other payers may reimburse on codes listed above.

Medicare Edits

	Fac RVU	Non-Fac RVU	FUD	Assist
11420	2.35	3.44	10	N/A
11421	3.21	4.47	10	N/A
11422	3.9	4.98	10	N/A
11423	4.54	5.77	10	N/A
11424	5.19	6.64	10	N/A
11426	7.91	9.49	10	N/A

Medicare References: 100-2,15,260; 100-4,12,30; 100-4,12,90.3; 100-4,14,10

11600-11606

11600	Excision, malignant lesion including margins, trunk, arms, or legs; excised diameter 0.5 cm or less
11601	excised diameter 0.6 to 1.0 cm
11602	excised diameter 1.1 to 2.0 cm
11603	excised diameter 2.1 to 3.0 cm
11604	excised diameter 3.1 to 4.0 cm
11606	excised diameter over 4.0 cm

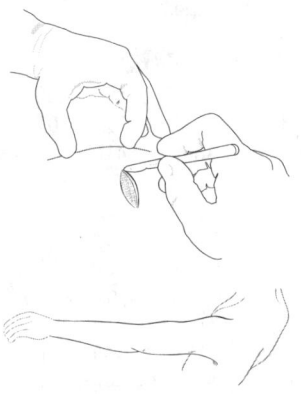

Codes 11600 through 11606 report excisions of malignant lesions that occur on the arms (and elsewhere) and are reported according to the diameter of the excision. Report 11600 for excisions 0.5 cm or less; 11601 for excisions 0.6 to 1.0 cm; 11602 for excisions 1.1 to 2.0 cm; 11603 for excisions 2.1 to 3.0 cm; 11604 for excisions 3.1 to 4.0 cm; and 11606 for excisions greater than 4.0 cm in diameter

Explanation

The physician removes a malignant lesion, including the margins, from the trunk or arms. After administering a local anesthetic, the physician makes a full-thickness incision through the skin, usually in an elliptical shape around and under the lesion. The lesion and a rim of normal tissue are removed. The skin incision is sutured simply. Complex or layered closure is reported separately, if required. Immediate reconstruction with local flaps may be necessary and is also reported separately. Report 11600 for an excised diameter 0.5 cm or less; 11601 for 0.6 cm to 1 cm; 11602 for 1.1 cm to 2 cm; 11603 for 2.1 cm to 3 cm; 11604 for 3.1 cm to 4 cm; and 11606 if the excised diameter is greater than 4 cm.

Coding Tips

When these procedures are performed with another separately identifiable procedure, the highest dollar value code is listed as the primary procedure and subsequent procedures are appended with modifier 51. If significant additional time and effort is documented, append modifier 22 and submit a cover letter and operative report. If specimen is transported to an outside laboratory, report 99000 for handling or conveyance. Prior to local infiltration, clinical lesion diameter is determined by measurement at the greatest diameter of the lesion plus the narrowest margins required for adequate removal of entire lesion. If intermediate (layered) or complex closure is necessary, see 12031–12037 or 13100–13122. For closure requiring skin grafts, see 15002–15261. For excision of benign lesions of the trunk, arms, or legs, see 11400–11406. For destruction of pre-malignant lesions, by any method, including laser, see 17000–17004. For destruction of benign lesions, by any method, including laser, see 17110–17111. For destruction of malignant lesions, by any method, see 17260–17266. Surgical trays, A4550, are not separately reimbursed by Medicare; however, other third-party payers may cover them. Check with the specific payer to determine coverage.

ICD-9-CM Procedural

86.3	Other local excision or destruction of lesion or tissue of skin and subcutaneous tissue

Anesthesia

00300, 00400

ICD-9-CM Diagnostic

172.5	Malignant melanoma of skin of trunk, except scrotum
172.6	Malignant melanoma of skin of upper limb, including shoulder
172.8	Malignant melanoma of other specified sites of skin
173.5	Other malignant neoplasm of skin of trunk, except scrotum
173.6	Other malignant neoplasm of skin of upper limb, including shoulder
173.8	Other malignant neoplasm of other specified sites of skin
195.4	Malignant neoplasm of upper limb
198.2	Secondary malignant neoplasm of skin
209.33	Merkel cell carcinoma of the upper limb
209.75	Secondary Merkel cell carcinoma
232.5	Carcinoma in situ of skin of trunk, except scrotum
232.6	Carcinoma in situ of skin of upper limb, including shoulder
238.2	Neoplasm of uncertain behavior of skin

CCI Version 16.3

00400, 0213T, 0216T, 0228T, 0230T, 11100, 11900-11901, 12001-12007, 12011-12018, 17250, 19120❖, 36000, 36400-36410, 36420-36430, 36440, 36600, 36640, 37202, 43752, 51701-51703, 62310-62319, 64400-64435, 64445-64450, 64479, 64483, 64490, 64493, 64505-64530, 69990, 93000-93010, 93040-93042, 93318, 94002, 94200, 94250, 94680-94690, 94770, 95812-95816, 95819, 95822, 95829, 95955, 96360, 96365, 96372, 96374-96376, 99148-99149, 99150, G0168, J0670, J2001

Also not with 11600: 10061❖, 17262-17266❖, 17271-17276❖, 17281-17286❖

Also not with 11601: 10061❖, 17264-17266❖, 17273-17276❖, 17282-17286❖

Also not with 11602: 10061❖, 17266❖, 17274-17276❖, 17283-17286❖

Also not with 11603: 10061❖, 17274-17276❖, 17283-17286❖

Also not with 11604: 17274-17276❖, 17283-17286❖

Also not with 11606: 15002❖, 15004❖, 17286❖

Note: These CCI edits are used for Medicare. Other payers may reimburse on codes listed above.

Medicare Edits

	Fac RVU	Non-Fac RVU	FUD	Assist
11600	3.42	5.38	10	N/A
11601	4.35	6.53	10	N/A
11602	4.79	7.15	10	N/A
11603	5.69	8.12	10	N/A
11604	6.26	9.0	10	N/A
11606	9.25	12.75	10	N/A

Medicare References: 100-2,15,260; 100-4,12,30; 100-4,12,40.2; 100-4,12,90.3; 100-4,14,10

11620-11626

11620	Excision, malignant lesion including margins, scalp, neck, hands, feet, genitalia; excised diameter 0.5 cm or less
11621	excised diameter 0.6 to 1.0 cm
11622	excised diameter 1.1 to 2.0 cm
11623	excised diameter 2.1 to 3.0 cm
11624	excised diameter 3.1 to 4.0 cm
11626	excised diameter over 4.0 cm

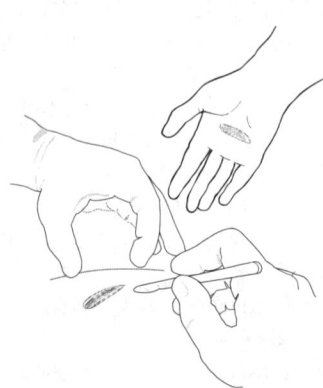

Codes 11620 through 11626 report excisions of malignant lesions that occur on the hands (and elsewhere) and are reported according to the diameter of the excision. Report 11620 for excisions 0.5 cm or less; 11621 for excisions 0.6 to 1.0 cm; 11622 for excisions 1.1 to 2.0 cm; 11623 for excisions 2.1 to 3.0 cm; 11624 for excisions 3.1 to 4.0 cm; and 11626 for excisions greater than 4.0 cm in diameter

Explanation

The physician removes a malignant lesion, including the margins, from the scalp, neck, hands, feet, or genitalia. After administering a local anesthetic, the physician makes a full-thickness incision through the skin, usually in an elliptical shape around and under the lesion. The lesion and a rim of normal tissue are removed. The skin incision is sutured simply. Complex or layered closure is reported separately, if required. Immediate reconstruction with local flaps may be necessary and is also reported separately. Report 11620 for an excised diameter 0.5 cm or less; 11621 for 0.6 cm to 1 cm; 11622 for 1.1 cm to 2 cm; 11623 for 2.1 cm to 3 cm; 11624 for 3.1 cm to 4 cm; and 11626 if the excised diameter is greater than 4 cm.

Coding Tips

Prior to local infiltration, clinical lesion diameter is determined by measurement at the greatest diameter of the lesion plus the narrowest margins required for adequate removal of the entire lesion. These procedures often require a larger excision than a similarly sized benign lesion. Excision of a malignant lesion requires a full-thickness incision and removal of the lesion and a rim of normal tissue margins. Local anesthesia is included in the service. It includes simple (non-layered) repair of the skin and/or subcutaneous tissues. If intermediate repair involving layered closure of deeper subcutaneous or non-muscle fascia is required, it is reported separately. For destruction of a lesion by electrosurgical or other methods, see 17000 et seq. For excision of a benign lesion, see 11420–11426. Surgical trays, A4550, are not separately reimbursed by Medicare; however, other third-party payers may cover them. Check with the specific payer to determine coverage.

ICD-9-CM Procedural

86.3	Other local excision or destruction of lesion or tissue of skin and subcutaneous tissue

Anesthesia

00300, 00400

ICD-9-CM Diagnostic

171.2	Malignant neoplasm of connective and other soft tissue of upper limb, including shoulder
171.8	Malignant neoplasm of other specified sites of connective and other soft tissue
172.4	Malignant melanoma of skin of scalp and neck
172.6	Malignant melanoma of skin of upper limb, including shoulder
172.8	Malignant melanoma of other specified sites of skin
173.4	Other malignant neoplasm of scalp and skin of neck
173.5	Other malignant neoplasm of skin of trunk, except scrotum
173.6	Other malignant neoplasm of skin of upper limb, including shoulder
195.4	Malignant neoplasm of upper limb
198.2	Secondary malignant neoplasm of skin
209.33	Merkel cell carcinoma of the upper limb
209.36	Merkel cell carcinoma of other sites
209.75	Secondary Merkel cell carcinoma
232.4	Carcinoma in situ of scalp and skin of neck
232.6	Carcinoma in situ of skin of upper limb, including shoulder
232.8	Carcinoma in situ of other specified sites of skin

Terms To Know

carcinoma in situ. Malignancy that arises from the cells of the vessel, gland, or organ of origin that remains confined to that site or has not invaded neighboring tissue. Carcinoma in situ codes are found in their own subchapter of neoplasms according to site.

malignant. Any condition tending to progress toward death, specifically an invasive tumor with a loss of cellular differentiation that has the ability to spread or metastasize to other areas in the body.

CCI Version 16.3

00400, 0213T, 0216T, 0228T, 0230T, 11100, 11900-11901, 12001-12007, 12011-12018, 17250, 36000, 36400-36410, 36420-36430, 36440, 36600, 36640, 37202, 43752, 51701-51703, 62310-62319, 64400-64435, 64445-64450, 64479, 64483, 64490, 64493, 64505-64530, 69990, 93000-93010, 93040-93042, 93318, 94002, 94200, 94250, 94680-94690, 94770, 95812-95816, 95819, 95822, 95829, 95955, 96360, 96365, 96372, 96374-96376, 99148-99149, 99150, G0168, J0670, J2001

Also not with 11620: 10061❖, 17262-17266❖, 17271-17276❖, 17281-17286❖

Also not with 11621: 10061❖, 17266❖, 17273-17276❖, 17282-17286❖

Also not with 11622: 10061❖, 17274-17276❖, 17283-17286❖

Also not with 11623: 17276❖, 17284-17286❖

Also not with 11624: 17286❖

Also not with 11626: 15002❖, 17286❖

Note: These CCI edits are used for Medicare. Other payers may reimburse on codes listed above.

Medicare Edits

	Fac RVU	Non-Fac RVU	FUD	Assist
11620	3.48	5.47	10	N/A
11621	4.39	6.59	10	N/A
11622	5.06	7.42	10	N/A
11623	6.22	8.67	10	N/A
11624	7.04	9.74	10	N/A
11626	8.68	11.77	10	N/A

Medicare References: 100-2,15,260; 100-4,12,30; 100-4,12,90.3; 100-4,14,10

11719

11719 Trimming of nondystrophic nails, any number

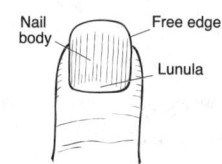
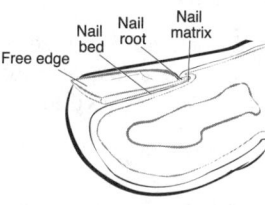

The free edge of any number of non-diseased nails are trimmed

Explanation
A physician trims a fingernail, usually with scissors, nail cutters, or other instruments. This code is used when the nails are not defective from nutritional or metabolic abnormalities. It is used for one or more nails.

Coding Tips
This code is used for one or more nails. For debridement of nails, see 11720–11721. This code is reported only once regardless of the number of nails that are trimmed. For the trimming of dystrophic nails, see G0127. Some non-Medicare payers may require that HCPCS Level II code S0390 be reported for this service when provided as routine foot care or as preventive maintenance in specific medical conditions. For diabetic patients with diabetic sensory neuropathy resulting in a loss of protective sensation (LOPS), see G0247. Medicare requires the use of specific HCPCS Level II modifiers Q7–Q9 to indicate clinical findings indicative of severe peripheral involvement that warrant the medical necessity of a podiatrist providing foot care such as nail debridement or trimming that would usually be considered routine and for which benefits would not be provided.

ICD-9-CM Procedural
89.01 Interview and evaluation, described as brief

Anesthesia
11719 N/A

ICD-9-CM Diagnostic
249.70 Secondary diabetes mellitus with peripheral circulatory disorders, not stated as uncontrolled, or unspecified — (Use additional code to identify manifestation: 443.81, 785.4) (Use additional code to identify any associated insulin use: V58.67)
249.71 Secondary diabetes mellitus with peripheral circulatory disorders, uncontrolled — (Use additional code to identify manifestation: 443.81, 785.4) (Use additional code to identify any associated insulin use: V58.67)
249.80 Secondary diabetes mellitus with other specified manifestations, not stated as uncontrolled, or unspecified — (Use additional code to identify manifestation: 707.10-707.9, 731.8) (Use additional code to identify any associated insulin use: V58.67)
250.70 Diabetes with peripheral circulatory disorders, type II or unspecified type, not stated as uncontrolled — (Use additional code to identify manifestation: 443.81, 785.4)
250.71 Diabetes with peripheral circulatory disorders, type I [juvenile type], not stated as uncontrolled — (Use additional code to identify manifestation: 443.81, 785.4)
250.72 Diabetes with peripheral circulatory disorders, type II or unspecified type, uncontrolled — (Use additional code to identify manifestation: 443.81, 785.4)
250.73 Diabetes with peripheral circulatory disorders, type I [juvenile type], uncontrolled — (Use additional code to identify manifestation: 443.81, 785.4)
342.01 Flaccid hemiplegia affecting dominant side
342.11 Spastic hemiplegia affecting dominant side
342.81 Other specified hemiplegia affecting dominant side
342.91 Unspecified hemiplegia affecting dominant side
344.00 Unspecified quadriplegia
344.01 Quadriplegia and quadriparesis, C1-C4, complete
344.02 Quadriplegia and quadriparesis, C1-C4, incomplete
344.03 Quadriplegia and quadriparesis, C5-C7, complete
344.04 C5-C7, incomplete
344.1 Paraplegia
344.2 Diplegia of upper limbs
344.41 Monoplegia of upper limb affecting dominant side
438.20 Hemiplegia affecting unspecified side due to cerebrovascular disease — (Use additional code to identify presence of hypertension)
438.31 Monoplegia of upper limb affecting dominant side due to cerebrovascular disease — (Use additional code to identify presence of hypertension)
438.51 Other paralytic syndrome affecting dominant side due to cerebrovascular disease — (Use additional code to identify presence of hypertension. Use additional code to identify type of paralytic syndrome: 344.00-344.09, 344.81)
438.84 Ataxia as late effect of cerebrovascular disease — (Use additional code to identify presence of hypertension)
443.81 Peripheral angiopathy in diseases classified elsewhere — (Code first underlying disease: 249.7, 250.7)

CCI Version 16.3
0213T, 0216T, 0228T, 0230T, 11720-11721❖, 29075-29086, 29125-29131, 29280, 29440, 29450, 29515, 36000, 36400-36410, 36420-36430, 36440, 36600, 36640, 37202, 43752, 51701-51703, 62310-62319, 64400-64435, 64445-64450, 64479, 64483, 64490, 64493, 64505-64530, 69990, 93000-93010, 93040-93042, 93318, 94002, 94200, 94250, 94680-94690, 94770, 95812-95816, 95819, 95822, 95829, 95955, 96360, 96365, 96372, 96374-96376, 97022, 97597-97598, 97602-97606, 99148-99149, 99150, 99203-99223❖, 99231-99239❖, 99281-99285❖, 99304-99310❖, 99315-99318❖, 99324-99328❖, 99334-99337❖, 99341-99350❖, 99354-99357❖, G0127❖, G0168, G0380-G0384❖, G0406-G0408❖, G0425-G0427❖

Note: These CCI edits are used for Medicare. Other payers may reimburse on codes listed above.

Medicare Edits

	Fac RVU	Non-Fac RVU	FUD	Assist
11719	0.24	0.62	0	N/A

Medicare References: 100-2,15,290; 100-3,70.2.1; 100-4,12,30

11720-11721

11720 Debridement of nail(s) by any method(s); 1 to 5
11721 6 or more

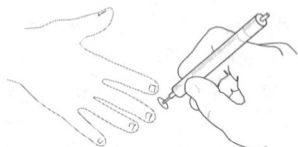

Nails are debrided using any of a number of methods. Report code 11720 for up to an initial five nails. Report 11721 when six or more nails are debrided

Explanation

The physician debrides fingernails or toenails, including tops and exposed undersides, by any method. The cleaning is performed manually with cleaning solutions, abrasive materials, and tools. The nails are shortened and shaped. Report 11720 for one to five nails and 11721 for six or more.

Coding Tips

For trimming of nondystrophic nails, see 11719.

ICD-9-CM Procedural

86.27 Debridement of nail, nail bed, or nail fold

Anesthesia

N/A

ICD-9-CM Diagnostic

110.1 Dermatophytosis of nail — (Use additional code to identify manifestation: 321.0-321.1, 380.15, 711.6)
249.70 Secondary diabetes mellitus with peripheral circulatory disorders, not stated as uncontrolled, or unspecified — (Use additional code to identify manifestation: 443.81, 785.4) (Use additional code to identify any associated insulin use: V58.67)
249.71 Secondary diabetes mellitus with peripheral circulatory disorders, uncontrolled — (Use additional code to identify manifestation: 443.81, 785.4) (Use additional code to identify any associated insulin use: V58.67)
249.80 Secondary diabetes mellitus with other specified manifestations, not stated as uncontrolled, or unspecified — (Use additional code to identify manifestation: 707.10-707.9, 731.8) (Use additional code to identify any associated insulin use: V58.67)
249.81 Secondary diabetes mellitus with other specified manifestations, uncontrolled — (Use additional code to identify manifestation: 707.10-707.9, 731.8) (Use additional code to identify any associated insulin use: V58.67)
249.90 Secondary diabetes mellitus with unspecified complication, not stated as uncontrolled, or unspecified — (Use additional code to identify any associated insulin use: V58.67)
249.91 Secondary diabetes mellitus with unspecified complication, uncontrolled — (Use additional code to identify any associated insulin use: V58.67)
250.70 Diabetes with peripheral circulatory disorders, type II or unspecified type, not stated as uncontrolled — (Use additional code to identify manifestation: 443.81, 785.4)
250.71 Diabetes with peripheral circulatory disorders, type I [juvenile type], not stated as uncontrolled — (Use additional code to identify manifestation: 443.81, 785.4)
250.72 Diabetes with peripheral circulatory disorders, type II or unspecified type, uncontrolled — (Use additional code to identify manifestation: 443.81, 785.4)
250.73 Diabetes with peripheral circulatory disorders, type I [juvenile type], uncontrolled — (Use additional code to identify manifestation: 443.81, 785.4)
443.81 Peripheral angiopathy in diseases classified elsewhere — (Code first underlying disease: 249.7, 250.7)
443.89 Other peripheral vascular disease
681.00 Unspecified cellulitis and abscess of finger — (Use additional code to identify organism: 041.1)
681.02 Onychia and paronychia of finger — (Use additional code to identify organism: 041.1)
681.9 Cellulitis and abscess of unspecified digit — (Use additional code to identify organism: 041.1)
703.0 Ingrowing nail
703.8 Other specified disease of nail
729.5 Pain in soft tissues of limb
757.5 Specified congenital anomalies of nails
991.1 Frostbite of hand

Terms To Know

abscess. Circumscribed collection of pus resulting from bacteria, frequently associated with swelling and other signs of inflammation.

cellulitis. Sudden, severe, suppurative inflammation and edema in subcutaneous tissue or muscle, most often caused by bacterial infection secondary to a cutaneous lesion.

debridement. Removal of dead or contaminated tissue and foreign matter from a wound.

onychia. Inflammation or infection of the nail matrix leading to a loss of the nail.

paronychia. Infection of nail structures.

CCI Version 16.3

0183T, 0213T, 0216T, 0228T, 0230T, 29075-29086, 29125-29131, 29280, 29440, 29450, 29515, 29550, 36000, 36400-36410, 36420-36430, 36440, 36600, 36640, 37202, 43752, 51701-51703, 62310-62319, 64400-64435, 64445-64450, 64479, 64483, 64490, 64493, 64505-64530, 69990, 93000-93010, 93040-93042, 93318, 94002, 94200, 94250, 94680-94690, 94770, 95812-95816, 95819, 95822, 95829, 95955, 96360, 96365, 96372, 96374-96376, 97022, 99148-99149, 99150, 99203-99223, 99231-99239, 99281-99285, 99304-99310, 99315-99318, 99324-99328, 99334-99337, 99341-99350, 99354-99357, G0127, G0168, G0380-G0384, G0406-G0408, G0425-G0427

Also not with 11720: 11755
Also not with 11721: 11720, 11740

Note: These CCI edits are used for Medicare. Other payers may reimburse on codes listed above.

Medicare Edits

	Fac RVU	Non-Fac RVU	FUD	Assist
11720	0.45	0.9	0	N/A
11721	0.76	1.23	0	N/A

Medicare References: 100-2,15,290; 100-3,70.2.1; 100-4,12,30

11730-11732

11730 Avulsion of nail plate, partial or complete, simple; single

11732 each additional nail plate (List separately in addition to code for primary procedure)

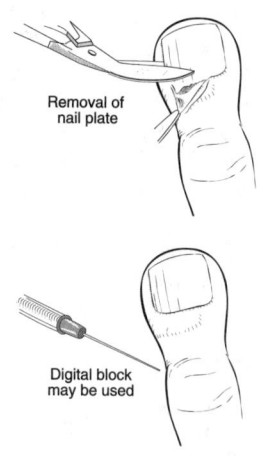

Removal of nail plate

Digital block may be used

A nail plate is avulsed, either partially or completely. A nerve block may be used. The affected area is dissected free and the nail plate is exposed. The nail is then cut free of the bed. Report code 11732 for each additional nail plate that is removed

Explanation

The physician avulses a nail plate partially or completely. A digital nerve block is used to numb the top of the digit. The physician bluntly dissects the nail plate from the nail bed. Any bleeding is cauterized. The digit is bandaged. Report 11730 if only one nail plate is removed. Report 11732 for each additional nail plate removed.

Coding Tips

Use 11732 in conjunction with 11730. As an "add-on" code, 11732 is not subject to multiple procedure rules. No reimbursement reduction or modifier 51 is applied. "Add-on" codes describe additional intra-service work associated with the primary procedure. They are performed by the same physician on the same date of service as the primary service/procedure, and must never be reported as a stand-alone code. Surgical trays, A4550, are not separately reimbursed by Medicare; however, other third-party payers may cover them. Check with the specific payer to determine coverage.

ICD-9-CM Procedural

86.23 Removal of nail, nailbed, or nail fold

Anesthesia

11730 00400
11732 N/A

ICD-9-CM Diagnostic

249.70 Secondary diabetes mellitus with peripheral circulatory disorders, not stated as uncontrolled, or unspecified — (Use additional code to identify manifestation: 443.81, 785.4) (Use additional code to identify any associated insulin use: V58.67)

249.71 Secondary diabetes mellitus with peripheral circulatory disorders, uncontrolled — (Use additional code to identify manifestation: 443.81, 785.4) (Use additional code to identify any associated insulin use: V58.67)

249.80 Secondary diabetes mellitus with other specified manifestations, not stated as uncontrolled, or unspecified — (Use additional code to identify manifestation: 707.10-707.9, 731.8) (Use additional code to identify any associated insulin use: V58.67)

249.81 Secondary diabetes mellitus with other specified manifestations, uncontrolled — (Use additional code to identify manifestation: 707.10-707.9, 731.8) (Use additional code to identify any associated insulin use: V58.67)

250.70 Diabetes with peripheral circulatory disorders, type II or unspecified type, not stated as uncontrolled — (Use additional code to identify manifestation: 443.81, 785.4)

250.71 Diabetes with peripheral circulatory disorders, type I [juvenile type], not stated as uncontrolled — (Use additional code to identify manifestation: 443.81, 785.4)

250.72 Diabetes with peripheral circulatory disorders, type II or unspecified type, uncontrolled — (Use additional code to identify manifestation: 443.81, 785.4)

250.73 Diabetes with peripheral circulatory disorders, type I [juvenile type], uncontrolled — (Use additional code to identify manifestation: 443.81, 785.4)

443.0 Raynaud's syndrome — (Use additional code to identify gangrene: 785.4)

443.81 Peripheral angiopathy in diseases classified elsewhere — (Code first underlying disease: 249.7, 250.7)

443.89 Other peripheral vascular disease

681.00 Unspecified cellulitis and abscess of finger — (Use additional code to identify organism: 041.1)

681.02 Onychia and paronychia of finger — (Use additional code to identify organism: 041.1)

681.9 Cellulitis and abscess of unspecified digit — (Use additional code to identify organism: 041.1)

682.8 Cellulitis and abscess of other specified site — (Use additional code to identify organism, such as 041.1, etc.)

703.0 Ingrowing nail

703.8 Other specified disease of nail

757.5 Specified congenital anomalies of nails

785.4 Gangrene — (Code first any associated underlying condition)

816.02 Closed fracture of distal phalanx or phalanges of hand

816.03 Closed fracture of multiple sites of phalanx or phalanges of hand

816.12 Open fracture of distal phalanx or phalanges of hand

816.13 Open fractures of multiple sites of phalanx or phalanges of hand

883.0 Open wound of finger(s), without mention of complication

883.1 Open wound of finger(s), complicated

883.2 Open wound of finger(s), with tendon involvement

CCI Version 16.3

Also not with 11730: 0213T, 0216T, 0228T, 0230T, 10160, 11000, 11040-11041, 11719-11721, 11740, 11755, 11765, 11900-11901, 17250, 29075-29086, 29125-29131, 29280, 29440, 29450, 29515, 29550-29581, 36000, 36400-36410, 36420-36430, 36440, 36600, 36640, 37202, 43752, 51701-51703, 62310-62319, 64400-64435, 64445-64450, 64479, 64483, 64490, 64493, 64505-64530, 69990, 93000-93010, 93040-93042, 93318, 94002, 94200, 94250, 94680-94690, 94770, 95812-95816, 95819, 95822, 95829, 95955, 96360, 96365, 96372, 96374-96376, 96405-96406, 97597-97598, 97602-97606, 99148-99149, 99150, G0127, G0168, J0670, J2001

Also not with 11732: 29580-29581

Note: These CCI edits are used for Medicare. Other payers may reimburse on codes listed above.

Medicare Edits

	Fac RVU	Non-Fac RVU	FUD	Assist
11730	1.54	2.77	0	N/A
11732	0.8	1.26	N/A	N/A

Medicare References: 100-2,15,290; 100-3,70.2.1; 100-4,12,30

11740

11740 Evacuation of subungual hematoma

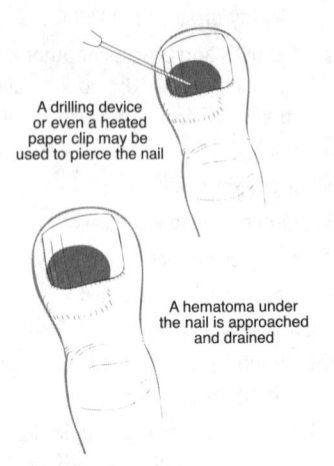

A drilling device or even a heated paper clip may be used to pierce the nail

A hematoma under the nail is approached and drained

A hematoma under a nail is drained. The nail is pierced and blood is drained from under the nail plate

Explanation

The physician evacuates blood from a hematoma located beneath a fingernail. The physician uses an electrocautery needle to pierce the nail plate so a hematoma can drain. Pressure may be applied to the nail bed to force the blood from beneath the nail plate. A loose dressing is applied so the area can continue to drain.

Coding Tips

Some payers may require the use of HCPCS Level II modifiers FA-F9 to identify the specific finger involved. Surgical trays, A4550, are not separately reimbursed by Medicare; however, other third-party payers may cover them. Check with the specific payer to determine coverage.

ICD-9-CM Procedural

86.04 Other incision with drainage of skin and subcutaneous tissue

Anesthesia

11740 00400

ICD-9-CM Diagnostic

816.02 Closed fracture of distal phalanx or phalanges of hand
816.03 Closed fracture of multiple sites of phalanx or phalanges of hand
816.12 Open fracture of distal phalanx or phalanges of hand
816.13 Open fractures of multiple sites of phalanx or phalanges of hand
883.0 Open wound of finger(s), without mention of complication
883.1 Open wound of finger(s), complicated
923.20 Contusion of hand(s)
923.3 Contusion of finger
927.3 Crushing injury of finger(s) — (Use additional code to identify any associated injuries: 800-829, 850.0-854.1, 860.0-869.1)
959.5 Injury, other and unspecified, finger
998.12 Hematoma complicating a procedure

Terms To Know

aspiration. Drawing fluid out by suction.

closed fracture. Break in a bone without a concomitant opening in the skin. A closed fracture is coded when the type of fracture is not specified.

contusion. Superficial injury (bruising) produced by impact without a break in the skin.

distal. Located farther away from a specified reference point.

electrocautery. Division or cutting of tissue using high-frequency electrical current to produce heat, which destroys cells.

fracture. Break in bone or cartilage.

hematoma. Tumor-like collection of blood in some part of the body caused by a break in a blood vessel wall, usually as a result of trauma.

incision and drainage. Cutting open body tissue for the removal of tissue fluids or infected discharge from a wound or cavity.

open fracture. Exposed break in a bone, always considered compound due to its high risk of infection from the open wound leading to the fracture. Broken bone ends may protrude through the skin and contaminants or foreign bodies are often embedded in the tissues.

phalanx. Bones of the digits (fingers or toes).

subcutaneous tissue. Sheet or wide band of adipose (fat) and areolar connective tissue in two layers attached to the dermis.

subungual. Under the nail.

CCI Version 16.3

0213T, 0216T, 0228T, 0230T, 10140, 10160, 11055-11057, 11719-11720, 11755, 11900-11901, 17250, 29075-29086, 29125-29131, 29280, 29440, 29450, 29515, 29540-29581, 36000, 36400-36410, 36420-36430, 36440, 36600, 36640, 37202, 43752, 51701-51703, 62310-62319, 64400-64435, 64445-64450, 64479, 64483, 64490, 64493, 64505-64530, 69990, 93000-93010, 93040-93042, 93318, 94002, 94200, 94250, 94680-94690, 94770, 95812-95816, 95819, 95822, 95829, 95955, 96360, 96365, 96372, 96374-96376, 96405-96406, 97597-97598, 97602-97606, 99148-99149, 99150, G0127, G0168, J0670, J2001

Note: These CCI edits are used for Medicare. Other payers may reimburse on codes listed above.

Medicare Edits

	Fac RVU	Non-Fac RVU	FUD	Assist
11740	0.92	1.34	0	N/A

Medicare References: 100-2,15,290; 100-4,12,30

11750-11752

11750 Excision of nail and nail matrix, partial or complete (eg, ingrown or deformed nail), for permanent removal;

11752 with amputation of tuft of distal phalanx

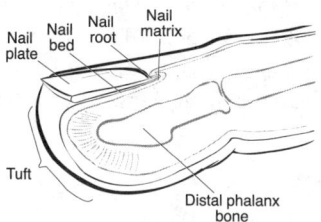

A nail and its matrix are removed. The matrix is the tissue from which the nail grows and removal effects permanent removal of the nail. Report 11752 when the tuft, or fleshy part, of the distal phalanx is amputated during the session

Explanation

The physician removes all or part of a fingernail, including the nail plate and matrix. In 11750, the physician bluntly dissects the nail plate away from the nail bed. The germ matrix is destroyed using electrocautery or excision. Bleeding is stopped with electrocautery and the wound is dressed. In 11752, the entire tuft of the distal phalanx is removed.

Coding Tips

Codes 11750 and 11752 may be reported only once per digit. Some payers may require the use of HCPCS Level II modifiers FA–F9 to identify the specific finger involved. A partial excision, even when the partial excision requires two incisions (medial and lateral aspects) of the nail, does not count as two separate procedures. When a skin graft is required, see 15050. For wedge excision of the skin of a nail fold (e.g., ingrown toenail), see 11765. Surgical trays, A4550, are not separately reimbursed by Medicare; however, other third-party payers may cover them. Check with the specific payer to determine coverage.

ICD-9-CM Procedural

86.23 Removal of nail, nailbed, or nail fold

Anesthesia

00400

ICD-9-CM Diagnostic

249.70 Secondary diabetes mellitus with peripheral circulatory disorders, not stated as uncontrolled, or unspecified — (Use additional code to identify manifestation: 443.81, 785.4) (Use additional code to identify any associated insulin use: V58.67)

249.71 Secondary diabetes mellitus with peripheral circulatory disorders, uncontrolled — (Use additional code to identify manifestation: 443.81, 785.4) (Use additional code to identify any associated insulin use: V58.67)

249.80 Secondary diabetes mellitus with other specified manifestations, not stated as uncontrolled, or unspecified — (Use additional code to identify manifestation: 707.10-707.9, 731.8) (Use additional code to identify any associated insulin use: V58.67)

249.81 Secondary diabetes mellitus with other specified manifestations, uncontrolled — (Use additional code to identify manifestation: 707.10-707.9, 731.8) (Use additional code to identify any associated insulin use: V58.67)

250.70 Diabetes with peripheral circulatory disorders, type II or unspecified type, not stated as uncontrolled — (Use additional code to identify manifestation: 443.81, 785.4)

250.71 Diabetes with peripheral circulatory disorders, type I [juvenile type], not stated as uncontrolled — (Use additional code to identify manifestation: 443.81, 785.4)

250.72 Diabetes with peripheral circulatory disorders, type II or unspecified type, uncontrolled — (Use additional code to identify manifestation: 443.81, 785.4)

250.73 Diabetes with peripheral circulatory disorders, type I [juvenile type], uncontrolled — (Use additional code to identify manifestation: 443.81, 785.4)

443.0 Raynaud's syndrome — (Use additional code to identify gangrene: 785.4)

443.81 Peripheral angiopathy in diseases classified elsewhere — (Code first underlying disease: 249.7, 250.7)

443.89 Other peripheral vascular disease

681.02 Onychia and paronychia of finger — (Use additional code to identify organism: 041.1)

703.0 Ingrowing nail

703.8 Other specified disease of nail

785.4 Gangrene — (Code first any associated underlying condition)

883.0 Open wound of finger(s), without mention of complication

883.1 Open wound of finger(s), complicated

927.3 Crushing injury of finger(s) — (Use additional code to identify any associated injuries: 800-829, 850.0-854.1, 860.0-869.1)

Terms To Know

amputation. Removal of all or part of a limb or digit through the shaft or body of a bone.

electrocautery. Division or cutting of tissue using high-frequency electrical current to produce heat, which destroys cells.

onychia. Inflammation or infection of the nail matrix leading to a loss of the nail.

paronychia. Infection of nail structures.

CCI Version 16.3

0213T, 0216T, 0228T, 0230T, 11000, 11040-11042, 11755-11760, 11765, 11900-11901, 13131, 17250, 20550-20553, 29075-29086, 29125-29131, 29280, 29440, 29450, 29515, 29540-29581, 36000, 36400-36410, 36420-36430, 36440, 36600, 36640, 37202, 43752, 51701-51703, 62310-62319, 64400-64435, 64445-64450, 64479, 64483, 64490, 64493, 64505-64530, 69990, 93000-93010, 93040-93042, 93318, 94002, 94200, 94250, 94680-94690, 94770, 95812-95816, 95819, 95822, 95829, 95955, 96360, 96365, 96372, 96374-96376, 96405-96406, 97597-97598, 97602-97606, 99148-99149, 99150, J0670, J2001

Also not with 11750: 10060, 11055-11057, 11719-11730, 11740, 15852, 87070, 87076-87077, 87102, G0127, G0168

Also not with 11752: 10060-10061, 11720-11730, 11740-11750, 12032

Note: These CCI edits are used for Medicare. Other payers may reimburse on codes listed above.

Medicare Edits

	Fac RVU	Non-Fac RVU	FUD	Assist
11750	5.03	6.26	10	N/A
11752	7.61	9.02	10	N/A

Medicare References: 100-2,15,290; 100-3,70.2.1; 100-4,12,30

11755

11755 Biopsy of nail unit (eg, plate, bed, matrix, hyponychium, proximal and lateral nail folds) (separate procedure)

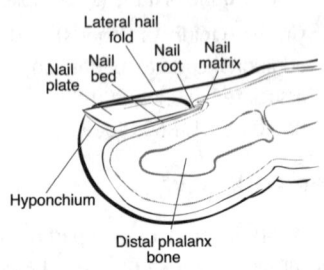
Any nail specimen is collected for biopsy, any method

Explanation
The physician removes a portion of the nail unit for a biopsy sample. Sections may be taken from the hard nail itself, the nail bed, lateral skin, or underlying soft tissue. The specimen is excised by clippers or with a scalpel.

Coding Tips
This separate procedure by definition is usually a component of a more complex service and is not identified separately. When performed alone or with other unrelated procedures/services it may be reported. If performed alone, list the code; if performed with other procedures/services, list the code and append modifier 59. An excisional biopsy is not reported separately when a therapeutic excision is performed during the same surgical session. Some payers may require the use of HCPCS Level II modifiers FA–F9 to identify the specific finger involved. Surgical trays, A4550, are not separately reimbursed by Medicare; however, other third-party payers may cover them. Check with the specific payer to determine coverage.

ICD-9-CM Procedural
86.11 Closed biopsy of skin and subcutaneous tissue

Anesthesia
11755 00400

ICD-9-CM Diagnostic
- 110.1 Dermatophytosis of nail — (Use additional code to identify manifestation: 321.0-321.1, 380.15, 711.6)
- 173.6 Other malignant neoplasm of skin of upper limb, including shoulder
- 198.2 Secondary malignant neoplasm of skin
- 216.6 Benign neoplasm of skin of upper limb, including shoulder
- 216.9 Benign neoplasm of skin, site unspecified
- 232.6 Carcinoma in situ of skin of upper limb, including shoulder
- 238.2 Neoplasm of uncertain behavior of skin
- 239.2 Neoplasms of unspecified nature of bone, soft tissue, and skin
- 697.0 Lichen planus
- 703.8 Other specified disease of nail

Terms To Know
benign. Mild or nonmalignant in nature.

biopsy. Tissue or fluid removed for diagnostic purposes through analysis of the cells in the biopsy material.

carcinoma in situ. Malignancy that arises from the cells of the vessel, gland, or organ of origin that remains confined to that site or has not invaded neighboring tissue.

excision. Surgical removal of an organ or tissue.

lateral. To/on the side.

malignant. Any condition tending to progress toward death, specifically an invasive tumor with a loss of cellular differentiation that has the ability to spread or metastasize to other areas in the body.

neoplasm. New abnormal growth, tumor.

proximal. Located closest to a specified reference point, usually the midline.

secondary. Second in order of occurrence or importance, or appearing during the course of another disease or condition.

soft tissue. Nonepithelial tissues outside of the skeleton that includes subcutaneous adipose tissue, fibrous tissue, fascia, muscles, blood and lymph vessels, and peripheral nervous system tissue.

subcutaneous tissue. Sheet or wide band of adipose (fat) and areolar connective tissue in two layers attached to the dermis.

therapeutic. Act meant to alleviate a medical or mental condition.

CCI Version 16.3
0213T, 0216T, 0228T, 0230T, 11055-11057, 11719, 11900-11901, 29075-29086, 29125-29131, 29280, 29440, 29450, 29515, 29550-29581, 36000, 36400-36410, 36420-36430, 36440, 36600, 36640, 37202, 43752, 51701-51703, 62310-62319, 64400-64435, 64445-64450, 64479, 64483, 64490, 64493, 64505-64530, 69990, 93000-93010, 93040-93042, 93318, 94002, 94200, 94250, 94680-94690, 94770, 95812-95816, 95819, 95822, 95829, 95955, 96360, 96365, 96372, 96374-96376, 96405-96406, 97597-97598, 97602-97606, 99148-99149, 99150, G0127, J0670, J2001

Note: These CCI edits are used for Medicare. Other payers may reimburse on codes listed above.

Medicare Edits

	Fac RVU	Non-Fac RVU	FUD	Assist
11755	2.36	3.82	0	80

Medicare References: 100-2,15,290; 100-4,12,30

11760

11760 Repair of nail bed

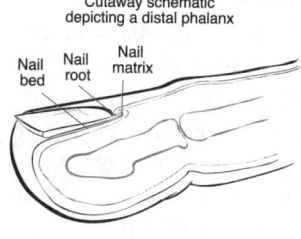

Code 11760 reports repair to the nail bed

Explanation

The physician repairs a damaged nail bed. The physician removes the damaged and surrounding nail from the nail bed. The nail bed is sutured into the correct position. Bleeding is controlled through electrocautery and the wound is dressed.

Coding Tips

Local anesthesia is included in this procedure. Some payers may require the use of HCPCS Level II modifiers FA–F9 to identify the specific finger involved. For reconstruction of a nail bed with a graft, see 11762. Surgical trays, A4550, are not separately reimbursed by Medicare; however, other third-party payers may cover them. Check with the specific payer to determine coverage.

ICD-9-CM Procedural

86.86 Onychoplasty

Anesthesia

11760 00400

ICD-9-CM Diagnostic

816.12 Open fracture of distal phalanx or phalanges of hand
816.13 Open fractures of multiple sites of phalanx or phalanges of hand
883.0 Open wound of finger(s), without mention of complication
883.1 Open wound of finger(s), complicated
927.3 Crushing injury of finger(s) — (Use additional code to identify any associated injuries: 800-829, 850.0-854.1, 860.0-869.1)

Terms To Know

distal. Located farther away from a specified reference point.

electrocautery. Division or cutting of tissue using high-frequency electrical current to produce heat, which destroys cells.

fracture. Break in bone or cartilage.

open fracture. Exposed break in a bone, always considered compound due to its high risk of infection from the open wound leading to the fracture. Broken bone ends may protrude through the skin and contaminants or foreign bodies are often embedded in the tissues.

open wound. Opening or break of the skin.

phalanx. Bones of the digits (fingers or toes).

reconstruction. Recreating, restoring, or rebuilding a body part or organ.

suture. Numerous stitching techniques employed in wound closure.

buried suture. Continuous or interrupted suture placed under the skin for a layered closure.

continuous suture. Running stitch with tension evenly distributed across a single strand to provide a leakproof closure line.

interrupted suture. Series of single stitches with tension isolated at each stitch, in which all stitches are not affected if one becomes loose, and the isolated sutures cannot act as a wick to transport an infection.

purse-string suture. Continuous suture placed around a tubular structure and tightened, to reduce or close the lumen.

retention suture. Secondary stitching that bridges the primary suture, providing support for the primary repair; a plastic or rubber bolster may be placed over the primary repair and under the retention sutures.

wound repair. Surgical closure of a wound is divided into three categories: simple, intermediate, and complex. **simple repair:** Surgical closure of a superficial wound, requiring single layer suturing of the skin epidermis, dermis, or subcutaneous tissue. **intermediate repair:** Surgical closure of a wound requiring closure of one or more of the deeper subcutaneous tissue and non-muscle fascia layers in addition to suturing the skin; contaminated wounds with single layer closure that need extensive cleaning or foreign body removal. **complex repair:** Repair of wounds requiring more than layered closure (debridement, scar revision, stents, retention sutures).

CCI Version 16.3

0213T, 0216T, 0228T, 0230T, 10060, 11000, 11040-11042, 11044, 11720-11730, 11740, 11755, 11762❖, 11900-11901, 12001-12005, 12011-12013, 12041-12044, 12047, 13101, 13131-13132, 17250, 20550-20553, 29075-29086, 29125-29131, 29280, 29440, 29450, 29515, 29540-29581, 36000, 36400-36410, 36420-36430, 36440, 36600, 36640, 37202, 43752, 51701-51703, 62310-62319, 64400-64435, 64445-64450, 64479, 64483, 64490, 64493, 64505-64530, 69990, 93000-93010, 93040-93042, 93318, 94002, 94200, 94250, 94680-94690, 94770, 95812-95816, 95819, 95822, 95829, 95955, 96360, 96365, 96372, 96374-96376, 96405-96406, 97597-97598, 97602-97606, 99148-99149, 99150, G0168, J0670, J2001

Note: These CCI edits are used for Medicare. Other payers may reimburse on codes listed above.

Medicare Edits

	Fac RVU	Non-Fac RVU	FUD	Assist
11760	3.84	6.21	10	N/A

Medicare References: 100-2,15,290; 100-4,12,30

11762

11762 Reconstruction of nail bed with graft

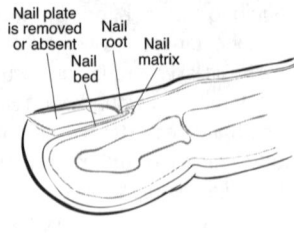

Cutaway schematic depicting a distal phalanx

Nail plate is removed or absent; Nail root; Nail matrix; Nail bed

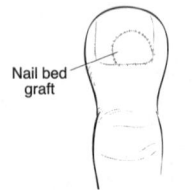

Nail bed graft

An area of the nail bed that has been injured, or otherwise disrupted, is reconstructed by suturing a piece of skin over the defect

Explanation

The physician repairs a damaged nail bed using a skin graft. The physician cleans the nail bed and prepares it for the graft. The graft is obtained and sutured into place. Hemostasis is achieved and a dressing is applied.

Coding Tips

This procedure is usually performed under local or regional anesthesia. However, this procedure may be performed under general anesthesia, depending on the age and/or condition of the patient. Some payers may require the use of HCPCS Level II modifiers FA–F9 to identify the specific finger involved. For repair of a nail bed, see 11760. Surgical trays, A4550, are not separately reimbursed by Medicare; however, other third-party payers may cover them. Check with the specific payer to determine coverage.

ICD-9-CM Procedural

86.86 Onychoplasty

Anesthesia

11762 00400

ICD-9-CM Diagnostic

- 171.2 Malignant neoplasm of connective and other soft tissue of upper limb, including shoulder
- 172.6 Malignant melanoma of skin of upper limb, including shoulder
- 173.6 Other malignant neoplasm of skin of upper limb, including shoulder
- 232.6 Carcinoma in situ of skin of upper limb, including shoulder
- 757.5 Specified congenital anomalies of nails
- 816.12 Open fracture of distal phalanx or phalanges of hand
- 816.13 Open fractures of multiple sites of phalanx or phalanges of hand
- 883.0 Open wound of finger(s), without mention of complication
- 883.1 Open wound of finger(s), complicated
- 906.1 Late effect of open wound of extremities without mention of tendon injury
- 906.7 Late effect of burn of other extremities
- 927.3 Crushing injury of finger(s) — (Use additional code to identify any associated injuries: 800-829, 850.0-854.1, 860.0-869.1)
- 944.01 Burn of unspecified degree of single digit [finger (nail)] other than thumb
- 944.02 Burn of unspecified degree of thumb (nail)
- 944.03 Burn of unspecified degree of two or more digits of hand, not including thumb
- 944.04 Burn of unspecified degree of two or more digits of hand, including thumb
- 944.20 Blisters with epidermal loss due to burn (second degree) of unspecified site of hand
- 944.21 Blisters with epidermal loss due to burn (second degree) of single digit [finger (nail)] other than thumb
- 944.23 Blisters with epidermal loss due to burn (second degree) of two or more digits of hand, not including thumb
- 944.24 Blisters with epidermal loss due to burn (second degree) of two or more digits of hand including thumb
- 944.28 Blisters with epidermal loss due to burn (second degree) of multiple sites of wrist(s) and hand(s)
- 944.30 Full-thickness skin loss due to burn (third degree NOS) of unspecified site of hand
- 944.31 Full-thickness skin loss due to burn (third degree NOS) of single digit [finger (nail)] other than thumb
- 944.32 Full-thickness skin loss due to burn (third degree NOS) of thumb (nail)
- 944.33 Full-thickness skin loss due to burn (third degree NOS) of two or more digits of hand, not including thumb
- 944.34 Full-thickness skin loss due to burn (third degree NOS) of two or more digits of hand including thumb
- 944.38 Full-thickness skin loss due to burn (third degree NOS) of multiple sites of wrist(s) and hand(s)
- 944.41 Deep necrosis of underlying tissues due to burn (deep third degree) of single digit [finger (nail)] other than thumb, without mention of loss of a body part
- 944.42 Deep necrosis of underlying tissues due to burn (deep third degree) of thumb (nail), without mention of loss of a body part
- 944.43 Deep necrosis of underlying tissues due to burn (deep third degree) of two or more digits of hand, not including thumb, without mention of loss of a body part
- 944.44 Deep necrosis of underlying tissues due to burn (deep third degree) of two or more digits of hand including thumb, without mention of loss of a body part
- 944.48 Deep necrosis of underlying tissues due to burn (deep third degree) of multiple sites of wrist(s) and hand(s), without mention of loss of a body part

Terms To Know

graft. Tissue implant from another part of the body or another person.

CCI Version 16.3

0213T, 0216T, 0228T, 0230T, 10060-10061, 11000, 11040-11042, 11044, 11720-11730, 11740-11755, 11900-11901, 20550-20553, 29075-29086, 29125-29131, 29280, 29440, 29450, 29515, 29540-29581, 36000, 36400-36410, 36420-36430, 36440, 36600, 36640, 37202, 43752, 51701-51703, 62310-62319, 64400-64435, 64445-64450, 64479, 64483, 64490, 64493, 64505-64530, 69990, 93000-93010, 93040-93042, 93318, 94002, 94200, 94250, 94680-94690, 94770, 95812-95816, 95819, 95822, 95829, 95955, 96360, 96365, 96372, 96374-96376, 96405-96406, 97597-97598, 97602-97606, 99148-99149, 99150, J0670, J2001

Note: These CCI edits are used for Medicare. Other payers may reimburse on codes listed above.

Medicare Edits

	Fac RVU	Non-Fac RVU	FUD	Assist
11762	5.5	7.81	10	N/A

Medicare References: 100-2,15,290; 100-4,12,30

11765

11765 Wedge excision of skin of nail fold (eg, for ingrown toenail)

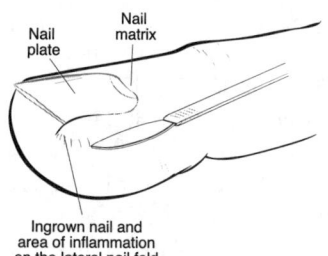

A wedge excision of the skin overlapping a nail is performed. The lateral nail fold is excised along its length and the incision may extend to include a portion of the nail matrix. Closure usually involves sutures

Explanation
The physician excises a wedge of restrictive skin in the nail fold to free an ingrown nail. The physician performs a wedge excision of the skin overlapping the lateral nail. The nail is examined and trimmed to encourage straight growth. The wound is dressed.

Coding Tips
Some payers may require the use of HCPCS Level II modifiers FA–F9 to identify the specific finger involved. For excision of a nail and nail matrix, partial or complete, for permanent removal, see 11750–11752. Surgical trays, A4550, are not separately reimbursed by Medicare; however, other third-party payers may cover them. Check with the specific payer to determine coverage.

ICD-9-CM Procedural
86.23 Removal of nail, nailbed, or nail fold

Anesthesia
11765 00400

ICD-9-CM Diagnostic
681.02 Onychia and paronychia of finger — (Use additional code to identify organism: 041.1)
686.1 Pyogenic granuloma of skin and subcutaneous tissue — (Use additional code to identify any infectious organism: 041.0-041.8)
703.0 Ingrowing nail

Terms To Know
lateral. To/on the side.

nail fold. Nail wall at the side and proximal end of the nail plate covered by a skin fold.

onychia. Inflammation or infection of the nail matrix leading to a loss of the nail.

paronychia. Infection of nail structures.

pyogenic granuloma. Small, erythematous papule on the skin and oral or gingival mucosa that increases in size and may become pendulum-like, infected, and/or ulcerated.

subcutaneous tissue. Sheet or wide band of adipose (fat) and areolar connective tissue in two layers attached to the dermis.

wedge excision. Surgical removal of a section of tissue that is thick at one edge and tapers to a thin edge.

CCI Version 16.3
0213T, 0216T, 0228T, 0230T, 11056-11057❖, 11740, 11755, 11900-11901, 13131, 17250, 20550-20553, 29075-29086, 29125-29131, 29280, 29440, 29450, 29515, 29540-29581, 36000, 36400-36410, 36420-36430, 36440, 36600, 36640, 37202, 43752, 51701-51703, 62310-62319, 64400-64435, 64445-64450, 64479, 64483, 64490, 64493, 64505-64530, 69990, 93000-93010, 93040-93042, 93318, 94002, 94200, 94250, 94680-94690, 94770, 95812-95816, 95819, 95822, 95829, 95955, 96360, 96365, 96372, 96374-96376, 96405-96406, 97597-97598, 97602-97606, 99148-99149, 99150, J0670, J2001

Note: These CCI edits are used for Medicare. Other payers may reimburse on codes listed above.

Medicare Edits

	Fac RVU	Non-Fac RVU	FUD	Assist
11765	1.99	3.94	10	N/A

Medicare References: 100-2,15,290; 100-4,12,30

12001-12007

12001 Simple repair of superficial wounds of scalp, neck, axillae, external genitalia, trunk and/or extremities (including hands and feet); 2.5 cm or less
12002 2.6 cm to 7.5 cm
12004 7.6 cm to 12.5 cm
12005 12.6 cm to 20.0 cm
12006 20.1 cm to 30.0 cm
12007 over 30.0 cm

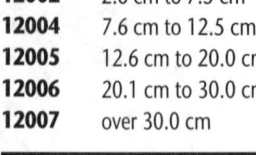

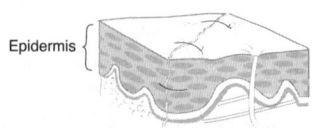

Example of a simple closure involving only one skin layer

12001: 2.5 cm or less
12002: 2.6 to 7.5 cm
12004: 7.6 to 12.5 cm
12005: 12.6 to 20.0 cm
12006: 20.1 to 30.0 cm
12007: more than 30.0 cm

A simple wound of the extremities, including the hands and elsewhere, is repaired. Report wounds according to the length of the lesion. Wounds of similar complexity in the same anatomical area may be summed and reported as a total length

Explanation

The physician sutures superficial lacerations of the scalp, neck, axillae, external genitalia, trunk, or extremities. A local anesthetic is injected around the laceration and the wound is cleansed, explored, and often irrigated with a saline solution. The physician performs a simple, one-layer repair of the epidermis, dermis, or subcutaneous tissues with sutures. With multiple wounds of the same complexity and in the same anatomical area, the length of all wounds sutured is summed and reported as one total length. Report 12001 for a total length of 2.5 cm or less; 12002 for 2.6 cm to 7.5 cm; 12004 for 7.6 cm to 12.5 cm; 12005 for 12.6 cm to 20 cm; 12006 for 20.1 cm to 30 cm; and 12007 if the total length is greater than 30 cm.

Coding Tips

Wounds treated with tissue glue or staples qualify as a simple repair even if they are not closed with sutures. When multiple wounds are repaired, add together the lengths of those in the same classification and report as a single item. Intermediate repair is used when layered closure of one or more of the deeper layers of subcutaneous tissue and superficial fascia, in addition to the skin, require closure.

Intermediate repair is also reported for single-layer closure of heavily contaminated wounds that have required extensive cleaning or removal of particulate matter. Medicare and some other payers may require G0168 be reported for wound closure by tissue adhesives only. Surgical trays, A4550, are not separately reimbursed by Medicare; however, other third-party payers may cover them. Check with the specific payer to determine coverage.

ICD-9-CM Procedural

86.59 Closure of skin and subcutaneous tissue of other sites

Anesthesia
00300, 00400

ICD-9-CM Diagnostic

873.0 Open wound of scalp, without mention of complication
874.8 Open wound of other and unspecified parts of neck, without mention of complication
879.6 Open wound of other and unspecified parts of trunk, without mention of complication
880.00 Open wound of shoulder region, without mention of complication
880.01 Open wound of scapular region, without mention of complication
880.02 Open wound of axillary region, without mention of complication
880.03 Open wound of upper arm, without mention of complication
880.09 Open wound of multiple sites of shoulder and upper arm, without mention of complication
881.00 Open wound of forearm, without mention of complication
881.01 Open wound of elbow, without mention of complication
881.02 Open wound of wrist, without mention of complication
882.0 Open wound of hand except finger(s) alone, without mention of complication
883.0 Open wound of finger(s), without mention of complication
884.0 Multiple and unspecified open wound of upper limb, without mention of complication

Terms To Know

simple repair. Surgical closure of a superficial wound, requiring single layer suturing of the skin (epidermis, dermis, or subcutaneous tissue).

CCI Version 16.3

0213T, 0216T, 0228T, 0230T, 11100, 11900-11901, 36000, 36400-36410, 36420-36430, 36440, 36600, 36640, 37202, 43752, 51701-51703, 62310-62319, 64400-64435, 64445-64450, 64479, 64483, 64490, 64493, 64505-64530, 69990, 93000-93010, 93040-93042, 93318, 94002, 94200, 94250, 94680-94690, 94770, 95812-95816, 95819, 95822, 95829, 95955, 96360, 96365, 96372, 96374-96376, 97597-97598, 97602-97606, 99148-99149, 99150, G0168, J0670, J2001

Also not with 12001: 11040-11042, 11055-11056, 11719, 11740-11750, 12011❖

Also not with 12002: 11040-11042, 11740, 12001, 12013-12014❖

Also not with 12004: 11040-11042, 12001-12002, 12015❖

Also not with 12005: 11040-11043, 12001-12004, 12016❖

Also not with 12006: 11042-11043, 12001-12005, 12017❖

Also not with 12007: 12001-12006, 12018❖

Note: These CCI edits are used for Medicare. Other payers may reimburse on codes listed above.

Medicare Edits

	Fac RVU	Non-Fac RVU	FUD	Assist
12001	1.62	2.82	0	N/A
12002	2.08	3.31	0	N/A
12004	2.53	3.93	0	N/A
12005	3.33	5.06	0	N/A
12006	4.07	6.11	0	N/A
12007	4.9	7.12	0	N/A

Medicare References: 100-2,15,260; 100-4,12,30; 100-4,12,90.3; 100-4,14,10

12020-12021

12020 Treatment of superficial wound dehiscence; simple closure
12021 with packing

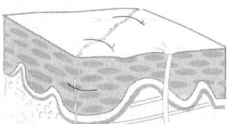

Example of a simple closure involving only one skin layer

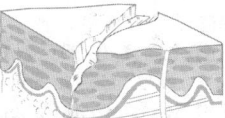

Example of wound with packing

Dehiscence is a failure of a wound to heal. In some instances, the wound will be a sutured surgical site. Others may be unstitched trauma sites. The margins of the wound tend to gape open. Report 12020 for treatment of the wound and simple closure. Report 12021 when packing is placed in the wound to allow healing

Explanation
There has been a breakdown of the healing skin either before or after suture removal. The skin margins have opened. The physician cleanses the wound with irrigation and antimicrobial solutions. The skin margins may be trimmed to initiate bleeding surfaces. Report 12020 if the wound is sutured in a single layer. Report 12021 if the wound is left open and packed with gauze strips due to the presence of infection. This allows infection to drain from the wound and the skin closure will be delayed until the infection is resolved.

Coding Tips
For extensive or complicated secondary closure of surgical wound or dehiscence, see 13160. Medicare and some other payers may require G0168 be reported for wound closure by tissue adhesives only. Surgical trays, A4550, are not separately reimbursed by Medicare; however, other third-party payers may cover them. Check with the specific payer to determine coverage.

ICD-9-CM Procedural
86.59 Closure of skin and subcutaneous tissue of other sites
96.59 Other irrigation of wound

Anesthesia
00300, 00400

ICD-9-CM Diagnostic
780.62 Postprocedural fever
998.30 Disruption of wound, unspecified
998.32 Disruption of external operation (surgical) wound
998.33 Disruption of traumatic injury wound repair
998.59 Other postoperative infection — (Use additional code to identify infection)
998.83 Non-healing surgical wound

Terms To Know
dehiscence. Complication of healing in which the surgical wound ruptures or bursts open, superficially or through multiple layers.

infection. Presence of microorganisms in body tissues that may result in cellular damage.

irrigation. To wash out or cleanse a body cavity, wound, or tissue with water or other fluid.

packing. Material placed into a cavity or wound, such as gels, gauze, pads, and sponges.

subcutaneous tissue. Sheet or wide band of adipose (fat) and areolar connective tissue in two layers attached to the dermis.

superficial. On the skin surface or near the surface of any involved structure or field of interest.

suture. Numerous stitching techniques employed in wound closure.

buried suture. Continuous or interrupted suture placed under the skin for a layered closure.

continuous suture. Running stitch with tension evenly distributed across a single strand to provide a leakproof closure line.

interrupted suture. Series of single stitches with tension isolated at each stitch, in which all stitches are not affected if one becomes loose, and the isolated sutures cannot act as a wick to transport an infection.

purse-string suture. Continuous suture placed around a tubular structure and tightened, to reduce or close the lumen.

retention suture. Secondary stitching that bridges the primary suture, providing support for the primary repair; a plastic or rubber bolster may be placed over the primary repair and under the retention sutures.

CCI Version 16.3
0213T, 0216T, 0228T, 0230T, 11100, 11900-11901, 36000, 36400-36410, 36420-36430, 36440, 36600, 36640, 37202, 43752, 51701-51703, 62310-62319, 64400-64435, 64445-64450, 64479, 64483, 64490, 64493, 64505-64530, 69990, 93000-93010, 93040-93042, 93318, 94002, 94200, 94250, 94680-94690, 94770, 95812-95816, 95819, 95822, 95829, 95955, 96360, 96365, 96372, 96374-96376, 97597-97598, 97602-97606, 99148-99149, 99150, G0168, J2001

Also not with 12020: 11041-11043, 12021, J0670

Also not with 12021: 11041-11042

Note: These CCI edits are used for Medicare. Other payers may reimburse on codes listed above.

Medicare Edits

	Fac RVU	Non-Fac RVU	FUD	Assist
12020	5.43	7.82	10	N/A
12021	4.0	4.65	10	N/A

Medicare References: 100-2,15,260; 100-4,12,30; 100-4,12,90.3; 100-4,14,10

12031-12037

12031 Repair, intermediate, wounds of scalp, axillae, trunk and/or extremities (excluding hands and feet); 2.5 cm or less
12032 2.6 cm to 7.5 cm
12034 7.6 cm to 12.5 cm
12035 12.6 cm to 20.0 cm
12036 20.1 cm to 30.0 cm
12037 over 30.0 cm

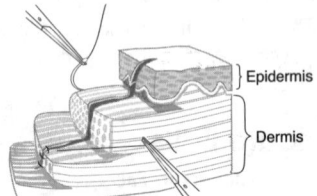

Schematic of layered closure

A layered closure of a wound of the arm, or elsewhere, but excluding the hands is performed

12031: 2.5 cm or less
12032: 2.6 to 7.5 cm
12034: 7.6 to 12.5 cm
12035: 12.6 to 20.0 cm
12036: 20.1 to 30.0 cm
12037: larger than 30.0 cm

Explanation

The physician performs an intermediate repair of a laceration of the scalp, axillae, trunk, and/or extremities (except hands and feet) using layered closure. A local anesthetic is injected around the laceration, and the wound is cleansed, explored, and often irrigated with a saline solution. Due to deeper or more complex lacerations, deep subcutaneous or layered suturing techniques are required. The physician closes tissue layers under the skin with dissolvable sutures before suturing the skin. Extensive cleaning or removal of foreign matter from a heavily contaminated wound that is closed with a single layer may also be reported as an intermediate repair. With multiple wounds of the same complexity and in the same anatomical area, the length of all wounds sutured is summed and reported as one total length. Report 12031 for a total length of 2.5 cm or less; 12032 for 2.6 cm to 7.5 cm; 12034 for 7.6 cm to 12.5 cm; 12035 for 12.6 cm to 20 cm; 12036 for 20.1 cm to 30 cm; and 12037 if the total length is greater than 30 cm.

Coding Tips

Intermediate repair includes the repair of wounds that require layered closure of one or more of the deeper layers of subcutaneous tissue and superficial fascia, in addition to skin closure. Single-layer closure of heavily contaminated wounds that require extensive cleaning or removal of foreign matter also constitute intermediate repair. For simple repairs, see 12001–12007; complex repairs, see 13100–13153. These procedures are usually performed using local anesthesia. However, these procedures may be performed under general anesthesia, depending on the age and/or condition of the patient. Medicare and some other payers may require G0168 be reported for wound closure by tissue adhesives only. Surgical trays, A4550, are not separately reimbursed by Medicare; however, other third-party payers may cover them. Check with the specific payer to determine coverage.

ICD-9-CM Procedural

86.59 Closure of skin and subcutaneous tissue of other sites

Anesthesia
00300, 00400

ICD-9-CM Diagnostic

172.6 Malignant melanoma of skin of upper limb, including shoulder
173.5 Other malignant neoplasm of skin of trunk, except scrotum
173.6 Other malignant neoplasm of skin of upper limb, including shoulder
209.33 Merkel cell carcinoma of the upper limb
216.5 Benign neoplasm of skin of trunk, except scrotum
216.6 Benign neoplasm of skin of upper limb, including shoulder
232.5 Carcinoma in situ of skin of trunk, except scrotum
232.6 Carcinoma in situ of skin of upper limb, including shoulder
686.1 Pyogenic granuloma of skin and subcutaneous tissue — (Use additional code to identify any infectious organism: 041.0-041.8)
702.0 Actinic keratosis
702.11 Inflamed seborrheic keratosis
706.2 Sebaceous cyst
709.1 Vascular disorder of skin
709.2 Scar condition and fibrosis of skin
757.32 Congenital vascular hamartomas
875.0 Open wound of chest (wall), without mention of complication
876.0 Open wound of back, without mention of complication
880.00 Open wound of shoulder region, without mention of complication
880.03 Open wound of upper arm, without mention of complication
881.00 Open wound of forearm, without mention of complication
881.01 Open wound of elbow, without mention of complication
881.02 Open wound of wrist, without mention of complication
884.0 Multiple and unspecified open wound of upper limb, without mention of complication

CCI Version 16.3

0213T, 0216T, 0228T, 0230T, 11100, 11900-11901, 36000, 36400-36410, 36420-36430, 36440, 36600, 36640, 37202, 43752, 51701-51703, 62310-62319, 64400-64435, 64445-64450, 64479, 64483, 64490, 64493, 64505-64530, 69990, 93000-93010, 93040-93042, 93318, 94002, 94200, 94250, 94680-94690, 94770, 95812-95816, 95819, 95822, 95829, 95955, 96360, 96365, 96372, 96374-96376, 97597-97598, 97602-97606, 99148-99149, 99150, G0168, J0670, J2001

Also not with 12031: 11041-11042, 11055-11056, 12041❖, 12051❖

Also not with 12032: 11040-11043, 12031, 12042❖, 12052-12053❖

Also not with 12034: 11042-11043, 12031-12032, 12044❖, 12054❖

Also not with 12035: 11042-11044, 12031-12034, 12045❖, 12055❖

Also not with 12036: 11043, 12031-12035, 12046❖, 12056❖

Also not with 12037: 11043-11044, 12031-12036, 12057❖

Note: These CCI edits are used for Medicare. Other payers may reimburse on codes listed above.

Medicare Edits

	Fac RVU	Non-Fac RVU	FUD	Assist
12031	4.75	7.08	10	N/A
12032	5.74	8.91	10	N/A
12034	5.99	8.89	10	N/A
12035	6.93	10.79	10	N/A
12036	7.92	11.78	10	N/A
12037	9.2	13.21	10	80

Medicare References: 100-2,15,260; 100-4,12,30; 100-4,12,90.3; 100-4,14,10

12041-12047

12041	Repair, intermediate, wounds of neck, hands, feet and/or external genitalia; 2.5 cm or less
12042	2.6 cm to 7.5 cm
12044	7.6 cm to 12.5 cm
12045	12.6 cm to 20.0 cm
12046	20.1 cm to 30.0 cm
12047	over 30.0 cm

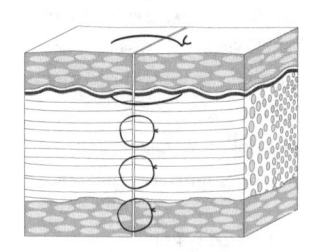

Example of layered sutures involving deeper tissues

For layered closure of wounds of the hands, or elsewhere
- 12041: 2.5 cm or less
- 12042: 2.6 to 7.5 cm
- 12033: 7.5 to 12.5 cm
- 12045: 12.6 to 20.0 cm
- 12046: 20.1 to 30.0 cm
- 12047: larger than 30.0 cm

Explanation

The physician performs an intermediate repair of a laceration of the neck, hands, feet, and/or external genitalia using layered closure. A local anesthetic is injected around the laceration, and the wound is cleansed, explored, and often irrigated with a saline solution. Due to deeper or more complex lacerations, deep subcutaneous or layered suturing techniques are required. The physician closes tissue layers under the skin with dissolvable sutures before suturing the skin. Extensive cleaning or removal of foreign matter from a heavily contaminated wound that is closed with a single layer may also be reported as an intermediate repair. With multiple wounds of the same complexity and in the same anatomical area, the length of all wounds sutured is summed and reported as one total length. Report 12041 for a total length of 2.5 cm or less; 12042 for 2.6 cm to 7.5 cm; 12044 for 7.6 cm to 12.5 cm; 12045 for 12.6 cm to 20 cm; 12046 for 20.1 cm to 30 cm; and 12047 if the total length is greater than 30 cm.

Coding Tips

A wound requiring a rubber drain, removal of foreign matter, or extensive cleansing and removal of damaged tissue is classified as intermediate repair even though it may be closed by a single layer of skin sutures. These procedures are usually performed using local anesthesia. However, these procedures may be performed under general anesthesia, depending on the age and/or condition of the patient. Medicare and some other payers may require G0168 be reported for wound closure by tissue adhesives only. Surgical trays, A4550, are not separately reimbursed by Medicare; however, other third-party payers may cover them. Check with the specific payer to determine coverage.

ICD-9-CM Procedural

- 86.59 Closure of skin and subcutaneous tissue of other sites

Anesthesia

00300, 00400

ICD-9-CM Diagnostic

- 172.4 Malignant melanoma of skin of scalp and neck
- 172.6 Malignant melanoma of skin of upper limb, including shoulder
- 173.4 Other malignant neoplasm of scalp and skin of neck
- 173.6 Other malignant neoplasm of skin of upper limb, including shoulder
- 198.2 Secondary malignant neoplasm of skin
- 209.33 Merkel cell carcinoma of the upper limb
- 214.1 Lipoma of other skin and subcutaneous tissue
- 216.4 Benign neoplasm of scalp and skin of neck
- 216.6 Benign neoplasm of skin of upper limb, including shoulder
- 216.8 Benign neoplasm of other specified sites of skin
- 228.01 Hemangioma of skin and subcutaneous tissue
- 232.4 Carcinoma in situ of scalp and skin of neck
- 232.6 Carcinoma in situ of skin of upper limb, including shoulder
- 448.1 Nevus, non-neoplastic
- 686.1 Pyogenic granuloma of skin and subcutaneous tissue — (Use additional code to identify any infectious organism: 041.0-041.8)
- 702.8 Other specified dermatoses
- 706.2 Sebaceous cyst
- 709.1 Vascular disorder of skin
- 709.2 Scar condition and fibrosis of skin
- 709.9 Unspecified disorder of skin and subcutaneous tissue
- 757.32 Congenital vascular hamartomas
- 757.33 Congenital pigmentary anomaly of skin
- 757.39 Other specified congenital anomaly of skin
- 782.2 Localized superficial swelling, mass, or lump
- 874.8 Open wound of other and unspecified parts of neck, without mention of complication
- 882.0 Open wound of hand except finger(s) alone, without mention of complication
- 882.1 Open wound of hand except finger(s) alone, complicated
- 883.0 Open wound of finger(s), without mention of complication
- 883.1 Open wound of finger(s), complicated

CCI Version 16.3

0213T, 0216T, 0228T, 0230T, 11100, 11900-11901, 36000, 36400-36410, 36420-36430, 36440, 36600, 36640, 37202, 43752, 51701-51703, 62310-62319, 64400-64435, 64445-64450, 64479, 64483, 64490, 64493, 64505-64530, 69990, 93000-93010, 93040-93042, 93318, 94002, 94200, 94250, 94680-94690, 94770, 95812-95816, 95819, 95822, 95829, 95955, 96360, 96365, 96372, 96374-96376, 97597-97598, 97602-97606, 99148-99149, 99150, G0168, J0670, J2001

Also not with 12041: 11055-11056, 11740, 12051❖

Also not with 12042: 11040-11042, 11740, 12041

Also not with 12044: 11043-11044, 12041-12042, 12054❖

Also not with 12045: 11042, 12041-12044, 12055❖

Also not with 12046: 11043-11044, 12041-12045, 12056❖

Also not with 12047: 12037-12046, 12057❖

Note: These CCI edits are used for Medicare. Other payers may reimburse on codes listed above.

Medicare Edits

	Fac RVU	Non-Fac RVU	FUD	Assist
12041	5.04	7.39	10	N/A
12042	5.87	8.46	10	N/A
12044	6.24	10.03	10	N/A
12045	7.09	10.74	10	N/A
12046	8.43	12.75	10	80
12047	9.08	13.84	10	80

Medicare References: 100-2,15,260; 100-4,12,30; 100-4,12,90.3; 100-4,14,10

13120-13122

13120 Repair, complex, scalp, arms, and/or legs; 1.1 cm to 2.5 cm
13121 2.6 cm to 7.5 cm
13122 each additional 5 cm or less (List separately in addition to code for primary procedure)

A complex wound 1.1 cm to 2.5 cm is debrided, irrigated, and a layered closure reported (13120)

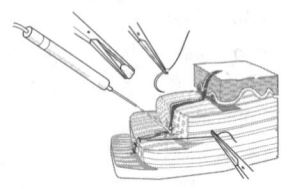

A larger wound, 2.6 cm to 7.5 cm, is reported by 13121. Report 13122 for each additional 5.0 cm or less beyond that coded by 13121

The wound is irrigated, debrided of fragments and damaged tissues, and a layered closure is performed

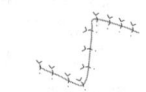

A local flap, scar revision, or other reconstructive efforts may also be required

Explanation

The physician repairs complex wounds of the scalp, arms, and/or legs. The physician performs complex, layered suturing of torn, crushed, or deeply lacerated tissue. The physician debrides the wound by removing foreign material or damaged tissue. Irrigation of the wound is performed and antimicrobial solutions are used to decontaminate and cleanse the wound. The physician may trim skin margins with a scalpel or scissors to allow for proper closure. The wound is closed in layers. The physician may perform scar revision, which creates a complex defect requiring repair. Stents or retention sutures may also be used in complex repair of a wound. Reconstructive procedures, such as utilization of local flaps, may be required and are reported separately. Report 13120 for wounds 1.1 cm to 2.5 cm; 13121 for 2.6 cm to 7.5 cm; and 13122 for each additional 5 cm or less.

Coding Tips

Complex repair is defined as the repair of wounds requiring more than layered closure. Examples include repairs requiring scar revision, debridement, extensive undermining, stents, or retention sutures. Use 13122 in conjunction with 13121. As an "add-on" code, 13122 is not subject to multiple procedure rules. No reimbursement reduction or modifier 51 is applied. "Add-on" codes describe additional intra-service work associated with the primary procedure. They are performed by the same physician on the same date of service as the primary service/procedure, and must never be reported as a stand-alone code. These procedures are usually performed using local anesthesia. However, these procedures may be performed under general anesthesia, depending on the age and/or condition of the patient. For wounds 1 cm or less, see simple or intermediate repair codes. Medicare and some other payers may require G0168 be reported for wound closure by tissue adhesives only. Surgical trays, A4550, are not separately reimbursed by Medicare; however, other third-party payers may cover them. Check with the specific payer to determine coverage.

ICD-9-CM Procedural

86.59 Closure of skin and subcutaneous tissue of other sites
86.89 Other repair and reconstruction of skin and subcutaneous tissue

Anesthesia

13120 00300, 00400
13121 00300, 00400
13122 N/A

ICD-9-CM Diagnostic

172.6 Malignant melanoma of skin of upper limb, including shoulder
173.6 Other malignant neoplasm of skin of upper limb, including shoulder
195.4 Malignant neoplasm of upper limb
198.2 Secondary malignant neoplasm of skin
209.33 Merkel cell carcinoma of the upper limb
214.1 Lipoma of other skin and subcutaneous tissue
216.6 Benign neoplasm of skin of upper limb, including shoulder
228.01 Hemangioma of skin and subcutaneous tissue
232.6 Carcinoma in situ of skin of upper limb, including shoulder
686.1 Pyogenic granuloma of skin and subcutaneous tissue — (Use additional code to identify any infectious organism: 041.0-041.8)
706.2 Sebaceous cyst
709.4 Foreign body granuloma of skin and subcutaneous tissue — (Use additional code to identify foreign body (V90.01-V90.9))
782.2 Localized superficial swelling, mass, or lump
880.03 Open wound of upper arm, without mention of complication
880.13 Open wound of upper arm, complicated
881.00 Open wound of forearm, without mention of complication
881.01 Open wound of elbow, without mention of complication
881.02 Open wound of wrist, without mention of complication
881.10 Open wound of forearm, complicated
881.11 Open wound of elbow, complicated
881.12 Open wound of wrist, complicated
884.0 Multiple and unspecified open wound of upper limb, without mention of complication
884.1 Multiple and unspecified open wound of upper limb, complicated

CCI Version 16.3

11100, 11900-11901, 13160❖, 69990

Also not with 13120: 0213T, 0216T, 0228T, 0230T, 11000, 11010-11012, 11040-11044, 13122, 36000, 36400-36410, 36420-36430, 36440, 36600, 36640, 37202, 43752, 51701-51703, 62310-62319, 64400-64435, 64445-64450, 64479, 64483, 64490, 64493, 64505-64530, 93000-93010, 93040-93042, 93318, 94002, 94200, 94250, 94680-94690, 94770, 95812-95816, 95819, 95822, 95829, 95955, 96360, 96365, 96372, 96374-96376, 97597-97598, 97602-97606, 99148-99149, 99150, G0168, J0670, J2001

Also not with 13121: 0213T, 0216T, 0228T, 0230T, 11000, 11010-11012, 11040-11044, 13120, 36000, 36400-36410, 36420-36430, 36440, 36600, 36640, 37202, 43752, 51701-51703, 62310-62319, 64400-64435, 64445-64450, 64479, 64483, 64490, 64493, 64505-64530, 93000-93010, 93040-93042, 93318, 94002, 94200, 94250, 94680-94690, 94770, 95812-95816, 95819, 95822, 95829, 95955, 96360, 96365, 96372, 96374-96376, 97597-97598, 97602-97606, 99148-99149, 99150, G0168, J0670, J2001

Note: These CCI edits are used for Medicare. Other payers may reimburse on codes listed above.

Medicare Edits

	Fac RVU	Non-Fac RVU	FUD	Assist
13120	7.24	9.5	10	N/A
13121	9.67	12.94	10	N/A
13122	2.55	3.49	N/A	N/A

Medicare References: 100-2,15,260; 100-4,12,30; 100-4,12,90.3; 100-4,14,10

13131-13133

13131 Repair, complex, forehead, cheeks, chin, mouth, neck, axillae, genitalia, hands and/or feet; 1.1 cm to 2.5 cm
13132 2.6 cm to 7.5 cm
13133 each additional 5 cm or less (List separately in addition to code for primary procedure)

Schematic of complex layered suturing of torn or deeply lacerated tissue

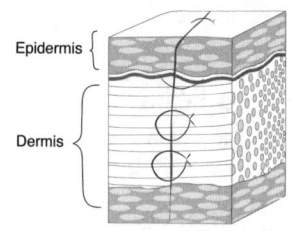

Repairs of the hand are included in the code descriptions. Report 13131 for length of repairs for the same group of anatomic sites that sum 1.1 cm to 2.5 cm. Report 13132 for those measuring a sum of 2.6 cm to 7.5 cm. Report 13133 for each additional 5.0 cm or less of a complex repair beyond that reported by 13132

Explanation

The physician repairs complex wounds of the forehead, cheeks, chin, mouth, neck, axillae, genitalia, hands, and/or feet. The physician performs complex, layered suturing of torn, crushed, or deeply lacerated tissue. The physician debrides the wound by removing foreign material or damaged tissue. Irrigation of the wound is performed and antimicrobial solutions are used to decontaminate and cleanse the wound. The physician may trim skin margins with a scalpel or scissors to allow for proper closure. The wound is closed in layers. The physician may perform scar revision, which creates a complex defect requiring repair. Stents or retention sutures may also be used in complex repair of a wound. Reconstructive procedures, such as utilization of local flaps, may be required and are reported separately. Report 13131 for wounds 1.1 cm to 2.5 cm; 13132 for 2.6 cm to 7.5 cm; and 13133 for each additional 5 cm or less.

Coding Tips

Complex repair is defined as the repair of wounds requiring more than layered closure. Examples include repairs requiring scar revision, debridement, extensive undermining, stents, or retention sutures. Use 13133 in conjunction with 13132. As an "add-on" code, 13133 is not subject to multiple procedure rules. No reimbursement reduction or modifier 51 is applied. "Add-on" codes describe additional intra-service work associated with the primary procedure. They are performed by the same physician on the same date of service as the primary service/procedure, and must never be reported as a stand-alone code. These procedures are usually performed using local anesthesia. However, these procedures may be performed under general anesthesia, depending on the age and/or condition of the patient. For wounds 1 cm or less, see simple or intermediate repair codes. Medicare and some other payers may require G0168 be reported for wound closure by tissue adhesives only. Surgical trays, A4550, are not separately reimbursed by Medicare; however, other third-party payers may cover them. Check with the specific payer to determine coverage.

ICD-9-CM Procedural

- 86.59 Closure of skin and subcutaneous tissue of other sites
- 86.89 Other repair and reconstruction of skin and subcutaneous tissue

Anesthesia

13131 00300, 00400
13132 00300, 00400
13133 N/A

ICD-9-CM Diagnostic

- 172.6 Malignant melanoma of skin of upper limb, including shoulder
- 173.4 Other malignant neoplasm of scalp and skin of neck
- 173.6 Other malignant neoplasm of skin of upper limb, including shoulder
- 195.4 Malignant neoplasm of upper limb
- 209.33 Merkel cell carcinoma of the upper limb
- 209.75 Secondary Merkel cell carcinoma
- 214.0 Lipoma of skin and subcutaneous tissue of face
- 214.1 Lipoma of other skin and subcutaneous tissue
- 216.6 Benign neoplasm of skin of upper limb, including shoulder
- 228.01 Hemangioma of skin and subcutaneous tissue
- 448.1 Nevus, non-neoplastic
- 686.1 Pyogenic granuloma of skin and subcutaneous tissue — (Use additional code to identify any infectious organism: 041.0-041.8)
- 709.4 Foreign body granuloma of skin and subcutaneous tissue — (Use additional code to identify foreign body (V90.01-V90.9))
- 880.02 Open wound of axillary region, without mention of complication
- 880.12 Open wound of axillary region, complicated
- 882.0 Open wound of hand except finger(s) alone, without mention of complication
- 882.1 Open wound of hand except finger(s) alone, complicated
- 883.0 Open wound of finger(s), without mention of complication
- 883.1 Open wound of finger(s), complicated

CCI Version 16.3

11100, 11900-11901, 13160❖, 69990

Also not with 13131: 0213T, 0216T, 0228T, 0230T, 11000, 11010-11012, 11040-11044, 13133, 36000, 36400-36410, 36420-36430, 36440, 36600, 36640, 37202, 43752, 51701-51703, 62310-62319, 64400-64435, 64445-64450, 64479, 64483, 64490, 64493, 64505-64530, 93000-93010, 93040-93042, 93318, 94002, 94200, 94250, 94680-94690, 94770, 95812-95816, 95819, 95822, 95829, 95955, 96360, 96365, 96372, 96374-96376, 97597-97598, 97602-97606, 99148-99149, 99150, G0168, J0670, J2001

Also not with 13132: 0213T, 0216T, 0228T, 0230T, 11000, 11010-11012, 11040-11044, 11056, 13131, 36000, 36400-36410, 36420-36430, 36440, 36600, 36640, 37202, 43752, 51701-51703, 62310-62319, 64400-64435, 64445-64450, 64479, 64483, 64490, 64493, 64505-64530, 93000-93010, 93040-93042, 93318, 94002, 94200, 94250, 94680-94690, 94770, 95812-95816, 95819, 95822, 95829, 95955, 96360, 96365, 96372, 96374-96376, 97597-97598, 97602-97606, 99148-99149, 99150, G0168, J0670, J2001

Note: These CCI edits are used for Medicare. Other payers may reimburse on codes listed above.

Medicare Edits

	Fac RVU	Non-Fac RVU	FUD	Assist
13131	8.15	10.49	10	N/A
13132	13.93	17.0	10	N/A
13133	3.94	4.93	N/A	N/A

Medicare References: 100-2,15,260; 100-4,12,30; 100-4,12,90.3; 100-4,14,10

13160

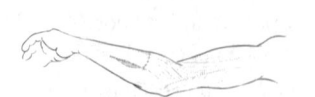

13160 Secondary closure of surgical wound or dehiscence, extensive or complicated

An extensive or complicated surgical wound is closed secondarily or extensive or complicated dehiscence is closed in the arm/shoulder area

Explanation

The physician secondarily repairs a surgical skin closure after an infectious breakdown of the healing skin. After resolution of the infection, the wound is ready for closure. The physician uses a scalpel to excise granulation and scar tissue. Skin margins are trimmed to bleeding edges. The wound is sutured in several layers.

Coding Tips

If incision and drainage of a hematoma, seroma, or fluid collection is performed, see 10140. This procedure is usually performed using local anesthesia. However, this procedure may be performed under general anesthesia, depending on the age and/or condition of the patient. For treatment of superficial wound dehiscence, with simple closure, see 12020; with packing, see 12021.

ICD-9-CM Procedural

54.62 Delayed closure of granulating abdominal wound

Anesthesia

13160 00300, 00400

ICD-9-CM Diagnostic

958.3 Posttraumatic wound infection not elsewhere classified
998.30 Disruption of wound, unspecified
998.31 Disruption of internal operation (surgical) wound
998.32 Disruption of external operation (surgical) wound
998.83 Non-healing surgical wound
V58.41 Planned postoperative wound closure — (This code should be used in conjunction with other aftercare codes to fully identify the reason for the aftercare encounter)

Terms To Know

dehiscence. Complication of healing in which the surgical wound ruptures or bursts open, superficially or through multiple layers.

excise. Remove or cut out.

granulation tissue. Loose collection of fibroblasts, inflammatory cells, and new vessels in an edematous fleshy projection that forms at the base of open wounds over which new skin forms, unless excessive granulation tissue, or proud flesh, rises above the wound surface.

infection. Presence of microorganisms in body tissues that may result in cellular damage.

secondary. Second in order of occurrence or importance, or appearing during the course of another disease or condition.

suture. Numerous stitching techniques employed in wound closure.

buried suture. Continuous or interrupted suture placed under the skin for a layered closure.

continuous suture. Running stitch with tension evenly distributed across a single strand to provide a leakproof closure line.

interrupted suture. Series of single stitches with tension isolated at each stitch, in which all stitches are not affected if one becomes loose, and the isolated sutures cannot act as a wick to transport an infection.

purse-string suture. Continuous suture placed around a tubular structure and tightened, to reduce or close the lumen.

retention suture. Secondary stitching that bridges the primary suture, providing support for the primary repair; a plastic or rubber bolster may be placed over the primary repair and under the retention sutures.

CCI Version 16.3

0213T, 0216T, 0228T, 0230T, 10180, 11000, 11010-11012, 11040-11044, 11100, 11900-11901, 12020-12021, 36000, 36400-36410, 36420-36430, 36440, 36600, 36640, 37202, 43752, 51701-51703, 62310-62319, 64400-64435, 64445-64450, 64479, 64483, 64490, 64493, 64505-64530, 69990, 93000-93010, 93040-93042, 93318, 94002, 94200, 94250, 94680-94690, 94770, 95812-95816, 95819, 95822, 95829, 95955, 96360, 96365, 96372, 96374-96376, 97597-97598, 97602-97606, 99148-99149, 99150, G0168

Note: These CCI edits are used for Medicare. Other payers may reimburse on codes listed above.

Medicare Edits

	Fac RVU	Non-Fac RVU	FUD	Assist
13160	23.72	23.72	90	N/A

Medicare References: 100-2,15,260; 100-4,12,30; 100-4,12,90.3; 100-4,14,10

14000-14001

14000 Adjacent tissue transfer or rearrangement, trunk; defect 10 sq cm or less
14001 defect 10.1 sq cm to 30.0 sq cm

Example of common Z-plasty. Lesion is removed with oval-shaped incision

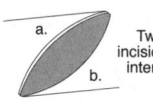

Two additional incisions (a. and b.) intersect the area

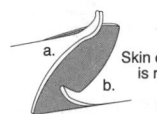

Skin of each incision is reflected back

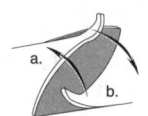

The flaps are then transposed and the repair is closed

An adjacent flap, or other rearrangement flap, is performed to repair a defect of 10 sq cm or less (14000); a larger defect (up to 30 sq cm) is coded 14001

Explanation
The physician transfers or rearranges adjacent tissue to repair traumatic or surgical wounds of the trunk. This includes, but is not limited to, such rearrangement procedures as Z-plasty, W-plasty, ZY-plasty, or tissue transfers such as rotational or advancement flaps. Report 14000 for defects that are 10 sq cm or less and 14001 for defects that are 10.1 sq cm to 30 sq cm.

Coding Tips
Excision of a lesion or a defect is included in adjacent tissue transfer or rearrangement procedures and is not reported separately. When these codes are used for the repair of traumatic wounds, the procedure must have been previously planned and developed by the physician to effect this particular repair configuration. These codes do not apply when direct closure or rearrangement of traumatized tissue incidentally results in these configurations. If a skin graft is required to close a secondary defect, it is reported as an additional procedure by appending modifier 51. For an intralesional injection to limit scarring, see 11900. Surgical trays, A4550, are not separately reimbursed by Medicare; however, other third-party payers may cover them. Check with the specific payer to determine coverage.

ICD-9-CM Procedural
- 86.3 Other local excision or destruction of lesion or tissue of skin and subcutaneous tissue
- 86.70 Pedicle or flap graft, not otherwise specified
- 86.71 Cutting and preparation of pedicle grafts or flaps
- 86.72 Advancement of pedicle graft
- 86.74 Attachment of pedicle or flap graft to other sites
- 86.84 Relaxation of scar or web contracture of skin
- 86.89 Other repair and reconstruction of skin and subcutaneous tissue

Anesthesia
00300, 00400

ICD-9-CM Diagnostic
- 172.5 Malignant melanoma of skin of trunk, except scrotum
- 173.5 Other malignant neoplasm of skin of trunk, except scrotum
- 216.5 Benign neoplasm of skin of trunk, except scrotum
- 228.01 Hemangioma of skin and subcutaneous tissue
- 232.5 Carcinoma in situ of skin of trunk, except scrotum
- 238.2 Neoplasm of uncertain behavior of skin
- 701.4 Keloid scar
- 706.2 Sebaceous cyst
- 707.01 Pressure ulcer, elbow — (Use additional code to identify pressure ulcer stage: 707.20-707.25)
- 707.02 Pressure ulcer, upper back — (Use additional code to identify pressure ulcer stage: 707.20-707.25)
- 707.03 Pressure ulcer, lower back — (Use additional code to identify pressure ulcer stage: 707.20-707.25)
- 707.8 Chronic ulcer of other specified site
- 709.2 Scar condition and fibrosis of skin
- 875.0 Open wound of chest (wall), without mention of complication
- 875.1 Open wound of chest (wall), complicated
- 876.0 Open wound of back, without mention of complication
- 876.1 Open wound of back, complicated
- 879.3 Open wound of abdominal wall, anterior, complicated
- 879.4 Open wound of abdominal wall, lateral, without mention of complication
- 879.5 Open wound of abdominal wall, lateral, complicated
- 906.0 Late effect of open wound of head, neck, and trunk
- 909.3 Late effect of complications of surgical and medical care
- 942.00 Burn of unspecified degree of trunk, unspecified site
- 942.01 Burn of trunk, unspecified degree of breast
- 942.02 Burn of trunk, unspecified degree of chest wall, excluding breast and nipple
- 942.04 Burn of trunk, unspecified degree of back (any part)
- 942.09 Burn of trunk, unspecified degree of other and multiple sites
- 942.34 Full-thickness skin loss due to burn (third degree NOS) of back (any part)
- 998.32 Disruption of external operation (surgical) wound

CCI Version 16.3
0213T, 0216T, 0228T, 0230T, 11000, 11040-11042, 11100, 11400-11471, 11600-11606, 11620-11646, 12001-12007, 12011-12037, 13100-13101, 20550-20553, 36000, 36400-36410, 36420-36430, 36440, 36600, 36640, 37202, 43752, 51701-51703, 62310-62319, 64400-64435, 64445-64450, 64479, 64483, 64490, 64493, 64505-64530, 69990, 93000-93010, 93040-93042, 93318, 94002, 94200, 94250, 94680-94690, 94770, 95812-95816, 95819, 95822, 95829, 95955, 96360, 96365, 96372, 96374-96376, 97597-97598, 97602-97606, 99148-99149, 99150, G0168, J0670, J2001

Also not with 14001: 14000

Note: These CCI edits are used for Medicare. Other payers may reimburse on codes listed above.

Medicare Edits

	Fac RVU	Non-Fac RVU	FUD	Assist
14000	14.91	18.19	90	N/A
14001	19.57	23.48	90	N/A

Medicare References: 100-2,15,260; 100-4,12,30; 100-4,12,90.3; 100-4,14,10

14020-14021

14020 Adjacent tissue transfer or rearrangement, scalp, arms and/or legs; defect 10 sq cm or less

14021 defect 10.1 sq cm to 30.0 sq cm

Example of common Z-plasty. Lesion is removed with oval-shaped incision

Skin of each incision is reflected back

The flaps are then transposed and the repair is closed

Two additional incisions (a. and b.) intersect the area

An adjacent flap, or other rearrangement flap of the upper extremity, is performed to repair a defect of 10.0 sq cm or less (14020); a larger defect (up to 30.0 sq cm) is reported with 14021

Explanation
The physician transfers or rearranges adjacent tissue to repair traumatic or surgical wounds of the scalp, arms, and/or legs. This includes, but is not limited to, such rearrangement procedures as Z-plasty, W-plasty, ZY-plasty, or tissue transfers such as rotational or advancement flaps. Report 14020 for defects that are 10 sq cm or less and 14021 for defects that are 10.1 sq cm to 30 sq cm.

Coding Tips
When adjacent tissue transfer or rearrangement is performed in conjunction with excision of a lesion, the lesion excision is not reported separately. When these codes are used to report repair of traumatic wounds, the procedure must have been previously planned and developed by the physician to effect the repair. These codes do not apply when direct closure or rearrangement of traumatized tissue incidentally results in these configurations. Any skin grafting required to close the secondary defect is reported separately. For an intralesional injection to limit scarring, see 11900. Surgical trays, A4550, are not separately reimbursed by Medicare; however, other third-party payers may cover them. Check with the specific payer to determine coverage.

ICD-9-CM Procedural
- 86.3 Other local excision or destruction of lesion or tissue of skin and subcutaneous tissue
- 86.70 Pedicle or flap graft, not otherwise specified
- 86.71 Cutting and preparation of pedicle grafts or flaps
- 86.72 Advancement of pedicle graft
- 86.74 Attachment of pedicle or flap graft to other sites
- 86.84 Relaxation of scar or web contracture of skin
- 86.89 Other repair and reconstruction of skin and subcutaneous tissue

Anesthesia
00300, 00400

ICD-9-CM Diagnostic
- 172.6 Malignant melanoma of skin of upper limb, including shoulder
- 173.6 Other malignant neoplasm of skin of upper limb, including shoulder
- 209.33 Merkel cell carcinoma of the upper limb
- 209.75 Secondary Merkel cell carcinoma
- 216.6 Benign neoplasm of skin of upper limb, including shoulder
- 232.6 Carcinoma in situ of skin of upper limb, including shoulder
- 707.01 Pressure ulcer, elbow — (Use additional code to identify pressure ulcer stage: 707.20-707.25)
- 709.2 Scar condition and fibrosis of skin
- 709.4 Foreign body granuloma of skin and subcutaneous tissue — (Use additional code to identify foreign body (V90.01-V90.9))
- 785.4 Gangrene — (Code first any associated underlying condition)
- 880.03 Open wound of upper arm, without mention of complication
- 880.13 Open wound of upper arm, complicated
- 881.00 Open wound of forearm, without mention of complication
- 881.01 Open wound of elbow, without mention of complication
- 881.02 Open wound of wrist, without mention of complication
- 881.10 Open wound of forearm, complicated
- 881.11 Open wound of elbow, complicated
- 881.12 Open wound of wrist, complicated
- 884.0 Multiple and unspecified open wound of upper limb, without mention of complication
- 884.1 Multiple and unspecified open wound of upper limb, complicated
- 906.1 Late effect of open wound of extremities without mention of tendon injury
- 906.6 Late effect of burn of wrist and hand
- 906.7 Late effect of burn of other extremities

Terms To Know
excision. Surgical removal of an organ or tissue.

neoplasm. New abnormal growth, tumor.

z-plasty. Plastic surgery technique used primarily to release tension or elongate contracted scar tissue in which a Z-shaped incision is made with the middle line of the Z crossing the area of greatest tension. The triangular flaps are then rotated so that they cross the incision line in the opposite direction, creating a reversed Z.

CCI Version 16.3
0213T, 0216T, 0228T, 0230T, 11000, 11040-11042, 11100, 11400-11471, 11600-11606, 11620-11646, 12001-12007, 12011-12037, 13120-13121, 20550-20553, 36000, 36400-36410, 36420-36430, 36440, 36600, 36640, 37202, 43752, 51701-51703, 62310-62319, 64400-64435, 64445-64450, 64479, 64483, 64490, 64493, 64505-64530, 69990, 93000-93010, 93040-93042, 93318, 94002, 94200, 94250, 94680-94690, 94770, 95812-95816, 95819, 95822, 95829, 95955, 96360, 96365, 96372, 96374-96376, 97597-97598, 97602-97606, 99148-99149, 99150, G0168, J0670, J2001

Also not with 14021: 14020, 29515

Note: These CCI edits are used for Medicare. Other payers may reimburse on codes listed above.

Medicare Edits

	Fac RVU	Non-Fac RVU	FUD	Assist
14020	16.96	20.42	90	N/A
14021	21.66	25.66	90	N/A

Medicare References: 100-2,15,260; 100-4,12,30; 100-4,12,90.3; 100-4,14,10

14040-14041

14040 Adjacent tissue transfer or rearrangement, forehead, cheeks, chin, mouth, neck, axillae, genitalia, hands and/or feet; defect 10 sq cm or less

14041 defect 10.1 sq cm to 30.0 sq cm

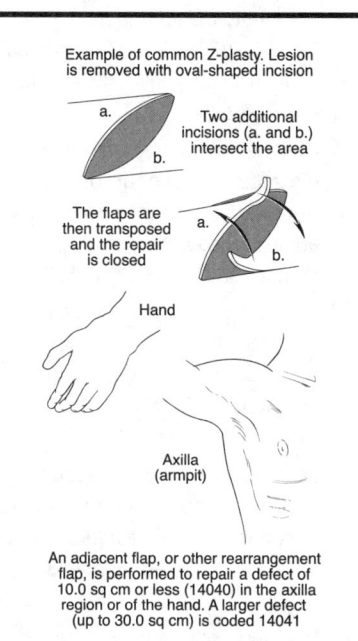

Example of common Z-plasty. Lesion is removed with oval-shaped incision

Two additional incisions (a. and b.) intersect the area

The flaps are then transposed and the repair is closed

Hand

Axilla (armpit)

An adjacent flap, or other rearrangement flap, is performed to repair a defect of 10.0 sq cm or less (14040) in the axilla region or of the hand. A larger defect (up to 30.0 sq cm) is coded 14041

Explanation

The physician transfers or rearranges adjacent tissue to repair traumatic or surgical wounds on the forehead, cheeks, chin, mouth, neck, axillae, genitalia, hands, and/or feet. This includes, but is not limited to, such rearrangement procedures as Z-plasty, W-plasty, ZY-plasty, or tissue transfers such as rotational flaps or advancement flaps. Report 14040 for defects that are 10 sq cm or less and 14041 for defects that are 10.1 sq cm to 30 sq cm.

Coding Tips

When adjacent tissue transfer or rearrangement is performed in conjunction with excision of a lesion, the lesion excision is not reported separately. When these codes are used to report repair of traumatic wounds, the procedure must have been previously planned and developed by the physician to effect the repair. These codes do not apply when direct closure or rearrangement of traumatized tissue incidentally results in these configurations. Any skin grafting required to close the secondary defect is reported separately. For an intralesional injection to limit scarring, see 11900. Surgical trays, A4550, are not separately reimbursed by Medicare; however, other third-party payers may cover them. Check with the specific payer to determine coverage.

ICD-9-CM Procedural

- 86.3 Other local excision or destruction of lesion or tissue of skin and subcutaneous tissue
- 86.70 Pedicle or flap graft, not otherwise specified
- 86.71 Cutting and preparation of pedicle grafts or flaps
- 86.72 Advancement of pedicle graft
- 86.73 Attachment of pedicle or flap graft to hand
- 86.74 Attachment of pedicle or flap graft to other sites
- 86.84 Relaxation of scar or web contracture of skin
- 86.89 Other repair and reconstruction of skin and subcutaneous tissue

Anesthesia
00300, 00400

ICD-9-CM Diagnostic

- 171.2 Malignant neoplasm of connective and other soft tissue of upper limb, including shoulder
- 172.6 Malignant melanoma of skin of upper limb, including shoulder
- 195.4 Malignant neoplasm of upper limb
- 198.2 Secondary malignant neoplasm of skin
- 209.33 Merkel cell carcinoma of the upper limb
- 214.1 Lipoma of other skin and subcutaneous tissue
- 215.2 Other benign neoplasm of connective and other soft tissue of upper limb, including shoulder
- 228.01 Hemangioma of skin and subcutaneous tissue
- 701.4 Keloid scar
- 701.5 Other abnormal granulation tissue
- 709.2 Scar condition and fibrosis of skin
- 709.4 Foreign body granuloma of skin and subcutaneous tissue — (Use additional code to identify foreign body (V90.01-V90.9))
- 757.32 Congenital vascular hamartomas
- 880.02 Open wound of axillary region, without mention of complication
- 880.12 Open wound of axillary region, complicated
- 882.0 Open wound of hand except finger(s) alone, without mention of complication
- 882.1 Open wound of hand except finger(s) alone, complicated
- 883.0 Open wound of finger(s), without mention of complication
- 883.1 Open wound of finger(s), complicated
- 884.0 Multiple and unspecified open wound of upper limb, without mention of complication
- 884.1 Multiple and unspecified open wound of upper limb, complicated
- 906.1 Late effect of open wound of extremities without mention of tendon injury
- 906.6 Late effect of burn of wrist and hand
- 996.92 Complications of reattached hand
- 996.93 Complications of reattached finger(s)
- 998.32 Disruption of external operation (surgical) wound
- 998.59 Other postoperative infection — (Use additional code to identify infection)
- 998.83 Non-healing surgical wound

CCI Version 16.3

0213T, 0216T, 0228T, 0230T, 11000, 11040-11042, 11100, 11400-11471, 11600-11606, 11620-11646, 12001-12007, 12011-12057, 13131-13132, 25259, 26340, 29086, 36000, 36400-36410, 36420-36430, 36440, 36600, 36640, 37202, 43752, 51701-51703, 62310-62319, 64400-64435, 64445-64450, 64479, 64483, 64490, 64493, 64505-64530, 69990, 93000-93010, 93040-93042, 93318, 94002, 94200, 94250, 94680-94690, 94770, 95812-95816, 95819, 95822, 95829, 95955, 96360, 96365, 96372, 96374-96376, 97597-97598, 97602-97606, 99148-99149, 99150, G0168, J0670, J2001

Also not with 14040: 11055-11056, 15852, 20526-20553

Also not with 14041: 14040, 20526, 20551-20553

Note: These CCI edits are used for Medicare. Other payers may reimburse on codes listed above.

Medicare Edits

	Fac RVU	Non-Fac RVU	FUD	Assist
14040	19.08	22.51	90	N/A
14041	23.51	27.91	90	N/A

Medicare References: 100-2,15,260; 100-4,12,30; 100-4,12,90.3; 100-4,14,10

14301-14302

14301 Adjacent tissue transfer or rearrangement, any area; defect 30.1 sq cm to 60.0 sq cm

14302 each additional 30.0 sq cm, or part thereof (List separately in addition to code for primary procedure)

Example of common Z-plasty

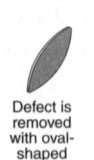

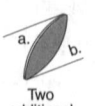

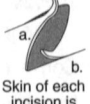

Defect is removed with oval-shaped incision

Two additional incisions intersect the removal area

Skin of each incision is reflected back

The flaps are transposed

And the repair is closed

Report 14301 when the defect is 30.0 to 60.0 sq cm and 14301 for each additional 30.0 sq cm

Explanation

The physician transfers or rearranges adjacent tissue of any area to repair traumatic or surgical wounds. This includes, but is not limited to, such rearrangement procedures as Z-plasty, W-plasty, ZY-plasty, or tissue transfers such as rotational flaps or advancement flaps. Report 14301 for defects 30.1 sq cm to 60 sq cm. Report 14302 for each additional 30 sq cm or part thereof.

Coding Tips

As an "add-on" code, 14301 is not subject to multiple procedure rules. No reimbursement reduction or modifier 51 is applied. Add-on codes describe additional intra-service work associated with the primary procedure. They are performed by the same physician on the same date of service as the primary service/procedure, and must never be reported as a stand-alone code. Report any skin grafts to close secondary defects separately. For an intralesional injection to limit scarring, see 11900.

ICD-9-CM Procedural

- 86.3 Other local excision or destruction of lesion or tissue of skin and subcutaneous tissue
- 86.70 Pedicle or flap graft, not otherwise specified
- 86.71 Cutting and preparation of pedicle grafts or flaps
- 86.72 Advancement of pedicle graft
- 86.73 Attachment of pedicle or flap graft to hand
- 86.74 Attachment of pedicle or flap graft to other sites
- 86.84 Relaxation of scar or web contracture of skin
- 86.89 Other repair and reconstruction of skin and subcutaneous tissue

Anesthesia

14301 00300, 00400
14302 N/A

ICD-9-CM Diagnostic

- 172.6 Malignant melanoma of skin of upper limb, including shoulder
- 172.8 Malignant melanoma of other specified sites of skin
- 173.6 Other malignant neoplasm of skin of upper limb, including shoulder
- 173.8 Other malignant neoplasm of other specified sites of skin
- 176.0 Kaposi's sarcoma of skin
- 195.4 Malignant neoplasm of upper limb
- 198.2 Secondary malignant neoplasm of skin
- 214.1 Lipoma of other skin and subcutaneous tissue
- 215.2 Other benign neoplasm of connective and other soft tissue of upper limb, including shoulder
- 215.4 Other benign neoplasm of connective and other soft tissue of thorax
- 228.01 Hemangioma of skin and subcutaneous tissue
- 232.6 Carcinoma in situ of skin of upper limb, including shoulder
- 239.2 Neoplasms of unspecified nature of bone, soft tissue, and skin
- 249.70 Secondary diabetes mellitus with peripheral circulatory disorders, not stated as uncontrolled, or unspecified — (Use additional code to identify manifestation: 443.81, 785.4) (Use additional code to identify any associated insulin use: V58.67)
- 249.71 Secondary diabetes mellitus with peripheral circulatory disorders, uncontrolled — (Use additional code to identify manifestation: 443.81, 785.4) (Use additional code to identify any associated insulin use: V58.67)
- 249.80 Secondary diabetes mellitus with other specified manifestations, not stated as uncontrolled, or unspecified — (Use additional code to identify manifestation: 707.10-707.9, 731.8) (Use additional code to identify any associated insulin use: V58.67)
- 249.81 Secondary diabetes mellitus with other specified manifestations, uncontrolled — (Use additional code to identify manifestation: 707.10-707.9, 731.8) (Use additional code to identify any associated insulin use: V58.67)
- 250.70 Diabetes with peripheral circulatory disorders, type II or unspecified type, not stated as uncontrolled — (Use additional code to identify manifestation: 443.81, 785.4)
- 250.71 Diabetes with peripheral circulatory disorders, type I [juvenile type], not stated as uncontrolled — (Use additional code to identify manifestation: 443.81, 785.4)
- 250.72 Diabetes with peripheral circulatory disorders, type II or unspecified type, uncontrolled — (Use additional code to identify manifestation: 443.81, 785.4)
- 443.0 Raynaud's syndrome — (Use additional code to identify gangrene: 785.4)

CCI Version 16.3

0213T, 0216T, 0228T, 0230T, 36000, 36400-36410, 36420-36430, 36440, 36600, 36640, 37202, 43752, 51701-51703, 62310-62319, 64400-64435, 64445-64450, 64479, 64483, 64490, 64493, 64505-64530, 69990, 93000-93010, 93040-93042, 93318, 94002, 94200, 94250, 94680-94690, 94770, 95812-95816, 95819, 95822, 95829, 95955, 96360, 96365, 96372, 96374-96376, 99148-99149, 99150

Also not with 14301: 11000, 11040-11042, 11100, 11400-11471, 11600-11606, 11620-11646, 12001-12007, 12011-12057, 13100-13101, 13120-13121, 13131-13132, 13150-13152, 14000-14001, 14020-14061✥, 20526-20553, 97597-97598, 97602-97606, G0168, J0670, J2001

Note: These CCI edits are used for Medicare. Other payers may reimburse on codes listed above.

Medicare Edits

	Fac RVU	Non-Fac RVU	FUD	Assist
14301	27.08	32.33	90	80
14302	6.9	6.9	N/A	80

Medicare References: None

14350

14350 Filleted finger or toe flap, including preparation of recipient site

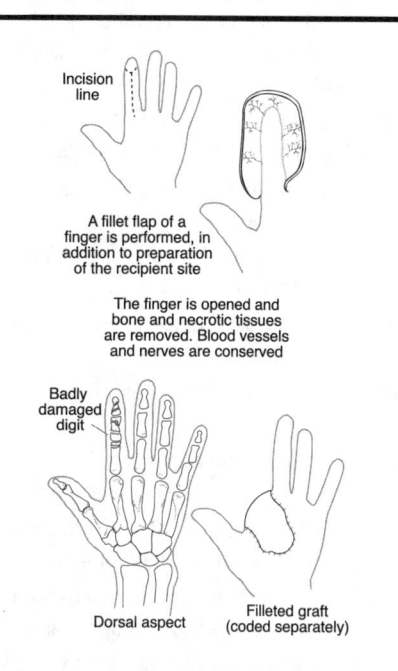

Incision line

A fillet flap of a finger is performed, in addition to preparation of the recipient site

The finger is opened and bone and necrotic tissues are removed. Blood vessels and nerves are conserved

Badly damaged digit

Dorsal aspect   *Filleted graft (coded separately)*

Explanation

The physician creates a filleted finger to repair a large deficit on the hand. The physician makes a bilateral longitudinal incision and dissects the tissue away from the bone, protecting vascular integrity. The recipient site is prepared and the flap is rotated into place. Excess tissue is excised and the wound is closed in sutured layers.

Coding Tips

When this code is used to report repair of traumatic wounds, the procedure must have been previously planned and developed by the physician to effect the repair. This code does not apply when direct closure or rearrangement of traumatized tissue incidentally results in these configurations. Preparation of the recipient site is included and should not be reported separately. Any skin grafting required to close the secondary defect is reported separately. Some payers may require the use of HCPCS Level II modifiers FA–F9 to identify the specific finger involved. For an intralesional injection to limit scarring, see 11900. Surgical trays, A4550, are not separately reimbursed by Medicare; however, other third-party payers may cover them. Check with the specific payer to determine coverage.

ICD-9-CM Procedural

86.3 Other local excision or destruction of lesion or tissue of skin and subcutaneous tissue

86.71 Cutting and preparation of pedicle grafts or flaps
86.72 Advancement of pedicle graft
86.73 Attachment of pedicle or flap graft to hand
86.74 Attachment of pedicle or flap graft to other sites

Anesthesia
14350 00400

ICD-9-CM Diagnostic

249.70 Secondary diabetes mellitus with peripheral circulatory disorders, not stated as uncontrolled, or unspecified — (Use additional code to identify manifestation: 443.81, 785.4) (Use additional code to identify any associated insulin use: V58.67)
249.71 Secondary diabetes mellitus with peripheral circulatory disorders, uncontrolled — (Use additional code to identify manifestation: 443.81, 785.4) (Use additional code to identify any associated insulin use: V58.67)
250.70 Diabetes with peripheral circulatory disorders, type II or unspecified type, not stated as uncontrolled — (Use additional code to identify manifestation: 443.81, 785.4)
250.71 Diabetes with peripheral circulatory disorders, type I [juvenile type], not stated as uncontrolled — (Use additional code to identify manifestation: 443.81, 785.4)
250.72 Diabetes with peripheral circulatory disorders, type II or unspecified type, uncontrolled — (Use additional code to identify manifestation: 443.81, 785.4)
250.73 Diabetes with peripheral circulatory disorders, type I [juvenile type], uncontrolled — (Use additional code to identify manifestation: 443.81, 785.4)
816.10 Open fracture of phalanx or phalanges of hand, unspecified
816.11 Open fracture of middle or proximal phalanx or phalanges of hand
816.12 Open fracture of distal phalanx or phalanges of hand
816.13 Open fractures of multiple sites of phalanx or phalanges of hand
885.0 Traumatic amputation of thumb (complete) (partial), without mention of complication
885.1 Traumatic amputation of thumb (complete) (partial), complicated
886.0 Traumatic amputation of other finger(s) (complete) (partial), without mention of complication
886.1 Traumatic amputation of other finger(s) (complete) (partial), complicated
944.31 Full-thickness skin loss due to burn (third degree NOS) of single digit [finger (nail)] other than thumb
944.32 Full-thickness skin loss due to burn (third degree NOS) of thumb (nail)
944.33 Full-thickness skin loss due to burn (third degree NOS) of two or more digits of hand, not including thumb
944.41 Deep necrosis of underlying tissues due to burn (deep third degree) of single digit [finger (nail)] other than thumb, without mention of loss of a body part
944.42 Deep necrosis of underlying tissues due to burn (deep third degree) of thumb (nail), without mention of loss of a body part
944.43 Deep necrosis of underlying tissues due to burn (deep third degree) of two or more digits of hand, not including thumb, without mention of loss of a body part

CCI Version 16.3

0213T, 0216T, 0228T, 0230T, 11000, 11040-11042, 11100, 11400-11471, 11600-11606, 11620-11646, 12001-12007, 12011-12021, 12041-12047, 13131-13132, 36000, 36400-36410, 36420-36430, 36440, 36600, 36640, 37202, 43752, 51701-51703, 62310-62319, 64400-64435, 64445-64450, 64479, 64483, 64490, 64493, 64505-64530, 69990, 93000-93010, 93040-93042, 93318, 94002, 94200, 94250, 94680-94690, 94770, 95812-95816, 95819, 95822, 95829, 95955, 96360, 96365, 96372, 96374-96376, 97597-97598, 97602-97606, 99148-99149, 99150, G0168

Note: These CCI edits are used for Medicare. Other payers may reimburse on codes listed above.

Medicare Edits

	Fac RVU	Non-Fac RVU	FUD	Assist
14350	21.21	21.21	90	80

Medicare References: 100-2,15,260; 100-4,12,30; 100-4,12,90.3; 100-4,14,10

15002-15003

15002 Surgical preparation or creation of recipient site by excision of open wounds, burn eschar, or scar (including subcutaneous tissues), or incisional release of scar contracture, trunk, arms, legs; first 100 sq cm or 1% of body area of infants and children

15003 each additional 100 sq cm, or part thereof, or each additional 1% of body area of infants and children (List separately in addition to code for primary procedure)

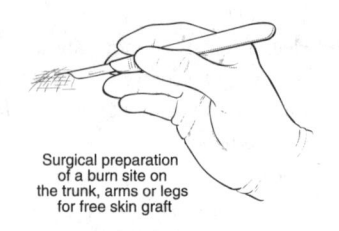

Surgical preparation of a burn site on the trunk, arms or legs for free skin graft

A recipient site is surgically prepared through excision of tissues. Report code 15002 for the first 100 sq cm and 15003 for each additional 100 sq cm

Explanation
The physician prepares tissue to receive a free skin graft needed to close or repair a defect. Skin, subcutaneous tissue, scars, burn eschar, and lesions are excised to provide a healthy, vascular tissue bed (where new vessels have been formed) onto which a skin graft will be placed. Alternatively, the physician may prepare tissue by incising or excising a scar contracture that is causing excessive tightening of the skin. Simple debridement of granulations or of recent avulsion is included. Report 15002 for the first 100 sq cm or 1 percent of body area of infants and children for grafts of the trunk arms and legs. Report 15003 for each additional 100 sq cm of graft area or each additional 1 percent of surface body area in infants and children within the same areas.

Coding Tips
As an "add-on" code, 15003 is not subject to multiple procedure rules. No reimbursement reduction or modifier 51 is applied. Add-on codes describe additional intra-service work associated with the primary procedure. They are performed by the same physician on the same date of service as the primary service/procedure, and must never be reported as a stand-alone code. Use 15003 in conjunction with 15002. These procedures are for preparation or creation of the recipient site. Free grafts should be listed by the appropriate code number when the graft, immediate or delayed, is applied. Identify by size and location of the defect (recipient area) and the type of graft. Surgical trays, A4550, are not separately reimbursed by Medicare; however, other third-party payers may cover them. Check with the specific payer to determine coverage.

ICD-9-CM Procedural
- 86.3 Other local excision or destruction of lesion or tissue of skin and subcutaneous tissue

Anesthesia
15002 00300, 00400, 01951, 01952
15003 N/A

ICD-9-CM Diagnostic
- 172.6 Malignant melanoma of skin of upper limb, including shoulder
- 173.6 Other malignant neoplasm of skin of upper limb, including shoulder
- 195.4 Malignant neoplasm of upper limb
- 209.33 Merkel cell carcinoma of the upper limb
- 216.5 Benign neoplasm of skin of trunk, except scrotum
- 216.6 Benign neoplasm of skin of upper limb, including shoulder
- 228.01 Hemangioma of skin and subcutaneous tissue
- 232.6 Carcinoma in situ of skin of upper limb, including shoulder
- 250.80 Diabetes with other specified manifestations, type II or unspecified type, not stated as uncontrolled — (Use additional code to identify manifestation: 707.10-707.9, 731.8)
- 250.81 Diabetes with other specified manifestations, type I [juvenile type], not stated as uncontrolled — (Use additional code to identify manifestation: 707.10-707.9, 731.8)
- 250.82 Diabetes with other specified manifestations, type II or unspecified type, uncontrolled — (Use additional code to identify manifestation: 707.10-707.9, 731.8)
- 250.83 Diabetes with other specified manifestations, type I [juvenile type], uncontrolled — (Use additional code to identify manifestation: 707.10-707.9, 731.8)
- 440.23 Atherosclerosis of native arteries of the extremities with ulceration — (Use additional code for any associated ulceration: 707.10-707.9)
- 785.4 Gangrene — (Code first any associated underlying condition)
- 880.10 Open wound of shoulder region, complicated
- 880.11 Open wound of scapular region, complicated
- 880.12 Open wound of axillary region, complicated
- 880.13 Open wound of upper arm, complicated
- 880.19 Open wound of multiple sites of shoulder and upper arm, complicated
- 943.31 Full-thickness skin loss due to burn (third degree NOS) of forearm
- 943.33 Full-thickness skin loss due to burn (third degree NOS) of upper arm
- 943.35 Full-thickness skin loss due to burn (third degree NOS) of shoulder
- 943.36 Full-thickness skin loss due to burn (third degree NOS) of scapular region
- 944.37 Full-thickness skin loss due to burn (third degree NOS) of wrist

CCI Version 16.3
Also not with 15002: 01951-01952, 0213T, 0216T, 0228T, 0230T, 11000❖, 11040-11044, 11100, 11400-11421❖, 11423-11444❖, 11450❖, 11600-11604❖, 11620-11624❖, 11640-11643❖, 12001-12007, 12011-12018, 12031-12057, 13100-13101, 13120-13121, 13131-13132, 13150-13152, 36000, 36400-36410, 36420-36430, 36440, 36600, 36640, 37202, 43752, 51701-51703, 62310-62319, 64400-64435, 64445-64450, 64479, 64483, 64490, 64493, 64505-64530, 69990, 93000-93010, 93040-93042, 93318, 94002, 94200, 94250, 94680-94690, 94770, 95812-95816, 95819, 95822, 95829, 95955, 96360, 96365, 96372, 96374-96376, 99148-99149, 99150, G0168, J0670, J2001

Note: These CCI edits are used for Medicare. Other payers may reimburse on codes listed above.

Medicare Edits

	Fac RVU	Non-Fac RVU	FUD	Assist
15002	6.67	9.8	0	80
15003	1.34	2.13	N/A	80

Medicare References: 100-2,15,260; 100-3,270.5; 100-4,3,20.1.2.8; 100-4,12,90.3; 100-4,14,10

15004-15005

15004 Surgical preparation or creation of recipient site by excision of open wounds, burn eschar, or scar (including subcutaneous tissues), or incisional release of scar contracture, face, scalp, eyelids, mouth, neck, ears, orbits, genitalia, hands, feet and/or multiple digits; first 100 sq cm or 1% of body area of infants and children

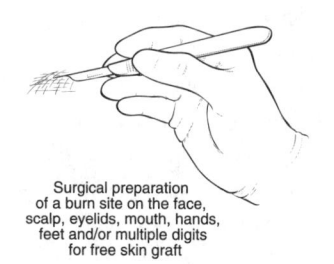

15005 each additional 100 sq cm, or part thereof, or each additional 1% of body area of infants and children (List separately in addition to code for primary procedure)

Surgical preparation of a burn site on the face, scalp, eyelids, mouth, hands, feet and/or multiple digits for free skin graft

A recipient site is surgically prepared through excision of tissues. Report code 15004 for the first 100 sq cm and 15005 for each additional 100 sq cm

Explanation

The physician prepares tissue to receive a free skin graft needed to close or repair a defect. Skin, subcutaneous tissue, scars, burn eschar, and lesions are excised to provide a healthy, vascular tissue bed (where new vessels have been formed) onto which a skin graft will be placed. Alternatively, the physician may prepare tissue by incising or excising a scar contracture that is causing excessive tightening of the skin. Simple debridement of granulations or of recent avulsion is included. Report 15004 for the first 100 sq cm or 1 percent of body area in infants and children of the face, scalp, eyelids, mouth, neck, ears, orbits, genitalia, hands, and/or feet. Report 15005 for each additional 100 sq cm or each additional 1 percent of body area in infants and children.

Coding Tips

As an "add-on" code, 15005 is not subject to multiple procedure rules. No reimbursement reduction or modifier 51 is applied. Add-on codes describe additional intra-service work associated with the primary procedure. They are performed by the same physician on the same date of service as the primary service/procedure, and must never be reported as a stand-alone code. Use 15005 in conjunction with 15004. These procedures are for preparation or creation of the recipient site. Free grafts should be listed by the appropriate code number when the graft, immediate or delayed, is applied. Identify by size and location of the defect (recipient area) and the type of graft. Surgical trays, A4550, are not separately reimbursed by Medicare; however, other third-party payers may cover them. Check with the specific payer to determine coverage. Check with the specific payer to determine coverage.

ICD-9-CM Procedural

- 86.3 Other local excision or destruction of lesion or tissue of skin and subcutaneous tissue

Anesthesia

- **15004** 00300, 00400, 00920, 01951, 01952, 01953
- **15005** N/A

ICD-9-CM Diagnostic

- 176.0 Kaposi's sarcoma of skin
- 198.2 Secondary malignant neoplasm of skin
- 209.33 Merkel cell carcinoma of the upper limb
- 209.75 Secondary Merkel cell carcinoma
- 214.1 Lipoma of other skin and subcutaneous tissue
- 443.0 Raynaud's syndrome — (Use additional code to identify gangrene: 785.4)
- 701.4 Keloid scar
- 709.2 Scar condition and fibrosis of skin
- 709.4 Foreign body granuloma of skin and subcutaneous tissue — (Use additional code to identify foreign body (V90.01-V90.9))
- 728.86 Necrotizing fasciitis — (Use additional code to identify infectious organism, 041.00-041.89, 785.4, if applicable)
- 785.4 Gangrene — (Code first any associated underlying condition)
- 874.8 Open wound of other and unspecified parts of neck, without mention of complication
- 874.9 Open wound of other and unspecified parts of neck, complicated
- 882.1 Open wound of hand except finger(s) alone, complicated
- 883.1 Open wound of finger(s), complicated
- 906.0 Late effect of open wound of head, neck, and trunk
- 906.5 Late effect of burn of eye, face, head, and neck
- 941.32 Full-thickness skin loss due to burn (third degree NOS) of eye (with other parts of face, head, and neck)
- 944.30 Full-thickness skin loss due to burn (third degree NOS) of unspecified site of hand
- 991.1 Frostbite of hand
- 996.52 Mechanical complication due to other tissue graft, not elsewhere classified
- 998.30 Disruption of wound, unspecified
- 998.32 Disruption of external operation (surgical) wound
- 998.33 Disruption of traumatic injury wound repair
- 998.59 Other postoperative infection — (Use additional code to identify infection)

CCI Version 16.3

Also not with 15004: 01951-01952, 0213T, 0216T, 0228T, 0230T, 11000❖, 11040-11044, 11100, 11400-11421❖, 11423-11450❖, 11462❖, 11470❖, 11600-11604❖, 11620-11644❖, 12001-12007, 12011-12018, 12031-12057, 13100-13101, 13120-13121, 13131-13132, 13150-13152, 36000, 36400-36410, 36420-36430, 36440, 36600, 36640, 37202, 51701-51703, 62310-62319, 64400-64435, 64445-64450, 64479, 64483, 64490, 64493, 64505-64530, 69990, 93000-93010, 93040-93042, 93318, 94002, 94200, 94250, 94680-94690, 94770, 95812-95816, 95819, 95822, 95829, 95955, 96360, 96365, 96372, 96374-96376, 99148-99149, 99150, G0168, J0670, J2001

Note: These CCI edits are used for Medicare. Other payers may reimburse on codes listed above.

Medicare Edits

	Fac RVU	Non-Fac RVU	FUD	Assist
15004	8.07	11.52	0	80
15005	2.67	3.54	N/A	80

Medicare References: 100-2,15,260; 100-4,3,20.1.2.8; 100-4,12,90.3; 100-4,14,10

15050

15050 Pinch graft, single or multiple, to cover small ulcer, tip of digit, or other minimal open area (except on face), up to defect size 2 cm diameter

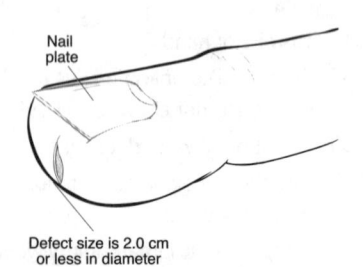

Nail plate

Defect size is 2.0 cm or less in diameter

A pinch graft, or series of pinch grafts, is taken and placed to cover a small defect such as on the tips of a digit

Explanation

The physician obtains one or more pinch grafts to cover a 2 cm or less open area, such as an ulcer of the toe or fingertip. The physician incises the skin to obtain a split thickness skin graft. The donor site is closed. The recipient site is cleaned and prepared. The graft is sewn into place.

Coding Tips

Some payers may require the use of HCPCS Level II modifiers FA–F9 to identify the specific finger involved. Preparation of the recipient site is reported separately, see 15002–15005. When this procedure is performed with another separately identifiable procedure, the highest dollar value code is listed as the primary procedure and subsequent procedures are appended with modifier 51. Surgical trays, A4550, are not separately reimbursed by Medicare; however, other third-party payers may cover them. Check with the specific payer to determine coverage.

ICD-9-CM Procedural

- 86.60 Free skin graft, not otherwise specified
- 86.62 Other skin graft to hand

Anesthesia

15050 00300, 00400

ICD-9-CM Diagnostic

- 171.2 Malignant neoplasm of connective and other soft tissue of upper limb, including shoulder
- 172.6 Malignant melanoma of skin of upper limb, including shoulder
- 173.6 Other malignant neoplasm of skin of upper limb, including shoulder
- 209.33 Merkel cell carcinoma of the upper limb
- 249.70 Secondary diabetes mellitus with peripheral circulatory disorders, not stated as uncontrolled, or unspecified — (Use additional code to identify manifestation: 443.81, 785.4) (Use additional code to identify any associated insulin use: V58.67)
- 249.71 Secondary diabetes mellitus with peripheral circulatory disorders, uncontrolled — (Use additional code to identify manifestation: 443.81, 785.4) (Use additional code to identify any associated insulin use: V58.67)
- 250.70 Diabetes with peripheral circulatory disorders, type II or unspecified type, not stated as uncontrolled — (Use additional code to identify manifestation: 443.81, 785.4)
- 250.71 Diabetes with peripheral circulatory disorders, type I [juvenile type], not stated as uncontrolled — (Use additional code to identify manifestation: 443.81, 785.4)
- 250.72 Diabetes with peripheral circulatory disorders, type II or unspecified type, uncontrolled — (Use additional code to identify manifestation: 443.81, 785.4)
- 250.73 Diabetes with peripheral circulatory disorders, type I [juvenile type], uncontrolled — (Use additional code to identify manifestation: 443.81, 785.4)
- 440.23 Atherosclerosis of native arteries of the extremities with ulceration — (Use additional code for any associated ulceration: 707.10-707.9)
- 443.81 Peripheral angiopathy in diseases classified elsewhere — (Code first underlying disease: 249.7, 250.7)
- 681.01 Felon — (Use additional code to identify organism: 041.1)
- 816.12 Open fracture of distal phalanx or phalanges of hand
- 882.0 Open wound of hand except finger(s) alone, without mention of complication
- 882.1 Open wound of hand except finger(s) alone, complicated
- 882.2 Open wound of hand except finger(s) alone, with tendon involvement
- 883.0 Open wound of finger(s), without mention of complication
- 883.1 Open wound of finger(s), complicated
- 883.2 Open wound of finger(s), with tendon involvement
- 885.0 Traumatic amputation of thumb (complete) (partial), without mention of complication
- 885.1 Traumatic amputation of thumb (complete) (partial), complicated
- 886.0 Traumatic amputation of other finger(s) (complete) (partial), without mention of complication
- 886.1 Traumatic amputation of other finger(s) (complete) (partial), complicated
- 906.4 Late effect of crushing
- 906.6 Late effect of burn of wrist and hand
- 927.3 Crushing injury of finger(s) — (Use additional code to identify any associated injuries: 800-829, 850.0-854.1, 860.0-869.1)

Terms To Know

graft. Tissue implant from another part of the body or another person.

CCI Version 16.3

01951-01952, 0213T, 0216T, 0228T, 0230T, 11000, 11040-11042, 11100, 12001-12007, 12011-12057, 13100-13101, 13120-13121, 13131-13132, 13150-13152, 15852, 16020-16030, 29000-29200, 29240-29450, 29505-29590, 36000, 36400-36410, 36420-36430, 36440, 36600, 36640, 37202, 43752, 51701-51703, 62310-62319, 64400-64435, 64445-64450, 64479, 64483, 64490, 64493, 64505-64530, 69990, 93000-93010, 93040-93042, 93318, 94002, 94200, 94250, 94680-94690, 94770, 95812-95816, 95819, 95822, 95829, 95955, 96360, 96365, 96372, 96374-96376, 97597-97598, 97602-97606, 99148-99149, 99150, G0168, J0670, J2001

Note: These CCI edits are used for Medicare. Other payers may reimburse on codes listed above.

Medicare Edits

	Fac RVU	Non-Fac RVU	FUD	Assist
15050	13.14	16.28	90	N/A

Medicare References: 100-2,15,260; 100-4,3,20.1.2.8; 100-4,12,30; 100-4,12,90.3; 100-4,14,10

15100-15101

15100 Split-thickness autograft, trunk, arms, legs; first 100 sq cm or less, or 1% of body area of infants and children (except 15050)

15101 each additional 100 sq cm, or each additional 1% of body area of infants and children, or part thereof (List separately in addition to code for primary procedure)

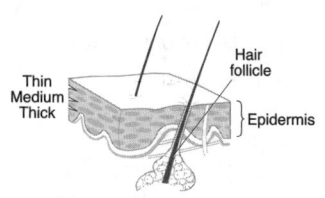

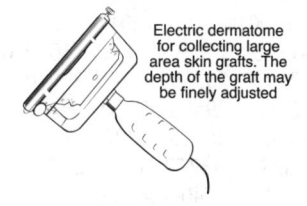

A split thickness skin graft is harvested and applied to an upper extremity, except the hands. Report 15100 for the first 100.0 sq cm or less. Report 15101 for each additional 100.0 sq cm

Explanation
The physician takes a split-thickness skin autograft from one area of the body and grafts it to an area needing repair. This procedure is performed when direct wound closure or adjacent tissue transfer is not possible. The physician harvests a split-thickness skin graft with a dermatome. The epidermis or top layer of skin is taken, along with a small portion of the dermis or bottom layer of the skin. This graft is applied to the recipient area on the trunk, arms, or legs. Report 15100 for the first 100 sq cm or less in adults or 1 percent of the total body area of infants and children. Report 15101 for each additional 100 sq cm or each additional 1 percent of the total body area in infants and children.

Coding Tips
As an "add-on" code, 15101 is not subject to multiple procedure rules. No reimbursement reduction or modifier 51 is applied. "Add-on" codes describe additional intra-service work associated with the primary procedure. They are performed by the same physician on the same date of service as the primary service/procedure, and must never be reported as a stand-alone code. Use 15101 in conjunction with 15100. Surgical trays, A4550, are not separately reimbursed by Medicare; however, other third-party payers may cover them. Check with the specific payer to determine coverage.

ICD-9-CM Procedural
86.60 Free skin graft, not otherwise specified
86.69 Other skin graft to other sites

Anesthesia
15100 00300, 00400
15101 N/A

ICD-9-CM Diagnostic
172.6 Malignant melanoma of skin of upper limb, including shoulder
173.6 Other malignant neoplasm of skin of upper limb, including shoulder
195.4 Malignant neoplasm of upper limb
209.33 Merkel cell carcinoma of the upper limb
249.70 Secondary diabetes mellitus with peripheral circulatory disorders, not stated as uncontrolled, or unspecified — (Use additional code to identify manifestation: 443.81, 785.4) (Use additional code to identify any associated insulin use: V58.67)
249.71 Secondary diabetes mellitus with peripheral circulatory disorders, uncontrolled — (Use additional code to identify manifestation: 443.81, 785.4) (Use additional code to identify any associated insulin use: V58.67)
250.70 Diabetes with peripheral circulatory disorders, type II or unspecified type, not stated as uncontrolled — (Use additional code to identify manifestation: 443.81, 785.4)
250.71 Diabetes with peripheral circulatory disorders, type I [juvenile type], not stated as uncontrolled — (Use additional code to identify manifestation: 443.81, 785.4)
250.72 Diabetes with peripheral circulatory disorders, type II or unspecified type, uncontrolled — (Use additional code to identify manifestation: 443.81, 785.4)
250.73 Diabetes with peripheral circulatory disorders, type I [juvenile type], uncontrolled — (Use additional code to identify manifestation: 443.81, 785.4)
709.4 Foreign body granuloma of skin and subcutaneous tissue — (Use additional code to identify foreign body (V90.01-V90.9))
880.00 Open wound of shoulder region, without mention of complication
880.01 Open wound of scapular region, without mention of complication
880.02 Open wound of axillary region, without mention of complication
880.03 Open wound of upper arm, without mention of complication
881.00 Open wound of forearm, without mention of complication
881.10 Open wound of forearm, complicated
881.12 Open wound of wrist, complicated
881.20 Open wound of forearm, with tendon involvement
881.22 Open wound of wrist, with tendon involvement
887.0 Traumatic amputation of arm and hand (complete) (partial), unilateral, below elbow, without mention of complication
887.2 Traumatic amputation of arm and hand (complete) (partial), unilateral, at or above elbow, without mention of complication

CCI Version 16.3
Also not with 15100: 01951-01952, 0213T, 0216T, 0228T, 0230T, 11000, 11040-11042, 11100, 12001-12007, 12020-12037, 12047, 13100-13133, 13153, 15050, 15852, 16020-16030, 29000-29085, 29105-29200, 29240-29450, 29505-29590, 36000, 36400-36410, 36420-36430, 36440, 36600, 36640, 37202, 43752, 51701-51703, 62310-62319, 64400-64435, 64445-64450, 64479, 64483, 64490, 64493, 64505-64530, 69990, 93000-93010, 93040-93042, 93318, 94002, 94200, 94250, 94680-94690, 94770, 95812-95816, 95819, 95822, 95829, 95955, 96360, 96365, 96372, 96374-96376, 97597-97598, 97602-97606, 99148-99149, 99150, G0168, J0670, J2001

Note: These CCI edits are used for Medicare. Other payers may reimburse on codes listed above.

Medicare Edits

	Fac RVU	Non-Fac RVU	FUD	Assist
15100	21.1	25.14	90	N/A
15101	3.29	5.43	N/A	N/A

Medicare References: 100-2,15,260; 100-4,3,20.1.2.8; 100-4,12,30; 100-4,12,90.3; 100-4,14,10

15120-15121

15120 Split-thickness autograft, face, scalp, eyelids, mouth, neck, ears, orbits, genitalia, hands, feet, and/or multiple digits; first 100 sq cm or less, or 1% of body area of infants and children (except 15050)

15121 each additional 100 sq cm, or each additional 1% of body area of infants and children, or part thereof (List separately in addition to code for primary procedure)

Schematic showing epidermal layer of skin

Thin / Medium / Thick

Hair follicle

Electric dermatome for collecting large area skin grafts. The depth of the graft may be finely adjusted

Report 15121 for each additional 100.0 sq cm or each additional one percent of body area for infants and children

A split thickness graft (thin graft of epidermis) is harvested, usually by dermatome, from a suitable area. The graft is then applied to the defect, which has been carefully prepared, and is the first 100.0 sq cm or less in an adult or one percent of body area in child or infant (15120)

Explanation

The physician takes a split-thickness skin autograft from one area of the body and grafts it to an area needing repair. This procedure is performed when direct wound closure or adjacent tissue transfer is not possible. The physician harvests a split-thickness skin graft with a dermatome. The epidermis or top layer of skin is taken, along with a small portion of the dermis or bottom layer of the skin. This graft is sutured or stapled onto the recipient area on the face, scalp, eyelids, neck, ears, orbits, mouth, genitalia, hands, feet, and/or multiple digits. Report 15120 for the first 100 sq cm or less in adults or children age 10 or over or 1 percent of the total body area of infants and children younger than age 10. Report 15121 for each additional 100 sq cm and each additional 1 percent of total body area of infants and children.

Coding Tips

Preparation of the recipient site is reported separately; see 15004–15005. Repair of the donor site requiring skin graft or local flaps is to be added as an additional procedure. Local anesthesia is included in these services; however, these procedures may be performed with the patient under general anesthesia. If specimen is transported to an outside laboratory, report 99000 for handling or conveyance. As an "add-on" code, 15121 is not subject to multiple procedure rules. No reimbursement reduction or modifier 51 is applied. Add-on codes describe additional intra-service work associated with the primary procedure. They are performed by the same physician on the same date of service as the primary service/procedure, and must never be reported as a stand-alone code. Use 15121 in conjunction with 15120. Surgical trays, A4550, are not separately reimbursed by Medicare; however, other third-party payers may cover them. Check with the specific payer to determine coverage.

ICD-9-CM Procedural

- 86.62 Other skin graft to hand
- 86.69 Other skin graft to other sites

Anesthesia

15120 00300, 00400
15121 N/A

ICD-9-CM Diagnostic

- 172.6 Malignant melanoma of skin of upper limb, including shoulder
- 173.6 Other malignant neoplasm of skin of upper limb, including shoulder
- 195.4 Malignant neoplasm of upper limb
- 209.33 Merkel cell carcinoma of the upper limb
- 209.75 Secondary Merkel cell carcinoma
- 682.4 Cellulitis and abscess of hand, except fingers and thumb — (Use additional code to identify organism, such as 041.1, etc.)
- 701.5 Other abnormal granulation tissue
- 701.9 Unspecified hypertrophic and atrophic condition of skin
- 709.2 Scar condition and fibrosis of skin
- 709.3 Degenerative skin disorder
- 874.8 Open wound of other and unspecified parts of neck, without mention of complication
- 882.0 Open wound of hand except finger(s) alone, without mention of complication
- 882.1 Open wound of hand except finger(s) alone, complicated
- 882.2 Open wound of hand except finger(s) alone, with tendon involvement
- 883.0 Open wound of finger(s), without mention of complication
- 883.1 Open wound of finger(s), complicated
- 883.2 Open wound of finger(s), with tendon involvement
- 885.0 Traumatic amputation of thumb (complete) (partial), without mention of complication
- 885.1 Traumatic amputation of thumb (complete) (partial), complicated
- 886.0 Traumatic amputation of other finger(s) (complete) (partial), without mention of complication
- 886.1 Traumatic amputation of other finger(s) (complete) (partial), complicated
- 906.6 Late effect of burn of wrist and hand
- 991.1 Frostbite of hand

CCI Version 16.3

Also not with 15120: 01951-01952, 0213T, 0216T, 0228T, 0230T, 11000, 11040-11042, 11100, 12001-12007, 12011-12057, 13102-13153, 15050, 15852, 16020-16030, 20526-20553, 25259, 26340, 29000-29200, 29240-29450, 29505-29590, 36000, 36400-36410, 36420-36430, 36440, 36600, 36640, 37202, 43752, 51701-51703, 62310-62319, 64400-64435, 64445-64450, 64479, 64483, 64490, 64493, 64505-64530, 69990, 93000-93010, 93040-93042, 93318, 94002, 94200, 94250, 94680-94690, 94770, 95812-95816, 95819, 95822, 95829, 95955, 96360, 96365, 96372, 96374-96376, 97597-97598, 97602-97606, 99148-99149, 99150, G0168, J0670, J2001

Note: These CCI edits are used for Medicare. Other payers may reimburse on codes listed above.

Medicare Edits

	Fac RVU	Non-Fac RVU	FUD	Assist
15120	23.26	27.78	90	N/A
15121	5.05	7.77	N/A	N/A

Medicare References: 100-2,15,260; 100-4,3,20.1.2.8; 100-4,12,30; 100-4,12,90.3; 100-4,14,10

15220-15221

15220 Full thickness graft, free, including direct closure of donor site, scalp, arms, and/or legs; 20 sq cm or less

15221 each additional 20 sq cm, or part thereof (List separately in addition to code for primary procedure)

Schematic showing layers of the skin

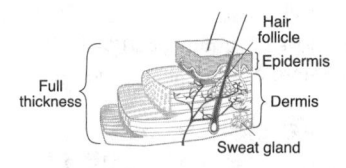

A full thickness graft (epidermis and dermis) is harvested, usually by dermatome, from a suitable area. The graft is then applied to the defect, which measures 20.0 sq cm or less

Report 15221 for each additional 20.0 sq cm

Explanation
The physician harvests a full-thickness skin graft with a scalpel from one area of the body and grafts it to an area needing repair. A full-thickness skin graft consists of both the superficial and deeper layers of skin (epidermis and dermis). The resulting surgical wound at the donor site is closed by lifting the remaining skin edges and placing sutures for direct closure. Fat is removed from the graft, which is sutured onto the recipient bed to cover a defect of the scalp, arms, and/or legs of no more than 20 sq cm. Report 15221 for each additional 20 sq cm or part thereof.

Coding Tips
As an "add-on" code, 15221 is not subject to multiple procedure rules. No reimbursement reduction or modifier 51 is applied. Add-on codes describe additional intra-service work associated with the primary procedure. They are performed by the same physician on the same date of service as the primary service/procedure, and must never be reported as a stand-alone code. Use 15221 in conjunction with 15220. This procedure may be performed during multiple surgical sessions as a staged procedure. To indicate that this is a staged or related procedure performed during the postoperative period by the same physician, append modifier 58. Preparation of the recipient site is reported separately; see 15002–15005. Free skin grafts are selected based on the size and location of the defect (recipient area) and the type of graft (split or full-thickness). Harvesting of keratinocytes is included and should not be reported separately. For adults and children age 10 and older, the code should be reported using the sq cm criteria. For children younger than age 10, use percent of body surface area. Repair of the donor site requiring a skin graft or local flaps is to be added as an additional procedure. Simple debridement of granulations or recent avulsion is also included. Use 15220–15221 for autogenous skin grafts.

ICD-9-CM Procedural
86.63 Full-thickness skin graft to other sites

Anesthesia
15220 00300, 00400
15221 N/A

ICD-9-CM Diagnostic
249.70 Secondary diabetes mellitus with peripheral circulatory disorders, not stated as uncontrolled, or unspecified — (Use additional code to identify manifestation: 443.81, 785.4) (Use additional code to identify any associated insulin use: V58.67)

249.71 Secondary diabetes mellitus with peripheral circulatory disorders, uncontrolled — (Use additional code to identify manifestation: 443.81, 785.4) (Use additional code to identify any associated insulin use: V58.67)

250.70 Diabetes with peripheral circulatory disorders, type II or unspecified type, not stated as uncontrolled — (Use additional code to identify manifestation: 443.81, 785.4)

250.71 Diabetes with peripheral circulatory disorders, type I [juvenile type], not stated as uncontrolled — (Use additional code to identify manifestation: 443.81, 785.4)

250.72 Diabetes with peripheral circulatory disorders, type II or unspecified type, uncontrolled — (Use additional code to identify manifestation: 443.81, 785.4)

250.73 Diabetes with peripheral circulatory disorders, type I [juvenile type], uncontrolled — (Use additional code to identify manifestation: 443.81, 785.4)

785.4 Gangrene — (Code first any associated underlying condition)

880.01 Open wound of scapular region, without mention of complication
880.02 Open wound of axillary region, without mention of complication
880.03 Open wound of upper arm, without mention of complication
881.00 Open wound of forearm, without mention of complication
881.01 Open wound of elbow, without mention of complication
881.02 Open wound of wrist, without mention of complication
887.0 Traumatic amputation of arm and hand (complete) (partial), unilateral, below elbow, without mention of complication
887.1 Traumatic amputation of arm and hand (complete) (partial), unilateral, below elbow, complicated
887.2 Traumatic amputation of arm and hand (complete) (partial), unilateral, at or above elbow, without mention of complication
887.3 Traumatic amputation of arm and hand (complete) (partial), unilateral, at or above elbow, complicated

CCI Version 16.3
Also not with 15220: 01951-01952, 0213T, 0216T, 0228T, 0230T, 11000, 11040-11042, 11100, 12001-12007, 12020-12037, 12045, 13120-13121, 13132, 15852, 16020-16030, 20550-20553, 29000-29200, 29240-29450, 29505-29590, 36000, 36400-36410, 36420-36430, 36440, 36600, 36640, 37202, 43752, 51701-51703, 62310-62319, 64400-64435, 64445-64450, 64479, 64483, 64490, 64493, 64505-64530, 69990, 93000-93010, 93040-93042, 93318, 94002, 94200, 94250, 94680-94690, 94770, 95812-95816, 95819, 95822, 95829, 95955, 96360, 96365, 96372, 96374-96376, 97597-97598, 97602-97606, 99148-99149, 99150, G0168, J0670, J2001

Note: These CCI edits are used for Medicare. Other payers may reimburse on codes listed above.

Medicare Edits

	Fac RVU	Non-Fac RVU	FUD	Assist
15220	18.31	22.49	90	N/A
15221	2.16	4.01	N/A	N/A

Medicare References: 100-2,15,260; 100-4,3,20.1.2.8; 100-4,12,30; 100-4,12,90.3; 100-4,14,10

15240-15241

15240 Full thickness graft, free, including direct closure of donor site, forehead, cheeks, chin, mouth, neck, axillae, genitalia, hands, and/or feet; 20 sq cm or less

15241 each additional 20 sq cm, or part thereof (List separately in addition to code for primary procedure)

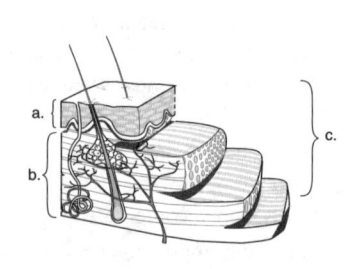

a. Epidermis   b. Dermis
c. Full thickness (epidermis and all of dermis) harvested in one cut

15240 reports grafts of 20.0 sq cm or less; 15241 reports each additional 20.0 sq cm

Explanation
The physician harvests a full-thickness skin graft with a scalpel from one area of the body and grafts it to an area needing repair. A full-thickness skin graft consists of both the superficial and deeper layers of skin (epidermis and dermis). The resulting surgical wound at the donor site is closed by lifting the remaining skin edges and placing sutures for direct closure. Fat is removed from the graft, which is sutured onto the recipient bed to cover a defect of the forehead, cheeks, chin, mouth, neck, axillae, genitalia, hands, and/or feet of 20 sq cm or less. Report 15241 for each additional 20 sq cm or part thereof.

Coding Tips
As an "add-on" code, 15241 is not subject to multiple procedure rules. No reimbursement reduction or modifier 51 is applied. Add-on codes describe additional intra-service work associated with the primary procedure. They are performed by the same physician on the same date of service as the primary service/procedure, and must never be reported as a stand-alone code. Use 15241 in conjunction with 15240. This procedure may be performed during multiple surgical sessions as a staged procedure. To indicate that this is a staged or related procedure performed during the postoperative period by the same physician, append modifier 58. Preparation of the recipient site is reported separately; see 15002–15005. Free skin grafts are selected based on the size and location of the defect (recipient area) and the type of graft (split or full-thickness). Harvesting of keratinocytes is included and should not be reported separately. For adults and children age 10 and older, the code should be reported using the sq cm criteria. For children younger than age 10, use percent of body surface area. Repair of the donor site requiring a skin graft or local flaps is to be added as an additional procedure. Simple debridement of granulations or recent avulsion is also included. Use 15240–15241 for autogenous skin grafts.

ICD-9-CM Procedural
- 86.61 Full-thickness skin graft to hand
- 86.63 Full-thickness skin graft to other sites

Anesthesia
15240 00300, 00400
15241 N/A

ICD-9-CM Diagnostic
- 232.6 Carcinoma in situ of skin of upper limb, including shoulder
- 880.12 Open wound of axillary region, complicated
- 882.1 Open wound of hand except finger(s) alone, complicated
- 883.1 Open wound of finger(s), complicated
- 885.1 Traumatic amputation of thumb (complete) (partial), complicated
- 886.1 Traumatic amputation of other finger(s) (complete) (partial), complicated
- 944.31 Full-thickness skin loss due to burn (third degree NOS) of single digit [finger (nail)] other than thumb
- 944.32 Full-thickness skin loss due to burn (third degree NOS) of thumb (nail)
- 944.33 Full-thickness skin loss due to burn (third degree NOS) of two or more digits of hand, not including thumb
- 944.34 Full-thickness skin loss due to burn (third degree NOS) of two or more digits of hand including thumb
- 944.35 Full-thickness skin loss due to burn (third degree NOS) of palm of hand
- 944.36 Full-thickness skin loss due to burn (third degree NOS) of back of hand
- 944.37 Full-thickness skin loss due to burn (third degree NOS) of wrist
- 944.38 Full-thickness skin loss due to burn (third degree NOS) of multiple sites of wrist(s) and hand(s)
- 944.55 Deep necrosis of underlying tissues due to burn (deep third degree) of palm of hand, with loss of a body part
- 944.56 Deep necrosis of underlying tissues due to burn (deep third degree) of back of hand, with loss of a body part
- 991.1 Frostbite of hand
- 998.83 Non-healing surgical wound

Terms To Know
free graft. Unattached piece of skin and tissue moved to another part of the body and sutured into place to repair a defect.

CCI Version 16.3
Also not with 15240: 01951-01952, 0213T, 0216T, 0228T, 0230T, 11000, 11040-11042, 11100, 12001-12007, 12016, 12020-12052, 12054, 13131-13132, 15852, 16020-16030, 20526, 20551-20553, 25259, 26340, 29000-29200, 29240-29450, 29505-29590, 36000, 36400-36410, 36420-36430, 36440, 36600, 36640, 37202, 43752, 51701-51703, 62310-62319, 64400-64435, 64445-64450, 64479, 64483, 64490, 64493, 64505-64530, 69990, 93000-93010, 93040-93042, 93318, 94002, 94200, 94250, 94680-94690, 94770, 95812-95816, 95819, 95822, 95829, 95955, 96360, 96365, 96372, 96374-96376, 97597-97598, 97602-97606, 99148-99149, 99150, G0168, J0670, J2001

Note: These CCI edits are used for Medicare. Other payers may reimburse on codes listed above.

Medicare Edits

	Fac RVU	Non-Fac RVU	FUD	Assist
15240	23.68	27.19	90	N/A
15241	3.38	5.4	N/A	N/A

Medicare References: 100-2,15,260; 100-4,3,20.1.2.8; 100-4,12,30; 100-4,12,90.3; 100-4,14,10

15400-15401

15400 Xenograft, skin (dermal), for temporary wound closure, trunk, arms, legs; first 100 sq cm or less, or 1% of body area of infants and children

15401 each additional 100 sq cm, or each additional 1% of body area of infants and children, or part thereof (List separately in addition to code for primary procedure)

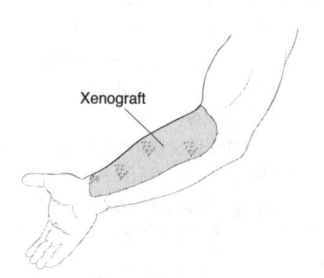

Xenograft

A xenograft is applied. Report 15400 when the application is up to, and including, 100.0 sq cm. Report code 15401 for each additional 100.0 sq cm

Explanation

The physician applies a xenograft to cover a wound on the patient. Xenograft dermal (skin) tissue is harvested from a non-human species (usually porcine) and used to cover a skin defect in humans. The physician covers the recipient site with this temporary resurfacing material to maintain viability of the tissue underneath the wound until a future transplant of appropriate skin graft material can be done. This procedure is often performed on burn patients when autografting is not feasible. Report 15400 for the first 100 sq cm or less in adults or children age 10 or older or 1 percent of body area of infants and children younger than age 10. Report 15401 for each additional 100 sq cm in adults or each additional 1 percent of body area in infants and children.

Coding Tips

Use 15401 in conjunction with 15400. As an "add-on" code, 15401 is not subject to multiple procedure rules. No reimbursement reduction or modifier 51 is applied. Add-on codes describe additional intra-service work associated with the primary procedure. They are performed by the same physician on the same date of service as the primary service/procedure, and must never be reported as a stand-alone code. If significant additional time and effort is documented, append modifier 22 and submit a cover letter and operative report.

ICD-9-CM Procedural

- 86.65 Heterograft to skin
- 86.71 Cutting and preparation of pedicle grafts or flaps
- 86.74 Attachment of pedicle or flap graft to other sites

Anesthesia

15400 00300, 00400
15401 N/A

ICD-9-CM Diagnostic

- 172.6 Malignant melanoma of skin of upper limb, including shoulder
- 173.6 Other malignant neoplasm of skin of upper limb, including shoulder
- 198.2 Secondary malignant neoplasm of skin
- 232.6 Carcinoma in situ of skin of upper limb, including shoulder
- 249.70 Secondary diabetes mellitus with peripheral circulatory disorders, not stated as uncontrolled, or unspecified — (Use additional code to identify manifestation: 443.81, 785.4) (Use additional code to identify any associated insulin use: V58.67)
- 249.71 Secondary diabetes mellitus with peripheral circulatory disorders, uncontrolled — (Use additional code to identify manifestation: 443.81, 785.4) (Use additional code to identify any associated insulin use: V58.67)
- 250.70 Diabetes with peripheral circulatory disorders, type II or unspecified type, not stated as uncontrolled — (Use additional code to identify manifestation: 443.81, 785.4)
- 250.71 Diabetes with peripheral circulatory disorders, type I [juvenile type], not stated as uncontrolled — (Use additional code to identify manifestation: 443.81, 785.4)
- 443.81 Peripheral angiopathy in diseases classified elsewhere — (Code first underlying disease: 249.7, 250.7)
- 681.01 Felon — (Use additional code to identify organism: 041.1)
- 681.02 Onychia and paronychia of finger — (Use additional code to identify organism: 041.1)
- 682.3 Cellulitis and abscess of upper arm and forearm — (Use additional code to identify organism, such as 041.1, etc.)
- 682.4 Cellulitis and abscess of hand, except fingers and thumb — (Use additional code to identify organism, such as 041.1, etc.)
- 709.2 Scar condition and fibrosis of skin
- 728.86 Necrotizing fasciitis — (Use additional code to identify infectious organism, 041.00-041.89, 785.4, if applicable)
- 785.4 Gangrene — (Code first any associated underlying condition)
- 880.00 Open wound of shoulder region, without mention of complication
- 880.03 Open wound of upper arm, without mention of complication
- 881.00 Open wound of forearm, without mention of complication
- 881.01 Open wound of elbow, without mention of complication
- 881.02 Open wound of wrist, without mention of complication
- 882.0 Open wound of hand except finger(s) alone, without mention of complication
- 882.1 Open wound of hand except finger(s) alone, complicated

CCI Version 16.3

Also not with 15400: 01951-01952, 0213T, 0216T, 0228T, 0230T, 11000, 11040-11042, 12001-12007, 12011-12057, 13100-13101, 13120-13121, 13131-13132, 13150-13152, 15852, 16020-16030, 29000-29200, 29240-29450, 29505-29590, 36000, 36400-36410, 36420-36430, 36440, 36600, 36640, 37202, 43752, 51701-51703, 62310-62319, 64400-64435, 64445-64450, 64479, 64483, 64490, 64493, 64505-64530, 69990, 93000-93010, 93040-93042, 93318, 94002, 94200, 94250, 94680-94690, 94770, 95812-95816, 95819, 95822, 95829, 95955, 96360, 96365, 96372, 96374-96376, 97597-97598, 97602-97606, 99148-99149, 99150, G0168, J0670, J2001

Note: These CCI edits are used for Medicare. Other payers may reimburse on codes listed above.

Medicare Edits

	Fac RVU	Non-Fac RVU	FUD	Assist
15400	10.4	11.78	90	N/A
15401	1.7	2.65	N/A	N/A

Medicare References: 100-2,15,260; 100-3,270.5; 100-4,3,20.1.2.8; 100-4,12,30; 100-4,12,90.3; 100-4,14,10

15732

15732 Muscle, myocutaneous, or fasciocutaneous flap; head and neck (eg, temporalis, masseter muscle, sternocleidomastoid, levator scapulae)

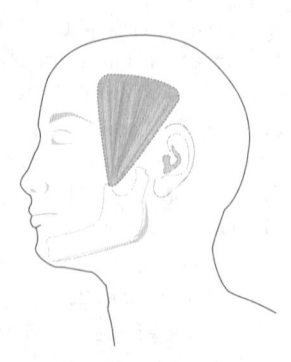

Temporalis muscle is an example of donor tissue

Tissue may be used to reconstruct a variety of defects in the head/neck area

Explanation

The physician repairs a defect area using a muscle, muscle and skin, or a fascia and skin flap. The physician rotates the prepared flap from the donor area to the site needing repair, suturing the flap in place. The donor area is closed primarily with sutures. If a skin graft or flap is used to repair the donor site, it is considered an additional procedure and is reported separately. Report 15732 for a muscle, myocutaneous, or fasciocutaneous flap of the head and neck.

Coding Tips

Reporting of a muscle, myocutaneous, or fasciocutaneous flap differs from that of other flaps as the procedure is always identified by the donor site never by the recipient site. Extensive immobilization and/or repair of the donor site is reported separately. When 15732 is performed with another separately identifiable procedure, the highest dollar value code is listed as the primary procedure and subsequent procedures are appended with modifier 51. If significant additional time and effort is documented, append modifier 22 and submit a cover letter and operative report.

ICD-9-CM Procedural

- 83.82 Graft of muscle or fascia
- 86.71 Cutting and preparation of pedicle grafts or flaps
- 86.74 Attachment of pedicle or flap graft to other sites

Anesthesia

15732 00300

ICD-9-CM Diagnostic

- 170.0 Malignant neoplasm of bones of skull and face, except mandible
- 170.1 Malignant neoplasm of mandible
- 171.0 Malignant neoplasm of connective and other soft tissue of head, face, and neck
- 172.4 Malignant melanoma of skin of scalp and neck
- 173.4 Other malignant neoplasm of scalp and skin of neck
- 195.0 Malignant neoplasm of head, face, and neck
- 209.75 Secondary Merkel cell carcinoma
- 215.0 Other benign neoplasm of connective and other soft tissue of head, face, and neck
- 234.8 Carcinoma in situ of other specified sites
- 238.0 Neoplasm of uncertain behavior of bone and articular cartilage
- 238.1 Neoplasm of uncertain behavior of connective and other soft tissue
- 238.2 Neoplasm of uncertain behavior of skin
- 874.8 Open wound of other and unspecified parts of neck, without mention of complication
- 874.9 Open wound of other and unspecified parts of neck, complicated
- 905.0 Late effect of fracture of skull and face bones
- 906.5 Late effect of burn of eye, face, head, and neck
- 909.2 Late effect of radiation
- 909.3 Late effect of complications of surgical and medical care
- 925.1 Crushing injury of face and scalp — (Use additional code to identify any associated injuries, such as: 800-829, 850.0-854.1, 860.0-869.1)
- 925.2 Crushing injury of neck — (Use additional code to identify any associated injuries, such as: 800-829, 850.0-854.1, 860.0-869.1)
- 941.38 Full-thickness skin loss due to burn (third degree NOS) of neck
- 941.48 Deep necrosis of underlying tissues due to burn (deep third degree) of neck, without mention of loss of a body part
- 959.01 Head injury, unspecified
- 959.09 Injury of face and neck, other and unspecified
- V51.8 Other aftercare involving the use of plastic surgery

Terms To Know

fascia. Fibrous sheet or band of tissue that envelops organs, muscles, and groupings of muscles.

CCI Version 16.3

01951-01952, 0213T, 0216T, 0228T, 0230T, 15731❖, 36000, 36400-36410, 36420-36430, 36440, 36600, 36640, 37202, 43752, 51701-51703, 62310-62319, 64400-64435, 64445-64450, 64479, 64483, 64490, 64493, 64505-64530, 69990, 93000-93010, 93040-93042, 93318, 94002, 94200, 94250, 94680-94690, 94770, 95812-95816, 95819, 95822, 95829, 95955, 96360, 96365, 96372, 96374-96376, 99148-99149, 99150, J0670, J2001

Note: These CCI edits are used for Medicare. Other payers may reimburse on codes listed above.

Medicare Edits

	Fac RVU	Non-Fac RVU	FUD	Assist
15732	39.41	44.07	90	N/A

Medicare References: 100-2,15,260; 100-4,3,20.1.2.8; 100-4,12,30; 100-4,12,90.3; 100-4,14,10

15734

15734 Muscle, myocutaneous, or fasciocutaneous flap; trunk

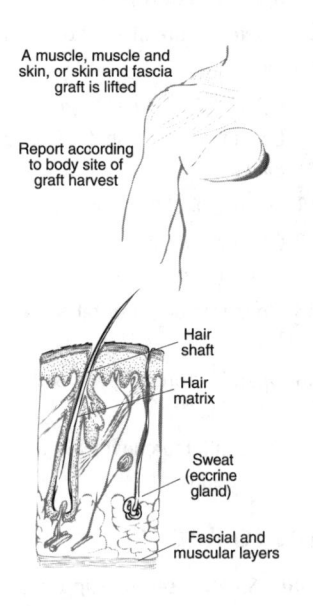

Explanation

The physician repairs a defect area using a muscle and skin or a fascia and skin flap. The physician rotates the prepared flap from the donor area to the site needing repair, suturing the flap in place. The donor area is closed primarily with sutures. If a skin graft or flap is used to repair the donor site, it is considered an additional procedure and is reported separately.

Coding Tips

Repair of the donor site that requires a skin graft or local flaps is considered an additional, separate procedure and should be coded separately. Extensive immobilization and/or repair of the donor site is reported separately. When 15734 is performed with another separately identifiable procedure, the highest dollar value code is listed as the primary procedure and subsequent procedures are appended with modifier 51. If significant additional time and effort is documented, append modifier 22 and submit a cover letter and operative report. For other flaps of the trunk, see 15570 and 15600; other flaps, see 15740–15758.

ICD-9-CM Procedural

- 83.82 Graft of muscle or fascia
- 86.71 Cutting and preparation of pedicle grafts or flaps
- 86.74 Attachment of pedicle or flap graft to other sites

Anesthesia
15734 00300, 00400

ICD-9-CM Diagnostic

- 171.4 Malignant neoplasm of connective and other soft tissue of thorax
- 171.7 Malignant neoplasm of connective and other soft tissue of trunk, unspecified site
- 171.8 Malignant neoplasm of other specified sites of connective and other soft tissue
- 172.5 Malignant melanoma of skin of trunk, except scrotum
- 198.2 Secondary malignant neoplasm of skin
- 209.35 Merkel cell carcinoma of the trunk
- 209.75 Secondary Merkel cell carcinoma
- 232.5 Carcinoma in situ of skin of trunk, except scrotum
- 238.2 Neoplasm of uncertain behavior of skin
- 239.2 Neoplasms of unspecified nature of bone, soft tissue, and skin
- 519.2 Mediastinitis — (Use additional code to identify infectious organism)
- 810.11 Open fracture of sternal end of clavicle
- 810.12 Open fracture of shaft of clavicle
- 810.13 Open fracture of acromial end of clavicle
- 811.10 Open fracture of unspecified part of scapula
- 811.11 Open fracture of acromial process of scapula
- 811.13 Open fracture of glenoid cavity and neck of scapula
- 811.19 Open fracture of other part of scapula
- 875.1 Open wound of chest (wall), complicated
- 876.0 Open wound of back, without mention of complication
- 876.1 Open wound of back, complicated
- 879.5 Open wound of abdominal wall, lateral, complicated
- 906.0 Late effect of open wound of head, neck, and trunk
- 908.4 Late effect of injury to blood vessel of thorax, abdomen, and pelvis
- 926.11 Crushing injury of back — (Use additional code to identify any associated injuries: 800-829, 850.0-854.1, 860.0-869.1)
- 942.33 Full-thickness skin loss due to burn (third degree NOS) of abdominal wall
- 942.34 Full-thickness skin loss due to burn (third degree NOS) of back (any part)
- 942.42 Deep necrosis of underlying tissues due to burn (deep third degree) of chest wall, excluding breast and nipple, without mention of loss of a body part
- 942.43 Deep necrosis of underlying tissues due to burn (deep third degree) of abdominal wall, without mention of loss of a body part
- 942.44 Deep necrosis of underlying tissues due to burn (deep third degree) of back (any part), without mention of loss of a body part
- 942.52 Deep necrosis of underlying tissues due to burn (deep third degree) of chest wall, excluding breast and nipple, with loss of a body part
- 942.53 Deep necrosis of underlying tissues due to burn (deep third degree) of abdominal wall with loss of a body part

CCI Version 16.3

01951-01952, 0213T, 0216T, 0228T, 0230T, 36000, 36400-36410, 36420-36430, 36440, 36600, 36640, 37202, 43752, 51701-51703, 62310-62319, 64400-64435, 64445-64450, 64479, 64483, 64490, 64493, 64505-64530, 69990, 93000-93010, 93040-93042, 93318, 94002, 94200, 94250, 94680-94690, 94770, 95812-95816, 95819, 95822, 95829, 95955, 96360, 96365, 96372, 96374-96376, 99148-99149, 99150, J0670, J2001

Note: These CCI edits are used for Medicare. Other payers may reimburse on codes listed above.

Medicare Edits

	Fac RVU	Non-Fac RVU	FUD	Assist
15734	39.79	44.78	90	80

Medicare References: 100-2,15,260; 100-4,3,20.1.2.8; 100-4,12,30; 100-4,12,90.3; 100-4,14,10

15736

15736 Muscle, myocutaneous, or fasciocutaneous flap; upper extremity

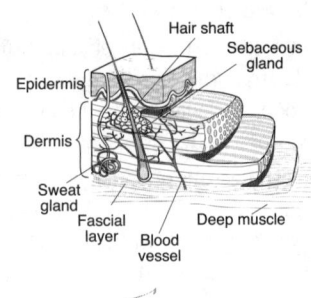

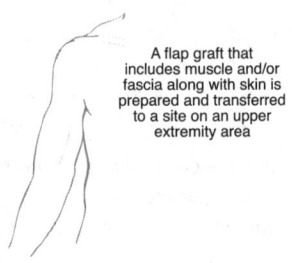

Explanation

The physician repairs a defect area using a muscle, muscle and skin, or a fascia and skin flap. The physician rotates the prepared flap from the donor area to the site needing repair, suturing the flap in place. The donor area is closed primarily with sutures. If a skin graft or flap is used to repair the donor site, it is considered an additional procedure and is reported separately.

Coding Tips

Reporting of a muscle, myocutaneous, or fasciocutaneous flap differs from that of other flaps as the procedure is always identified by the donor site never by the recipient site. Extensive immobilization and/or repair of the donor site is reported separately. When 15736 is performed with another separately identifiable procedure, the highest dollar value code is listed as the primary procedure and subsequent procedures are appended with modifier 51. If significant additional time and effort is documented, append modifier 22 and submit a cover letter and operative report.

ICD-9-CM Procedural

- 83.82 Graft of muscle or fascia
- 86.71 Cutting and preparation of pedicle grafts or flaps
- 86.74 Attachment of pedicle or flap graft to other sites

Anesthesia

15736 01610, 01710, 01810

ICD-9-CM Diagnostic

- 171.2 Malignant neoplasm of connective and other soft tissue of upper limb, including shoulder
- 172.6 Malignant melanoma of skin of upper limb, including shoulder
- 173.6 Other malignant neoplasm of skin of upper limb, including shoulder
- 198.2 Secondary malignant neoplasm of skin
- 209.33 Merkel cell carcinoma of the upper limb
- 209.75 Secondary Merkel cell carcinoma
- 232.6 Carcinoma in situ of skin of upper limb, including shoulder
- 232.8 Carcinoma in situ of other specified sites of skin
- 682.3 Cellulitis and abscess of upper arm and forearm — (Use additional code to identify organism, such as 041.1, etc.)
- 682.4 Cellulitis and abscess of hand, except fingers and thumb — (Use additional code to identify organism, such as 041.1, etc.)
- 701.5 Other abnormal granulation tissue
- 709.2 Scar condition and fibrosis of skin
- 728.82 Foreign body granuloma of muscle — (Use additional code to identify foreign body (V90.01-V90.9))
- 728.86 Necrotizing fasciitis — (Use additional code to identify infectious organism, 041.00-041.89, 785.4, if applicable)
- 728.88 Rhabdomyolysis
- 812.12 Open fracture of anatomical neck of humerus
- 812.13 Open fracture of greater tuberosity of humerus
- 812.19 Other open fracture of upper end of humerus
- 812.31 Open fracture of shaft of humerus
- 812.51 Open fracture of supracondylar humerus
- 812.52 Open fracture of lateral condyle of humerus
- 812.53 Open fracture of medial condyle of humerus
- 812.59 Other open fracture of lower end of humerus
- 813.11 Open fracture of olecranon process of ulna
- 813.12 Open fracture of coronoid process of ulna
- 813.13 Open Monteggia's fracture
- 813.15 Open fracture of head of radius
- 813.16 Open fracture of neck of radius
- 813.18 Open fracture of radius with ulna, upper end (any part)
- 813.31 Open fracture of shaft of radius (alone)
- 813.32 Open fracture of shaft of ulna (alone)
- 813.33 Open fracture of shaft of radius with ulna
- 813.51 Open Colles' fracture
- 813.52 Other open fractures of distal end of radius (alone)
- 813.53 Open fracture of distal end of ulna (alone)
- 813.54 Open fracture of lower end of radius with ulna
- V51.8 Other aftercare involving the use of plastic surgery

Terms To Know

cellulitis. Sudden, severe, suppurative inflammation and edema in subcutaneous tissue or muscle, most often caused by bacterial infection secondary to a cutaneous lesion.

CCI Version 16.3

01951-01952, 0213T, 0216T, 0228T, 0230T, 36000, 36400-36410, 36420-36430, 36440, 36600, 36640, 37202, 43752, 51701-51703, 62310-62319, 64400-64435, 64445-64450, 64479, 64483, 64490, 64493, 64505-64530, 69990, 93000-93010, 93040-93042, 93318, 94002, 94200, 94250, 94680-94690, 94770, 95812-95816, 95819, 95822, 95829, 95955, 96360, 96365, 96372, 96374-96376, 99148-99149, 99150, J0670, J2001

Note: These CCI edits are used for Medicare. Other payers may reimburse on codes listed above.

Medicare Edits

	Fac RVU	Non-Fac RVU	FUD	Assist
15736	34.26	39.41	90	N/A

Medicare References: 100-2,15,260; 100-4,3,20.1.2.8; 100-4,12,30; 100-4,12,90.3; 100-4,14,10

15740

15740 Flap; island pedicle

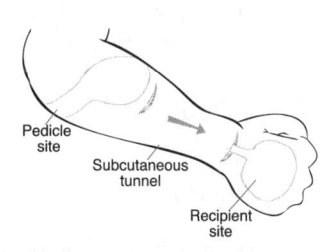

Enlarged schematic of island pedicle

An island pedicle flap is prepared

Skin and subcutaneous tissue containing a vascular link are trimmed for use as an island pedicle flap. The pedicle is devested of extra tissue so that the connection to the donor site is little more than an artery and vein. The flap is rotated and passed through a subcutaneous tunnel to the recipient site.

Explanation

The physician forms an island pedicle flap. A defect is being covered by elevation of a flap of skin and subcutaneous tissue. The original blood supply to the pedicle remains intact across the debulked pedicle. This can consist of an island of skin, muscle, fascia, or subcutaneous tissue. The flap is rotated into a nearby but not immediately adjacent defect. Often this flap will be transferred through a tunnel underneath the skin and sutured into its new position. The donor site is closed directly.

Coding Tips

Repair of the donor site that requires a skin graft or local flaps is considered an additional, separate procedure and should be coded separately. When 15740 is performed with another separately identifiable procedure, the highest dollar value code is listed as the primary procedure and subsequent procedures are appended with modifier 51. If significant additional time and effort is documented, append modifier 22 and submit a cover letter and operative report.

ICD-9-CM Procedural

- 86.70 Pedicle or flap graft, not otherwise specified

Anesthesia

15740 00300, 00400

ICD-9-CM Diagnostic

- 172.6 Malignant melanoma of skin of upper limb, including shoulder
- 198.2 Secondary malignant neoplasm of skin
- 209.32 Merkel cell carcinoma of the scalp and neck
- 209.33 Merkel cell carcinoma of the upper limb
- 209.35 Merkel cell carcinoma of the trunk
- 209.36 Merkel cell carcinoma of other sites
- 209.75 Secondary Merkel cell carcinoma
- 216.6 Benign neoplasm of skin of upper limb, including shoulder
- 232.6 Carcinoma in situ of skin of upper limb, including shoulder
- 707.01 Pressure ulcer, elbow — (Use additional code to identify pressure ulcer stage: 707.20-707.25)
- 757.33 Congenital pigmentary anomaly of skin
- 785.4 Gangrene — (Code first any associated underlying condition)
- 880.12 Open wound of axillary region, complicated
- 882.1 Open wound of hand except finger(s) alone, complicated
- 882.2 Open wound of hand except finger(s) alone, with tendon involvement
- 883.1 Open wound of finger(s), complicated
- 883.2 Open wound of finger(s), with tendon involvement
- 884.1 Multiple and unspecified open wound of upper limb, complicated
- 885.0 Traumatic amputation of thumb (complete) (partial), without mention of complication
- 885.1 Traumatic amputation of thumb (complete) (partial), complicated
- 886.0 Traumatic amputation of other finger(s) (complete) (partial), without mention of complication
- 886.1 Traumatic amputation of other finger(s) (complete) (partial), complicated
- 906.6 Late effect of burn of wrist and hand
- 944.31 Full-thickness skin loss due to burn (third degree NOS) of single digit [finger (nail)] other than thumb
- 944.32 Full-thickness skin loss due to burn (third degree NOS) of thumb (nail)
- 944.35 Full-thickness skin loss due to burn (third degree NOS) of palm of hand
- 944.36 Full-thickness skin loss due to burn (third degree NOS) of back of hand
- 944.37 Full-thickness skin loss due to burn (third degree NOS) of wrist
- 944.41 Deep necrosis of underlying tissues due to burn (deep third degree) of single digit [finger (nail)] other than thumb, without mention of loss of a body part
- 944.42 Deep necrosis of underlying tissues due to burn (deep third degree) of thumb (nail), without mention of loss of a body part
- 944.45 Deep necrosis of underlying tissues due to burn (deep third degree) of palm of hand, without mention of loss of a body part
- 944.46 Deep necrosis of underlying tissues due to burn (deep third degree) of back of hand, without mention of loss of a body part
- 944.47 Deep necrosis of underlying tissues due to burn (deep third degree) of wrist, without mention of loss of a body part
- 991.1 Frostbite of hand

Terms To Know

graft. Tissue implant from another part of the body or another person.

pedicle flap. Full-thickness skin and subcutaneous tissue for grafting that remains partially attached to the donor site by a pedicle or stem in which the blood vessels supplying the flap remain intact.

CCI Version 16.3

01951-01952, 0213T, 0216T, 0228T, 0230T, 36000, 36400-36410, 36420-36430, 36440, 36600, 36640, 37202, 43752, 51701-51703, 62310-62319, 64400-64435, 64445-64450, 64479, 64483, 64490, 64493, 64505-64530, 69990, 93000-93010, 93040-93042, 93318, 94002, 94200, 94250, 94680-94690, 94770, 95812-95816, 95819, 95822, 95829, 95955, 96360, 96365, 96372, 96374-96376, 99148-99149, 99150, J0670, J2001

Note: These CCI edits are used for Medicare. Other payers may reimburse on codes listed above.

Medicare Edits

	Fac RVU	Non-Fac RVU	FUD	Assist
15740	25.74	30.05	90	N/A

Medicare References: 100-2,15,260; 100-4,3,20.1.2.8; 100-4,12,30; 100-4,12,90.3; 100-4,14,10

15750

15750 Flap; neurovascular pedicle

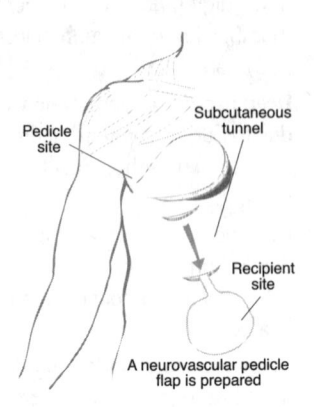

Skin and subcutaneous tissue containing a neurovascular link is trimmed for use as an island pedicle flap. The pedicle is devested of extra tissue so that the connection to the donor site is little more than an innervated artery and vein. The flap is rotated and passed through a subcutaneous tunnel to the recipient site

Explanation

The physician forms a neurovascular pedicle flap. A defect is being covered by elevation of a flap of skin and subcutaneous tissue with its nerve and blood supply intact. The flap is rotated into a nearby but not immediately adjacent defect. Often this flap will be transferred through a tunnel underneath the skin and sutured into its new position. The donor site is closed directly.

Coding Tips

A neurovascular pedicle flap is a type of graft where the pedicle consists of the artery and vein that provide the blood supply and includes the nerve as well. Repair of the donor site requiring a skin graft or local flap is reported as an additional procedure.

ICD-9-CM Procedural

- 04.5 Cranial or peripheral nerve graft
- 86.70 Pedicle or flap graft, not otherwise specified

Anesthesia

15750 00300, 00400

ICD-9-CM Diagnostic

- 171.2 Malignant neoplasm of connective and other soft tissue of upper limb, including shoulder
- 172.6 Malignant melanoma of skin of upper limb, including shoulder
- 198.2 Secondary malignant neoplasm of skin
- 209.32 Merkel cell carcinoma of the scalp and neck
- 209.33 Merkel cell carcinoma of the upper limb
- 209.35 Merkel cell carcinoma of the trunk
- 209.36 Merkel cell carcinoma of other sites
- 209.75 Secondary Merkel cell carcinoma
- 232.6 Carcinoma in situ of skin of upper limb, including shoulder
- 682.3 Cellulitis and abscess of upper arm and forearm — (Use additional code to identify organism, such as 041.1, etc.)
- 682.4 Cellulitis and abscess of hand, except fingers and thumb — (Use additional code to identify organism, such as 041.1, etc.)
- 728.86 Necrotizing fasciitis — (Use additional code to identify infectious organism, 041.00-041.89, 785.4, if applicable)
- 874.8 Open wound of other and unspecified parts of neck, without mention of complication
- 875.1 Open wound of chest (wall), complicated
- 876.0 Open wound of back, without mention of complication
- 876.1 Open wound of back, complicated
- 879.5 Open wound of abdominal wall, lateral, complicated
- 880.03 Open wound of upper arm, without mention of complication
- 880.09 Open wound of multiple sites of shoulder and upper arm, without mention of complication
- 880.13 Open wound of upper arm, complicated
- 880.19 Open wound of multiple sites of shoulder and upper arm, complicated
- 880.23 Open wound of upper arm, with tendon involvement
- 942.30 Full-thickness skin loss due to burn (third degree NOS) of unspecified site of trunk
- 942.33 Full-thickness skin loss due to burn (third degree NOS) of abdominal wall
- 942.34 Full-thickness skin loss due to burn (third degree NOS) of back (any part)
- 942.40 Deep necrosis of underlying tissues due to burn (deep third degree) of trunk, unspecified site, without mention of loss of a body part
- 942.42 Deep necrosis of underlying tissues due to burn (deep third degree) of chest wall, excluding breast and nipple, without mention of loss of a body part
- 942.43 Deep necrosis of underlying tissues due to burn (deep third degree) of abdominal wall, without mention of loss of a body part
- 942.44 Deep necrosis of underlying tissues due to burn (deep third degree) of back (any part), without mention of loss of a body part
- 998.83 Non-healing surgical wound

Terms To Know

flap graft. Mass of flesh and skin partially excised from its location but retaining its blood supply, grafted onto another site to repair adjacent or distant defects.

harvest. Removal of cells or tissue from their native site to be used as a graft or transplant to another part of the donor's body or placed into another person.

island pedicle. Flap consisting of full-thickness skin and subcutaneous tissue that remains attached to its nutrient supply of blood vessels.

CCI Version 16.3

01951-01952, 0213T, 0216T, 0228T, 0230T, 36000, 36400-36410, 36420-36430, 36440, 36600, 36640, 37202, 43752, 51701-51703, 62310-62319, 64400-64435, 64445-64450, 64479, 64483, 64490, 64493, 64505-64530, 69990, 93000-93010, 93040-93042, 93318, 94002, 94200, 94250, 94680-94690, 94770, 95812-95816, 95819, 95822, 95829, 95955, 96360, 96365, 96372, 96374-96376, 99148-99149, 99150

Note: These CCI edits are used for Medicare. Other payers may reimburse on codes listed above.

Medicare Edits

	Fac RVU	Non-Fac RVU	FUD	Assist
15750	27.0	27.0	90	80

Medicare References: 100-2,15,260; 100-4,3,20.1.2.8; 100-4,12,30; 100-4,12,90.3; 100-4,14,10

15756

15756 Free muscle or myocutaneous flap with microvascular anastomosis

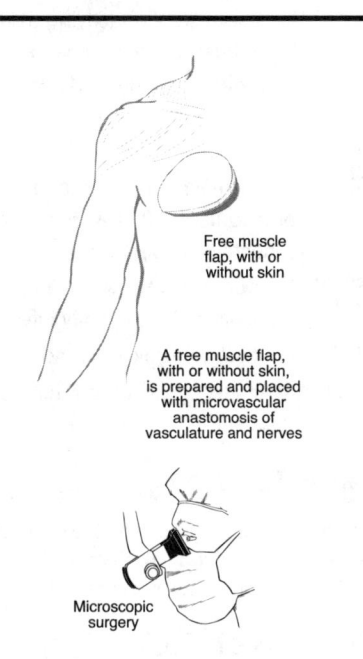

Free muscle flap, with or without skin

A free muscle flap, with or without skin, is prepared and placed with microvascular anastomosis of vasculature and nerves

Microscopic surgery

Explanation

The physician implants a free muscle flap with microvascular anastomosis. With the patient under general anesthesia, the physician prepares and irrigates the wound. The new muscle is completely removed from the donor site and prepared. The physician inserts the new muscle and uses half-mattress sutures to secure the section. Using microscopy, the physician joins the vessels, uniting the new muscle to the site. Before all are joined, the physician may inject fluorescein dye in the vascular system and check the area for fluorescence under an ultraviolet light. Adjustments and corrections to the vascular connections are made and the physician sutures the skin. Light dressing is applied and, in many cases, the flap is splinted to help prevent shrinkage. The donor site is sutured and covered with a light dressing.

Coding Tips

Repair of the donor site requiring a skin graft or local flap is reported as an additional procedure. Do not report the use of an operating microscope separately (69990) as it is included in any microvascular repair. This code reports either a free myofascial flap or a myocutaneous flap, as the amount of work associated with these two procedures is not appreciably different. If a myocutaneous free flap is combined with a bone graft, codes in the family 20970 through 20972 should be used, not 15756 or 15757.

ICD-9-CM Procedural

39.31	Suture of artery
39.32	Suture of vein
82.72	Plastic operation on hand with graft of muscle or fascia
83.77	Muscle transfer or transplantation
86.61	Full-thickness skin graft to hand
86.63	Full-thickness skin graft to other sites

Anesthesia

15756 00300, 00400

ICD-9-CM Diagnostic

171.2	Malignant neoplasm of connective and other soft tissue of upper limb, including shoulder
172.6	Malignant melanoma of skin of upper limb, including shoulder
209.32	Merkel cell carcinoma of the scalp and neck
209.33	Merkel cell carcinoma of the upper limb
209.35	Merkel cell carcinoma of the trunk
209.36	Merkel cell carcinoma of other sites
209.75	Secondary Merkel cell carcinoma
810.11	Open fracture of sternal end of clavicle
810.12	Open fracture of shaft of clavicle
810.13	Open fracture of acromial end of clavicle
813.10	Unspecified open fracture of upper end of forearm
813.11	Open fracture of olecranon process of ulna
813.12	Open fracture of coronoid process of ulna
813.13	Open Monteggia's fracture
813.15	Open fracture of head of radius
813.16	Open fracture of neck of radius
813.17	Other and unspecified open fractures of proximal end of radius (alone)
813.18	Open fracture of radius with ulna, upper end (any part)
813.30	Unspecified open fracture of shaft of radius or ulna
813.31	Open fracture of shaft of radius (alone)
813.32	Open fracture of shaft of ulna (alone)
813.33	Open fracture of shaft of radius with ulna
813.50	Unspecified open fracture of lower end of forearm
813.51	Open Colles' fracture
813.52	Other open fractures of distal end of radius (alone)
813.53	Open fracture of distal end of ulna (alone)
813.54	Open fracture of lower end of radius with ulna
880.10	Open wound of shoulder region, complicated
880.11	Open wound of scapular region, complicated
880.12	Open wound of axillary region, complicated
880.13	Open wound of upper arm, complicated
881.10	Open wound of forearm, complicated
881.11	Open wound of elbow, complicated
881.12	Open wound of wrist, complicated
882.1	Open wound of hand except finger(s) alone, complicated
998.83	Non-healing surgical wound
V51.8	Other aftercare involving the use of plastic surgery

CCI Version 16.3

01951-01952, 0213T, 0216T, 0228T, 0230T, 12001-12007, 12031-12047, 15050-15100, 15120, 15200, 15220, 15240, 15260, 15400, 15920❖, 19366, 23395-23397, 35201, 35207, 35226, 36000, 36400-36410, 36420-36430, 36440, 36600, 36640, 37202, 43752, 51701-51703, 62310-62319, 64400-64435, 64445-64450, 64479, 64483, 64490, 64493, 64505-64530, 69990, 93000-93010, 93040-93042, 93318, 94002, 94200, 94250, 94680-94690, 94770, 95812-95816, 95819, 95822, 95829, 95955, 96360, 96365, 96372, 96374-96376, 99148-99149, 99150

Note: These CCI edits are used for Medicare. Other payers may reimburse on codes listed above.

Medicare Edits

	Fac RVU	Non-Fac RVU	FUD	Assist
15756	69.92	69.92	90	80

Medicare References: None

15757

15757 Free skin flap with microvascular anastomosis

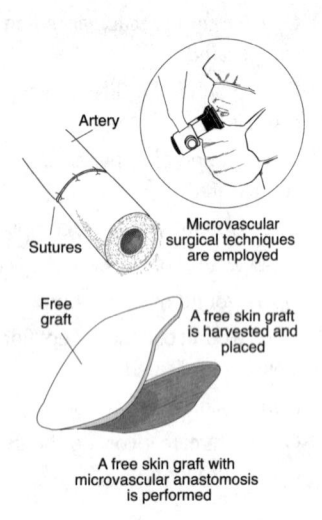

Explanation

The physician implants a free skin flap with microvascular anastomosis. With the patient under general anesthesia, the physician prepares and irrigates the wound. The new skin is completely removed from the donor site with blood vessels and prepared. The physician inserts the new skin and uses half-mattress sutures to secure the section. Using microscopy, the physician joins the vessels and nerves uniting the new skin to the site. Before all are joined, the physician may inject fluorescein dye in the vascular system and check the area for fluorescence under an ultraviolet light. Adjustments and corrections to the vascular connections are made and the physician sutures the skin. Light dressing is applied and, in many cases, the flap is splinted to help prevent shrinkage. The donor site is sutured and covered with a light dressing.

Coding Tips

Repair of the donor site requiring a skin graft or local flap is reported as an additional procedure. Do not report the use of an operating microscope separately (69990) as it is included in any microvascular repair.

ICD-9-CM Procedural

- 39.31 Suture of artery
- 39.32 Suture of vein
- 86.70 Pedicle or flap graft, not otherwise specified
- 86.71 Cutting and preparation of pedicle grafts or flaps
- 86.73 Attachment of pedicle or flap graft to hand
- 86.74 Attachment of pedicle or flap graft to other sites
- 86.75 Revision of pedicle or flap graft

Anesthesia

15757 00300, 00400

ICD-9-CM Diagnostic

- 172.6 Malignant melanoma of skin of upper limb, including shoulder
- 198.2 Secondary malignant neoplasm of skin
- 209.32 Merkel cell carcinoma of the scalp and neck
- 209.33 Merkel cell carcinoma of the upper limb
- 209.35 Merkel cell carcinoma of the trunk
- 209.36 Merkel cell carcinoma of other sites
- 209.75 Secondary Merkel cell carcinoma
- 216.6 Benign neoplasm of skin of upper limb, including shoulder
- 232.6 Carcinoma in situ of skin of upper limb, including shoulder
- 728.86 Necrotizing fasciitis — (Use additional code to identify infectious organism, 041.00-041.89, 785.4, if applicable)
- 785.4 Gangrene — (Code first any associated underlying condition)
- 880.12 Open wound of axillary region, complicated
- 882.1 Open wound of hand except finger(s) alone, complicated
- 882.2 Open wound of hand except finger(s) alone, with tendon involvement
- 883.1 Open wound of finger(s), complicated
- 883.2 Open wound of finger(s), with tendon involvement
- 884.1 Multiple and unspecified open wound of upper limb, complicated
- 884.2 Multiple and unspecified open wound of upper limb, with tendon involvement
- 944.35 Full-thickness skin loss due to burn (third degree NOS) of palm of hand
- 944.36 Full-thickness skin loss due to burn (third degree NOS) of back of hand
- 944.37 Full-thickness skin loss due to burn (third degree NOS) of wrist
- 944.45 Deep necrosis of underlying tissues due to burn (deep third degree) of palm of hand, without mention of loss of a body part
- 944.46 Deep necrosis of underlying tissues due to burn (deep third degree) of back of hand, without mention of loss of a body part
- 944.47 Deep necrosis of underlying tissues due to burn (deep third degree) of wrist, without mention of loss of a body part
- 991.1 Frostbite of hand
- 997.69 Other late amputation stump complication — (Use additional code to identify complications)
- 998.59 Other postoperative infection — (Use additional code to identify infection)
- 998.83 Non-healing surgical wound
- V51.8 Other aftercare involving the use of plastic surgery

Terms To Know

anastomosis. Surgically created connection between ducts, blood vessels, or bowel segments to allow flow from one to the other.

CCI Version 16.3

01951-01952, 0213T, 0216T, 0228T, 0230T, 12001-12007, 12031-12047, 15756, 19366, 35201, 35207, 35226, 36000, 36400-36410, 36420-36430, 36440, 36600, 36640, 37202, 43752, 51701-51703, 62310-62319, 64400-64435, 64445-64450, 64479, 64483, 64490, 64493, 64505-64530, 69990, 93000-93010, 93040-93042, 93318, 94002, 94200, 94250, 94680-94690, 94770, 95812-95816, 95819, 95822, 95829, 95955, 96360, 96365, 96372, 96374-96376, 99148-99149, 99150

Note: These CCI edits are used for Medicare. Other payers may reimburse on codes listed above.

Medicare Edits

	Fac RVU	Non-Fac RVU	FUD	Assist
15757	69.22	69.22	90	80

Medicare References: 100-4,12,30

15758

15758 Free fascial flap with microvascular anastomosis

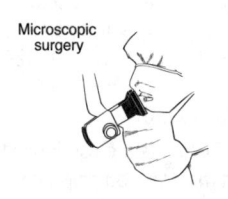

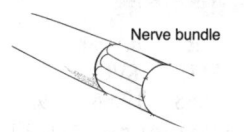

Explanation
The physician implants a free fascial flap with microvascular anastomosis. With the patient under general anesthesia, the physician prepares and irrigates the wound. The new fascia is removed from the donor site and prepared. The physician inserts the new fascia and uses sutures to secure the section. Using microscopy, the physician joins the vessels and nerves uniting the new fascia to the site. Before all are joined, the physician may inject fluorescein dye in the vascular system and check the area for fluorescence under an ultraviolet light. Adjustments and corrections to the vascular connections are made and the physician sutures the skin. A light dressing is applied and, in many cases, the flap is splinted to help prevent shrinkage. The donor site is sutured and covered with a light dressing.

Coding Tips
Repair of the donor site requiring a skin graft or local flap is reported as an additional procedure. Do not report the use of an operating microscope separately (69990) as it is included in any microvascular repair.

ICD-9-CM Procedural
- 39.31 Suture of artery
- 39.32 Suture of vein
- 82.72 Plastic operation on hand with graft of muscle or fascia
- 83.82 Graft of muscle or fascia

Anesthesia
15758 01610, 01710, 01810

ICD-9-CM Diagnostic
- 881.10 Open wound of forearm, complicated
- 881.11 Open wound of elbow, complicated
- 881.12 Open wound of wrist, complicated
- 881.20 Open wound of forearm, with tendon involvement
- 881.21 Open wound of elbow, with tendon involvement
- 881.22 Open wound of wrist, with tendon involvement
- 882.1 Open wound of hand except finger(s) alone, complicated
- 882.2 Open wound of hand except finger(s) alone, with tendon involvement
- 883.1 Open wound of finger(s), complicated
- 883.2 Open wound of finger(s), with tendon involvement
- 906.1 Late effect of open wound of extremities without mention of tendon injury
- 906.4 Late effect of crushing
- 906.6 Late effect of burn of wrist and hand
- 927.10 Crushing injury of forearm — (Use additional code to identify any associated injuries: 800-829, 850.0-854.1, 860.0-869.1)
- 927.11 Crushing injury of elbow — (Use additional code to identify any associated injuries: 800-829, 850.0-854.1, 860.0-869.1)
- 927.20 Crushing injury of hand(s) — (Use additional code to identify any associated injuries: 800-829, 850.0-854.1, 860.0-869.1)
- 927.21 Crushing injury of wrist — (Use additional code to identify any associated injuries: 800-829, 850.0-854.1, 860.0-869.1)
- 943.31 Full-thickness skin loss due to burn (third degree NOS) of forearm
- 943.41 Deep necrosis of underlying tissues due to burn (deep third degree) of forearm, without mention of loss of a body part
- 944.35 Full-thickness skin loss due to burn (third degree NOS) of palm of hand
- 944.36 Full-thickness skin loss due to burn (third degree NOS) of back of hand
- 944.37 Full-thickness skin loss due to burn (third degree NOS) of wrist
- 944.45 Deep necrosis of underlying tissues due to burn (deep third degree) of palm of hand, without mention of loss of a body part
- 944.46 Deep necrosis of underlying tissues due to burn (deep third degree) of back of hand, without mention of loss of a body part
- 944.47 Deep necrosis of underlying tissues due to burn (deep third degree) of wrist, without mention of loss of a body part

Terms To Know

anastomosis. Surgically created connection between ducts, blood vessels, or bowel segments to allow flow from one to the other.

fascia. Fibrous sheet or band of tissue that envelops organs, muscles, and groupings of muscles.

CCI Version 16.3
01951-01952, 0213T, 0216T, 0228T, 0230T, 12001-12007, 12031-12047, 15050-15100, 15120, 15200, 15220, 15240, 15260, 15400, 15756-15757, 19366, 35201, 35207, 35226, 36000, 36400-36410, 36420-36430, 36440, 36600, 36640, 37202, 43752, 51701-51703, 62310-62319, 64400-64435, 64445-64450, 64479, 64483, 64490, 64493, 64505-64530, 69990, 93000-93010, 93040-93042, 93318, 94002, 94200, 94250, 94680-94690, 94770, 95812-95816, 95819, 95822, 95829, 95955, 96360, 96365, 96372, 96374-96376, 99148-99149, 99150

Note: These CCI edits are used for Medicare. Other payers may reimburse on codes listed above.

Medicare Edits

	Fac RVU	Non-Fac RVU	FUD	Assist
15758	68.92	68.92	90	80

Medicare References: 100-4,12,30

15770

15770 Graft; derma-fat-fascia

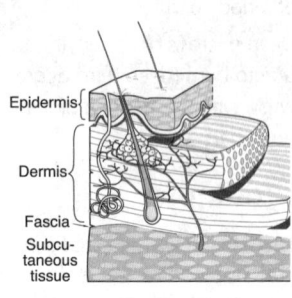

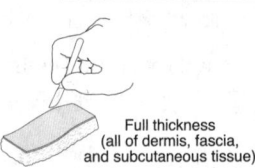

Explanation
The physician takes a graft composed of derma, fat, and fascia to repair and blend in defects left behind by atrophy, surgical excisions, or other fleshy defects, much like a composite graft. The derma-fat-fascia graft may be a continuous piece of all three of these layers, individual sections done layer by layer, or graft pieces laid in the recipient bed as combinations, such as a fascia-fat layer, followed by a dermal layer. The graft is used on defects much like a composite graft to maintain support for the continuity of the local flesh. The graft is laid in the recipient area so as to fill and blend in pockets of defects to restore the surrounding area to normal positioning and to maintain the continuity of the local flesh.

Coding Tips
Repair of the donor site requiring a skin graft or local flap is reported as an additional procedure.

ICD-9-CM Procedural
- 83.82 Graft of muscle or fascia
- 86.69 Other skin graft to other sites
- 86.71 Cutting and preparation of pedicle grafts or flaps

Anesthesia
15770 00300, 00400, 00700, 00730, 00800, 00820

ICD-9-CM Diagnostic
The application of this code is too broad to adequately present ICD-9-CM diagnostic code links here. Refer to your ICD-9-CM book.

Terms To Know

dermis. Skin layer found under the epidermis that contains a papillary upper layer and the deep reticular layer of collagen, vascular bed, and nerves.

epidermis. Outermost, nonvascular layer of skin that contains four to five differentiated layers depending on its body location: stratum corneum, lucidum, granulosum, spinosum, and basale.

fascia. Fibrous sheet or band of tissue that envelops organs, muscles, and groupings of muscles.

graft. Tissue implant from another part of the body or another person.

harvest. Removal of cells or tissue from their native site to be used as a graft or transplant to another part of the donor's body or placed into another person.

subcutaneous tissue. Sheet or wide band of adipose (fat) and areolar connective tissue in two layers attached to the dermis.

suture. Numerous stitching techniques employed in wound closure.

buried suture. Continuous or interrupted suture placed under the skin for a layered closure.

continuous suture. Running stitch with tension evenly distributed across a single strand to provide a leakproof closure line.

interrupted suture. Series of single stitches with tension isolated at each stitch, in which all stitches are not affected if one becomes loose, and the isolated sutures cannot act as a wick to transport an infection.

purse-string suture. Continuous suture placed around a tubular structure and tightened, to reduce or close the lumen.

retention suture. Secondary stitching that bridges the primary suture, providing support for the primary repair; a plastic or rubber bolster may be placed over the primary repair and under the retention sutures.

CCI Version 16.3
01951-01952, 0213T, 0216T, 0228T, 0230T, 36000, 36400-36410, 36420-36430, 36440, 36600, 36640, 37202, 43752, 51701-51703, 62310-62319, 64400-64435, 64445-64450, 64479, 64483, 64490, 64493, 64505-64530, 69990, 93000-93010, 93040-93042, 93318, 94002, 94200, 94250, 94680-94690, 94770, 95812-95816, 95819, 95822, 95829, 95955, 96360, 96365, 96372, 96374-96376, 99148-99149, 99150

Note: These CCI edits are used for Medicare. Other payers may reimburse on codes listed above.

Medicare Edits

	Fac RVU	Non-Fac RVU	FUD	Assist
15770	19.68	19.68	90	80

Medicare References: 100-2,15,260; 100-4,3,20.1.2.8; 100-4,12,30; 100-4,12,90.3; 100-4,14,10

15850-15851

15850 Removal of sutures under anesthesia (other than local), same surgeon
15851 Removal of sutures under anesthesia (other than local), other surgeon

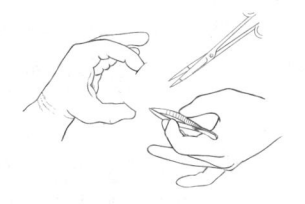

Sutures are removed under anesthesia

Explanation
The physician who completed the surgery on the patient now removes sutures on that patient with the aid of sedation or general anesthesia. Report 15851 for removal of sutures by another surgeon under anesthesia (not local).

Coding Tips
Removal of sutures from surgery are usually in the postoperative period and should not be reported apart from the surgical procedure.

ICD-9-CM Procedural
- 97.38 Removal of sutures from head and neck
- 97.43 Removal of sutures from thorax
- 97.84 Removal of sutures from trunk, not elsewhere classified
- 97.89 Removal of other therapeutic device

Anesthesia
00300, 00400

ICD-9-CM Diagnostic
- 729.90 Disorders of soft tissue, unspecified
- 729.91 Post-traumatic seroma
- 998.30 Disruption of wound, unspecified
- 998.31 Disruption of internal operation (surgical) wound
- 998.32 Disruption of external operation (surgical) wound
- 998.33 Disruption of traumatic injury wound repair
- 998.51 Infected postoperative seroma — (Use additional code to identify organism)
- 998.59 Other postoperative infection — (Use additional code to identify infection)
- V58.32 Encounter for removal of sutures

Terms To Know
absorbable sutures. Strands prepared from collagen or a synthetic polymer and capable of being absorbed by tissue over time.

anesthesia. Loss of feeling or sensation, usually induced to permit the performance of surgery or other painful procedures.

infected postoperative seroma. Infection within a tumor-like growth of serum following surgery.

nonabsorbable sutures. Strands of natural or synthetic material that resist absorption into living tissue and are removed once healing is under way. Nonabsorbable sutures are commonly used to close skin wounds and repair tendons or collagenous tissue.

suture. Numerous stitching techniques employed in wound closure.

buried suture. Continuous or interrupted suture placed under the skin for a layered closure.

continuous suture. Running stitch with tension evenly distributed across a single strand to provide a leakproof closure line.

interrupted suture. Series of single stitches with tension isolated at each stitch, in which all stitches are not affected if one becomes loose, and the isolated sutures cannot act as a wick to transport an infection.

purse-string suture. Continuous suture placed around a tubular structure and tightened, to reduce or close the lumen.

retention suture. Secondary stitching that bridges the primary suture, providing support for the primary repair; a plastic or rubber bolster may be placed over the primary repair and under the retention sutures.

CCI Version 16.3
Also not with 15851: 0213T, 0216T, 0228T, 0230T, 36000, 36400-36410, 36420-36430, 36440, 36600, 36640, 37202, 43752, 51701-51703, 62310-62319, 64400-64435, 64445-64450, 64479, 64483, 64490, 64493, 64505-64530, 69990, 93000-93010, 93040-93042, 93318, 94002, 94200, 94250, 94680-94690, 94770, 95812-95816, 95819, 95822, 95829, 95955, 96360, 96365, 96372, 96374-96376, 97597-97598, 97602-97606, 99148-99149, 99150, J0670, J2001

Note: These CCI edits are used for Medicare. Other payers may reimburse on codes listed above.

Medicare Edits

	Fac RVU	Non-Fac RVU	FUD	Assist
15850	1.17	2.51	N/A	N/A
15851	1.35	2.76	0	N/A

Medicare References: 100-4,12,30

15852

15852 Dressing change (for other than burns) under anesthesia (other than local)

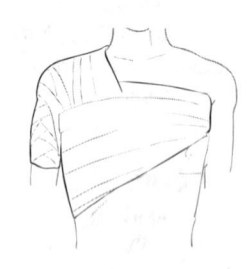

A dressing for a condition other than burn is changed under anesthesia

Explanation

The physician changes a dressing on a wound other than a burn while the patient is under sedation or general anesthesia. This is commonly done for severe crush injuries where serial tissue debridement is required and also for certain types of infection.

Coding Tips

For dressing changes for burns, see 16000–16030.

ICD-9-CM Procedural

93.57 Application of other wound dressing

Anesthesia

15852 00300, 00400

ICD-9-CM Diagnostic

- 707.01 Pressure ulcer, elbow — (Use additional code to identify pressure ulcer stage: 707.20-707.25)
- 785.4 Gangrene — (Code first any associated underlying condition)
- 880.12 Open wound of axillary region, complicated
- 882.1 Open wound of hand except finger(s) alone, complicated
- 882.2 Open wound of hand except finger(s) alone, with tendon involvement
- 883.1 Open wound of finger(s), complicated
- 883.2 Open wound of finger(s), with tendon involvement
- 884.1 Multiple and unspecified open wound of upper limb, complicated
- 884.2 Multiple and unspecified open wound of upper limb, with tendon involvement
- 926.11 Crushing injury of back — (Use additional code to identify any associated injuries: 800-829, 850.0-854.1, 860.0-869.1)
- 926.19 Crushing injury of other specified sites of trunk — (Use additional code to identify any associated injuries: 800-829, 850.0-854.1, 860.0-869.1)
- 926.8 Crushing injury of multiple sites of trunk — (Use additional code to identify any associated injuries: 800-829, 850.0-854.1, 860.0-869.1)
- 926.9 Crushing injury of unspecified site of trunk — (Use additional code to identify any associated injuries: 800-829, 850.0-854.1, 860.0-869.1)
- 927.00 Crushing injury of shoulder region — (Use additional code to identify any associated injuries: 800-829, 850.0-854.1, 860.0-869.1)
- 927.01 Crushing injury of scapular region — (Use additional code to identify any associated injuries: 800-829, 850.0-854.1, 860.0-869.1)
- 927.02 Crushing injury of axillary region — (Use additional code to identify any associated injuries: 800-829, 850.0-854.1, 860.0-869.1)
- 927.03 Crushing injury of upper arm — (Use additional code to identify any associated injuries: 800-829, 850.0-854.1, 860.0-869.1)
- 927.09 Crushing injury of multiple sites of upper arm — (Use additional code to identify any associated injuries: 800-829, 850.0-854.1, 860.0-869.1)
- 927.10 Crushing injury of forearm — (Use additional code to identify any associated injuries: 800-829, 850.0-854.1, 860.0-869.1)
- 927.11 Crushing injury of elbow — (Use additional code to identify any associated injuries: 800-829, 850.0-854.1, 860.0-869.1)
- 927.20 Crushing injury of hand(s) — (Use additional code to identify any associated injuries: 800-829, 850.0-854.1, 860.0-869.1)
- 927.21 Crushing injury of wrist — (Use additional code to identify any associated injuries: 800-829, 850.0-854.1, 860.0-869.1)
- 927.3 Crushing injury of finger(s) — (Use additional code to identify any associated injuries: 800-829, 850.0-854.1, 860.0-869.1)
- 927.8 Crushing injury of multiple sites of upper limb — (Use additional code to identify any associated injuries: 800-829, 850.0-854.1, 860.0-869.1)
- 927.9 Crushing injury of unspecified site of upper limb — (Use additional code to identify any associated injuries: 800-829, 850.0-854.1, 860.0-869.1)
- 998.32 Disruption of external operation (surgical) wound
- 998.51 Infected postoperative seroma — (Use additional code to identify organism)
- 998.59 Other postoperative infection — (Use additional code to identify infection)
- 998.6 Persistent postoperative fistula, not elsewhere classified
- V58.31 Encounter for change or removal of surgical wound dressing

Terms To Know

debridement. Removal of dead or contaminated tissue and foreign matter from a wound.

CCI Version 16.3

0213T, 0216T, 0228T, 0230T, 36000, 36400-36410, 36420-36430, 36440, 36600, 36640, 37202, 43752, 51701-51703, 62310-62319, 64400-64435, 64445-64450, 64479, 64483, 64490, 64493, 64505-64530, 69990, 93000-93010, 93040-93042, 93318, 94002, 94200, 94250, 94680-94690, 94770, 95812-95816, 95819, 95822, 95829, 95955, 96360, 96365, 96372, 96374-96376, 97597-97598, 97602-97606, 99148-99149, 99150, J2001

Note: These CCI edits are used for Medicare. Other payers may reimburse on codes listed above.

Medicare Edits

	Fac RVU	Non-Fac RVU	FUD	Assist
15852	1.39	1.39	0	N/A

Medicare References: 100-4,12,30

15860

15860 Intravenous injection of agent (eg, fluorescein) to test vascular flow in flap or graft

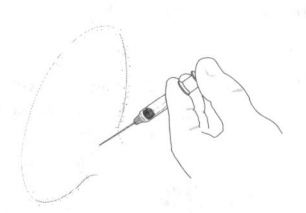

The results may be viewed directly or interpreted through a separately reported imaging study

A placed graft is intravenously injected to test blood flow

Explanation
The physician injects a dye such as fluorescein or methylene blue to test the viability of blood vessels in a flap or graft. The agent is injected intravenously.

Coding Tips
Fluorescein injection to test blood flow in a flap or graft may be reported additionally when performed at the time of flap or graft attachment.

ICD-9-CM Procedural
- 86.89 Other repair and reconstruction of skin and subcutaneous tissue

Anesthesia
15860 N/A

ICD-9-CM Diagnostic
- 172.6 Malignant melanoma of skin of upper limb, including shoulder
- 198.2 Secondary malignant neoplasm of skin
- 209.33 Merkel cell carcinoma of the upper limb
- 209.35 Merkel cell carcinoma of the trunk
- 209.75 Secondary Merkel cell carcinoma
- 216.6 Benign neoplasm of skin of upper limb, including shoulder
- 232.6 Carcinoma in situ of skin of upper limb, including shoulder
- 239.2 Neoplasms of unspecified nature of bone, soft tissue, and skin
- 443.0 Raynaud's syndrome — (Use additional code to identify gangrene: 785.4)
- 728.86 Necrotizing fasciitis — (Use additional code to identify infectious organism, 041.00-041.89, 785.4, if applicable)
- 757.33 Congenital pigmentary anomaly of skin
- 785.4 Gangrene — (Code first any associated underlying condition)
- 880.12 Open wound of axillary region, complicated
- 882.1 Open wound of hand except finger(s) alone, complicated
- 882.2 Open wound of hand except finger(s) alone, with tendon involvement
- 883.1 Open wound of finger(s), complicated
- 884.1 Multiple and unspecified open wound of upper limb, complicated
- 884.2 Multiple and unspecified open wound of upper limb, with tendon involvement
- 885.0 Traumatic amputation of thumb (complete) (partial), without mention of complication
- 885.1 Traumatic amputation of thumb (complete) (partial), complicated
- 906.6 Late effect of burn of wrist and hand
- 943.54 Deep necrosis of underlying tissues due to burn (deep third degree) of axilla, with loss of a body part
- 944.30 Full-thickness skin loss due to burn (third degree NOS) of unspecified site of hand
- 944.31 Full-thickness skin loss due to burn (third degree NOS) of single digit [finger (nail)] other than thumb
- 944.32 Full-thickness skin loss due to burn (third degree NOS) of thumb (nail)
- 944.33 Full-thickness skin loss due to burn (third degree NOS) of two or more digits of hand, not including thumb
- 944.34 Full-thickness skin loss due to burn (third degree NOS) of two or more digits of hand including thumb
- 944.35 Full-thickness skin loss due to burn (third degree NOS) of palm of hand
- 944.36 Full-thickness skin loss due to burn (third degree NOS) of back of hand
- 944.37 Full-thickness skin loss due to burn (third degree NOS) of wrist
- 944.45 Deep necrosis of underlying tissues due to burn (deep third degree) of palm of hand, without mention of loss of a body part
- 944.46 Deep necrosis of underlying tissues due to burn (deep third degree) of back of hand, without mention of loss of a body part
- 944.47 Deep necrosis of underlying tissues due to burn (deep third degree) of wrist, without mention of loss of a body part
- 944.48 Deep necrosis of underlying tissues due to burn (deep third degree) of multiple sites of wrist(s) and hand(s), without mention of loss of a body part

Terms To Know
graft. Tissue implant from another part of the body or another person.

injection. Forcing a liquid substance into a body part such as a joint or muscle.

intravenous. Within a vein or veins.

vascular. Pertaining to blood vessels.

CCI Version 16.3
0213T, 0216T, 0228T, 0230T, 36000, 36400-36410, 36420-36430, 36440, 36600, 36640, 37202, 43752, 51701-51703, 62310-62319, 64400-64435, 64445-64450, 64479, 64483, 64490, 64493, 64505-64530, 69990, 93000-93010, 93040-93042, 93318, 94002, 94200, 94250, 94680-94690, 94770, 95812-95816, 95819, 95822, 95829, 95955, 96360, 96365, 96372, 96374-96376, 99148-99149, 99150

Note: These CCI edits are used for Medicare. Other payers may reimburse on codes listed above.

Medicare Edits

	Fac RVU	Non-Fac RVU	FUD	Assist
15860	3.23	3.23	0	80

Medicare References: None

15931-15933

15931 Excision, sacral pressure ulcer, with primary suture;
15933 with ostectomy

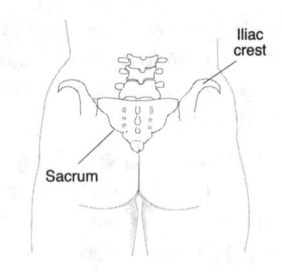

A sacral pressure ulcer is excised and a primary closure completes the procedure. Report 15933 when sacral bone removal is required at the site.

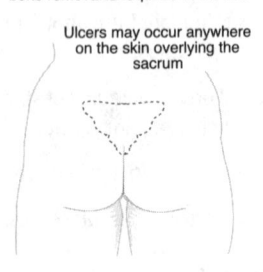

Ulcers may occur anywhere on the skin overlying the sacrum

Explanation
The physician excises a sacral pressure ulcer. The patient is positioned prone (face down) and the physician makes an elliptical incision over the sacrum, removing the strip of skin that contains the pressure sore. The wound is irrigated and the soft tissue is brought back together and closed with sutures. Report 15933 if bone below the wound is removed before the soft tissue is brought back together and closed.

Coding Tips
For a free skin graft to close an ulcer or a donor site, see 15002 et seq. If an autogenous bone graft is obtained through a separate incision, report 20900 or 20902 in addition to 15933. Report 15931 if no bone is excised from the ulcer site. Report 15933 if bone below the wound is removed.

ICD-9-CM Procedural
- 77.89 Other partial ostectomy of other bone, except facial bones
- 86.3 Other local excision or destruction of lesion or tissue of skin and subcutaneous tissue
- 86.4 Radical excision of skin lesion

Anesthesia
15931 00300
15933 01120

ICD-9-CM Diagnostic
- 707.03 Pressure ulcer, lower back — (Use additional code to identify pressure ulcer stage: 707.20-707.25)
- 707.20 Pressure ulcer, unspecified stage — (Code first site of pressure ulcer: 707.00-707.09)
- 707.21 Pressure ulcer, stage I — (Code first site of pressure ulcer: 707.00-707.09)
- 707.22 Pressure ulcer stage II — (Code first site of pressure ulcer: 707.00-707.09)
- 707.23 Pressure ulcer stage III — (Code first site of pressure ulcer: 707.00-707.09)
- 707.24 Pressure ulcer stage IV — (Code first site of pressure ulcer: 707.00-707.09)
- 707.25 Pressure ulcer, unstageable — (Code first site of pressure ulcer: 707.00-707.09)
- 730.18 Chronic osteomyelitis, other specified sites — (Use additional code to identify organism: 041.1. Use additional code to identify major osseous defect, if applicable: 731.3)
- 785.4 Gangrene — (Code first any associated underlying condition)

Terms To Know
decubitus ulcer. Progressively eroding skin lesion produced by inflamed necrotic tissue as it sloughs off caused by continual pressure to a localized area, especially over bony areas, where blood circulation is cut off when a patient lies still for too long without changing position.

gangrene. Death of tissue, usually resulting from a loss of vascular supply, followed by a bacterial attack or onset of disease.

lesion. Area of damaged tissue that has lost continuity or function, due to disease or trauma. Lesions may be located on internal structures such as the brain, nerves, or kidneys, or visible on the skin.

osteomyelitis. Inflammation of bone that may remain localized or spread to the marrow, cortex, or periosteum, in response to an infecting organism, usually bacterial and pyogenic.

soft tissue. Nonepithelial tissues outside of the skeleton that includes subcutaneous adipose tissue, fibrous tissue, fascia, muscles, blood and lymph vessels, and peripheral nervous system tissue.

subcutaneous tissue. Sheet or wide band of adipose (fat) and areolar connective tissue in two layers attached to the dermis.

CCI Version 16.3
0213T, 0216T, 0228T, 0230T, 11010-11012, 11100, 15756-15757❖, 15936-15937❖, 36000, 36400-36410, 36420-36430, 36440, 36600, 36640, 37202, 43752, 51701-51703, 62310-62319, 64400-64435, 64445-64450, 64479, 64483, 64490, 64493, 64505-64530, 69990, 93000-93010, 93040-93042, 93318, 94002, 94200, 94250, 94680-94690, 94770, 95812-95816, 95819, 95822, 95829, 95955, 96360, 96365, 96372, 96374-96376, 99148-99149, 99150

Also not with 15933: 15931

Note: These CCI edits are used for Medicare. Other payers may reimburse on codes listed above.

Medicare Edits

	Fac RVU	Non-Fac RVU	FUD	Assist
15931	19.65	19.65	90	N/A
15933	24.35	24.35	90	80

Medicare References: 100-2,15,260; 100-3,270.5; 100-4,12,30; 100-4,12,90.3; 100-4,14,10

15934-15935

15934 Excision, sacral pressure ulcer, with skin flap closure;
15935 with ostectomy

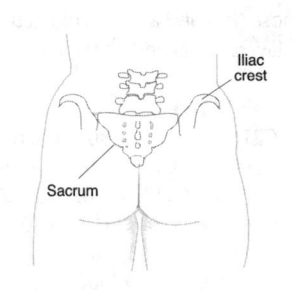

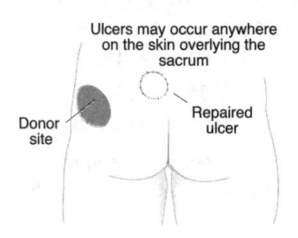

Explanation

The physician excises a sacral pressure ulcer. The patient is positioned prone (face down) and the physician makes a 15 cm elliptical incision over the sacrum, removing the strip of skin that contains the pressure sore. The wound is irrigated and closed using a skin flap from the groin or other donor site. The flap is sutured in place and covered with mesh petroleum gauze and loose bandages. Report 15935 if bone below the wound is removed before the wound is repaired with a skin flap.

Coding Tips

For a free skin graft to close an ulcer or a donor site, see 15002 et seq. If an autogenous bone graft is obtained through a separate incision, report 20900 or 20902 in addition to 15935. Report 15934 if no excision of bone is required. Report 15935 if bone below the wound is removed.

ICD-9-CM Procedural

- 77.89 Other partial ostectomy of other bone, except facial bones
- 86.3 Other local excision or destruction of lesion or tissue of skin and subcutaneous tissue
- 86.4 Radical excision of skin lesion
- 86.74 Attachment of pedicle or flap graft to other sites

Anesthesia

- **15934** 00300
- **15935** 01120

ICD-9-CM Diagnostic

- 707.03 Pressure ulcer, lower back — (Use additional code to identify pressure ulcer stage: 707.20-707.25)
- 707.20 Pressure ulcer, unspecified stage — (Code first site of pressure ulcer: 707.00-707.09)
- 707.21 Pressure ulcer, stage I — (Code first site of pressure ulcer: 707.00-707.09)
- 707.22 Pressure ulcer stage II — (Code first site of pressure ulcer: 707.00-707.09)
- 707.23 Pressure ulcer stage III — (Code first site of pressure ulcer: 707.00-707.09)
- 707.24 Pressure ulcer stage IV — (Code first site of pressure ulcer: 707.00-707.09)
- 707.25 Pressure ulcer, unstageable — (Code first site of pressure ulcer: 707.00-707.09)
- 730.18 Chronic osteomyelitis, other specified sites — (Use additional code to identify organism: 041.1. Use additional code to identify major osseous defect, if applicable: 731.3)
- 785.4 Gangrene — (Code first any associated underlying condition)

Terms To Know

decubitus ulcer. Progressively eroding skin lesion produced by inflamed necrotic tissue as it sloughs off caused by continual pressure to a localized area, especially over bony areas, where blood circulation is cut off when a patient lies still for too long without changing position.

gangrene. Death of tissue, usually resulting from a loss of vascular supply, followed by a bacterial attack or onset of disease.

lesion. Area of damaged tissue that has lost continuity or function, due to disease or trauma. Lesions may be located on internal structures such as the brain, nerves, or kidneys, or visible on the skin.

osteomyelitis. Inflammation of bone that may remain localized or spread to the marrow, cortex, or periosteum, in response to an infecting organism, usually bacterial and pyogenic.

subcutaneous tissue. Sheet or wide band of adipose (fat) and areolar connective tissue in two layers attached to the dermis.

CCI Version 16.3

0213T, 0216T, 0228T, 0230T, 11010-11012, 11100, 15756-15757❖, 36000, 36400-36410, 36420-36430, 36440, 36600, 36640, 37202, 43752, 51701-51703, 62310-62319, 64400-64435, 64445-64450, 64479, 64483, 64490, 64493, 64505-64530, 69990, 93000-93010, 93040-93042, 93318, 94002, 94200, 94250, 94680-94690, 94770, 95812-95816, 95819, 95822, 95829, 95955, 96360, 96365, 96372, 96374-96376, 99148-99149, 99150

Also not with 15934: 15937❖
Also not with 15935: 15934

Note: These CCI edits are used for Medicare. Other payers may reimburse on codes listed above.

Medicare Edits

	Fac RVU	Non-Fac RVU	FUD	Assist
15934	27.06	27.06	90	N/A
15935	32.05	32.05	90	80

Medicare References: 100-2,15,260; 100-3,270.5; 100-4,12,30; 100-4,12,90.3; 100-4,14,10

15936-15937

15936 Excision, sacral pressure ulcer, in preparation for muscle or myocutaneous flap or skin graft closure;
15937 with ostectomy

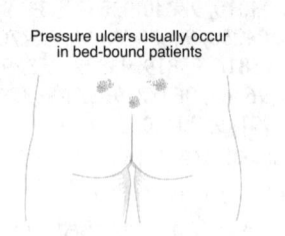

Pressure ulcers usually occur in bed-bound patients

A sacral pressure ulcer is excised in preparation for muscle or myocutaneous flap or skin graft closure. Report 15937 when sacral bone is also removed

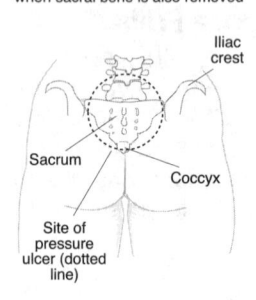

Iliac crest · Sacrum · Coccyx · Site of pressure ulcer (dotted line)

Explanation

The physician excises a sacral ulcer to prepare for muscle or myocutaneous flap or skin graft closure. The physician makes an incision around the pressure sore that lies over the sacrum. The infected wound is removed and the area is irrigated. The space that remains is filled with a muscle flap graft, usually taken from the latissimus dorsi muscle and the overlying skin. The donor site is prepared and the incision is made for the appropriate size of graft to be taken. Once the portion of the muscle is removed, the overlying skin is removed and the wound is sutured closed. The graft is sutured in place and a soft dressing is applied. Report 15937 if the underlying bone is removed before the wound is repaired with the flap or graft.

Coding Tips

Report 15734 or 15738, based on the donor site of the flap used for closure, with 15936. If closed via a skin graft, report 15100 and 15101 with 15936.

ICD-9-CM Procedural

- **77.89** Other partial ostectomy of other bone, except facial bones
- **83.82** Graft of muscle or fascia
- **86.3** Other local excision or destruction of lesion or tissue of skin and subcutaneous tissue
- **86.4** Radical excision of skin lesion
- **86.74** Attachment of pedicle or flap graft to other sites

Anesthesia

- **15936** 00300
- **15937** 01120

ICD-9-CM Diagnostic

- **707.03** Pressure ulcer, lower back — (Use additional code to identify pressure ulcer stage: 707.20-707.25)
- **707.20** Pressure ulcer, unspecified stage — (Code first site of pressure ulcer: 707.00-707.09)
- **707.21** Pressure ulcer, stage I — (Code first site of pressure ulcer: 707.00-707.09)
- **707.22** Pressure ulcer stage II — (Code first site of pressure ulcer: 707.00-707.09)
- **707.23** Pressure ulcer stage III — (Code first site of pressure ulcer: 707.00-707.09)
- **707.24** Pressure ulcer stage IV — (Code first site of pressure ulcer: 707.00-707.09)
- **707.25** Pressure ulcer, unstageable — (Code first site of pressure ulcer: 707.00-707.09)
- **730.18** Chronic osteomyelitis, other specified sites — (Use additional code to identify organism: 041.1. Use additional code to identify major osseous defect, if applicable: 731.3)
- **785.4** Gangrene — (Code first any associated underlying condition)

Terms To Know

decubitus ulcer. Progressively eroding skin lesion produced by inflamed necrotic tissue as it sloughs off caused by continual pressure to a localized area, especially over bony areas, where blood circulation is cut off when a patient lies still for too long without changing position.

fascia. Fibrous sheet or band of tissue that envelops organs, muscles, and groupings of muscles.

gangrene. Death of tissue, usually resulting from a loss of vascular supply, followed by a bacterial attack or onset of disease.

lesion. Area of damaged tissue that has lost continuity or function, due to disease or trauma. Lesions may be located on internal structures such as the brain, nerves, or kidneys, or visible on the skin.

osteomyelitis. Inflammation of bone that may remain localized or spread to the marrow, cortex, or periosteum, in response to an infecting organism, usually bacterial and pyogenic.

subcutaneous tissue. Sheet or wide band of adipose (fat) and areolar connective tissue in two layers attached to the dermis.

CCI Version 16.3

0213T, 0216T, 0228T, 0230T, 11010-11012, 11100, 36000, 36400-36410, 36420-36430, 36440, 36600, 36640, 37202, 43752, 51701-51703, 62310-62319, 64400-64435, 64445-64450, 64479, 64483, 64490, 64493, 64505-64530, 69990, 93000-93010, 93040-93042, 93318, 94002, 94200, 94250, 94680-94690, 94770, 95812-95816, 95819, 95822, 95829, 95955, 96360, 96365, 96372, 96374-96376, 99148-99149, 99150

Also not with 15936: 15934-15935❖

Also not with 15937: 15935-15936

Note: These CCI edits are used for Medicare. Other payers may reimburse on codes listed above.

Medicare Edits

	Fac RVU	Non-Fac RVU	FUD	Assist
15936	26.12	26.12	90	N/A
15937	30.58	30.58	90	N/A

Medicare References: 100-2,15,260; 100-3,270.5; 100-4,12,30; 100-4,12,90.3; 100-4,14,10

17260-17266

17260 Destruction, malignant lesion (eg, laser surgery, electrosurgery, cryosurgery, chemosurgery, surgical curettement), trunk, arms or legs; lesion diameter 0.5 cm or less
17261 lesion diameter 0.6 to 1.0 cm
17262 lesion diameter 1.1 to 2.0 cm
17263 lesion diameter 2.1 to 3.0 cm
17264 lesion diameter 3.1 to 4.0 cm
17266 lesion diameter over 4.0 cm

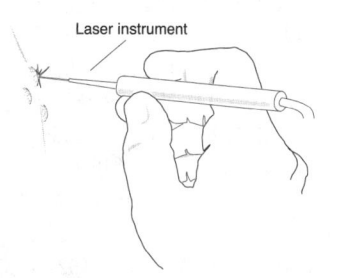

Malignant lesions of the arms are destroyed by any number of methods. Lasers may be used as well as electrocautery or cryotherapy. Once destroyed, a curette may be used to remove the dead tissue

17260: 0.5 cm diameter lesion or less
17261: 0.6 cm to 1.0 cm diameter
17262: 1.1 to 2.0 cm diameter
17263: 2.1 to 3.0 cm diameter
17264: 3.1 to 4.0 cm diameter
17266: larger than 4.0 cm diameter

Report 17260-17266 regardless of method

Explanation

The physician destroys a malignant lesion of the trunk, arms, and legs. Destruction may be accomplished by using a laser or electrocautery to burn the lesion, cryotherapy to freeze the lesion, chemicals to destroy the lesion, or surgical curettement to remove the lesion. Report 17260 for a lesion diameter 0.5 cm or less; 17261 for 0.6 cm to 1 cm; 17262 for 1.1 cm to 2 cm; 17263 for 2.1 cm to 3 cm; 17264 for 3.1 cm to 4 cm; and 17266 if the lesion diameter is greater than 4 cm.

Coding Tips

Local anesthesia is included in these services. For excision of a malignant lesion, see 11600–11606.

ICD-9-CM Procedural

86.3 Other local excision or destruction of lesion or tissue of skin and subcutaneous tissue

Anesthesia

00300, 00400

ICD-9-CM Diagnostic

173.5 Other malignant neoplasm of skin of trunk, except scrotum
173.6 Other malignant neoplasm of skin of upper limb, including shoulder
209.33 Merkel cell carcinoma of the upper limb
209.35 Merkel cell carcinoma of the trunk
209.75 Secondary Merkel cell carcinoma
232.5 Carcinoma in situ of skin of trunk, except scrotum
232.6 Carcinoma in situ of skin of upper limb, including shoulder
238.2 Neoplasm of uncertain behavior of skin

Terms To Know

carcinoma in situ. Malignancy that arises from the cells of the vessel, gland, or organ of origin that remains confined to that site or has not invaded neighboring tissue.

lesion. Area of damaged tissue that has lost continuity or function, due to disease or trauma. Lesions may be located on internal structures such as the brain, nerves, or kidneys, or visible on the skin.

malignant. Any condition tending to progress toward death, specifically an invasive tumor with a loss of cellular differentiation that has the ability to spread or metastasize to other areas in the body.

neoplasm. New abnormal growth, tumor.

subcutaneous tissue. Sheet or wide band of adipose (fat) and areolar connective tissue in two layers attached to the dermis.

CCI Version 16.3

0213T, 0216T, 0228T, 0230T, 11100, 11900-11901, 36000, 36400-36410, 36420-36430, 36440, 36600, 36640, 37202, 43752, 51701-51703, 62310-62319, 64400-64435, 64445-64450, 64479, 64483, 64490, 64493, 64505-64530, 69990, 93000-93010, 93040-93042, 93318, 94002, 94200, 94250, 94680-94690, 94770, 95812-95816, 95819, 95822, 95829, 95955, 96360, 96365, 96372, 96374-96376, 99148-99149, 99150, J0670, J2001

Also not with 17260: 11057❖, 11600-11606❖, 11620-11646❖

Also not with 17261: 11600-11606❖, 11620-11646❖

Also not with 17262: 11601-11606❖, 11621-11626❖, 11641-11646❖

Also not with 17263: 11601-11606❖, 11621-11626❖, 11641-11646❖

Also not with 17264: 11602-11606❖, 11621-11626❖, 11641-11646❖

Also not with 17266: 11603-11606❖, 11622-11626❖, 11641-11646❖

Note: These CCI edits are used for Medicare. Other payers may reimburse on codes listed above.

Medicare Edits

	Fac RVU	Non-Fac RVU	FUD	Assist
17260	2.0	2.77	10	N/A
17261	2.73	4.19	10	N/A
17262	3.47	5.07	10	N/A
17263	3.84	5.59	10	N/A
17264	4.1	5.98	10	N/A
17266	4.77	6.78	10	N/A

Medicare References: 100-3,140.5; 100-4,12,30

17270-17276

17270 Destruction, malignant lesion (eg, laser surgery, electrosurgery, cryosurgery, chemosurgery, surgical curettement), scalp, neck, hands, feet, genitalia; lesion diameter 0.5 cm or less
17271 lesion diameter 0.6 to 1.0 cm
17272 lesion diameter 1.1 to 2.0 cm
17273 lesion diameter 2.1 to 3.0 cm
17274 lesion diameter 3.1 to 4.0 cm
17276 lesion diameter over 4.0 cm

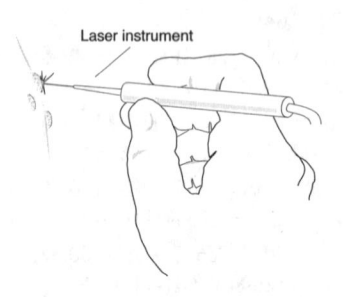

Malignant lesions of the hands are destroyed by any number of methods. Lasers may be used as well as electrocautery or cryotherapy. Once destroyed, a curette may be used to remove dead tissue

17270: 0.5 cm diameter lesion or less
17271: 0.6 cm to 1.0 cm diameter
17272: 1.1 to 2.0 cm diameter
17273: 2.1 to 3.0 cm diameter
17274: 3.1 to 4.0 cm diameter
17276: larger than 4.0 cm diameter

Code 17270-17276 regardless of method

Explanation
The physician destroys a malignant lesion of the scalp, neck, hands, feet, or genitalia. Destruction may be accomplished by using a laser or electrocautery to burn the lesion, cryotherapy to freeze the lesion, chemicals to destroy the lesion, or surgical curettement to remove the lesion. Report 17270 for a lesion diameter 0.5 cm or less; 17271 for 0.6 cm to 1 cm; 17272 for 1.1 cm to 2 cm; 17273 for 2.1 cm to 3 cm; 17274 for 3.1 cm to 4 cm; and 17276 if the lesion diameter is greater than 4 cm.

Coding Tips
Local anesthesia is included in these services. For excision of a malignant lesion, see 11620–11626.

ICD-9-CM Procedural
86.3 Other local excision or destruction of lesion or tissue of skin and subcutaneous tissue

Anesthesia
00300, 00400

ICD-9-CM Diagnostic
173.6 Other malignant neoplasm of skin of upper limb, including shoulder
209.33 Merkel cell carcinoma of the upper limb
209.36 Merkel cell carcinoma of other sites
209.75 Secondary Merkel cell carcinoma
232.6 Carcinoma in situ of skin of upper limb, including shoulder
232.8 Carcinoma in situ of other specified sites of skin
238.2 Neoplasm of uncertain behavior of skin

Terms To Know
carcinoma in situ. Malignancy that arises from the cells of the vessel, gland, or organ of origin that remains confined to that site or has not invaded neighboring tissue.

lesion. Area of damaged tissue that has lost continuity or function, due to disease or trauma. Lesions may be located on internal structures such as the brain, nerves, or kidneys, or visible on the skin.

malignant. Any condition tending to progress toward death, specifically an invasive tumor with a loss of cellular differentiation that has the ability to spread or metastasize to other areas in the body.

neoplasm. New abnormal growth, tumor.

subcutaneous tissue. Sheet or wide band of adipose (fat) and areolar connective tissue in two layers attached to the dermis.

CCI Version 16.3
0213T, 0216T, 0228T, 0230T, 11100, 11900-11901, 36000, 36400-36410, 36420-36430, 36440, 36600, 36640, 37202, 43752, 51701-51703, 62310-62319, 64400-64435, 64445-64450, 64479, 64483, 64490, 64493, 64505-64530, 69990, 93000-93010, 93040-93042, 93318, 94002, 94200, 94250, 94680-94690, 94770, 95812-95816, 95819, 95822, 95829, 95955, 96360, 96365, 96372, 96374-96376, 99148-99149, 99150, J0670, J2001

Also not with 17270: 11600-11606❖, 11620-11646❖

Also not with 17271: 11601-11606❖, 11621-11646❖

Also not with 17272: 11601-11606❖, 11621-11626❖, 11641-11646❖

Also not with 17273: 11602-11606❖, 11622-11626❖, 11641-11646❖

Also not with 17274: 11606❖, 11623-11626❖, 11642-11646❖

Also not with 17276: 11606❖, 11624-11626❖, 11643-11646❖

Note: These CCI edits are used for Medicare. Other payers may reimburse on codes listed above.

Medicare Edits

	Fac RVU	Non-Fac RVU	FUD	Assist
17270	2.96	4.36	10	N/A
17271	3.31	4.79	10	N/A
17272	3.82	5.46	10	N/A
17273	4.31	6.09	10	N/A
17274	5.26	7.18	10	N/A
17276	6.3	8.31	10	N/A

Medicare References: 100-3,140.5

20005

20005 Incision and drainage of soft tissue abscess, subfascial (ie, involves the soft tissue below the deep fascia)

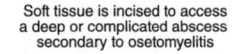

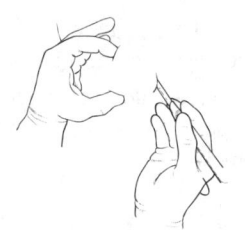

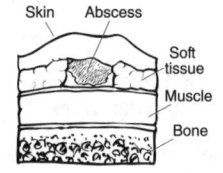

Explanation
The physician makes an incision through skin and fascia directly over an abscessed area involving the soft tissue below the deep fascia. The abscess cavity is explored, debrided, and drained. Depending on the appearance of the area, the physician may place a drain or packing after copious irrigation of the area.

Coding Tips
This code has been revised for 2011 in the official CPT description. For a sequestrectomy for osteomyelitis and drainage of a bone abscess, see the appropriate anatomical area. For cutaneous or subcutaneous incision and drainage procedures, see 10060–10061. Surgical trays, A4550, are not separately reimbursed by Medicare; however, other third-party payers may cover them. Check with the specific payer to determine coverage.

ICD-9-CM Procedural
83.09   Other incision of soft tissue

Anesthesia
20005   00300, 00400

ICD-9-CM Diagnostic
682.1   Cellulitis and abscess of neck — (Use additional code to identify organism, such as 041.1, etc.)
682.2   Cellulitis and abscess of trunk — (Use additional code to identify organism, such as 041.1, etc.)
682.3   Cellulitis and abscess of upper arm and forearm — (Use additional code to identify organism, such as 041.1, etc.)
682.4   Cellulitis and abscess of hand, except fingers and thumb — (Use additional code to identify organism, such as 041.1, etc.)
730.01   Acute osteomyelitis, shoulder region — (Use additional code to identify organism: 041.1. Use additional code to identify major osseous defect, if applicable: 731.3)
730.02   Acute osteomyelitis, upper arm — (Use additional code to identify organism: 041.1. Use additional code to identify major osseous defect, if applicable: 731.3)
730.03   Acute osteomyelitis, forearm — (Use additional code to identify organism: 041.1. Use additional code to identify major osseous defect, if applicable: 731.3)
730.04   Acute osteomyelitis, hand — (Use additional code to identify organism: 041.1. Use additional code to identify major osseous defect, if applicable: 731.3)
730.11   Chronic osteomyelitis, shoulder region — (Use additional code to identify organism: 041.1. Use additional code to identify major osseous defect, if applicable: 731.3)
730.12   Chronic osteomyelitis, upper arm — (Use additional code to identify organism: 041.1. Use additional code to identify major osseous defect, if applicable: 731.3)
730.13   Chronic osteomyelitis, forearm — (Use additional code to identify organism: 041.1. Use additional code to identify major osseous defect, if applicable: 731.3)
730.14   Chronic osteomyelitis, hand — (Use additional code to identify organism: 041.1. Use additional code to identify major osseous defect, if applicable: 731.3)
730.31   Periostitis, without mention of osteomyelitis, shoulder region — (Use additional code to identify organism: 041.1)
730.32   Periostitis, without mention of osteomyelitis, upper arm — (Use additional code to identify organism: 041.1)
730.33   Periostitis, without mention of osteomyelitis, forearm — (Use additional code to identify organism: 041.1)
730.34   Periostitis, without mention of osteomyelitis, hand — (Use additional code to identify organism: 041.1)
730.38   Periostitis, without mention of osteomyelitis, other specified sites — (Use additional code to identify organism: 041.1)
730.81   Other infections involving bone diseases classified elsewhere, shoulder region — (Use additional code to identify organism: 041.1. Code first underlying disease: 002.0, 015.0-015.9)
730.84   Other infections involving diseases classified elsewhere, hand bone — (Use additional code to identify organism: 041.1. Code first underlying disease: 002.0, 015.0-015.9)
996.66   Infection and inflammatory reaction due to internal joint prosthesis — (Use additional code to identify specified infections. Use additional code to identify infected prosthetic joint: V43.60-V43.69)

CCI Version 16.3
0213T, 0216T, 0228T, 0230T, 11040-11043, 20000, 20500, 36000, 36400-36410, 36420-36430, 36440, 36600, 36640, 37202, 43752, 51701-51703, 62310-62319, 64400-64435, 64445-64450, 64479, 64483, 64490, 64493, 64505-64530, 69990, 93000-93010, 93040-93042, 93318, 94002, 94200, 94250, 94680-94690, 94770, 95812-95816, 95819, 95822, 95829, 95955, 96360, 96365, 96372, 96374-96376, 97597-97598, 97602-97606, 99148-99149, 99150, J0670, J2001

Note: These CCI edits are used for Medicare. Other payers may reimburse on codes listed above.

Medicare Edits

	Fac RVU	Non-Fac RVU	FUD	Assist
20005	6.78	8.7	10	N/A

Medicare References: 100-2,15,260; 100-4,12,30; 100-4,12,90.3; 100-4,14,10

20102-20103

20102 Exploration of penetrating wound (separate procedure); abdomen/flank/back
20103 extremity

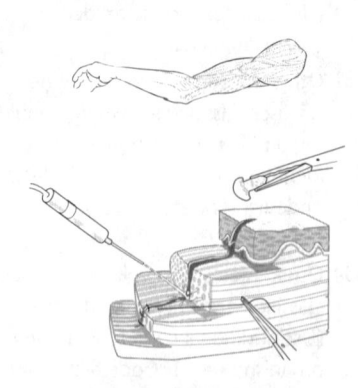

Fragments such as bullets or metal debris are removed from the extremity

A penetrating wound of an extremity is explored. The depth of the wound is assessed and the tissues debrided of fragments. Repairs and closures are made as needed

Explanation

The physician explores a penetrating wound in the operating room, such as a gunshot or stab wound, to help identify damaged structures. Nerve, organ, and blood vessel integrity is assessed. The wound may be enlarged to help assess the damage. Debridement, removal of foreign bodies, and ligation or coagulation of minor blood vessels in the subcutaneous tissues, fascia, and muscle are also included in this range of codes. Damaged tissues are debrided and repaired when possible. The wound is closed (if clean) or packed open if contaminated by the penetrating body. Report 20100 for exploration of a neck wound. Report 20101 for exploration of a chest wound. Report 20102 for exploration of an abdomen, flank, or back wound. Report 20103 for exploration of a wound to an extremity.

Coding Tips

These separate procedures by definition are usually a component of a more complex service and are not identified separately. When performed alone or with other unrelated procedures/services they may be reported. If performed alone, list the code; if performed with other procedures/services, list the code and append modifier 59. These codes report surgical exploration and enlargement of the wound, extension of dissection, debridement, removal of foreign bodies, and ligation of minor blood vessels. If repair of major blood vessels is required, the major blood vessel repair should be reported instead of these codes. Repair not requiring enlargement of the wound or extension of dissection should be reported with repair codes: see 12001-12007 for simple repair; 12031-12037 for intermediate repair; or 13120-13122 and 13131-13133 for complex repair.

ICD-9-CM Procedural

82.02 Myotomy of hand
83.02 Myotomy
83.09 Other incision of soft tissue
83.65 Other suture of muscle or fascia
84.99 Other operations on musculoskeletal system
86.05 Incision with removal of foreign body or device from skin and subcutaneous tissue
86.09 Other incision of skin and subcutaneous tissue
86.22 Excisional debridement of wound, infection, or burn
86.28 Nonexcisional debridement of wound, infection, or burn

Anesthesia

20102 00700
20103 00400

ICD-9-CM Diagnostic

880.00 Open wound of shoulder region, without mention of complication
880.01 Open wound of scapular region, without mention of complication
880.02 Open wound of axillary region, without mention of complication
880.03 Open wound of upper arm, without mention of complication
880.09 Open wound of multiple sites of shoulder and upper arm, without mention of complication
880.10 Open wound of shoulder region, complicated
880.11 Open wound of scapular region, complicated
880.12 Open wound of axillary region, complicated
880.13 Open wound of upper arm, complicated
880.19 Open wound of multiple sites of shoulder and upper arm, complicated
881.00 Open wound of forearm, without mention of complication
881.01 Open wound of elbow, without mention of complication
881.02 Open wound of wrist, without mention of complication
881.10 Open wound of forearm, complicated
881.11 Open wound of elbow, complicated
881.12 Open wound of wrist, complicated
882.0 Open wound of hand except finger(s) alone, without mention of complication
882.1 Open wound of hand except finger(s) alone, complicated
883.0 Open wound of finger(s), without mention of complication
883.1 Open wound of finger(s), complicated
884.0 Multiple and unspecified open wound of upper limb, without mention of complication

Terms To Know

exploration. Examination for diagnostic purposes.

ligation. Tying off a blood vessel or duct with a suture or a soft, thin wire.

penetrating wound. Wounds resulting from a traumatic injury piercing the skin to the inside of the body such as a gunshot or stab wound.

CCI Version 16.3

0213T, 0216T, 0228T, 0230T, 11000, 13160, 36000, 36400-36410, 36420-36430, 36440, 36600, 36640, 37202, 43752, 51701-51703, 62310-62319, 64400-64435, 64445-64450, 64479, 64483, 64490, 64493, 64505-64530, 69990, 93000-93010, 93040-93042, 93318, 94002, 94200, 94250, 94680-94690, 94770, 95812-95816, 95819, 95822, 95829, 95955, 96360, 96365, 96372, 96374-96376, 97597-97598, 97602-97606, 99148-99149, 99150, G0168, J0670, J2001

Also not with 20102: 11041-11044, 12001-12007, 12020-12037, 13100-13102, 13122, 13133

Also not with 20103: 11010-11011, 11040-11044, 12001-12002, 12005-12007, 12020-12047, 13102-13133, 24300, 25259, 26340, 29105, 29515, 64704

Note: These CCI edits are used for Medicare. Other payers may reimburse on codes listed above.

Medicare Edits

	Fac RVU	Non-Fac RVU	FUD	Assist
20102	7.36	13.75	10	N/A
20103	10.26	16.54	10	80

Medicare References: None

20200-20205

20200 Biopsy, muscle; superficial
20205 deep

A biopsy sample is taken from muscle tissue of the upper extremity, by incision or percutaneously. Report 20200 for superficial incisional biopsy. Report 20205 when the biopsy is from deep muscle tissue.

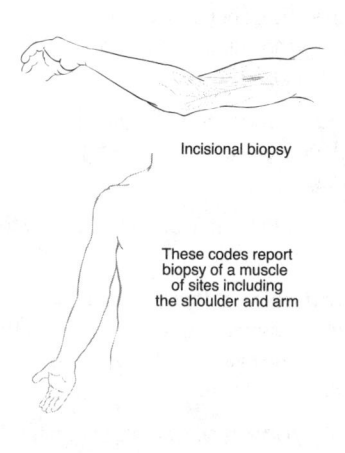

Incisional biopsy

These codes report biopsy of a muscle of sites including the shoulder and arm

Explanation

The physician secures a sample of tissue from a muscle for biopsy. The physician incises the overlying skin and bluntly dissects to the suspect muscle. The muscle tissue is obtained. Bleeding is controlled and the wound is sutured in layers. Report 20200 if the muscle site sampled is superficial and 20205 if the muscle site sampled is deep.

Coding Tips

Local anesthesia is included in these procedures. For excision of a deep muscle tumor, see the specific anatomic section. Surgical trays, A4550, are not separately reimbursed by Medicare; however, other third-party payers may cover them. Check with the specific payer to determine coverage.

ICD-9-CM Procedural

83.21 Open biopsy of soft tissue

Anesthesia

00300, 00400, 01610, 01710, 01810

ICD-9-CM Diagnostic

135	Sarcoidosis
171.0	Malignant neoplasm of connective and other soft tissue of head, face, and neck
171.2	Malignant neoplasm of connective and other soft tissue of upper limb, including shoulder
171.4	Malignant neoplasm of connective and other soft tissue of thorax
171.5	Malignant neoplasm of connective and other soft tissue of abdomen
171.7	Malignant neoplasm of connective and other soft tissue of trunk, unspecified site
171.8	Malignant neoplasm of other specified sites of connective and other soft tissue
198.89	Secondary malignant neoplasm of other specified sites
215.0	Other benign neoplasm of connective and other soft tissue of head, face, and neck
215.2	Other benign neoplasm of connective and other soft tissue of upper limb, including shoulder
215.4	Other benign neoplasm of connective and other soft tissue of thorax
215.5	Other benign neoplasm of connective and other soft tissue of abdomen
215.7	Other benign neoplasm of connective and other soft tissue of trunk, unspecified
215.8	Other benign neoplasm of connective and other soft tissue of other specified sites
229.8	Benign neoplasm of other specified sites
239.2	Neoplasms of unspecified nature of bone, soft tissue, and skin
277.30	Amyloidosis, unspecified — (Use additional code to identify any associated mental retardation)
277.31	Familial Mediterranean fever — (Use additional code to identify any associated mental retardation)
359.0	Congenital hereditary muscular dystrophy
359.1	Hereditary progressive muscular dystrophy
359.6	Symptomatic inflammatory myopathy in diseases classified elsewhere — (Code first underlying disease: 135, 140.0-208.9, 277.30-277.39, 446.0, 710.0, 710.1, 710.2, 714.0)
728.0	Infective myositis
728.19	Other muscular calcification and ossification
728.79	Other fibromatoses of muscle, ligament, and fascia
728.81	Interstitial myositis
728.88	Rhabdomyolysis
729.1	Unspecified myalgia and myositis

Terms To Know

biopsy. Tissue or fluid removed for diagnostic purposes through analysis of the cells in the biopsy material.

myositis. Inflammation of a muscle with voluntary movement.

polyarteritis nodosa. Systemic necrotizing vasculitis of small and medium arteries that results in the infarction and scarring within the affected organs.

superficial. On the skin surface or near the surface of any involved structure or field of interest.

CCI Version 16.3

0213T, 0216T, 0228T, 0230T, 10021-10022, 20103, 20206, 24300, 25259, 26340, 36000, 36400-36410, 36420-36430, 36440, 36600, 36640, 37202, 43752, 51701-51703, 62310-62319, 64400-64435, 64445-64450, 64479, 64483, 64490, 64493, 64505-64530, 69990, 93000-93010, 93040-93042, 93318, 94002, 94200, 94250, 94680-94690, 94770, 95812-95816, 95819, 95822, 95829, 95955, 96360, 96365, 96372, 96374-96376, 99148-99149, 99150, J0670, J2001

Also not with 20205: 12001-12007, 12020-12047, 13100-13101, 13120-13121, 13131-13132, 20200, 49000-49002, 95900

Note: These CCI edits are used for Medicare. Other payers may reimburse on codes listed above.

Medicare Edits

	Fac RVU	Non-Fac RVU	FUD	Assist
20200	2.76	5.75	0	N/A
20205	4.46	7.91	0	N/A

Medicare References: 100-2,15,260; 100-4,12,30; 100-4,12,90.3; 100-4,13,80.2; 100-4,14,10

20206

20206 Biopsy, muscle, percutaneous needle

Biopsy syringe

Detail of biopsy needle

Muscle tissue biopsy specimens are collected using a percutaneous needle approach

Explanation
The physician removes a sample of muscle tissue using a percutaneous needle. The physician applies a local anesthetic to the skin. The physician uses a bore needle to pierce the skin, fascia, and muscle, obtaining a sample of muscle tissue. The needle is withdrawn. No repair is usually necessary. Radiologic supervision, if necessary, is reported separately.

Coding Tips
Local anesthesia is included in this procedure. For radiological guidance for needle placement, see 76942, 77012, and 77021. For open biopsy of a muscle, see 20200–20205. Surgical trays, A4550, are not separately reimbursed by Medicare; however, other third-party payers may cover them. Check with the specific payer to determine coverage.

ICD-9-CM Procedural
83.21 Open biopsy of soft tissue

Anesthesia
20206 00300, 00400, 01610, 01710, 01810

ICD-9-CM Diagnostic
- 171.0 Malignant neoplasm of connective and other soft tissue of head, face, and neck
- 171.2 Malignant neoplasm of connective and other soft tissue of upper limb, including shoulder
- 171.4 Malignant neoplasm of connective and other soft tissue of thorax
- 171.5 Malignant neoplasm of connective and other soft tissue of abdomen
- 171.7 Malignant neoplasm of connective and other soft tissue of trunk, unspecified site
- 171.8 Malignant neoplasm of other specified sites of connective and other soft tissue
- 198.89 Secondary malignant neoplasm of other specified sites
- 215.0 Other benign neoplasm of connective and other soft tissue of head, face, and neck
- 215.2 Other benign neoplasm of connective and other soft tissue of upper limb, including shoulder
- 215.4 Other benign neoplasm of connective and other soft tissue of thorax
- 215.5 Other benign neoplasm of connective and other soft tissue of abdomen
- 215.7 Other benign neoplasm of connective and other soft tissue of trunk, unspecified
- 215.8 Other benign neoplasm of connective and other soft tissue of other specified sites
- 229.8 Benign neoplasm of other specified sites
- 238.1 Neoplasm of uncertain behavior of connective and other soft tissue
- 239.2 Neoplasms of unspecified nature of bone, soft tissue, and skin
- 277.30 Amyloidosis, unspecified — (Use additional code to identify any associated mental retardation)
- 277.31 Familial Mediterranean fever — (Use additional code to identify any associated mental retardation)
- 277.39 Other amyloidosis — (Use additional code to identify any associated mental retardation)
- 359.0 Congenital hereditary muscular dystrophy
- 359.1 Hereditary progressive muscular dystrophy
- 359.6 Symptomatic inflammatory myopathy in diseases classified elsewhere — (Code first underlying disease: 135, 140.0-208.9, 277.30-277.39, 446.0, 710.0, 710.1, 710.2, 714.0)
- 359.81 Critical illness myopathy
- 359.89 Other myopathies
- 728.0 Infective myositis
- 728.19 Other muscular calcification and ossification
- 728.79 Other fibromatoses of muscle, ligament, and fascia
- 728.81 Interstitial myositis
- 728.88 Rhabdomyolysis
- 729.1 Unspecified myalgia and myositis

Terms To Know
biopsy. Tissue or fluid removed for diagnostic purposes through analysis of the cells in the biopsy material.

fascia. Fibrous sheet or band of tissue that envelops organs, muscles, and groupings of muscles.

myositis. Inflammation of a muscle with voluntary movement.

polyarteritis nodosa. Systemic necrotizing vasculitis of small and medium arteries that results in the infarction and scarring within the affected organs.

sicca syndrome. Complex of symptoms of unknown source in middle-aged women in which the following triad exists: keratoconjunctivitis sicca, zerostomia, and connective tissue disease (usually rheumatoid arthritis but sometimes systemic lupus erythematosus).

systemic sclerosis. Systemic disease characterized by excess fibrotic collagen build-up, turning the skin thickened and hard. Fibrotic changes also occur in various organs and cause vascular abnormalities and affect more women than men.

CCI Version 16.3
0213T, 0216T, 0228T, 0230T, 10021-10022, 24300, 25259, 26340, 36000, 36400-36410, 36420-36430, 36440, 36600, 36640, 37202, 43752, 51701-51703, 62310-62319, 64400-64435, 64445-64450, 64479, 64483, 64490, 64493, 64505-64530, 69990, 76000-76001, 77002, 93000-93010, 93040-93042, 93318, 94002, 94200, 94250, 94680-94690, 94770, 95812-95816, 95819, 95822, 95829, 95900, 95955, 96360, 96365, 96372, 96374-96376, 99148-99149, 99150, J0670, J2001

Note: These CCI edits are used for Medicare. Other payers may reimburse on codes listed above.

Medicare Edits

	Fac RVU	Non-Fac RVU	FUD	Assist
20206	1.78	7.3	0	N/A

Medicare References: 100-2,15,260; 100-4,12,30; 100-4,12,90.3; 100-4,13,80.1; 100-4,14,10

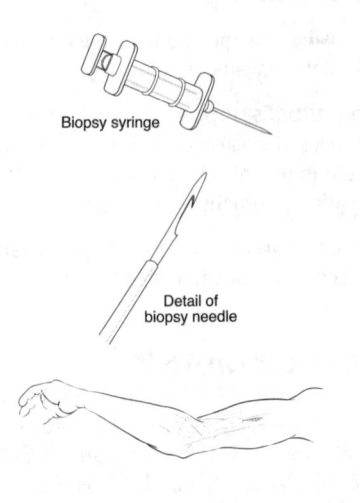

20220-20225

20220 Biopsy, bone, trocar, or needle; superficial (eg, ilium, sternum, spinous process, ribs)
20225 deep (eg, vertebral body, femur)

A trocar or needle is used to biopsy a bone of the upper extremity, or elsewhere. Report 20220 for a superficial biopsy. Report 20225 if the biopsy is deep.

Explanation

The physician usually performs a biopsy on bone to confirm a suspected growth, disease, or infection. The physician normally uses local anesthesia; however, general anesthesia may be used. The physician places a large needle into the spinous process or other superficial bone to obtain the sample in 20220. For sampling a deeper lying bone, such as a vertebra in 20225, an exploring needle is passed through a larger needle to the desired depth and a piece of tissue is removed for testing. Different approaches are taken for vertebral biopsies, based on differing levels of vertebrae. The top three cervical vertebrae are approached from a pharyngeal or anterior approach. The lower four cervical vertebrae are approached from a lateral direction. Thoracic and lumbar vertebra are approached from behind and to the right to avoid major arteries. Radiographs are sometimes used to confirm the placement of the needle.

Coding Tips

If multiple areas are biopsied, report 20220 or 20225 for each site taken and append modifier 51 to the second and subsequent codes. A needle biopsy is not reported separately if a therapeutic excision is performed on the same site during the same surgical session. For an excisional biopsy of bone, superficial (e.g., spinous process), see 20240. For biopsy, vertebral body, open thoracic, see 20250; lumbar or cervical, see 20251. For a bone marrow biopsy, see 38221.

For radiology supervision and interpretation, see 77002, 77012, and 77021. Surgical trays, A4550, are not separately reimbursed by Medicare; however, other third-party payers may cover them. Check with the specific payer to determine coverage.

ICD-9-CM Procedural

- 77.40 Biopsy of bone, unspecified site
- 77.41 Biopsy of scapula, clavicle, and thorax (ribs and sternum)
- 77.42 Biopsy of humerus
- 77.43 Biopsy of radius and ulna
- 77.44 Biopsy of carpals and metacarpals
- 77.49 Biopsy of other bone, except facial bones

Anesthesia

20220 00454, 00640, 01620, 01730, 01820
20225 00620, 00630

ICD-9-CM Diagnostic

- 170.2 Malignant neoplasm of vertebral column, excluding sacrum and coccyx
- 170.3 Malignant neoplasm of ribs, sternum, and clavicle
- 170.4 Malignant neoplasm of scapula and long bones of upper limb
- 170.5 Malignant neoplasm of short bones of upper limb
- 198.5 Secondary malignant neoplasm of bone and bone marrow
- 213.3 Benign neoplasm of ribs, sternum, and clavicle
- 213.4 Benign neoplasm of scapula and long bones of upper limb
- 213.5 Benign neoplasm of short bones of upper limb
- 730.11 Chronic osteomyelitis, shoulder region — (Use additional code to identify organism: 041.1. Use additional code to identify major osseous defect, if applicable: 731.3)
- 730.12 Chronic osteomyelitis, upper arm — (Use additional code to identify organism: 041.1. Use additional code to identify major osseous defect, if applicable: 731.3)
- 730.13 Chronic osteomyelitis, forearm — (Use additional code to identify organism: 041.1. Use additional code to identify major osseous defect, if applicable: 731.3)
- 730.14 Chronic osteomyelitis, hand — (Use additional code to identify organism: 041.1. Use additional code to identify major osseous defect, if applicable: 731.3)
- 730.21 Unspecified osteomyelitis, shoulder region — (Use additional code to identify organism: 041.1. Use additional code to identify major osseous defect, if applicable: 731.3)
- 730.22 Unspecified osteomyelitis, upper arm — (Use additional code to identify organism: 041.1. Use additional code to identify major osseous defect, if applicable: 731.3)
- 730.23 Unspecified osteomyelitis, forearm — (Use additional code to identify organism: 041.1. Use additional code to identify major osseous defect, if applicable: 731.3)
- 730.24 Unspecified osteomyelitis, hand — (Use additional code to identify organism: 041.1. Use additional code to identify major osseous defect, if applicable: 731.3)
- 730.81 Other infections involving bone diseases classified elsewhere, shoulder region — (Use additional code to identify organism: 041.1. Code first underlying disease: 002.0, 015.0-015.9)

CCI Version 16.3

0213T, 0216T, 0228T, 0230T, 24300, 25259, 26340, 36000, 36400-36410, 36420-36430, 36440, 36600, 36640, 37202, 43752, 51701-51703, 62310-62319, 64400-64435, 64445-64450, 64479, 64483, 64490, 64493, 64505-64530, 69990, 93000-93010, 93040-93042, 93318, 94002, 94200, 94250, 94680-94690, 94770, 95812-95816, 95819, 95822, 95829, 95955, 96360, 96365, 96372, 96374-96376, 99148-99149, 99150, G0364, J0670, J2001

Also not with 20220: 21750, 38220, 76000-76001

Also not with 20225: 20220, 38220-38221, 49010

Note: These CCI edits are used for Medicare. Other payers may reimburse on codes listed above.

Medicare Edits

	Fac RVU	Non-Fac RVU	FUD	Assist
20220	2.2	4.8	0	N/A
20225	3.35	17.99	0	N/A

Medicare References: 100-2,15,260; 100-4,12,30; 100-4,12,90.3; 100-4,13,80.1; 100-4,13,80.2; 100-4,14,10

20240-20245

20240 Biopsy, bone, open; superficial (eg, ilium, sternum, spinous process, ribs, trochanter of femur)
20245 deep (eg, humerus, ischium, femur)

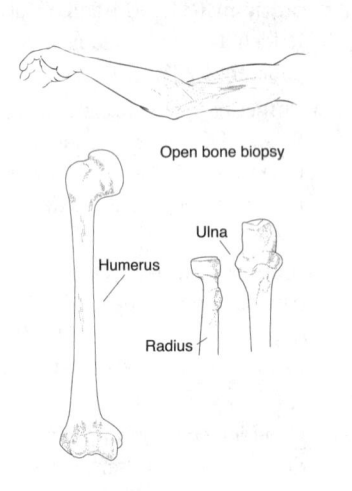

Open bone biopsy

Humerus
Ulna
Radius

A bone biopsy of an upper extremity, or elsewhere, is collected by open approach. Report 20240 for superficial biopsy. And report 20245 for deep biopsy (e.g., humerus)

Explanation

The physician performs an open biopsy on bone to confirm a suspected growth, disease, or infection. With the patient under general anesthesia, and placed in the appropriate position, the physician makes an incision overlying the biopsy site and carries it down through the tissue to the level of the bone being biopsied. A piece of bone tissue is removed and sent for examination. The wound is sutured closed and the patient is moved to the recovery area. Report 20240 if the biopsy is of a superficial bone such as the ribs, ilium, sternum, or spinous process; report 20245 if the bone biopsied lies deep, such as the femur or ischium.

Coding Tips

If multiple areas are biopsied, report 20240 or 20245 for each site taken and append modifier 51 to the second and subsequent codes. An excisional biopsy is not reported separately if a therapeutic excision is performed during the same surgical session. Surgical trays, A4550, are not separately reimbursed by Medicare; however, other third-party payers may cover them. Check with the specific payer to determine coverage.

ICD-9-CM Procedural

77.40 Biopsy of bone, unspecified site
77.41 Biopsy of scapula, clavicle, and thorax (ribs and sternum)
77.42 Biopsy of humerus
77.43 Biopsy of radius and ulna
77.44 Biopsy of carpals and metacarpals
77.49 Biopsy of other bone, except facial bones

Anesthesia
20240 00470, 00620, 00630
20245 01740, 01758

ICD-9-CM Diagnostic

170.2 Malignant neoplasm of vertebral column, excluding sacrum and coccyx
170.3 Malignant neoplasm of ribs, sternum, and clavicle
170.4 Malignant neoplasm of scapula and long bones of upper limb
170.5 Malignant neoplasm of short bones of upper limb
198.5 Secondary malignant neoplasm of bone and bone marrow
213.3 Benign neoplasm of ribs, sternum, and clavicle
213.4 Benign neoplasm of scapula and long bones of upper limb
213.5 Benign neoplasm of short bones of upper limb
730.12 Chronic osteomyelitis, upper arm — (Use additional code to identify organism: 041.1. Use additional code to identify major osseous defect, if applicable: 731.3)
730.13 Chronic osteomyelitis, forearm — (Use additional code to identify organism: 041.1. Use additional code to identify major osseous defect, if applicable: 731.3)
730.14 Chronic osteomyelitis, hand — (Use additional code to identify organism: 041.1. Use additional code to identify major osseous defect, if applicable: 731.3)
730.21 Unspecified osteomyelitis, shoulder region — (Use additional code to identify organism: 041.1. Use additional code to identify major osseous defect, if applicable: 731.3)
730.22 Unspecified osteomyelitis, upper arm — (Use additional code to identify organism: 041.1. Use additional code to identify major osseous defect, if applicable: 731.3)
730.23 Unspecified osteomyelitis, forearm — (Use additional code to identify organism: 041.1. Use additional code to identify major osseous defect, if applicable: 731.3)
730.24 Unspecified osteomyelitis, hand — (Use additional code to identify organism: 041.1. Use additional code to identify major osseous defect, if applicable: 731.3)
730.81 Other infections involving bone diseases classified elsewhere, shoulder region — (Use additional code to identify organism: 041.1. Code first underlying disease: 002.0, 015.0-015.9)
730.82 Other infections involving bone diseases classified elsewhere, upper arm — (Use additional code to identify organism: 041.1. Code first underlying disease: 002.0, 015.0-015.9)
730.83 Other infections involving bone in diseases classified elsewhere, forearm — (Use additional code to identify organism: 041.1. Code first underlying disease: 002.0, 015.0-015.9)
730.84 Other infections involving diseases classified elsewhere, hand bone — (Use additional code to identify organism: 041.1. Code first underlying disease: 002.0, 015.0-015.9)
731.0 Osteitis deformans without mention of bone tumor

CCI Version 16.3

0213T, 0216T, 0228T, 0230T, 20200-20206, 20220-20225, 24300, 25259, 26340, 36000, 36400-36410, 36420-36430, 36440, 36600, 36640, 37202, 38220-38221, 43752, 51701-51703, 62310-62319, 64400-64435, 64445-64450, 64479, 64483, 64490, 64493, 64505-64530, 69990, 93000-93010, 93040-93042, 93318, 94002, 94200, 94250, 94680-94690, 94770, 95812-95816, 95819, 95822, 95829, 95955, 96360, 96365, 96372, 96374-96376, 99148-99149, 99150, G0364

Also not with 20240: 21750, 32100, 64718
Also not with 20245: 20240, 26262, 28175, 29105

Note: These CCI edits are used for Medicare. Other payers may reimburse on codes listed above.

Medicare Edits

	Fac RVU	Non-Fac RVU	FUD	Assist
20240	6.57	6.57	10	N/A
20245	18.46	18.46	10	N/A

Medicare References: 100-2,15,260; 100-4,3,20.2.1; 100-4,12,30; 100-4,12,90.3; 100-4,14,10

20250-20251

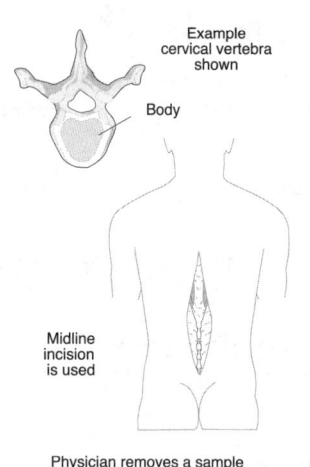

20250 Biopsy, vertebral body, open; thoracic
20251 lumbar or cervical

Explanation

These procedures are used to confirm a suspected growth, disease, or infection. The patient is placed in a prone position. A midline incision is made overlying the vertebrae to be biopsied. The incision is carried down and the fascia is incised. Paravertebral muscles are retracted and the vertebral area to be biopsied is identified. A piece of tissue is then excised or a needle is used to extract a sample of tissue for evaluation. The paravertebral muscles are replaced in their anatomical position and the incision is closed in layers. Report 20250 for a thoracic biopsy; 20251 for a lumbar or cervical biopsy.

Coding Tips

If multiple areas are biopsied, report 20250 or 20251 for each site taken and append modifier 51 to the second and subsequent codes. An excisional biopsy is not reported separately if a therapeutic excision is performed during the same surgical session. For an excisional biopsy, superficial (e.g., spinous process), see 20240. For a needle biopsy of bone, superficial (e.g., spinous process), see 20220; deep (e.g., vertebral body), see 20225. For partial excision of an intrinsic bony lesion, posterior vertebral component (spinous process, lamina, facet), see 22100–22103; vertebral body, see 22110–22116.

ICD-9-CM Procedural

77.49 Biopsy of other bone, except facial bones

Anesthesia

20250 00620
20251 00600, 00630

ICD-9-CM Diagnostic

170.2 Malignant neoplasm of vertebral column, excluding sacrum and coccyx
198.5 Secondary malignant neoplasm of bone and bone marrow
198.89 Secondary malignant neoplasm of other specified sites
209.73 Secondary neuroendocrine tumor of bone
213.2 Benign neoplasm of vertebral column, excluding sacrum and coccyx
237.70 Neurofibromatosis, unspecified
237.71 Neurofibromatosis, Type 1 (von Recklinghausen's disease)
237.72 Neurofibromatosis, Type 2 (acoustic neurofibromatosis)
237.73 Schwannomatosis
237.79 Other neurofibromatosis
238.0 Neoplasm of uncertain behavior of bone and articular cartilage
239.2 Neoplasms of unspecified nature of bone, soft tissue, and skin
277.5 Mucopolysaccharidosis — (Use additional code to identify any associated mental retardation)
356.1 Peroneal muscular atrophy
720.81 Inflammatory spondylopathies in diseases classified elsewhere — (Code first underlying disease: 015.0)
720.89 Other inflammatory spondylopathies
723.4 Brachial neuritis or radiculitis nos.
724.4 Thoracic or lumbosacral neuritis or radiculitis, unspecified
730.18 Chronic osteomyelitis, other specified sites — (Use additional code to identify organism: 041.1. Use additional code to identify major osseous defect, if applicable: 731.3)
730.28 Unspecified osteomyelitis, other specified sites — (Use additional code to identify organism: 041.1. Use additional code to identify major osseous defect, if applicable: 731.3)
730.80 Other infections involving bone in diseases classified elsewhere, site unspecified — (Use additional code to identify organism: 041.1. Code first underlying disease: 002.0, 015.0-015.9)
730.88 Other infections involving bone diseases classified elsewhere, other specified sites — (Use additional code to identify organism: 041.1. Code first underlying disease: 002.0, 015.0-015.9)
731.0 Osteitis deformans without mention of bone tumor
733.00 Unspecified osteoporosis — (Use additional code to identify major osseous defect, if applicable: 731.3) (Use additional code to identify personal history of pathologic (healed) fracture: V13.51)
733.01 Senile osteoporosis — (Use additional code to identify major osseous defect, if applicable: 731.3) (Use additional code to identify personal history of pathologic (healed) fracture: V13.51)
733.02 Idiopathic osteoporosis — (Use additional code to identify major osseous defect, if applicable: 731.3) (Use additional code to identify personal history of pathologic (healed) fracture: V13.51)
733.03 Disuse osteoporosis — (Use additional code to identify major osseous defect, if applicable: 731.3) (Use additional code to identify personal history of pathologic (healed) fracture: V13.51)

CCI Version 16.3

0213T, 0216T, 0228T, 0230T, 20220-20225, 36000, 36400-36410, 36420-36430, 36440, 36600, 36640, 37202, 38220-38221, 43752, 51701-51703, 62310-62319, 64400-64435, 64445-64450, 64479, 64483, 64490, 64493, 64505-64530, 69990, 93000-93010, 93040-93042, 93318, 94002, 94200, 94250, 94680-94690, 94770, 95812-95816, 95819, 95822, 95829, 95955, 96360, 96365, 96372, 96374-96376, 99148-99149, 99150, G0364
Also not with 20250: 32100, 32601, 95900
Also not with 20251: 37615, 37617, 49010
Note: These CCI edits are used for Medicare. Other payers may reimburse on codes listed above.

Medicare Edits

	Fac RVU	Non-Fac RVU	FUD	Assist
20250	11.1	11.1	10	N/A
20251	12.14	12.14	10	80

Medicare References: 100-2,15,260; 100-4,3,20.2.1; 100-4,12,30; 100-4,12,90.3; 100-4,14,10

20520-20525

20520 Removal of foreign body in muscle or tendon sheath; simple
20525 deep or complicated

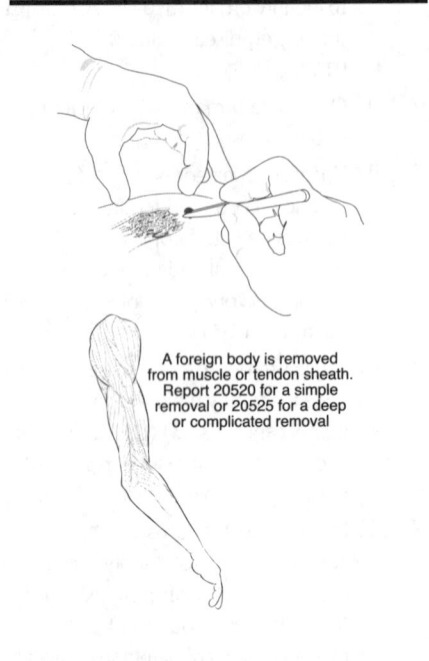

A foreign body is removed from muscle or tendon sheath. Report 20520 for a simple removal or 20525 for a deep or complicated removal

Explanation

The physician removes a foreign body in a muscle or tendon sheath. The physician incises the skin and dissects to the muscle or sheath. The foreign body is isolated by palpation or radiographic imagery (separately reported) and removed. The incision may be closed if clean or packed if contaminated by the object. Report 20520 if the removal is simple; report 20525 if the foreign object lies deep or requires a complicated procedure to remove it.

Coding Tips

For incision and removal of a foreign body from subcutaneous tissues, see 10120 and 10121. Surgical trays, A4550, are not separately reimbursed by Medicare; however, other third-party payers may cover them. Check with the specific payer to determine coverage.

ICD-9-CM Procedural

- 82.01 Exploration of tendon sheath of hand
- 82.02 Myotomy of hand
- 83.01 Exploration of tendon sheath
- 83.02 Myotomy
- 98.25 Removal of other foreign body without incision from trunk except scrotum, penis, or vulva
- 98.26 Removal of foreign body from hand without incision
- 98.27 Removal of foreign body without incision from upper limb, except hand

Anesthesia

00300, 00700, 00730, 01610, 01710, 01810

ICD-9-CM Diagnostic

- 709.4 Foreign body granuloma of skin and subcutaneous tissue — (Use additional code to identify foreign body (V90.01-V90.9))
- 728.82 Foreign body granuloma of muscle — (Use additional code to identify foreign body (V90.01-V90.9))
- 729.6 Residual foreign body in soft tissue — (Use additional code to identify foreign body (V90.01-V90.9))
- 875.1 Open wound of chest (wall), complicated
- 876.1 Open wound of back, complicated
- 879.3 Open wound of abdominal wall, anterior, complicated
- 879.5 Open wound of abdominal wall, lateral, complicated
- 879.9 Open wound(s) (multiple) of unspecified site(s), complicated
- 880.10 Open wound of shoulder region, complicated
- 880.11 Open wound of scapular region, complicated
- 880.12 Open wound of axillary region, complicated
- 880.13 Open wound of upper arm, complicated
- 880.19 Open wound of multiple sites of shoulder and upper arm, complicated
- 880.20 Open wound of shoulder region, with tendon involvement
- 880.21 Open wound of scapular region, with tendon involvement
- 880.22 Open wound of axillary region, with tendon involvement
- 880.23 Open wound of upper arm, with tendon involvement
- 880.29 Open wound of multiple sites of shoulder and upper arm, with tendon involvement
- 881.10 Open wound of forearm, complicated
- 881.11 Open wound of elbow, complicated
- 881.12 Open wound of wrist, complicated
- 881.20 Open wound of forearm, with tendon involvement
- 881.21 Open wound of elbow, with tendon involvement
- 881.22 Open wound of wrist, with tendon involvement
- 882.1 Open wound of hand except finger(s) alone, complicated
- 882.2 Open wound of hand except finger(s) alone, with tendon involvement
- 883.1 Open wound of finger(s), complicated
- 883.2 Open wound of finger(s), with tendon involvement

Terms To Know

dissect. Cut apart or separate tissue for surgical purposes or for visual or microscopic study.

incision. Act of cutting into tissue or an organ.

palpate. Examination by feeling with the hand.

CCI Version 16.3

0213T, 0216T, 0228T, 0230T, 11040-11043, 20103, 20200-20205, 20526-20553, 24300, 25259, 25295, 26340, 27680-27681, 36000, 36400-36410, 36420-36430, 36440, 36600, 36640, 37202, 43752, 51701-51703, 62310-62319, 64400-64435, 64445-64450, 64479, 64483, 64490, 64493, 64505-64530, 69990, 93000-93010, 93040-93042, 93318, 94002, 94200, 94250, 94680-94690, 94770, 95812-95816, 95819, 95822, 95829, 95955, 96360, 96365, 96372, 96374-96376, 99148-99149, 99150, J0670, J2001

Also not with 20520: 12001, G0168

Also not with 20525: 12001-12007, 12011-12057, 13100-13101, 13120-13121, 13131-13132, 13150-13152, 20000-20005, 20520, 21501, 23030, 25028, 26440-26449, 26990, 27301, 27603, 28220-28226, 29125, 49000-49002, 77002, 87102

Note: These CCI edits are used for Medicare. Other payers may reimburse on codes listed above.

Medicare Edits

	Fac RVU	Non-Fac RVU	FUD	Assist
20520	4.19	5.65	10	N/A
20525	7.25	13.68	10	N/A

Medicare References: 100-2,15,260; 100-4,12,30; 100-4,12,90.3; 100-4,14,10

20526

20526 Injection, therapeutic (eg, local anesthetic, corticosteroid), carpal tunnel

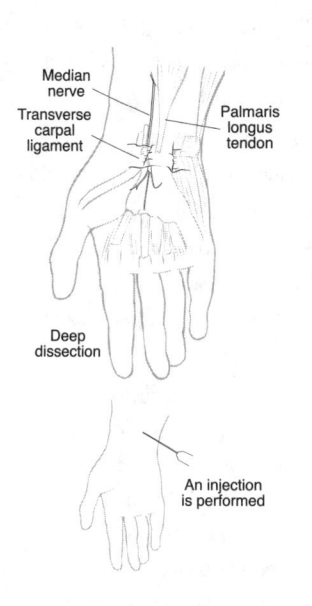

Explanation

A physician administers a single therapeutic injection of corticosteroid or anesthetic, 4 cm proximal to the wrist crease between the tendons of the radial flexor and the long palmar muscles on the lateral side of the forearm. This procedure is performed for therapeutic relief of the persistent symptoms of carpal tunnel syndrome.

Coding Tips

This is a unilateral procedure. If performed bilaterally, some payers require that the service be reported twice with modifier 50 appended to the second code, while others require identification of the service only once with modifier 50 appended. Check with individual payers. Modifier 50 identifies a procedure performed identically on the opposite side of the body (mirror image). Local anesthesia is included in this service. For injection into a tendon sheath or ligament, see 20550. For injection of a ganglion cyst, see 20612. Supplies used when providing this procedure may be reported with J0702, J1020, J1030, J1040, J1094, J1100, J1700, J1710, J1720, J2920, J2930, J3301–J3303, or S0020. Check with the specific payer to determine coverage.

ICD-9-CM Procedural

99.23 Injection of steroid
99.29 Injection or infusion of other therapeutic or prophylactic substance
99.77 Application or administration of adhesion barrier substance

Anesthesia

20526 N/A

ICD-9-CM Diagnostic

354.0 Carpal tunnel syndrome

Terms To Know

carpal tunnel. Anatomical landmark referring to the space in the wrist on the palmar side that houses the median nerve and all nine of the flexor tendons serving the fingers and thumb. The space is created by the bones of the wrist on either side and a thick ligament called the transverse carpal ligament.

carpal tunnel syndrome. Swelling and inflammation in the tendons or bursa surrounding the median nerve caused by repetitive activity. The resulting compression on the nerve causes pain, numbness, and tingling especially to the palm, index, middle finger, and thumb.

flexor. Muscle/tendon that bends or flexes a limb or part as opposed to extending it.

lateral. To/on the side.

muscle tissue. Network of specialized cells for performing contraction to produce voluntary or involuntary movement of body parts, and skeletal, cardiac, or visceral muscles.

proximal. Located closest to a specified reference point, usually the midline.

tendon. Fibrous tissue that connects muscle to bone, consisting primarily of collagen and containing little vasculature.

CCI Version 16.3

0213T, 0216T, 0228T, 0230T, 10160, 11900-11901, 20500, 29075, 29105-29125, 29260, 29590, 36000, 36400-36410, 36420-36430, 36440, 36600, 36640, 37202, 43752, 51701-51703, 64400-64435, 64445-64449, 64479, 64483, 64490, 64493, 64505-64530, 69990, 76000-76001, 93000-93010, 93040-93042, 93318, 94002, 94200, 94250, 94680-94690, 94770, 95812-95816, 95819, 95822, 95829, 95955, 96360, 96365, 96372, 96374-96376, 99148-99149, 99150, J0670, J2001

Note: These CCI edits are used for Medicare. Other payers may reimburse on codes listed above.

Medicare Edits

	Fac RVU	Non-Fac RVU	FUD	Assist
20526	1.67	2.18	0	N/A

Medicare References: 100-4,12,30

20550

20550 Injection(s); single tendon sheath, or ligament, aponeurosis (eg, plantar "fascia")

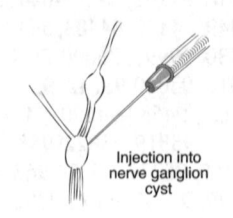

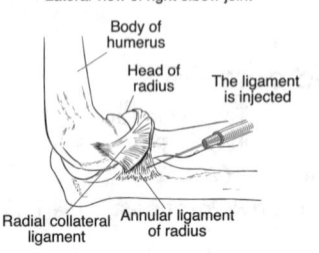

Explanation

The physician injects a therapeutic agent into a single tendon sheath, or ligament, aponeurosis such as the plantar fascia. The physician identifies the injection site by palpation or radiographs (reported separately) and marks the injection site. The needle is inserted and the medicine is injected. After withdrawing the needle, the patient is monitored for reactions to the therapeutic agent.

Coding Tips

When multiple, separate tendon sheaths are injected in the same encounter, each injection is reported separately. Report 20550 and append modifier 59 for the second and subsequent sites. For injection or aspiration of a ganglion cyst, see 20612. For injection of trigger points, see 20552 and 20553. Supplies used when providing this procedure may be reported with J0702, J1020–J1040, J1094, J1100, J1700–J1720, J2920, J2930, and S0020. Check with the specific payer to determine coverage.

ICD-9-CM Procedural

- 81.92 Injection of therapeutic substance into joint or ligament
- 83.97 Injection of therapeutic substance into tendon

Anesthesia

20550 N/A

ICD-9-CM Diagnostic

- 353.0 Brachial plexus lesions
- 353.1 Lumbosacral plexus lesions
- 353.2 Cervical root lesions, not elsewhere classified
- 353.3 Thoracic root lesions, not elsewhere classified
- 353.4 Lumbosacral root lesions, not elsewhere classified
- 353.8 Other nerve root and plexus disorders
- 354.1 Other lesion of median nerve
- 354.2 Lesion of ulnar nerve
- 354.3 Lesion of radial nerve
- 354.5 Mononeuritis multiplex
- 354.8 Other mononeuritis of upper limb
- 357.1 Polyneuropathy in collagen vascular disease — (Code first underlying disease: 446.0, 710.0, 714.0)
- 359.6 Symptomatic inflammatory myopathy in diseases classified elsewhere — (Code first underlying disease: 135, 140.0-208.9, 277.30-277.39, 446.0, 710.0, 710.1, 710.2, 714.0)
- 714.0 Rheumatoid arthritis — (Use additional code to identify manifestation: 357.1, 359.6)
- 715.00 Generalized osteoarthrosis, unspecified site
- 715.04 Generalized osteoarthrosis, involving hand
- 715.09 Generalized osteoarthrosis, involving multiple sites
- 716.50 Unspecified polyarthropathy or polyarthritis, site unspecified
- 716.51 Unspecified polyarthropathy or polyarthritis, shoulder region
- 716.52 Unspecified polyarthropathy or polyarthritis, upper arm
- 716.53 Unspecified polyarthropathy or polyarthritis, forearm
- 716.54 Unspecified polyarthropathy or polyarthritis, hand
- 716.58 Unspecified polyarthropathy or polyarthritis, other specified sites
- 716.59 Unspecified polyarthropathy or polyarthritis, multiple sites
- 716.60 Unspecified monoarthritis, site unspecified
- 716.61 Unspecified monoarthritis, shoulder region
- 716.62 Unspecified monoarthritis, upper arm
- 716.63 Unspecified monoarthritis, forearm
- 716.64 Unspecified monoarthritis, hand
- 716.68 Unspecified monoarthritis, other specified sites
- 716.90 Unspecified arthropathy, site unspecified
- 716.91 Unspecified arthropathy, shoulder region
- 716.92 Unspecified arthropathy, upper arm
- 716.93 Unspecified arthropathy, forearm
- 716.94 Unspecified arthropathy, hand
- 716.99 Unspecified arthropathy, multiple sites
- 719.40 Pain in joint, site unspecified
- 719.41 Pain in joint, shoulder region
- 719.42 Pain in joint, upper arm
- 719.43 Pain in joint, forearm
- 719.44 Pain in joint, hand
- 719.48 Pain in joint, other specified sites
- 719.49 Pain in joint, multiple sites
- 720.0 Ankylosing spondylitis
- 726.10 Unspecified disorders of bursae and tendons in shoulder region
- 726.32 Lateral epicondylitis of elbow
- 727.00 Unspecified synovitis and tenosynovitis
- 727.03 Trigger finger (acquired)
- 727.04 Radial styloid tenosynovitis
- 727.05 Other tenosynovitis of hand and wrist
- 727.09 Other synovitis and tenosynovitis
- 727.2 Specific bursitides often of occupational origin
- 727.3 Other bursitis disorders
- 729.4 Unspecified fasciitis
- 729.5 Pain in soft tissues of limb

CCI Version 16.3

10160, 11010❖, 11900-11901, 12032, 12042, 20500, 20526, 20551-20553❖, 29075, 29105-29125, 29130, 29260, 29405-29425, 29450, 29515, 29530-29590, 36000, 36400-36410, 36420-36430, 36440, 36600, 36640, 37202, 43752, 51701-51703, 62310-62319, 64408-64410, 64435, 64455, 64505-64550, 64714, 69990, 72240, 72265, 72295, 76000-76001, 87076-87077, 87102, 93000-93010, 93040-93042, 93318, 94002, 94200, 94250, 94680-94690, 94770, 95812-95816, 95819, 95822, 95829, 95900, 95955, 96360, 96365, 96372, 96374-96376, 99148-99149, 99150, J0670, J2001

Note: These CCI edits are used for Medicare. Other payers may reimburse on codes listed above.

Medicare Edits

	Fac RVU	Non-Fac RVU	FUD	Assist
20550	1.2	1.66	0	N/A

Medicare References: 100-3,150.7; 100-4,12,30; 100-4,13,80.1; 100-4,13,80.2

20551

20551 Injection(s); single tendon origin/insertion

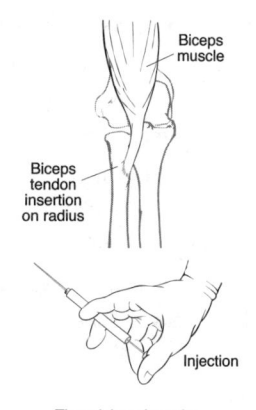

The origin or insertion of a tendon is injected

Insertion is the attachment of a tendon to the bone that it moves. The origin is the attachment of a tendon to the bone that anchors the movement

Explanation

The physician injects a therapeutic agent into a tendon origin/insertion. The physician identifies the injection site by palpation or radiographs (reported separately), marks the injection site, and inserts the needle. After withdrawing the needle, the patient is monitored for reactions to the therapeutic agent.

Coding Tips

When multiple, separate tendon origins/insertions are injected in the same encounter, each injection is reported separately. Report 20551 and append modifier 59 for the second and subsequent sites. Local anesthesia is included in this service. If imaging guidance is performed, see 76942, 77002, and 77021. Supplies used when providing this procedure may be reported with J0702, J1020–J1040, J1094, J1100, J1700–J1720, J2920, J2930, and S0020. Check with the specific payer to determine coverage.

ICD-9-CM Procedural

82.95	Injection of therapeutic substance into tendon of hand
83.97	Injection of therapeutic substance into tendon

Anesthesia

20551 N/A

ICD-9-CM Diagnostic

353.0	Brachial plexus lesions
353.1	Lumbosacral plexus lesions
353.2	Cervical root lesions, not elsewhere classified
353.3	Thoracic root lesions, not elsewhere classified
353.4	Lumbosacral root lesions, not elsewhere classified
353.8	Other nerve root and plexus disorders
354.1	Other lesion of median nerve
354.2	Lesion of ulnar nerve
354.3	Lesion of radial nerve
354.5	Mononeuritis multiplex
354.8	Other mononeuritis of upper limb
355.9	Mononeuritis of unspecified site
357.1	Polyneuropathy in collagen vascular disease — (Code first underlying disease: 446.0, 710.0, 714.0)
359.6	Symptomatic inflammatory myopathy in diseases classified elsewhere — (Code first underlying disease: 135, 140.0-208.9, 277.30-277.39, 446.0, 710.0, 710.1, 710.2, 714.0)
714.0	Rheumatoid arthritis — (Use additional code to identify manifestation: 357.1, 359.6)
715.00	Generalized osteoarthrosis, unspecified site
715.04	Generalized osteoarthrosis, involving hand
715.09	Generalized osteoarthrosis, involving multiple sites
715.18	Primary localized osteoarthrosis, other specified sites
715.38	Localized osteoarthrosis not specified whether primary or secondary, other specified sites
716.51	Unspecified polyarthropathy or polyarthritis, shoulder region
716.52	Unspecified polyarthropathy or polyarthritis, upper arm
716.53	Unspecified polyarthropathy or polyarthritis, forearm
716.54	Unspecified polyarthropathy or polyarthritis, hand
716.58	Unspecified polyarthropathy or polyarthritis, other specified sites
716.59	Unspecified polyarthropathy or polyarthritis, multiple sites
716.61	Unspecified monoarthritis, shoulder region
716.62	Unspecified monoarthritis, upper arm
716.63	Unspecified monoarthritis, forearm
716.64	Unspecified monoarthritis, hand
716.68	Unspecified monoarthritis, other specified sites
716.91	Unspecified arthropathy, shoulder region
716.92	Unspecified arthropathy, upper arm
716.93	Unspecified arthropathy, forearm
716.94	Unspecified arthropathy, hand
716.99	Unspecified arthropathy, multiple sites
719.41	Pain in joint, shoulder region
719.42	Pain in joint, upper arm
719.43	Pain in joint, forearm
719.44	Pain in joint, hand
719.48	Pain in joint, other specified sites
719.49	Pain in joint, multiple sites
720.0	Ankylosing spondylitis
726.10	Unspecified disorders of bursae and tendons in shoulder region
726.32	Lateral epicondylitis of elbow
727.00	Unspecified synovitis and tenosynovitis
727.02	Giant cell tumor of tendon sheath
727.03	Trigger finger (acquired)
727.04	Radial styloid tenosynovitis
727.05	Other tenosynovitis of hand and wrist
727.09	Other synovitis and tenosynovitis
727.2	Specific bursitides often of occupational origin
727.3	Other bursitis disorders
729.4	Unspecified fasciitis
729.5	Pain in soft tissues of limb

CCI Version 16.3

10160, 11900-11901, 20500, 20526, 20552-20553❖, 29075, 29105-29125, 29130, 29260, 29405-29425, 29450, 29515, 29530-29590, 36000, 36400-36410, 36420-36430, 36440, 36600, 36640, 37202, 43752, 51701-51703, 62310-62319, 64408-64410, 64435, 64455, 64505-64530, 69990, 76000-76001, 93000-93010, 93040-93042, 93318, 94002, 94200, 94250, 94680-94690, 94770, 95812-95816, 95819, 95822, 95829, 95955, 96360, 96365, 96372, 96374-96376, 99148-99149, 99150, J0670, J2001

Note: These CCI edits are used for Medicare. Other payers may reimburse on codes listed above.

Medicare Edits

	Fac RVU	Non-Fac RVU	FUD	Assist
20551	1.24	1.68	0	N/A

Medicare References: 100-3,150.7

20552-20553

20552 Injection(s); single or multiple trigger point(s), 1 or 2 muscle(s)
20553 single or multiple trigger point(s), 3 or more muscle(s)

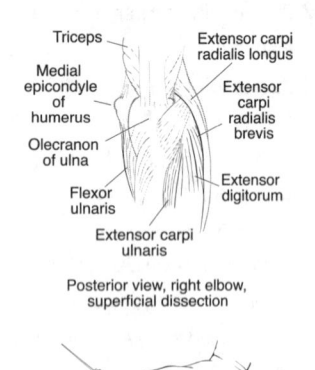

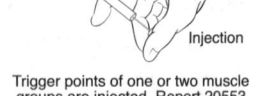

Trigger points of one or two muscle groups are injected. Report 20553 when a third or more groups are treated

Explanation

The physician injects a therapeutic agent into a single or multiple trigger points of one or two muscles in 20552 and into a single or multiple trigger points for three or more muscles in 20553. Trigger points are focal, discrete spots of hypersensitive irritability identified within bands of muscle. These points cause local or referred pain. Trigger points may be formed by acute or repetitive trauma to the muscle tissue, which puts too much stress on the fibers. The physician identifies the trigger point injection site by palpation or radiographic imaging and marks the injection site. The needle is inserted and the medicine is injected into the trigger point. The injection may be done under separately reportable image guidance. After withdrawing the needle, the patient is monitored for reactions to the therapeutic agent. The injection procedure is repeated at the other trigger points for multiple sites.

Coding Tips

Local anesthesia is included in this service. Supplies used when providing this procedure may be reported with J0702, J1020, J1030, J1040, J1094, J1100, J1700, J1710, J1720, J2920, J2930, or S0020. Check with the specific payer to determine coverage. If imaging guidance is performed see 76942, 77002, and 77021. For therapeutic injection of carpal tunnel, see 20526. For injection tendon sheath, or ligament, see 20550. For injection of tendon origin/insertion, see 20551.

ICD-9-CM Procedural

83.98 Injection of locally acting therapeutic substance into other soft tissue

Anesthesia
N/A

ICD-9-CM Diagnostic

- 353.8 Other nerve root and plexus disorders
- 354.5 Mononeuritis multiplex
- 354.8 Other mononeuritis of upper limb
- 357.1 Polyneuropathy in collagen vascular disease — (Code first underlying disease: 446.0, 710.0, 714.0)
- 359.6 Symptomatic inflammatory myopathy in diseases classified elsewhere — (Code first underlying disease: 135, 140.0-208.9, 277.30-277.39, 446.0, 710.0, 710.1, 710.2, 714.0)
- 714.0 Rheumatoid arthritis — (Use additional code to identify manifestation: 357.1, 359.6)
- 715.04 Generalized osteoarthrosis, involving hand
- 715.09 Generalized osteoarthrosis, involving multiple sites
- 715.18 Primary localized osteoarthrosis, other specified sites
- 715.38 Localized osteoarthrosis not specified whether primary or secondary, other specified sites
- 716.50 Unspecified polyarthropathy or polyarthritis, site unspecified
- 716.51 Unspecified polyarthropathy or polyarthritis, shoulder region
- 716.52 Unspecified polyarthropathy or polyarthritis, upper arm
- 716.53 Unspecified polyarthropathy or polyarthritis, forearm
- 716.54 Unspecified polyarthropathy or polyarthritis, hand
- 716.58 Unspecified polyarthropathy or polyarthritis, other specified sites
- 716.60 Unspecified monoarthritis, site unspecified
- 716.61 Unspecified monoarthritis, shoulder region
- 716.62 Unspecified monoarthritis, upper arm
- 716.63 Unspecified monoarthritis, forearm
- 716.64 Unspecified monoarthritis, hand
- 716.68 Unspecified monoarthritis, other specified sites
- 716.91 Unspecified arthropathy, shoulder region
- 716.92 Unspecified arthropathy, upper arm
- 716.93 Unspecified arthropathy, forearm
- 716.94 Unspecified arthropathy, hand
- 716.99 Unspecified arthropathy, multiple sites
- 719.41 Pain in joint, shoulder region
- 719.42 Pain in joint, upper arm
- 719.43 Pain in joint, forearm
- 719.44 Pain in joint, hand
- 719.48 Pain in joint, other specified sites
- 720.0 Ankylosing spondylitis
- 720.2 Sacroiliitis, not elsewhere classified
- 724.1 Pain in thoracic spine
- 724.2 Lumbago
- 724.3 Sciatica
- 724.4 Thoracic or lumbosacral neuritis or radiculitis, unspecified
- 726.10 Unspecified disorders of bursae and tendons in shoulder region
- 726.32 Lateral epicondylitis of elbow
- 727.00 Unspecified synovitis and tenosynovitis
- 727.03 Trigger finger (acquired)
- 727.04 Radial styloid tenosynovitis
- 727.05 Other tenosynovitis of hand and wrist
- 727.09 Other synovitis and tenosynovitis
- 729.2 Unspecified neuralgia, neuritis, and radiculitis
- 729.4 Unspecified fasciitis
- 729.5 Pain in soft tissues of limb

CCI Version 16.3

01991-01992, 10160, 11900-11901, 20500, 20526, 29075, 29105-29125, 29130, 29260, 29405-29425, 29450, 29515, 29530-29590, 36000, 36400-36410, 36420-36430, 36440, 36600, 36640, 37202, 43752, 51701-51703, 62310-62319, 64408-64410, 64435, 64455, 64505-64530, 69990, 76000-76001, 93000-93010, 93040-93042, 93318, 94002, 94200, 94250, 94680-94690, 94770, 95812-95816, 95819, 95822, 95829, 95955, 96360, 96365, 96372, 96374-96376, 99148-99149, 99150, J0670, J2001

Also not with 20553: 20552

Note: These CCI edits are used for Medicare. Other payers may reimburse on codes listed above.

Medicare Edits

	Fac RVU	Non-Fac RVU	FUD	Assist
20552	1.08	1.54	0	N/A
20553	1.21	1.75	0	N/A

Medicare References: 100-3, 150.7

20600-20610

20600 Arthrocentesis, aspiration and/or injection; small joint or bursa (eg, fingers, toes)
20605 intermediate joint or bursa (eg, temporomandibular, acromioclavicular, wrist, elbow or ankle, olecranon bursa)
20610 major joint or bursa (eg, shoulder, hip, knee joint, subacromial bursa)

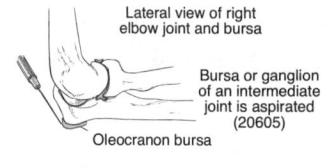

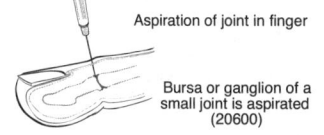

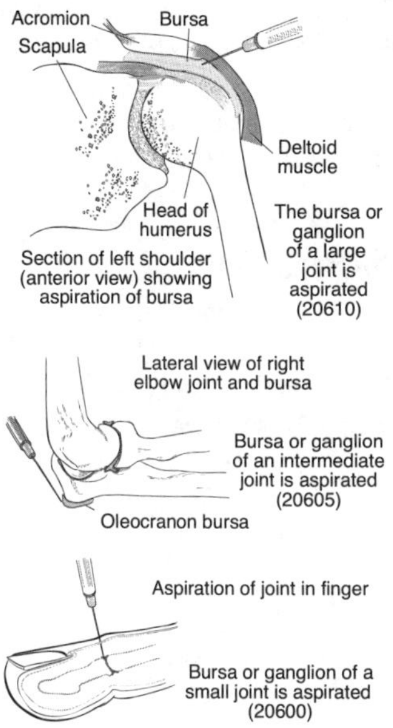

Explanation

After administering a local anesthetic, the physician inserts a needle through the skin and into a joint or bursa. A fluid sample may be removed from the joint or a fluid may be injected for lavage or drug therapy. The needle is withdrawn and pressure is applied to stop any bleeding. Report 20600 for arthrocentesis of a small joint or bursa, such as of the fingers or toes; 20605 for an intermediate joint or bursa, such as the wrist, elbow, ankle, olecranon bursa, or temporomandibular or acromioclavicular area. Report 20610 for a major joint or bursa injection or aspiration, such as of the shoulder, hip, knee joint, or subacromial bursa.

Coding Tips

These codes should be reported only once even if an aspiration and injection are performed during the same session. Local anesthesia is included in these services. To report imaging guidance, see 76942, 77002, 77012, and 77021. For aspiration or injection of a ganglion cyst, see 20612. Supplies used when providing this procedure may be reported with J0702, J1020–J1040, J1094, J1100, J1700–J1720, J2920, J2930, and J3301–J3303. Check with the specific payer to determine coverage.

ICD-9-CM Procedural

- 81.91 Arthrocentesis
- 81.92 Injection of therapeutic substance into joint or ligament
- 82.92 Aspiration of bursa of hand
- 82.94 Injection of therapeutic substance into bursa of hand
- 82.95 Injection of therapeutic substance into tendon of hand
- 83.94 Aspiration of bursa
- 83.96 Injection of therapeutic substance into bursa

Anesthesia

N/A

ICD-9-CM Diagnostic

- 274.00 Gouty arthropathy, unspecified
- 274.01 Acute gouty arthropathy
- 274.02 Chronic gouty arthropathy without mention of tophus (tophi)
- 274.03 Chronic gouty arthropathy with tophus (tophi)
- 338.0 Central pain syndrome — (Use additional code to identify pain associated with psychological factors: 307.89)
- 354.0 Carpal tunnel syndrome
- 354.2 Lesion of ulnar nerve
- 354.3 Lesion of radial nerve
- 354.5 Mononeuritis multiplex
- 354.8 Other mononeuritis of upper limb
- 357.1 Polyneuropathy in collagen vascular disease — (Code first underlying disease: 446.0, 710.0, 714.0)
- 712.24 Chondrocalcinosis due to pyrophosphate crystals, hand — (Code first underlying disease: 275.4)
- 714.0 Rheumatoid arthritis — (Use additional code to identify manifestation: 357.1, 359.6)
- 715.00 Generalized osteoarthrosis, unspecified site
- 715.04 Generalized osteoarthrosis, involving hand
- 719.00 Effusion of joint, site unspecified
- 719.04 Effusion of hand joint
- 727.00 Unspecified synovitis and tenosynovitis
- 727.03 Trigger finger (acquired)
- 727.05 Other tenosynovitis of hand and wrist

CCI Version 16.3

00400, 01380, 10060-10061, 10140, 10160, 11010✦, 25259, 26340, 29065-29085, 29505-29515, 36000, 36400-36410, 36420-36430, 36440, 36600, 36640, 37202, 43752, 51701-51703, 64400-64435, 64445-64450, 69990, 76000-76001, 93000-93010, 93040-93042, 93318, 94002, 94200, 94250, 94680-94690, 94770, 95812-95816, 95819, 95822, 95829, 95900, 95955, 96360, 96365, 96372, 96374-96376, 99148-99149, 99150, J0670, J2001

Also not with 20600: 0228T, 0230T, 11719, 20500, 20526-20553, 29105-29125, 29130, 29260-29280, 29365-29425, 29540-29590, 62310-62319, 64479, 64483, 64505-64530, 64704-64708, 72240, 72265, G0127

Also not with 20605: 11900, 12011, 15852, 20526-20553, 24300, 29105-29126, 29240-29260, 29405-29425, 29445, 29540, 29580-29590, 29705, 64505-64550, 64704

Also not with 20610: 11900, 12001-12002, 12020, 12031, 12044, 15851, 20500-20501, 20550-20553, 24300, 29105-29125, 29130, 29240-29260, 29345-29355, 29365-29425, 29530-29540, 29580-29581, 64505-64553, 64718, 72255, 72265, 72295, 76080, G0168

Note: These CCI edits are used for Medicare. Other payers may reimburse on codes listed above.

Medicare Edits

	Fac RVU	Non-Fac RVU	FUD	Assist
20600	1.14	1.57	0	N/A
20605	1.2	1.7	0	N/A
20610	1.46	2.27	0	N/A

Medicare References: 100-3,150.6; 100-3,150.7; 100-4,12,30; 100-4,13,80.1; 100-4,13,80.2

20612

20612 Aspiration and/or injection of ganglion cyst(s) any location

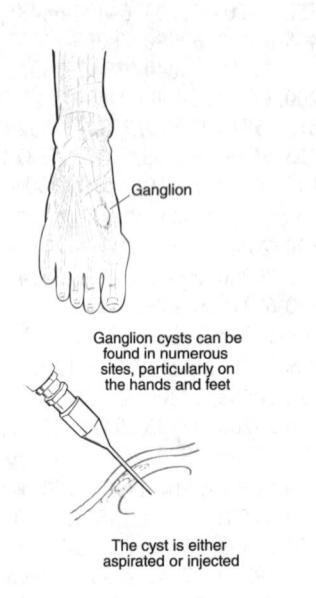

Explanation
The physician aspirates and/or injects a ganglion cyst. After administering a local anesthetic, the physician inserts a needle through the skin and into the ganglion cyst. A ganglion cyst is a benign mass consisting of a thin capsule containing clear, mucinous fluid arising from an aponeurosis or tendon sheath, such as on the back of the wrist or foot. A fluid sample may be withdrawn from the cyst or a medicinal substance may be injected for therapy. The needle is withdrawn and pressure is applied to stop any bleeding.

Coding Tips
To report multiple ganglion cyst aspirations/injections, use 20612 with modifier 59 appended. For excision of a ganglion cyst, see 25111–25112. Surgical trays, A4550, are not separately reimbursed by Medicare; however, other third-party payers may cover them. Check with the specific payer to determine coverage. Supplies used when providing this procedure may be reported with J0702, J1020–J1040, and S0020. Check with the specific payer to determine coverage.

ICD-9-CM Procedural
05.39 Other injection into sympathetic nerve or ganglion

Anesthesia
20612 N/A

ICD-9-CM Diagnostic
727.40 Unspecified synovial cyst
727.41 Ganglion of joint
727.42 Ganglion of tendon sheath
727.43 Unspecified ganglion
727.49 Other ganglion and cyst of synovium, tendon, and bursa

Terms To Know
anesthesia. Loss of feeling or sensation, usually induced to permit the performance of surgery or other painful procedures.

aponeurosis. Flat expansion of white, ribbon-like tendinous tissue that functions as the connection of a muscle to its moving part.

aspiration. Drawing fluid out by suction.

benign. Mild or nonmalignant in nature.

cyst. Elevated encapsulated mass containing fluid, semisolid, or solid material with a membranous lining.

excision. Surgical removal of an organ or tissue.

ganglion. Fluid-filled, benign cyst appearing on a tendon sheath or aponeurosis, frequently found in the hand, wrist, or foot and connecting to an underlying joint.

injection. Forcing a liquid substance into a body part such as a joint or muscle.

joint capsule. Sac-like enclosure enveloping the synovial joint cavity with a fibrous membrane attached to the articular ends of the bones in the joint.

synovia. Clear fluid lubricant of joints, bursae, and tendon sheaths, secreted by the synovial membrane.

tendon. Fibrous tissue that connects muscle to bone, consisting primarily of collagen and containing little vasculature.

therapeutic. Act meant to alleviate a medical or mental condition.

CCI Version 16.3
00400, 01820, 0213T, 0216T, 0228T, 0230T, 10060-10061, 10140, 10160, 20500, 20526-20553, 36000, 36400-36410, 36420-36430, 36440, 36600, 36640, 37202, 43752, 51701-51703, 62310-62319, 64400-64435, 64445-64450, 64479, 64483, 64490, 64493, 64505-64530, 69990, 76000-76001, 77002, 93000-93010, 93040-93042, 93318, 94002, 94200, 94250, 94680-94690, 94770, 95812-95816, 95819, 95822, 95829, 95955, 96360, 96365, 96372, 96374-96376, 99148-99149, 99150, J0670, J2001

Note: These CCI edits are used for Medicare. Other payers may reimburse on codes listed above.

Medicare Edits

	Fac RVU	Non-Fac RVU	FUD	Assist
20612	1.22	1.69	0	N/A

Medicare References: 100-4,12,30

20615

20615 Aspiration and injection for treatment of bone cyst

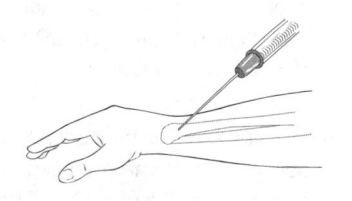

Fluid is aspirated from a cyst or fluid may be injected

Explanation
After administering a local anesthetic, the physician inserts a needle through the skin and into a bone cyst. A fluid sample is removed from the cyst and medication injected for lavage or drug therapy. The needle is withdrawn and pressure is applied to stop any bleeding.

Coding Tips
For arthrocentesis, see 20600–20610. Surgical trays, A4550, are not separately reimbursed by Medicare; however, other third-party payers may cover them. Check with the specific payer to determine coverage.

ICD-9-CM Procedural
- 78.40 Other repair or plastic operations on bone, unspecified site
- 78.41 Other repair or plastic operations on scapula, clavicle, and thorax (ribs and sternum)
- 78.43 Other repair or plastic operations on radius and ulna
- 78.44 Other repair or plastic operations on carpals and metacarpals
- 78.49 Other repair or plastic operations on other bone, except facial bones

Anesthesia
20615 00640, 01620, 01730, 01820

ICD-9-CM Diagnostic
- 733.20 Unspecified cyst of bone (localized)
- 733.21 Solitary bone cyst
- 733.22 Aneurysmal bone cyst
- 733.29 Other cyst of bone

Terms To Know
aneurysmal bone cyst. Solitary bone lesion that bulges into the periosteum, marked by a calcified rim.

aspiration. Drawing fluid out by suction.

cyst. Elevated encapsulated mass containing fluid, semisolid, or solid material with a membranous lining.

lavage. Washing.

CCI Version 16.3
0213T, 0216T, 0228T, 0230T, 11010❖, 20526, 29365, 36000, 36400-36410, 36420-36430, 36440, 36600, 36640, 37202, 43752, 51701-51703, 62310-62319, 64400-64435, 64445-64450, 64479, 64483, 64490, 64493, 64505-64530, 69990, 93000-93010, 93040-93042, 93318, 94002, 94200, 94250, 94680-94690, 94770, 95812-95816, 95819, 95822, 95829, 95955, 96360, 96365, 96372, 96374-96376, 99148-99149, 99150, J2001

Note: These CCI edits are used for Medicare. Other payers may reimburse on codes listed above.

Medicare Edits

	Fac RVU	Non-Fac RVU	FUD	Assist
20615	4.62	6.31	10	N/A

Medicare References: None

20650

20650 Insertion of wire or pin with application of skeletal traction, including removal (separate procedure)

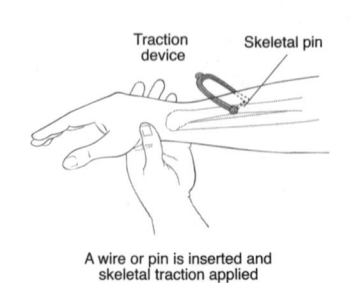

Traction device / Skeletal pin

A wire or pin is inserted and skeletal traction applied

Explanation
The physician makes a small skin incision laterally or medially over the affected bone. A Steinmann pin is drilled transversely through the bone so that an end protrudes through the skin from either side. An apparatus with a weight is attached to the pin, providing a traction force to reduce (reposition) and align the fracture as a temporary measure to stabilize it until the fracture itself can be addressed.

Coding Tips
This separate procedure by definition is usually a component of a more complex service and is not identified separately. When performed alone or with other unrelated procedures/services it may be reported. If performed alone, list the code; if performed with other procedures/services, list the code and append modifier 59. Surgical trays, A4550, are not separately reimbursed by Medicare; however, other third-party payers may cover them. Check with the specific payer to determine coverage.

ICD-9-CM Procedural
93.44 Other skeletal traction

Anesthesia
20650 01120, 01220, 01340, 01390, 01462, 01620, 01630, 01740, 01820, 01830

ICD-9-CM Diagnostic
- 733.95 Stress fracture of other bone — (Use additional external cause code(s) to identify the cause of the stress fracture)
- 812.00 Closed fracture of unspecified part of upper end of humerus
- 812.01 Closed fracture of surgical neck of humerus
- 812.02 Closed fracture of anatomical neck of humerus
- 812.03 Closed fracture of greater tuberosity of humerus
- 812.09 Other closed fractures of upper end of humerus
- 812.10 Open fracture of unspecified part of upper end of humerus
- 812.11 Open fracture of surgical neck of humerus
- 812.12 Open fracture of anatomical neck of humerus
- 812.13 Open fracture of greater tuberosity of humerus
- 812.20 Closed fracture of unspecified part of humerus
- 812.21 Closed fracture of shaft of humerus
- 812.30 Open fracture of unspecified part of humerus
- 812.31 Open fracture of shaft of humerus
- 812.40 Closed fracture of unspecified part of lower end of humerus
- 812.41 Closed fracture of supracondylar humerus
- 812.42 Closed fracture of lateral condyle of humerus
- 812.43 Closed fracture of medial condyle of humerus
- 812.44 Closed fracture of unspecified condyle(s) of humerus
- 812.49 Other closed fracture of lower end of humerus
- 812.50 Open fracture of unspecified part of lower end of humerus
- 812.51 Open fracture of supracondylar humerus
- 812.52 Open fracture of lateral condyle of humerus
- 812.53 Open fracture of medial condyle of humerus
- 812.54 Open fracture of unspecified condyle(s) of humerus
- 812.59 Other open fracture of lower end of humerus
- 813.07 Other and unspecified closed fractures of proximal end of radius (alone)
- 813.17 Other and unspecified open fractures of proximal end of radius (alone)
- 996.40 Unspecified mechanical complication of internal orthopedic device, implant, and graft — (Use additional code to identify prosthetic joint with mechanical complication, V43.60-V43.69)
- 996.49 Other mechanical complication of other internal orthopedic device, implant, and graft — (Use additional code to identify prosthetic joint with mechanical complication, V43.60-V43.69)
- 996.67 Infection and inflammatory reaction due to other internal orthopedic device, implant, and graft — (Use additional code to identify specified infections)
- 996.78 Other complications due to other internal orthopedic device, implant, and graft — (Use additional code to identify complication: 338.18-338.19, 338.28-338.29)

Terms To Know
skeletal traction. Applying a pulling force directly on the long axis of bones by inserted wires or pins and using weights and pulleys to keep the bone in proper alignment.

CCI Version 16.3
0213T, 0216T, 0228T, 0230T, 11010❖, 20103, 20670-20680, 24300, 25259, 26340, 29075, 29405-29425, 29740, 36000, 36400-36410, 36420-36430, 36440, 36600, 36640, 37202, 43752, 51701-51703, 62310-62319, 64400-64435, 64445-64450, 64479, 64483, 64490, 64493, 64505-64530, 69990, 93000-93010, 93040-93042, 93318, 94002, 94200, 94250, 94680-94690, 94770, 95812-95816, 95819, 95822, 95829, 95955, 96360, 96365, 96372, 96374-96376, 99148-99149, 99150, J0670, J2001

Note: These CCI edits are used for Medicare. Other payers may reimburse on codes listed above.

Medicare Edits

	Fac RVU	Non-Fac RVU	FUD	Assist
20650	4.46	5.72	10	N/A

Medicare References: 100-2,15,260; 100-4,12,30; 100-4,12,90.3; 100-4,14,10

20660

20660 Application of cranial tongs, caliper, or stereotactic frame, including removal (separate procedure)

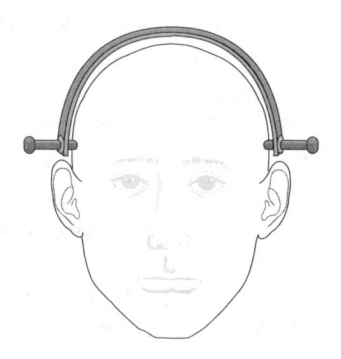

Cranial tongs (shown) applied for traction of cervical spine

Physician applies cranial tongs, caliper, or frame to perform procedure

Explanation
The physician applies cranial tongs, a caliper, or a stereotactic frame to stabilize an injured cervical spine for radiography, a stretch test, surgery, or spinal realignment. The physician places the patient supine with the head supported just over the end of the table. The physician applies Betadine solution with sponges to the hair above the ears. The physician separates or removes hair 1 cm above the ears slightly posterior to the midlateral line. A local anesthetic is injected into the areas selected for pin insertion. Tongs are held in the appropriate position while both skull pins are inserted simultaneously, keeping the tongs equidistant from the skull on either side. The pins are advanced until the indicator button on one pin protrudes 2 to 3 mm. Lock nuts are applied and the pins are checked every two to three hours for proper tightness.

Coding Tips
This separate procedure by definition is usually a component of a more complex service and is not identified separately. When performed alone or with other unrelated procedures/services, it may be reported. If performed alone, list the code; if performed with other procedures/services, list the code and append modifier 59. This procedure includes removal of the device by the same physician. For removal of tongs or a halo applied by another physician, see 20665. For application of a halo, including removal, cranial, see 20661.

ICD-9-CM Procedural
- 02.94 Insertion or replacement of skull tongs or halo traction device
- 02.95 Removal of skull tongs or halo traction device
- 93.41 Spinal traction using skull device

Anesthesia
20660 00190

ICD-9-CM Diagnostic
- 805.01 Closed fracture of first cervical vertebra without mention of spinal cord injury
- 805.02 Closed fracture of second cervical vertebra without mention of spinal cord injury
- 805.03 Closed fracture of third cervical vertebra without mention of spinal cord injury
- 805.04 Closed fracture of fourth cervical vertebra without mention of spinal cord injury
- 805.05 Closed fracture of fifth cervical vertebra without mention of spinal cord injury
- 805.06 Closed fracture of sixth cervical vertebra without mention of spinal cord injury
- 805.07 Closed fracture of seventh cervical vertebra without mention of spinal cord injury
- 805.11 Open fracture of first cervical vertebra without mention of spinal cord injury
- 805.12 Open fracture of second cervical vertebra without mention of spinal cord injury
- 805.13 Open fracture of third cervical vertebra without mention of spinal cord injury
- 805.14 Open fracture of fourth cervical vertebra without mention of spinal cord injury
- 805.15 Open fracture of fifth cervical vertebra without mention of spinal cord injury
- 805.16 Open fracture of sixth cervical vertebra without mention of spinal cord injury
- 805.17 Open fracture of seventh cervical vertebra without mention of spinal cord injury
- 806.01 Closed fracture of C1-C4 level with complete lesion of cord
- 806.02 Closed fracture of C1-C4 level with anterior cord syndrome
- 806.03 Closed fracture of C1-C4 level with central cord syndrome
- 806.04 Closed fracture of C1-C4 level with other specified spinal cord injury
- 806.06 Closed fracture of C5-C7 level with complete lesion of cord
- 806.07 Closed fracture of C5-C7 level with anterior cord syndrome
- 806.08 Closed fracture of C5-C7 level with central cord syndrome
- 806.11 Open fracture of C1-C4 level with complete lesion of cord
- 806.12 Open fracture of C1-C4 level with anterior cord syndrome
- 806.13 Open fracture of C1-C4 level with central cord syndrome
- 806.16 Open fracture of C5-C7 level with complete lesion of cord
- 806.17 Open fracture of C5-C7 level with anterior cord syndrome
- 806.18 Open fracture of C5-C7 level with central cord syndrome

CCI Version 16.3
0213T, 0216T, 0228T, 0230T, 11010❖, 29540, 36000, 36400-36410, 36420-36430, 36440, 36600, 36640, 37202, 43752, 51701-51703, 62310-62319, 64400-64435, 64445-64450, 64479, 64483, 64490, 64493, 64505-64530, 69990, 92585, 93000-93010, 93040-93042, 93318, 94002, 94200, 94250, 94680-94690, 94770, 95812-95816, 95819, 95822, 95829, 95860-95861, 95867-95868, 95870, 95900, 95904, 95920, 95925-95934, 95936-95937, 95955, 96360, 96365, 96372, 96374-96376, 99148-99149, 99150

Note: These CCI edits are used for Medicare. Other payers may reimburse on codes listed above.

Medicare Edits
	Fac RVU	Non-Fac RVU	FUD	Assist
20660	7.2	7.2	0	N/A

Medicare References: 100-4,12,30

20661

20661 Application of halo, including removal; cranial

The physician places halo on patient's head

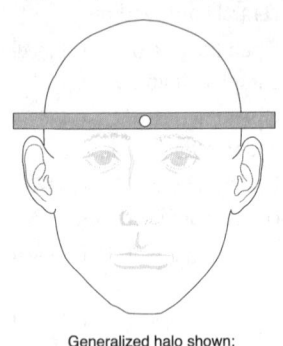

Generalized halo shown; several brands, styles of halos used

Halo stabilizes cervical spine or provides traction

A variety of hardware, vests, or traction can be connected to the halo

Explanation

The physician applies a cranial halo to stabilize an injured cervical spine for radiography, traction, or to facilitate surgery. The physician places the patient supine (lying on the back) with the head supported just over the end of the stretcher. Skin and scalp are sterilized with a povidone-iodine solution. The halo is positioned about the patient's head below the area of greatest skull diameter. A local anesthetic is injected into the areas selected for frame pin insertion. The anterior pins are inserted first, followed by the posterior pins. Two diagonally opposed pins are tightened simultaneously until all four engage the skin and bone. Using a torque screwdriver, all are tightened and secured with nuts or set screws before attachment to a traction setup or to a halo vest or cast.

Coding Tips

This procedure includes removal of the device by the same physician. For application of a halo, including removal, cranial, six or more pins placed, for thin skull osteology, see 20664. For removal of tongs or a halo applied by another physician, see 20665. For application of cranial tongs, a caliper, or a stereotactic head frame, including removal, see 20660.

ICD-9-CM Procedural

- 02.94 Insertion or replacement of skull tongs or halo traction device
- 02.95 Removal of skull tongs or halo traction device
- 93.41 Spinal traction using skull device

Anesthesia
20661 00190

ICD-9-CM Diagnostic

- 805.01 Closed fracture of first cervical vertebra without mention of spinal cord injury
- 805.02 Closed fracture of second cervical vertebra without mention of spinal cord injury
- 805.03 Closed fracture of third cervical vertebra without mention of spinal cord injury
- 805.04 Closed fracture of fourth cervical vertebra without mention of spinal cord injury
- 805.05 Closed fracture of fifth cervical vertebra without mention of spinal cord injury
- 805.06 Closed fracture of sixth cervical vertebra without mention of spinal cord injury
- 805.07 Closed fracture of seventh cervical vertebra without mention of spinal cord injury
- 805.08 Closed fracture of multiple cervical vertebrae without mention of spinal cord injury
- 805.10 Open fracture of cervical vertebra, unspecified level without mention of spinal cord injury
- 805.11 Open fracture of first cervical vertebra without mention of spinal cord injury
- 805.12 Open fracture of second cervical vertebra without mention of spinal cord injury
- 805.13 Open fracture of third cervical vertebra without mention of spinal cord injury
- 805.14 Open fracture of fourth cervical vertebra without mention of spinal cord injury
- 805.15 Open fracture of fifth cervical vertebra without mention of spinal cord injury
- 805.16 Open fracture of sixth cervical vertebra without mention of spinal cord injury
- 805.17 Open fracture of seventh cervical vertebra without mention of spinal cord injury
- 806.01 Closed fracture of C1-C4 level with complete lesion of cord
- 806.02 Closed fracture of C1-C4 level with anterior cord syndrome
- 806.03 Closed fracture of C1-C4 level with central cord syndrome
- 806.05 Closed fracture of C5-C7 level with unspecified spinal cord injury
- 806.06 Closed fracture of C5-C7 level with complete lesion of cord
- 806.07 Closed fracture of C5-C7 level with anterior cord syndrome
- 806.08 Closed fracture of C5-C7 level with central cord syndrome
- 806.11 Open fracture of C1-C4 level with complete lesion of cord
- 806.12 Open fracture of C1-C4 level with anterior cord syndrome
- 806.13 Open fracture of C1-C4 level with central cord syndrome
- 806.15 Open fracture of C5-C7 level with unspecified spinal cord injury
- 806.16 Open fracture of C5-C7 level with complete lesion of cord
- 806.17 Open fracture of C5-C7 level with anterior cord syndrome
- 806.18 Open fracture of C5-C7 level with central cord syndrome

CCI Version 16.3

0213T, 0216T, 0228T, 0230T, 12002, 20660, 20665, 29000, 29020, 29035, 36000, 36400-36410, 36420-36430, 36440, 36600, 36640, 37202, 43752, 51701-51703, 62310-62319, 64400-64435, 64445-64450, 64479, 64483, 64490, 64493, 64505-64530, 69990, 93000-93010, 93040-93042, 93318, 94002, 94200, 94250, 94680-94690, 94770, 95812-95816, 95819, 95822, 95829, 95955, 96360, 96365, 96372, 96374-96376, 99148-99149, 99150

Note: These CCI edits are used for Medicare. Other payers may reimburse on codes listed above.

Medicare Edits

	Fac RVU	Non-Fac RVU	FUD	Assist
20661	14.26	14.26	90	N/A

Medicare References: 100-4,12,30

20664

20664 Application of halo, including removal, cranial, 6 or more pins placed, for thin skull osteology (eg, pediatric patients, hydrocephalus, osteogenesis imperfecta)

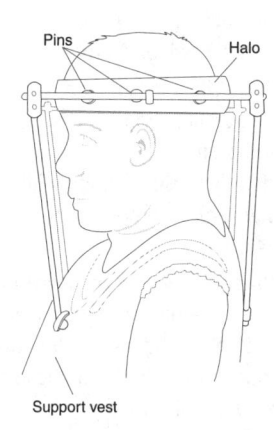

Pins — Halo — Support vest

The halo is mounted to provide support and traction for a condition known as thin skull osteology

Explanation
The physician places a cranial halo on the skull of a child whose skull is unusually thin because of a congenital or developmental problem. The physician sterilizes the skin and scalp with a povidone-iodine solution. The halo is positioned on the patient's head with six or more pins, which are advanced until firm, but not to the tension allowed by a normal skull. Diagonally opposed pins are tightened simultaneously. All are secured with nuts. This code includes the removal of the halo.

Coding Tips
This code has been revised for 2011 in the official CPT description. Report 20664 for patients with thin skull osteology where additional pins (six or more) are required for halo application. This procedure includes removal of the device. For application of a cranial halo with fewer than six pins, see 20661.

ICD-9-CM Procedural
- 02.94 Insertion or replacement of skull tongs or halo traction device
- 02.95 Removal of skull tongs or halo traction device
- 93.41 Spinal traction using skull device

Anesthesia
20664 00190

ICD-9-CM Diagnostic
- 741.01 Spina bifida with hydrocephalus, cervical region
- 741.02 Spina bifida with hydrocephalus, dorsal (thoracic) region
- 741.03 Spina bifida with hydrocephalus, lumbar region
- 742.3 Congenital hydrocephalus
- 756.0 Congenital anomalies of skull and face bones
- 756.51 Osteogenesis imperfecta
- 805.01 Closed fracture of first cervical vertebra without mention of spinal cord injury
- 805.02 Closed fracture of second cervical vertebra without mention of spinal cord injury
- 805.03 Closed fracture of third cervical vertebra without mention of spinal cord injury
- 805.04 Closed fracture of fourth cervical vertebra without mention of spinal cord injury
- 805.05 Closed fracture of fifth cervical vertebra without mention of spinal cord injury
- 805.06 Closed fracture of sixth cervical vertebra without mention of spinal cord injury
- 805.07 Closed fracture of seventh cervical vertebra without mention of spinal cord injury
- 805.08 Closed fracture of multiple cervical vertebrae without mention of spinal cord injury
- 805.11 Open fracture of first cervical vertebra without mention of spinal cord injury
- 805.12 Open fracture of second cervical vertebra without mention of spinal cord injury
- 805.13 Open fracture of third cervical vertebra without mention of spinal cord injury
- 805.14 Open fracture of fourth cervical vertebra without mention of spinal cord injury
- 805.15 Open fracture of fifth cervical vertebra without mention of spinal cord injury
- 805.16 Open fracture of sixth cervical vertebra without mention of spinal cord injury
- 805.17 Open fracture of seventh cervical vertebra without mention of spinal cord injury
- 806.01 Closed fracture of C1-C4 level with complete lesion of cord
- 806.02 Closed fracture of C1-C4 level with anterior cord syndrome
- 806.03 Closed fracture of C1-C4 level with central cord syndrome
- 806.06 Closed fracture of C5-C7 level with complete lesion of cord
- 806.07 Closed fracture of C5-C7 level with anterior cord syndrome
- 806.08 Closed fracture of C5-C7 level with central cord syndrome
- 806.11 Open fracture of C1-C4 level with complete lesion of cord
- 806.12 Open fracture of C1-C4 level with anterior cord syndrome
- 806.13 Open fracture of C1-C4 level with central cord syndrome
- 806.16 Open fracture of C5-C7 level with complete lesion of cord
- 806.17 Open fracture of C5-C7 level with anterior cord syndrome
- 806.18 Open fracture of C5-C7 level with central cord syndrome
- 996.40 Unspecified mechanical complication of internal orthopedic device, implant, and graft — (Use additional code to identify prosthetic joint with mechanical complication, V43.60-V43.69)
- 996.67 Infection and inflammatory reaction due to other internal orthopedic device, implant, and graft — (Use additional code to identify specified infections)

CCI Version 16.3
0213T, 0216T, 0228T, 0230T, 36000, 36400-36410, 36420-36430, 36440, 36600, 36640, 37202, 43752, 51701-51703, 62310-62319, 64400-64435, 64445-64450, 64479, 64483, 64490, 64493, 64505-64530, 69990, 93000-93010, 93040-93042, 93318, 94002, 94200, 94250, 94680-94690, 94770, 95812-95816, 95819, 95822, 95829, 95955, 96360, 96365, 96372, 96374-96376, 99148-99149, 99150

Note: These CCI edits are used for Medicare. Other payers may reimburse on codes listed above.

Medicare Edits

	Fac RVU	Non-Fac RVU	FUD	Assist
20664	23.82	23.82	90	N/A

Medicare References: None

20665

20665 Removal of tongs or halo applied by another physician

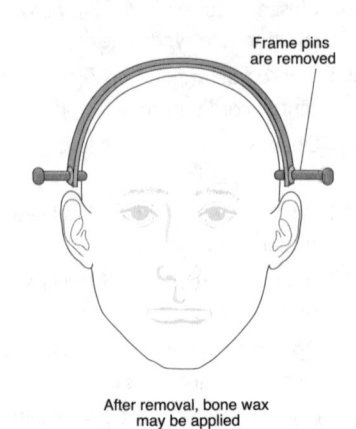

Frame pins are removed

After removal, bone wax may be applied

In 20665, physician removes tongs applied by another physician

Explanation

The physician removes tongs or a halo applied by another physician. Maintaining alignment of the cervical spine, the physician unscrews the frame pins from the skull and removes the tongs or halo. Bone wax may be applied to the wounds to promote healing of the skull. Dressing may be applied to the skin wounds, and the skin may be sutured.

Coding Tips

Removal of tongs or a halo is included in the basic procedure when performed by the same physician. Code 20665 is only used when the removal is performed by another physician. For application of cranial tongs, a caliper, or a stereotactic frame, see 20660. For application of a halo, including removal, cranial, see 20661. For application of a halo, cranial, six or more pins placed, for thin skull osteology, see 20664.

ICD-9-CM Procedural

02.95 Removal of skull tongs or halo traction device

Anesthesia

20665 00190, 01120, 01340

ICD-9-CM Diagnostic

- 805.01 Closed fracture of first cervical vertebra without mention of spinal cord injury
- 805.02 Closed fracture of second cervical vertebra without mention of spinal cord injury
- 805.03 Closed fracture of third cervical vertebra without mention of spinal cord injury
- 805.04 Closed fracture of fourth cervical vertebra without mention of spinal cord injury
- 805.05 Closed fracture of fifth cervical vertebra without mention of spinal cord injury
- 805.06 Closed fracture of sixth cervical vertebra without mention of spinal cord injury
- 805.07 Closed fracture of seventh cervical vertebra without mention of spinal cord injury
- 805.11 Open fracture of first cervical vertebra without mention of spinal cord injury
- 805.12 Open fracture of second cervical vertebra without mention of spinal cord injury
- 805.13 Open fracture of third cervical vertebra without mention of spinal cord injury
- 805.14 Open fracture of fourth cervical vertebra without mention of spinal cord injury
- 805.15 Open fracture of fifth cervical vertebra without mention of spinal cord injury
- 805.16 Open fracture of sixth cervical vertebra without mention of spinal cord injury
- 805.17 Open fracture of seventh cervical vertebra without mention of spinal cord injury
- 806.01 Closed fracture of C1-C4 level with complete lesion of cord
- 806.02 Closed fracture of C1-C4 level with anterior cord syndrome
- 806.03 Closed fracture of C1-C4 level with central cord syndrome
- 806.05 Closed fracture of C5-C7 level with unspecified spinal cord injury
- 806.06 Closed fracture of C5-C7 level with complete lesion of cord
- 806.07 Closed fracture of C5-C7 level with anterior cord syndrome
- 806.08 Closed fracture of C5-C7 level with central cord syndrome
- 806.11 Open fracture of C1-C4 level with complete lesion of cord
- 806.12 Open fracture of C1-C4 level with anterior cord syndrome
- 806.13 Open fracture of C1-C4 level with central cord syndrome
- 806.15 Open fracture of C5-C7 level with unspecified spinal cord injury
- 806.16 Open fracture of C5-C7 level with complete lesion of cord
- 806.17 Open fracture of C5-C7 level with anterior cord syndrome
- 806.18 Open fracture of C5-C7 level with central cord syndrome
- 996.40 Unspecified mechanical complication of internal orthopedic device, implant, and graft — (Use additional code to identify prosthetic joint with mechanical complication, V43.60-V43.69)
- 996.49 Other mechanical complication of other internal orthopedic device, implant, and graft — (Use additional code to identify prosthetic joint with mechanical complication, V43.60-V43.69)
- 996.67 Infection and inflammatory reaction due to other internal orthopedic device, implant, and graft — (Use additional code to identify specified infections)
- V54.01 Encounter for removal of internal fixation device
- V54.17 Aftercare for healing traumatic fracture of vertebrae
- V54.89 Other orthopedic aftercare
- V67.4 Treatment of healed fracture follow-up examination

CCI Version 16.3

0213T, 0216T, 0228T, 0230T, 11010❖, 36000, 36400-36410, 36420-36430, 36440, 36600, 36640, 37202, 43752, 51701-51703, 62310-62319, 64400-64435, 64445-64450, 64479, 64483, 64490, 64493, 64505-64530, 69990, 93000-93010, 93040-93042, 93318, 94002, 94200, 94250, 94680-94690, 94770, 95812-95816, 95819, 95822, 95829, 95955, 96360, 96365, 96372, 96374-96376, 99148-99149, 99150

Note: These CCI edits are used for Medicare. Other payers may reimburse on codes listed above.

Medicare Edits

	Fac RVU	Non-Fac RVU	FUD	Assist
20665	2.72	3.22	10	80

Medicare References: None

20670

20670 Removal of implant; superficial (eg, buried wire, pin or rod) (separate procedure)

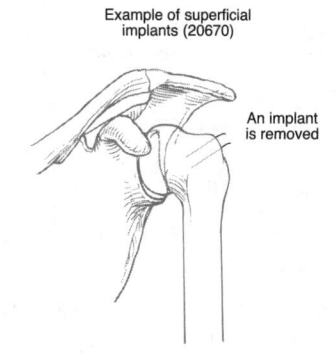

Example of superficial implants (20670)

An implant is removed

Explanation

The physician makes a small incision overlying the site of the implant. The implant is located. The physician removes the implant by pulling or unscrewing it. The incision is closed with sutures and/or Steri-strips.

Coding Tips

This separate procedure by definition is usually a component of a more complex service and is not identified separately. When performed alone or with other unrelated procedures/services, it may be reported. If performed alone, list the code; if performed with other procedures/services, list the code and append modifier 59. Surgical trays, A4550, are not separately reimbursed by Medicare; however, other third-party payers may cover them. Check with the specific payer to determine coverage.

ICD-9-CM Procedural

- 78.60 Removal of implanted device, unspecified site
- 78.61 Removal of implanted device from scapula, clavicle, and thorax (ribs and sternum)
- 78.62 Removal of implanted device from humerus
- 78.63 Removal of implanted device from radius and ulna
- 78.64 Removal of implanted device from carpals and metacarpals
- 78.69 Removal of implanted device from other bone
- 80.02 Arthrotomy for removal of prosthesis without replacement, elbow
- 84.57 Removal of (cement) spacer

Anesthesia

20670 00300, 00400, 01620, 01630, 01740, 01820, 01830

ICD-9-CM Diagnostic

- 996.40 Unspecified mechanical complication of internal orthopedic device, implant, and graft — (Use additional code to identify prosthetic joint with mechanical complication, V43.60-V43.69)
- 996.49 Other mechanical complication of other internal orthopedic device, implant, and graft — (Use additional code to identify prosthetic joint with mechanical complication, V43.60-V43.69)
- 996.67 Infection and inflammatory reaction due to other internal orthopedic device, implant, and graft — (Use additional code to identify specified infections)
- 996.78 Other complications due to other internal orthopedic device, implant, and graft — (Use additional code to identify complication: 338.18-338.19, 338.28-338.29)
- V54.01 Encounter for removal of internal fixation device
- V54.10 Aftercare for healing traumatic fracture of arm, unspecified
- V54.11 Aftercare for healing traumatic fracture of upper arm
- V54.12 Aftercare for healing traumatic fracture of lower arm
- V54.19 Aftercare for healing traumatic fracture of other bone
- V54.20 Aftercare for healing pathologic fracture of arm, unspecified
- V54.21 Aftercare for healing pathologic fracture of upper arm
- V54.22 Aftercare for healing pathologic fracture of lower arm
- V54.29 Aftercare for healing pathologic fracture of other bone
- V54.81 Aftercare following joint replacement — (Use additional code to identify joint replacement site: V43.60-V43.69)
- V54.89 Other orthopedic aftercare
- V67.4 Treatment of healed fracture follow-up examination

Terms To Know

complication. Condition arising after the beginning of observation and treatment that modifies the course of the patient's illness or the medical care required, or an undesired result or misadventure in medical care.

implant. Material or device inserted or placed within the body for therapeutic, reconstructive, or diagnostic purposes.

internal skeletal fixation. Repair involving wires, pins, screws, and/or plates placed through or within the fractured area to stabilize and immobilize the injury.

CCI Version 16.3

0213T, 0216T, 0228T, 0230T, 11010❖, 11040-11044, 20526, 20680❖, 24300, 25259, 26340, 29075, 29125, 29358, 29405, 29550, 29705, 36000, 36400-36410, 36420-36430, 36440, 36600, 36640, 37202, 43752, 51701-51703, 62310-62319, 64400-64435, 64445-64450, 64479, 64483, 64490, 64493, 64505-64530, 69990, 76000-76001, 93000-93010, 93040-93042, 93318, 94002, 94200, 94250, 94680-94690, 94770, 95812-95816, 95819, 95822, 95829, 95955, 96360, 96365, 96372, 96374-96376, 99148-99149, 99150, J0670, J2001

Note: These CCI edits are used for Medicare. Other payers may reimburse on codes listed above.

Medicare Edits

	Fac RVU	Non-Fac RVU	FUD	Assist
20670	4.33	11.25	10	N/A

Medicare References: 100-2,15,260; 100-4,12,30; 100-4,12,90.3; 100-4,14,10

20680

20680 Removal of implant; deep (eg, buried wire, pin, screw, metal band, nail, rod or plate)

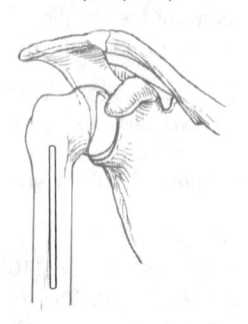

Example of a deep implant (20680)

Explanation

The physician makes an incision overlying the site of the implant. Deep dissection is carried down to visualize the implant, which is usually below the muscle level and within bone. The physician uses instruments to remove the implant from the bone. The incision is repaired in multiple layers using sutures, staples, and/or Steri-strips.

Coding Tips

This is a unilateral procedure. If performed bilaterally, some payers require that the service be reported twice with modifier 50 appended to the second code, while others require identification of the service only once with modifier 50 appended. Check with individual payers. Modifier 50 identifies a procedure performed identically on the opposite side of the body (mirror image). When 20680 is performed with another separately identifiable procedure, the highest dollar value code is listed as the primary procedure and subsequent procedures are appended with modifier 51. If two separate, unrelated incisions are performed to remove different implants, report 20680 twice and append modifier 59 to the second procedure. For removal of an implant, superficial, see 20670. Surgical trays, A4550, are not separately reimbursed by Medicare; however, other third-party payers may cover them. Check with the specific payer to determine coverage.

ICD-9-CM Procedural

- 78.60 Removal of implanted device, unspecified site
- 78.61 Removal of implanted device from scapula, clavicle, and thorax (ribs and sternum)
- 78.62 Removal of implanted device from humerus
- 78.63 Removal of implanted device from radius and ulna
- 78.64 Removal of implanted device from carpals and metacarpals
- 78.69 Removal of implanted device from other bone
- 80.02 Arthrotomy for removal of prosthesis without replacement, elbow
- 84.57 Removal of (cement) spacer

Anesthesia

20680 00600, 00620, 00630, 01120, 01170, 01630, 01740, 01830

ICD-9-CM Diagnostic

- 996.40 Unspecified mechanical complication of internal orthopedic device, implant, and graft — (Use additional code to identify prosthetic joint with mechanical complication, V43.60-V43.69)
- 996.49 Other mechanical complication of other internal orthopedic device, implant, and graft — (Use additional code to identify prosthetic joint with mechanical complication, V43.60-V43.69)
- 996.67 Infection and inflammatory reaction due to other internal orthopedic device, implant, and graft — (Use additional code to identify specified infections)
- 996.78 Other complications due to other internal orthopedic device, implant, and graft — (Use additional code to identify complication: 338.18-338.19, 338.28-338.29)
- V54.01 Encounter for removal of internal fixation device
- V54.10 Aftercare for healing traumatic fracture of arm, unspecified
- V54.11 Aftercare for healing traumatic fracture of upper arm
- V54.12 Aftercare for healing traumatic fracture of lower arm
- V54.19 Aftercare for healing traumatic fracture of other bone
- V54.20 Aftercare for healing pathologic fracture of arm, unspecified
- V54.21 Aftercare for healing pathologic fracture of upper arm
- V54.22 Aftercare for healing pathologic fracture of lower arm
- V54.29 Aftercare for healing pathologic fracture of other bone
- V54.81 Aftercare following joint replacement — (Use additional code to identify joint replacement site: V43.60-V43.69)
- V54.89 Other orthopedic aftercare
- V67.4 Treatment of healed fracture follow-up examination

Terms To Know

dissection. Separating by cutting tissue or body structures apart.

implant. Material or device inserted or placed within the body for therapeutic, reconstructive, or diagnostic purposes.

prosthesis. Man-made substitute for a missing body part.

CCI Version 16.3

0213T, 0216T, 0228T, 0230T, 11000, 11010❖, 11040-11044, 12001-12007, 12011-12057, 13100-13101, 13120-13121, 13131-13132, 13150-13152, 20526-20553, 24300, 25259, 26340, 27704❖, 29075, 29105-29125, 29345, 29405-29425, 29515, 29847❖, 36000, 36400-36410, 36420-36430, 36440, 36600, 36640, 37202, 43752, 51701-51703, 62310-62319, 64400-64435, 64445-64450, 64479, 64483, 64490, 64493, 64505-64530, 64708, 64714, 64718, 64722, 69990, 76000-76001, 93000-93010, 93040-93042, 93318, 94002, 94200, 94250, 94680-94690, 94770, 95812-95816, 95819, 95822, 95829, 95955, 96360, 96365, 96372, 96374-96376, 99148-99149, 99150, J0670, J2001

Note: These CCI edits are used for Medicare. Other payers may reimburse on codes listed above.

Medicare Edits

	Fac RVU	Non-Fac RVU	FUD	Assist
20680	12.38	17.69	90	80

Medicare References: 100-2,15,260; 100-4,12,30; 100-4,12,90.3; 100-4,14,10

20690-20692

20690 Application of a uniplane (pins or wires in 1 plane), unilateral, external fixation system

20692 Application of a multiplane (pins or wires in more than 1 plane), unilateral, external fixation system (eg, Ilizarov, Monticelli type)

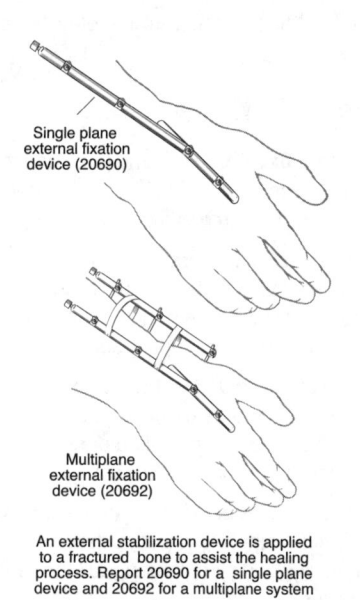

Single plane external fixation device (20690)

Multiplane external fixation device (20692)

An external stabilization device is applied to a fractured bone to assist the healing process. Report 20690 for a single plane device and 20692 for a multiplane system

Explanation

The physician applies an external fixation system to help a fracture or joint injury heal. These procedures are performed in addition to a coded treatment of fracture or joint injury unless listed as part of the basic procedure. These procedures involve the use of an external fixator to stabilize an injury such as a simple fracture. One or more pins or wires may by used. Small stab incisions are made in the skin and a drill is used to make a hole into the bone. Each pin or wire is inserted into the bone through the drill holes and secured to an external fixation device. This holds the fracture or joint in a stable position. Report 20690 if uniplane fixation is applied and 20692 if multiplane fixation is applied.

Coding Tips

Do not report separately if the primary procedure specifically includes the application of an external fixation in the code description. For adjustment/revision of an external fixation system requiring anesthesia, see 20693. For removal of an external fixation system requiring anesthesia, see 20694. Surgical trays, A4450, are not separately reimbursed by Medicare; however, other third-party payers may cover them. Check with the specific payer to determine coverage.

ICD-9-CM Procedural

78.10 Application of external fixator device, unspecified site
78.11 Application of external fixator device, scapula, clavicle, and thorax [ribs and sternum]
78.12 Application of external fixator device, humerus
78.13 Application of external fixator device, radius and ulna
78.14 Application of external fixator device, carpals and metacarpals
78.19 Application of external fixator device, other

Anesthesia
01170, 01630, 01740, 01830

ICD-9-CM Diagnostic
This is designated as an add-on code by Ingenix only. Refer to the corresponding primary procedure code for ICD-9-CM diagnosis code links.

Terms To Know

fracture. Break in bone or cartilage.

incision. Act of cutting into tissue or an organ.

multiplane external fixation device. Stabilization device that uses more than one external fixation system to stabilize a fracture.

unilateral. Located on or affecting one side.

CCI Version 16.3
0213T, 0216T, 0228T, 0230T, 20526, 20650, 24300, 25259, 26340, 36000, 36400-36410, 36420-36430, 36440, 36600, 36640, 37202, 43752, 51701-51703, 62310-62319, 64400-64435, 64445-64450, 64479, 64483, 64490, 64493, 64505-64530, 69990, 93000-93010, 93040-93042, 93318, 94002, 94200, 94250, 94680-94690, 94770, 95812-95816, 95819, 95822, 95829, 95955, 96360, 96365, 96372, 96374-96376, 99148-99149, 99150

Also not with 20690: 11010❖

Also not with 20692: 20690

Note: These CCI edits are used for Medicare. Other payers may reimburse on codes listed above.

Medicare Edits

	Fac RVU	Non-Fac RVU	FUD	Assist
20690	16.81	16.81	90	N/A
20692	31.6	31.6	90	80

Medicare References: 100-2,15,260; 100-4,12,30; 100-4,12,90.3; 100-4,14,10

20693

20693 Adjustment or revision of external fixation system requiring anesthesia (eg, new pin[s] or wire[s] and/or new ring[s] or bar[s])

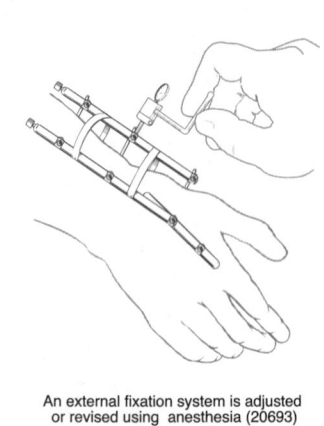

An external fixation system is adjusted or revised using anesthesia (20693)

Explanation

The physician performs an adjustment or revision of an external fixation to allow for healing, development of neurovascular problems, infections, loosening of pins, or failure of the bone fracture to heal. The physician places the patient under anesthesia. If additional pins are needed or must be moved, the physician drills a hole through the bone and inserts the pin, which is attached to external frame devices.

Coding Tips

If multiple pins, wires, rings, and/or bars are adjusted or replaced on one injury site on the same extremity, 20693 should be reported only once. Adjustment/revision not requiring anesthesia is not reported. For application of an external fixation system, see 20690–20692. For removal of an external fixation system requiring anesthesia, see 20694.

ICD-9-CM Procedural

93.44 Other skeletal traction

Anesthesia

20693 01630, 01740, 01830

ICD-9-CM Diagnostic

733.95 Stress fracture of other bone — (Use additional external cause code(s) to identify the cause of the stress fracture)

812.01 Closed fracture of surgical neck of humerus
812.02 Closed fracture of anatomical neck of humerus
812.11 Open fracture of surgical neck of humerus
812.12 Open fracture of anatomical neck of humerus
812.13 Open fracture of greater tuberosity of humerus
812.19 Other open fracture of upper end of humerus
812.21 Closed fracture of shaft of humerus
812.31 Open fracture of shaft of humerus
812.41 Closed fracture of supracondylar humerus
812.42 Closed fracture of lateral condyle of humerus
812.43 Closed fracture of medial condyle of humerus
812.44 Closed fracture of unspecified condyle(s) of humerus
812.51 Open fracture of supracondylar humerus
812.52 Open fracture of lateral condyle of humerus
812.53 Open fracture of medial condyle of humerus
812.54 Open fracture of unspecified condyle(s) of humerus
813.01 Closed fracture of olecranon process of ulna
813.02 Closed fracture of coronoid process of ulna
813.03 Closed Monteggia's fracture
813.05 Closed fracture of head of radius
813.06 Closed fracture of neck of radius
813.11 Open fracture of olecranon process of ulna
813.12 Open fracture of coronoid process of ulna
813.13 Open Monteggia's fracture
813.15 Open fracture of head of radius
813.16 Open fracture of neck of radius
813.21 Closed fracture of shaft of radius (alone)
813.22 Closed fracture of shaft of ulna (alone)
813.23 Closed fracture of shaft of radius with ulna
813.31 Open fracture of shaft of radius (alone)
813.32 Open fracture of shaft of ulna (alone)
813.33 Open fracture of shaft of radius with ulna
813.41 Closed Colles' fracture
813.43 Closed fracture of distal end of ulna (alone)
813.44 Closed fracture of lower end of radius with ulna
813.45 Torus fracture of radius (alone)
813.46 Torus fracture of ulna (alone)
813.51 Open Colles' fracture
816.13 Open fractures of multiple sites of phalanx or phalanges of hand
V53.7 Fitting and adjustment of orthopedic device

Terms To Know

external fixation. Rods and pins connected in a lattice to secure bone. There are several indications for external fixation:

acute fractures: External fixation may be required when a limb fracture is complicated by severe bony comminution, extensive soft tissue damage, or multiple trauma.

failure of previous treatment: External fixation may also be used after acute injury when there is delayed healing or nonunion of the fracture or when infection is present.

other uses include: Fixation in major pelvic disruption, joint fusion (arthrodesis), osteotomy, bone lengthening, or shortening procedures.

CCI Version 16.3

0213T, 0216T, 0228T, 0230T, 20526-20553, 20650, 20690, 20692❖, 24300, 25259, 26340, 29740, 36000, 36400-36410, 36420-36430, 36440, 36600, 36640, 37202, 43752, 51701-51703, 62310-62319, 64400-64435, 64445-64450, 64479, 64483, 64490, 64493, 64505-64530, 69990, 93000-93010, 93040-93042, 93318, 94002, 94200, 94250, 94680-94690, 94770, 95812-95816, 95819, 95822, 95829, 95955, 96360, 96365, 96372, 96374-96376, 99148-99149, 99150

Note: These CCI edits are used for Medicare. Other payers may reimburse on codes listed above.

Medicare Edits

	Fac RVU	Non-Fac RVU	FUD	Assist
20693	13.3	13.3	90	N/A

Medicare References: 100-2,15,260; 100-4,12,30; 100-4,12,90.3; 100-4,14,10

20694

20694 Removal, under anesthesia, of external fixation system

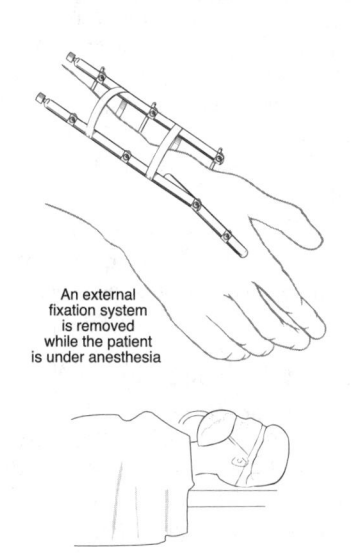

An external fixation system is removed while the patient is under anesthesia

The patient is under anesthesia

Explanation

The physician removes the external fixation frame and pulls pins out manually while the patient is under anesthesia. Incisions are closed with sutures and Steri-strips.

Coding Tips

For adjustment/revision of an external fixation system requiring anesthesia, see 20693. For application of an external fixation system, see 20690–20692.

ICD-9-CM Procedural

- 78.60 Removal of implanted device, unspecified site
- 78.61 Removal of implanted device from scapula, clavicle, and thorax (ribs and sternum)
- 78.62 Removal of implanted device from humerus
- 78.63 Removal of implanted device from radius and ulna
- 78.64 Removal of implanted device from carpals and metacarpals
- 78.69 Removal of implanted device from other bone

Anesthesia

20694 01630, 01740, 01830

ICD-9-CM Diagnostic

- 733.95 Stress fracture of other bone — (Use additional external cause code(s) to identify the cause of the stress fracture)
- 812.01 Closed fracture of surgical neck of humerus
- 812.02 Closed fracture of anatomical neck of humerus
- 812.11 Open fracture of surgical neck of humerus
- 812.12 Open fracture of anatomical neck of humerus
- 812.13 Open fracture of greater tuberosity of humerus
- 812.21 Closed fracture of shaft of humerus
- 812.31 Open fracture of shaft of humerus
- 812.41 Closed fracture of supracondylar humerus
- 812.42 Closed fracture of lateral condyle of humerus
- 812.43 Closed fracture of medial condyle of humerus
- 812.49 Other closed fracture of lower end of humerus
- 812.51 Open fracture of supracondylar humerus
- 812.52 Open fracture of lateral condyle of humerus
- 812.53 Open fracture of medial condyle of humerus
- 812.59 Other open fracture of lower end of humerus
- 813.01 Closed fracture of olecranon process of ulna
- 813.02 Closed fracture of coronoid process of ulna
- 813.03 Closed Monteggia's fracture
- 813.05 Closed fracture of head of radius
- 813.06 Closed fracture of neck of radius
- 813.07 Other and unspecified closed fractures of proximal end of radius (alone)
- 813.11 Open fracture of olecranon process of ulna
- 813.12 Open fracture of coronoid process of ulna
- 813.13 Open Monteggia's fracture
- 813.15 Open fracture of head of radius
- 813.16 Open fracture of neck of radius
- 813.17 Other and unspecified open fractures of proximal end of radius (alone)
- 813.21 Closed fracture of shaft of radius (alone)
- 813.22 Closed fracture of shaft of ulna (alone)
- 813.23 Closed fracture of shaft of radius with ulna
- 813.31 Open fracture of shaft of radius (alone)
- 813.32 Open fracture of shaft of ulna (alone)
- 813.33 Open fracture of shaft of radius with ulna
- 813.41 Closed Colles' fracture
- 813.42 Other closed fractures of distal end of radius (alone)
- 813.43 Closed fracture of distal end of ulna (alone)
- 813.44 Closed fracture of lower end of radius with ulna
- 813.51 Open Colles' fracture
- 813.52 Other open fractures of distal end of radius (alone)
- 813.53 Open fracture of distal end of ulna (alone)
- 813.54 Open fracture of lower end of radius with ulna
- 814.10 Unspecified open fracture of carpal bone
- 815.00 Closed fracture of metacarpal bone(s), site unspecified
- 815.10 Open fracture of metacarpal bone(s), site unspecified
- 816.03 Closed fracture of multiple sites of phalanx or phalanges of hand
- V54.89 Other orthopedic aftercare
- V67.4 Treatment of healed fracture follow-up examination

CCI Version 16.3

0213T, 0216T, 0228T, 0230T, 11010❖, 12002, 20526-20553, 20650, 24300, 25259, 26340, 29065-29085, 29405-29435, 29515, 36000, 36400-36410, 36420-36430, 36440, 36600, 36640, 37202, 43752, 51701-51703, 62310-62319, 64400-64435, 64445-64450, 64479, 64483, 64490, 64493, 64505-64530, 69990, 76000-76001, 93000-93010, 93040-93042, 93318, 94002, 94200, 94250, 94680-94690, 94770, 95812-95816, 95819, 95822, 95829, 95955, 96360, 96365, 96372, 96374-96376, 99148-99149, 99150, J0670, J2001

Note: These CCI edits are used for Medicare. Other payers may reimburse on codes listed above.

Medicare Edits

	Fac RVU	Non-Fac RVU	FUD	Assist
20694	9.82	12.3	90	N/A

Medicare References: 100-2,15,260; 100-4,12,30; 100-4,12,90.3; 100-4,14,10

20696-20697

20696 Application of multiplane (pins or wires in more than 1 plane), unilateral, external fixation with stereotactic computer-assisted adjustment (eg, spatial frame), including imaging; initial and subsequent alignment(s), assessment(s), and computation(s) of adjustment schedule(s)

20697 exchange (ie, removal and replacement) of strut, each

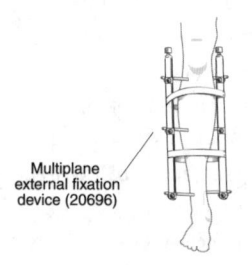

Multiplane external fixation device (20696)

An external stabilization device is applied utilizing stereotactic computer assistance. Report 20696 for assessment and computation of fixation system. Report 20697 for exchange of each strut.

Explanation

Using stereotactic computer-assisted adjustment, such as a spatial frame, the physician applies a unilateral external fixation system with pins or wires in more than one plane (multiplane) to help a fracture or joint injury heal. This procedure is performed in addition to a coded treatment of fracture or joint injury unless listed as part of the basic procedure. This procedure uses an external fixator to stabilize an injury such as a simple fracture. Small stab incisions are made in the skin, and a drill is used to make a hole into the bone. Each pin or wire is inserted into the bone through the drill holes and secured to an external fixation device. This holds the fracture or joint in a stable position. Report 20696 for the application, including imaging, initial and subsequent alignments, assessments, and computations of adjustment schedules. Report 20697 for the removal and replacement of each strut.

Coding Tips

As exempt from modifier 51, 20697 has not been designated in CPT as an add-on service/procedure. However, codes identified as exempt from modifier 51 are not subject to multiple procedure rules. No reimbursement reduction or modifier 51 is applied. Do not report 20696 or 20697 with 20692. Do not report 20697 with 20696. For application of a multiplane, unilateral, external fixation system, see 20692. For adjustment/revision of an external fixation system requiring anesthesia, see 20693. For removal of an external fixation system requiring anesthesia, see 20694.

ICD-9-CM Procedural

00.39	Other computer assisted surgery
78.10	Application of external fixator device, unspecified site
78.11	Application of external fixator device, scapula, clavicle, and thorax [ribs and sternum]
78.12	Application of external fixator device, humerus
78.13	Application of external fixator device, radius and ulna
78.14	Application of external fixator device, carpals and metacarpals
78.19	Application of external fixator device, other

Anesthesia

20696 N/A
20697 01830

ICD-9-CM Diagnostic

The application of this code is too broad to adequately present ICD-9-CM diagnostic code links here. Refer to your ICD-9-CM book.

Terms To Know

multiplane external fixation device. Stabilization device that uses more than one external fixation system to stabilize a fracture.

stereotaxis. Three-dimensional method for precisely locating structures.

unilateral. Located on or affecting one side.

CCI Version 16.3

0213T, 0216T, 11010❖, 20526, 20650, 20690, 20692-20693❖, 24300, 25259, 26340, 36000, 36410, 37202, 51701-51703, 61795, 62318-62319, 64415-64417, 64450, 64490, 64493, 69990, 73000-73040, 73050-73085, 73090-73115, 73120-73223, 73500-73525, 73530-73580, 73590-73615, 73620-73725, 76000-76001, 76942, 76998, 77002, 77011-77012, 77021, 77031, 96360, 96365, 96372, 96374-96376, 99148-99149, 99150

Also not with 20697: 20696

Note: These CCI edits are used for Medicare. Other payers may reimburse on codes listed above.

Medicare Edits

	Fac RVU	Non-Fac RVU	FUD	Assist
20696	31.5	31.5	90	80
20697	49.49	49.49	0	80

Medicare References: None

20802

20802 Replantation, arm (includes surgical neck of humerus through elbow joint), complete amputation

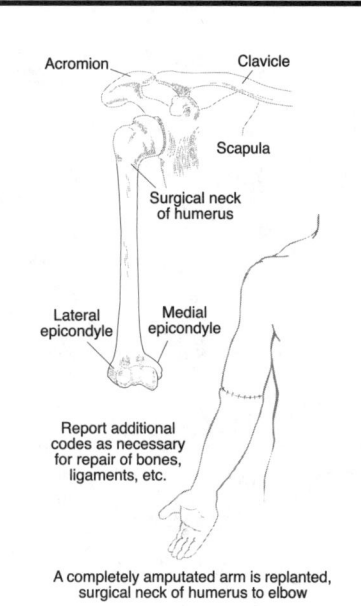

A completely amputated arm is replanted, surgical neck of humerus to elbow

Explanation

The physician replants an arm following a complete amputation. The physician reattaches the upper extremity at a level between the elbow and shoulder. With the patient under anesthesia, the physician identifies the severed neurovascular structures, muscles, bone, and tendons. Each tissue is systematically reattached using sutures, wires, plates, or other fixation devices. Dead tissue is debrided. The skin is joined and closed with sutures after thorough cleaning and irrigation.

Coding Tips

Partial amputation is reported with specific codes for repair of bone, ligament, tendon, nerve, and/or blood vessels. When repair of these structures involves less work than normally associated with the code reported, append modifier 52. If significant additional time and effort is documented, append modifier 22 and submit a cover letter and operative report.

ICD-9-CM Procedural

84.24 Upper arm reattachment

Anesthesia

20802 01770

ICD-9-CM Diagnostic

887.2 Traumatic amputation of arm and hand (complete) (partial), unilateral, at or above elbow, without mention of complication
887.3 Traumatic amputation of arm and hand (complete) (partial), unilateral, at or above elbow, complicated
887.6 Traumatic amputation of arm and hand (complete) (partial), bilateral (any level), without mention of complication
887.7 Traumatic amputation of arm and hand (complete) (partial), bilateral (any level), complicated

Terms To Know

bilateral. Consisting of or affecting two sides.

tendon. Fibrous tissue that connects muscle to bone, consisting primarily of collagen and containing little vasculature.

traumatic amputation. Removal of a part or limb from accidental injury.

unilateral. Located on or affecting one side.

CCI Version 16.3

0213T, 0216T, 0228T, 0230T, 20103, 20550-20553, 20650, 20690, 20692, 20696-20697, 23615, 24006, 24300, 24342, 24515-24516, 24545, 35206, 36000, 36400-36410, 36420-36430, 36440, 36600, 36640, 37202, 43752, 51701-51703, 62310-62319, 64400-64435, 64445-64450, 64479, 64483, 64490, 64493, 64505-64530, 64856-64857, 69990, 93000-93010, 93040-93042, 93318, 94002, 94200, 94250, 94680-94690, 94770, 95812-95816, 95819, 95822, 95829, 95955, 96360, 96365, 96372, 96374-96376, 97597-97598, 97602-97606, 99148-99149, 99150

Note: These CCI edits are used for Medicare. Other payers may reimburse on codes listed above.

Medicare Edits

	Fac RVU	Non-Fac RVU	FUD	Assist
20802	67.79	67.79	90	80

Medicare References: 100-4,12,30

20805

20805 Replantation, forearm (includes radius and ulna to radial carpal joint), complete amputation

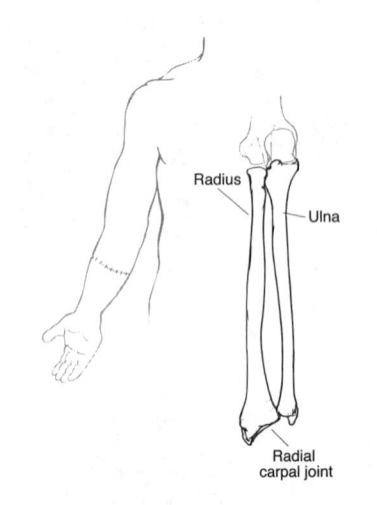

A completely amputated arm is replanted, radius and ulna to radial carpal joint

Explanation

The physician reattaches a severed forearm at a level between the wrist and the elbow. With the patient under anesthesia, the physician identifies each structure that has been cut or separated. The nerves, blood vessels, tendons, and bone are each reattached using sutures, wires, plates or other fixation devices. Dead tissue is debrided. The skin is joined and closed with sutures after thorough cleaning and irrigation.

Coding Tips

Partial amputation is reported with specific codes for repair of bone, ligament, tendon, nerve, and/or blood vessels. When repair of these structures involves less work than normally associated with the code reported, append modifier 52. If significant additional time and effort is documented, append modifier 22 and submit a cover letter and operative report.

ICD-9-CM Procedural

84.23 Forearm, wrist, or hand reattachment

Anesthesia

20805 01840

ICD-9-CM Diagnostic

887.0 Traumatic amputation of arm and hand (complete) (partial), unilateral, below elbow, without mention of complication
887.1 Traumatic amputation of arm and hand (complete) (partial), unilateral, below elbow, complicated
887.6 Traumatic amputation of arm and hand (complete) (partial), bilateral (any level), without mention of complication
887.7 Traumatic amputation of arm and hand (complete) (partial), bilateral (any level), complicated

Terms To Know

bilateral. Consisting of or affecting two sides.

tendon. Fibrous tissue that connects muscle to bone, consisting primarily of collagen and containing little vasculature.

traumatic amputation. Removal of a part or limb from accidental injury.

unilateral. Located on or affecting one side.

CCI Version 16.3

0213T, 0216T, 0228T, 0230T, 20103, 20526, 20650, 20690, 20692, 20696-20697, 24300, 25259-25260, 25270, 25575, 25606-25609, 26340, 35206, 36000, 36400-36410, 36420-36430, 36440, 36600, 36640, 37202, 43752, 51701-51703, 62310-62319, 64400-64435, 64445-64450, 64479, 64483, 64490, 64493, 64505-64530, 64856-64857, 69990, 93000-93010, 93040-93042, 93318, 94002, 94200, 94250, 94680-94690, 94770, 95812-95816, 95819, 95822, 95829, 95955, 96360, 96365, 96372, 96374-96376, 97597-97598, 97602-97606, 99148-99149, 99150

Note: These CCI edits are used for Medicare. Other payers may reimburse on codes listed above.

Medicare Edits

	Fac RVU	Non-Fac RVU	FUD	Assist
20805	83.85	83.85	90	80

Medicare References: None

20808

20808 Replantation, hand (includes hand through metacarpophalangeal joints), complete amputation

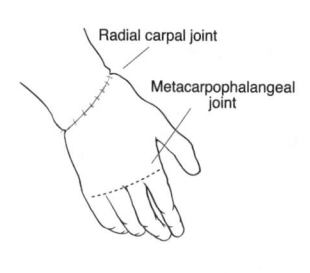

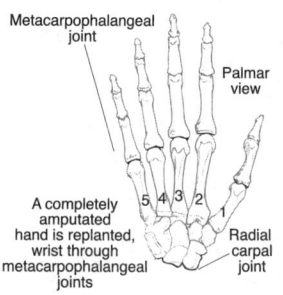

Explanation
The physician reattaches a hand that has been completely severed from the forearm between the wrist and the fingers. With the patient under anesthesia, the physician identifies the nerves, blood vessels, tendon, and bones. Each structure is reattached in a systematic fashion with debridement of dead tissue. Sutures, wires, plates, or other devices may be used. Copious irrigation is required. The overlying soft tissues and skin are joined with sutures in layers.

Coding Tips
Partial amputation is reported with specific codes for repair of bone, ligament, tendon, nerve, and/or blood vessels. When repair of these structures involves less work than normally associated with the code reported, append modifier 52. If significant additional time and effort is documented, append modifier 22 and submit a cover letter and operative report.

ICD-9-CM Procedural
84.23 Forearm, wrist, or hand reattachment

Anesthesia
20808 01840

ICD-9-CM Diagnostic
887.0 Traumatic amputation of arm and hand (complete) (partial), unilateral, below elbow, without mention of complication
887.1 Traumatic amputation of arm and hand (complete) (partial), unilateral, below elbow, complicated
887.4 Traumatic amputation of arm and hand (complete) (partial), unilateral, level not specified, without mention of complication
887.5 Traumatic amputation of arm and hand (complete) (partial), unilateral, level not specified, complicated
887.6 Traumatic amputation of arm and hand (complete) (partial), bilateral (any level), without mention of complication
887.7 Traumatic amputation of arm and hand (complete) (partial), bilateral (any level), complicated

Terms To Know
bilateral. Consisting of or affecting two sides.

soft tissue. Nonepithelial tissues outside of the skeleton that includes subcutaneous adipose tissue, fibrous tissue, fascia, muscles, blood and lymph vessels, and peripheral nervous system tissue.

tendon. Fibrous tissue that connects muscle to bone, consisting primarily of collagen and containing little vasculature.

traumatic amputation. Removal of a part or limb from accidental injury.

unilateral. Located on or affecting one side.

CCI Version 16.3
0213T, 0216T, 0228T, 0230T, 20103, 20526-20553, 20650, 20690, 20692, 20696-20697, 26340-26350, 26410, 26418, 26615, 26665, 26686, 26746, 26841, 26850, 35206-35207, 36000, 36400-36410, 36420-36430, 36440, 36600, 36640, 37202, 43752, 51701-51703, 62310-62319, 64400-64435, 64445-64450, 64479, 64483, 64490, 64493, 64505-64530, 64831, 64834-64835, 64856, 69990, 93000-93010, 93040-93042, 93318, 94002, 94200, 94250, 94680-94690, 94770, 95812-95816, 95819, 95822, 95829, 95955, 96360, 96365, 96372, 96374-96376, 97597-97598, 97602-97606, 99148-99149, 99150

Note: These CCI edits are used for Medicare. Other payers may reimburse on codes listed above.

Medicare Edits

	Fac RVU	Non-Fac RVU	FUD	Assist
20808	122.72	122.72	90	80

Medicare References: None

20816

20816 Replantation, digit, excluding thumb (includes metacarpophalangeal joint to insertion of flexor sublimis tendon), complete amputation

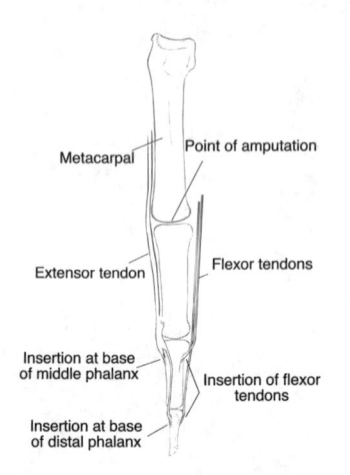

A completely amputated digit is reimplanted. Flexor tendons used in grasping are reattached, typically at the distal metacarpal joint, the site of the amputation

Explanation

The physician reattaches one of the four fingers, excluding the thumb, that has been completely severed from the hand at or near its articulation with its specific metacarpal bone. With the patient under anesthesia, the physician identifies the nerves, tendons, and bones. Dead tissue is debrided and the wound is irrigated thoroughly. Each tissue is systematically reattached using sutures, wires, plates, or other devices. Skin is joined and sutured closed.

Coding Tips

Partial amputation is reported with specific codes for repair of bone, ligament, tendon, nerve, and/or blood vessels. When repair of these structures involves less work than normally associated with the code reported, append modifier 52.

ICD-9-CM Procedural

84.22 Finger reattachment

Anesthesia

20816 01830, 01840

ICD-9-CM Diagnostic

886.0 Traumatic amputation of other finger(s) (complete) (partial), without mention of complication

886.1 Traumatic amputation of other finger(s) (complete) (partial), complicated

Terms To Know

distal. Located farther away from a specified reference point.

tendon. Fibrous tissue that connects muscle to bone, consisting primarily of collagen and containing little vasculature.

traumatic amputation. Removal of a part or limb from accidental injury.

CCI Version 16.3

0213T, 0216T, 0228T, 0230T, 20103, 20526-20553, 20650, 20690, 20692, 20696-20697, 26340-26350, 26356, 26370, 26410, 26418, 26615, 26735, 26746, 26776, 26850, 26860, 26910-26952, 35206-35207, 36000, 36400-36410, 36420-36430, 36440, 36600, 36640, 37202, 43752, 51701-51703, 62310-62319, 64400-64435, 64445-64450, 64479, 64483, 64490, 64493, 64505-64530, 64831, 64834, 69990, 93000-93010, 93040-93042, 93318, 94002, 94200, 94250, 94680-94690, 94770, 95812-95816, 95819, 95822, 95829, 95955, 96360, 96365, 96372, 96374-96376, 97597-97598, 97602-97606, 99148-99149, 99150

Note: These CCI edits are used for Medicare. Other payers may reimburse on codes listed above.

Medicare Edits

	Fac RVU	Non-Fac RVU	FUD	Assist
20816	63.16	63.16	90	80

Medicare References: None

20822

20822 Replantation, digit, excluding thumb (includes distal tip to sublimis tendon insertion), complete amputation

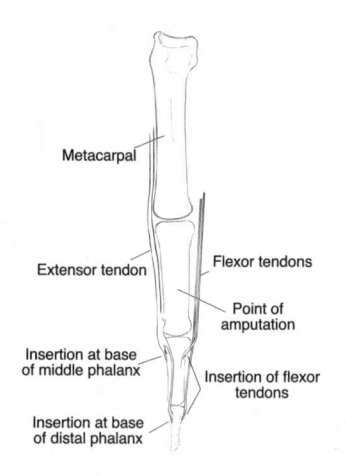

A completely amputated digit is reimplanted. Flexor tendons used in grasping are reattached, typically at the proximal or middle phalanx, the site of the amputation

Explanation

The physician reattaches one of the four fingers, excluding the thumb, which has been completely severed from the hand at a level between the fingertip and the attachment of the finger to the hand itself. With the patient under anesthesia, the physician identifies severed structures, including nerves, blood vessels, tendons, and bones. Dead tissue is debrided and the wound is thoroughly irrigated. Each tissue is reattached using sutures, wires, plates, or other devices. Skin is joined in layers with sutures.

Coding Tips

Partial amputation is reported with specific codes for repair of bone, ligament, tendon, nerve, and/or blood vessels. When repair of these structures involves less work than normally associated with the code reported, append modifier 52. If significant additional time and effort is documented, append modifier 22 and submit a cover letter and operative report.

ICD-9-CM Procedural

84.22 Finger reattachment

Anesthesia

20822 01840

ICD-9-CM Diagnostic

886.0 Traumatic amputation of other finger(s) (complete) (partial), without mention of complication

886.1 Traumatic amputation of other finger(s) (complete) (partial), complicated

Terms To Know

proximal. Located closest to a specified reference point, usually the midline.

tendon. Fibrous tissue that connects muscle to bone, consisting primarily of collagen and containing little vasculature.

traumatic amputation. Removal of a part or limb from accidental injury.

CCI Version 16.3

0213T, 0216T, 0228T, 0230T, 20103, 20526-20553, 20650, 20690, 20692, 20696-20697, 26340-26350, 26356, 26370, 26410, 26418, 26735, 26746, 26765, 26776, 26850, 26860, 26910-26952, 35206-35207, 36000, 36400-36410, 36420-36430, 36440, 36600, 36640, 37202, 43752, 51701-51703, 62310-62319, 64400-64435, 64445-64450, 64479, 64483, 64490, 64493, 64505-64530, 64831, 69990, 93000-93010, 93040-93042, 93318, 94002, 94200, 94250, 94680-94690, 94770, 95812-95816, 95819, 95822, 95829, 95955, 96360, 96365, 96372, 96374-96376, 97597-97598, 97602-97606, 99148-99149, 99150

Note: These CCI edits are used for Medicare. Other payers may reimburse on codes listed above.

Medicare Edits

	Fac RVU	Non-Fac RVU	FUD	Assist
20822	55.81	55.81	90	80

Medicare References: None

20824

20824 Replantation, thumb (includes carpometacarpal joint to MP joint), complete amputation

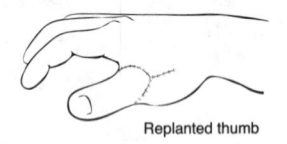

Replanted thumb

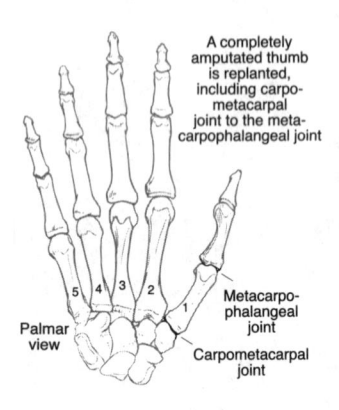

A completely amputated thumb is replanted, including carpometacarpal joint to the metacarpophalangeal joint

Palmar view
Metacarpophalangeal joint
Carpometacarpal joint

Explanation

The physician reattaches the thumb that has been completely severed from the hand at the attachment of the thumb to the hand itself. With the patient under anesthesia, the physician identifies severed structures, including nerves, blood vessels, tendons, and bones. Dead tissue is debrided and the wound is thoroughly irrigated. Each tissue is reattached using sutures, wires, plates, or other devices. Skin is joined in layers with sutures.

Coding Tips

Partial amputation is reported with specific codes for repair of bone, ligament, tendon, nerve, and/or blood vessels. When repair of these structures involves less work than normally associated with the code reported, append modifier 52. If significant additional time and effort is documented, append modifier 22 and submit a cover letter and operative report.

ICD-9-CM Procedural

84.21 Thumb reattachment

Anesthesia

20824 01840

ICD-9-CM Diagnostic

885.0 Traumatic amputation of thumb (complete) (partial), without mention of complication
885.1 Traumatic amputation of thumb (complete) (partial), complicated

Terms To Know

tendon. Fibrous tissue that connects muscle to bone, consisting primarily of collagen and containing little vasculature.

traumatic amputation. Removal of a part or limb from accidental injury.

CCI Version 16.3

0213T, 0216T, 0228T, 0230T, 20103, 20526-20553, 20650, 20690, 20692, 20696-20697, 26340-26350, 26356, 26410, 26418, 26591, 26615, 26665, 26746, 26765, 26841, 26850, 35207, 36000, 36400-36410, 36420-36430, 36440, 36600, 36640, 37202, 43752, 51701-51703, 62310-62319, 64400-64435, 64445-64450, 64479, 64483, 64490, 64493, 64505-64530, 64831, 64834-64835, 69990, 93000-93010, 93040-93042, 93318, 94002, 94200, 94250, 94680-94690, 94770, 95812-95816, 95819, 95822, 95829, 95955, 96360, 96365, 96372, 96374-96376, 97597-97598, 97602-97606, 99148-99149, 99150

Note: These CCI edits are used for Medicare. Other payers may reimburse on codes listed above.

Medicare Edits

	Fac RVU	Non-Fac RVU	FUD	Assist
20824	63.84	63.84	90	80

Medicare References: None

20827

20827 Replantation, thumb (includes distal tip to MP joint), complete amputation

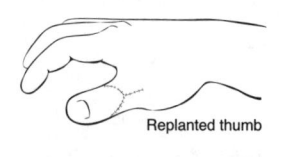

Replanted thumb

A completely amputated thumb is replanted, including metacarpophalangeal joint to the distal tip of the thumb

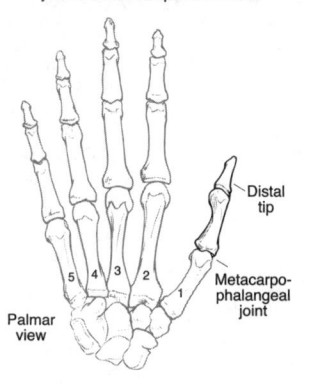

Palmar view — Distal tip, Metacarpophalangeal joint

Explanation
The physician reattaches a thumb that has been completely severed from the hand at a point distal to where the thumb attaches to the hand. With the patient under anesthesia, the physician carefully identifies severed tissues, including nerves, blood vessels, tendons, and bones. Dead tissue is debrided and the wound is thoroughly irrigated. Each tissue is reattached using sutures, wires, plates, or other devices. Skin is joined in layers with sutures.

Coding Tips
Partial amputation is reported with specific codes for repair of bone, ligament, tendon, nerve, and/or blood vessels. When repair of these structures involves less work than normally associated with the code reported, append modifier 52. If significant additional time and effort is documented, append modifier 22 and submit a cover letter and operative report.

ICD-9-CM Procedural
84.21 Thumb reattachment

Anesthesia
20827 01840

ICD-9-CM Diagnostic
885.0 Traumatic amputation of thumb (complete) (partial), without mention of complication
885.1 Traumatic amputation of thumb (complete) (partial), complicated

Terms To Know
debridement. Removal of dead or contaminated tissue and foreign matter from a wound.

distal. Located farther away from a specified reference point.

tendon. Fibrous tissue that connects muscle to bone, consisting primarily of collagen and containing little vasculature.

traumatic amputation. Removal of a part or limb from accidental injury.

CCI Version 16.3
0213T, 0216T, 0228T, 0230T, 20103, 20526-20553, 20650, 20690, 20692, 20696-20697, 26340-26350, 26356, 26410, 26418, 26735, 26746, 26765, 26850, 26860, 35207, 36000, 36400-36410, 36420-36430, 36440, 36600, 36640, 37202, 43752, 51701-51703, 62310-62319, 64400-64435, 64445-64450, 64479, 64483, 64490, 64493, 64505-64530, 64831, 69990, 93000-93010, 93040-93042, 93318, 94002, 94200, 94250, 94680-94690, 94770, 95812-95816, 95819, 95822, 95829, 95955, 96360, 96365, 96372, 96374-96376, 97597-97598, 97602-97606, 99148-99149, 99150

Note: These CCI edits are used for Medicare. Other payers may reimburse on codes listed above.

Medicare Edits

	Fac RVU	Non-Fac RVU	FUD	Assist
20827	57.95	57.95	90	80

Medicare References: None

20900-20902

20900 Bone graft, any donor area; minor or small (eg, dowel or button)
20902 major or large

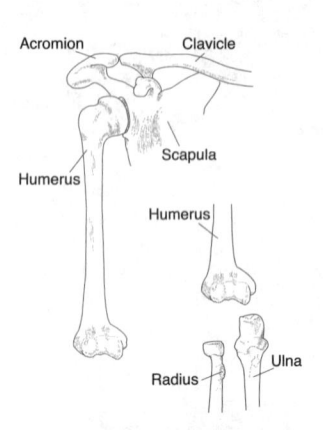

A bone graft is harvested from any donor area, including an upper extremity. Report 20900 for minor or small grafts, such as a dowel or button. Report 20902 for major or large grafts

Explanation

Bone grafts offer physicians excellent building blocks when repairing skeletal problems. The physician makes an incision overlying the rib, ilium, fibula, or other site from which the autograft will be harvested. Fascia and muscles are incised and retracted. A knife, chisel, cutter, or saw may be used to obtain the bone graft, which will be prepared as needed for implantation. Cancellous bone chips may be obtained, as well. The incision is closed with sutures. Report 20900 if the graft is small. Report 20902 if the graft is larger than a dowel or a button.

Coding Tips

The harvest of autogenous bone through a separate incision is to be reported only when a graft is not already listed as part of the basic procedure. Local anesthesia is included in this service.

ICD-9-CM Procedural

77.70	Excision of bone for graft, unspecified site
77.71	Excision of scapula, clavicle, and thorax (ribs and sternum) for graft
77.72	Excision of humerus for graft
77.73	Excision of radius and ulna for graft
77.74	Excision of carpals and metacarpals for graft
77.79	Excision of other bone for graft, except facial bones

Anesthesia

20900 01830
20902 01120

ICD-9-CM Diagnostic

This is designated as an add-on code by Ingenix only. Refer to the corresponding primary procedure code for ICD-9-CM diagnosis code links.

Terms To Know

autograft. Any tissue harvested from one anatomical site of a person and grafted to another anatomical site of the same person. Most commonly, blood vessels, skin, tendons, fascia, and bone are used as autografts.

cancellous bone graft. Highly porous, spongy bone composed of a lattice-like or trabecular meshwork structure, found in the interior of bones and harvested primarily from the iliac crest or rib to be tapped into place as a bone filler.

fascia. Fibrous sheet or band of tissue that envelops organs, muscles, and groupings of muscles.

graft. Tissue implant from another part of the body or another person.

incision. Act of cutting into tissue or an organ.

CCI Version 16.3

0213T, 0216T, 0228T, 0230T, 36000, 36400-36410, 36420-36430, 36440, 36600, 36640, 37202, 38220-38221, 43752, 51701-51703, 62310-62319, 64400-64435, 64445-64450, 64479, 64483, 64490, 64493, 64505-64530, 69990, 93000-93010, 93040-93042, 93318, 94002, 94200, 94250, 94680-94690, 94770, 95812-95816, 95819, 95822, 95829, 95955, 96360, 96365, 96372, 96374-96376, 99148-99149, 99150, G0364

Also not with 20900: J0670, J2001

Also not with 20902: 13152, 20900, 25430, 29105, 29345, 32100, 64704, 64718, 76000-76001

Note: These CCI edits are used for Medicare. Other payers may reimburse on codes listed above.

Medicare Edits

	Fac RVU	Non-Fac RVU	FUD	Assist
20900	6.81	12.06	0	80
20902	9.62	9.62	0	80

Medicare References: 100-2,15,260; 100-4,12,30; 100-4,12,90.3; 100-4,14,10

20910

20910 Cartilage graft; costochondral

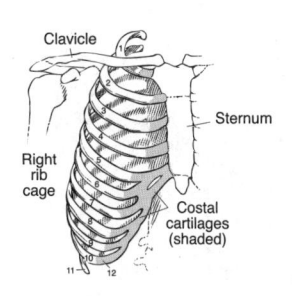

A costochondral cartilage graft is harvested

Explanation
The physician takes a cartilage graft from the rib for later use in reconstructing areas of the lower face such as the temporomandibular joint (TMJ). The physician makes a small incision in the skin through the pectoralis muscle and dissects adjacent tissues away near the sternum. The rib is exposed where the bone and cartilage meet. The cartilage is then removed. After the cartilage is harvested, the donor site is closed with layered sutures.

Coding Tips
The harvest of autogenous bone, cartilage, tendon, fascia lata grafts, or other tissues through separate incisions is to be reported only when a graft is not already listed as part of the basic procedure. Local anesthesia is included in the service. For a fascia lata graft, see 20920–20922.

ICD-9-CM Procedural
80.49 Division of joint capsule, ligament, or cartilage of other specified site
81.99 Other operations on joint structures

Anesthesia
20910 00470

ICD-9-CM Diagnostic
This is designated as an add-on code by Ingenix only. Refer to the corresponding primary procedure code for ICD-9-CM diagnosis code links.

Terms To Know
cartilage. Variety of fibrous connective tissue that is inherently nonvascular. Usually found in the joints, it aids in movement and provides a cushion to absorb jolts and shocks.

costochondral. Pertaining to the ribs and the scapula.

dissect. Cut apart or separate tissue for surgical purposes or for visual or microscopic study.

graft. Tissue implant from another part of the body or another person.

reconstruction. Recreating, restoring, or rebuilding a body part or organ.

suture. Stitching technique employed in wound closure.

CCI Version 16.3
0213T, 0216T, 0228T, 0230T, 36000, 36400-36410, 36420-36430, 36440, 36600, 36640, 37202, 43752, 51701-51703, 62310-62319, 64400-64435, 64445-64450, 64479, 64483, 64490, 64493, 64505-64530, 69990, 93000-93010, 93040-93042, 93318, 94002, 94200, 94250, 94680-94690, 94770, 95812-95816, 95819, 95822, 95829, 95955, 96360, 96365, 96372, 96374-96376, 99148-99149, 99150, J2001

Note: These CCI edits are used for Medicare. Other payers may reimburse on codes listed above.

Medicare Edits

	Fac RVU	Non-Fac RVU	FUD	Assist
20910	12.4	12.4	90	80

Medicare References: 100-2,15,260; 100-4,12,30; 100-4,12,90.3; 100-4,14,10

20920-20922

20920 Fascia lata graft; by stripper
20922 by incision and area exposure, complex or sheet

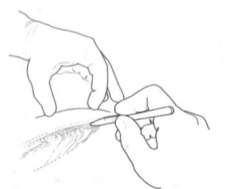

Report 20922 for an incision with exposure, complex or sheet procedure

A graft of the fascia lata muscle is harvested by a stripper (20920). Report 20922 when the graft is by incision with exposure, complex or sheet

Explanation

The physician harvests fascia lata by making a small incision over the lateral aspect of the lower thigh. A stripper instrument is advanced upward underneath the fascia as the physician maintains downward pressure on the cut end of fascia lata. Once the desired graft length is obtained, the cutting mechanism on the stripper is used to release the fascia from above. The stripper and graft are then removed together and the wound is sutured. A compressive dressing is also applied. In 20922, the physician incises skin and subcutaneous tissue, then elevates the flap off the fascia lata. The amount of connective tissue is then acquired by incising and elevating the fascia of the thigh musculature. A small strip or patch may be obtained in this manner. The wound is closed primarily.

Coding Tips

For a costochondral cartilage graft, see 20910.

ICD-9-CM Procedural

83.43 Excision of muscle or fascia for graft

Anesthesia

01250

ICD-9-CM Diagnostic

This is designated as an add-on code by Ingenix only. Refer to the corresponding primary procedure code for ICD-9-CM diagnosis code links.

Terms To Know

excision. Surgical removal of an organ or tissue.

fascia. Fibrous sheet or band of tissue that envelops organs, muscles, and groupings of muscles.

graft. Tissue implant from another part of the body or another person.

incision. Act of cutting into tissue or an organ.

subcutaneous tissue. Sheet or wide band of adipose (fat) and areolar connective tissue in two layers attached to the dermis.

CCI Version 16.3

0213T, 0216T, 0228T, 0230T, 12001-12007, 12011-12047, 35206, 36000, 36400-36410, 36420-36430, 36440, 36600, 36640, 37202, 43752, 51701-51703, 62310-62319, 64400-64435, 64445-64450, 64479, 64483, 64490, 64493, 64505-64530, 69990, 93000-93010, 93040-93042, 93318, 94002, 94200, 94250, 94680-94690, 94770, 95812-95816, 95819, 95822, 95829, 95955, 96360, 96365, 96372, 96374-96376, 99148-99149, 99150

Also not with 20922: 20920, J0670, J2001

Note: These CCI edits are used for Medicare. Other payers may reimburse on codes listed above.

Medicare Edits

	Fac RVU	Non-Fac RVU	FUD	Assist
20920	11.81	11.81	90	N/A
20922	14.49	17.49	90	80

Medicare References: 100-2,15,260; 100-4,12,30; 100-4,12,90.3; 100-4,14,10

20924

20924 Tendon graft, from a distance (eg, palmaris, toe extensor, plantaris)

Subfascial structures, palmar view

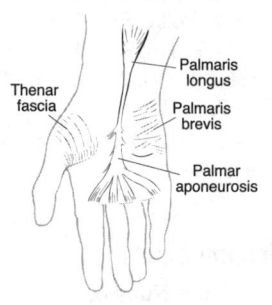

- Thenar fascia
- Palmaris longus
- Palmaris brevis
- Palmar aponeurosis

The tendonous portion of the palmaris longus, or other suitable tendon, is excised and used as a graft in a distant area

A tendon is harvested for graft purposes, from a distance

Explanation
The physician decides on a donor site and makes a cut down to the desired tendon. The tendon is severed and one end held with a hemostat. Dissection is carried to the muscular origin and the tendon is removed. A pressure dressing is applied.

Coding Tips
Codes for obtaining tendon grafts are reported only when the graft is not listed as included in the primary procedure.

ICD-9-CM Procedural
- 82.32 Excision of tendon of hand for graft
- 82.53 Reattachment of tendon of hand
- 82.99 Other operations on muscle, tendon, and fascia of hand
- 83.41 Excision of tendon for graft
- 83.73 Reattachment of tendon
- 83.75 Tendon transfer or transplantation

Anesthesia
20924 00400, 01470, 01710, 01810

ICD-9-CM Diagnostic
This is designated as an add-on code by Ingenix only. Refer to the corresponding primary procedure code for ICD-9-CM diagnosis code links.

Terms To Know

dissection. Separating by cutting tissue or body structures apart.

extensor. Any muscle that extends a joint.

fascia. Fibrous sheet or band of tissue that envelops organs, muscles, and groupings of muscles.

graft. Tissue implant from another part of the body or another person.

tendon. Fibrous tissue that connects muscle to bone, consisting primarily of collagen and containing little vasculature.

CCI Version 16.3
0213T, 0216T, 0228T, 0230T, 29085, 36000, 36400-36410, 36420-36430, 36440, 36600, 36640, 37202, 43752, 51701-51703, 62310-62319, 64400-64435, 64445-64450, 64479, 64483, 64490, 64493, 64505-64530, 69990, 93000-93010, 93040-93042, 93318, 94002, 94200, 94250, 94680-94690, 94770, 95812-95816, 95819, 95822, 95829, 95955, 96360, 96365, 96372, 96374-96376, 99148-99149, 99150

Note: These CCI edits are used for Medicare. Other payers may reimburse on codes listed above.

Medicare Edits

	Fac RVU	Non-Fac RVU	FUD	Assist
20924	14.76	14.76	90	80

Medicare References: 100-2,15,260; 100-4,12,30; 100-4,12,90.3; 100-4,14,10

20926

20926 Tissue grafts, other (eg, paratenon, fat, dermis)

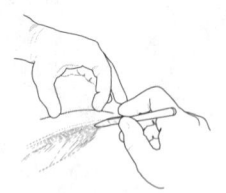

A tissue graft such as paratenon, fat, or skin is obtained

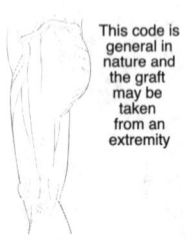

This code is general in nature and the graft may be taken from an extremity

A tissue graft not previously described is obtained through a separate incision

Explanation

The physician obtains a paratenon, fat, or dermis graft. The physician incises the skin and retracts the skin flap to expose the underlying connective tissue. The tissue is incised to the required layer. The graft is lifted and implanted in the recipient site in a separately reportable procedure. The donor site is closed in sutured layers.

Coding Tips

Codes for obtaining tissue grafts are reported only when the graft is not listed as included in the primary procedure.

ICD-9-CM Procedural

The ICD-9-CM procedural code(s) would be the same as the actual procedure performed because these are in-addition-to codes.

Anesthesia

20926 00400

ICD-9-CM Diagnostic

This is designated as an add-on code by Ingenix only. Refer to the corresponding primary procedure code for ICD-9-CM diagnosis code links.

Terms To Know

connective tissue. Body tissue made from fibroblasts, collagen, and elastic fibrils that connects, supports, and holds together other tissues and cells and includes cartilage, collagenous, fibrous, elastic, and osseous tissue.

dermis. Skin layer found under the epidermis that contains a papillary upper layer and the deep reticular layer of collagen, vascular bed, and nerves.

graft. Tissue implant from another part of the body or another person.

incise. To cut open or into.

paratenon. Fatty tissue filling the gaps or space within a tendon sheath or compartment.

suture. Numerous stitching techniques employed in wound closure.

buried suture. Continuous or interrupted suture placed under the skin for a layered closure.

continuous suture. Running stitch with tension evenly distributed across a single strand to provide a leakproof closure line.

interrupted suture. Series of single stitches with tension isolated at each stitch, in which all stitches are not affected if one becomes loose, and the isolated sutures cannot act as a wick to transport an infection.

purse-string suture. Continuous suture placed around a tubular structure and tightened, to reduce or close the lumen.

retention suture. Secondary stitching that bridges the primary suture, providing support for the primary repair; a plastic or rubber bolster may be placed over the primary repair and under the retention sutures.

CCI Version 16.3

0213T, 0216T, 0228T, 0230T, 12001-12007, 12011-12057, 13100-13101, 13120-13121, 13131-13132, 13150-13152, 36000, 36400-36410, 36420-36430, 36440, 36600, 36640, 37202, 43752, 51701-51703, 62310-62319, 64400-64435, 64445-64450, 64479, 64483, 64490, 64493, 64505-64530, 64713, 69990, 93000-93010, 93040-93042, 93318, 94002, 94200, 94250, 94680-94690, 94770, 95812-95816, 95819, 95822, 95829, 95955, 96360, 96365, 96372, 96374-96376, 99148-99149, 99150

Note: These CCI edits are used for Medicare. Other payers may reimburse on codes listed above.

Medicare Edits

	Fac RVU	Non-Fac RVU	FUD	Assist
20926	12.78	12.78	90	N/A

Medicare References: 100-2,15,260; 100-4,12,30; 100-4,12,90.3; 100-4,14,10

20930-20931

20930 Allograft, morselized, or placement of osteopromotive material, for spine surgery only (List separately in addition to code for primary procedure)

20931 Allograft, structural, for spine surgery only (List separately in addition to code for primary procedure)

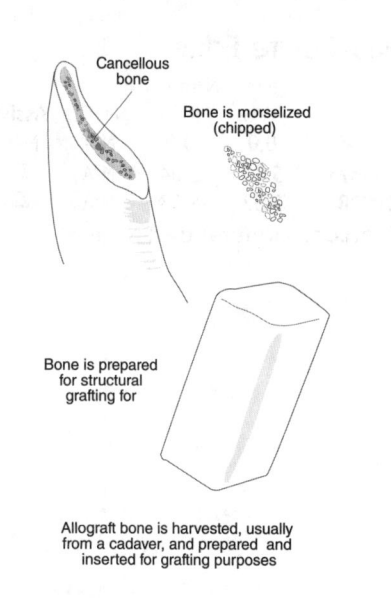

Explanation
In 20930, the physician inserts an osteopromotive material, such as bone morphogenetic protein (BMP), autogenous growth factor concentrate, bovine bone-derived osteoinductive protein, or recombinant human MP52, to promote bone healing and enhance fusion rates in patients undergoing spinal surgery. Alternately, the physician may use an allograft (a graft from the same species) that has been prepared as cancellous chips (morselized). The physician obtains a bone graft from a cadaver donor that is frozen or freeze dried until used. The physician prepares and inserts the allograft in a separately reportable spinal procedure. In 20931, the physician inserts an allograft that has been prepared in a bicortical or tricortical shape for structural use.

Coding Tips
These codes have been revised for 2011 in the official CPT description. As "add-on" codes, 20930 and 20931 are not subject to multiple procedure rules. No reimbursement reduction or modifier 51 is applied. Add-on codes describe additional intra-service work associated with the primary procedure. They are performed by the same physician on the same date of service as the primary service/procedure, and must never be reported as a stand-alone code. Report 20930 and 20931 in conjunction with 22319, 22532, 22533, 22548-22558, 22590-22612, 22630, and 22800-22812. Code 20930 can also be reported in conjunction with 0195T and 0196T. Report only one bone graft code per operative session. Do not report bone graft procedures 20930–20931 with modifier 62.

ICD-9-CM Procedural
The ICD-9-CM procedural code(s) would be the same as the actual procedure performed because these are in-addition-to codes.

Anesthesia
N/A

ICD-9-CM Diagnostic
The ICD-9-CM diagnostic code(s) would be the same as the actual procedure performed because these are in-addition-to codes.

Terms To Know
allograft. Graft from one individual to another of the same species.

autograft. Any tissue harvested from one anatomical site of a person and grafted to another anatomical site of the same person. Most commonly, blood vessels, skin, tendons, fascia, and bone are used as autografts.

bones. Hard, rigid tissue of the skeletal system made of both living organic cells and inorganic mineral components.

cadaver. Dead body.

cancellous bone. Bone found mostly in the midshaft of long bones that is spongy and porous with a lattice-like construction.

cortical bone. Thin, superficial layer of dense, compact bone that covers the cancellous bone and makes up most of the diaphysis (shaft) of the long bones, providing strength to the long bones of the body.

fusion. Union of adjacent tissues, especially bone.

harvest. Removal of cells or tissue from their native site to be used as a graft or transplant to another part of the donor's body or placed into another person.

xenograft. Tissue that is nonhuman and harvested from one species and grafted to another. Pigskin is the most common xenograft for human skin and is applied to a wound as a temporary closure until a permanent option is performed.

CCI Version 16.3
Also not with 20931: 11010❖, 92585, 95822, 95860-95861, 95867-95868, 95870, 95900, 95904, 95920, 95925-95934, 95936-95937

Note: These CCI edits are used for Medicare. Other payers may reimburse on codes listed above.

Medicare Edits

	Fac RVU	Non-Fac RVU	FUD	Assist
20930	0.0	0.0	N/A	N/A
20931	3.36	3.36	N/A	N/A

Medicare References: None

20936-20938

20936 Autograft for spine surgery only (includes harvesting the graft); local (eg, ribs, spinous process, or laminar fragments) obtained from same incision (List separately in addition to code for primary procedure)

20937 morselized (through separate skin or fascial incision) (List separately in addition to code for primary procedure)

20938 structural, bicortical or tricortical (through separate skin or fascial incision) (List separately in addition to code for primary procedure)

Example of structural autograft with plate

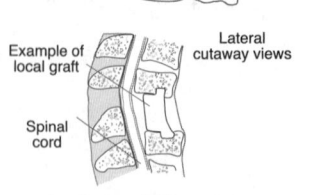

Lateral cutaway views

Example of local graft

Spinal cord

Local autograft is harvested, processed, and placed

In 20936, grafts are typically harvested from costal area of ribs, spinous processes, or laminae and are always taken through the main surgical incision

Graft may be morselized (chipped) in 20937, or fashioned into a structural graft in 20938; harvest is via separate surgical incision

Autografts are typically harvested from the iliac crest or fibula as well as other sites; a separate surgical access incision is made

Explanation

During a vertebral fusion or other spinal procedure, the physician may choose to use bone fragments taken from the vertebral bodies adjacent to the affected disc, from the spinous process, or laminar fragment. Some of these may have been removed during the surgery or as part of the surgical approach. In 20936, a local graft is taken from the same incision. Local grafts prevent extra morbidity caused by obtaining an iliac or a tibial graft and lessen the possibility of cadaver-borne transmittable diseases. When grafts are harvested, they are obtained through the use of power tools or special chisels. The grafts may be morselized, carved into pegs, or shaped as bars. This code is listed in addition to the primary procedure. In 20937 and 20938, the graft is taken through a separate incision. The physician makes an incision over the ilium, fibula, or other site from which the autograft will be obtained. Fascia and muscles are incised and retracted. A knife, chisel, cutter, or saw may be used to obtain the autograft, which will be prepared as needed for implantation in the spine. In 20937, cancellous bone chips (morselized) are obtained. In 20938, structural bicortical or tricortical grafts are obtained. The incision is closed with sutures.

Coding Tips

As "add-on" codes, 20936, 20937, and 20938 are not subject to multiple procedure rules. No reimbursement reduction or modifier 51 is applied. Add-on codes describe additional intra-service work associated with the primary procedure. They are performed by the same physician on the same date of service as the primary service/procedure, and must never be reported as a stand-alone code. Codes 20936–20938 should only be used to report grafts for spinal surgery. For bone grafts to other sites, see 20900–20902. Do not report bone graft procedures 20936–20938 with modifier 62.

ICD-9-CM Procedural

77.70 Excision of bone for graft, unspecified site

77.79 Excision of other bone for graft, except facial bones

Anesthesia
N/A

ICD-9-CM Diagnostic

The ICD-9-CM diagnostic code(s) would be the same as the actual procedure performed because these are in-addition-to codes.

Terms To Know

autograft. Any tissue harvested from one anatomical site of a person and grafted to another anatomical site of the same person. Most commonly, blood vessels, skin, tendons, fascia, and bone are used as autografts.

fascia. Fibrous sheet or band of tissue that envelops organs, muscles, and groupings of muscles.

CCI Version 16.3

Also not with 20937: 11010❖, 38220-38221, 92585, 95822, 95860-95861, 95867-95868, 95870, 95900, 95904, 95920, 95925-95934, 95936-95937, G0364

Also not with 20938: 11010-11012❖, 38220-38221, G0364

Note: These CCI edits are used for Medicare. Other payers may reimburse on codes listed above.

Medicare Edits

	Fac RVU	Non-Fac RVU	FUD	Assist
20936	0.0	0.0	N/A	N/A
20937	5.04	5.04	N/A	80
20938	5.53	5.53	N/A	80

Medicare References: None

20950

20950 Monitoring of interstitial fluid pressure (includes insertion of device, eg, wick catheter technique, needle manometer technique) in detection of muscle compartment syndrome

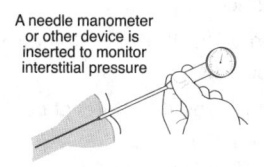

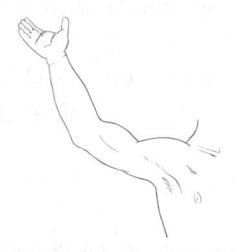

Explanation

The physician inserts an interstitial fluid pressure monitoring device into a muscle compartment using a wick catheter, needle, or other method. The physician checks the monitoring device for escalation of pressure, which indicates developing compartment syndrome and tissue ischemia. Once the data has been gathered, the catheter or needle is removed.

Coding Tips

This code is used to report monitoring by a slit catheter or side-ported needle. Any medical or surgical treatment of compartment syndrome is reported additionally. Surgical trays, A4550, are not separately reimbursed by Medicare; however, other third-party payers may cover them. Check with the specific payer to determine coverage.

ICD-9-CM Procedural

83.29 Other diagnostic procedures on muscle, tendon, fascia, and bursa, including that of hand

Anesthesia

20950 01610, 01710, 01810

ICD-9-CM Diagnostic

286.6 Defibrination syndrome
443.0 Raynaud's syndrome — (Use additional code to identify gangrene: 785.4)
728.86 Necrotizing fasciitis — (Use additional code to identify infectious organism, 041.00-041.89, 785.4, if applicable)
729.71 Nontraumatic compartment syndrome of upper extremity — (Code first, if applicable, postprocedural complication: 998.89)
785.4 Gangrene — (Code first any associated underlying condition)
925.2 Crushing injury of neck — (Use additional code to identify any associated injuries, such as: 800-829, 850.0-854.1, 860.0-869.1)
926.11 Crushing injury of back — (Use additional code to identify any associated injuries: 800-829, 850.0-854.1, 860.0-869.1)
926.19 Crushing injury of other specified sites of trunk — (Use additional code to identify any associated injuries: 800-829, 850.0-854.1, 860.0-869.1)
926.8 Crushing injury of multiple sites of trunk — (Use additional code to identify any associated injuries: 800-829, 850.0-854.1, 860.0-869.1)
927.00 Crushing injury of shoulder region — (Use additional code to identify any associated injuries: 800-829, 850.0-854.1, 860.0-869.1)
927.01 Crushing injury of scapular region — (Use additional code to identify any associated injuries: 800-829, 850.0-854.1, 860.0-869.1)
927.02 Crushing injury of axillary region — (Use additional code to identify any associated injuries: 800-829, 850.0-854.1, 860.0-869.1)
927.03 Crushing injury of upper arm — (Use additional code to identify any associated injuries: 800-829, 850.0-854.1, 860.0-869.1)
927.09 Crushing injury of multiple sites of upper arm — (Use additional code to identify any associated injuries: 800-829, 850.0-854.1, 860.0-869.1)
927.10 Crushing injury of forearm — (Use additional code to identify any associated injuries: 800-829, 850.0-854.1, 860.0-869.1)
927.11 Crushing injury of elbow — (Use additional code to identify any associated injuries: 800-829, 850.0-854.1, 860.0-869.1)
927.3 Crushing injury of finger(s) — (Use additional code to identify any associated injuries: 800-829, 850.0-854.1, 860.0-869.1)
927.8 Crushing injury of multiple sites of upper limb — (Use additional code to identify any associated injuries: 800-829, 850.0-854.1, 860.0-869.1)
958.91 Traumatic compartment syndrome of upper extremity

Terms To Know

axillary region. Pertaining to the area immediately surrounding the armpit.

gangrene. Death of tissue, usually resulting from a loss of vascular supply, followed by a bacterial attack or onset of disease.

infection. Presence of microorganisms in body tissues that may result in cellular damage.

ischemia. Deficiency in blood supply causing tissues to be deprived of oxygen, resulting from trauma, mechanical or functional constriction of blood vessels, or a physical obstruction.

scapular region. Pertaining to the shoulder blade area.

wick catheter. Device used to monitor interstitial fluid pressure, and sometimes used intraoperatively during fasciotomy procedures to evaluate the effectiveness of the decompression.

CCI Version 16.3

0213T, 0216T, 0228T, 0230T, 11010-11012❖, 36000, 36400-36410, 36420-36430, 36440, 36600, 36640, 37202, 43752, 51701-51703, 62310-62319, 64400-64435, 64445-64450, 64479, 64483, 64490, 64493, 64505-64530, 69990, 93000-93010, 93040-93042, 93318, 94002, 94200, 94250, 94680-94690, 94770, 95812-95816, 95819, 95822, 95829, 95900, 95955, 96360, 96365, 96372, 96374-96376, 99148-99149, 99150

Note: These CCI edits are used for Medicare. Other payers may reimburse on codes listed above.

Medicare Edits

	Fac RVU	Non-Fac RVU	FUD	Assist
20950	2.65	7.17	0	80

Medicare References: 100-4,12,30

20974-20975

20974 Electrical stimulation to aid bone healing; noninvasive (nonoperative)
20975 invasive (operative)

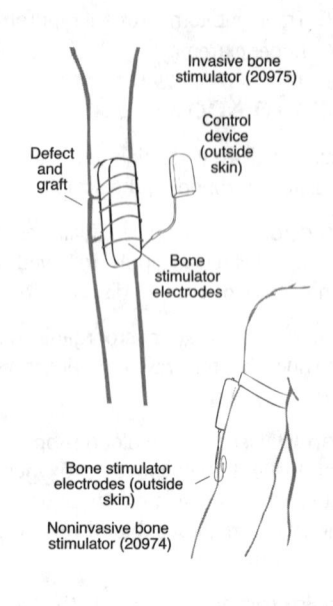

Explanation

The physician performs electrical stimulation of bone. The physician places electrodes over the skin surface along the region of a fracture or defect and then administers a low voltage current. This is a non-surgical technique used to stimulate bone healing. Report 20975 if invasive.

Coding Tips

As "exempt from modifier 51," 20974–20975 have not been designated in CPT as "add-on" services/procedures. However, codes identified as exempt from modifier 51 are not subject to multiple procedure rules. No reimbursement reduction or modifier 51 is applied. For noninvasive low intensity ultrasound stimulation for bone healing, see 20979.

ICD-9-CM Procedural

- 78.90 Insertion of bone growth stimulator, unspecified site
- 78.91 Insertion of bone growth stimulator into scapula, clavicle and thorax (ribs and sternum)
- 78.92 Insertion of bone growth stimulator into humerus
- 78.93 Insertion of bone growth stimulator into radius and ulna
- 78.94 Insertion of bone growth stimulator into carpals and metacarpals
- 78.99 Insertion of bone growth stimulator into other bone
- 83.92 Insertion or replacement of skeletal muscle stimulator
- 99.86 Non-invasive placement of bone growth stimulator

Anesthesia

20974 00300, 00400
20975 01830

ICD-9-CM Diagnostic

- 733.82 Nonunion of fracture
- 805.01 Closed fracture of first cervical vertebra without mention of spinal cord injury
- 805.02 Closed fracture of second cervical vertebra without mention of spinal cord injury
- 805.03 Closed fracture of third cervical vertebra without mention of spinal cord injury
- 805.04 Closed fracture of fourth cervical vertebra without mention of spinal cord injury
- 805.05 Closed fracture of fifth cervical vertebra without mention of spinal cord injury
- 805.06 Closed fracture of sixth cervical vertebra without mention of spinal cord injury
- 805.07 Closed fracture of seventh cervical vertebra without mention of spinal cord injury
- 805.11 Open fracture of first cervical vertebra without mention of spinal cord injury
- 805.12 Open fracture of second cervical vertebra without mention of spinal cord injury
- 805.13 Open fracture of third cervical vertebra without mention of spinal cord injury
- 805.14 Open fracture of fourth cervical vertebra without mention of spinal cord injury
- 805.15 Open fracture of fifth cervical vertebra without mention of spinal cord injury
- 805.16 Open fracture of sixth cervical vertebra without mention of spinal cord injury
- 805.17 Open fracture of seventh cervical vertebra without mention of spinal cord injury
- 805.2 Closed fracture of dorsal (thoracic) vertebra without mention of spinal cord injury
- 805.3 Open fracture of dorsal (thoracic) vertebra without mention of spinal cord injury
- 805.4 Closed fracture of lumbar vertebra without mention of spinal cord injury
- 805.5 Open fracture of lumbar vertebra without mention of spinal cord injury
- 812.01 Closed fracture of surgical neck of humerus
- 812.02 Closed fracture of anatomical neck of humerus
- 812.09 Other closed fractures of upper end of humerus
- 812.12 Open fracture of anatomical neck of humerus
- 812.13 Open fracture of greater tuberosity of humerus
- 812.31 Open fracture of shaft of humerus
- 812.41 Closed fracture of supracondylar humerus
- 812.52 Open fracture of lateral condyle of humerus
- 812.53 Open fracture of medial condyle of humerus

CCI Version 16.3

0213T, 0216T, 0228T, 0230T, 11010-11012❖, 36000, 36400-36410, 36420-36430, 36440, 36600, 36640, 37202, 43752, 51701-51703, 62310-62319, 64400-64435, 64445-64450, 64479, 64483, 64490, 64493, 64505-64530, 69990, 93000-93010, 93040-93042, 93318, 94002, 94200, 94250, 94680-94690, 94770, 95812-95816, 95819, 95822, 95829, 95955, 96360, 96365, 96372, 96374-96376, 97032, 99148-99149, 99150

Also not with 20974: G0281, G0283
Also not with 20975: 20974

Note: These CCI edits are used for Medicare. Other payers may reimburse on codes listed above.

Medicare Edits

	Fac RVU	Non-Fac RVU	FUD	Assist
20974	1.42	2.03	0	N/A
20975	5.19	5.19	0	80

Medicare References: 100-2,15,260; 100-3,150.2; 100-4,12,30; 100-4,12,90.3; 100-4,14,10

20979

20979 Low intensity ultrasound stimulation to aid bone healing, noninvasive (nonoperative)

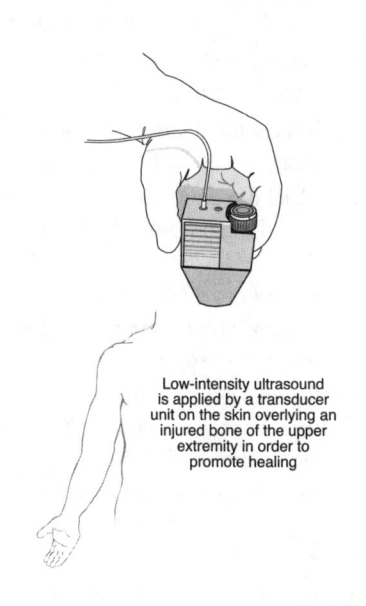

Low-intensity ultrasound is applied by a transducer unit on the skin overlying an injured bone of the upper extremity in order to promote healing

Explanation

A rehabilitation specialist or physical therapist applies low-intensity ultrasound to a bone by placing a transducer on the skin to stimulate bone healing.

Coding Tips

For electrical stimulation to aid bone healing, see 20974–20975.

ICD-9-CM Procedural

93.35 Other heat therapy

Anesthesia

20979 N/A

ICD-9-CM Diagnostic

733.82 Nonunion of fracture
805.01 Closed fracture of first cervical vertebra without mention of spinal cord injury
805.02 Closed fracture of second cervical vertebra without mention of spinal cord injury
805.03 Closed fracture of third cervical vertebra without mention of spinal cord injury
805.04 Closed fracture of fourth cervical vertebra without mention of spinal cord injury
805.05 Closed fracture of fifth cervical vertebra without mention of spinal cord injury
805.06 Closed fracture of sixth cervical vertebra without mention of spinal cord injury
805.07 Closed fracture of seventh cervical vertebra without mention of spinal cord injury
805.08 Closed fracture of multiple cervical vertebrae without mention of spinal cord injury
805.11 Open fracture of first cervical vertebra without mention of spinal cord injury
805.12 Open fracture of second cervical vertebra without mention of spinal cord injury
805.13 Open fracture of third cervical vertebra without mention of spinal cord injury
805.14 Open fracture of fourth cervical vertebra without mention of spinal cord injury
805.15 Open fracture of fifth cervical vertebra without mention of spinal cord injury
805.16 Open fracture of sixth cervical vertebra without mention of spinal cord injury
805.17 Open fracture of seventh cervical vertebra without mention of spinal cord injury
805.18 Open fracture of multiple cervical vertebrae without mention of spinal cord injury
805.2 Closed fracture of dorsal (thoracic) vertebra without mention of spinal cord injury
805.3 Open fracture of dorsal (thoracic) vertebra without mention of spinal cord injury
805.4 Closed fracture of lumbar vertebra without mention of spinal cord injury
805.5 Open fracture of lumbar vertebra without mention of spinal cord injury
810.02 Closed fracture of shaft of clavicle
810.12 Open fracture of shaft of clavicle
811.01 Closed fracture of acromial process of scapula
812.01 Closed fracture of surgical neck of humerus
812.02 Closed fracture of anatomical neck of humerus
812.09 Other closed fractures of upper end of humerus
812.11 Open fracture of surgical neck of humerus
812.12 Open fracture of anatomical neck of humerus
812.13 Open fracture of greater tuberosity of humerus
812.20 Closed fracture of unspecified part of humerus
812.31 Open fracture of shaft of humerus
812.44 Closed fracture of unspecified condyle(s) of humerus
812.49 Other closed fracture of lower end of humerus
812.52 Open fracture of lateral condyle of humerus
812.53 Open fracture of medial condyle of humerus
812.54 Open fracture of unspecified condyle(s) of humerus
812.59 Other open fracture of lower end of humerus
817.0 Multiple closed fractures of hand bones
817.1 Multiple open fractures of hand bones

CCI Version 16.3

0213T, 0216T, 0228T, 0230T, 36000, 36400-36410, 36420-36430, 36440, 36600, 36640, 37202, 43752, 51701-51703, 62310-62319, 64400-64435, 64445-64450, 64479, 64483, 64490, 64493, 64505-64530, 93000-93010, 93040-93042, 93318, 94002, 94200, 94250, 94680-94690, 94770, 95812-95816, 95819, 95822, 95829, 95955, 96360, 96365, 96372, 96374-96376, 99148-99149, 99150

Note: These CCI edits are used for Medicare. Other payers may reimburse on codes listed above.

Medicare Edits

	Fac RVU	Non-Fac RVU	FUD	Assist
20979	0.99	1.52	0	N/A

Medicare References: 100-3,220.5; 100-4,12,30

20982

20982 Ablation, bone tumor(s) (eg, osteoid osteoma, metastasis) radiofrequency, percutaneous, including computed tomographic guidance

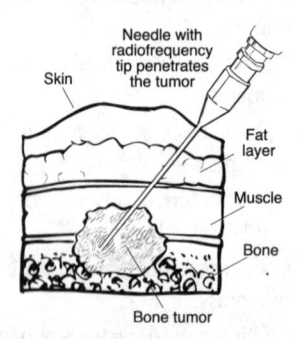

Explanation

Percutaneous radiofrequency ablation of bone tumors may be done as a safe and effective alternative or adjunct to radiation/chemotherapy for metastatic bone cancer lesions and as an effective alternative/adjunct to surgical treatment for benign, but painful, osteoid osteomas. Tumors are destroyed using heat energy, basically "cooking" tumors through a needle. This procedure is performed under conscious sedation or general anesthesia. The patient is connected to an electrical circuit by placing grounding pads on the thighs. A tiny needle-electrode with an insulated shaft, and an uninsulated tip is inserted through the skin, directly into the tumor. Ultrasound, CT scan, or MRI may be used to guide the needle. This code includes CT guidance. The appropriate amount of wattage and current are sent through the needle from a generator. Active ablation is done for about 10 to 15 minutes. The energy leads to cell death and coagulation, resulting in a sphere of dead tissue after every treatment session. A small margin of normal tissue next to tumors is also burned, to try to leave no single tumor cell behind.

Coding Tips

When 20982 is performed with another separately identifiable procedure, the highest dollar value code is listed as the primary procedure and subsequent procedures are appended with modifier 51. Conscious sedation performed with 20982 is considered to be an integral part of the procedure and is not reported separately. However, anesthesia services (00100–01999) may be billed separately when performed by a physician (or other qualified provider) other than the physician performing the procedure.

ICD-9-CM Procedural

01.6	Excision of lesion of skull
76.2	Local excision or destruction of lesion of facial bone
77.60	Local excision of lesion or tissue of bone, unspecified site
77.61	Local excision of lesion or tissue of scapula, clavicle, and thorax (ribs and sternum)
77.62	Local excision of lesion or tissue of humerus
77.63	Local excision of lesion or tissue of radius and ulna
77.64	Local excision of lesion or tissue of carpals and metacarpals
77.69	Local excision of lesion or tissue of other bone, except facial bones

Anesthesia
20982 00450, 00640, 01620, 01730, 01820

ICD-9-CM Diagnostic

170.0	Malignant neoplasm of bones of skull and face, except mandible
170.1	Malignant neoplasm of mandible
170.2	Malignant neoplasm of vertebral column, excluding sacrum and coccyx
170.3	Malignant neoplasm of ribs, sternum, and clavicle
170.4	Malignant neoplasm of scapula and long bones of upper limb
170.5	Malignant neoplasm of short bones of upper limb
170.9	Malignant neoplasm of bone and articular cartilage, site unspecified
198.5	Secondary malignant neoplasm of bone and bone marrow
209.73	Secondary neuroendocrine tumor of bone
213.0	Benign neoplasm of bones of skull and face
213.1	Benign neoplasm of lower jaw bone
213.2	Benign neoplasm of vertebral column, excluding sacrum and coccyx
213.3	Benign neoplasm of ribs, sternum, and clavicle
213.4	Benign neoplasm of scapula and long bones of upper limb
213.5	Benign neoplasm of short bones of upper limb
213.9	Benign neoplasm of bone and articular cartilage, site unspecified
238.0	Neoplasm of uncertain behavior of bone and articular cartilage
239.2	Neoplasms of unspecified nature of bone, soft tissue, and skin
731.3	Major osseous defects — (Code first underlying disease: 170.0-170.9, 730.00-730.29, 733.00-733.09, 733.40-733.49, 996.45)
V10.90	Personal history of unspecified malignant neoplasm
V10.91	Personal history of malignant neuroendocrine tumor — (Code first any continuing functional activity, such as: carcinoid syndrome (259.2))

Terms To Know

ablation. Removal or destruction of a body part or tissue or its function. Ablation may be performed by surgical means, hormones, drugs, radiofrequency, heat, chemical application, or other methods.

coagulation. Clot formation.

percutaneous. Through the skin.

tumor. Pathological swelling or enlargement; a neoplastic growth of uncontrolled, abnormal multiplication of cells.

ultrasound. Imaging using ultra-high sound frequency bounced off body structures.

CCI Version 16.3

0213T, 0216T, 0228T, 0230T, 36000, 36400-36410, 36420-36430, 36440, 36600, 36640, 37202, 43752, 51701-51703, 62310-62319, 64400-64435, 64445-64450, 64479, 64483, 64490, 64493, 64505-64530, 69990, 76000-76001, 76940, 76998, 77002, 77012-77013, 77021-77022, 93000-93010, 93040-93042, 93318, 94002, 94200, 94250, 94680-94690, 94770, 95812-95816, 95819, 95822, 95829, 95955, 96360, 96365, 96372, 96374-96376, 99143-99149, 99150, J0670, J2001

Note: These CCI edits are used for Medicare. Other payers may reimburse on codes listed above.

Medicare Edits

	Fac RVU	Non-Fac RVU	FUD	Assist
20982	11.38	105.58	0	N/A

Medicare References: 100-4,12,30; 100-4,12,40.7

20985

20985 Computer-assisted surgical navigational procedure for musculoskeletal procedures, image-less (List separately in addition to code for primary procedure)

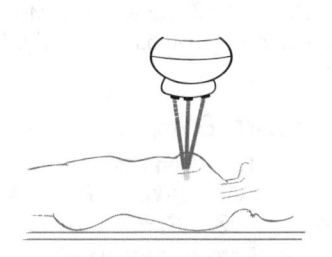

Surgical navigation is aided by computer assistance

Explanation
Imageless computer-assisted surgery (CAS) is an adjunct process used in conjunction with certain orthopaedic procedures. Using such tools as markers, reference frames, intraoperative sensing, and computer workstations, imageless computer-assisted navigational procedures increase visualization of the surgical field and aid in precise navigation with minimally invasive approaches. Imageless navigation uses angles and measurements (kinematics) for anatomy determination. Through direct imageless applications, landmarks are established on a universal limb model. This application requires touch-pointing the anatomic landmarks, which are then registered in the computer for use in accurate navigation and measurement in relation to any bone or instrument movement as the surgery is performed. This application provides a way to establish coordinates as an aid for precisely locating anatomical structures in open or percutaneous procedures without the use of preoperative or intraoperative images. Code 20985 is reported in addition to the procedure code when the physician uses an imageless system to help determine coordinates.

Coding Tips
As an "add-on" code, 20985 is not subject to multiple procedure rules. No reimbursement reduction or modifier 51 is applied. Add-on codes describe additional intra-service work associated with the primary procedure. They are performed by the same physician on the same date of service as the primary service/procedure, and must never be reported as a stand-alone code. Do not report 20985 with 61795. For computer-assisted navigational procedures with image guidance, see 0054T and 0055T.

ICD-9-CM Procedural
00.34   Imageless computer assisted surgery

Anesthesia
20985   N/A

ICD-9-CM Diagnostic
The ICD-9-CM diagnostic code(s) would be the same as the actual procedure performed because these are in-addition-to codes.

Terms To Know
fluoroscopy. Radiology technique that allows visual examination of part of the body or a function of an organ using a device that projects an x-ray image on a fluorescent screen.

ultrasound. Imaging using ultra-high sound frequency bounced off body structures.

CCI Version 16.3
0213T, 0216T, 36000, 36410, 37202, 62318-62319, 64415-64417, 64450, 64490, 64493, 69990, 76000-76001, 76380, 76942, 76970, 76998, 77002, 77011-77012, 77021, 96360, 96365, 96372, 96374-96376

Note: These CCI edits are used for Medicare. Other payers may reimburse on codes listed above.

Medicare Edits

	Fac RVU	Non-Fac RVU	FUD	Assist
20985	4.39	4.39	N/A	80

Medicare References: None

21550

21550 Biopsy, soft tissue of neck or thorax

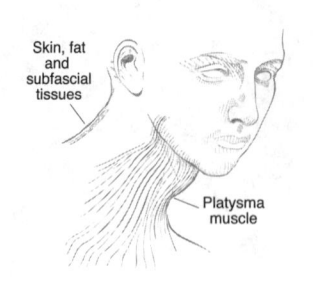

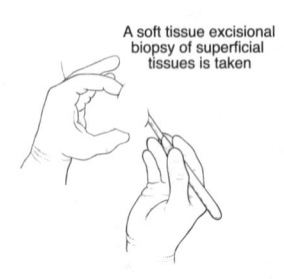

Skin, fat and subfascial tissues

Platysma muscle

A soft tissue excisional biopsy of superficial tissues is taken

Explanation

The physician performs a biopsy of the soft tissues of the neck or thorax. With proper anesthesia administered, the physician identifies the mass through palpation and x-ray (reported separately), if needed. An incision is made over the site and dissection is taken down to the subcutaneous fat or further into the fascia or muscle to reach the lesion. A portion of the tissue mass is excised and submitted for pathology. The area is irrigated and the incision is closed with layered sutures.

Coding Tips

Note that 21550 is for an incisional biopsy. For a needle biopsy of muscle, see 20206. A biopsy is not reported separately when followed by an excisional removal during the same operative session. When 21550 is performed with another separately identifiable procedure, the highest dollar value code is listed as the primary procedure and subsequent procedures are appended with modifier 51. Surgical trays, A4550, are not separately reimbursed by Medicare; however, other third-party payers may cover them. Check with the specific payer to determine coverage.

ICD-9-CM Procedural

- 34.23 Biopsy of chest wall
- 83.21 Open biopsy of soft tissue

Anesthesia

21550 00300

ICD-9-CM Diagnostic

- 171.0 Malignant neoplasm of connective and other soft tissue of head, face, and neck
- 171.4 Malignant neoplasm of connective and other soft tissue of thorax
- 195.0 Malignant neoplasm of head, face, and neck
- 195.1 Malignant neoplasm of thorax
- 198.89 Secondary malignant neoplasm of other specified sites
- 215.0 Other benign neoplasm of connective and other soft tissue of head, face, and neck
- 215.4 Other benign neoplasm of connective and other soft tissue of thorax
- 229.8 Benign neoplasm of other specified sites
- 234.8 Carcinoma in situ of other specified sites
- 238.1 Neoplasm of uncertain behavior of connective and other soft tissue
- 239.89 Neoplasms of unspecified nature, other specified sites
- 709.9 Unspecified disorder of skin and subcutaneous tissue
- 782.2 Localized superficial swelling, mass, or lump
- 784.2 Swelling, mass, or lump in head and neck

Terms To Know

benign. Mild or nonmalignant in nature.

carcinoma in situ. Malignancy that arises from the cells of the vessel, gland, or organ of origin that remains confined to that site or has not invaded neighboring tissue.

malignant. Any condition tending to progress toward death, specifically an invasive tumor with a loss of cellular differentiation that has the ability to spread or metastasize to other areas in the body.

neoplasm. New abnormal growth, tumor.

secondary. Second in order of occurrence or importance, or appearing during the course of another disease or condition.

soft tissue. Nonepithelial tissues outside of the skeleton that includes subcutaneous adipose tissue, fibrous tissue, fascia, muscles, blood and lymph vessels, and peripheral nervous system tissue.

subcutaneous tissue. Sheet or wide band of adipose (fat) and areolar connective tissue in two layers attached to the dermis.

CCI Version 16.3

0213T, 0216T, 0228T, 0230T, 10021-10022, 10060, 10140, 10160, 20100, 36000, 36400-36410, 36420-36430, 36440, 36600, 36640, 37202, 38500, 43752, 51701-51703, 62310-62319, 64400-64435, 64445-64450, 64479, 64483, 64490, 64493, 64505-64530, 69990, 93000-93010, 93040-93042, 93318, 94002, 94200, 94250, 94680-94690, 94770, 95812-95816, 95819, 95822, 95829, 95955, 96360, 96365, 96372, 96374-96376, 99148-99149, 99150, J0670, J2001

Note: These CCI edits are used for Medicare. Other payers may reimburse on codes listed above.

Medicare Edits

	Fac RVU	Non-Fac RVU	FUD	Assist
21550	4.65	7.52	10	N/A

Medicare References: None

21555-21556 (21552, 21554)

21555 Excision, tumor, soft tissue of neck or anterior thorax, subcutaneous; less than 3 cm
21552 3 cm or greater
21556 Excision, tumor, soft tissue of neck or anterior thorax, subfascial (eg, intramuscular); less than 5 cm
21554 5 cm or greater

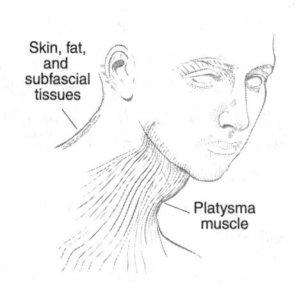

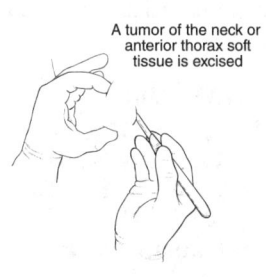

Explanation

The physician removes a tumor from the soft tissue of the neck or anterior thorax (chest) that is located in the subcutaneous tissue in 21552 or 21555 and in the deep soft tissue, below the fascial plane or within the muscle, in 21554 or 21556. With the proper anesthesia administered, the physician makes an incision in the skin overlying the mass and dissects down to the tumor. The extent of the tumor is identified and a dissection is undertaken all the way around the tumor. A portion of neighboring soft tissue may also be removed to ensure adequate removal of all tumor tissue. A drain may be inserted and the incision is repaired with layers of sutures, staples, or Steri-strips. Report 21555 for excision of subcutaneous tumors less than 3 cm and 21552 for excision of subcutaneous tumors 3 cm or greater. Report 21556 for excision of subfascial or intramuscular tumors less than 5 cm and 21554 for excision of subfascial or intramuscular tumors 5 cm or greater.

Coding Tips

Codes 21552 and 21554 are resequenced codes and will not display in numeric order. When any of these procedures is performed with another separately identifiable procedure, the highest dollar value code is listed as the primary procedure and subsequent procedures are appended with modifier 51. If significant additional time and effort is documented, append modifier 22 and submit a cover letter and operative report. An excisional biopsy is not reported separately when a therapeutic excision is performed during the same surgical session. Report any free grafts or flaps separately. Surgical trays, A4550, are not separately reimbursed by Medicare; however, other third-party payers may cover them. Check with the specific payer to determine coverage.

ICD-9-CM Procedural

83.32	Excision of lesion of muscle
83.39	Excision of lesion of other soft tissue
83.49	Other excision of soft tissue
86.3	Other local excision or destruction of lesion or tissue of skin and subcutaneous tissue
86.4	Radical excision of skin lesion

Anesthesia

21552 00300, 00400
21554 00300, 00400
21555 00300
21556 00300

ICD-9-CM Diagnostic

171.0	Malignant neoplasm of connective and other soft tissue of head, face, and neck
171.4	Malignant neoplasm of connective and other soft tissue of thorax
171.8	Malignant neoplasm of other specified sites of connective and other soft tissue
195.0	Malignant neoplasm of head, face, and neck
195.1	Malignant neoplasm of thorax
198.89	Secondary malignant neoplasm of other specified sites
199.0	Disseminated malignant neoplasm
199.1	Other malignant neoplasm of unspecified site
209.32	Merkel cell carcinoma of the scalp and neck
209.35	Merkel cell carcinoma of the trunk
209.75	Secondary Merkel cell carcinoma
214.1	Lipoma of other skin and subcutaneous tissue
214.8	Lipoma of other specified sites
215.0	Other benign neoplasm of connective and other soft tissue of head, face, and neck
215.4	Other benign neoplasm of connective and other soft tissue of thorax
229.8	Benign neoplasm of other specified sites
234.8	Carcinoma in situ of other specified sites
238.1	Neoplasm of uncertain behavior of connective and other soft tissue
239.2	Neoplasms of unspecified nature of bone, soft tissue, and skin
782.2	Localized superficial swelling, mass, or lump
784.2	Swelling, mass, or lump in head and neck
786.6	Swelling, mass, or lump in chest

CCI Version 16.3

0228T, 0230T, 10021-10022, 10060, 10140, 10160, 11010-11012❖, 11040-11044, 12001-12007, 12020-12047, 13100-13101, 13131-13132, 36000, 36400-36410, 36420-36430, 36440, 36600, 36640, 37202, 38500-38520❖, 38542-38555❖, 38700❖, 38720❖, 38724❖, 43752, 51701-51703, 62310-62319, 64400-64435, 64445-64450, 64479, 64483, 64505-64530, 69990, 93000-93010, 93040-93042, 93318, 94002, 94200, 94250, 94680-94690, 94770, 95812-95816, 95819, 95822, 95829, 95955, 96360, 96365, 96372, 96374-96376, 99148-99149, 99150

Also not with 21552: 0213T, 0216T, 21501, 21550, 21555, 64490, 64493, J2001

Also not with 21554: 0213T, 0216T, 21501, 21550-21552, 21555-21556, 64490, 64493

Also not with 21555: 21550, J0670, J2001

Also not with 21556: 21501, 21550-21552, 21555

Note: These CCI edits are used for Medicare. Other payers may reimburse on codes listed above.

Medicare Edits

	Fac RVU	Non-Fac RVU	FUD	Assist
21552	13.41	13.41	90	80
21554	22.0	22.0	90	80
21555	9.02	11.98	90	N/A
21556	15.15	15.15	90	N/A

Medicare References: 100-2,15,260; 100-4,12,30; 100-4,12,90.3; 100-4,14,10

21557-21558

21557 Radical resection of tumor (eg, malignant neoplasm), soft tissue of neck or anterior thorax; less than 5 cm
21558 5 cm or greater

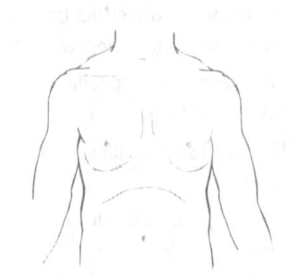

Radical resection of soft tissue tumor of the neck or anterior thorax is reported with 21557 if less than 5 cm and with 21558 if greater than 5 cm

Explanation

The physician performs a radical resection of a malignant soft tissue tumor from the neck or anterior thorax, not involving bone. An incision is made over the tumor and dissection exposes it. The tumor and any adjacent tissue that may be affected by the spread of the neoplasm are excised. Large resections may be needed. The type and stage of the lesion determines the extent of the tumor margin resection area. Muscle or fascia may need to be repaired and drains may be placed. The surgical wound is repaired by intermediate or complex closure, adjacent tissue transfer, or graft. Report 21557 for excision of tumors less than 5 cm and 21558 for excision of tumors 5 cm or greater.

Coding Tips

An excisional biopsy is not reported separately when a therapeutic excision is performed during the same surgical session. Report any free grafts or flaps separately.

ICD-9-CM Procedural

- 83.32 Excision of lesion of muscle
- 83.39 Excision of lesion of other soft tissue
- 83.49 Other excision of soft tissue
- 86.3 Other local excision or destruction of lesion or tissue of skin and subcutaneous tissue
- 86.4 Radical excision of skin lesion

Anesthesia

21557 00300
21558 00300, 00400

ICD-9-CM Diagnostic

- 171.0 Malignant neoplasm of connective and other soft tissue of head, face, and neck
- 171.4 Malignant neoplasm of connective and other soft tissue of thorax
- 171.8 Malignant neoplasm of other specified sites of connective and other soft tissue
- 195.0 Malignant neoplasm of head, face, and neck
- 195.1 Malignant neoplasm of thorax
- 198.89 Secondary malignant neoplasm of other specified sites
- 199.0 Disseminated malignant neoplasm
- 199.1 Other malignant neoplasm of unspecified site
- 209.32 Merkel cell carcinoma of the scalp and neck
- 209.35 Merkel cell carcinoma of the trunk
- 209.75 Secondary Merkel cell carcinoma
- 214.1 Lipoma of other skin and subcutaneous tissue
- 214.8 Lipoma of other specified sites
- 215.0 Other benign neoplasm of connective and other soft tissue of head, face, and neck
- 215.4 Other benign neoplasm of connective and other soft tissue of thorax
- 229.8 Benign neoplasm of other specified sites
- 234.8 Carcinoma in situ of other specified sites
- 238.1 Neoplasm of uncertain behavior of connective and other soft tissue
- 239.2 Neoplasms of unspecified nature of bone, soft tissue, and skin
- 782.2 Localized superficial swelling, mass, or lump
- 784.2 Swelling, mass, or lump in head and neck
- 786.6 Swelling, mass, or lump in chest

Terms To Know

radical resection. Removal of an entire tumor (e.g., malignant neoplasm) along with a large area of surrounding tissue, including adjacent lymph nodes that may have been infiltrated.

soft tissue. Nonepithelial tissues outside of the skeleton that includes subcutaneous adipose tissue, fibrous tissue, fascia, muscles, blood and lymph vessels, and peripheral nervous system tissue.

CCI Version 16.3

0213T, 0216T, 0228T, 0230T, 10060, 10140, 10160, 11010-11012❖, 11040-11044, 12001-12007, 12020-12047, 13100-13101, 13131-13132, 21501, 36000, 36400-36410, 36420-36430, 36440, 36600, 36640, 37202, 38500-38520❖, 38542-38555❖, 38700❖, 38720❖, 38724❖, 43752, 51701-51703, 62310-62319, 64400-64435, 64445-64450, 64479, 64483, 64490, 64493, 64505-64530, 69990, 93000-93010, 93040-93042, 93318, 94002, 94200, 94250, 94680-94690, 94770, 95812-95816, 95819, 95822, 95829, 95955, 96360, 96365, 96372, 96374-96376, 99148-99149, 99150

Also not with 21557: 21550-21556
Also not with 21558: 21550-21557

Note: These CCI edits are used for Medicare. Other payers may reimburse on codes listed above.

Medicare Edits

	Fac RVU	Non-Fac RVU	FUD	Assist
21557	26.26	26.26	90	80
21558	40.9	40.9	90	80

Medicare References: None

21600

21600 Excision of rib, partial

Typical access incisions for partial rib removal

A portion of a single rib is surgically removed

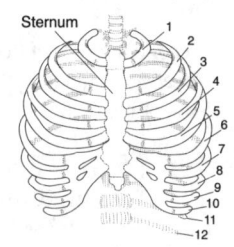

The ribs are the framework of the thoracic cage. Ten pairs connect anteriorly to the sternum and two pairs (11 and 12) float. Ribs numbered 7 to 10 fuse to form the costal margin before attaching to the sternum

Explanation

The physician removes part of one rib. With the patient under anesthesia, the physician makes an incision in the skin of the chest overlying the rib. The tissues are dissected deep to the rib itself. The rib is identified. The physician removes the desired part of the rib using a saw and other instruments. The remaining pieces of the rib and the wound itself are irrigated and debrided. The incision is sutured in layers.

Coding Tips

If this procedure is a component of a more complex service, it is not reported separately. When 21600 is performed with another separately identifiable procedure, the highest dollar value code is listed as the primary procedure, and subsequent procedures are appended with modifier 51. For excision of the first and/or cervical rib, see 21615–21616. For resection of the cervical rib with division of scalenus anticus, see 21705. For an excision of a chest wall tumor involving the ribs, see 19260–19272. For radical chest wall or rib cage debridement due to an injury, see 11042–11047.

ICD-9-CM Procedural

77.81 Other partial ostectomy of scapula, clavicle, and thorax (ribs and sternum)

Anesthesia

21600 00470

ICD-9-CM Diagnostic

170.3 Malignant neoplasm of ribs, sternum, and clavicle
198.5 Secondary malignant neoplasm of bone and bone marrow
209.73 Secondary neuroendocrine tumor of bone
213.3 Benign neoplasm of ribs, sternum, and clavicle
229.8 Benign neoplasm of other specified sites
238.0 Neoplasm of uncertain behavior of bone and articular cartilage
239.2 Neoplasms of unspecified nature of bone, soft tissue, and skin
730.18 Chronic osteomyelitis, other specified sites — (Use additional code to identify organism: 041.1. Use additional code to identify major osseous defect, if applicable: 731.3)
730.88 Other infections involving bone diseases classified elsewhere, other specified sites — (Use additional code to identify organism: 041.1. Code first underlying disease: 002.0, 015.0-015.9)
731.3 Major osseous defects — (Code first underlying disease: 170.0-170.9, 730.00-730.29, 733.00-733.09, 733.40-733.49, 996.45)
756.2 Cervical rib
756.3 Other congenital anomaly of ribs and sternum
V10.90 Personal history of unspecified malignant neoplasm
V10.91 Personal history of malignant neuroendocrine tumor — (Code first any continuing functional activity, such as: carcinoid syndrome (259.2))

Terms To Know

benign. Mild or nonmalignant in nature.

chronic. Persistent, continuing, or recurring.

congenital. Present at birth, occurring through heredity or an influence during gestation up to the moment of birth.

malignant. Any condition tending to progress toward death, specifically an invasive tumor with a loss of cellular differentiation that has the ability to spread or metastasize to other areas in the body.

neoplasm. New abnormal growth, tumor.

osteomyelitis. Inflammation of bone that may remain localized or spread to the marrow, cortex, or periosteum, in response to an infecting organism, usually bacterial and pyogenic.

secondary. Second in order of occurrence or importance, or appearing during the course of another disease or condition.

CCI Version 16.3

0213T, 0216T, 0228T, 0230T, 11012❖, 21610, 35820, 36000, 36400-36410, 36420-36430, 36440, 36600, 36640, 37202, 43752, 49010, 51701-51703, 62310-62319, 64400-64435, 64445-64450, 64479, 64483, 64490, 64493, 64505-64530, 69990, 93000-93010, 93040-93042, 93318, 94002, 94200, 94250, 94680-94690, 94770, 95812-95816, 95819, 95822, 95829, 95955, 96360, 96365, 96372, 96374-96376, 99148-99149, 99150

Note: These CCI edits are used for Medicare. Other payers may reimburse on codes listed above.

Medicare Edits

	Fac RVU	Non-Fac RVU	FUD	Assist
21600	16.52	16.52	90	80

Medicare References: 100-2,15,260; 100-4,12,30; 100-4,12,90.3; 100-4,14,10

21610

21610 Costotransversectomy (separate procedure)

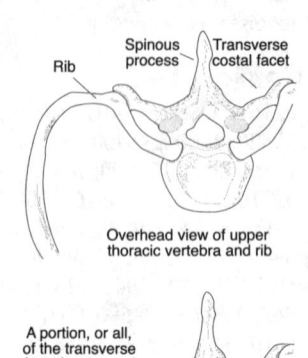

Spinous process, Transverse costal facet, Rib
Overhead view of upper thoracic vertebra and rib

A portion, or all, of the transverse facet is removed along with the part of the rib
Vertebral body

Explanation
The physician resects the costovertebral joint. The physician makes a posterior incision overlying the joint. The tissues are dissected from the joint and the transverse process is cut from the vertebral body. The physician removes all or a portion of the adjacent rib. The incision is closed in sutured layers.

Coding Tips
This separate procedure by definition is usually a component of a more complex service and is not identified separately. When performed alone or with other unrelated procedures/services it may be reported. If performed alone, list the code; if performed with other procedures/services, list the code and append modifier 59.

ICD-9-CM Procedural
77.91 Total ostectomy of scapula, clavicle, and thorax (ribs and sternum)

Anesthesia
21610 00470

ICD-9-CM Diagnostic
170.2 Malignant neoplasm of vertebral column, excluding sacrum and coccyx
170.3 Malignant neoplasm of ribs, sternum, and clavicle
198.5 Secondary malignant neoplasm of bone and bone marrow
209.73 Secondary neuroendocrine tumor of bone
213.2 Benign neoplasm of vertebral column, excluding sacrum and coccyx
213.3 Benign neoplasm of ribs, sternum, and clavicle
229.8 Benign neoplasm of other specified sites
238.0 Neoplasm of uncertain behavior of bone and articular cartilage
239.2 Neoplasms of unspecified nature of bone, soft tissue, and skin
715.09 Generalized osteoarthrosis, involving multiple sites
715.18 Primary localized osteoarthrosis, other specified sites
715.98 Osteoarthrosis, unspecified whether generalized or localized, other specified sites
730.18 Chronic osteomyelitis, other specified sites — (Use additional code to identify organism: 041.1. Use additional code to identify major osseous defect, if applicable: 731.3)
730.88 Other infections involving bone diseases classified elsewhere, other specified sites — (Use additional code to identify organism: 041.1. Code first underlying disease: 002.0, 015.0-015.9)
731.3 Major osseous defects — (Code first underlying disease: 170.0-170.9, 730.00-730.29, 733.00-733.09, 733.40-733.49, 996.45)
756.3 Other congenital anomaly of ribs and sternum
V10.90 Personal history of unspecified malignant neoplasm
V10.91 Personal history of malignant neuroendocrine tumor — (Code first any continuing functional activity, such as: carcinoid syndrome (259.2))

Terms To Know
benign. Mild or nonmalignant in nature.

chronic. Persistent, continuing, or recurring.

malignant. Any condition tending to progress toward death, specifically an invasive tumor with a loss of cellular differentiation that has the ability to spread or metastasize to other areas in the body.

neoplasm. New abnormal growth, tumor.

osteoarthrosis. Most common form of a noninflammatory degenerative joint disease with degenerating articular cartilage, bone enlargement, and synovial membrane changes.

osteomyelitis. Inflammation of bone that may remain localized or spread to the marrow, cortex, or periosteum, in response to an infecting organism, usually bacterial and pyogenic.

posterior. Located in the back part or caudal end of the body.

secondary. Second in order of occurrence or importance, or appearing during the course of another disease or condition.

CCI Version 16.3
0213T, 0216T, 0228T, 0230T, 20101, 36000, 36400-36410, 36420-36430, 36440, 36600, 36640, 37202, 37616, 43752, 51701-51703, 62310-62319, 64400-64435, 64445-64450, 64479, 64483, 64490, 64493, 64505-64530, 69990, 93000-93010, 93040-93042, 93318, 94002, 94200, 94250, 94680-94690, 94770, 95812-95816, 95819, 95822, 95829, 95955, 96360, 96365, 96372, 96374-96376, 99148-99149, 99150

Note: These CCI edits are used for Medicare. Other payers may reimburse on codes listed above.

Medicare Edits

	Fac RVU	Non-Fac RVU	FUD	Assist
21610	34.1	34.1	90	80

Medicare References: 100-2,15,260; 100-4,12,30; 100-4,12,90.3; 100-4,14,10

21615-21616

21615 Excision first and/or cervical rib;
21616 with sympathectomy

Sympathetic nerve pathways serve the thoracic region and a concurrent interruption of these nerves is reported with 21616

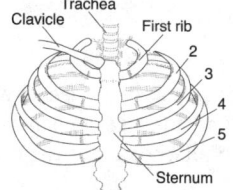

A superior view of C7 showing cervical rib; attachment anteriorly may be to the first rib, or its costal cartilage (Type II), or even the sternum (Type IV); no anterior attachment is also found (Type I)

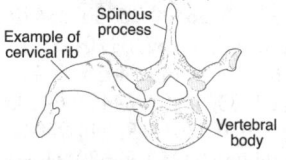

A cervical rib is present on the seventh vertebra in about 1 percent of the population. Removal of the first and/or supernumerary cervical rib is reported with 21615 or 21616

Explanation

The physician performs surgery to remove the first rib and/or an extraneous cervical rib. With the patient under anesthesia, the physician makes an incision in the skin just above the clavicle on the affected side. Tissues are dissected deep to the rib. The rib is identified and the attached soft tissues are carefully debrided. The physician excises the rib using a saw and other surgical instruments. The rib is freed from its articulation and removed. The wound is irrigated thoroughly and closed in layers. A dressing is applied. Report 21616 if a sympathectomy is performed during the procedure.

Coding Tips

These are unilateral procedures. If performed bilaterally, some payers require that the service be reported twice with modifier 50 appended to the second code while others require identification of the service only once with modifier 50 appended. Check with individual payers. Modifier 50 identifies a procedure performed identically on the opposite side of the body (mirror image). For cervical or cervicothoracic sympathectomy not requiring excision of the cervical rib, see 64802–64804.

ICD-9-CM Procedural

05.22   Cervical sympathectomy
77.91   Total ostectomy of scapula, clavicle, and thorax (ribs and sternum)

Anesthesia
00470

ICD-9-CM Diagnostic

353.0   Brachial plexus lesions
443.0   Raynaud's syndrome — (Use additional code to identify gangrene: 785.4)
444.21 Embolism and thrombosis of arteries of upper extremity
723.1   Cervicalgia
723.4   Brachial neuritis or radiculitis nos.
756.2   Cervical rib
786.52 Painful respiration
786.6   Swelling, mass, or lump in chest

Terms To Know

brachial plexus lesions. Acquired defect in tissues along the network of nerves in the shoulder, causing corresponding motor and sensory dysfunction.

cervicalgia. Pain localized to the cervical region, generally referring to the posterior or lateral regions of the neck.

embolism. Obstruction of a blood vessel resulting from a clot or foreign substance.

gangrene. Death of tissue, usually resulting from a loss of vascular supply, followed by a bacterial attack or onset of disease.

lesion. Area of damaged tissue that has lost continuity or function, due to disease or trauma. Lesions may be located on internal structures such as the brain, nerves, or kidneys, or visible on the skin.

neuritis. Inflammation of a nerve or group of nerves, often manifested by loss of function and reflexes, pain, and numbness or tingling.

radiculitis. Pain along an inflamed nerve, with inflammation of the root of the associated spinal nerve.

Raynaud's phenomenon. Vascular disorder resulting in bilateral decreased circulation of the fingers and toes causing a pale or bluish appearance, numbness, tingling, and pain brought on by cold or emotions and relieved with heat.

sympathectomy. Surgical interruption or transection of a sympathetic nervous system pathway.

thrombosis. Condition arising from the presence or formation of blood clots within a blood vessel that may cause vascular obstruction and insufficient oxygenation.

CCI Version 16.3

0213T, 0216T, 0228T, 0230T, 20101, 36000, 36400-36410, 36420-36430, 36440, 36600, 36640, 37202, 43752, 51701-51703, 62310-62319, 64400-64435, 64445-64450, 64479, 64483, 64490, 64493, 64505-64530, 69990, 93000-93010, 93040-93042, 93318, 94002, 94200, 94250, 94680-94690, 94770, 95812-95816, 95819, 95822, 95829, 95955, 96360, 96365, 96372, 96374-96376, 99148-99149, 99150

Also not with 21615: 21600-21610
Also not with 21616: 21600-21615

Note: These CCI edits are used for Medicare. Other payers may reimburse on codes listed above.

Medicare Edits

	Fac RVU	Non-Fac RVU	FUD	Assist
21615	19.58	19.58	90	80
21616	23.91	23.91	90	80

Medicare References: 100-4,12,30

21620

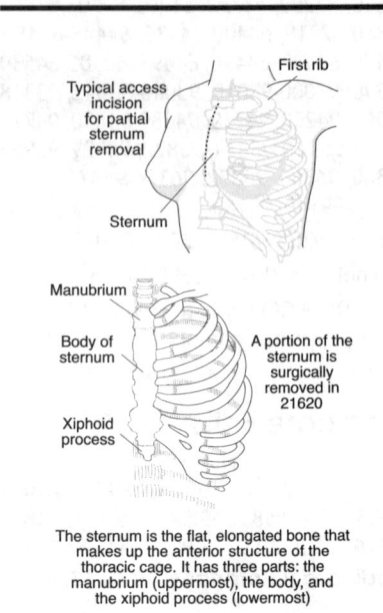

21620 Ostectomy of sternum, partial

Explanation

The physician removes a portion of the sternum from the chest. With the patient under anesthesia, the physician makes an incision in the skin overlying the sternum. This is carried deep through the subcutaneous tissues to the bone. The sternum is identified and soft tissues are debrided. The physician marks the portion of the sternum to be removed. The bone is cut in the appropriate places using a saw and other surgical instruments. The remaining portion of the bone is irrigated and smoothed as needed. The wound is closed in layers and a dressing is applied.

Coding Tips

For sternal debridement, see 21627; for radical resection of the sternum, see 21630–21632. If significant additional time and effort is documented, append modifier 22 and submit a cover letter and operative report. When 21620 is performed with another separately identifiable procedure, the highest dollar value code is listed as the primary procedure, and subsequent procedures are appended with modifier 51.

ICD-9-CM Procedural

77.81 Other partial ostectomy of scapula, clavicle, and thorax (ribs and sternum)

Anesthesia

21620 00470

ICD-9-CM Diagnostic

- 170.3 Malignant neoplasm of ribs, sternum, and clavicle
- 198.5 Secondary malignant neoplasm of bone and bone marrow
- 209.73 Secondary neuroendocrine tumor of bone
- 213.3 Benign neoplasm of ribs, sternum, and clavicle
- 238.0 Neoplasm of uncertain behavior of bone and articular cartilage
- 239.2 Neoplasms of unspecified nature of bone, soft tissue, and skin
- 519.2 Mediastinitis — (Use additional code to identify infectious organism)
- 730.18 Chronic osteomyelitis, other specified sites — (Use additional code to identify organism: 041.1. Use additional code to identify major osseous defect, if applicable: 731.3)
- 730.28 Unspecified osteomyelitis, other specified sites — (Use additional code to identify organism: 041.1. Use additional code to identify major osseous defect, if applicable: 731.3)
- 730.88 Other infections involving bone diseases classified elsewhere, other specified sites — (Use additional code to identify organism: 041.1. Code first underlying disease: 002.0, 015.0-015.9)
- 731.3 Major osseous defects — (Code first underlying disease: 170.0-170.9, 730.00-730.29, 733.00-733.09, 733.40-733.49, 996.45)
- 733.49 Aseptic necrosis of other bone site — (Use additional code to identify major osseous defect, if applicable: 731.3)
- 733.99 Other disorders of bone and cartilage
- V10.90 Personal history of unspecified malignant neoplasm
- V10.91 Personal history of malignant neuroendocrine tumor — (Code first any continuing functional activity, such as: carcinoid syndrome (259.2))

Terms To Know

aseptic necrosis. Death of bone tissue resulting from a disruption in the vascular supply, caused by a noninfectious disease process, such as a fracture or the administration of immunosuppressive drugs.

benign. Mild or nonmalignant in nature.

chronic. Persistent, continuing, or recurring.

malignant. Any condition tending to progress toward death, specifically an invasive tumor with a loss of cellular differentiation that has the ability to spread or metastasize to other areas in the body.

osteomyelitis. Inflammation of bone that may remain localized or spread to the marrow, cortex, or periosteum, in response to an infecting organism, usually bacterial and pyogenic.

subcutaneous tissue. Sheet or wide band of adipose (fat) and areolar connective tissue in two layers attached to the dermis.

CCI Version 16.3

00550, 0213T, 0216T, 0228T, 0230T, 11012❖, 20101, 21750, 35820, 36000, 36400-36410, 36420-36430, 36440, 36600, 36640, 37202, 43752, 51701-51703, 62310-62319, 64400-64435, 64445-64450, 64479, 64483, 64490, 64493, 64505-64530, 69990, 93000-93010, 93040-93042, 93318, 94002, 94200, 94250, 94680-94690, 94770, 95812-95816, 95819, 95822, 95829, 95955, 96360, 96365, 96372, 96374-96376, 99148-99149, 99150

Note: These CCI edits are used for Medicare. Other payers may reimburse on codes listed above.

Medicare Edits

	Fac RVU	Non-Fac RVU	FUD	Assist
21620	15.48	15.48	90	80

Medicare References: None

21627

21627 Sternal debridement

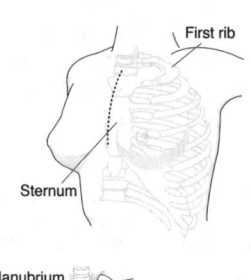

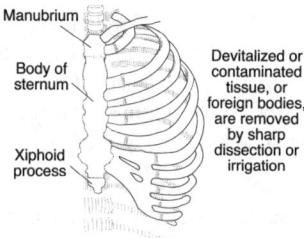

Explanation
The physician performs a debridement of the sternum. With the patient under anesthesia, the physician makes an incision in the skin overlying the sternum. The incision is carried deep to the bone. The sternum is debrided as warranted using any of a variety of hand or powered surgical instruments. Irrigation is used so that debridement can be completed as extensively as indicated. The wound is closed in layers and a dressing is applied.

Coding Tips
This procedure is usually performed to treat postoperative infection following open thoracic surgery. It may also be performed following open injury complicated by infection. For closure of sternotomy separation with debridement, see 21750.

ICD-9-CM Procedural
- 77.61 Local excision of lesion or tissue of scapula, clavicle, and thorax (ribs and sternum)

Anesthesia
21627 00550

ICD-9-CM Diagnostic
- 170.3 Malignant neoplasm of ribs, sternum, and clavicle
- 198.5 Secondary malignant neoplasm of bone and bone marrow
- 209.73 Secondary neuroendocrine tumor of bone
- 213.3 Benign neoplasm of ribs, sternum, and clavicle
- 238.0 Neoplasm of uncertain behavior of bone and articular cartilage
- 239.2 Neoplasms of unspecified nature of bone, soft tissue, and skin
- 519.2 Mediastinitis — (Use additional code to identify infectious organism)
- 730.18 Chronic osteomyelitis, other specified sites — (Use additional code to identify organism: 041.1. Use additional code to identify major osseous defect, if applicable: 731.3)
- 730.28 Unspecified osteomyelitis, other specified sites — (Use additional code to identify organism: 041.1. Use additional code to identify major osseous defect, if applicable: 731.3)
- 730.88 Other infections involving bone diseases classified elsewhere, other specified sites — (Use additional code to identify organism: 041.1. Code first underlying disease: 002.0, 015.0-015.9)
- 731.3 Major osseous defects — (Code first underlying disease: 170.0-170.9, 730.00-730.29, 733.00-733.09, 733.40-733.49, 996.45)
- 733.49 Aseptic necrosis of other bone site — (Use additional code to identify major osseous defect, if applicable: 731.3)
- 875.1 Open wound of chest (wall), complicated
- 998.51 Infected postoperative seroma — (Use additional code to identify organism)
- 998.59 Other postoperative infection — (Use additional code to identify infection)
- 998.83 Non-healing surgical wound

Terms To Know

aseptic necrosis. Death of bone tissue resulting from a disruption in the vascular supply, caused by a noninfectious disease process, such as a fracture or the administration of immunosuppressive drugs.

benign. Mild or nonmalignant in nature.

foreign body. Any object or substance found in an organ and tissue that does not belong under normal circumstances.

infected postoperative seroma. Infection within a tumor-like growth of serum following surgery.

malignant. Any condition tending to progress toward death, specifically an invasive tumor with a loss of cellular differentiation that has the ability to spread or metastasize to other areas in the body.

osteomyelitis. Inflammation of bone that may remain localized or spread to the marrow, cortex, or periosteum, in response to an infecting organism, usually bacterial and pyogenic.

secondary. Second in order of occurrence or importance, or appearing during the course of another disease or condition.

seroma. Tumor-like swelling caused by the collection of serum, or clear fluid, in the tissues.

soft tissue. Nonepithelial tissues outside of the skeleton that includes subcutaneous adipose tissue, fibrous tissue, fascia, muscles, blood and lymph vessels, and peripheral nervous system tissue.

CCI Version 16.3
00550, 0213T, 0216T, 0228T, 0230T, 11012❖, 20101, 20500, 20670-20680, 35820, 36000, 36400-36410, 36420-36430, 36440, 36600, 36640, 37202, 43752, 51701-51703, 62310-62319, 64400-64435, 64445-64450, 64479, 64483, 64490, 64493, 64505-64530, 69990, 93000-93010, 93040-93042, 93318, 94002, 94200, 94250, 94680-94690, 94770, 95812-95816, 95819, 95822, 95829, 95955, 96360, 96365, 96372, 96374-96376, 99148-99149, 99150

Note: These CCI edits are used for Medicare. Other payers may reimburse on codes listed above.

Medicare Edits

	Fac RVU	Non-Fac RVU	FUD	Assist
21627	16.21	16.21	90	80

Medicare References: None

21630-21632

21630 Radical resection of sternum;
21632 with mediastinal lymphadenectomy

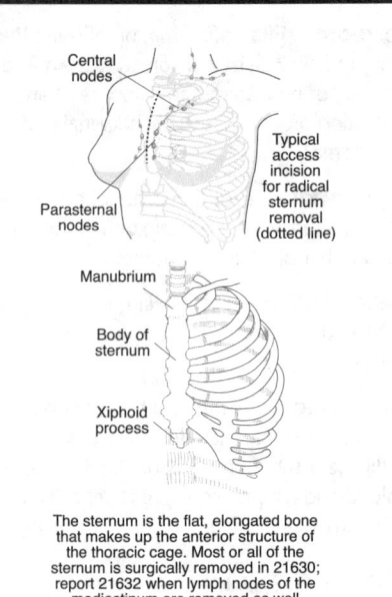

The sternum is the flat, elongated bone that makes up the anterior structure of the thoracic cage. Most or all of the sternum is surgically removed in 21630; report 21632 when lymph nodes of the mediastinum are removed as well

Explanation

The physician removes most or all of the sternum from the chest. With the patient under anesthesia, the physician makes a long incision overlying the sternum and anterior chest. This is carried deep to the bone. Dissection is performed around the sternum. Ribs are disarticulated as needed and thorough debridement is accomplished. Using saws and other surgical instruments, the physician removes the bone. Internal fixation devices (reported separately) are often needed to support the ribs and chest wall. The wound is thoroughly irrigated and closed in layers. Report 21632 if a mediastinal lymphadenectomy is performed during the procedure.

Coding Tips

Debridement, irrigation, and closure are not reported separately. If significant additional time and effort are documented, append modifier 22 and submit a cover letter and operative report. When 21630 or 21632 is performed with another separately identifiable procedure, the highest dollar value code is listed as the primary procedure, and subsequent procedures are appended with modifier 51. If internal fixation devices are necessary, report separately; see 21825.

ICD-9-CM Procedural

- 40.22 Excision of internal mammary lymph node
- 40.3 Regional lymph node excision
- 40.59 Radical excision of other lymph nodes
- 77.81 Other partial ostectomy of scapula, clavicle, and thorax (ribs and sternum)
- 77.91 Total ostectomy of scapula, clavicle, and thorax (ribs and sternum)

Anesthesia
00474

ICD-9-CM Diagnostic

- 170.3 Malignant neoplasm of ribs, sternum, and clavicle
- 196.1 Secondary and unspecified malignant neoplasm of intrathoracic lymph nodes
- 197.1 Secondary malignant neoplasm of mediastinum
- 198.5 Secondary malignant neoplasm of bone and bone marrow
- 209.73 Secondary neuroendocrine tumor of bone
- 213.3 Benign neoplasm of ribs, sternum, and clavicle
- 238.0 Neoplasm of uncertain behavior of bone and articular cartilage
- 730.18 Chronic osteomyelitis, other specified sites — (Use additional code to identify organism: 041.1. Use additional code to identify major osseous defect, if applicable: 731.3)
- 730.28 Unspecified osteomyelitis, other specified sites — (Use additional code to identify organism: 041.1. Use additional code to identify major osseous defect, if applicable: 731.3)
- 730.88 Other infections involving bone diseases classified elsewhere, other specified sites — (Use additional code to identify organism: 041.1. Code first underlying disease: 002.0, 015.0-015.9)
- 731.3 Major osseous defects — (Code first underlying disease: 170.0-170.9, 730.00-730.29, 733.00-733.09, 733.40-733.49, 996.45)
- 733.49 Aseptic necrosis of other bone site — (Use additional code to identify major osseous defect, if applicable: 731.3)
- 875.1 Open wound of chest (wall), complicated
- 998.59 Other postoperative infection — (Use additional code to identify infection)
- V10.90 Personal history of unspecified malignant neoplasm
- V10.91 Personal history of malignant neuroendocrine tumor — (Code first any continuing functional activity, such as: carcinoid syndrome (259.2))

Terms To Know

aseptic necrosis. Death of bone tissue resulting from a disruption in the vascular supply, caused by a noninfectious disease process, such as a fracture or the administration of immunosuppressive drugs.

benign. Mild or nonmalignant in nature.

chronic. Persistent, continuing, or recurring.

malignant. Any condition tending to progress toward death, specifically an invasive tumor with a loss of cellular differentiation that has the ability to spread or metastasize to other areas in the body.

osteomyelitis. Inflammation of bone that may remain localized or spread to the marrow, cortex, or periosteum, in response to an infecting organism, usually bacterial and pyogenic.

secondary. Second in order of occurrence or importance, or appearing during the course of another disease or condition.

CCI Version 16.3

00550, 0213T, 0216T, 0228T, 0230T, 10060, 10140, 10160, 20101, 20670-20680, 21600, 21750, 36000, 36400-36410, 36420-36430, 36440, 36600, 36640, 37202, 43752, 51701-51703, 62310-62319, 64400-64435, 64445-64450, 64479, 64483, 64490, 64493, 64505-64530, 69990, 93000-93010, 93040-93042, 93318, 94002, 94200, 94250, 94680-94690, 94770, 95812-95816, 95819, 95822, 95829, 95955, 96360, 96365, 96372, 96374-96376, 99148-99149, 99150

Also not with 21630: 12001-12007, 12020-12037, 13100-13101, 21620-21627, 35820

Also not with 21632: 21620-21630

Note: These CCI edits are used for Medicare. Other payers may reimburse on codes listed above.

Medicare Edits

	Fac RVU	Non-Fac RVU	FUD	Assist
21630	37.5	37.5	90	80
21632	37.31	37.31	90	80

Medicare References: None

21685

21685 Hyoid myotomy and suspension

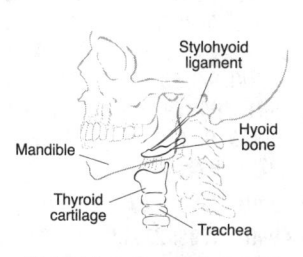

The hyoid bone is surgically exposed by a neck incision. Fascial or synthetic fibers are used to suspend the hyoid bone forward, often from the mandible

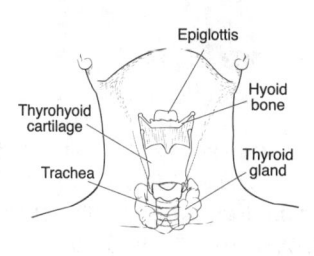

Explanation

The hyoid bone is a small C-shaped bone in the neck above the Adam's apple, or thyroid cartilage, with muscles of the tongue and throat attached to it. Hyoid myotomy and suspension is done to open the oro-hypopharyngeal airway for correcting breathing in sleep apnea. It involves repositioning and fixating the hyoid bone to improve the airway. A submental incision is made to expose the hyoid bone in the neck. The muscles below the hyoid are transected and separated to expose a small, isolated, mid-portion of the hyoid bone. Strips of fascia lata (bands of fibrous tissue), nonresorbable suture, or other strong materials are wrapped around the body of the hyoid and used to pull it forward and secure it to the inferior mandibular border. An alternative method pulls the hyoid downward to the voicebox cartilage for thyro-hyoid suspension, and secures it there.

Coding Tips

When 21685 is performed with another separately identifiable procedure, the highest dollar value code is listed as the primary procedure and subsequent procedures are appended with modifier 51.

ICD-9-CM Procedural

83.02 Myotomy

Anesthesia

21685   00300, 00320

ICD-9-CM Diagnostic

327.20   Organic sleep apnea, unspecified
327.23   Obstructive sleep apnea (adult) (pediatric)
327.29   Other organic sleep apnea
780.50   Unspecified sleep disturbance
780.51   Insomnia with sleep apnea, unspecified
780.53   Hypersomnia with sleep apnea, unspecified
780.57   Unspecified sleep apnea

Terms To Know

cartilage. Variety of fibrous connective tissue that is inherently nonvascular. Usually found in the joints, it aids in movement and provides a cushion to absorb jolts and shocks.

epiglottis. Lid-like cartilaginous tissue that covers the entrance to the larynx and blocks food from entering the trachea.

fascia. Fibrous sheet or band of tissue that envelops organs, muscles, and groupings of muscles.

hyoid bone. Single, U-shaped bone palpable in the neck above the larynx and below the mandible (lower jaw) with various muscles attached but not articulating with any other bone.

hypersomnia. Disorder identified by the need for excessive sleep.

insomnia. Inability to sleep.

mandible. Lower jawbone giving structure to the floor of the oral cavity.

sleep apnea. Intermittent cessation of breathing during sleep that may cause hypoxemia and pulmonary arterial hypertension.

trachea. Tube descending from the larynx and branching into the right and left main bronchi.

CCI Version 16.3

0213T, 0216T, 0228T, 0230T, 31505, 31525, 31575, 36000, 36400-36410, 36420-36430, 36440, 36600, 36640, 37202, 43752, 51701-51703, 62310-62319, 64400-64435, 64445-64450, 64479, 64483, 64490, 64493, 64505-64530, 69990, 92502, 93000-93010, 93040-93042, 93318, 94002, 94200, 94250, 94680-94690, 94770, 95812-95816, 95819, 95822, 95829, 95955, 96360, 96365, 96372, 96374-96376, 99148-99149, 99150, J0670, J2001

Note: These CCI edits are used for Medicare. Other payers may reimburse on codes listed above.

Medicare Edits

	Fac RVU	Non-Fac RVU	FUD	Assist
21685	29.71	29.71	90	80

Medicare References: None

21700-21705

21700 Division of scalenus anticus; without resection of cervical rib
21705 with resection of cervical rib

Numerous structures cross or attach to the first rib, including the anterior scalenus

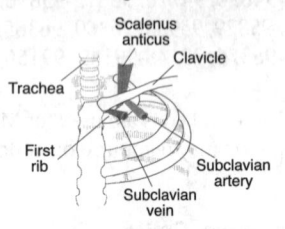

Superior view of C7 showing cervical rib, which usually occurs bilaterally

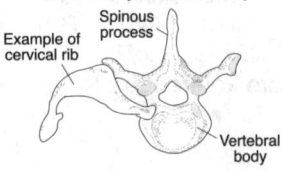

Report 21700 for scalenus anticus division alone; 21705 when a cervical rib is removed in addition to scalenus anticus division

Explanation

The physician performs a surgical procedure where the scalenus anticus muscle is divided usually for the purpose of treating thoracic outlet syndrome. With the patient under anesthesia, the physician makes an incision overlying the scalene muscle. This incision is carried deep to the muscle. The muscle is exposed and identified. A dissection of the muscle is performed in line of the fibers. This relieves the pressure on the neurovascular structures. The wound is thoroughly irrigated and closed in layers. Report 21700 if the procedure does not include resection of the cervical rib. Report 21705 if resection of the cervical rib is performed during the procedure.

Coding Tips

When 21700 or 21705 is performed with another separately identifiable procedure, the highest dollar value code is listed as the primary procedure, and subsequent procedures are appended with modifier 51. For resection of the cervical rib without division of scalenus anticus, see 21615–21616.

ICD-9-CM Procedural

77.81 Other partial ostectomy of scapula, clavicle, and thorax (ribs and sternum)
83.19 Other division of soft tissue

Anesthesia

21700 00300
21705 00470

ICD-9-CM Diagnostic

353.0 Brachial plexus lesions
728.85 Spasm of muscle
756.2 Cervical rib

Terms To Know

bilateral. Consisting of or affecting two sides.

dissection. Separating by cutting tissue or body structures apart.

lesion. Area of damaged tissue that has lost continuity or function, due to disease or trauma. Lesions may be located on internal structures such as the brain, nerves, or kidneys, or visible on the skin.

muscle tissue. Network of specialized cells for performing contraction to produce voluntary or involuntary movement of body parts, and skeletal, cardiac, or visceral muscles.

soft tissue. Nonepithelial tissues outside of the skeleton that includes subcutaneous adipose tissue, fibrous tissue, fascia, muscles, blood and lymph vessels, and peripheral nervous system tissue.

spasm. Involuntary muscle contraction.

thoracic outlet syndrome. Constellation of symptoms resulting from compression of nerves and/or blood vessels, due to insufficient space in the thoracic outlet between the base of the neck and the axilla. Since the thoracic outlet is bordered by muscle, bone, and other tissues, any condition causing enlargement or displacement of the tissues near the thoracic outlet can result in thoracic outlet syndrome. Symptoms range in location and severity and may include pain in the neck and shoulder, arm numbness, or impaired circulation.

trachea. Tube descending from the larynx and branching into the right and left main bronchi.

CCI Version 16.3

0213T, 0216T, 0228T, 0230T, 36000, 36400-36410, 36420-36430, 36440, 36600, 36640, 37202, 43752, 51701-51703, 62310-62319, 64400-64435, 64445-64450, 64479, 64483, 64490, 64493, 64505-64530, 69990, 93000-93010, 93040-93042, 93318, 94002, 94200, 94250, 94680-94690, 94770, 95812-95816, 95819, 95822, 95829, 95955, 96360, 96365, 96372, 96374-96376, 99148-99149, 99150

Also not with 21700: 11012❖, J2001
Also not with 21705: 21700

Note: These CCI edits are used for Medicare. Other payers may reimburse on codes listed above.

Medicare Edits

	Fac RVU	Non-Fac RVU	FUD	Assist
21700	12.68	12.68	90	80
21705	17.95	17.95	90	80

Medicare References: 100-2,15,260; 100-4,12,30; 100-4,12,90.3; 100-4,14,10

21720-21725

21720 Division of sternocleidomastoid for torticollis, open operation; without cast application
21725 with cast application

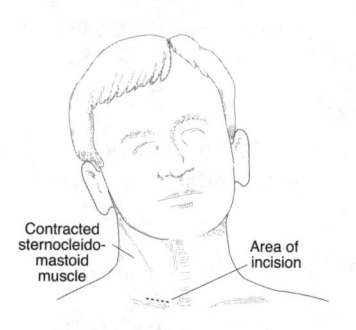

Contracted sternocleidomastoid muscle
Area of incision

Torticollis may be a congenital condition, (birth trauma to the sternocleidomastoid muscle), or a result of injury or trauma. The muscle is always contracted, drawing down the head of the affected side while the face turns to the unaffected side, giving a "wry-neck" appearance

Surgery typically involves accessing the sternocleidomastoid attachment near the collarbone. Muscle and tendon is divided to relieve contraction in 21720. Report 21725 when a cast is applied following closure

Explanation

Torticollis is a dysfunction of the neck with congenital or traumatic onset. The head becomes inclined toward the affected side and the face toward the opposite side. The physician makes an incision 5 cm long above and parallel to the medial end of the collarbone to access the tendons of the sternocleidomastoid muscle. A blunt instrument is placed behind the tendons to protect vital structures in the neck. The muscle's tendons attach just behind the ear and to the collarbone. The physician splits the tendons further up the muscle to release the restriction. The physician probes the wound to identify remaining tight muscles or fascia, which are cut until full motion is obtained. The physician closes the incision with sutures and Steri-strips. A cervical collar is applied for six weeks in 21720 and a cast is applied to hold the neck in place in 21725.

Coding Tips

When any of these procedures is performed with another separately identifiable procedure, the highest dollar value code is listed as the primary procedure and subsequent procedures are appended with modifier 51.

ICD-9-CM Procedural

83.19 Other division of soft tissue
93.52 Application of neck support
93.53 Application of other cast

Anesthesia
00300

ICD-9-CM Diagnostic

333.83 Spasmodic torticollis — (Use additional E code to identify drug, if drug-induced)
723.5 Torticollis, unspecified
754.1 Congenital musculoskeletal deformity of sternocleidomastoid muscle
781.93 Ocular torticollis

Terms To Know

congenital. Present at birth, occurring through heredity or an influence during gestation up to the moment of birth.

fascia. Fibrous sheet or band of tissue that envelops organs, muscles, and groupings of muscles.

medial. Middle or midline.

soft tissue. Nonepithelial tissues outside of the skeleton that includes subcutaneous adipose tissue, fibrous tissue, fascia, muscles, blood and lymph vessels, and peripheral nervous system tissue.

tendon. Fibrous tissue that connects muscle to bone, consisting primarily of collagen and containing little vasculature.

torticollis. Twisted, unnatural position of the neck due to contracted cervical muscles that pull the head to one side.

CCI Version 16.3

0213T, 0216T, 0228T, 0230T, 11012❖, 36000, 36400-36410, 36420-36430, 36440, 36600, 36640, 37202, 43752, 51701-51703, 62310-62319, 64400-64435, 64445-64450, 64479, 64483, 64490, 64493, 64505-64530, 69990, 93000-93010, 93040-93042, 93318, 94002, 94200, 94250, 94680-94690, 94770, 95812-95816, 95819, 95822, 95829, 95955, 96360, 96365, 96372, 96374-96376, 99148-99149, 99150

Also not with 21720: J2001
Also not with 21725: 21720

Note: These CCI edits are used for Medicare. Other payers may reimburse on codes listed above.

Medicare Edits

	Fac RVU	Non-Fac RVU	FUD	Assist
21720	13.19	13.19	90	80
21725	15.62	15.62	90	80

Medicare References: 100-2,15,260; 100-4,12,30; 100-4,12,90.3; 100-4,14,10

21750

21750 Closure of median sternotomy separation with or without debridement (separate procedure)

The sternotomy edges may be debrided

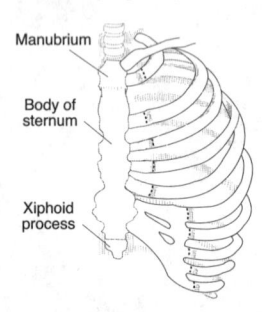

- Manubrium
- Body of sternum
- Xiphoid process

Internal fixation may be required

Surgical closure of a sternotomy separation is reported with 21750

Explanation

The physician performs surgery on the sternum bone to put the bone back together following previous surgical separation. With the patient under anesthesia, the physician makes an incision overlying the sternum. The incision is carried deep to the bone and the separated pieces are identified. The physician debrides soft tissue or bone. The bony fragments are manipulated back together and held in place. The physician uses wire or other internal fixation devices to maintain the bone in the appropriate position. The wound is irrigated and closed in layers.

Coding Tips

This separate procedure by definition is usually a component of a more complex service and is not identified separately. When performed alone or with other unrelated procedures/services, it may be reported. If performed alone, list the code; if performed with other procedures/services, list the code and append modifier 59. Sternal debridement is included in this procedure and should not be reported separately. For sternal debridement only, see 21627. When 21750 is performed with another separately identifiable procedure, the highest dollar value code is listed as the primary procedure, and subsequent procedures are appended with modifier 51.

ICD-9-CM Procedural

- 77.61 Local excision of lesion or tissue of scapula, clavicle, and thorax (ribs and sternum)
- 78.49 Other repair or plastic operations on other bone, except facial bones
- 84.94 Insertion of sternal fixation device with rigid plates

Anesthesia

21750 00400, 00540, 00550

ICD-9-CM Diagnostic

- 733.81 Malunion of fracture
- 733.82 Nonunion of fracture
- 998.31 Disruption of internal operation (surgical) wound
- 998.59 Other postoperative infection — (Use additional code to identify infection)
- 998.83 Non-healing surgical wound

Terms To Know

fracture. Break in bone or cartilage.

lesion. Area of damaged tissue that has lost continuity or function, due to disease or trauma. Lesions may be located on internal structures such as the brain, nerves, or kidneys, or visible on the skin.

malunion. Fracture that has united in a faulty position due to inadequate reduction of the original fracture, insufficient holding of a previously well-reduced fracture, contracture of the soft tissues, or comminuted or osteoporotic bone causing a slow disintegration of the fracture.

nonunion. Failure of two ends of a fracture to mend or completely heal.

soft tissue. Nonepithelial tissues outside of the skeleton that includes subcutaneous adipose tissue, fibrous tissue, fascia, muscles, blood and lymph vessels, and peripheral nervous system tissue.

CCI Version 16.3

00550, 0213T, 0216T, 0228T, 0230T, 20670-20680, 21627, 35820, 36000, 36400-36410, 36420-36430, 36440, 36600, 36640, 37202, 43752, 51701-51703, 62310-62319, 64400-64435, 64445-64450, 64479, 64483, 64490, 64493, 64505-64530, 69990, 93000-93010, 93040-93042, 93318, 94002, 94200, 94250, 94680-94690, 94770, 95812-95816, 95819, 95822, 95829, 95955, 96360, 96365, 96372, 96374-96376, 99148-99149, 99150

Note: These CCI edits are used for Medicare. Other payers may reimburse on codes listed above.

Medicare Edits

	Fac RVU	Non-Fac RVU	FUD	Assist
21750	20.96	20.96	90	80

Medicare References: None

21800

21800 Closed treatment of rib fracture, uncomplicated, each

Report 21800 for each rib fracture that can be reduced without surgery

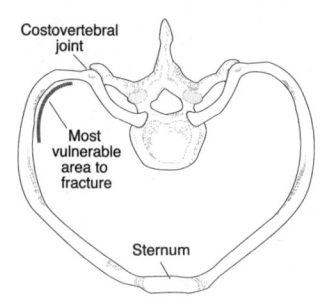

Superior schematic showing a thoracic rib and its attachments. Ribs are most vulnerable to fracture at the area of greatest curvature

Explanation
Closed treatment of an uncomplicated rib fracture is performed. The rib fracture may be diagnosed by examination alone or with separately reportable x-rays. If the fracture is nondisplaced and stable, closed treatment is initiated. Closed treatment involves management of the rib fracture directed at protecting the underlying lung and ensuring adequate oxygenation and ventilation, evaluation to exclude complications, pain control, patient education, and routine follow-up. Braces or splints are not used as they restrict normal chest expansion and can lead to pulmonary complications. The patient's activity is modified while the fracture heals.

Coding Tips
For open treatment of a rib fracture, see 21805. Supplies used when providing this procedure may be reported with the appropriate HCPCS Level II code. Check with the specific payer to determine coverage.

ICD-9-CM Procedural
79.09 Closed reduction of fracture of other specified bone, except facial bones, without internal fixation

Anesthesia
21800 00520

ICD-9-CM Diagnostic
786.52 Painful respiration

807.00 Closed fracture of rib(s), unspecified
807.01 Closed fracture of one rib
807.02 Closed fracture of two ribs
807.03 Closed fracture of three ribs
807.04 Closed fracture of four ribs
807.05 Closed fracture of five ribs
807.06 Closed fracture of six ribs
807.07 Closed fracture of seven ribs
807.08 Closed fracture of eight or more ribs
807.09 Closed fracture of multiple ribs, unspecified

Terms To Know
closed fracture. Break in a bone without a concomitant opening in the skin. A closed fracture is coded when the type of fracture is not specified.

fracture. Break in bone or cartilage.

CCI Version 16.3
0213T, 0216T, 0228T, 0230T, 12001-12002, 12011-12014, 12032, 21810❖, 29200, 29240, 29700-29715, 36000, 36400-36410, 36420-36430, 36440, 36600, 36640, 37202, 43752, 51701-51703, 62310-62319, 64400-64435, 64445-64450, 64479, 64483, 64490, 64493, 64505-64530, 69990, 93000-93010, 93040-93042, 93318, 94002, 94200, 94250, 94680-94690, 94770, 95812-95816, 95819, 95822, 95829, 95955, 96360, 96365, 96372, 96374-96376, 97597-97598, 97602-97606, 99148-99149, 99150, G0168

Note: These CCI edits are used for Medicare. Other payers may reimburse on codes listed above.

Medicare Edits

	Fac RVU	Non-Fac RVU	FUD	Assist
21800	3.04	2.97	90	N/A

Medicare References: 100-2,15,260; 100-4,12,30; 100-4,12,90.3; 100-4,14,10

21805

21805 Open treatment of rib fracture without fixation, each

Report 21805 for each fracture that requires open surgical reduction

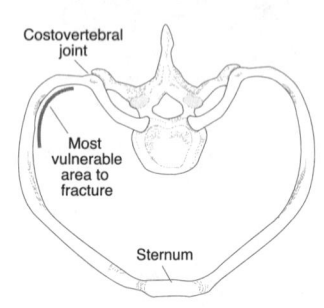

Superior schematic showing a thoracic rib and its attachments. Ribs are most vulnerable to fracture at the area of greatest curvature

Explanation

The physician performs surgery on a fractured rib without the need for any internal or external fixation devices. With the patient under anesthesia, the physician makes an incision overlying the fractured rib. This is carried deep to the bone. The fracture is found and the pieces are identified. Dead tissue is debrided as needed. The physician manipulates the fracture fragments into an acceptable position and alignment. The wound is irrigated thoroughly and closed in layers.

Coding Tips

This code is reported for each rib treated. For closed treatment of a rib fracture, see 21800.

ICD-9-CM Procedural

79.29 Open reduction of fracture of other specified bone, except facial bones, without internal fixation

Anesthesia

21805   00470

ICD-9-CM Diagnostic

807.01 Closed fracture of one rib
807.02 Closed fracture of two ribs
807.03 Closed fracture of three ribs
807.04 Closed fracture of four ribs
807.05 Closed fracture of five ribs
807.06 Closed fracture of six ribs
807.07 Closed fracture of seven ribs
807.08 Closed fracture of eight or more ribs
807.11 Open fracture of one rib
807.12 Open fracture of two ribs
807.13 Open fracture of three ribs
807.14 Open fracture of four ribs
807.15 Open fracture of five ribs
807.16 Open fracture of six ribs
807.17 Open fracture of seven ribs
807.18 Open fracture of eight or more ribs

Terms To Know

alignment. Establishment of a straight line or harmonious relationship between structures.

closed fracture. Break in a bone without a concomitant opening in the skin. A closed fracture is coded when the type of fracture is not specified.

fracture. Break in bone or cartilage.

open fracture. Exposed break in a bone, always considered compound due to its high risk of infection from the open wound leading to the fracture. Broken bone ends may protrude through the skin and contaminants or foreign bodies are often embedded in the tissues.

CCI Version 16.3

0213T, 0216T, 0228T, 0230T, 21800, 29200, 29700-29715, 36000, 36400-36410, 36420-36430, 36440, 36600, 36640, 37202, 43752, 51701-51703, 62310-62319, 64400-64435, 64445-64450, 64479, 64483, 64490, 64493, 64505-64530, 69990, 93000-93010, 93040-93042, 93318, 94002, 94200, 94250, 94680-94690, 94770, 95812-95816, 95819, 95822, 95829, 95955, 96360, 96365, 96372, 96374-96376, 97597-97598, 97602-97606, 99148-99149, 99150

Note: These CCI edits are used for Medicare. Other payers may reimburse on codes listed above.

Medicare Edits

	Fac RVU	Non-Fac RVU	FUD	Assist
21805	7.7	7.7	90	80

Medicare References: 100-2,15,260; 100-4,12,30; 100-4,12,90.3; 100-4,14,10

21810

21810 Treatment of rib fracture requiring external fixation (flail chest)

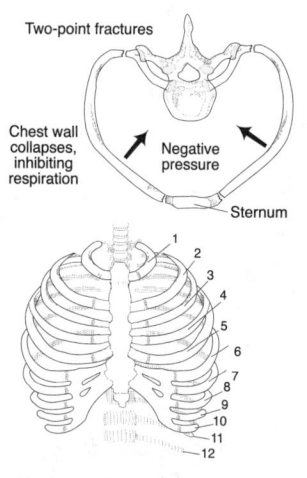

Explanation

The physician treats a rib fracture that results in a so-called "flail chest" using external fixation devices. A flail chest inhibits proper pulmonary function. With the patient under anesthesia, the physician makes an incision overlying the fractured rib. The physician identifies the rib involved. Using external fixation and other devices such as pins, screws, or sandbags, the physician stabilizes the rib fracture and the chest wall. The wound is closed with layered sutures.

Coding Tips

For open treatment of a rib fracture without internal fixation, see 21805.

ICD-9-CM Procedural

- 78.11 Application of external fixator device, scapula, clavicle, and thorax [ribs and sternum]
- 79.09 Closed reduction of fracture of other specified bone, except facial bones, without internal fixation

Anesthesia
21810 00472

ICD-9-CM Diagnostic
807.4 Flail chest

Terms To Know

flail chest. Instability of the chest wall resulting from a fracture of the sternum or ribs.

fracture. Break in bone or cartilage.

CCI Version 16.3

0213T, 0216T, 0228T, 0230T, 20650, 20690, 20692, 20696-20697, 21805, 29700-29715, 36000, 36400-36410, 36420-36430, 36440, 36600, 36640, 37202, 43752, 51701-51703, 62310-62319, 64400-64435, 64445-64450, 64479, 64483, 64490, 64493, 64505-64530, 69990, 93000-93010, 93040-93042, 93318, 94002, 94200, 94250, 94680-94690, 94770, 95812-95816, 95819, 95822, 95829, 95955, 96360, 96365, 96372, 96374-96376, 97597-97598, 97602-97606, 99148-99149, 99150

Note: These CCI edits are used for Medicare. Other payers may reimburse on codes listed above.

Medicare Edits

	Fac RVU	Non-Fac RVU	FUD	Assist
21810	15.31	15.31	90	80

Medicare References: None

21820

21820 Closed treatment of sternum fracture

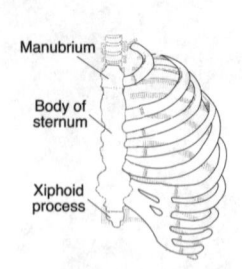

Fractures often occur at or near the juncture of the manubrium and the body of the sternum

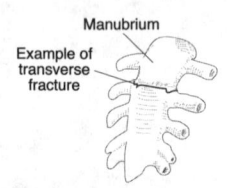

Example of transverse fracture

Fractures of the sternum often occur as a result of blows to the chest (such as impact from an auto steering wheel)

Explanation

Separately reportable x-rays are used to identify if a fracture of the sternum is present. If the fracture is non-displaced and stable, closed treatment is initiated. Braces or splints are not used. The patient's activity is modified while the fracture heals.

Coding Tips

For open treatment of a sternum fracture with or without internal fixation, see 21825.

ICD-9-CM Procedural

79.09 Closed reduction of fracture of other specified bone, except facial bones, without internal fixation

Anesthesia

21820 00470, 00520

ICD-9-CM Diagnostic

807.2 Closed fracture of sternum

Terms To Know

closed fracture. Break in a bone without a concomitant opening in the skin. A closed fracture is coded when the type of fracture is not specified.

CCI Version 16.3

00550, 0213T, 0216T, 0228T, 0230T, 21750, 29200, 29700-29715, 36000, 36400-36410, 36420-36430, 36440, 36600, 36640, 37202, 43752, 51701-51703, 62310-62319, 64400-64435, 64445-64450, 64479, 64483, 64490, 64493, 64505-64530, 69990, 93000-93010, 93040-93042, 93318, 94002, 94200, 94250, 94680-94690, 94770, 95812-95816, 95819, 95822, 95829, 95955, 96360, 96365, 96372, 96374-96376, 97597-97598, 97602-97606, 99148-99149, 99150

Note: These CCI edits are used for Medicare. Other payers may reimburse on codes listed above.

Medicare Edits

	Fac RVU	Non-Fac RVU	FUD	Assist
21820	4.02	3.95	90	N/A

Medicare References: 100-2,15,260; 100-4,12,30; 100-4,12,90.3; 100-4,14,10

21825

21825 Open treatment of sternum fracture with or without skeletal fixation

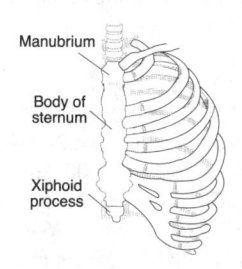

Fractures often occur at or near the juncture of the manubrium and the body of the sternum

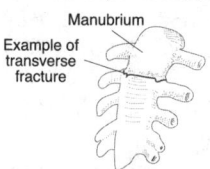

Example of transverse fracture

Fractures of the sternum often occur as a result of blows to the chest (such as impact from an auto steering wheel). Code 21825 for open surgical reduction and or those that require fixation. Report accompanying broken ribs separately

Explanation

The physician performs an open surgical reduction of a sternum fracture. The patient is positioned supine on the operating table. A longitudinal incision is made along the midportion of the sternum. Dissection exposes the fractured sternum. The surgeon reduces the fracture. If fixation is needed to keep the fracture stable, the physician drills holes on either side of the fracture. Wire is passed through the holes and around the fracture and the wire ends are twisted together to immobilize the fracture. The incision is repaired in layers with sutures, staples, or Steri-strips.

Coding Tips

Any wiring or internal fixation is not reported separately. Report treatment of any rib fractures separately; see 21805–21810. When 21825 is performed with another separately identifiable procedure, the highest dollar value code is listed as the primary procedure, and subsequent procedures are appended with modifier 51. For closed treatment of a sternum fracture, see 21820.

ICD-9-CM Procedural

79.29	Open reduction of fracture of other specified bone, except facial bones, without internal fixation
79.39	Open reduction of fracture of other specified bone, except facial bones, with internal fixation
84.94	Insertion of sternal fixation device with rigid plates

Anesthesia

21825   00472

ICD-9-CM Diagnostic

733.81	Malunion of fracture
733.82	Nonunion of fracture
807.2	Closed fracture of sternum
807.3	Open fracture of sternum

Terms To Know

closed fracture. Break in a bone without a concomitant opening in the skin. A closed fracture is coded when the type of fracture is not specified.

malunion. Fracture that has united in a faulty position due to inadequate reduction of the original fracture, insufficient holding of a previously well-reduced fracture, contracture of the soft tissues, or comminuted or osteoporotic bone causing a slow disintegration of the fracture.

nonunion. Failure of two ends of a fracture to mend or completely heal.

open fracture. Exposed break in a bone, always considered compound due to its high risk of infection from the open wound leading to the fracture. Broken bone ends may protrude through the skin and contaminants or foreign bodies are often embedded in the tissues.

supine. Lying on the back.

CCI Version 16.3

00550, 0213T, 0216T, 0228T, 0230T, 20690, 20692, 20696-20697, 21750, 21820, 29200, 29700-29715, 36000, 36400-36410, 36420-36430, 36440, 36600, 36640, 37202, 43752, 51701-51703, 62310-62319, 64400-64435, 64445-64450, 64479, 64483, 64490, 64493, 64505-64530, 69990, 93000-93010, 93040-93042, 93318, 94002, 94200, 94250, 94680-94690, 94770, 95812-95816, 95819, 95822, 95829, 95955, 96360, 96365, 96372, 96374-96376, 97597-97598, 97602-97606, 99148-99149, 99150

Note: These CCI edits are used for Medicare. Other payers may reimburse on codes listed above.

Medicare Edits

	Fac RVU	Non-Fac RVU	FUD	Assist
21825	16.68	16.68	90	80

Medicare References: 100-4,12,30

21920-21925

21920 Biopsy, soft tissue of back or flank; superficial
21925 deep

Incisional biopsy

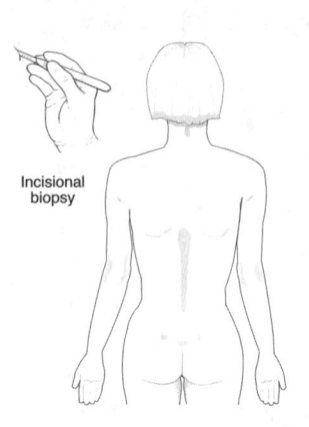

The soft tissue of the back or flank is biopsied through a superficial open incision (21920). A deep biopsy is performed in 21925

Explanation
The physician performs a biopsy of the soft tissues of the back or flank. The patient is positioned lying on the side or prone. With proper anesthesia administered, an incision is made over the biopsy area. Dissection is carried down within the superficial soft tissue layers in 21920, usually the subcutaneous fat to the uppermost fascial layer. In 21925, dissection is taken down deep within the soft tissue, such as into the fascial layer or within the muscle. A portion of the tissue is excised and submitted for pathology. The area is irrigated and the incision is closed with layered sutures, staples, or Steri-strips.

Coding Tips
Note that these codes report an incisional biopsy. For a needle biopsy of muscle, see 20206. A biopsy is not reported separately when followed by an excisional removal during the same operative session. When these procedures are performed with another separately identifiable procedure, the highest dollar value code is listed as the primary procedure and subsequent procedures are appended with modifier 51. Surgical trays, A4550, are not separately reimbursed by Medicare; however, other third-party payers may cover them. Check with the specific payer to determine coverage.

ICD-9-CM Procedural
83.21 Open biopsy of soft tissue

Anesthesia
00300, 00730, 00820

ICD-9-CM Diagnostic
- 171.7 Malignant neoplasm of connective and other soft tissue of trunk, unspecified site
- 195.8 Malignant neoplasm of other specified sites
- 198.89 Secondary malignant neoplasm of other specified sites
- 214.1 Lipoma of other skin and subcutaneous tissue
- 215.7 Other benign neoplasm of connective and other soft tissue of trunk, unspecified
- 229.8 Benign neoplasm of other specified sites
- 238.1 Neoplasm of uncertain behavior of connective and other soft tissue
- 238.8 Neoplasm of uncertain behavior of other specified sites
- 239.2 Neoplasms of unspecified nature of bone, soft tissue, and skin
- 239.89 Neoplasms of unspecified nature, other specified sites
- 782.2 Localized superficial swelling, mass, or lump

Terms To Know
benign. Mild or nonmalignant in nature.

cyst. Elevated encapsulated mass containing fluid, semisolid, or solid material with a membranous lining.

fascia. Fibrous sheet or band of tissue that envelops organs, muscles, and groupings of muscles.

lipoma. Benign tumor containing fat cells and the most common of soft tissue lesions, which are usually painless and asymptomatic, with the exception of an angiolipoma.

malignant. Any condition tending to progress toward death, specifically an invasive tumor with a loss of cellular differentiation that has the ability to spread or metastasize to other areas in the body.

secondary. Second in order of occurrence or importance, or appearing during the course of another disease or condition.

soft tissue. Nonepithelial tissues outside of the skeleton that includes subcutaneous adipose tissue, fibrous tissue, fascia, muscles, blood and lymph vessels, and peripheral nervous system tissue.

superficial. On the skin surface or near the surface of any involved structure or field of interest.

tumor. Pathological swelling or enlargement; a neoplastic growth of uncontrolled, abnormal multiplication of cells.

CCI Version 16.3
0213T, 0216T, 0228T, 0230T, 10060, 10140, 10160, 20102, 36000, 36400-36410, 36420-36430, 36440, 36600, 36640, 37202, 43752, 51701-51703, 62310-62319, 64400-64435, 64445-64450, 64479, 64483, 64490, 64493, 64505-64530, 69990, 93000-93010, 93040-93042, 93318, 94002, 94200, 94250, 94680-94690, 94770, 95812-95816, 95819, 95822, 95829, 95955, 96360, 96365, 96372, 96374-96376, 99148-99149, 99150, J0670, J2001

Also not with 21920: 11010-11012❖, 11900, 12001, 38500, G0168

Also not with 21925: 11011-11012❖, 20200, 21920, 49010

Note: These CCI edits are used for Medicare. Other payers may reimburse on codes listed above.

Medicare Edits

	Fac RVU	Non-Fac RVU	FUD	Assist
21920	4.75	7.53	10	N/A
21925	10.05	12.52	90	N/A

Medicare References: 100-2,15,260; 100-4,12,30; 100-4,12,90.3; 100-4,14,10

21930-21933

21930	Excision, tumor, soft tissue of back or flank, subcutaneous; less than 3 cm
21931	3 cm or greater
21932	Excision, tumor, soft tissue of back or flank, subfascial (eg, intramuscular); less than 5 cm
21933	5 cm or greater

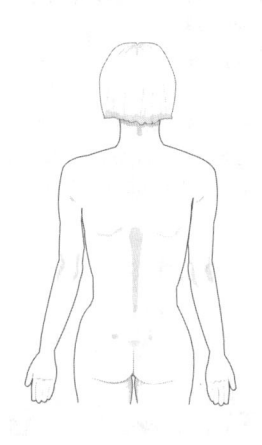

Report 21930 or 21931 for subcutaneous excision and 21932 or 21933 for subfascial excision of a soft tissue tumor of the back or flank

Explanation

The physician removes a tumor from the soft tissue of the back or flank that is located in the subcutaneous tissue in 21930-21931 and in the deep soft tissue, below the fascial plane or within the muscle, in 21932-21933. The patient is positioned lying on the side or prone. With the proper anesthesia administered, the physician makes an incision in the skin overlying the mass and dissects down to the tumor. The extent of the tumor is identified and a dissection is undertaken all the way around the tumor. A portion of neighboring soft tissue may also be removed to ensure adequate removal of all tumor tissue. A drain may be inserted and the incision is repaired with layers of sutures, staples, or Steri-strips. Report 21930 for excision of subcutaneous tumors less than 3 cm and 21931 for excision of subcutaneous tumors 3 cm or greater. Report 21932 for excision of subfascial or intramuscular tumors less than 5 cm and 21933 for excision of subfascial or intramuscular tumors 5 cm or greater.

Coding Tips

When any of these procedures is performed with another separately identifiable procedure, the highest dollar value code is listed as the primary procedure and subsequent procedures are appended with modifier 51. If significant additional time and effort is documented, append modifier 22 and submit a cover letter and operative report. An excisional biopsy is not reported separately when a therapeutic excision is performed during the same surgical session. Report any free grafts or flaps separately.

ICD-9-CM Procedural

83.32	Excision of lesion of muscle
83.39	Excision of lesion of other soft tissue
83.49	Other excision of soft tissue
86.3	Other local excision or destruction of lesion or tissue of skin and subcutaneous tissue
86.4	Radical excision of skin lesion

Anesthesia
00300, 00730, 00820

ICD-9-CM Diagnostic

171.7	Malignant neoplasm of connective and other soft tissue of trunk, unspecified site
172.5	Malignant melanoma of skin of trunk, except scrotum
195.8	Malignant neoplasm of other specified sites
198.89	Secondary malignant neoplasm of other specified sites
209.35	Merkel cell carcinoma of the trunk
209.75	Secondary Merkel cell carcinoma
214.1	Lipoma of other skin and subcutaneous tissue
215.7	Other benign neoplasm of connective and other soft tissue of trunk, unspecified
228.01	Hemangioma of skin and subcutaneous tissue
238.1	Neoplasm of uncertain behavior of connective and other soft tissue
239.2	Neoplasms of unspecified nature of bone, soft tissue, and skin
782.2	Localized superficial swelling, mass, or lump

Terms To Know

hemangioma. Benign neoplasm arising from vascular tissue or malformations of vascular structures. It is most commonly seen in children and infants as a tumor of newly formed blood vessels due to malformed fetal angioblastic tissues.

lipoma. Benign tumor containing fat cells and the most common of soft tissue lesions, which are usually painless and asymptomatic, with the exception of an angiolipoma.

malignant. Any condition tending to progress toward death, specifically an invasive tumor with a loss of cellular differentiation that has the ability to spread or metastasize to other areas in the body.

secondary. Second in order of occurrence or importance, or appearing during the course of another disease or condition.

soft tissue. Nonepithelial tissues outside of the skeleton that includes subcutaneous adipose tissue, fibrous tissue, fascia, muscles, blood and lymph vessels, and peripheral nervous system tissue.

subcutaneous tissue. Sheet or wide band of adipose (fat) and areolar connective tissue in two layers attached to the dermis.

tumor. Pathological swelling or enlargement; a neoplastic growth of uncontrolled, abnormal multiplication of cells.

CCI Version 16.3

0228T, 0230T, 10060, 10140, 10160, 11010-11012❖, 11040-11044, 12001-12007, 12020-12037, 13100-13101, 20102, 36000, 36400-36410, 36420-36430, 36440, 36600, 36640, 37202, 38500, 43752, 49010, 51701-51703, 62310-62319, 64400-64435, 64445-64450, 64479, 64483, 64505-64530, 69990, 93000-93010, 93040-93042, 93318, 94002, 94200, 94250, 94680-94690, 94770, 95812-95816, 95819, 95822, 95829, 95955, 96360, 96365, 96372, 96374-96376, 99148-99149, 99150, J2001

Also not with 21930: 21920-21925, J0670

Also not with 21931: 0213T, 0216T, 21920-21930, 64490, 64493

Also not with 21932: 0213T, 0216T, 21920-21931, 64490, 64493

Also not with 21933: 0213T, 0216T, 21920-21932, 64490, 64493

Note: These CCI edits are used for Medicare. Other payers may reimburse on codes listed above.

Medicare Edits

	Fac RVU	Non-Fac RVU	FUD	Assist
21930	10.64	13.52	90	N/A
21931	13.99	13.99	90	80
21932	19.98	19.98	90	80
21933	22.01	22.01	90	80

Medicare References: 100-2,15,260; 100-4,12,30; 100-4,12,90.3; 100-4,14,10

21935-21936

21935 Radical resection of tumor (eg, malignant neoplasm), soft tissue of back or flank; less than 5 cm

21936 5 cm or greater

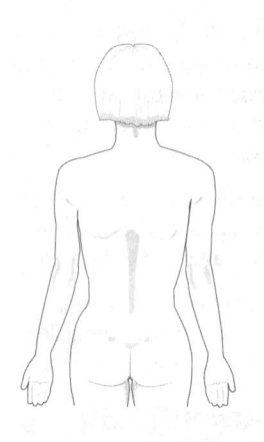

Radical resection of a soft tissue tumor of the back or flank is reported with 21935 if less than 5 cm and 21936 of 5 cm or greater

Explanation

The physician performs a radical resection of a malignant soft tissue tumor from the back or flank, not involving bone. An incision is made over the tumor and dissection exposes it. The tumor and any adjacent tissue that may be affected by the spread of the neoplasm are excised. Large resections may be needed. The type and stage of the lesion determines the extent of the tumor margin resection area. Muscle or fascia may need to be repaired and drains may be placed. The surgical wound is repaired by intermediate or complex closure, adjacent tissue transfer, or graft. Report 21935 for excision of tumors less than 5 cm and 21936 for excision of tumors 5 cm or greater.

Coding Tips

An excisional biopsy is not reported separately when a therapeutic excision is performed during the same surgical session. Report any free grafts or flaps separately.

ICD-9-CM Procedural

- 83.32 Excision of lesion of muscle
- 83.39 Excision of lesion of other soft tissue
- 83.49 Other excision of soft tissue
- 86.3 Other local excision or destruction of lesion or tissue of skin and subcutaneous tissue
- 86.4 Radical excision of skin lesion

Anesthesia

00300, 00730, 00820

ICD-9-CM Diagnostic

- 171.7 Malignant neoplasm of connective and other soft tissue of trunk, unspecified site
- 172.5 Malignant melanoma of skin of trunk, except scrotum
- 195.8 Malignant neoplasm of other specified sites
- 198.89 Secondary malignant neoplasm of other specified sites
- 209.35 Merkel cell carcinoma of the trunk
- 209.75 Secondary Merkel cell carcinoma
- 214.1 Lipoma of other skin and subcutaneous tissue
- 215.7 Other benign neoplasm of connective and other soft tissue of trunk, unspecified
- 228.01 Hemangioma of skin and subcutaneous tissue
- 238.1 Neoplasm of uncertain behavior of connective and other soft tissue
- 239.2 Neoplasms of unspecified nature of bone, soft tissue, and skin
- 782.2 Localized superficial swelling, mass, or lump

Terms To Know

radical resection. Removal of an entire tumor (e.g., malignant neoplasm) along with a large area of surrounding tissue, including adjacent lymph nodes that may have been infiltrated.

soft tissue. Nonepithelial tissues outside of the skeleton.

CCI Version 16.3

0228T, 0230T, 10060, 10140, 10160, 11010-11012❖, 11040-11044, 12001-12007, 12020-12037, 13100-13101, 20102, 36000, 36400-36410, 36420-36430, 36440, 36600, 36640, 37202, 43752, 49010, 51701-51703, 62310-62319, 64400-64435, 64445-64450, 64479, 64483, 64505-64530, 69990, 93000-93010, 93040-93042, 93318, 94002, 94200, 94250, 94680-94690, 94770, 95812-95816, 95819, 95822, 95829, 95955, 96360, 96365, 96372, 96374-96376, 99148-99149, 99150

Also not with 21935: 21920-21933

Also not with 21936: 0213T, 0216T, 21920-21935, 64490, 64493

Note: These CCI edits are used for Medicare. Other payers may reimburse on codes listed above.

Medicare Edits

	Fac RVU	Non-Fac RVU	FUD	Assist
21935	30.33	30.33	90	N/A
21936	42.64	42.64	90	80

Medicare References: 100-2,15,260; 100-4,12,30; 100-4,12,90.3; 100-4,14,10

22010-22015

22010 Incision and drainage, open, of deep abscess (subfascial), posterior spine; cervical, thoracic, or cervicothoracic

22015 lumbar, sacral, or lumbosacral

Open treatment of a deep abscess of the posterior spine requires that vessels, muscle and other tissue be deflected away from the spinous process. In 22010, the site is cervical or thoracic; in 22015, the site is lumbar or sacral

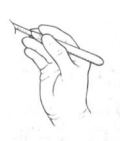

Necrotic tissue and debris may be removed

Explanation

The physician performs an open incision and drainage of a deep abscess of the posterior spine. Once a paraspinal soft tissue abscess or a lumbar psoas muscle abscess is identified by MRI or CT scan, an aspiration biopsy may be performed prior to open surgical drainage. The extent of the surgery depends on the size of the abscess and the area affected. The deep fascia is incised and the wound opened, irrigated, and debrided. Necrotic tissue and debris are removed and the cavity is irrigated with antibiotic solution. The wound is closed in layers and a drain or wound vacuum device may be placed. Report 22010 for incision and drainage of a deep abscess in the cervical, thoracic, or cervicothoracic region of the posterior spine and 22015 for the lumbar, sacral, or lumbosacral region.

Coding Tips

Local anesthesia is included in these services. Do not report 22015 in conjunction with 22010 unless a separate anatomical area is treated. Append modifier 59 as needed. Incision and drainage performed at the thoracolumbar junction should be reported separately. For posterior instrumentation removal, see 22850 and 22852. For incision and drainage of a superficial abscess, hematoma, or fluid collection, see 10060 and 10140.

ICD-9-CM Procedural

- 77.10 Other incision of bone without division, unspecified site
- 77.19 Other incision of other bone, except facial bones, without division
- 83.09 Other incision of soft tissue

Anesthesia

22010 00300, 00600, 00604, 00620
22015 00630

ICD-9-CM Diagnostic

- 324.9 Intracranial and intraspinal abscess of unspecified site
- 682.1 Cellulitis and abscess of neck — (Use additional code to identify organism, such as 041.1, etc.)
- 682.2 Cellulitis and abscess of trunk — (Use additional code to identify organism, such as 041.1, etc.)
- 682.8 Cellulitis and abscess of other specified site — (Use additional code to identify organism, such as 041.1, etc.)
- 728.86 Necrotizing fasciitis — (Use additional code to identify infectious organism, 041.00-041.89, 785.4, if applicable)
- 728.89 Other disorder of muscle, ligament, and fascia — (Use additional E code to identify drug, if drug-induced)
- 730.08 Acute osteomyelitis, other specified site — (Use additional code to identify organism: 041.1. Use additional code to identify major osseous defect, if applicable: 731.3)
- 731.3 Major osseous defects — (Code first underlying disease: 170.0-170.9, 730.00-730.29, 733.00-733.09, 733.40-733.49, 996.45)
- 996.63 Infection and inflammatory reaction due to nervous system device, implant, and graft — (Use additional code to identify specified infections)
- 996.67 Infection and inflammatory reaction due to other internal orthopedic device, implant, and graft — (Use additional code to identify specified infections)
- 996.78 Other complications due to other internal orthopedic device, implant, and graft — (Use additional code to identify complication: 338.18-338.19, 338.28-338.29)
- 998.59 Other postoperative infection — (Use additional code to identify infection)

Terms To Know

aspiration. Drawing fluid out by suction.

biopsy. Tissue or fluid removed for diagnostic purposes through analysis of the cells in the biopsy material.

blunt dissection. Surgical technique used to expose an underlying area by separating along natural cleavage lines of tissue, without cutting.

CCI Version 16.3

00600-00604, 00620, 00625-00626, 0213T, 0216T, 0228T, 0230T, 10060, 10140, 10160-10180, 22505, 36000, 36400-36410, 36420-36430, 36440, 36600, 36640, 37202, 43752, 51701-51703, 62310-62319, 64400-64435, 64445-64450, 64479, 64483, 64490, 64493, 64505-64530, 69990, 76000-76001, 93000-93010, 93040-93042, 93318, 94002, 94200, 94250, 94680-94690, 94770, 95812-95816, 95819, 95822, 95829, 95955, 96360, 96365, 96372, 96374-96376, 97597-97598, 97602-97606, 99148-99149, 99150

Also not with 22010: 22015

Note: These CCI edits are used for Medicare. Other payers may reimburse on codes listed above.

Medicare Edits

	Fac RVU	Non-Fac RVU	FUD	Assist
22010	27.4	27.4	90	80
22015	26.96	26.96	90	N/A

Medicare References: None

22100-22103

22100 Partial excision of posterior vertebral component (eg, spinous process, lamina or facet) for intrinsic bony lesion, single vertebral segment; cervical
22101 thoracic
22102 lumbar
22103 each additional segment (List separately in addition to code for primary procedure)

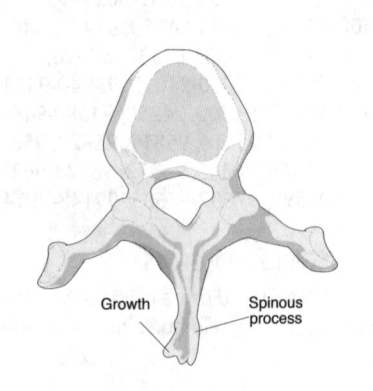

Physician removes growths from the spinous process of a cervical vertebra (22100) of a thoracic vertebra (22101) or lumbar vertebra (22102) or additional segment (22103)

Explanation

The physician removes spurs, other growths, or bone disease by partial resection of a posterior vertebral component such as the spinous process, lamina, or facet. The patient is placed prone and an incision is made overlying the affected vertebra and taken down to the level of the fascia. The fascia is incised and the paravertebral muscles are retracted. The physician removes the affected part of the spinous process, lamina, or facet. Paravertebral muscles are repositioned and the tissue and skin is closed with layered sutures. Report 22100 for a cervical vertebral segment; 22101 for a thoracic vertebral segment; and 22102 for a lumbar vertebral segment. Report 22103 for each additional segment in conjunction with the code for the primary procedure.

Coding Tips

An excisional biopsy is not reported separately if a therapeutic excision is performed during the same surgical session. Use 22103 in conjunction with 22100–22102. As an "add-on" code, 22103 is not subject to multiple procedure rules. No reimbursement reduction or modifier 51 is applied. Add-on codes describe additional intra-service work associated with the primary procedure. They are performed by the same physician on the same date of service as the primary service/procedure, and must never be reported as a stand-alone code. For partial excision of vertebral body, for intrinsic bony lesion, without decompression of the spinal cord and/or nerve root, see 22110–22116. For complete or near complete resection of the vertebral body, see vertebral corpectomy codes 63081–63091.

ICD-9-CM Procedural

77.89 Other partial ostectomy of other bone, except facial bones

Anesthesia

22100 00600, 00604, 00670
22101 00620, 00670
22102 00630, 00635, 00640, 00670
22103 N/A

ICD-9-CM Diagnostic

170.2 Malignant neoplasm of vertebral column, excluding sacrum and coccyx
198.5 Secondary malignant neoplasm of bone and bone marrow
213.2 Benign neoplasm of vertebral column, excluding sacrum and coccyx
720.0 Ankylosing spondylitis
720.1 Spinal enthesopathy
720.81 Inflammatory spondylopathies in diseases classified elsewhere — (Code first underlying disease: 015.0)
720.89 Other inflammatory spondylopathies
720.9 Unspecified inflammatory spondylopathy
721.0 Cervical spondylosis without myelopathy
721.1 Cervical spondylosis with myelopathy
721.2 Thoracic spondylosis without myelopathy
721.3 Lumbosacral spondylosis without myelopathy
721.41 Spondylosis with myelopathy, thoracic region
721.42 Spondylosis with myelopathy, lumbar region
721.5 Kissing spine
721.8 Other allied disorders of spine
723.0 Spinal stenosis in cervical region
730.18 Chronic osteomyelitis, other specified sites — (Use additional code to identify organism: 041.1. Use additional code to identify major osseous defect, if applicable: 731.3)
733.13 Pathologic fracture of vertebrae
733.20 Unspecified cyst of bone (localized)
733.21 Solitary bone cyst
733.22 Aneurysmal bone cyst
738.5 Other acquired deformity of back or spine
756.15 Congenital fusion of spine (vertebra)

CCI Version 16.3

92585, 95822, 95860-95861, 95867-95868, 95900, 95904, 95920, 95936-95937

Also not with 22100: 0213T, 0216T, 0228T, 0230T, 10060, 10140, 10160, 22505, 36000, 36400-36410, 36420-36430, 36440, 36600, 36640, 37202, 43752, 51701-51703, 62310-62319, 64400-64435, 64445-64450, 64479, 64483, 64490, 64493, 64505-64530, 69990, 76000-76001, 93000-93010, 93040-93042, 93318, 94002, 94200, 94250, 94680-94690, 94770, 95812-95816, 95819, 95829, 95870, 95925-95934, 95955, 96360, 96365, 96372, 96374-96376, 99148-99149, 99150

Also not with 22101: 0213T, 0216T, 0228T, 0230T, 10060, 10140, 10160, 22100, 22505, 36000, 36400-36410, 36420-36430, 36440, 36600, 36640, 37202, 43752, 51701-51703, 62310-62319, 64400-64435, 64445-64450, 64479, 64483, 64490, 64493, 64505-64530, 69990, 76000-76001, 93000-93010, 93040-93042, 93318, 94002, 94200, 94250, 94680-94690, 94770, 95812-95816, 95819, 95829, 95870, 95925-95934, 95955, 96360, 96365, 96372, 96374-96376, 99148-99149, 99150

Also not with 22102: 0171T❖, 0213T, 0216T, 0228T, 0230T, 10060, 10140, 10160, 22101, 22505, 36000, 36400-36410, 36420-36430, 36440, 36600, 36640, 37202, 43752, 51701-51703, 62310-62319, 64400-64435, 64445-64450, 64479, 64483, 64490, 64493, 64505-64530, 64712, 69990, 76000-76001, 93000-93010, 93040-93042, 93318, 94002, 94200, 94250, 94680-94690, 94770, 95812-95816, 95819, 95829, 95870, 95925-95934, 95955, 96360, 96365, 96372, 96374-96376, 99148-99149, 99150

Also not with 22103: 95925-95927, 95930-95934

Note: These CCI edits are used for Medicare. Other payers may reimburse on codes listed above.

Medicare Edits

	Fac RVU	Non-Fac RVU	FUD	Assist
22100	25.56	25.56	90	80
22101	25.03	25.03	90	80
22102	24.04	24.04	90	80
22103	4.3	4.3	N/A	80

Medicare References: None

22110-22116

22110 Partial excision of vertebral body, for intrinsic bony lesion, without decompression of spinal cord or nerve root(s), single vertebral segment; cervical
22112 thoracic
22114 lumbar
22116 each additional vertebral segment (List separately in addition to code for primary procedure)

Explanation
The physician removes spurs, other growths, or bone disease by partial resection of a vertebral body. With the patient stabilized by a halo or cranial tongs, the physician makes an anterior incision to reach the vertebral body. Lower cervical vertebrae are approached above the clavicle, dividing the superficial muscles and fascia and retracting the trachea, esophagus, and thyroid medially. After blunt division of the deep fascia and paravertebral muscles, the anterior aspect of the cervical spine is exposed. The bony lesion is identified and excised from the affected vertebral body. Once the lesion is removed, a drain is placed and the incision is closed in layered sutures. The halo or tongs are attached to a body jacket to assure stabilization of the spine. Report 22110 for a cervical segment; 22112 for a thoracic segment; and 22114 for a lumbar vertebral segment. Report 22116 for each additional segment in conjunction with the code for the primary procedure.

Coding Tips
An excisional biopsy is not reported separately if a therapeutic excision is performed during the same surgical session. Use 22116 in conjunction with 22110–22114. As an "add-on" code, 22116 is not subject to multiple procedure rules. No reimbursement reduction or modifier 51 is applied. Add-on codes describe additional intra-service work associated with the primary procedure. They are performed by the same physician on the same date of service as the primary service/procedure, and must never be reported as a stand-alone code. For partial resection of a posterior vertebral component (spinous processes, lamina or facet), for an intrinsic bony lesion, see 22100–22103. For complete or near complete resection of the vertebral body, see vertebral corpectomy codes 63081–63091. For a bone graft for spinal procedures, see 20930–20938.

ICD-9-CM Procedural
77.89 Other partial ostectomy of other bone, except facial bones

Anesthesia
22110 00600, 00604, 00670
22112 00620, 00625, 00626, 00670
22114 00630, 00670
22116 N/A

ICD-9-CM Diagnostic
094.0 Tabes dorsalis — (Use additional code to identify any associated mental disorder. Use additional code to identify manifestation: 713.5)
098.53 Gonococcal spondylitis
170.2 Malignant neoplasm of vertebral column, excluding sacrum and coccyx
198.5 Secondary malignant neoplasm of bone and bone marrow
213.2 Benign neoplasm of vertebral column, excluding sacrum and coccyx
238.0 Neoplasm of uncertain behavior of bone and articular cartilage
721.5 Kissing spine
722.31 Schmorl's nodes, thoracic region
722.32 Schmorl's nodes, lumbar region
722.39 Schmorl's nodes, other spinal region
723.0 Spinal stenosis in cervical region
724.01 Spinal stenosis of thoracic region
724.02 Spinal stenosis of lumbar region, without neurogenic claudication
724.03 Spinal stenosis of lumbar region, with neurogenic claudication
730.18 Chronic osteomyelitis, other specified sites — (Use additional code to identify organism: 041.1. Use additional code to identify major osseous defect, if applicable: 731.3)
731.3 Major osseous defects — (Code first underlying disease: 170.0-170.9, 730.00-730.29, 733.00-733.09, 733.40-733.49, 996.45)
733.21 Solitary bone cyst
733.22 Aneurysmal bone cyst
733.29 Other cyst of bone

CCI Version 16.3
92585, 95822, 95860-95861, 95867-95868, 95900, 95904, 95920, 95936-95937

Also not with 22110: 0213T, 0216T, 0228T, 0230T, 10060, 10140, 10160, 22505, 36000, 36400-36410, 36420-36430, 36440, 36600, 36640, 37202, 43752, 51701-51703, 62310-62319, 64400-64435, 64445-64450, 64479, 64483, 64490, 64493, 64505-64530, 69990, 76000-76001, 93000-93010, 93040-93042, 93318, 94002, 94200, 94250, 94680-94690, 94770, 95812-95816, 95819, 95829, 95870, 95925-95934, 95955, 96360, 96365, 96372, 96374-96376, 99148-99149, 99150

Also not with 22112: 0213T, 0216T, 0228T, 0230T, 10060, 10140, 10160, 22101, 22110, 22505, 36000, 36400-36410, 36420-36430, 36440, 36600, 36640, 37202, 43752, 51701-51703, 62310-62319, 64400-64435, 64445-64450, 64479, 64483, 64490, 64493, 64505-64530, 69990, 76000-76001, 93000-93010, 93040-93042, 93318, 94002, 94200, 94250, 94680-94690, 94770, 95812-95816, 95819, 95829, 95870, 95925-95934, 95955, 96360, 96365, 96372, 96374-96376, 99148-99149, 99150

Also not with 22114: 0213T, 0216T, 0228T, 0230T, 10060, 10140, 10160, 22102, 22112, 22505, 36000, 36400-36410, 36420-36430, 36440, 36600, 36640, 37202, 43752, 49000-49010, 51701-51703, 62310-62319, 64400-64435, 64445-64450, 64479, 64483, 64490, 64493, 64505-64530, 69990, 76000-76001, 93000-93010, 93040-93042, 93318, 94002, 94200, 94250, 94680-94690, 94770, 95812-95816, 95819, 95829, 95870, 95925-95934, 95955, 96360, 96365, 96372, 96374-96376, 99148-99149, 99150

Also not with 22116: 95925-95927, 95930-95934

Note: These CCI edits are used for Medicare. Other payers may reimburse on codes listed above.

Medicare Edits

	Fac RVU	Non-Fac RVU	FUD	Assist
22110	31.43	31.43	90	80
22112	30.99	30.99	90	80
22114	29.0	29.0	90	80
22116	4.19	4.19	N/A	80

Medicare References: None

22206-22208

22206 Osteotomy of spine, posterior or posterolateral approach, 3 columns, 1 vertebral segment (eg, pedicle/vertebral body subtraction); thoracic
22207 lumbar
22208 each additional vertebral segment (List separately in addition to code for primary procedure)

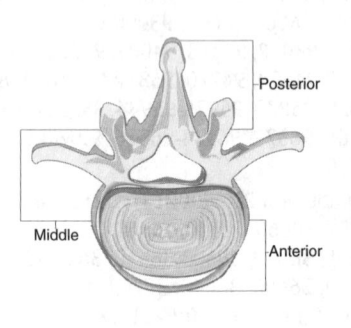

Spinal Columns — Posterior, Middle, Anterior

Explanation
Three-column spinal osteotomy is performed to correct moderate to severe spinal deformities that result in limited flexibility. Also known as pedicle subtraction osteotomy, it involves cutting and removing one or more portions of the vertebral segment in order to prepare for spinal realignment. The three columns consist of the anterior (anterior two-thirds of the vertebral body), the middle (posterior third of the vertebral body and the pedicle), and the posterior (articular facets, lamina, and spinous process). Using a posterior or posterolateral approach, the surgeon excises all posterior elements at the site of the correction, including the pedicles and the adjacent facet joints (inferior and superior). The physician then removes a posterior wedge of cancellous bone from the vertebral body to achieve the desired correction. The entire posterior and lateral vertebral body walls may also be removed. The osteotomy is closed by extending the patient's position on the operative frame or through instrumentation compression. Report 22206 if the procedure is performed on a thoracic vertebral segment and 22207 if the segment is lumbar. Report 22208 for each additional vertebral segment in conjunction with the code for the primary procedure.

Coding Tips
As an "add-on" code, 22208 is not subject to multiple procedure rules. No reimbursement reduction or modifier 51 is applied. Add-on codes describe additional intra-service work associated with the primary procedure. They are performed by the same physician on the same date of service as the primary service/procedure, and must never be reported as a stand-alone code. Use 22208 in conjunction with 22206–22207. Do not report 22206–22207 in conjunction with 22210–22226, 22830, 63001–63048, 63055–63066, 63075–63091, or 63101–63103 when performed at the same level. For arthrodesis performed with an osteotomy of the spine, see 22590–22632. Spinal instrumentation is reported separately, see 22840–22847. Bone graft for spinal procedures is also reported separately, see 20930–20938.

ICD-9-CM Procedural
77.29 Wedge osteotomy of other bone, except facial bones
77.39 Other division of other bone, except facial bones

Anesthesia
22206 00620, 00670
22207 00630, 00670
22208 N/A

ICD-9-CM Diagnostic
237.71 Neurofibromatosis, Type 1 (von Recklinghausen's disease)
237.73 Schwannomatosis
268.1 Rickets, late effect — (Use additional code to identify the nature of late effect)
720.0 Ankylosing spondylitis
721.7 Traumatic spondylopathy
731.0 Osteitis deformans without mention of bone tumor
732.0 Juvenile osteochondrosis of spine
733.13 Pathologic fracture of vertebrae
737.10 Kyphosis (acquired) (postural)
737.11 Kyphosis due to radiation
737.12 Kyphosis, postlaminectomy
737.19 Other kyphosis (acquired)
737.20 Lordosis (acquired) (postural)
737.30 Scoliosis (and kyphoscoliosis), idiopathic
737.41 Kyphosis associated with other condition — (Code first associated condition: 015.0, 138, 237.7, 252.01, 277.5, 356.1, 731.0, 733.00-733.09)
738.5 Other acquired deformity of back or spine
756.12 Congenital spondylolisthesis
756.15 Congenital fusion of spine (vertebra)
756.19 Other congenital anomaly of spine
805.00 Closed fracture of cervical vertebra, unspecified level without mention of spinal cord injury

CCI Version 16.3
Also not with 22206: 0213T, 0216T, 0228T, 0230T, 11010-11012❖, 22100❖, 22112❖, 22114❖, 22207, 22212-22214, 22220-22224, 22505, 22830, 36000, 36400-36410, 36420-36430, 36440, 36600, 36640, 37202, 43752, 62310-62319, 63001-63005, 63011-63020, 63040, 63042, 63045-63046, 63055-63056, 63064, 63075, 63077, 63081, 63085, 63087, 63090, 63101-63102, 63170-63191❖, 63194-63200❖, 63265-63283❖, 63295-63305❖, 63307❖, 64400-64435, 64445-64450, 64479, 64483, 64490, 64493, 64505-64530, 69990, 76000-76001, 92585, 93000-93010, 93040-93042, 93318, 94002, 94200, 94250, 94680-94690, 94770, 95812-95816, 95819, 95822, 95829, 95860-95861, 95867-95868, 95870, 95900, 95904, 95920, 95925-95934, 95936-95937, 95955, 96360, 96365, 96372, 96374-96376, 99148-99149, 99150

Also not with 22207: 0213T, 0216T, 0228T, 0230T, 11010-11012❖, 22100❖, 22112❖, 22114❖, 22210-22214, 22220-22224, 22505, 22830, 36000, 36400-36410, 36420-36430, 36440, 36600, 36640, 37202, 43752, 62310-62319, 63001-63005, 63011-63020, 63030, 63040, 63042, 63045-63047, 63055-63056, 63064, 63075, 63077, 63081, 63085, 63087, 63090, 63101-63102, 63170-63191❖, 63194-63200❖, 63265-63283❖, 63295-63307❖, 64400-64435, 64445-64450, 64479, 64483, 64490, 64493, 64505-64530, 69990, 76000-76001, 92585, 93000-93010, 93040-93042, 93318, 94002, 94200, 94250, 94680-94690, 94770, 95812-95816, 95819, 95822, 95829, 95860-95861, 95867-95868, 95870, 95900, 95904, 95920, 95925-95934, 95936-95937, 95955, 96360, 96365, 96372, 96374-96376, 99148-99149, 99150

Note: These CCI edits are used for Medicare. Other payers may reimburse on codes listed above.

Medicare Edits

	Fac RVU	Non-Fac RVU	FUD	Assist
22206	69.19	69.19	90	80
22207	70.3	70.3	90	80
22208	17.51	17.51	N/A	80

Medicare References: 100-4,12,40.8

22210-22216

22210 Osteotomy of spine, posterior or posterolateral approach, 1 vertebral segment; cervical
22212 thoracic
22214 lumbar
22216 each additional vertebral segment (List separately in addition to primary procedure)

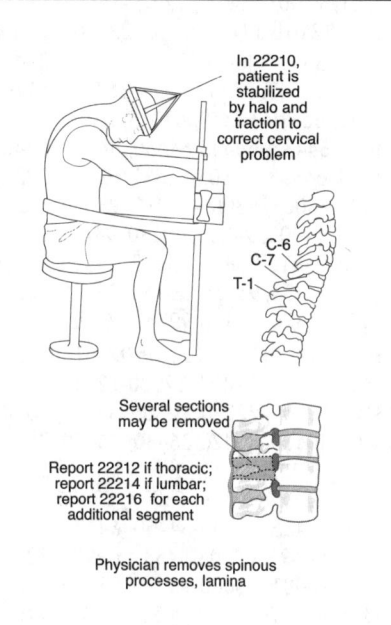

Explanation

These procedures are performed to correct spinal deformities. The patient is placed in a sitting position with the head supported by a halo. In 22210, a posterior midline incision is made over the cervicothoracic junction. The physician exposes the spine from C5 to T1. The posterior elements of C7 are removed as are the caudal half of C6 and cephalad half of T1. The osteotomy continues laterally. The patient is placed under general anesthesia and the forward parts of the vertebrae are fractured. The resected bone is placed laterally and the muscles are reattached with sutures. The wound is closed with layered sutures. The angle of the neck is adjusted using the halo and a halo vest. Report 22210 if the site is cervical; 22212 if the site is thoracic; 22214 if the site is lumbar; and 22216 for each additional segment.

Coding Tips

Codes 22210–22216 report an osteotomy performed by a posterior or posterolateral approach; if performed by anterior approach, see 22220–22226. Use 22216 in conjunction with 22210–22214. As an "add-on" code, 22216 is not subject to multiple procedure rules. No reimbursement reduction or modifier 51 is applied. Add-on codes describe additional intra-service work associated with the primary procedure. They are performed by the same physician on the same date of service as the primary service/procedure, and must never be reported as a stand-alone code. If arthrodesis is performed with an osteotomy of the spine, it is reported separately; see 22590–22632. Note that arthrodesis codes are also assigned by approach. Any spinal instrumentation is reported separately; see 22840–22847. Bone graft for spinal procedures is also reported separately; see 20930–20938. For vertebral corpectomy, see 63081–63091.

ICD-9-CM Procedural

77.29 Wedge osteotomy of other bone, except facial bones
77.39 Other division of other bone, except facial bones

Anesthesia

22210 00600, 00670
22212 00620, 00670
22214 00630, 00670
22216 N/A

ICD-9-CM Diagnostic

237.71 Neurofibromatosis, Type 1 (von Recklinghausen's disease)
237.73 Schwannomatosis
237.79 Other neurofibromatosis
720.0 Ankylosing spondylitis
721.7 Traumatic spondylopathy
731.0 Osteitis deformans without mention of bone tumor
732.0 Juvenile osteochondrosis of spine
733.13 Pathologic fracture of vertebrae
737.10 Kyphosis (acquired) (postural)
737.11 Kyphosis due to radiation
737.12 Kyphosis, postlaminectomy
737.19 Other kyphosis (acquired)
737.20 Lordosis (acquired) (postural)
737.30 Scoliosis (and kyphoscoliosis), idiopathic
737.41 Kyphosis associated with other condition — (Code first associated condition: 015.0, 138, 237.7, 252.01, 277.5, 356.1, 731.0, 733.00-733.09)
738.5 Other acquired deformity of back or spine
756.12 Congenital spondylolisthesis
756.15 Congenital fusion of spine (vertebra)
756.19 Other congenital anomaly of spine
805.00 Closed fracture of cervical vertebra, unspecified level without mention of spinal cord injury
805.10 Open fracture of cervical vertebra, unspecified level without mention of spinal cord injury

CCI Version 16.3

92585, 95822, 95860-95861, 95867-95868, 95900, 95904, 95920, 95936-95937

Also not with 22210: 0213T, 0216T, 0228T, 0230T, 12001-12007, 12020-12047, 13100-13101, 13131-13132, 22212, 22505, 36000, 36400-36410, 36420-36430, 36440, 36600, 36640, 37202, 43752, 51701-51703, 62310-62319, 63020, 63045, 64400-64435, 64445-64450, 64479, 64483, 64490, 64493, 64505-64530, 69990, 76000-76001, 93000-93010, 93040-93042, 93318, 94002, 94200, 94250, 94680-94690, 94770, 95812-95816, 95819, 95829, 95870, 95925-95934, 95955, 96360, 96365, 96372, 96374-96376, 99148-99149, 99150

Also not with 22212: 0213T, 0216T, 0228T, 0230T, 12001-12007, 12020-12037, 13100-13101, 22222❖, 22505, 36000, 36440, 36400-36410, 36420-36430, 36600, 36640, 37202, 43752, 51701-51703, 62310-62319, 64400-64435, 64445-64450, 64479, 64483, 64490, 64493, 64505-64530, 76000-76001, 93000-93010, 93040-93042, 93318, 94002, 94200, 94250, 94680-94690, 94770, 95812-95816, 95819, 95829, 95870, 95925-95934, 95955, 96360, 96365, 96372, 96374-96376, 99148-99149, 99150

Also not with 22214: 0171T❖, 0213T, 0216T, 0228T, 0230T, 12001-12007, 12020-12037, 13100-13101, 22212, 22224❖, 22505, 36000, 36400-36410, 36420-36430, 36440, 36600, 36640, 37202, 43752, 51701-51703, 62310-62319, 63030, 63047, 64400-64435, 64445-64450, 64479, 64483, 64490, 64493, 64505-64530, 69990, 76000-76001, 93000-93010, 93040-93042, 93318, 94002, 94200, 94250, 94680-94690, 94770, 95812-95816, 95819, 95829, 95870, 95925-95934, 95955, 96360, 96365, 96372, 96374-96376, 99148-99149, 99150

Also not with 22216: 95925-95927, 95930-95934

Note: These CCI edits are used for Medicare. Other payers may reimburse on codes listed above.

Medicare Edits

	Fac RVU	Non-Fac RVU	FUD	Assist
22210	51.85	51.85	90	80
22212	42.98	42.98	90	80
22214	43.26	43.26	90	80
22216	10.93	10.93	N/A	80

Medicare References: 100-4,12,40.8

22220-22226

22220 Osteotomy of spine, including discectomy, anterior approach, single vertebral segment; cervical
22222 thoracic
22224 lumbar
22226 each additional vertebral segment (List separately in addition to code for primary procedure)

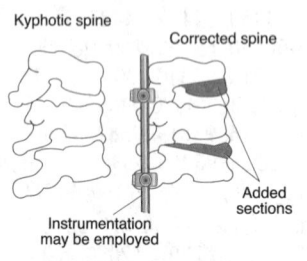

Kyphotic spine
Corrected spine
Added sections
Instrumentation may be employed
Physician corrects kyphosis by adding grafts to anterior body
Report 22220 if cervical; report 22222 if thoracic; report 22224 if lumbar; report 22226 for each additional segment
Sections removed
Spine extended

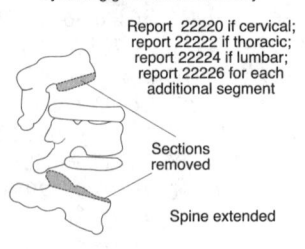

Explanation

Spinal osteotomy is performed to correct spinal deformities. In this procedure, the physician uses an anterior approach to reach the involved vertebrae. For a cervical vertebral segment in 22220, an incision is made through the neck, avoiding the esophagus, trachea, and thyroid. For a thoracic vertebral segment in 22222, an incision is made through the chest, with possible detachment of the clavicle, costal cartilage, and manubrium. For a lumbar vertebral segment in 22224, an incision is made through the tenth rib, into the chest cavity with rib spreaders, and dissection of abdominal contents away from the diaphragm. Retractors separate the intervertebral muscles. A marker is inserted in the affected vertebral segment and the location is confirmed by separately reportable x-ray. With a rongeur, the physician cleans out the intervertebral disc space between the concerned vertebral bone and its neighboring vertebrae. An osteotomy of the single vertebral segment is carried out by removing a wedge of bone from the middle portion of the vertebral body. The spine is extended to achieve correction and separately reportable bone grafts and/or spinal instrumentation may need to be placed to maintain the spine in the straightened position. The muscles are reattached and the wound is closed with layered sutures. Report 22226 for each additional vertebral segment in conjunction with the code for the primary procedure.

Coding Tips

Codes 22220–22226 report an osteotomy performed by an anterior approach. If performed by a posterior or posterolateral approach, see 22210–22216. Use 22226 in conjunction with 22220–22224. As an "add-on" code, 22226 is not subject to multiple procedure rules. No reimbursement reduction or modifier 51 is applied. Add-on codes describe additional intra-service work associated with the primary procedure. They are performed by the same physician on the same date of service as the primary service/procedure, and must never be reported as a stand-alone code.

ICD-9-CM Procedural

- 77.29 Wedge osteotomy of other bone, except facial bones
- 77.39 Other division of other bone, except facial bones
- 80.51 Excision of intervertebral disc

Anesthesia

22220 00600, 00670
22222 00620, 00625, 00626
22224 00630, 00670
22226 N/A

ICD-9-CM Diagnostic

- 237.70 Neurofibromatosis, unspecified
- 237.73 Schwannomatosis
- 722.0 Displacement of cervical intervertebral disc without myelopathy
- 722.10 Displacement of lumbar intervertebral disc without myelopathy
- 722.11 Displacement of thoracic intervertebral disc without myelopathy
- 722.4 Degeneration of cervical intervertebral disc
- 722.51 Degeneration of thoracic or thoracolumbar intervertebral disc
- 722.52 Degeneration of lumbar or lumbosacral intervertebral disc
- 722.71 Intervertebral cervical disc disorder with myelopathy, cervical region
- 722.72 Intervertebral thoracic disc disorder with myelopathy, thoracic region
- 722.73 Intervertebral lumbar disc disorder with myelopathy, lumbar region
- 737.10 Kyphosis (acquired) (postural)
- 737.12 Kyphosis, postlaminectomy
- 737.20 Lordosis (acquired) (postural)
- 737.30 Scoliosis (and kyphoscoliosis), idiopathic
- 756.12 Congenital spondylolisthesis
- 756.15 Congenital fusion of spine (vertebra)

CCI Version 16.3

92585, 95822, 95860-95861, 95867-95868, 95900, 95904, 95920, 95936-95937

Also not with 22220: 0213T, 0216T, 0228T, 0230T, 12001-12007, 12020-12047, 13100-13101, 13131-13132, 22210❖, 22505, 36000, 36400-36410, 36420-36430, 36440, 36600, 36640, 37202, 43752, 51701-51703, 62291, 62310-62319, 63075, 63081, 64400-64435, 64445-64450, 64479, 64483, 64490, 64493, 64505-64530, 69990, 72285, 76000-76001, 93000-93010, 93040-93042, 93318, 94002, 94200, 94250, 94680-94690, 94770, 95812-95816, 95819, 95829, 95870, 95925-95934, 95955, 96360, 96365, 96372, 96374-96376, 99148-99149, 99150

Also not with 22222: 0213T, 0216T, 0228T, 0230T, 12001-12007, 12020-12037, 13100-13101, 22220, 22505, 32100, 36000, 36400-36410, 36420-36430, 36440, 36600, 36640, 37202, 43752, 49010, 51701-51703, 62291, 62310-62319, 63077, 63085, 64400-64435, 64445-64450, 64479, 64483, 64490, 64493, 64505-64530, 69990, 72285, 76000-76001, 93000-93010, 93040-93042, 93318, 94002, 94200, 94250, 94680-94690, 94770, 95812-95816, 95819, 95829, 95870, 95925-95934, 95955, 96360, 96365, 96372, 96374-96376, 99148-99149, 99150

Also not with 22224: 0213T, 0216T, 0228T, 0230T, 12001-12007, 12020-12037, 13100-13101, 22222, 22505, 22857❖, 36000, 36400-36410, 36420-36430, 36440, 36600, 36640, 37202, 43752, 49000-49010, 51701-51703, 62267❖, 62290, 62310-62319, 63087, 63090, 64400-64435, 64445-64450, 64479, 64483, 64490, 64493, 64505-64530, 69990, 72295, 76000-76001, 93000-93010, 93040-93042, 93318, 94002, 94200, 94250, 94680-94690, 94770, 95812-95816, 95819, 95829, 95870, 95925-95934, 95955, 96360, 96365, 96372, 96374-96376, 99148-99149, 99150

Also not with 22226: 95925-95927, 95930-95934

Note: These CCI edits are used for Medicare. Other payers may reimburse on codes listed above.

Medicare Edits

	Fac RVU	Non-Fac RVU	FUD	Assist
22220	47.19	47.19	90	80
22222	43.79	43.79	90	80
22224	46.24	46.24	90	80
22226	10.96	10.96	N/A	80

Medicare References: 100-4,12,40.8

22305

22305 Closed treatment of vertebral process fracture(s)

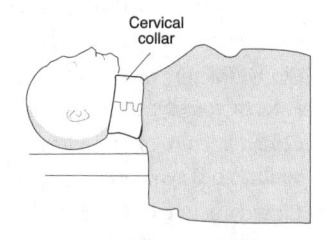

Cervical collar

Physician treats fractures passively with immobilization

Physician may choose sandbags or collar to immobilize cervical injuries and casting to immobilize other levels of the spine

Explanation

Closed treatment of a vertebral process fracture is only indicated if the spine is stable and the type of fracture does not require surgical intervention. In the case of the cervical spine, the physician initially immobilizes the patient's neck and spine with sandbags or a cervical collar as necessary. Use this code if the fracture is located in the vertebral processes.

Coding Tips

For closed treatment of a vertebral fracture and/or dislocation requiring casting or bracing, with or without anesthesia, by manipulation or traction, see 22315. When open treatment of a vertebral fracture and/or dislocation is performed, see 22325–22327. For decompression of the spine following a fracture, see 63001–63091. For arthrodesis of the spine following a fracture, see 22548–22650.

ICD-9-CM Procedural

- 03.53 Repair of vertebral fracture
- 79.09 Closed reduction of fracture of other specified bone, except facial bones, without internal fixation

Anesthesia

22305 00630, 00640

ICD-9-CM Diagnostic

- 336.9 Unspecified disease of spinal cord
- 731.3 Major osseous defects — (Code first underlying disease: 170.0-170.9, 730.00-730.29, 733.00-733.09, 733.40-733.49, 996.45)
- 733.01 Senile osteoporosis — (Use additional code to identify major osseous defect, if applicable: 731.3) (Use additional code to identify personal history of pathologic (healed) fracture: V13.51)
- 733.02 Idiopathic osteoporosis — (Use additional code to identify major osseous defect, if applicable: 731.3) (Use additional code to identify personal history of pathologic (healed) fracture: V13.51)
- 733.13 Pathologic fracture of vertebrae
- 733.95 Stress fracture of other bone — (Use additional external cause code(s) to identify the cause of the stress fracture)
- 805.01 Closed fracture of first cervical vertebra without mention of spinal cord injury
- 805.02 Closed fracture of second cervical vertebra without mention of spinal cord injury
- 805.03 Closed fracture of third cervical vertebra without mention of spinal cord injury
- 805.04 Closed fracture of fourth cervical vertebra without mention of spinal cord injury
- 805.05 Closed fracture of fifth cervical vertebra without mention of spinal cord injury
- 805.06 Closed fracture of sixth cervical vertebra without mention of spinal cord injury
- 805.07 Closed fracture of seventh cervical vertebra without mention of spinal cord injury
- 805.08 Closed fracture of multiple cervical vertebrae without mention of spinal cord injury
- 805.2 Closed fracture of dorsal (thoracic) vertebra without mention of spinal cord injury
- 805.4 Closed fracture of lumbar vertebra without mention of spinal cord injury
- 805.6 Closed fracture of sacrum and coccyx without mention of spinal cord injury
- 806.00 Closed fracture of C1-C4 level with unspecified spinal cord injury
- 806.01 Closed fracture of C1-C4 level with complete lesion of cord
- 806.02 Closed fracture of C1-C4 level with anterior cord syndrome
- 806.03 Closed fracture of C1-C4 level with central cord syndrome
- 806.04 Closed fracture of C1-C4 level with other specified spinal cord injury
- 806.05 Closed fracture of C5-C7 level with unspecified spinal cord injury
- 806.06 Closed fracture of C5-C7 level with complete lesion of cord
- 806.07 Closed fracture of C5-C7 level with anterior cord syndrome
- 806.08 Closed fracture of C5-C7 level with central cord syndrome
- 806.20 Closed fracture of T1-T6 level with unspecified spinal cord injury
- 806.21 Closed fracture of T1-T6 level with complete lesion of cord
- 806.22 Closed fracture of T1-T6 level with anterior cord syndrome
- 806.23 Closed fracture of T1-T6 level with central cord syndrome
- 806.24 Closed fracture of T1-T6 level with other specified spinal cord injury
- 806.25 Closed fracture of T7-T12 level with unspecified spinal cord injury
- 806.26 Closed fracture of T7-T12 level with complete lesion of cord
- 806.27 Closed fracture of T7-T12 level with anterior cord syndrome
- 806.28 Closed fracture of T7-T12 level with central cord syndrome
- 806.4 Closed fracture of lumbar spine with spinal cord injury

CCI Version 16.3

00640, 0213T, 0216T, 0228T, 0230T, 22110❖, 22310, 22505, 29010, 29020, 29035, 29200, 29700-29715, 36000, 36400-36410, 36420-36430, 36440, 36600, 36640, 37202, 43752, 51701-51703, 62310-62319, 64400-64435, 64445-64450, 64479, 64483, 64490, 64493, 64505-64530, 69990, 76000-76001, 92585, 93000-93010, 93040-93042, 93318, 94002, 94200, 94250, 94680-94690, 94770, 95812-95816, 95819, 95822, 95829, 95860-95861, 95867-95868, 95870, 95900, 95904, 95920, 95925-95934, 95936-95937, 95955, 96360, 96365, 96372, 96374-96376, 97597-97598, 97602-97606, 99148-99149, 99150

Note: These CCI edits are used for Medicare. Other payers may reimburse on codes listed above.

Medicare Edits

	Fac RVU	Non-Fac RVU	FUD	Assist
22305	4.98	5.43	90	N/A

Medicare References: 100-2,15,260; 100-4,12,30; 100-4,12,90.3; 100-4,14,10

22310

22310 Closed treatment of vertebral body fracture(s), without manipulation, requiring and including casting or bracing

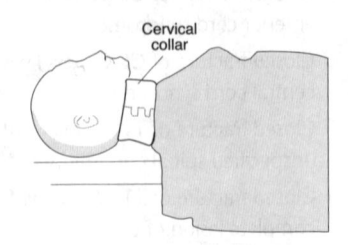

Cervical collar

Physician treats fractures passively with immobilization

Physician may choose sandbags or collar to immobilize cervical injuries and casting to immobilize other levels of the spine

Explanation

Closed treatment of a vertebral body fracture is only indicated if the spine is stable and the type of fracture does not require surgical intervention. In the case of the cervical spine, the physician initially immobilizes the patient's neck and spine with sandbags or a cervical collar as necessary. Use this code if the fracture is located in the vertebral body and treated without manipulation, but requiring and including casting or bracing.

Coding Tips

For closed treatment of a vertebral fracture and/or dislocation requiring casting or bracing, with or without anesthesia, by manipulation or traction, see 22315. When open treatment of a vertebral fracture and/or dislocation is performed, see 22325–22327. For decompression of the spine following a fracture, see 63001–63091. For arthrodesis of the spine following a fracture, see 22548–22650.

ICD-9-CM Procedural

- 03.53 Repair of vertebral fracture
- 79.09 Closed reduction of fracture of other specified bone, except facial bones, without internal fixation

Anesthesia

22310   00630, 00640

ICD-9-CM Diagnostic

- 336.9 Unspecified disease of spinal cord
- 731.3 Major osseous defects — (Code first underlying disease: 170.0-170.9, 730.00-730.29, 733.00-733.09, 733.40-733.49, 996.45)
- 733.13 Pathologic fracture of vertebrae
- 733.95 Stress fracture of other bone — (Use additional external cause code(s) to identify the cause of the stress fracture)
- 805.01 Closed fracture of first cervical vertebra without mention of spinal cord injury
- 805.02 Closed fracture of second cervical vertebra without mention of spinal cord injury
- 805.03 Closed fracture of third cervical vertebra without mention of spinal cord injury
- 805.04 Closed fracture of fourth cervical vertebra without mention of spinal cord injury
- 805.05 Closed fracture of fifth cervical vertebra without mention of spinal cord injury
- 805.06 Closed fracture of sixth cervical vertebra without mention of spinal cord injury
- 805.07 Closed fracture of seventh cervical vertebra without mention of spinal cord injury
- 805.08 Closed fracture of multiple cervical vertebrae without mention of spinal cord injury
- 805.2 Closed fracture of dorsal (thoracic) vertebra without mention of spinal cord injury
- 805.4 Closed fracture of lumbar vertebra without mention of spinal cord injury
- 805.6 Closed fracture of sacrum and coccyx without mention of spinal cord injury
- 806.00 Closed fracture of C1-C4 level with unspecified spinal cord injury
- 806.01 Closed fracture of C1-C4 level with complete lesion of cord
- 806.02 Closed fracture of C1-C4 level with anterior cord syndrome
- 806.03 Closed fracture of C1-C4 level with central cord syndrome
- 806.04 Closed fracture of C1-C4 level with other specified spinal cord injury
- 806.05 Closed fracture of C5-C7 level with unspecified spinal cord injury
- 806.06 Closed fracture of C5-C7 level with complete lesion of cord
- 806.07 Closed fracture of C5-C7 level with anterior cord syndrome
- 806.08 Closed fracture of C5-C7 level with central cord syndrome
- 806.09 Closed fracture of C5-C7 level with other specified spinal cord injury
- 806.20 Closed fracture of T1-T6 level with unspecified spinal cord injury
- 806.21 Closed fracture of T1-T6 level with complete lesion of cord
- 806.22 Closed fracture of T1-T6 level with anterior cord syndrome
- 806.23 Closed fracture of T1-T6 level with central cord syndrome
- 806.24 Closed fracture of T1-T6 level with other specified spinal cord injury
- 806.25 Closed fracture of T7-T12 level with unspecified spinal cord injury
- 806.26 Closed fracture of T7-T12 level with complete lesion of cord
- 806.27 Closed fracture of T7-T12 level with anterior cord syndrome
- 806.28 Closed fracture of T7-T12 level with central cord syndrome
- 806.29 Closed fracture of T7-T12 level with other specified spinal cord injury
- 806.4 Closed fracture of lumbar spine with spinal cord injury

CCI Version 16.3

00640, 0213T, 0216T, 0228T, 0230T, 22505, 29010, 29020, 29035, 29200, 29700-29715, 36000, 36400-36410, 36420-36430, 36440, 36600, 36640, 37202, 43752, 51701-51703, 62310-62319, 64400-64435, 64445-64450, 64479, 64483, 64490, 64493, 64505-64530, 69990, 76000-76001, 92585, 93000-93010, 93040-93042, 93318, 94002, 94200, 94250, 94680-94690, 94770, 95812-95816, 95819, 95822, 95829, 95860-95861, 95867-95868, 95870, 95900, 95904, 95920, 95925-95934, 95936-95937, 95955, 96360, 96365, 96372, 96374-96376, 97597-97598, 97602-97606, 99148-99149, 99150

Note: These CCI edits are used for Medicare. Other payers may reimburse on codes listed above.

Medicare Edits

	Fac RVU	Non-Fac RVU	FUD	Assist
22310	8.07	8.69	90	N/A

Medicare References: 100-2,15,260; 100-4,12,30; 100-4,12,90.3; 100-4,14,10

22315

22315 Closed treatment of vertebral fracture(s) and/or dislocation(s) requiring casting or bracing, with and including casting and/or bracing by manipulation or traction

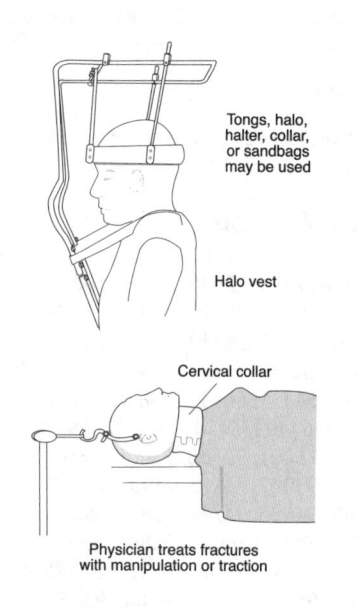

Tongs, halo, halter, collar, or sandbags may be used

Halo vest

Cervical collar

Physician treats fractures with manipulation or traction

Explanation

Following dislocation or traumatic or pathological fracture of the vertebrae, the physician decompresses the spine into proper alignment and immobilizes the vertebrae. The fracture or dislocation may be realigned by manual manipulation of the spine. If traction is employed, the patient is placed supine with a halo or tongs affixed to the skull. Traction is applied to the feet and to the halo or tongs, decompressing the vertebrae. As the traction is increased in stages, the physician assures that there is no additional neurological deficit. Traction is removed when the desired correction of the spine is accomplished. The patient is immobilized with bracing or casting, such as a halo cast.

Coding Tips

This code has been revised for 2011 in the official CPT description. Pay attention to diagnosis when assigning 22315. It is most often used for fractures and complete dislocations. However, it may be reported for subluxation (partial or incomplete dislocation) if casting or bracing is required. For treatment of subluxation with manipulation of the spine requiring anesthesia, but without casting or bracing, see 22505. For treatment of spinal subluxation with manipulation performed by a physician and not requiring general anesthesia and not using casting or bracing, see 97140. For open treatment of vertebral fractures and/or dislocations, see 22325–22328.

ICD-9-CM Procedural

03.53	Repair of vertebral fracture
79.09	Closed reduction of fracture of other specified bone, except facial bones, without internal fixation

Anesthesia

22315   00640

ICD-9-CM Diagnostic

336.9	Unspecified disease of spinal cord
731.3	Major osseous defects — (Code first underlying disease: 170.0-170.9, 730.00-730.29, 733.00-733.09, 733.40-733.49, 996.45)
733.13	Pathologic fracture of vertebrae
805.01	Closed fracture of first cervical vertebra without mention of spinal cord injury
805.02	Closed fracture of second cervical vertebra without mention of spinal cord injury
805.03	Closed fracture of third cervical vertebra without mention of spinal cord injury
805.04	Closed fracture of fourth cervical vertebra without mention of spinal cord injury
805.05	Closed fracture of fifth cervical vertebra without mention of spinal cord injury
805.06	Closed fracture of sixth cervical vertebra without mention of spinal cord injury
805.07	Closed fracture of seventh cervical vertebra without mention of spinal cord injury
805.2	Closed fracture of dorsal (thoracic) vertebra without mention of spinal cord injury
805.4	Closed fracture of lumbar vertebra without mention of spinal cord injury
806.02	Closed fracture of C1-C4 level with anterior cord syndrome
806.03	Closed fracture of C1-C4 level with central cord syndrome
806.06	Closed fracture of C5-C7 level with complete lesion of cord
806.07	Closed fracture of C5-C7 level with anterior cord syndrome
806.08	Closed fracture of C5-C7 level with central cord syndrome
806.22	Closed fracture of T1-T6 level with anterior cord syndrome
806.23	Closed fracture of T1-T6 level with central cord syndrome
806.26	Closed fracture of T7-T12 level with complete lesion of cord
806.27	Closed fracture of T7-T12 level with anterior cord syndrome
806.28	Closed fracture of T7-T12 level with central cord syndrome
806.4	Closed fracture of lumbar spine with spinal cord injury
839.01	Closed dislocation, first cervical vertebra
839.02	Closed dislocation, second cervical vertebra
839.03	Closed dislocation, third cervical vertebra
839.04	Closed dislocation, fourth cervical vertebra
839.05	Closed dislocation, fifth cervical vertebra
839.06	Closed dislocation, sixth cervical vertebra
839.07	Closed dislocation, seventh cervical vertebra
839.20	Closed dislocation, lumbar vertebra
839.21	Closed dislocation, thoracic vertebra

CCI Version 16.3

00640, 0213T, 0216T, 0228T, 0230T, 20650, 20690, 22305-22310, 22505, 29010, 29020, 29035, 29200, 29700-29715, 36000, 36400-36410, 36420-36430, 36440, 36600, 36640, 37202, 43752, 51701-51703, 62310-62319, 64400-64435, 64445-64450, 64479, 64483, 64490, 64493, 64505-64530, 69990, 76000-76001, 92585, 93000-93010, 93040-93042, 93318, 94002, 94200, 94250, 94680-94690, 94770, 95812-95816, 95819, 95822, 95829, 95860-95861, 95867-95868, 95870, 95900, 95904, 95920, 95925-95934, 95936-95937, 95955, 96360, 96365, 96372, 96374-96376, 97597-97598, 97602-97606, 99148-99149, 99150, J2001

Note: These CCI edits are used for Medicare. Other payers may reimburse on codes listed above.

Medicare Edits

	Fac RVU	Non-Fac RVU	FUD	Assist
22315	22.48	25.46	90	N/A

Medicare References: 100-2,15,260; 100-4,12,30; 100-4,12,90.3; 100-4,14,10

22318-22319

22318 Open treatment and/or reduction of odontoid fracture(s) and or dislocation(s) (including os odontoideum), anterior approach, including placement of internal fixation; without grafting

22319 with grafting

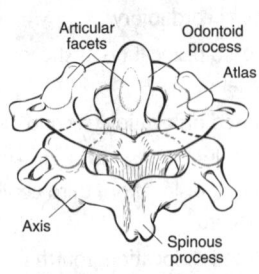

Posterior view of the first two vertebrae, the atlas (C-1) and the axis (C-2)

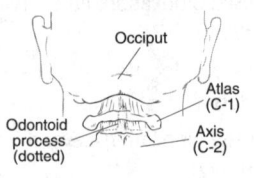

An odontoid fracture or dislocation is reduced and internal fixation may be placed. Report 22319 when grafts are used to stabilize the fracture

Explanation

The physician performs an open treatment and/or reduction of odontoid fracture and/or dislocation including the os odontoideum. The odontoid/os odontoideum (dens) is the tooth-like process located on the second cervical vertebra in the neck. The patient is placed in a supine position and the fracture/dislocation is reduced with skeletal traction. The physician then makes an anterior 6.0 to 7.0 cm transverse skin incision at the level of the C5-6 disc space. Dissection is carried down to the odontoid process by longitudinally splitting the muscle and by blunt careful dissection of the space between the carotid, trachea, and esophagus; a retractor is placed and the anterior longitudinal ligament is incised. The superior thyroid artery may be ligated. Using imaging intensification, guide wires are inserted into an area of the dens and screws are placed over the wires. In 22319, a bone graft is placed to stabilize the fracture/disclocation. When the procedure is complete, a drain may be placed and the wound is closed with layered sutures.

Coding Tips

Harvesting of grafts should not be reported separately for 22319. For open treatment of other cervical spine fractures, see 22326.

ICD-9-CM Procedural

- 03.53 Repair of vertebral fracture
- 78.09 Bone graft of other bone, except facial bones
- 78.59 Internal fixation of other bone, except facial bones, without fracture reduction
- 79.39 Open reduction of fracture of other specified bone, except facial bones, with internal fixation
- 79.89 Open reduction of dislocation of other specified site, except temporomandibular

Anesthesia

00600, 00670

ICD-9-CM Diagnostic

- 756.10 Congenital anomaly of spine, unspecified
- 805.02 Closed fracture of second cervical vertebra without mention of spinal cord injury
- 805.12 Open fracture of second cervical vertebra without mention of spinal cord injury
- 806.00 Closed fracture of C1-C4 level with unspecified spinal cord injury
- 806.01 Closed fracture of C1-C4 level with complete lesion of cord
- 806.02 Closed fracture of C1-C4 level with anterior cord syndrome
- 806.03 Closed fracture of C1-C4 level with central cord syndrome
- 806.04 Closed fracture of C1-C4 level with other specified spinal cord injury
- 806.10 Open fracture of C1-C4 level with unspecified spinal cord injury
- 806.11 Open fracture of C1-C4 level with complete lesion of cord
- 806.12 Open fracture of C1-C4 level with anterior cord syndrome
- 806.13 Open fracture of C1-C4 level with central cord syndrome
- 806.14 Open fracture of C1-C4 level with other specified spinal cord injury
- 839.02 Closed dislocation, second cervical vertebra
- 839.12 Open dislocation, second cervical vertebra

Terms To Know

anomaly. Irregularity in the structure or position of an organ or tissue.

closed dislocation. Simple displacement of a body part without an open wound.

congenital. Present at birth, occurring through heredity or an influence during gestation up to the moment of birth.

dissection. Separating by cutting tissue or body structures apart.

fracture. Break in bone or cartilage.

open dislocation. Displacement of a bone or joint with an open wound.

supine. Lying on the back.

transverse. Crosswise at right angles to the long axis of a structure or part.

CCI Version 16.3

0213T, 0216T, 0228T, 0230T, 20100, 20661, 22305-22315, 22505, 29000, 29015, 29025, 29040, 29700-29715, 36000, 36400-36410, 36420-36430, 36440, 36600, 36640, 37202, 43752, 51701-51703, 62310-62319, 64400-64435, 64445-64450, 64479, 64483, 64490, 64493, 64505-64530, 69990, 76000-76001, 92585, 93000-93010, 93040-93042, 93318, 94002, 94200, 94250, 94680-94690, 94770, 95812-95816, 95819, 95822, 95829, 95860-95861, 95867-95868, 95870, 95900, 95904, 95920, 95925-95934, 95936-95937, 95955, 96360, 96365, 96372, 96374-96376, 97597-97598, 97602-97606, 99148-99149, 99150

Also not with 22318: 20931, 20937-20938, 22319❖

Note: These CCI edits are used for Medicare. Other payers may reimburse on codes listed above.

Medicare Edits

	Fac RVU	Non-Fac RVU	FUD	Assist
22318	47.81	47.81	90	80
22319	53.26	53.26	90	80

Medicare References: None

22325-22328

22325 Open treatment and/or reduction of vertebral fracture(s) and/or dislocation(s), posterior approach, 1 fractured vertebra or dislocated segment; lumbar
22326 cervical
22327 thoracic
22328 each additional fractured vertebra or dislocated segment (List separately in addition to code for primary procedure)

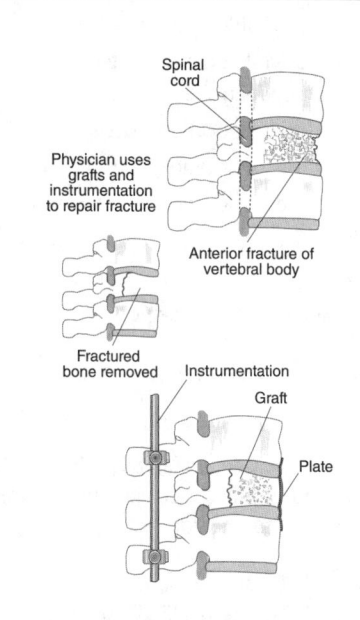

Explanation

The physician performs open treatment and/or reduction of a vertebral fracture or dislocation from a posterior approach. The patient is placed prone and the skin, fascia, and paravertebral muscles are incised and retracted to expose the fractured vertebra or dislocated segment. The proper rod (e.g., Harrington, Edwards) is selected and anatomic or C-shaped hooks are placed on vertebrae above and below the injury. The rod is inserted in the hooks and the spine is aligned. If fusion is desired, the physician may place separately reportable grafts between the vertebrae or place sleeves on the rod and position them to stabilize the injured vertebrae. The incision is closed by layered sutures. Report 22325 if the site is lumbar; 22326 if the site is cervical; and 22327 if the site is thoracic. Report 22328 for each additional fractured vertebra or dislocated segment in conjunction with the code for the primary procedure.

Coding Tips

Use 22328 in conjunction with 22325–22327. As an "add-on" code, 22328 is not subject to multiple procedure rules. No reimbursement reduction or modifier 51 is applied. Add-on codes describe additional intra-service work associated with the primary procedure. They are performed by the same physician on the same date of service as the primary service/procedure, and must never be reported as a stand-alone code. If spinal instrumentation is performed, it is listed separately; see 22840–22847. Any bone graft is also reported separately; see 20930–20938.

ICD-9-CM Procedural

03.53 Repair of vertebral fracture
79.29 Open reduction of fracture of other specified bone, except facial bones, without internal fixation

Anesthesia

22325 00630, 00670
22326 00600, 00604, 00670
22327 00620, 00670
22328 N/A

ICD-9-CM Diagnostic

805.13 Open fracture of third cervical vertebra without mention of spinal cord injury
805.14 Open fracture of fourth cervical vertebra without mention of spinal cord injury
805.15 Open fracture of fifth cervical vertebra without mention of spinal cord injury
805.16 Open fracture of sixth cervical vertebra without mention of spinal cord injury
805.17 Open fracture of seventh cervical vertebra without mention of spinal cord injury
805.5 Open fracture of lumbar vertebra without mention of spinal cord injury
806.16 Open fracture of C5-C7 level with complete lesion of cord
806.17 Open fracture of C5-C7 level with anterior cord syndrome
806.18 Open fracture of C5-C7 level with central cord syndrome
806.31 Open fracture of T1-T6 level with complete lesion of cord
806.32 Open fracture of T1-T6 level with anterior cord syndrome
806.33 Open fracture of T1-T6 level with central cord syndrome
806.36 Open fracture of T7-T12 level with complete lesion of cord
806.37 Open fracture of T7-T12 level with anterior cord syndrome
806.38 Open fracture of T7-T12 level with central cord syndrome

CCI Version 16.3

92585, 95822, 95860-95861, 95867-95868, 95900, 95904, 95920, 95936-95937

Also not with 22325: 0213T, 0216T, 0228T, 0230T, 20102, 22305-22315, 22505, 22521❖, 29010, 29020, 29035, 29700-29715, 36000, 36400-36410, 36420-36430, 36440, 36600, 36640, 37202, 43752, 51701-51703, 62310-62319, 64400-64435, 64445-64450, 64479, 64483, 64490, 64493, 64505-64530, 69990, 75822, 76000-76001, 93000-93010, 93040-93042, 93318, 94002, 94200, 94250, 94680-94690, 94770, 95812-95816, 95819, 95829, 95870, 95925-95934, 95955, 96360, 96365, 96372, 96374-96376, 97597-97598, 97602-97606, 99148-99149, 99150

Also not with 22326: 0213T, 0216T, 0228T, 0230T, 20100, 20102, 22305-22319❖, 22327, 22505, 29700-29715, 36000, 36400-36410, 36420-36430, 36440, 36600, 36640, 37202, 43752, 51701-51703, 62310-62319, 63045, 64400-64435, 64445-64450, 64479, 64483, 64490, 64493, 64505-64530, 69990, 76000-76001, 93000-93010, 93040-93042, 93318, 94002, 94200, 94250, 94680-94690, 94770, 95812-95816, 95819, 95829, 95870, 95925-95934, 95955, 96360, 96365, 96372, 96374-96376, 97597-97598, 97602-97606, 99148-99149, 99150

Also not with 22327: 0213T, 0216T, 0228T, 0230T, 20102, 22305-22315, 22325, 22505-22520❖, 22523❖, 29010, 29020, 29035, 29200, 29700-29715, 36000, 36400-36410, 36420-36430, 36440, 36600, 36640, 37202, 43752, 51701-51703, 62310-62319, 63046, 64400-64435, 64445-64450, 64479, 64483, 64490, 64493, 64505-64530, 69990, 76000-76001, 93000-93010, 93040-93042, 93318, 94002, 94200, 94250, 94680-94690, 94770, 95812-95816, 95819, 95829, 95870, 95925-95934, 95955, 96360, 96365, 96372, 96374-96376, 97597-97598, 97602-97606, 99148-99149, 99150

Also not with 22328: 95925-95927, 95930-95934

Note: These CCI edits are used for Medicare. Other payers may reimburse on codes listed above.

Medicare Edits

	Fac RVU	Non-Fac RVU	FUD	Assist
22325	41.79	41.79	90	80
22326	43.42	43.42	90	80
22327	43.12	43.12	90	80
22328	8.48	8.48	N/A	80

Medicare References: None

22505

22505 Manipulation of spine requiring anesthesia, any region

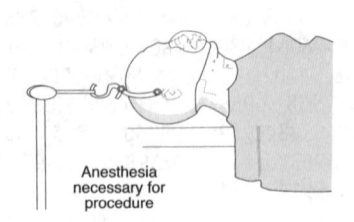

Anesthesia necessary for procedure

Halter, tong, or halo may be affixed
Physician performs correction requiring anesthesia

Explanation
Spinal manipulation under anesthesia (SMUA) is performed mostly by osteopaths although orthopedists may also use it to treat spinal dysfunction and alleviate neck and back pain. The induction of anesthesia reduces muscle tone and the natural reflex actions so that the spine can be manipulated more effectively to restore joint function and reduce pain. The manipulations are carried out so as to break up fibrotic adhesions of the soft tissues in and around to the spinal joints. SMUA is usually followed by a week of daily rehabilitative manipulation to maintain joint mobility and prevent re-adhesion of the fibrotic tissue.

Coding Tips
Report 22505 for treatment of subluxation (partial or incomplete dislocation) requiring general anesthesia but not requiring casting or bracing. For treatment of a fracture or dislocation requiring casting or bracing, see 22315. For treatment of spinal subluxation with manipulation performed by a physician and not requiring general anesthesia, see 97140. Manipulation of the spine may be performed during many procedures for varying reasons. It should not be reported separately when it is incidental to or inherent to the procedure being performed.

ICD-9-CM Procedural
- 93.29 Other forcible correction of musculoskeletal deformity

Anesthesia
- **22505** 00640

ICD-9-CM Diagnostic
- 720.2 Sacroiliitis, not elsewhere classified
- 722.0 Displacement of cervical intervertebral disc without myelopathy
- 722.10 Displacement of lumbar intervertebral disc without myelopathy
- 722.11 Displacement of thoracic intervertebral disc without myelopathy
- 722.2 Displacement of intervertebral disc, site unspecified, without myelopathy
- 722.4 Degeneration of cervical intervertebral disc
- 722.51 Degeneration of thoracic or thoracolumbar intervertebral disc
- 722.52 Degeneration of lumbar or lumbosacral intervertebral disc
- 722.90 Other and unspecified disc disorder of unspecified region
- 722.92 Other and unspecified disc disorder of thoracic region
- 722.93 Other and unspecified disc disorder of lumbar region
- 723.5 Torticollis, unspecified
- 724.00 Spinal stenosis, unspecified region other than cervical
- 724.01 Spinal stenosis of thoracic region
- 724.02 Spinal stenosis of lumbar region, without neurogenic claudication
- 724.03 Spinal stenosis of lumbar region, with neurogenic claudication
- 724.2 Lumbago
- 724.3 Sciatica
- 728.85 Spasm of muscle
- 729.2 Unspecified neuralgia, neuritis, and radiculitis
- 739.2 Nonallopathic lesion of thoracic region, not elsewhere classified
- 739.3 Nonallopathic lesion of lumbar region, not elsewhere classified
- 739.4 Nonallopathic lesion of sacral region, not elsewhere classified
- 781.93 Ocular torticollis
- 839.00 Closed dislocation, unspecified cervical vertebra
- 839.01 Closed dislocation, first cervical vertebra
- 839.02 Closed dislocation, second cervical vertebra
- 839.03 Closed dislocation, third cervical vertebra
- 839.04 Closed dislocation, fourth cervical vertebra
- 839.05 Closed dislocation, fifth cervical vertebra
- 839.06 Closed dislocation, sixth cervical vertebra
- 839.07 Closed dislocation, seventh cervical vertebra
- 839.08 Closed dislocation, multiple cervical vertebrae
- 839.20 Closed dislocation, lumbar vertebra
- 839.21 Closed dislocation, thoracic vertebra
- 839.40 Closed dislocation, vertebra, unspecified site
- 839.41 Closed dislocation, coccyx
- 839.42 Closed dislocation, sacrum
- 839.49 Closed dislocation, other vertebra
- 847.0 Neck sprain and strain
- 953.0 Injury to cervical nerve root
- 956.0 Injury to sciatic nerve

Terms To Know
supine. Lying on the back.

torticollis. Twisted, unnatural position of the neck due to contracted cervical muscles that pull the head to one side.

CCI Version 16.3
00640, 0213T, 0216T, 0228T, 0230T, 11010-11012❖, 36000, 36400-36410, 36420-36430, 36440, 36600, 36640, 37202, 43752, 51701-51703, 62310-62319, 64400-64435, 64445-64450, 64479, 64483, 64490, 64493, 64505-64530, 69990, 76000-76001, 92585, 93000-93010, 93040-93042, 93318, 94002, 94200, 94250, 94680-94690, 94770, 95812-95816, 95819, 95822, 95829, 95860-95861, 95867-95868, 95870, 95900, 95904, 95920, 95925-95934, 95936-95937, 95955, 96360, 96365, 96372, 96374-96376, 99148-99149, 99150

Note: These CCI edits are used for Medicare. Other payers may reimburse on codes listed above.

Medicare Edits

	Fac RVU	Non-Fac RVU	FUD	Assist
22505	3.47	3.47	10	N/A

Medicare References: 100-2,15;260; 100-4,12,30; 100-4,12,90.3; 100-4,14,10

22520-22522

22520 Percutaneous vertebroplasty, 1 vertebral body, unilateral or bilateral injection; thoracic
22521 lumbar
22522 each additional thoracic or lumbar vertebral body (List separately in addition to code for primary procedure)

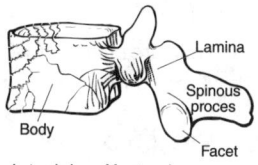

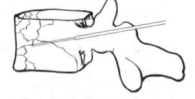

Explanation

Percutaneous vertebroplasty is performed by a one- or two-sided injection of a vertebral body. A local anesthetic is administered. In a separately reportable procedure, the radiologist uses imaging techniques, such as CT scanning and fluoroscopy, to guide percutaneous placement of the needle during the procedure and to monitor the injection procedure. Sterile biomaterial such as methyl methacrylate is injected from one side or both sides into the damaged vertebral body and acts as a bone cement to reinforce the fractured or collapsed vertebra. The procedure does not restore the original shape to the vertebra, but it does stabilize the bone, preventing further fracture or collapse. Following the procedure, the patient may experience significant, almost immediate, pain relief. Report 22520 for percutaneous vertebroplasty of one vertebral body at the thoracic level; 22521 for percutaneous vertebroplasty of one vertebral body at the lumbar level; and 22522 for each additional thoracic or lumbar vertebral body treated.

Coding Tips

As an "add-on" code, 22522 is not subject to multiple procedure rules. No reimbursement reduction or modifier 51 is applied. "Add-on" codes describe additional intra-service work associated with the primary procedure. They are performed by the same physician on the same date of service as the primary service/procedure, and must never be reported as a stand-alone code. Use 22522 in conjunction with 22520–22521. For radiological supervision and interpretation of the percutaneous vertebroplasty by fluoroscopy, see 72291; by CT, see 72292.

ICD-9-CM Procedural

81.65 Percutaneous vertebroplasty

Anesthesia

22520 01936
22521 01936
22522 N/A

ICD-9-CM Diagnostic

- 170.2 Malignant neoplasm of vertebral column, excluding sacrum and coccyx
- 198.5 Secondary malignant neoplasm of bone and bone marrow
- 203.00 Multiple myeloma, without mention of having achieved remission
- 203.01 Multiple myeloma in remission
- 203.02 Multiple myeloma, in relapse
- 209.73 Secondary neuroendocrine tumor of bone
- 213.2 Benign neoplasm of vertebral column, excluding sacrum and coccyx
- 238.0 Neoplasm of uncertain behavior of bone and articular cartilage
- 238.6 Neoplasm of uncertain behavior of plasma cells
- 239.2 Neoplasms of unspecified nature of bone, soft tissue, and skin
- 731.0 Osteitis deformans without mention of bone tumor
- 731.3 Major osseous defects — (Code first underlying disease: 170.0-170.9, 730.00-730.29, 733.00-733.09, 733.40-733.49, 996.45)
- 733.01 Senile osteoporosis — (Use additional code to identify major osseous defect, if applicable: 731.3) (Use additional code to identify personal history of pathologic (healed) fracture: V13.51)
- 733.02 Idiopathic osteoporosis — (Use additional code to identify major osseous defect, if applicable: 731.3) (Use additional code to identify personal history of pathologic (healed) fracture: V13.51)
- 733.03 Disuse osteoporosis — (Use additional code to identify major osseous defect, if applicable: 731.3) (Use additional code to identify personal history of pathologic (healed) fracture: V13.51)
- 733.13 Pathologic fracture of vertebrae
- 733.7 Algoneurodystrophy
- 733.95 Stress fracture of other bone — (Use additional external cause code(s) to identify the cause of the stress fracture)
- 805.2 Closed fracture of dorsal (thoracic) vertebra without mention of spinal cord injury
- 805.4 Closed fracture of lumbar vertebra without mention of spinal cord injury

CCI Version 16.3

92585, 95822, 95860-95861, 95867-95868, 95900, 95904, 95920, 95936-95937

Also not with 22520: 01935-01936, 0213T, 0228T, 0230T, 20220-20225, 20240, 20250, 22305-22315, 22505, 22521❖, 36000, 36005, 36400-36410, 36420-36430, 36440, 36600, 36640, 37202, 43752, 51701-51703, 61795, 62292, 62310-62318, 64400-64435, 64445-64450, 64479, 64483, 64490, 64505-64530, 69990, 72128-72130, 75872, 76000-76001, 77002-77003, 93000-93010, 93040-93042, 93318, 94002, 94200, 94250, 94680-94690, 94770, 95812-95816, 95819, 95829, 95870, 95925-95934, 95955, 96360, 96365, 96372, 96374-96376, 99143-99149, 99150, J0670, J2001

Also not with 22521: 0171T❖, 01935-01936, 0202T, 0216T, 0228T, 0230T, 20220-20225, 20240, 20251, 22305-22315, 22505, 36000, 36005, 36400-36410, 36420-36430, 36440, 36600, 36640, 37202, 43752, 51701-51703, 61795, 62292, 62310-62311, 62319, 64400-64435, 64445-64450, 64479, 64483, 64493, 64505-64530, 69990, 72131-72133, 75872, 76000-76001, 77002-77003, 93000-93010, 93040-93042, 93318, 94002, 94200, 94250, 94680-94690, 94770, 95812-95816, 95819, 95829, 95870, 95925-95934, 95955, 96360, 96365, 96372, 96374-96376, 99143-99149, 99150, J0670, J2001

Also not with 22522: 95925-95927, 95930-95934

Note: These CCI edits are used for Medicare. Other payers may reimburse on codes listed above.

Medicare Edits

	Fac RVU	Non-Fac RVU	FUD	Assist
22520	15.43	65.85	10	N/A
22521	14.58	64.59	10	N/A
22522	6.81	6.81	N/A	N/A

Medicare References: None

22523-22525

22523 Percutaneous vertebral augmentation, including cavity creation (fracture reduction and bone biopsy included when performed) using mechanical device, 1 vertebral body, unilateral or bilateral cannulation (eg, kyphoplasty); thoracic
22524 lumbar
22525 each additional thoracic or lumbar vertebral body (List separately in addition to code for primary procedure)

Physician injects contrast material into spine

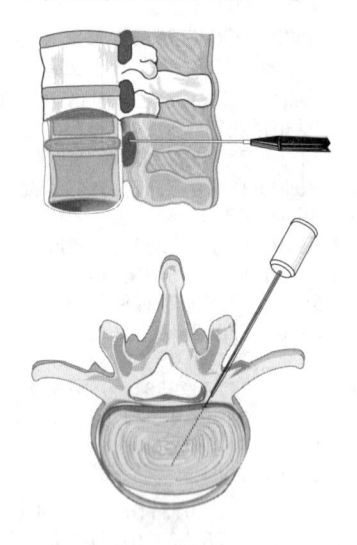

Explanation
The physician performs a percutaneous kyphoplasty, a modification of the percutaneous vertebroplasty, to reduce the pain associated with osteoporotic vertebral compression fractures. This procedure has the added advantage of restoring vertebral body. The procedure is performed under separately reported x-ray. The patient is placed in a prone, slightly flexed position. A 5 mm to 7 mm incision is made and small cannulas are inserted into the vertebral body from both sides. Balloon catheters, called "tamps," are inserted into the vertebra and inflated. The tamps create a void in the soft trabecular bone and restore vertebral alignment. The balloon is removed and bone cement is injected into the cavity. Report 22523 when the procedure is performed in the thoracic spine; 22524 when the procedure is performed in the lumbar spine; and 22525 for each additional vertebral body.

Coding Tips
Use 22525 in conjunction with 22523–22524. As an "add-on" code, 22525 is not subject to multiple procedure rules. No reimbursement reduction or modifier 51 is applied. Add-on codes describe additional intra-service work associated with the primary procedure. They are performed by the same physician on the same date of service as the primary service/procedure, and must never be reported as a stand-alone code. For radiological supervision and interpretation, see codes 72291–72292.

ICD-9-CM Procedural
81.66 Percutaneous vertebral augmentation

Anesthesia
22523 01936
22524 01936
22525 N/A

ICD-9-CM Diagnostic
170.2 Malignant neoplasm of vertebral column, excluding sacrum and coccyx
198.5 Secondary malignant neoplasm of bone and bone marrow
203.00 Multiple myeloma, without mention of having achieved remission
203.01 Multiple myeloma in remission
213.2 Benign neoplasm of vertebral column, excluding sacrum and coccyx
237.5 Neoplasm of uncertain behavior of brain and spinal cord
238.0 Neoplasm of uncertain behavior of bone and articular cartilage
239.2 Neoplasms of unspecified nature of bone, soft tissue, and skin
731.0 Osteitis deformans without mention of bone tumor
731.3 Major osseous defects — (Code first underlying disease: 170.0-170.9, 730.00-730.29, 733.00-733.09, 733.40-733.49, 996.45)
733.00 Unspecified osteoporosis — (Use additional code to identify major osseous defect, if applicable: 731.3) (Use additional code to identify personal history of pathologic (healed) fracture: V13.51)
733.01 Senile osteoporosis — (Use additional code to identify major osseous defect, if applicable: 731.3) (Use additional code to identify personal history of pathologic (healed) fracture: V13.51)
733.02 Idiopathic osteoporosis — (Use additional code to identify major osseous defect, if applicable: 731.3) (Use additional code to identify personal history of pathologic (healed) fracture: V13.51)
733.03 Disuse osteoporosis — (Use additional code to identify major osseous defect, if applicable: 731.3) (Use additional code to identify personal history of pathologic (healed) fracture: V13.51)
733.13 Pathologic fracture of vertebrae
733.95 Stress fracture of other bone — (Use additional external cause code(s) to identify the cause of the stress fracture)
805.2 Closed fracture of dorsal (thoracic) vertebra without mention of spinal cord injury
805.4 Closed fracture of lumbar vertebra without mention of spinal cord injury

CCI Version 16.3
Also not with 22523: 01935-01936, 0213T, 0228T, 0230T, 20220-20225, 20240, 20250, 22305-22315, 22505-22520❖, 22851❖, 36000, 36400-36410, 36420-36430, 36440, 36600, 36640, 37202, 43752, 51701-51703, 62292, 62310-62318, 64400-64435, 64445-64450, 64479, 64483, 64490, 64505-64530, 69990, 72128-72130, 75872, 76000-76001, 77002-77003, 93000-93010, 93040-93042, 93318, 94002, 94200, 94250, 94680-94690, 94770, 95812-95816, 95819, 95822, 95829, 95860-95861, 95870, 95900, 95904, 95920, 95925-95934, 95936-95937, 95955, 96360, 96365, 96372, 96374-96376, 99148-99149, 99150

Also not with 22524: 0171T❖, 01935-01936, 0202T, 0216T, 0228T, 0230T, 20220-20225, 20240, 20250, 22305-22315, 22505, 22521❖, 22851❖, 36000, 36400-36410, 36420-36430, 36440, 36600, 36640, 37202, 43752, 51701-51703, 62292, 62310-62311, 62319, 64400-64435, 64445-64450, 64479, 64483, 64493, 64505-64530, 69990, 72131-72133, 75872, 76000-76001, 77002-77003, 93000-93010, 93040-93042, 93318, 94002, 94200, 94250, 94680-94690, 94770, 95812-95816, 95819, 95822, 95829, 95860-95861, 95870, 95900, 95904, 95920, 95925-95934, 95936-95937, 95955, 96360, 96365, 96372, 96374-96376, 99148-99149, 99150

Note: These CCI edits are used for Medicare. Other payers may reimburse on codes listed above.

Medicare Edits

	Fac RVU	Non-Fac RVU	FUD	Assist
22523	17.3	17.3	10	N/A
22524	16.64	16.64	10	N/A
22525	7.77	7.77	N/A	N/A

Medicare References: None

22526-22527

22526 Percutaneous intradiscal electrothermal annuloplasty, unilateral or bilateral including fluoroscopic guidance; single level

22527 1 or more additional levels (List separately in addition to code for primary procedure)

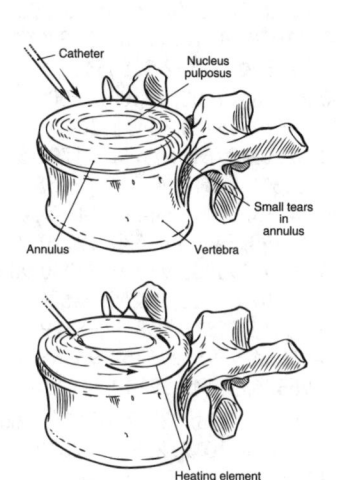

A hot needle treats small tears in the annulus
Report 22526 for one disc and 22527 for additional discs

Explanation
Percutaneous intradiscal annuloplasty is a minimally invasive technique performed under fluoroscopic guidance to treat small tears in the annulus without an associated disc protrusion. The most common technique is intradiscal electrothermal therapy (IDET). In IDET, the physician advances a needle into the disc using x-ray image guidance. The appropriate treatment catheter is selected and inserted through the needle. Once the catheter is in position, the temperature of the heating portion of the catheter is increased gradually, raising the temperature of the affected site. The increased heat contracts and thickens the collagen disc wall, which may result in contracture and closure of the tears in the annulus. The physician may perform the procedure on one (unilateral) or both sides of the disc. Report 22526 when a single disc is treated and 22527 for one or more additional discs.

Coding Tips
As an "add-on" code, 22527 is not subject to multiple procedure rules. No reimbursement reduction or modifier 51 is applied. Add-on codes describe additional intra-service work associated with the primary procedure. They are performed by the same physician on the same date of service as the primary service/procedure, and must never be reported as a stand-alone code. Moderate sedation performed with 22526, 22527 is considered to be an integral part of the procedure and is not reported separately. However, anesthesia services (00100–01999) may be reported separately when performed by an anesthesiologist (or qualified provider) other than the physician performing the procedure. If percutaneous intradiscal annuloplasty is performed using a method other than electrothermal, see 0062T, 0063T. Codes 22526, 22527 should not be reported with 77002, 77003.

ICD-9-CM Procedural
80.59 Other destruction of intervertebral disc

Anesthesia
22526 00640
22527 N/A

ICD-9-CM Diagnostic
721.0 Cervical spondylosis without myelopathy
721.1 Cervical spondylosis with myelopathy
721.2 Thoracic spondylosis without myelopathy
721.3 Lumbosacral spondylosis without myelopathy
721.41 Spondylosis with myelopathy, thoracic region
721.42 Spondylosis with myelopathy, lumbar region
721.8 Other allied disorders of spine
721.90 Spondylosis of unspecified site without mention of myelopathy
721.91 Spondylosis of unspecified site with myelopathy
722.0 Displacement of cervical intervertebral disc without myelopathy
722.10 Displacement of lumbar intervertebral disc without myelopathy
722.11 Displacement of thoracic intervertebral disc without myelopathy
722.2 Displacement of intervertebral disc, site unspecified, without myelopathy
722.30 Schmorl's nodes, unspecified region
722.31 Schmorl's nodes, thoracic region
722.32 Schmorl's nodes, lumbar region
722.39 Schmorl's nodes, other spinal region
722.4 Degeneration of cervical intervertebral disc
722.51 Degeneration of thoracic or thoracolumbar intervertebral disc
722.52 Degeneration of lumbar or lumbosacral intervertebral disc
722.6 Degeneration of intervertebral disc, site unspecified
722.70 Intervertebral disc disorder with myelopathy, unspecified region
722.71 Intervertebral cervical disc disorder with myelopathy, cervical region
722.72 Intervertebral thoracic disc disorder with myelopathy, thoracic region
722.73 Intervertebral lumbar disc disorder with myelopathy, lumbar region
724.4 Thoracic or lumbosacral neuritis or radiculitis, unspecified

Terms To Know
degeneration. Deterioration of an anatomic structure due to disease or other factors.

CCI Version 16.3
No CCI Edits apply to this code.

Medicare Edits

	Fac RVU	Non-Fac RVU	FUD	Assist
22526	9.57	61.76	10	N/A
22527	4.29	49.68	N/A	N/A

Medicare References: 100-3,150.11; 100-4,32,220.1; 100-4,32,220.2

22532-22534

22532 Arthrodesis, lateral extracavitary technique, including minimal discectomy to prepare interspace (other than for decompression); thoracic

22533 lumbar

22534 thoracic or lumbar, each additional vertebral segment (List separately in addition to code for primary procedure)

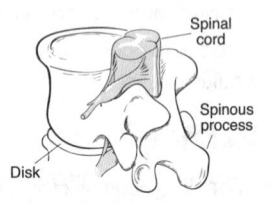

Posterior-lateral view of thoracic spine, spinal cord, and disk

Two spinal segments are fused (arthodesis) using an extracavitary lateral approach. Report 22532 for thoracic segments and 22533 for lumbar segments. Report 22534 for each additional fused segment

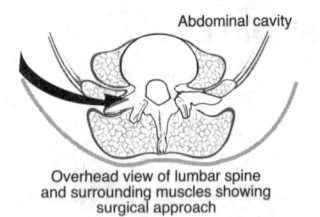

Overhead view of lumbar spine and surrounding muscles showing surgical approach

Explanation
Arthrodesis is performed by lateral extracavitary approach. A midline incision is made in the area of the fractured segment and inferiorly curved out to the lateral plane. The paraspinous muscles are exposed, lifted off the spinous processes, and divided and lifted off the ribs. Imaging must be used to identify the targeted interspace. The corresponding rib is dissected from the intercostal muscles and resected in one piece from the curve to the costovertebral connection. The appropriate transverse process and part of the facet and pedicle are removed with a drill from the lateral aspect. The dura and the vertebral body are exposed from the dorsolateral view. Further posterior and lateral access to the vertebral body is gained by gently retracting the nerve root and surrounding structures. A minimal discectomy is now done to prepare the interspace by removing the damaged tissue with curettes and rongeurs. Cartilage is scraped, bone is decorticated, and the arthrodesis is accomplished by tapping bone graft material into the vertebral endplates. A drain is placed and closure is done in layers. Report 22532 for thoracic arthrodesis; 22533 for lumbar arthrodesis; and 22534 for each additional thoracic or lumbar vertebral segment done by lateral extracavitary approach.

Coding Tips
Arthrodesis codes are assigned according to the surgical approach used (e.g., posterior, posterolateral, posterior interbody, lateral transverse process, lateral extracavitary, anterior interbody); if more than one approach is used, each is reported separately. Arthrodesis is frequently performed with other procedures on the spine, which should be reported separately. If spinal instrumentation is performed, it is listed separately; see 22840–22847. Any bone graft is also reported separately; see 20930–20938.

ICD-9-CM Procedural
81.00 Spinal fusion, not otherwise specified

Anesthesia
22532 00620, 00670
22533 00630, 00670
22534 N/A

ICD-9-CM Diagnostic
170.2 Malignant neoplasm of vertebral column, excluding sacrum and coccyx
198.5 Secondary malignant neoplasm of bone and bone marrow
213.2 Benign neoplasm of vertebral column, excluding sacrum and coccyx
721.41 Spondylosis with myelopathy, thoracic region
721.42 Spondylosis with myelopathy, lumbar region
722.0 Displacement of cervical intervertebral disc without myelopathy
722.10 Displacement of lumbar intervertebral disc without myelopathy
722.11 Displacement of thoracic intervertebral disc without myelopathy
722.31 Schmorl's nodes, thoracic region
722.4 Degeneration of cervical intervertebral disc
722.51 Degeneration of thoracic or thoracolumbar intervertebral disc
722.52 Degeneration of lumbar or lumbosacral intervertebral disc
722.71 Intervertebral cervical disc disorder with myelopathy, cervical region
722.72 Intervertebral thoracic disc disorder with myelopathy, thoracic region
722.73 Intervertebral lumbar disc disorder with myelopathy, lumbar region
723.0 Spinal stenosis in cervical region
724.01 Spinal stenosis of thoracic region
724.02 Spinal stenosis of lumbar region, without neurogenic claudication
731.0 Osteitis deformans without mention of bone tumor
733.13 Pathologic fracture of vertebrae
733.82 Nonunion of fracture

CCI Version 16.3
92585, 95822, 95860-95861, 95867-95868, 95900, 95904, 95920, 95936-95937

Also not with 22532: 0213T, 0216T, 0228T, 0230T, 11010-11012, 22505, 22830, 22849-22850❖, 22852-22855❖, 29000-29046, 29200, 32100, 36000, 36400-36410, 36420-36430, 36440, 36600, 36640, 37202, 37616, 43752, 51701-51703, 62291, 62310-62319, 63046, 63055, 64400-64435, 64445-64450, 64479, 64483, 64490, 64493, 64505-64530, 69990, 72285, 76000-76001, 93000-93010, 93040-93042, 93318, 94002, 94200, 94250, 94680-94690, 94770, 95812-95816, 95819, 95829, 95870, 95925-95934, 95955, 96360, 96365, 96372, 96374-96376, 99148-99149, 99150

Also not with 22533: 0213T, 0216T, 0228T, 0230T, 11010-11012, 22505, 22830, 22849-22850❖, 22852-22855❖, 29020-29025, 29044-29046, 32100, 36000, 36400-36410, 36420-36430, 36440, 36600, 36640, 37202, 37616-37617, 43752, 49000-49010, 51701-51703, 62267, 62287, 62290, 62310-62319, 63047, 63056, 64400-64435, 64445-64450, 64479, 64483, 64490, 64493, 64505-64530, 69990, 72295, 76000-76001, 93000-93010, 93040-93042, 93318, 94002, 94200, 94250, 94680-94690, 94770, 95812 95816, 95819, 95829, 95870, 95925-95934, 95955, 96360, 96365, 96372, 96374-96376, 99148-99149, 99150

Also not with 22534: 95925-95927, 95930-95934

Note: These CCI edits are used for Medicare. Other payers may reimburse on codes listed above.

Medicare Edits

	Fac RVU	Non-Fac RVU	FUD	Assist
22532	52.36	52.36	90	80
22533	49.35	49.35	90	80
22534	10.89	10.89	N/A	80

Medicare References: None

22548

22548 Arthrodesis, anterior transoral or extraoral technique, clivus-C1-C2 (atlas-axis), with or without excision of odontoid process

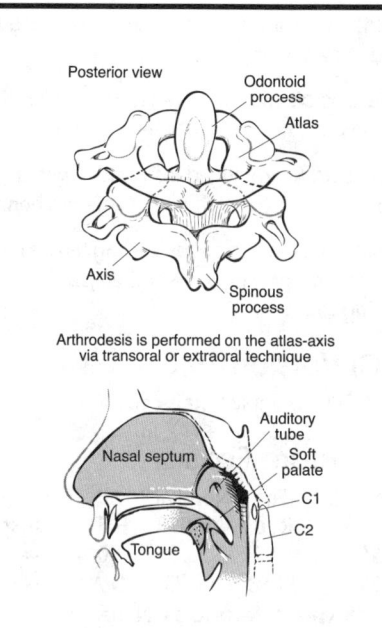

Explanation

Spinal arthrodesis, or fusion, may be done for conditions of herniated disc, degenerative, traumatic, and/or congenital lesions, or to stabilize fractures or dislocations of the spine. Skull tong traction is applied. Avoiding the esophagus, pharynx, or esophageal nerve, the physician may incise the back of the throat, but most often enters from the outside of the neck, left of the throat to reach the C1-C2 (atlas-axis) vertebrae. Retractors separate the intervertebral muscles. A drill is inserted in the affected vertebrae and the location confirmed by x-ray. The physician incises a trough in the front of the vertebrae with a drill or saw. The physician cleans out the intervertebral disc spaces with a rongeur and removes the cartilaginous plates above and below the vertebrae to be fused. The odontoid process (dens), the tooth-like projection located on the second cervical vertebra in the neck, may be excised. The physician obtains and packs separately reportable grafts of iliac or other donor bone into the spaces and trims them. Traction is gradually decreased to maintain the graft in its bed. The fascia is sutured. A drain is placed in the incision and the incision is sutured.

Coding Tips

Arthrodesis codes are assigned according to the surgical approach used (e.g., anterior interbody, posterior or posterolateral, posterior interbody, lateral transverse process); if more than one approach is used, each is reported separately. Arthrodesis is frequently performed with other procedures on the spine, which should be reported separately. If spinal instrumentation is performed, it is listed separately; see 22840–22847. Any bone graft is also reported separately; see 20930–20938. Report separately any laminotomy, laminectomy, corpectomy, exploration/decompression of neural elements, or excision of herniated intervertebral disc; see 63075–63076, 63081–63082, 63300, 63304, and 63308.

ICD-9-CM Procedural

- 81.01 Atlas-axis spinal fusion
- 81.31 Refusion of Atlas-axis spine
- 81.62 Fusion or refusion of 2-3 vertebrae

Anesthesia

22548 00670

ICD-9-CM Diagnostic

- 170.2 Malignant neoplasm of vertebral column, excluding sacrum and coccyx
- 198.5 Secondary malignant neoplasm of bone and bone marrow
- 209.73 Secondary neuroendocrine tumor of bone
- 213.2 Benign neoplasm of vertebral column, excluding sacrum and coccyx
- 238.0 Neoplasm of uncertain behavior of bone and articular cartilage
- 721.1 Cervical spondylosis with myelopathy
- 721.8 Other allied disorders of spine
- 723.2 Cervicocranial syndrome
- 723.3 Cervicobrachial syndrome (diffuse)
- 738.5 Other acquired deformity of back or spine
- 805.01 Closed fracture of first cervical vertebra without mention of spinal cord injury
- 805.02 Closed fracture of second cervical vertebra without mention of spinal cord injury
- 805.08 Closed fracture of multiple cervical vertebrae without mention of spinal cord injury
- 805.11 Open fracture of first cervical vertebra without mention of spinal cord injury
- 805.12 Open fracture of second cervical vertebra without mention of spinal cord injury
- 806.00 Closed fracture of C1-C4 level with unspecified spinal cord injury
- 806.01 Closed fracture of C1-C4 level with complete lesion of cord
- 806.02 Closed fracture of C1-C4 level with anterior cord syndrome
- 806.03 Closed fracture of C1-C4 level with central cord syndrome
- 806.04 Closed fracture of C1-C4 level with other specified spinal cord injury
- 806.10 Open fracture of C1-C4 level with unspecified spinal cord injury
- 806.11 Open fracture of C1-C4 level with complete lesion of cord
- 806.12 Open fracture of C1-C4 level with anterior cord syndrome
- 806.13 Open fracture of C1-C4 level with central cord syndrome
- 806.14 Open fracture of C1-C4 level with other specified spinal cord injury

CCI Version 16.3

0213T, 0216T, 0228T, 0230T, 22505, 22830, 29000, 29015, 29025, 29040, 36000, 36400-36410, 36420-36430, 36440, 36600, 36640, 37202, 43752, 51701-51703, 62310-62319, 64400-64435, 64445-64450, 64479, 64483, 64490, 64493, 64505-64530, 69990, 76000-76001, 92585, 93000-93010, 93040-93042, 93318, 94002, 94200, 94250, 94680-94690, 94770, 95812-95816, 95819, 95822, 95829, 95860-95861, 95867-95868, 95870, 95900, 95904, 95920, 95925-95934, 95936-95937, 95955, 96360, 96365, 96372, 96374-96376, 99148-99149, 99150

Note: These CCI edits are used for Medicare. Other payers may reimburse on codes listed above.

Medicare Edits

	Fac RVU	Non-Fac RVU	FUD	Assist
22548	57.1	57.1	90	80

Medicare References: 100-3, 150.2

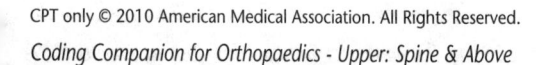

22551-22552

22551 Arthrodesis, anterior interbody, including disc space preparation, discectomy, osteophytectomy and decompression of spinal cord and/or nerve roots; cervical below C2

22552 cervical below C2, each additional interspace (List separately in addition to code for separate procedure)

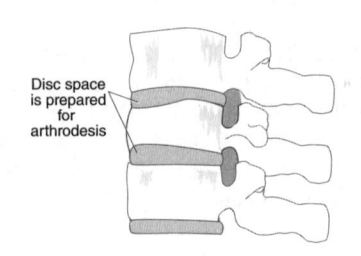

Disc space is prepared for arthrodesis

Explanation
The physician performs spinal fusion (arthrodesis) for indications such as herniated disc; degenerative, traumatic, and/or congenital lesions; or to stabilize fractures or dislocations of the spine. Skull tong traction is applied. The physician uses an anterior approach to reach the damaged vertebrae. An incision is made through the neck, avoiding the esophagus, trachea, and thyroid. Retractors separate the intervertebral muscles. The physician cleans out the intervertebral disc space with a rongeur, removing the cartilaginous material above and below the vertebra to be fused. Preparation includes discectomy and osteophytectomy for nerve root or spinal cord decompression. The physician obtains and packs separately reportable graft material of iliac or other donor bone into the spaces. Traction is gradually decreased to maintain the graft in its bed. The fascia is sutured. A drain is placed and the incision is sutured. Report 22551 for a single cervical interspace below C2. Report 22552 for each additional interspace below C2.

Coding Tips
These codes are new for 2011. As an "add-on" code, 22552 is not subject to multiple procedure rules. No reimbursement reduction or modifier 51 is applied. Add-on codes describe additional intra-service work associated with the primary procedure. They are performed by the same physician on the same date of service as the primary service/procedure, and must never be reported as a stand-alone code. Report 22552 in conjunction with 22551. Arthrodesis is frequently performed with other procedures on the spine, which should be reported separately. If spinal instrumentation is performed, it is listed separately; see 22840–22847. Any bone graft is reported separately; see 20930–20938. If complete discectomy is performed, report separately and append modifier 59. Documentation must support medical necessity and additional work; see 63075–63078. Report separately any corpectomy or removal of spinal lesion; see 63081–63091 and 63300–63308.

ICD-9-CM Procedural
- 81.00 Spinal fusion, not otherwise specified
- 81.02 Other cervical fusion of the anterior column, anterior technique
- 81.04 Dorsal and dorsolumbar fusion of the anterior column, anterior technique
- 81.06 Lumbar and lumbosacral fusion of the anterior column, anterior technique
- 81.32 Refusion of other cervical spine, anterior column, anterior technique
- 81.34 Refusion of dorsal and dorsolumbar spine, anterior column, anterior technique
- 81.36 Refusion of lumbar and lumbosacral spine, anterior column, anterior technique
- 81.62 Fusion or refusion of 2-3 vertebrae
- 81.63 Fusion or refusion of 4-8 vertebrae
- 81.64 Fusion or refusion of 9 or more vertebrae

Anesthesia
00600, 00670

ICD-9-CM Diagnostic
The application of this code is too broad to adequately present ICD-9-CM diagnostic code links here. Refer to your ICD-9-CM book.

Terms To Know
anterior. Situated in the front area or toward the belly surface of the body.

congenital. Present at birth, occurring through heredity or an influence during gestation up to the moment of birth.

decompression. Release of pressure.

fascia. Fibrous sheet or band of tissue that envelops organs, muscles, and groupings of muscles.

fusion. Union of adjacent tissues, especially bone.

graft. Tissue implant from another part of the body or another person.

interspace. Space between two similar objects.

rongeur. Sharp-edged instrument with a scoop-tip used to cut through tissue and bone.

traction. Drawing out or holding tension on an area by applying a direct therapeutic pulling force.

CCI Version 16.3
No CCI Edits apply to this code.

Medicare Edits

	Fac RVU	Non-Fac RVU	FUD	Assist
22551	51.2	51.2	90	80
22552	11.93	11.93	N/A	80

Medicare References: None

22554-22585

22554 Arthrodesis, anterior interbody technique, including minimal discectomy to prepare interspace (other than for decompression); cervical below C2
22556 thoracic
22558 lumbar
22585 each additional interspace (List separately in addition to code for primary procedure)

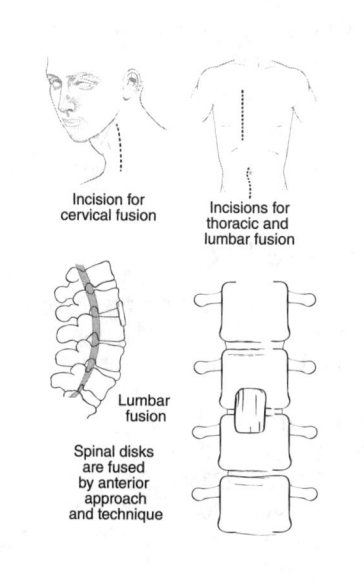

Explanation

Spinal arthrodesis, or fusion, may be done for conditions of herniated disc, degenerative, traumatic, and/or congenital lesions, or to stabilize fractures or dislocations of the spine. Skull tong traction is applied. The physician uses an anterior approach to reach the damaged vertebrae. For cervical vertebrae in 22554, an incision is made through the neck, avoiding the esophagus, trachea, and thyroid. Retractors separate the intervertebral muscles. A drill is inserted in the affected vertebrae and the location is confirmed by separately reportable x-ray. The physician incises a trough in the front of the vertebrae with a drill or saw. The physician cleans out the intervertebral disc spaces with a rongeur and removes the cartilaginous plates above and below the vertebrae to be fused. The physician obtains and packs separately reportable grafts of iliac or other donor bone into the spaces and trims them. Traction is gradually decreased to maintain the graft in its bed. The fascia is sutured. A drain is placed and the incision is sutured. Report 22556 if the spinal arthrodesis site is thoracic. Report 22558 if the spinal arthrodesis site is lumbar. Report 22585 for each additional interspace treated in conjunction with the code for the primary procedure.

Coding Tips

Arthrodesis codes are assigned according to the surgical approach used (e.g., anterior interbody, posterior or posterolateral, posterior interbody, lateral transverse process); if more than one approach is used, each is reported separately. As an "add-on" code, 22585 is not subject to multiple procedure rules. No reimbursement reduction or modifier 51 is applied. Add-on codes describe additional intra-service work associated with the primary procedure. They are performed by the same physician on the same date of service as the primary service/procedure, and must never be reported as a stand-alone code. Use 22585 in conjunction with 22554–22558. Do not report 32551 separately for tube thoracostomy, as it is integral to procedure 22556. Arthrodesis is frequently performed with other procedures on the spine, which should be reported separately. If spinal instrumentation is performed, it is listed separately; see 22840–22847. Any bone graft is reported separately; see 20930–20938. If complete discectomy is performed, report separately and append modifier 59. Documentation must support medical necessity and additional work; see 63075–63078. Report separately any corpectomy or removal of spinal lesion; see 63081–63091 and 63300–63308.

ICD-9-CM Procedural

- 81.00 Spinal fusion, not otherwise specified
- 81.02 Other cervical fusion of the anterior column, anterior technique
- 81.04 Dorsal and dorsolumbar fusion of the anterior column, anterior technique
- 81.06 Lumbar and lumbosacral fusion of the anterior column, anterior technique
- 81.32 Refusion of other cervical spine, anterior column, anterior technique
- 81.34 Refusion of dorsal and dorsolumbar spine, anterior column, anterior technique
- 81.36 Refusion of lumbar and lumbosacral spine, anterior column, anterior technique
- 81.62 Fusion or refusion of 2-3 vertebrae
- 81.63 Fusion or refusion of 4-8 vertebrae
- 81.64 Fusion or refusion of 9 or more vertebrae

Anesthesia

- **22554** 00600, 00670
- **22556** 00625, 00626
- **22558** 00630, 00670
- **22585** N/A

ICD-9-CM Diagnostic

The application of this code is too broad to adequately present ICD-9-CM diagnostic code links here. Refer to your ICD-9-CM book.

CCI Version 16.3

92585, 95822, 95860-95861, 95867-95868, 95900, 95904, 95920, 95936-95937

Also not with 22554: 0213T, 0216T, 0228T, 0230T, 12034, 22505, 22830, 29000, 29015, 29025, 29040, 36000, 36400-36410, 36420-36430, 36440, 36600, 36640, 37202, 43752, 51701-51703, 62291, 62310-62319, 64400-64435, 64445-64450, 64479, 64483, 64490, 64493, 64505-64530, 64718, 64722, 69990, 72285, 76000-76001, 93000-93010, 93040-93042, 93318, 94002, 94200, 94250, 94680-94690, 94770, 95812-95816, 95819, 95829, 95870, 95925-95934, 95955, 96360, 96365, 96372, 96374-96376, 99148-99149, 99150

Also not with 22556: 0213T, 0216T, 0228T, 0230T, 22505, 22554, 22558, 22830, 29000-29046, 29200, 32100, 36000, 36400-36410, 36420-36430, 36440, 36600, 36640, 37202, 37616, 43752, 51701-51703, 62291, 62310-62319, 64400-64435, 64445-64450, 64479, 64483, 64490, 64493, 64505-64530, 69990, 72285, 76000-76001, 93000-93010, 93040-93042, 93318, 94002, 94200, 94250, 94680-94690, 94770, 95812-95816, 95819, 95829, 95870, 95925-95934, 95955, 96360, 96365, 96372, 96374-96376, 99148-99149, 99150

Also not with 22558: 0195T, 0213T, 0216T, 0228T, 0230T, 22505, 22830, 29020-29025, 29044-29046, 32100, 36000, 36400-36410, 36420-36430, 36440, 36600, 36640, 37202, 37617, 43752, 49000-49010, 51701-51703, 62267❖, 62290, 62310-62319, 64400-64435, 64445-64450, 64479, 64483, 64490, 64493, 64505-64530, 69990, 72295, 76000-76001, 93000-93010, 93040-93042, 93318, 94002, 94200, 94250, 94680-94690, 94770, 95812-95816, 95819, 95829, 95870, 95925-95934, 95955, 96360, 96365, 96372, 96374-96376, 99148-99149, 99150

Also not with 22585: 95925-95927, 95930-95934

Note: These CCI edits are used for Medicare. Other payers may reimburse on codes listed above.

Medicare Edits

	Fac RVU	Non-Fac RVU	FUD	Assist
22554	37.43	37.43	90	80
22556	49.08	49.08	90	80
22558	45.37	45.37	90	80
22585	10.11	10.11	N/A	80

Medicare References: 100-3,150.2

22590

22590 Arthrodesis, posterior technique, craniocervical (occiput-C2)

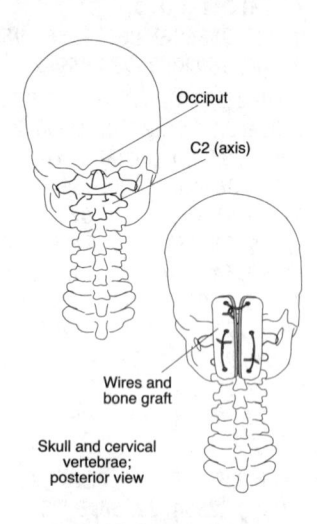

Occiput
C2 (axis)
Wires and bone graft
Skull and cervical vertebrae; posterior view

Physician fuses skull to C2 (axis) to stabilize cervical vertebrae; anchor holes are drilled in the occiput of the skull

Explanation

Spinal arthrodesis, or fusion, may be done for conditions of herniated disc, degenerative, traumatic, and/or congenital lesions, or to stabilize fractures or dislocations of the spine. The patient is placed in a Stryker frame with a previously applied halo vest. The physician incises the skin from the occiput to the C3 vertebra, opens the fascia, and retracts the paravertebral muscles. A horizontal hole is drilled in the occiput using a burr. A second hole is drilled in the base of C2. The physician places wires through these holes. A third wire is placed around the ring of C1. Separately reportable bone grafts are obtained from the iliac crest or other donor bone. They are prepared, positioned, and tied in place using the wires. The retractors are removed and the incision is closed over a drain.

Coding Tips

Arthrodesis codes are assigned according to the surgical approach used (e.g., posterior or posterolateral, posterior interbody, lateral transverse process, anterior interbody); if more than one approach is used, each is reported separately. Arthrodesis is frequently performed with other procedures on the spine, which should be reported separately. If spinal instrumentation is performed, it is listed separately, see 22840–22847. Any bone graft is also reported separately, see 20930–20938. Report separately any laminotomy, laminectomy, corpectomy, exploration/decompression of neural elements, or excision of herniated intervertebral disc, see 63020–63091.

ICD-9-CM Procedural

- 81.01 Atlas-axis spinal fusion
- 81.03 Other cervical fusion of the posterior column, posterior technique
- 81.31 Refusion of Atlas-axis spine
- 81.33 Refusion of other cervical spine, posterior column, posterior technique
- 81.62 Fusion or refusion of 2-3 vertebrae

Anesthesia

22590 00600, 00670

ICD-9-CM Diagnostic

- 170.2 Malignant neoplasm of vertebral column, excluding sacrum and coccyx
- 198.5 Secondary malignant neoplasm of bone and bone marrow
- 209.73 Secondary neuroendocrine tumor of bone
- 213.2 Benign neoplasm of vertebral column, excluding sacrum and coccyx
- 238.0 Neoplasm of uncertain behavior of bone and articular cartilage
- 721.1 Cervical spondylosis with myelopathy
- 721.8 Other allied disorders of spine
- 723.2 Cervicocranial syndrome
- 723.3 Cervicobrachial syndrome (diffuse)
- 733.81 Malunion of fracture
- 733.82 Nonunion of fracture
- 738.5 Other acquired deformity of back or spine
- 756.12 Congenital spondylolisthesis
- 805.01 Closed fracture of first cervical vertebra without mention of spinal cord injury
- 805.02 Closed fracture of second cervical vertebra without mention of spinal cord injury
- 805.11 Open fracture of first cervical vertebra without mention of spinal cord injury
- 805.12 Open fracture of second cervical vertebra without mention of spinal cord injury
- 806.00 Closed fracture of C1-C4 level with unspecified spinal cord injury
- 806.01 Closed fracture of C1-C4 level with complete lesion of cord
- 806.02 Closed fracture of C1-C4 level with anterior cord syndrome
- 806.03 Closed fracture of C1-C4 level with central cord syndrome
- 806.04 Closed fracture of C1-C4 level with other specified spinal cord injury
- 806.10 Open fracture of C1-C4 level with unspecified spinal cord injury
- 806.11 Open fracture of C1-C4 level with complete lesion of cord
- 806.12 Open fracture of C1-C4 level with anterior cord syndrome
- 806.13 Open fracture of C1-C4 level with central cord syndrome
- 806.14 Open fracture of C1-C4 level with other specified spinal cord injury
- 839.01 Closed dislocation, first cervical vertebra
- 839.02 Closed dislocation, second cervical vertebra
- 839.11 Open dislocation, first cervical vertebra
- 839.12 Open dislocation, second cervical vertebra

Terms To Know

cervicobrachial syndrome. Neuropathy of the brachial plexus causing pain leading from the neck and radiating down the arm.

CCI Version 16.3

0213T, 0216T, 0228T, 0230T, 20100, 22505, 22804-22808❖, 22830, 29000, 29015, 29025, 29040, 36000, 36400-36410, 36420-36430, 36440, 36600, 36640, 37202, 43752, 51701-51703, 61250, 61253, 62310-62319, 63295, 64400-64435, 64445-64450, 64479, 64483, 64490, 64493, 64505-64530, 69990, 76000-76001, 92585, 93000-93010, 93040-93042, 93318, 94002, 94200, 94250, 94680-94690, 94770, 95812-95816, 95819, 95822, 95829, 95860-95861, 95867-95868, 95870, 95900, 95904, 95920, 95925-95934, 95936-95937, 95955, 96360, 96365, 96372, 96374-96376, 99148-99149, 99150

Note: These CCI edits are used for Medicare. Other payers may reimburse on codes listed above.

Medicare Edits

	Fac RVU	Non-Fac RVU	FUD	Assist
22590	46.17	46.17	90	80

Medicare References: 100-3,150.2

22595

22595 Arthrodesis, posterior technique, atlas-axis (C1-C2)

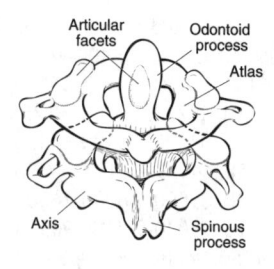

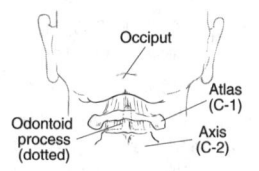

Explanation
Spinal arthrodesis, or fusion, may be done for conditions of herniated disc, degenerative, traumatic, and/or congenital lesions, or to stabilize fractures or dislocations of the spine. The patient is placed in a Stryker frame with a previously applied halo vest. The physician makes an incision from the occiput to the fourth or fifth vertebra. The physician exposes the posterior arch of the atlas (C1) and laminae of the axis (C2) and removes all soft tissue from bony surfaces. The upper arch of C1 is exposed and a wire loop is brought from below upward under the arch of the atlas and sutured. The physician passes the free ends through the loop, grasping the arch of C1. A graft taken from the iliac crest or other donor bone is placed against the lamina of the C2 and the arch of C1 beneath the wire. The physician passes one end of the wire through the spinous process of C2 and twists it securely into place. The retractors are removed and the incision is closed over a drain.

Coding Tips
Arthrodesis codes are assigned according to the surgical approach used (e.g., posterior or posterolateral, posterior interbody, lateral transverse process, anterior interbody); if more than one approach is used, each is reported separately. Arthrodesis is frequently performed with other procedures on the spine, which should be reported separately. If spinal instrumentation is performed, it is listed separately, see 22840–22847. Any bone graft is also reported separately, see 20930–20938.

Report separately any laminotomy, laminectomy, corpectomy, exploration/decompression of neural elements, or excision of herniated intervertebral disc, see 63020–63091.

ICD-9-CM Procedural
- 81.01 Atlas-axis spinal fusion
- 81.31 Refusion of Atlas-axis spine
- 81.62 Fusion or refusion of 2-3 vertebrae

Anesthesia
22595 00600, 00604, 00670

ICD-9-CM Diagnostic
- 170.2 Malignant neoplasm of vertebral column, excluding sacrum and coccyx
- 198.5 Secondary malignant neoplasm of bone and bone marrow
- 209.73 Secondary neuroendocrine tumor of bone
- 213.2 Benign neoplasm of vertebral column, excluding sacrum and coccyx
- 238.0 Neoplasm of uncertain behavior of bone and articular cartilage
- 721.8 Other allied disorders of spine
- 723.0 Spinal stenosis in cervical region
- 723.1 Cervicalgia
- 723.2 Cervicocranial syndrome
- 723.4 Brachial neuritis or radiculitis nos.
- 733.13 Pathologic fracture of vertebrae
- 733.81 Malunion of fracture
- 733.82 Nonunion of fracture
- 733.95 Stress fracture of other bone — (Use additional external cause code(s) to identify the cause of the stress fracture)
- 756.12 Congenital spondylolisthesis
- 756.19 Other congenital anomaly of spine
- 805.01 Closed fracture of first cervical vertebra without mention of spinal cord injury
- 805.02 Closed fracture of second cervical vertebra without mention of spinal cord injury
- 805.11 Open fracture of first cervical vertebra without mention of spinal cord injury
- 805.12 Open fracture of second cervical vertebra without mention of spinal cord injury
- 806.00 Closed fracture of C1-C4 level with unspecified spinal cord injury
- 806.01 Closed fracture of C1-C4 level with complete lesion of cord
- 806.02 Closed fracture of C1-C4 level with anterior cord syndrome
- 806.03 Closed fracture of C1-C4 level with central cord syndrome
- 806.04 Closed fracture of C1-C4 level with other specified spinal cord injury
- 806.10 Open fracture of C1-C4 level with unspecified spinal cord injury
- 806.11 Open fracture of C1-C4 level with complete lesion of cord
- 806.12 Open fracture of C1-C4 level with anterior cord syndrome
- 806.13 Open fracture of C1-C4 level with central cord syndrome
- 806.14 Open fracture of C1-C4 level with other specified spinal cord injury
- 839.01 Closed dislocation, first cervical vertebra
- 839.02 Closed dislocation, second cervical vertebra
- 839.11 Open dislocation, first cervical vertebra
- 839.12 Open dislocation, second cervical vertebra

CCI Version 16.3
0213T, 0216T, 0228T, 0230T, 20100, 22505, 22804-22808❖, 22830, 29000, 29015, 29025, 29040, 36000, 36400-36410, 36420-36430, 36440, 36600, 36640, 37202, 43752, 51701-51703, 61250, 61253, 62310-62319, 63295, 64400-64435, 64445-64450, 64479, 64483, 64490, 64493, 64505-64530, 69990, 76000-76001, 92585, 93000-93010, 93040-93042, 93318, 94002, 94200, 94250, 94680-94690, 94770, 95812-95816, 95819, 95822, 95829, 95860-95861, 95867-95868, 95870, 95900, 95904, 95920, 95925-95934, 95936-95937, 95955, 96360, 96365, 96372, 96374-96376, 99148-99149, 99150

Note: These CCI edits are used for Medicare. Other payers may reimburse on codes listed above.

Medicare Edits

	Fac RVU	Non-Fac RVU	FUD	Assist
22595	43.89	43.89	90	80

Medicare References: 100-3,150.2

22600-22614

22600 Arthrodesis, posterior or posterolateral technique, single level; cervical below C2 segment
22610 thoracic (with or without lateral transverse technique)
22612 lumbar (with or without lateral transverse technique)
22614 each additional vertebral segment (List separately in addition to code for primary procedure)

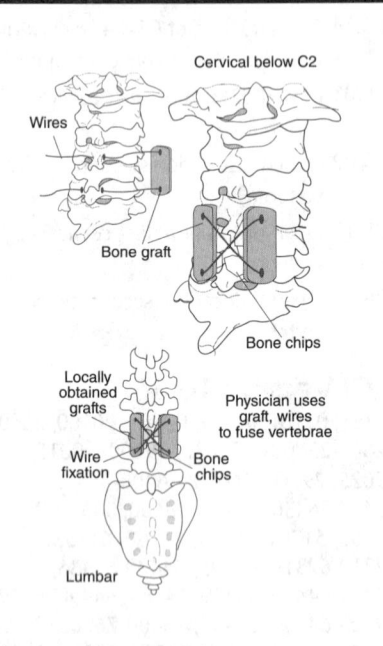

Explanation

Spinal arthrodesis, or fusion, may be done for conditions of herniated disc, degenerative, traumatic, and/or congenital lesions, or to stabilize fractures or dislocations of the spine. The physician makes an incision overlying the vertebrae and separates the fascia and the supraspinous ligaments in line with the incision. The physician prepares the vertebrae and lifts ligaments and muscles out of the way. A chisel elevator is used to strip away the capsules of the lateral articulations and the articular cartilage and cortical bone is excised. Separately reportable chips are cut from the fossa below the lateral articulations and from the laminae, or fragments of the spinous process are taken and used to fill the interlaminal space and the gap left by the articular cartilage removal. Additional bone grafts are taken from the ilium or other donor bone and are used to join the laminae. The periosteum, ligaments, and paravertebral muscles are sutured to secure the bone grafting. The skin and subcutaneous tissues are closed with sutures, as well. Report 22600 for cervical arthrodesis; 22610 for thoracic arthrodesis; 22612 for lumbar arthrodesis; and 22614 for each additional vertebral segment in conjunction with the code for the primary procedure.

Coding Tips

Arthrodesis codes are assigned according to the surgical approach used (e.g., posterior or posterolateral, posterior interbody, lateral transverse process, anterior interbody); if more than one approach is used, each is reported separately. Use 22614 in conjunction with 22600–22612. As an "add-on" code, 22614 is not subject to multiple procedure rules. No reimbursement reduction or modifier 51 is applied. Add-on codes describe additional intra-service work associated with the primary procedure. They are performed by the same physician on the same date of service as the primary service/procedure, and must never be reported as a stand-alone code. If spinal instrumentation is performed, it is listed separately in addition to the code for the arthrodesis; see 22840–22847.

ICD-9-CM Procedural

- 81.01 Atlas-axis spinal fusion
- 81.03 Other cervical fusion of the posterior column, posterior technique
- 81.05 Dorsal and dorsolumbar fusion of the posterior column, posterior technique
- 81.07 Lumbar and lumbosacral fusion of the posterior column, posterior technique
- 81.08 Lumbar and lumbosacral fusion of the anterior column, posterior technique
- 81.31 Refusion of Atlas-axis spine
- 81.33 Refusion of other cervical spine, posterior column, posterior technique
- 81.35 Refusion of dorsal and dorsolumbar spine, posterior column, posterior technique
- 81.37 Refusion of lumbar and lumbosacral spine, posterior column, posterior technique
- 81.38 Refusion of lumbar and lumbosacral spine, anterior column, posterior technique
- 81.62 Fusion or refusion of 2-3 vertebrae
- 81.63 Fusion or refusion of 4-8 vertebrae

Anesthesia

- **22600** 00600, 00604, 00670
- **22610** 00620
- **22612** 00630, 00670
- **22614** N/A

ICD-9-CM Diagnostic

The application of this code is too broad to adequately present ICD-9-CM diagnostic code links here. Refer to your ICD-9-CM book.

CCI Version 16.3

92585, 95822, 95860-95861, 95867-95868, 95900, 95904, 95920, 95936-95937

Also not with 22600: 0213T, 0216T, 0228T, 0230T, 12001-12007, 12020-12047, 13100-13101, 13131-13132, 22505, 22610, 22804-22808✦, 22830, 29000, 29015, 29025, 29040, 36000, 36400-36410, 36420-36430, 36440, 36600, 36640, 37202, 43752, 51701-51703, 61250, 61253, 62310-62319, 63295, 64400-64435, 64445-64450, 64479, 64483, 64490, 64493, 64505-64530, 69990, 76000-76001, 93000-93010, 93040-93042, 93318, 94002, 94200, 94250, 94680-94690, 94770, 95812-95816, 95819, 95829, 95870, 95925-95934, 95955, 96360, 96365, 96372, 96374-96376, 99148-99149, 99150

Also not with 22610: 0213T, 0216T, 0228T, 0230T, 12001-12007, 12020-12037, 13100-13101, 22505, 22804-22808✦, 22830, 29000-29046, 29200, 36000, 36400-36410, 36420-36430, 36440, 36600, 36640, 37202, 43752, 51701-51703, 62310-62319, 63050-63051, 63295, 64400-64435, 64445-64450, 64479, 64483, 64490, 64493, 64505-64530, 69990, 76000-76001, 93000-93010, 93040-93042, 93318, 94002, 94200, 94250, 94680-94690, 94770, 95812-95816, 95819, 95829, 95870, 95925-95934, 95955, 96360, 96365, 96372, 96374-96376, 99148-99149, 99150

Also not with 22612: 0171T✦, 0213T, 0216T, 0228T, 0230T, 12001-12007, 12020-12037, 13100-13101, 22505, 22610, 22804-22808✦, 22830, 22857✦, 29020-29025, 29044-29046, 36000, 36400-36410, 36420-36430, 36440, 36600, 36640, 37202, 43752, 49000-49002, 51701-51703, 62310-62319, 63050-63051, 63295, 64400-64435, 64445-64450, 64479, 64483, 64490, 64493, 64505-64530, 64712, 64714, 69990, 76000-76001, 93000-93010, 93040-93042, 93318, 94002, 94200, 94250, 94680-94690, 94770, 95812-95816, 95819, 95829, 95870, 95925-95934, 95955, 96360, 96365, 96372, 96374-96376, 99148-99149, 99150

Also not with 22614: 95925-95927, 95930-95934

Note: These CCI edits are used for Medicare. Other payers may reimburse on codes listed above.

Medicare Edits

	Fac RVU	Non-Fac RVU	FUD	Assist
22600	37.48	37.48	90	80
22610	36.72	36.72	90	80
22612	46.97	46.97	90	80
22614	11.77	11.77	N/A	80

Medicare References: 100-3, 150.2

22630-22632

22630 Arthrodesis, posterior interbody technique, including laminectomy and/or discectomy to prepare interspace (other than for decompression), single interspace; lumbar

22632 each additional interspace (List separately in addition to code for primary procedure)

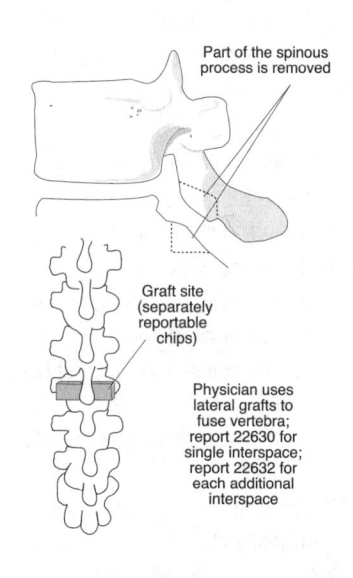

Part of the spinous process is removed

Graft site (separately reportable chips)

Physician uses lateral grafts to fuse vertebra; report 22630 for single interspace; report 22632 for each additional interspace

Explanation

Spinal arthrodesis, or fusion, may be done for conditions of herniated disc, degenerative, traumatic, and/or congenital lesions, or to stabilize fractures or dislocations of the spine. The physician makes an incision overlying the lumbar vertebrae and separates the fascia and the supraspinous ligaments in line with the incision. The physician prepares the vertebrae and lifts ligaments and muscles out of the way. A chisel elevator is used to strip away the capsules of the lateral articulations and the articular cartilage and cortical bone is excised. Separately reportable chips are cut from the fossa below the lateral articulations and from the laminae, or fragments of the spinous process are taken and used to fill the interlaminal space and the gap left by the articular cartilage removal. Part of the lamina may be removed on one side and/or part of the disc may be removed to facilitate preparation of the interspace for fusion. Additional bone grafts are taken from the ilium or other donor bone and are used to bridge the laminae. The periosteum, ligaments, and paravertebral muscles are sutured to secure the bone grafting. The skin and subcutaneous tissues are closed with sutures as well. Report 22632 for each additional interspace in conjunction with the code for the primary procedure.

Coding Tips

Arthrodesis codes are assigned according to the surgical approach used (e.g., posterior or posterolateral, posterior interbody, lateral transverse process, anterior interbody); if more than one approach is used, each is reported separately. Use 22632 in conjunction with 22630. As an "add-on" code, 22632 is not subject to multiple procedure rules. No reimbursement reduction or modifier 51 is applied. Arthrodesis is frequently performed with other procedures on the spine, which should be reported separately. If spinal instrumentation is performed, it is listed separately, see 22840–22855. Any bone graft is also reported separately, see 20930-20938. Report separately any laminotomy, laminectomy, corpectomy, exploration/decompression of neural elements, or excision of herniated intervertebral disc, see 63030–63035, 63042, 63044, 63047–63048, 63056–63057, 63200, 63252, 63267, 63272, 63277, 63282, 63287, and 63295.

ICD-9-CM Procedural

81.07	Lumbar and lumbosacral fusion of the posterior column, posterior technique
81.08	Lumbar and lumbosacral fusion of the anterior column, posterior technique
81.37	Refusion of lumbar and lumbosacral spine, posterior column, posterior technique
81.38	Refusion of lumbar and lumbosacral spine, anterior column, posterior technique
81.62	Fusion or refusion of 2-3 vertebrae
81.63	Fusion or refusion of 4-8 vertebrae
81.64	Fusion or refusion of 9 or more vertebrae

Anesthesia

22630 00630, 00670
22632 N/A

ICD-9-CM Diagnostic

170.2	Malignant neoplasm of vertebral column, excluding sacrum and coccyx
213.2	Benign neoplasm of vertebral column, excluding sacrum and coccyx
721.42	Spondylosis with myelopathy, lumbar region
722.52	Degeneration of lumbar or lumbosacral intervertebral disc
722.73	Intervertebral lumbar disc disorder with myelopathy, lumbar region
722.83	Postlaminectomy syndrome, lumbar region
724.02	Spinal stenosis of lumbar region, without neurogenic claudication
724.03	Spinal stenosis of lumbar region, with neurogenic claudication
724.2	Lumbago
724.3	Sciatica
731.0	Osteitis deformans without mention of bone tumor
805.5	Open fracture of lumbar vertebra without mention of spinal cord injury
806.4	Closed fracture of lumbar spine with spinal cord injury
806.5	Open fracture of lumbar spine with spinal cord injury
839.20	Closed dislocation, lumbar vertebra
839.30	Open dislocation, lumbar vertebra

Terms To Know

arthrodesis. Surgical fixation or fusion of a joint to reduce pain and improve stability, performed openly or arthroscopically.

fascia. Fibrous sheet or band of tissue that envelops organs, muscles, and groupings of muscles.

CCI Version 16.3

92585, 95822, 95860-95861, 95867-95868, 95900, 95904, 95920, 95936-95937

Also not with 22630: 0195T❖, 0213T, 0216T, 0228T, 0230T, 22224, 22505, 22558❖, 22804-22808❖, 22830, 22857❖, 29020-29025, 29044-29046, 36000, 36400-36410, 36420-36430, 36440, 36600, 36640, 37202, 43752, 51701-51703, 62267, 62287, 62310-62319, 63005, 63012, 63017, 63030, 63047, 63056, 63170, 63185-63191, 63200, 63267, 63277, 64400-64435, 64445-64450, 64479, 64483, 64490, 64493, 64505-64530, 69990, 76000-76001, 93000-93010, 93040-93042, 93318, 94002, 94200, 94250, 94680-94690, 94770, 95812-95816, 95819, 95829, 95870, 95925-95934, 95955, 96360, 96365, 96372, 96374-96376, 99148-99149, 99150

Also not with 22632: 95925-95927, 95930-95934

Note: These CCI edits are used for Medicare. Other payers may reimburse on codes listed above.

Medicare Edits

	Fac RVU	Non-Fac RVU	FUD	Assist
22630	45.26	45.26	90	80
22632	9.59	9.59	N/A	80

Medicare References: 100-3,150.2

22800-22804

22800 Arthrodesis, posterior, for spinal deformity, with or without cast; up to 6 vertebral segments
22802 7 to 12 vertebral segments
22804 13 or more vertebral segments

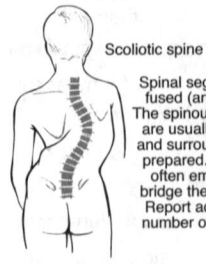

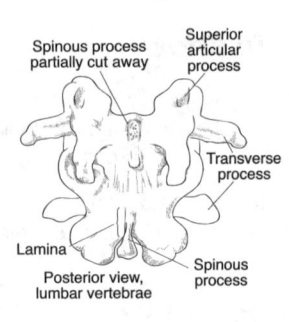

Explanation
Spinal arthrodesis, or fusion, is done here to correct a spinal deformity. The patient is placed prone. A midline posterior incision is made overlying the affected vertebrae. The fascia and the paravertebral muscles are incised and retracted. The physician uses a curette and rongeur to clean interspinous ligaments. One of several techniques may be used. In one, the spinous processes are split and removed and a curette is used to cut into the lateral articulations. Thin pieces of separately reportable iliac or other donor bone graft are placed in these slots. Grafts are obtained, prepared, and packed on both sides of the spinal curve, with more bone chips on the concave sides. Separately reportable instrumentation may be affixed to the spine. The incision is closed with layered sutures. A cast may be applied to stabilize the spine. Report 22800 for fusion of up to six vertebral segments; 22802 for fusion of seven to 12 vertebral segments; and 22804 for 13 or more vertebral segments.

Coding Tips
Only one spinal arthrodesis code is used per operative session. Codes 22800–22804 identify arthrodesis for spinal deformities by the approach used (e.g., posterior, anterior). The spinal deformity may be congenital (e.g., scoliosis) or acquired due to a disease or other process (e.g., kyphosis). These codes should not be used to report fusion for spinal deformity due to a fracture or previous arthrodesis. If spinal instrumentation is performed, it is listed separately in addition to the code for the arthrodesis, see 22840–22847. Any bone graft is also reported separately, see 20930–20938. If the services of two primary surgeons performing separate and distinct components of the arthrodesis are required, each surgeon should report the procedure code(s) for the cosurgery and append modifier 62.

ICD-9-CM Procedural
81.00	Spinal fusion, not otherwise specified
81.01	Atlas-axis spinal fusion
81.03	Other cervical fusion of the posterior column, posterior technique
81.05	Dorsal and dorsolumbar fusion of the posterior column, posterior technique
81.07	Lumbar and lumbosacral fusion of the posterior column, posterior technique
81.08	Lumbar and lumbosacral fusion of the anterior column, posterior technique
81.31	Refusion of Atlas-axis spine
81.33	Refusion of other cervical spine, posterior column, posterior technique
81.35	Refusion of dorsal and dorsolumbar spine, posterior column, posterior technique
81.37	Refusion of lumbar and lumbosacral spine, posterior column, posterior technique
81.38	Refusion of lumbar and lumbosacral spine, anterior column, posterior technique
81.62	Fusion or refusion of 2-3 vertebrae
81.63	Fusion or refusion of 4-8 vertebrae
81.64	Fusion or refusion of 9 or more vertebrae

Anesthesia
00670

ICD-9-CM Diagnostic
138	Late effects of acute poliomyelitis — (Note: This category is to be used to indicate conditions classifiable to 045 as the cause of late effects, which are themselves classified elsewhere. The "late effects" include those specified as such, as sequelae, or as due to old or inactive poliomyelitis, without evidence of active disease.)
237.71	Neurofibromatosis, Type 1 (von Recklinghausen's disease)
237.72	Neurofibromatosis, Type 2 (acoustic neurofibromatosis)
356.1	Peroneal muscular atrophy
731.0	Osteitis deformans without mention of bone tumor
732.0	Juvenile osteochondrosis of spine
733.01	Senile osteoporosis — (Use additional code to identify major osseous defect, if applicable: 731.3) (Use additional code to identify personal history of pathologic (healed) fracture: V13.51)
737.0	Adolescent postural kyphosis
737.10	Kyphosis (acquired) (postural)
737.20	Lordosis (acquired) (postural)
737.30	Scoliosis (and kyphoscoliosis), idiopathic
737.32	Progressive infantile idiopathic scoliosis
737.33	Scoliosis due to radiation
737.34	Thoracogenic scoliosis
737.8	Other curvatures of spine associated with other conditions
738.5	Other acquired deformity of back or spine
754.2	Congenital musculoskeletal deformity of spine
756.10	Congenital anomaly of spine, unspecified
756.12	Congenital spondylolisthesis

CCI Version 16.3
0213T, 0216T, 0228T, 0230T, 22505, 22830, 29000-29046, 29200, 36000, 36400-36410, 36420-36430, 36440, 36600, 36640, 37202, 43752, 51701-51703, 62310-62319, 64400-64435, 64445-64450, 64479, 64483, 64490, 64493, 64505-64530, 69990, 76000-76001, 92585, 93000-93010, 93040-93042, 93318, 94002, 94200, 94250, 94680-94690, 94770, 95812-95816, 95819, 95822, 95829, 95860-95861, 95867-95868, 95870, 95900, 95904, 95920, 95925-95934, 95936-95937, 95955, 96360, 96365, 96372, 96374-96376, 99148-99149, 99150

Also not with 22800: 22802❖, 22810-22812❖

Also not with 22802: 22856-22857❖, 22862-22864❖, 32100

Also not with 22804: 22800, 22802, 22856-22864❖, 32100

Note: These CCI edits are used for Medicare. Other payers may reimburse on codes listed above.

Medicare Edits

	Fac RVU	Non-Fac RVU	FUD	Assist
22800	39.76	39.76	90	80
22802	62.26	62.26	90	80
22804	71.74	71.74	90	80

Medicare References: 100-3,150.2

22808-22812

22808 Arthrodesis, anterior, for spinal deformity, with or without cast; 2 to 3 vertebral segments
22810 4 to 7 vertebral segments
22812 8 or more vertebral segments

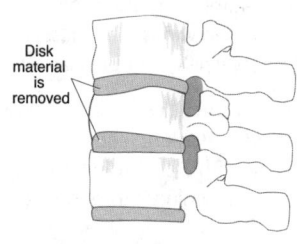

Disk material is removed

Physician fuses vertebrae to correct spinal deformity; several methods may be used

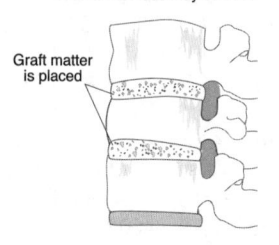

Graft matter is placed

Report 22808 for two to three vertebral segments; report 22810 for four to seven; report 22812 if eight or more

Explanation
Spinal arthrodesis, or fusion, is done here to correct a spinal deformity. An anterior approach is used. In the case of affected thoracolumbar vertebrae, the dissection is carried out through the abdominal muscles to the tenth rib, which is resected to allow access to the vertebrae in back. Dissection continues until the vertebral bodies are exposed. The physician cleans out the intervertebral disc spaces and removes the cartilaginous plates above and below the vertebrae to be fused. The physician obtains and packs separately reportable grafts of iliac or other donor bone into the spaces. Separately reportable instrumentation may be affixed to the spine. A drainage tube may be placed and the surgical wound is sutured closed. A cast may be applied to stabilize the spine. Report 22808 if two to three vertebral segments are fused; 22810 if four to seven vertebral segments are fused; and 22812 if eight or more vertebral segments are fused.

Coding Tips
Codes 22808–22812 identify arthrodesis for spinal deformities only. The spinal deformity may be congenital (e.g., scoliosis) or acquired due to a disease or other process (e.g., kyphosis). These codes should not be used to report fusion for spinal deformity due to a fracture or previous arthrodesis. Only one code from this range (22808–22812) may be reported. Arthrodesis codes are assigned according to the surgical approach used (anterior, posterior); if more than one approach is used, each is reported separately. If spinal instrumentation is performed, it is listed separately in addition to the code for the arthrodesis, see 22840–22847. Any bone graft is also reported separately, see 20930–20938. If the services of two primary surgeons performing separate and distinct components of the arthrodesis are required, each surgeon should report the procedure code(s) for the cosurgery and append modifier 62.

ICD-9-CM Procedural
- 81.00 Spinal fusion, not otherwise specified
- 81.01 Atlas-axis spinal fusion
- 81.02 Other cervical fusion of the anterior column, anterior technique
- 81.04 Dorsal and dorsolumbar fusion of the anterior column, anterior technique
- 81.06 Lumbar and lumbosacral fusion of the anterior column, anterior technique
- 81.31 Refusion of Atlas-axis spine
- 81.32 Refusion of other cervical spine, anterior column, anterior technique
- 81.34 Refusion of dorsal and dorsolumbar spine, anterior column, anterior technique
- 81.36 Refusion of lumbar and lumbosacral spine, anterior column, anterior technique
- 81.62 Fusion or refusion of 2-3 vertebrae
- 81.63 Fusion or refusion of 4-8 vertebrae
- 81.64 Fusion or refusion of 9 or more vertebrae

Anesthesia
00625, 00626, 00670

ICD-9-CM Diagnostic
- 237.71 Neurofibromatosis, Type 1 (von Recklinghausen's disease)
- 237.72 Neurofibromatosis, Type 2 (acoustic neurofibromatosis)
- 252.01 Primary hyperparathyroidism
- 356.1 Peroneal muscular atrophy
- 731.0 Osteitis deformans without mention of bone tumor
- 732.0 Juvenile osteochondrosis of spine
- 733.01 Senile osteoporosis — (Use additional code to identify major osseous defect, if applicable: 731.3) (Use additional code to identify personal history of pathologic (healed) fracture: V13.51)
- 733.02 Idiopathic osteoporosis — (Use additional code to identify major osseous defect, if applicable: 731.3) (Use additional code to identify personal history of pathologic (healed) fracture: V13.51)
- 737.0 Adolescent postural kyphosis
- 737.10 Kyphosis (acquired) (postural)
- 737.20 Lordosis (acquired) (postural)
- 737.30 Scoliosis (and kyphoscoliosis), idiopathic
- 737.32 Progressive infantile idiopathic scoliosis
- 737.33 Scoliosis due to radiation
- 737.34 Thoracogenic scoliosis
- 737.41 Kyphosis associated with other condition — (Code first associated condition: 015.0, 138, 237.7, 252.01, 277.5, 356.1, 731.0, 733.00-733.09)
- 737.42 Lordosis associated with other condition — (Code first associated condition: 015.0, 138, 237.7, 252.01, 277.5, 356.1, 731.0, 733.00-733.09)
- 754.2 Congenital musculoskeletal deformity of spine

CCI Version 16.3
0213T, 0216T, 0228T, 0230T, 22505, 22830, 29000-29046, 29200, 32100, 36000, 36400-36410, 36420-36430, 36440, 36600, 36640, 37202, 43752, 49000-49002, 51701-51703, 62310-62319, 63075, 63077, 64400-64435, 64445-64450, 64479, 64483, 64490, 64493, 64505-64530, 69990, 76000-76001, 92585, 93000-93010, 93040-93042, 93318, 94002, 94200, 94250, 94680-94690, 94770, 95812-95816, 95819, 95822, 95829, 95860-95861, 95867-95868, 95870, 95900, 95904, 95920, 95925-95934, 95936-95937, 95955, 96360, 96365, 96372, 96374-96376, 99148-99149, 99150

Also not with 22808: 22856-22857❖

Also not with 22810: 22802❖, 22808, 22856-22857❖, 22862-22864❖

Also not with 22812: 22802❖, 22808-22810❖, 22856-22864❖

Note: These CCI edits are used for Medicare. Other payers may reimburse on codes listed above.

Medicare Edits

	Fac RVU	Non-Fac RVU	FUD	Assist
22808	54.1	54.1	90	80
22810	60.2	60.2	90	80
22812	65.08	65.08	90	80

Medicare References: 100-3, 150.2

22818-22819

22818 Kyphectomy, circumferential exposure of spine and resection of vertebral segment(s) (including body and posterior elements); single or 2 segments

22819 3 or more segments

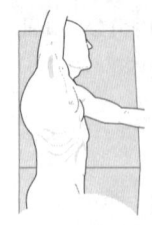

The thoracic spine is accessed and its circumference exposed. The spinal body and posterior processes are resected

Example of kyphotic spinal abnormality. The condition may be congenital or acquired

The physician accesses and removes a kyphotic segment of the spine. The entire circumference of the segment is exposed. The body and spinous process are cut away. Instrumentation and grafting may be required. Code 22818 for one or two segments and 22819 for three or more segments

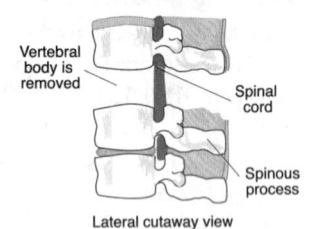

Vertebral body is removed — Spinal cord — Spinous process

Lateral cutaway view

Explanation

The physician performs this procedure for spinal deformities of kyphosis, a hunchback type increase in the convex curvature of the thoracic spine. The patient is placed prone. The physician makes a posterior midline incision, superior to the spinal abnormality, and dissects the periosteum of the normal vertebrae above and down into the lamina of the affected vertebrae, until the foramina are exposed on both sides of the spine. The nerve, artery, and vein within the foramina are divided, exposing the dural sac. The sac is dissected and the dura is closed with suture, leaving the sac remnant. Dissection is continued around the affected vertebral bodies and the intervertebral disc of the vertebra at the apex of the kyphosis is removed first, followed by the vertebra. Just enough vertebrae are removed to correct the kyphosis. The sac remnant that was left is used to cover the site of the resected vertebrae. Removed vertebral bodies are morselized and used for bone grafting. Rod instrumentation is applied and segmental wires are used to hold the rod in place. The wound is irrigated and closed with layered sutures over suction drains. A body jacket is applied. Report 22818 if a single or two-segment kyphectomy is performed. Report 22819 if a three or more segments kyphectomy is performed.

Coding Tips

Kyphectomy is frequently performed with other procedures on the spine, which should be reported separately. If spinal instrumentation is performed, it is listed separately, see 22840–22847. Any bone graft is also reported separately, see 20930–20938. To report arthrodesis, see 22800–22804 and use modifier 51. If the services of two primary surgeons performing separate and distinct components of the arthrodesis are required, each surgeon should report the procedure code(s) for the cosurgery and append modifier 62.

ICD-9-CM Procedural

77.99 Total ostectomy of other bone, except facial bones

Anesthesia

00670

ICD-9-CM Diagnostic

737.10 Kyphosis (acquired) (postural)

737.30 Scoliosis (and kyphoscoliosis), idiopathic

737.32 Progressive infantile idiopathic scoliosis

737.41 Kyphosis associated with other condition — (Code first associated condition: 015.0, 138, 237.7, 252.01, 277.5, 356.1, 731.0, 733.00-733.09)

737.43 Scoliosis associated with other condition — (Code first associated condition: 015.0, 138, 237.7, 252.01, 277.5, 356.1, 731.0, 733.00-733.09)

738.5 Other acquired deformity of back or spine

741.00 Spina bifida with hydrocephalus, unspecified region

741.02 Spina bifida with hydrocephalus, dorsal (thoracic) region

741.03 Spina bifida with hydrocephalus, lumbar region

741.90 Spina bifida without mention of hydrocephalus, unspecified region

741.92 Spina bifida without mention of hydrocephalus, dorsal (thoracic) region

741.93 Spina bifida without mention of hydrocephalus, lumbar region

742.59 Other specified congenital anomaly of spinal cord

754.2 Congenital musculoskeletal deformity of spine

756.19 Other congenital anomaly of spine

Terms To Know

kyphosis. Abnormal posterior convex curvature of the spine, usually in the thoracic region, resembling a hunchback.

scoliosis. Congenital condition of lateral curvature of the spine, often associated with other spinal column defects, congenital heart disease, or genitourinary abnormalities. It may also be associated with spinal muscular atrophy, cerebral palsy, or muscular dystrophy.

spina bifida cystica. Defective closure of the spinal column during early fetal development with a protrusion or herniation of the cord and meninges through the defect.

CCI Version 16.3

0213T, 0216T, 0228T, 0230T, 22101, 22505, 22856-22864❖, 29000-29046, 32100, 36000, 36400-36410, 36420-36430, 36440, 36600, 36640, 37202, 43752, 49000-49002, 51701-51703, 62310-62319, 63075, 63077, 63707, 64400-64435, 64445-64450, 64479, 64483, 64490, 64493, 64505-64530, 69990, 76000-76001, 92585, 93000-93010, 93040-93042, 93318, 94002, 94200, 94250, 94680-94690, 94770, 95812-95816, 95819, 95822, 95829, 95860-95861, 95867-95868, 95870, 95900, 95904, 95920, 95925-95934, 95936-95937, 95955, 96360, 96365, 96372, 96374-96376, 99148-99149, 99150

Also not with 22819: 22214, 22818

Note: These CCI edits are used for Medicare. Other payers may reimburse on codes listed above.

Medicare Edits

	Fac RVU	Non-Fac RVU	FUD	Assist
22818	64.35	64.35	90	80
22819	80.38	80.38	90	80

Medicare References: 100-3,150.2

22830

22830 Exploration of spinal fusion

Physician explores previously completed fusion

Midline incision

Instrumentation may be examined. Any removal or revision is reported separately

Explanation

The physician explores an existing fusion to diagnose and correct problems. The patient is placed in various positions depending on how the original fusion was performed (e.g., anterior, posterior, posterolateral). The physician makes an incision overlying the fused vertebrae. Fascia and paravertebral muscles are incised and retracted. The physician explores previous instrumentation, grafts, and wires. If any or all of the instrumentation is removed, replaced, or adjusted during the exploration, it is reported separately. When the exploration is complete, the fascia and vertebral muscles are repaired and returned to their anatomical positions. The incision is closed with layered sutures.

Coding Tips

Exploration of a spinal fusion may be reported with an arthrodesis if performed during the same operative session on the same level. Codes for removal, replacement, or reinsertion of spinal instrumentation are also reported separately, see 22849–22850 and 22852–22855. Add modifier 51 to 22830 when performed with any other definitive spinal procedure.

ICD-9-CM Procedural

03.09   Other exploration and decompression of spinal canal

Anesthesia

22830   00625, 00626, 00670

ICD-9-CM Diagnostic

324.1   Intraspinal abscess
722.81 Postlaminectomy syndrome, cervical region
722.82 Postlaminectomy syndrome, thoracic region
722.83 Postlaminectomy syndrome, lumbar region
724.4   Thoracic or lumbosacral neuritis or radiculitis, unspecified
733.13 Pathologic fracture of vertebrae
733.81 Malunion of fracture
733.82 Nonunion of fracture
733.95 Stress fracture of other bone — (Use additional external cause code(s) to identify the cause of the stress fracture)
996.40 Unspecified mechanical complication of internal orthopedic device, implant, and graft — (Use additional code to identify prosthetic joint with mechanical complication, V43.60-V43.69)
996.49 Other mechanical complication of other internal orthopedic device, implant, and graft — (Use additional code to identify prosthetic joint with mechanical complication, V43.60-V43.69)
996.67 Infection and inflammatory reaction due to other internal orthopedic device, implant, and graft — (Use additional code to identify specified infections)
996.78 Other complications due to other internal orthopedic device, implant, and graft — (Use additional code to identify complication: 338.18-338.19, 338.28-338.29)
V45.4   Arthrodesis status

Terms To Know

anterior. Situated in the front area or toward the belly surface of the body; an anatomical reference point used to show the position and relationship of one body structure to another.

fascia. Fibrous sheet or band of tissue that envelops organs, muscles, and groupings of muscles.

malunion. Fracture that has united in a faulty position due to inadequate reduction of the original fracture, insufficient holding of a previously well-reduced fracture, contracture of the soft tissues, or comminuted or osteoporotic bone causing a slow disintegration of the fracture.

posterior. Located in the back part or caudal end of the body.

posterolateral. Located in the back and off to the side.

CCI Version 16.3

0213T, 0216T, 0228T, 0230T, 13101, 13120, 22505, 29000-29046, 29200, 36000, 36400-36410, 36420-36430, 36440, 36600, 36640, 37202, 43752, 51701-51703, 62310-62319, 64400-64435, 64445-64450, 64479, 64483, 64490, 64493, 64505-64530, 69990, 76000-76001, 92585, 93000-93010, 93040-93042, 93318, 94002, 94200, 94250, 94680-94690, 94770, 95812-95816, 95819, 95822, 95829, 95860-95861, 95867-95868, 95870, 95900, 95904, 95920, 95925-95934, 95936-95937, 95955, 96360, 96365, 96372, 96374-96376, 99148-99149, 99150

Note: These CCI edits are used for Medicare. Other payers may reimburse on codes listed above.

Medicare Edits

	Fac RVU	Non-Fac RVU	FUD	Assist
22830	23.69	23.69	90	80

Medicare References: 100-3, 150.2

22840-22844

22840 Posterior non-segmental instrumentation (eg, Harrington rod technique, pedicle fixation across 1 interspace, atlantoaxial transarticular screw fixation, sublaminar wiring at C1, facet screw fixation) (List separately in addition to code for primary procedure)

22841 Internal spinal fixation by wiring of spinous processes (List separately in addition to code for primary procedure)

22842 Posterior segmental instrumentation (eg, pedicle fixation, dual rods with multiple hooks and sublaminar wires); 3 to 6 vertebral segments (List separately in addition to code for primary procedure)

22843 7 to 12 vertebral segments (List separately in addition to code for primary procedure)

22844 13 or more vertebral segments (List separately in addition to code for primary procedure)

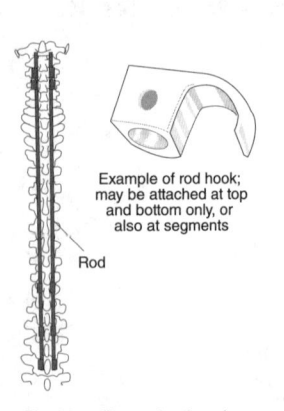

Example of rod hook; may be attached at top and bottom only, or also at segments

Rod

Physician affixes rod to the spine with hooks, clamps, wires, or screws; stylized rod shown

Explanation
The physician uses spinal instrumentation to correct a defect of the spine caused by disease, trauma, or congenital anomaly and to stabilize the spine to reduce risks of neurological damage or nonfusion after arthrodesis. Non-segmental instrumentation is a construct placed with fixation at either end only and not in the intervening levels. The physician makes a midline incision in the skin, fascia, and paravertebral muscles over the affected vertebrae. Upper and lower hooks or screws are introduced into the vertebral pedicles. A rod fashioned to fit the spinal contours is anchored to the screws or hooks. To achieve correction, distraction is applied with an instrument to increase the distance between the hooks at each end of the rod, which is secured in position. Another method of securing the rod is to use wires passed under prepared lamina and tightened around the rods. The minimal wiring inherent in this procedure should not be reported with 22841. The wound is closed with layered sutures. These Harrington rod instrumentation techniques have become outdated and are being replaced by more rigid, segmental fixation methods.

Coding Tips
As "add-on" codes, 22840–22844 are not subject to multiple procedure rules. No reimbursement reduction or modifier 51 is applied. Add-on codes describe additional intra-service work associated with the primary procedure. They are performed by the same physician on the same date of service as the primary service/procedure, and must never be reported as a stand-alone code. Any bone graft is reported separately; see 20930–20938. Report separately codes for treatment of a fracture/dislocation (22325–22328) and arthrodesis (22548–22812). It is inappropriate to append modifier 62 to spinal instrumentation codes.

ICD-9-CM Procedural
84.59   Insertion of other spinal devices

Anesthesia
00670

ICD-9-CM Diagnostic
The ICD-9-CM diagnostic code(s) would be the same as the actual procedure performed because these are in-addition-to codes.

Terms To Know
anomaly. Irregularity in the structure or position of an organ or tissue.

CCI Version 16.3
Also not with 22840: 0202T, 0228T, 22505, 22843-22844❖, 51701-51703, 62310, 62318, 63295, 64479, 92585, 95822, 95860-95861, 95867-95868, 95870, 95900, 95904, 95920, 95925-95934, 95936-95937

Also not with 22842: 0228T, 0230T, 22505, 51701-51703, 62310-62319, 63295, 64479, 64483, 76000-76001, 92585, 95822, 95860-95861, 95867-95868, 95870, 95900, 95904, 95920, 95925-95934, 95936-95937

Also not with 22843: 0228T, 0230T, 22505, 51701-51703, 62310-62319, 63295, 64479, 64483, 92585, 95822, 95860-95861, 95867-95868, 95870, 95900, 95904, 95920, 95925-95934, 95936-95937

Also not with 22844: 0228T, 0230T, 22505, 51701-51703, 62310-62319, 63295, 64479, 64483, 92585, 95822, 95860-95861, 95867-95868, 95870, 95900, 95904, 95920, 95925-95934, 95936-95937

Note: These CCI edits are used for Medicare. Other payers may reimburse on codes listed above.

Medicare Edits

	Fac RVU	Non-Fac RVU	FUD	Assist
22840	22.94	22.94	N/A	80
22841	0.0	0.0	N/A	N/A
22842	22.98	22.98	N/A	80
22843	24.39	24.39	N/A	80
22844	29.45	29.45	N/A	80

Medicare References: None

22845-22847

22845 Anterior instrumentation; 2 to 3 vertebral segments (List separately in addition to code for primary procedure)

22846 4 to 7 vertebral segments (List separately in addition to code for primary procedure)

22847 8 or more vertebral segments (List separately in addition to code for primary procedure)

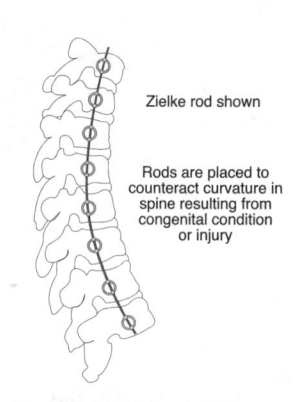

Zielke rod shown

Rods are placed to counteract curvature in spine resulting from congenital condition or injury

Physician uses rods installed in front to correct spinal deformities; Report 22845 for two to three vertebral segments; report 22846 for four to seven segments; report 22847 for eight or more

Explanation

Anterior instrumentation is reserved for flexible lumbar or thoracolumbar scoliotic curves. Several methods and types are available (e.g., Dwyer, Zielke, Scottish Rite) but all are based on a rod or cable fixated through large-headed, slotted, or cannulated screws. A thoracic or general surgeon assists for the intraoperative exposure, mainly thoracoabdominal or abdominal retroperitoneal. A hole is made in the vertebral body on the lateral side as posteriorly as possible. The screw is inserted across the midportion of the vertebra to the opposite cortex in a slight posteroanterior angle. A flexible threaded rod or cable is inserted in the angled screw heads. The spine is derotated and the rod is locked into its straighter position with nuts. The wound is closed in a routine manner. Report 22845 for two to three vertebral segments; 22846 for four to seven vertebral segments; and 22847 for eight or more vertebral segments.

Coding Tips

As "add-on" codes, 22845–22847 are not subject to multiple procedure rules. No reimbursement reduction or modifier 51 is applied. Add-on codes describe additional intra-service work associated with the primary procedure. They are performed by the same physician on the same date of service as the primary service/procedure, and must never be reported as a stand-alone code. Any bone graft is reported separately; see 20930–20938. Report separately codes for treatment of a fracture/dislocation (22325–22328) and arthrodesis (22548–22812). It is inappropriate to append modifier 62 to spinal instrumentation codes.

ICD-9-CM Procedural

84.59 Insertion of other spinal devices

Anesthesia

00670

ICD-9-CM Diagnostic

The ICD-9-CM diagnostic code(s) would be the same as the actual procedure performed because these are in-addition-to codes.

Terms To Know

anterior. Situated in the front area or toward the belly surface of the body; an anatomical reference point used to show the position and relationship of one body structure to another.

congenital. Present at birth, occurring through heredity or an influence during gestation up to the moment of birth.

deformity. Irregularity or malformation of the body.

dislocation. Displacement of a bone in relation to its neighboring tissue, especially a joint.

fracture. Break in bone or cartilage.

instrumentation. Use of a tool for therapeutic reasons.

internal skeletal fixation. Repair involving wires, pins, screws, and/or plates placed through or within the fractured area to stabilize and immobilize the injury.

posterior. Located in the back part or caudal end of the body.

scoliosis. Congenital condition of lateral curvature of the spine, often associated with other spinal column defects, congenital heart disease, or genitourinary abnormalities. It may also be associated with spinal muscular atrophy, cerebral palsy, or muscular dystrophy.

vertebra. Any one of the 33 bones composing the spinal column, generally having a disc-shaped body, two transverse processes, and a spinal process centered posteriorly. Vertebrae are connected by the laminae between them and are attached to the body by pedicles, forming an enclosed, protective ring around the vertebral foramen through which the spinal cord runs.

vertebral column. Thirty-three bones that house the spinal cord, consisting of seven cervical vertebrae, 12 thoracic vertebrae, five lumbar vertebrae, five fused vertebrae in the sacrum, and four fused vertebrae in the coccyx.

CCI Version 16.3

0228T, 0230T, 22505, 32100, 49000-49002, 51701-51703, 62310-62319, 64479, 64483, 92585, 95822, 95860-95861, 95867-95868, 95870, 95900, 95904, 95920, 95925-95934, 95936-95937

Note: These CCI edits are used for Medicare. Other payers may reimburse on codes listed above.

Medicare Edits

	Fac RVU	Non-Fac RVU	FUD	Assist
22845	22.12	22.12	N/A	80
22846	22.95	22.95	N/A	80
22847	26.23	26.23	N/A	80

Medicare References: None

22848

22848 Pelvic fixation (attachment of caudal end of instrumentation to pelvic bony structures) other than sacrum (List separately in addition to code for primary procedure)

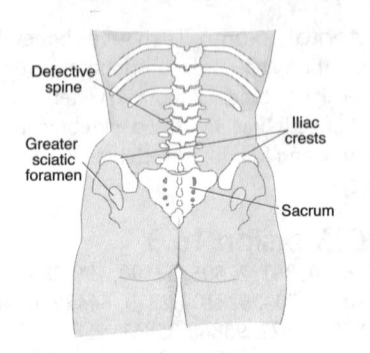

Posterior view of Galveston fixation

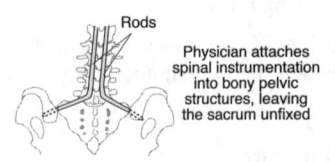

Rods are inserted into the iliac spine and contoured to correct and support spine; sacrum remains unfixed

Physician attaches spinal instrumentation into bony pelvic structures, leaving the sacrum unfixed

Explanation
The physician joins axial connectors, such as the tail end of spinal instrumentation devices, to a rod configured to fit along the flat of the sacrum and impacted longitudinally between the cornices of the ilium just above the greater sciatic notch. The rod is driven through the ilium and negates the need for anterior instrumentation. This procedure, usually called the "Galveston technique," often accompanies a procedure for scoliosis, myelomeningocele, or paralytic spinal defects where sacral fixation is not desirable.

Coding Tips
As an "add-on" code, 22848 is not subject to multiple procedure rules. No reimbursement reduction or modifier 51 is applied. Add-on codes describe additional intra-service work associated with the primary procedure. They are performed by the same physician on the same date of service as the primary service/procedure, and must never be reported as a stand-alone code. Any bone graft is reported separately; see 20930–20938. Report separately codes for treatment of a fracture/dislocation (22325–22328) and arthrodesis (22548–22812). It is inappropriate to append modifier 62 to spinal instrumentation codes.

ICD-9-CM Procedural
78.59 Internal fixation of other bone, except facial bones, without fracture reduction
84.59 Insertion of other spinal devices

Anesthesia
22848 00670

ICD-9-CM Diagnostic
The ICD-9-CM diagnostic code(s) would be the same as the actual procedure performed because these are in-addition-to codes.

Terms To Know

anterior. Situated in the front area or toward the belly surface of the body; an anatomical reference point used to show the position and relationship of one body structure to another.

instrumentation. Use of a tool for therapeutic reasons.

internal skeletal fixation. Repair involving wires, pins, screws, and/or plates placed through or within the fractured area to stabilize and immobilize the injury.

myelomeningocele. Congenital disorder in which the spinal cord and meninges herniate through a vertebral canal defect.

pelvic bones. Ilium, ischium, pubis, and sacrum together forming a bony circle to protect the pelvic contents, provide stability for the vertebral column (sacrum), and provide an appropriate surface for femoral articulation for ambulation.

pelvis. Distal anterior portion of the trunk that lies between the hipbones, sacrum, and coccyx bones; the inferior portion of the abdominal cavity.

sacrum. Lower portion of the spine composed of five fused vertebrae designated as S1-S5.

scoliosis. Congenital condition of lateral curvature of the spine, often associated with other spinal column defects, congenital heart disease, or genitourinary abnormalities. It may also be associated with spinal muscular atrophy, cerebral palsy, or muscular dystrophy.

vertebral body. Disc-shaped portion of a vertebra that is anteriorly located and bears weight.

CCI Version 16.3
0230T, 11012❖, 22505, 51701-51703, 62311, 62319, 64483, 92585, 95822, 95860-95861, 95867-95868, 95870, 95900, 95904, 95920, 95925-95934, 95936-95937

Note: These CCI edits are used for Medicare. Other payers may reimburse on codes listed above.

Medicare Edits

	Fac RVU	Non-Fac RVU	FUD	Assist
22848	10.79	10.79	N/A	80

Medicare References: None

22849

22849 Reinsertion of spinal fixation device

Detached hooks — *Corrected fixation*

Physician reinserts spinal fixation device following failure or reappearance of the deformity

Hook, screw, or wire loosened by spinal changes or event

Explanation
This code describes the procedures used following failure of devices such as wires, screws, cables, plates, or rods used in spinal fixation. The patient is placed in the position dictated by the failure. The physician makes a midline incision overlying the damaged section. The fascia, paravertebral muscles, and ligaments are retracted. A number of reparative techniques may be used, depending on the device and point of failure. In most cases, the device must be replaced. The physician closes the muscles, fascia, and skin with layered sutures.

Coding Tips
Report exploration of a spinal fusion separately; see 22830. Removal of instrumentation (22850, 22852, 22855) is not reported separately when performed with reinsertion of a spinal fixation device at the same spine levels. It is inappropriate to append modifier 62 to spinal instrumentation codes.

ICD-9-CM Procedural
- 78.59 Internal fixation of other bone, except facial bones, without fracture reduction
- 84.51 Insertion of interbody spinal fusion device
- 84.59 Insertion of other spinal devices

Anesthesia
22849 00670

ICD-9-CM Diagnostic
- 996.40 Unspecified mechanical complication of internal orthopedic device, implant, and graft — (Use additional code to identify prosthetic joint with mechanical complication, V43.60-V43.69)
- 996.49 Other mechanical complication of other internal orthopedic device, implant, and graft — (Use additional code to identify prosthetic joint with mechanical complication, V43.60-V43.69)
- 996.67 Infection and inflammatory reaction due to other internal orthopedic device, implant, and graft — (Use additional code to identify specified infections)
- 996.78 Other complications due to other internal orthopedic device, implant, and graft — (Use additional code to identify complication: 338.18-338.19, 338.28-338.29)
- V45.4 Arthrodesis status

Terms To Know
fascia. Fibrous sheet or band of tissue that envelops organs, muscles, and groupings of muscles.

incision. Act of cutting into tissue or an organ.

infection. Presence of microorganisms in body tissues that may result in cellular damage.

internal skeletal fixation. Repair involving wires, pins, screws, and/or plates placed through or within the fractured area to stabilize and immobilize the injury.

vertebral body. Disc-shaped portion of a vertebra that is anteriorly located and bears weight.

vertebral column. Thirty-three bones that house the spinal cord, consisting of seven cervical vertebrae, 12 thoracic vertebrae, five lumbar vertebrae, five fused vertebrae in the sacrum, and four fused vertebrae in the coccyx.

CCI Version 16.3
0213T, 0216T, 0228T, 0230T, 22505, 22850, 22852-22855, 29000-29046, 29200, 36000, 36400-36410, 36420-36430, 36440, 36600, 36640, 37202, 43752, 51701-51703, 62310-62319, 64400-64435, 64445-64450, 64479, 64483, 64490, 64493, 64505-64530, 76000-76001, 92585, 93000-93010, 93040-93042, 93318, 94002, 94200, 94250, 94680-94690, 94770, 95812-95816, 95819, 95822, 95829, 95860-95861, 95867-95868, 95870, 95900, 95904, 95920, 95925-95934, 95936-95937, 95955, 96360, 96365, 96372, 96374-96376, 99148-99149, 99150

Note: These CCI edits are used for Medicare. Other payers may reimburse on codes listed above.

Medicare Edits

	Fac RVU	Non-Fac RVU	FUD	Assist
22849	38.35	38.35	90	80

Medicare References: None

22850

22850 Removal of posterior nonsegmental instrumentation (eg, Harrington rod)

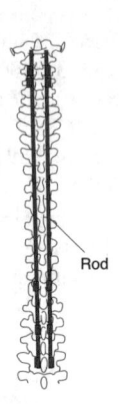

Rod

Report 22850 if instrumentation is nonsegmental

Physician removes posterior instrumentation no longer necessary or appropriate

Explanation
Previously applied posterior spinal nonsegmental instrumentation is removed. Instrumentation is sometimes removed when correction is complete and stable, when the patient is a growing juvenile, or when the instrumentation causes complications, such as infection or pain. The patient is placed prone. The physician makes an incision overlying the affected area through the skin, fascia, and paravertebral muscles. Collagen is removed. The instrumentation is exposed and the superior hook or screw is loosened. Using forceps, the upper and lower hooks are disconnected from the vertebra and the hardware is removed.

Coding Tips
Report exploration of a spinal fusion separately; see 22830. For removal of posterior segmental instrumentation, see 22852. For removal of anterior instrumentation, see 22855. Removal of instrumentation is not reported separately when performed in conjunction with reinsertion. It is inappropriate to append modifier 62 to spinal instrumentation codes.

ICD-9-CM Procedural
78.69 Removal of implanted device from other bone

Anesthesia
22850 00670

ICD-9-CM Diagnostic
- 996.40 Unspecified mechanical complication of internal orthopedic device, implant, and graft — (Use additional code to identify prosthetic joint with mechanical complication, V43.60-V43.69)
- 996.49 Other mechanical complication of other internal orthopedic device, implant, and graft — (Use additional code to identify prosthetic joint with mechanical complication, V43.60-V43.69)
- 996.67 Infection and inflammatory reaction due to other internal orthopedic device, implant, and graft — (Use additional code to identify specified infections)
- 996.78 Other complications due to other internal orthopedic device, implant, and graft — (Use additional code to identify complication: 338.18-338.19, 338.28-338.29)
- V45.4 Arthrodesis status
- V54.01 Encounter for removal of internal fixation device

Terms To Know
collagen. Protein based substance of strength and flexibility that is the major component of connective tissue, found in cartilage, bone, tendons, and skin.

complication. Condition arising after the beginning of observation and treatment that modifies the course of the patient's illness or the medical care required, or an undesired result or misadventure in medical care.

fascia. Fibrous sheet or band of tissue that envelops organs, muscles, and groupings of muscles.

infection. Presence of microorganisms in body tissues that may result in cellular damage.

instrumentation. Use of a tool for therapeutic reasons.

posterior. Located in the back part or caudal end of the body.

prone. Lying face downward.

vertebral column. Thirty-three bones that house the spinal cord, consisting of seven cervical vertebrae, 12 thoracic vertebrae, five lumbar vertebrae, five fused vertebrae in the sacrum, and four fused vertebrae in the coccyx.

CCI Version 16.3
0213T, 0216T, 0228T, 0230T, 22010, 22015, 22505, 22830, 29000-29046, 29200, 36000, 36400-36410, 36420-36430, 36440, 36600, 36640, 37202, 43752, 51701-51703, 62310-62319, 64400-64435, 64445-64450, 64479, 64483, 64490, 64493, 64505-64530, 76000-76001, 92585, 93000-93010, 93040-93042, 93318, 94002, 94200, 94250, 94680-94690, 94770, 95812-95816, 95819, 95822, 95829, 95860-95861, 95867-95868, 95870, 95900, 95904, 95920, 95925-95934, 95936-95937, 95955, 96360, 96365, 96372, 96374-96376, 99148-99149, 99150

Note: These CCI edits are used for Medicare. Other payers may reimburse on codes listed above.

Medicare Edits

	Fac RVU	Non-Fac RVU	FUD	Assist
22850	21.04	21.04	90	80

Medicare References: None

22851

22851 Application of intervertebral biomechanical device(s) (eg, synthetic cage(s), methylmethacrylate) to vertebral defect or interspace (List separately in addition to code for primary procedure)

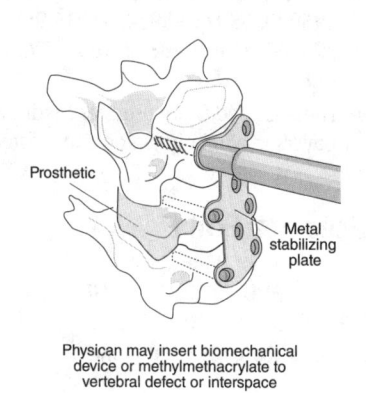

Prosthetic

Metal stabilizing plate

Physican may insert biomechanical device or methylmethacrylate to vertebral defect or interspace

Explanation
The physician replaces a vertebral body or partial vertebral body resected due to destruction by disease, trauma, or other processes. Once the vertebral body has been removed by a separately identifiable procedure, a hole is cored out of the vertebral bodies above and below the removed vertebrae to secure a biomechanical device (metal/synthetic cage or methylmethacrylate) into the resulting vertebral defect or interspace. The physician selects the biomechanical device best suited to the location and type of deformity being corrected. For example, to correct a deformity caused by a malignancy, the physician may elect to inject methylmethacrylate into the area and allow it to dry to replace the excised vertebral body. Screws, wires, or plates may be used to secure the device. Muscles are allowed to fall back into place and the wound is closed over a drain with layered sutures.

Coding Tips
This code has been revised for 2011 in the official CPT description. As an "add-on" code, 22851 is not subject to multiple procedure rules. No reimbursement reduction or modifier 51 is applied. Add-on codes describe additional intra-service work associated with the primary procedure. They are performed by the same physician on the same date of service as the primary service/procedure, and must never be reported as a stand-alone code. Report 22851 for each interspace treated. Any bone graft is reported separately; see 20930–20938. Report separately treatment of a fracture/dislocation (22325–22328) and arthrodesis (22548–22812). It is inappropriate to append modifier 62 to spinal instrumentation codes.

ICD-9-CM Procedural
- 84.51 Insertion of interbody spinal fusion device
- 84.56 Insertion or replacement of (cement) spacer
- 84.59 Insertion of other spinal devices

Anesthesia
22851 00670

ICD-9-CM Diagnostic
The ICD-9-CM diagnostic code(s) would be the same as the actual procedure performed because these are in-addition-to codes.

Terms To Know
defect. Imperfection, flaw, or absence.

graft. Tissue implant from another part of the body or another person.

malignant. Any condition tending to progress toward death, specifically an invasive tumor with a loss of cellular differentiation that has the ability to spread or metastasize to other areas in the body.

resect. Cutting out or removing a portion or all of a bone, organ, or other structure.

vertebral body. Disc-shaped portion of a vertebra that is anteriorly located and bears weight.

vertebral foramen. Space between the vertebral body and vertebra arch that contains the spinal cord.

vertebral interspace. Non-bony space between two adjacent vertebral bodies that contains the cushioning intervertebral disk.

CCI Version 16.3
01935-01936, 0202T, 0228T, 0230T, 11012❖, 22505-22521❖, 49000-49002, 51701-51703, 62310-62319, 64479, 64483, 76000-76001, 92585, 95822, 95860-95861, 95867-95868, 95870, 95900, 95904, 95920, 95925-95934, 95936-95937

Note: These CCI edits are used for Medicare. Other payers may reimburse on codes listed above.

Medicare Edits

	Fac RVU	Non-Fac RVU	FUD	Assist
22851	12.27	12.27	N/A	80

Medicare References: None

22852

22852 Removal of posterior segmental instrumentation

Example of segmental fixation hook
Rod

Growth, the healing process, and other factors may necessitate removal of segmental instrumentation by the physician

Explanation
Previously applied posterior spinal segmental instrumentation is removed. Instrumentation is sometimes removed when correction is complete and stable, when the patient is a growing juvenile, or when the instrumentation causes complications, such as infection or pain. The patient is placed prone. The physician makes a midline incision overlying the affected area through the skin, fascia, and paravertebral muscles. Collagen is removed. The instrumentation is exposed. Using forceps, the superior hook is loosened. The superior, inferior, and all segmental hooks between are disconnected from the vertebrae. The hardware is removed. The incision is closed with layered sutures.

Coding Tips
Report exploration of a spinal fusion separately; see 22830. For removal of posterior nonsegmental instrumentation (e.g., Harrington rod), see 22850. For removal of anterior instrumentation, see 22855. Removal of instrumentation is not reported separately when performed in conjunction with reinsertion (22849). It is inappropriate to append modifier 62 to spinal instrumentation codes.

ICD-9-CM Procedural
78.69 Removal of implanted device from other bone

Anesthesia
22852   00670

ICD-9-CM Diagnostic
- 996.40 Unspecified mechanical complication of internal orthopedic device, implant, and graft — (Use additional code to identify prosthetic joint with mechanical complication, V43.60-V43.69)
- 996.49 Other mechanical complication of other internal orthopedic device, implant, and graft — (Use additional code to identify prosthetic joint with mechanical complication, V43.60-V43.69)
- 996.67 Infection and inflammatory reaction due to other internal orthopedic device, implant, and graft — (Use additional code to identify specified infections)
- 996.78 Other complications due to other internal orthopedic device, implant, and graft — (Use additional code to identify complication: 338.18-338.19, 338.28-338.29)
- V45.4 Arthrodesis status
- V54.01 Encounter for removal of internal fixation device

Terms To Know
collagen. Protein based substance of strength and flexibility that is the major component of connective tissue, found in cartilage, bone, tendons, and skin.

complication. Condition arising after the beginning of observation and treatment that modifies the course of the patient's illness or the medical care required, or an undesired result or misadventure in medical care.

fascia. Fibrous sheet or band of tissue that envelops organs, muscles, and groupings of muscles.

infection. Presence of microorganisms in body tissues that may result in cellular damage.

posterior. Located in the back part or caudal end of the body.

CCI Version 16.3
0213T, 0216T, 0228T, 0230T, 22010, 22015, 22505, 22830, 29000-29046, 29200, 32100, 36000, 36400-36410, 36420-36430, 36440, 36600, 36640, 37202, 43752, 49010, 51701-51703, 62310-62319, 64400-64435, 64445-64450, 64479, 64483, 64490, 64493, 64505-64530, 76000-76001, 92585, 93000-93010, 93040-93042, 93318, 94002, 94200, 94250, 94680-94690, 94770, 95812-95816, 95819, 95822, 95829, 95860-95861, 95867-95868, 95870, 95900, 95904, 95920, 95925-95934, 95936-95937, 95955, 96360, 96365, 96372, 96374-96376, 99148-99149, 99150

Note: These CCI edits are used for Medicare. Other payers may reimburse on codes listed above.

Medicare Edits

	Fac RVU	Non-Fac RVU	FUD	Assist
22852	20.11	20.11	90	80

Medicare References: None

22855

22855 Removal of anterior instrumentation

Physician removes anterior rods no longer necessary; growth, the healing process, and other factors may eliminate the need for the rod

Explanation
Previously applied anterior spinal instrumentation is removed. Instrumentation is sometimes removed when correction is complete and stable, when the patient is a growing juvenile, or when the instrumentation causes complications, such as infection or pain. The patient is placed supine for the removal of anterior spinal fixation devices. The physician makes an abdominal retroperitoneal or thoracic incision to reach the affected area. Collagen is removed. The instrumentation is exposed and the superior hook or screw is loosened. Using forceps, the superior hook or screw is disconnected from the vertebra, as are the inferior and all segmental hooks or screws. The hardware is removed. The incision is closed with layered sutures.

Coding Tips
When an anterior approach to the thoracic cavity is performed, the negative pressure is lost and a thoracotomy tube is routinely inserted to help reestablish the normal negative pressure and re-inflate the lung(s) after closure. This is a life-sustaining measure that must be performed in order to complete the procedure and, as such, tube thoracostomy (32551) should not be reported separately. Removal of instrumentation is not reported separately when performed in conjunction with reinsertion (22849). Report exploration of a spinal fusion separately, see 22830. For removal of posterior nonsegmental instrumentation (e.g., Harrington rod), see 22850. For removal of posterior segmental fixation, see 22852.

ICD-9-CM Procedural
78.69 Removal of implanted device from other bone

Anesthesia
22855 00625, 00626, 00670

ICD-9-CM Diagnostic
996.40 Unspecified mechanical complication of internal orthopedic device, implant, and graft — (Use additional code to identify prosthetic joint with mechanical complication, V43.60-V43.69)
996.49 Other mechanical complication of other internal orthopedic device, implant, and graft — (Use additional code to identify prosthetic joint with mechanical complication, V43.60-V43.69)
996.67 Infection and inflammatory reaction due to other internal orthopedic device, implant, and graft — (Use additional code to identify specified infections)
996.78 Other complications due to other internal orthopedic device, implant, and graft — (Use additional code to identify complication: 338.18-338.19, 338.28-338.29)
V45.4 Arthrodesis status
V54.01 Encounter for removal of internal fixation device

Terms To Know
anterior. Situated in the front area or toward the belly surface of the body; an anatomical reference point used to show the position and relationship of one body structure to another.

collagen. Protein based substance of strength and flexibility that is the major component of connective tissue, found in cartilage, bone, tendons, and skin.

fascia. Fibrous sheet or band of tissue that envelops organs, muscles, and groupings of muscles.

infection. Presence of microorganisms in body tissues that may result in cellular damage.

CCI Version 16.3
0213T, 0216T, 0228T, 0230T, 22505, 22830, 29000-29046, 29200, 32100, 36000, 36400-36410, 36420-36430, 36440, 36600, 36640, 37202, 43752, 49000-49010, 51701-51703, 62310-62319, 64400-64435, 64445-64450, 64479, 64483, 64490, 64493, 64505-64530, 76000-76001, 92585, 93000-93010, 93040-93042, 93318, 94002, 94200, 94250, 94680-94690, 94770, 95812-95816, 95819, 95822, 95829, 95860-95861, 95867-95868, 95870, 95900, 95904, 95920, 95925-95934, 95936-95937, 95955, 96360, 96365, 96372, 96374-96376, 99148-99149, 99150

Note: These CCI edits are used for Medicare. Other payers may reimburse on codes listed above.

Medicare Edits

	Fac RVU	Non-Fac RVU	FUD	Assist
22855	32.84	32.84	90	80

Medicare References: None

22856-22857

22856 Total disc arthroplasty (artificial disc), anterior approach, including discectomy with end plate preparation (includes osteophytectomy for nerve root or spinal cord decompression and microdissection), single interspace, cervical

22857 Total disc arthroplasty (artificial disc), anterior approach, including discectomy to prepare interspace (other than for decompression), single interspace, lumbar

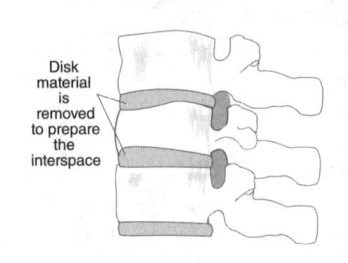

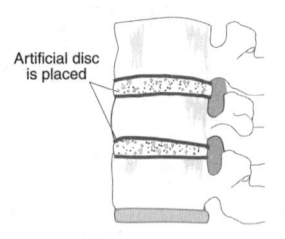

Total disc arthroplasty including end plate preparation, decompression, and microdissection for cervical interspace (22856) or lumbar interspace (22857)

Explanation
Total disc arthroplasty is performed to replace a severely damaged or diseased intervertebral disc, most often caused by degenerative disc disease. The physician uses an anterior approach to reach the damaged cervical vertebrae in 22856 by making an incision through the neck, avoiding the esophagus, trachea, and thyroid. In 22857, the physician uses an anterior approach to reach the damaged lumbar vertebrae by making an incision through the abdomen. Some implants require only minimal access, approximately 7 cm long, for a mini-retroperitoneal approach. Retractors separate the intervertebral muscles. The affected intervertebral disc location is confirmed by separately reportable x-ray. The physician cleans out the intervertebral disc space with a rongeur, removing the cartilaginous material to be replaced in preparation for inserting the implant. Preparation may include discectomy, osteophytectomy for nerve root or spinal cord decompression, and/or microdissection. One type of implant for total disc replacement has two endplates made of a metal alloy and a convex weight-bearing surface made of ultra high molecular weight polyethylene. The endplates are inserted in a collapsed form and seated into the vertebral bodies above and below the interspace. Minimal distraction is applied to open the intervertebral space, and the polyethylene disc material is snap-fitted into the lower endplate. With the disc assembly complete, the wound is closed, and a drain may be placed. Each of these codes reports a single interspace and includes fluoroscopy when performed.

Coding Tips
Do not report 22856 with 22554, 22845, 22851, or 63075 when performed at the same level. Do not report 22857 with 22558, 22845, 22851, or 49010 when performed at the same level. Use of an operating microscope is included in this procedure. Do not report 69990 separately. Fluoroscopy, when performed, is included and should not be reported separately. For additional total disc arthroplasty, cervical spine interspace, report 0092T. For additional total disc arthroplasty, lumbar spine interspace, report 0163T.

ICD-9-CM Procedural
- 84.62 Insertion of total spinal disc prosthesis, cervical
- 84.65 Insertion of total spinal disc prosthesis, lumbosacral

Anesthesia
00670

ICD-9-CM Diagnostic
- 198.5 Secondary malignant neoplasm of bone and bone marrow
- 213.2 Benign neoplasm of vertebral column, excluding sacrum and coccyx
- 238.0 Neoplasm of uncertain behavior of bone and articular cartilage
- 721.3 Lumbosacral spondylosis without myelopathy
- 721.42 Spondylosis with myelopathy, lumbar region
- 721.8 Other allied disorders of spine
- 722.10 Displacement of lumbar intervertebral disc without myelopathy
- 722.51 Degeneration of thoracic or thoracolumbar intervertebral disc
- 722.52 Degeneration of lumbar or lumbosacral intervertebral disc
- 722.73 Intervertebral lumbar disc disorder with myelopathy, lumbar region
- 722.83 Postlaminectomy syndrome, lumbar region
- 722.93 Other and unspecified disc disorder of lumbar region
- 724.02 Spinal stenosis of lumbar region, without neurogenic claudication
- 724.4 Thoracic or lumbosacral neuritis or radiculitis, unspecified
- 731.0 Osteitis deformans without mention of bone tumor
- 733.13 Pathologic fracture of vertebrae
- 733.82 Nonunion of fracture
- 738.5 Other acquired deformity of back or spine
- 756.11 Congenital spondylolysis, lumbosacral region
- 756.12 Congenital spondylolisthesis
- 756.19 Other congenital anomaly of spine
- 805.4 Closed fracture of lumbar vertebra without mention of spinal cord injury
- 805.5 Open fracture of lumbar vertebra without mention of spinal cord injury
- 806.4 Closed fracture of lumbar spine with spinal cord injury
- 806.5 Open fracture of lumbar spine with spinal cord injury
- 839.20 Closed dislocation, lumbar vertebra
- 839.30 Open dislocation, lumbar vertebra

CCI Version 16.3
0213T, 0216T, 22505, 22554, 22800❖, 22845, 22851, 36000, 37202, 51701-51703, 64490, 64493, 69990, 76000-76001, 92585, 95822, 95860-95861, 95867-95868, 95870, 95900, 95904, 95920, 95925-95934, 95936-95937, 96360, 96365, 96372, 96374-96376, 99148-99149, 99150

Also not with 22856: 22220❖, 22600❖, 29000, 29015, 29025, 29040, 36410, 62291, 62310, 62318-62319, 63075, 64415-64417, 64450

Also not with 22857: 0195T❖, 0202T, 0228T, 0230T, 22100, 22556-22558, 29020-29025, 29044-29046, 36400-36410, 36420-36430, 36440, 36600, 36640, 43752, 49000-49010, 62290, 62310-62319, 64400-64435, 64445-64450, 64479, 64483, 64505-64530, 72295, 93000-93010, 93040-93042, 93318, 94002, 94200, 94250, 94680-94690, 94770, 95812-95816, 95819, 95829, 95955

Note: These CCI edits are used for Medicare. Other payers may reimburse on codes listed above.

Medicare Edits

	Fac RVU	Non-Fac RVU	FUD	Assist
22856	48.79	48.79	90	80
22857	49.44	49.44	90	80

Medicare References: None

22861-22862

22861 Revision including replacement of total disc arthroplasty (artificial disc), anterior approach, single interspace; cervical
22862 lumbar

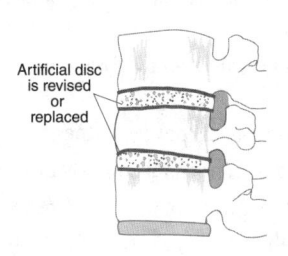

Explanation
The physician revises an artificial disc prosthesis placed during a previous disc arthroplasty through anterior approach. The prosthesis may be migrating from a lack of fixation and require components to be replaced or adjusted. The physician approaches the cervical vertebrae in 22861 by making an incision through the neck, avoiding the esophagus, trachea, and thyroid. The lumbar vertebrae (22862) are approached by making an incision through the abdomen. Retractors separate the intervertebral muscles. The implant is located, the area is explored, and any adhesions are freed. Distraction is applied to open the intervertebral space. The arthroplastic disc is removed, and the endplates of the vertebral body are reshaped and prepped for reinsertion. New height, depth, and width dimensions may also be taken with the vertebral body distracted in cases where another, more appropriately sized disc prosthesis is required. The components are reinserted, and the fascia and vertebral muscles are repaired and returned to their anatomical positions. The incision is closed. Each of these codes reports a single interspace and includes fluoroscopy when performed.

Coding Tips
Do not report 22861 with 22845, 22851, 22864, or 63075 when performed at the same level. Do not report 22862 with 22558, 22845, 22851, 22865 or 49010 when performed at the same level. Use of an operating microscope is included in 22861. Do not report 69990 separately. Fluoroscopy, when performed, is included and should not be reported separately. For revision of cervical total disc arthroplasty, additional interspaces, see 0098T. For revision of lumbar total disc arthroplasty, additional interspaces, see 0165T.

ICD-9-CM Procedural
- 84.66 Revision or replacement of artificial spinal disc prosthesis, cervical
- 84.68 Revision or replacement of artificial spinal disc prosthesis, lumbosacral
- 84.69 Revision or replacement of artificial spinal disc prosthesis, not otherwise specified

Anesthesia
00670

ICD-9-CM Diagnostic
- 170.2 Malignant neoplasm of vertebral column, excluding sacrum and coccyx
- 198.5 Secondary malignant neoplasm of bone and bone marrow
- 213.2 Benign neoplasm of vertebral column, excluding sacrum and coccyx
- 238.0 Neoplasm of uncertain behavior of bone and articular cartilage
- 336.9 Unspecified disease of spinal cord
- 721.0 Cervical spondylosis without myelopathy
- 721.1 Cervical spondylosis with myelopathy
- 721.3 Lumbosacral spondylosis without myelopathy
- 721.42 Spondylosis with myelopathy, lumbar region
- 721.8 Other allied disorders of spine
- 722.0 Displacement of cervical intervertebral disc without myelopathy
- 722.10 Displacement of lumbar intervertebral disc without myelopathy
- 722.4 Degeneration of cervical intervertebral disc
- 722.51 Degeneration of thoracic or thoracolumbar intervertebral disc
- 722.52 Degeneration of lumbar or lumbosacral intervertebral disc
- 722.71 Intervertebral cervical disc disorder with myelopathy, cervical region
- 722.73 Intervertebral lumbar disc disorder with myelopathy, lumbar region
- 722.81 Postlaminectomy syndrome, cervical region
- 722.83 Postlaminectomy syndrome, lumbar region
- 722.91 Other and unspecified disc disorder of cervical region
- 722.93 Other and unspecified disc disorder of lumbar region
- 723.0 Spinal stenosis in cervical region
- 723.8 Other syndromes affecting cervical region
- 724.02 Spinal stenosis of lumbar region, without neurogenic claudication
- 724.4 Thoracic or lumbosacral neuritis or radiculitis, unspecified
- 731.0 Osteitis deformans without mention of bone tumor
- 733.13 Pathologic fracture of vertebrae
- 733.82 Nonunion of fracture
- 738.5 Other acquired deformity of back or spine
- 756.11 Congenital spondylolysis, lumbosacral region
- 756.12 Congenital spondylolisthesis
- 756.19 Other congenital anomaly of spine

CCI Version 16.3
0213T, 0216T, 22505, 22800✦, 22845, 22851, 36000, 37202, 51701-51703, 64490, 64493, 69990, 76000-76001, 92585, 95822, 95860-95861, 95867-95868, 95870, 95900, 95904, 95920, 95925-95934, 95936-95937, 96360, 96365, 96372, 96374-96376, 99148-99149, 99150

Also not with 22861: 22220✦, 22554✦, 22600✦, 22802✦, 22808-22810✦, 22856✦, 22864, 29000, 29015, 29025, 29040, 36410, 62291, 62310, 62318-62319, 63075, 64415-64417, 64450

Also not with 22862: 0195T✦, 0228T, 0230T, 22224✦, 22558, 22612✦, 22630✦, 22808✦, 22857✦, 22865, 29020-29025, 29044-29046, 36400-36410, 36420-36430, 36440, 36600, 36640, 43752, 49000-49010, 62290, 62310-62319, 64400-64435, 64445-64450, 64479, 64483, 64505-64530, 72295, 93000-93010, 93040-93042, 93318, 94002, 94200, 94250, 94680-94690, 94770, 95812-95816, 95819, 95829, 95955

Note: These CCI edits are used for Medicare. Other payers may reimburse on codes listed above.

Medicare Edits

	Fac RVU	Non-Fac RVU	FUD	Assist
22861	59.51	59.51	90	80
22862	56.28	56.28	90	80

Medicare References: None

22864-22865

22864 Removal of total disc arthroplasty (artificial disc), anterior approach, single interspace; cervical
22865 lumbar

Artificial disc is removed

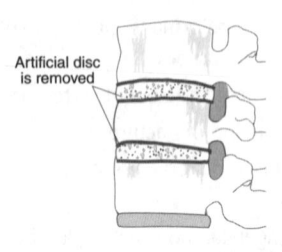

Removal of an artificial disc of the cervical interspace (22864) or the lumbar interspace (22865)

Explanation
The physician removes an artificial disc prosthesis placed during a previous disc arthroplasty by anterior approach. The physician approaches the cervical vertebrae in 22864 by making an incision through the neck, avoiding the esophagus, trachea, and thyroid. The lumbar vertebrae (22865) are approached by making an incision through the abdomen. Retractors separate the intervertebral muscles. The implant is located and any adhesions are freed. Distraction is applied to open the intervertebral space, and the implant is removed. The area is explored and debrided. When the procedure is complete, the fascia and vertebral muscles are repaired and returned to their anatomical positions, drains are placed, and the wound is closed. Each of these codes reports a single vertebral interspace and includes fluoroscopy when performed.

Coding Tips
Do not report 22864 with 22861. Do not report 22865 with 49010. Use of an operating microscope is included in 22864. Do not report 69990 separately. Fluoroscopy, when performed, is included and should not be reported separately. For removal of cervical total disc arthroplasty, additional interspaces, see 0095T. For removal of lumbar total disc arthroplasty, additional interspaces, see 0164T.

ICD-9-CM Procedural
- 84.66 Revision or replacement of artificial spinal disc prosthesis, cervical
- 84.68 Revision or replacement of artificial spinal disc prosthesis, lumbosacral
- 84.69 Revision or replacement of artificial spinal disc prosthesis, not otherwise specified

Anesthesia
00670

ICD-9-CM Diagnostic
- 170.2 Malignant neoplasm of vertebral column, excluding sacrum and coccyx
- 198.5 Secondary malignant neoplasm of bone and bone marrow
- 213.2 Benign neoplasm of vertebral column, excluding sacrum and coccyx
- 238.0 Neoplasm of uncertain behavior of bone and articular cartilage
- 336.9 Unspecified disease of spinal cord
- 721.0 Cervical spondylosis without myelopathy
- 721.1 Cervical spondylosis with myelopathy
- 721.3 Lumbosacral spondylosis without myelopathy
- 721.42 Spondylosis with myelopathy, lumbar region
- 721.8 Other allied disorders of spine
- 722.0 Displacement of cervical intervertebral disc without myelopathy
- 722.10 Displacement of lumbar intervertebral disc without myelopathy
- 722.4 Degeneration of cervical intervertebral disc
- 722.51 Degeneration of thoracic or thoracolumbar intervertebral disc
- 722.52 Degeneration of lumbar or lumbosacral intervertebral disc
- 722.71 Intervertebral cervical disc disorder with myelopathy, cervical region
- 722.73 Intervertebral lumbar disc disorder with myelopathy, lumbar region
- 722.81 Postlaminectomy syndrome, cervical region
- 722.83 Postlaminectomy syndrome, lumbar region
- 722.91 Other and unspecified disc disorder of cervical region
- 722.93 Other and unspecified disc disorder of lumbar region
- 723.0 Spinal stenosis in cervical region
- 723.8 Other syndromes affecting cervical region
- 724.02 Spinal stenosis of lumbar region, without neurogenic claudication
- 724.03 Spinal stenosis of lumbar region, with neurogenic claudication
- 724.4 Thoracic or lumbosacral neuritis or radiculitis, unspecified
- 731.0 Osteitis deformans without mention of bone tumor
- 733.13 Pathologic fracture of vertebrae
- 733.82 Nonunion of fracture
- 738.5 Other acquired deformity of back or spine
- 756.11 Congenital spondylolysis, lumbosacral region
- 756.12 Congenital spondylolisthesis
- 756.19 Other congenital anomaly of spine
- 805.00 Closed fracture of cervical vertebra, unspecified level without mention of spinal cord injury
- 805.01 Closed fracture of first cervical vertebra without mention of spinal cord injury

CCI Version 16.3
0213T, 0216T, 22505, 22851, 36000, 37202, 51701-51703, 64490, 64493, 69990, 76000-76001, 92585, 95822, 95860-95861, 95867-95868, 95870, 95900, 95904, 95920, 95925-95934, 95936-95937, 96360, 96365, 96372, 96374-96376, 99148-99149, 99150

Also not with 22864: 22220❖, 22554❖, 22600❖, 22800❖, 22808❖, 22845❖, 22856❖, 29000, 29015, 29025, 29040, 36410, 62291, 62310, 62318-62319, 63075, 64415-64417, 64450

Also not with 22865: 0195T❖, 0228T, 0230T, 22224❖, 22558❖, 22857❖, 29020-29025, 29044-29046, 36400-36410, 36420-36430, 36440, 36600, 36640, 43752, 49000-49010, 62290, 62310-62319, 64400-64435, 64445-64450, 64479, 64483, 64505-64530, 72295, 93000-93010, 93040-93042, 93318, 94002, 94200, 94250, 94680-94690, 94770, 95812-95816, 95819, 95829, 95955

Note: These CCI edits are used for Medicare. Other payers may reimburse on codes listed above.

Medicare Edits

	Fac RVU	Non-Fac RVU	FUD	Assist
22864	55.88	55.88	90	80
22865	59.74	59.74	90	80

Medicare References: None

23000

23000 Removal of subdeltoid calcareous deposits, open

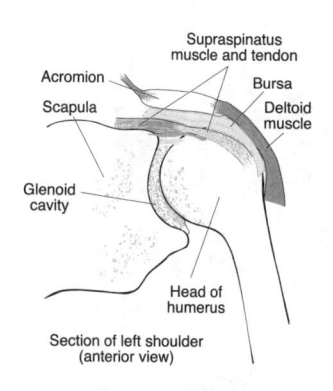

Section of left shoulder (anterior view)

Inflammatory cells from wear and tear cause calcareous (calcium) deposits to form in the supraspinatus tendon and deltoid muscle. The deposits are removed from sites under the tendon or from beneath the deltoid in the shoulder.

Explanation

The physician removes subdeltoid calcareous deposits by making a small incision over the deltoid muscle to expose the rotator cuff tendons. The raised area over the calcium deposits is incised in line with the axis of the fibers and the calcareous deposits are removed. A large cavity is made in the tendon with a curette to remove all damaged tissue. The opening is closed with side-to-side sutures. Once the tendon is repaired, the skin incision is closed and a soft dressing is applied.

Coding Tips

When the physician cannot complete the procedure through the arthroscope and an open procedure is performed, list the open procedure first, code the arthroscope as diagnostic, and append modifier 51. Medicare and some other third party payers do not allow a scope procedure when performed in conjunction with a related open procedure. Check with individual payers regarding their specific coding guidelines. For excisional biopsy of soft tissue of the shoulder, superficial, see 23065; deep, see 23066. For needle biopsy of muscle, see 20206.

ICD-9-CM Procedural

83.39 Excision of lesion of other soft tissue

Anesthesia

23000 01610

ICD-9-CM Diagnostic

- 712.11 Chondrocalcinosis due to dicalcium phosphate crystals, shoulder region — (Code first underlying disease: 275.4)
- 712.21 Chondrocalcinosis due to pyrophosphate crystals, shoulder region — (Code first underlying disease: 275.4)
- 712.31 Chondrocalcinosis, cause unspecified, involving shoulder region — (Code first underlying disease: 275.4)
- 712.81 Other specified crystal arthropathies, shoulder region
- 726.11 Calcifying tendinitis of shoulder
- 726.19 Other specified disorders of rotator cuff syndrome of shoulder and allied disorders
- 726.2 Other affections of shoulder region, not elsewhere classified
- 727.82 Calcium deposits in tendon and bursa
- 727.89 Other disorders of synovium, tendon, and bursa
- 728.11 Progressive myositis ossificans
- 728.12 Traumatic myositis ossificans
- 728.13 Postoperative heterotopic calcification
- 728.19 Other muscular calcification and ossification

Terms To Know

bursa. Cavity or sac containing fluid that occurs between articulating surfaces and serves to reduce friction from moving parts. An anatomical structure frequently referenced in orthopedic notes as it may become diseased or need removal.

calcifying tendinitis. Inflammation and hardening of tissue due to calcium salt deposits, occurring in the tendons and areas of tendonomuscular attachment.

myositis ossificans. Inflammatory disease of muscles due to bony deposits or conversion of muscle tissue to bony tissue.

ossification. Formation of bony growth or hardening into bone-like substance.

tendon. Fibrous tissue that connects muscle to bone, consisting primarily of collagen and containing little vasculature.

CCI Version 16.3

01610, 0213T, 0216T, 0228T, 0230T, 11010-11012❖, 23075, 24332, 36000, 36400-36410, 36420-36430, 36440, 36600, 36640, 37202, 43752, 51701-51703, 62310-62319, 64400-64435, 64445-64450, 64479, 64483, 64490, 64493, 64505-64530, 69990, 93000-93010, 93040-93042, 93318, 94002, 94200, 94250, 94680-94690, 94770, 95812-95816, 95819, 95822, 95829, 95955, 96360, 96365, 96372, 96374-96376, 99148-99149, 99150, J0670, J2001

Note: These CCI edits are used for Medicare. Other payers may reimburse on codes listed above.

Medicare Edits

	Fac RVU	Non-Fac RVU	FUD	Assist
23000	10.59	16.01	90	80

Medicare References: 100-2,15,260; 100-4,12,30; 100-4,12,90.3; 100-4,14,10

23020

23020 Capsular contracture release (eg, Sever type procedure)

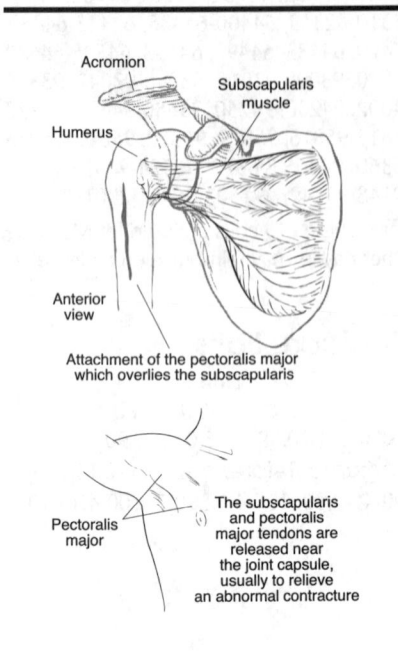

Anterior view: Acromion, Subscapularis muscle, Humerus, Attachment of the pectoralis major which overlies the subscapularis

Pectoralis major — The subscapularis and pectoralis major tendons are released near the joint capsule, usually to relieve an abnormal contracture

Explanation

Capsular contracture release is not commonly performed unless the shoulder is fixed in marked internal rotation and adduction. In this position, the arm is unable to move away from the body. The physician makes an incision at the front of the shoulder where the deltoid meets the pectoral muscle. The subscapularis tendon is removed from the glenoid rim. The anterior capsule is left intact. The pectoralis major tendon is severed from its attachment on the humerus. The skin incision is closed and a soft dressing is applied. The arm is positioned in abduction (arm elevated out to the side of the body).

Coding Tips

When 23020 is performed with another separately identifiable procedure, the highest dollar value code is listed as the primary procedure and subsequent procedures are appended with modifier 51. If significant additional time and effort is documented, append modifier 22 and submit a cover letter and operative report.

ICD-9-CM Procedural

80.41 Division of joint capsule, ligament, or cartilage of shoulder
83.19 Other division of soft tissue

Anesthesia

23020 01610

ICD-9-CM Diagnostic

718.41 Contracture of shoulder joint

Terms To Know

abduction. Pulling away from a central reference line, such as moving away from the midline of the body.

adduction. Pulling toward a central reference line, such as toward the midline of the body.

anterior. Situated in the front area or toward the belly surface of the body; an anatomical reference point used to show the position and relationship of one body structure to another.

contracture. Shortening of muscle or connective tissue.

soft tissue. Nonepithelial tissues outside of the skeleton that includes subcutaneous adipose tissue, fibrous tissue, fascia, muscles, blood and lymph vessels, and peripheral nervous system tissue.

tendon. Fibrous tissue that connects muscle to bone, consisting primarily of collagen and containing little vasculature.

CCI Version 16.3

01610, 0213T, 0216T, 0228T, 0230T, 23405, 23700, 36000, 36400-36410, 36420-36430, 36440, 36600, 36640, 37202, 43752, 51701-51703, 62310-62319, 64400-64435, 64445-64450, 64479, 64483, 64490, 64493, 64505-64530, 69990, 93000-93010, 93040-93042, 93318, 94002, 94200, 94250, 94680-94690, 94770, 95812-95816, 95819, 95822, 95829, 95955, 96360, 96365, 96372, 96374-96376, 99148-99149, 99150

Note: These CCI edits are used for Medicare. Other payers may reimburse on codes listed above.

Medicare Edits

	Fac RVU	Non-Fac RVU	FUD	Assist
23020	20.02	20.02	90	80

Medicare References: 100-2,15,260; 100-4,12,30; 100-4,12,90.3; 100-4,14,10

23030-23031

23030 Incision and drainage, shoulder area; deep abscess or hematoma
23031 infected bursa

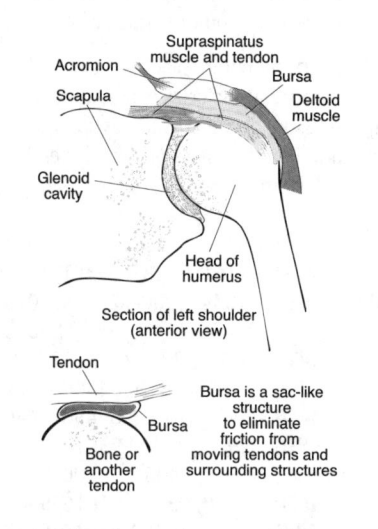

Explanation
The physician drains a deep abscess or hematoma in 23030 or an infected bursa in 23031 from the shoulder area. The physician makes an incision in the shoulder overlying the site of the abscess, hematoma, or bursa to be incised. Dissection is carried down through the deep subcutaneous tissues and may be continued into the fascia or muscle to expose the abscess or hematoma. The incision may be extended if the mass is larger than expected. When the infected bursa, abscess, or hematoma is identified, it is incised and the contents are drained. The area is irrigated and the incision is repaired in layers with sutures, staples, and/or Steri-strips; closed with drains in place; or simply left open to further facilitate drainage of infection.

Coding Tips
If significant additional time and effort is documented, append modifier 22 and submit a cover letter and operative report. For incision and drainage in the shoulder area, superficial, see 10060–10061.

ICD-9-CM Procedural
83.02   Myotomy

Anesthesia
01610

ICD-9-CM Diagnostic
682.3   Cellulitis and abscess of upper arm and forearm — (Use additional code to identify organism, such as 041.1, etc.)
711.41 Arthropathy associated with other bacterial diseases, shoulder region — (Code first underlying disease, such as diseases classifiable to 010-040 (except 036.82), 090-099 (except 098.50))
719.11 Hemarthrosis, shoulder region
726.10 Unspecified disorders of bursae and tendons in shoulder region
727.3   Other bursitis disorders
727.89 Other disorders of synovium, tendon, and bursa
729.92 Nontraumatic hematoma of soft tissue
730.11 Chronic osteomyelitis, shoulder region — (Use additional code to identify organism: 041.1. Use additional code to identify major osseous defect, if applicable: 731.3)
730.21 Unspecified osteomyelitis, shoulder region — (Use additional code to identify organism: 041.1. Use additional code to identify major osseous defect, if applicable: 731.3)
730.31 Periostitis, without mention of osteomyelitis, shoulder region — (Use additional code to identify organism: 041.1)
731.3   Major osseous defects — (Code first underlying disease: 170.0-170.9, 730.00-730.29, 733.00-733.09, 733.40-733.49, 996.45)
780.62 Postprocedural fever
923.00 Contusion of shoulder region
998.12 Hematoma complicating a procedure
998.51 Infected postoperative seroma — (Use additional code to identify organism)
998.59 Other postoperative infection — (Use additional code to identify infection)

Terms To Know

abscess. Circumscribed collection of pus resulting from bacteria, frequently associated with swelling and other signs of inflammation.

bursa. Cavity or sac containing fluid that occurs between articulating surfaces and serves to reduce friction from moving parts. An anatomical structure frequently referenced in orthopedic notes as it may become diseased or need removal.

contusion. Superficial injury (bruising) produced by impact without a break in the skin.

hemarthrosis. Occurrence of blood within a joint space.

hematoma. Tumor-like collection of blood in some part of the body caused by a break in a blood vessel wall, usually as a result of trauma.

infected postoperative seroma. Infection within a tumor-like growth of serum following surgery.

osteomyelitis. Inflammation of bone that may remain localized or spread to the marrow, cortex, or periosteum, in response to an infecting organism, usually bacterial and pyogenic.

periostitis. Inflammation of the outer layers of bone.

soft tissue. Nonepithelial tissues outside of the skeleton that includes subcutaneous adipose tissue, fibrous tissue, fascia, muscles, blood and lymph vessels, and peripheral nervous system tissue.

CCI Version 16.3
01610, 0213T, 0216T, 0228T, 0230T, 10060, 10140, 10160, 11043, 20103, 23035❖, 36000, 36400-36410, 36420-36430, 36440, 36600, 36640, 37202, 43752, 51701-51703, 62310-62319, 64400-64435, 64445-64450, 64479, 64483, 64490, 64493, 64505-64530, 69990, 93000-93010, 93040-93042, 93318, 94002, 94200, 94250, 94680-94690, 94770, 95812-95816, 95819, 95822, 95829, 95955, 96360, 96365, 96372, 96374-96376, 97597-97598, 97602-97606, 99148-99149, 99150, J0670, J2001

Also not with 23031: 11010-11012❖, 23030❖

Note: These CCI edits are used for Medicare. Other payers may reimburse on codes listed above.

Medicare Edits

	Fac RVU	Non-Fac RVU	FUD	Assist
23030	7.46	12.45	10	N/A
23031	6.25	11.59	10	N/A

Medicare References: 100-2,15,260; 100-4,12,30; 100-4,12,90.3; 100-4,14,10

23035

23035 Incision, bone cortex (eg, osteomyelitis or bone abscess), shoulder area

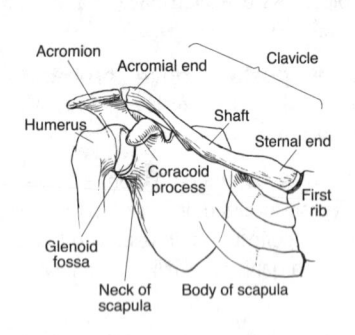

A bone in the shoulder area is incised to the cortex and an abscess or dead tissue is removed

Explanation

The physician incises bone cortex in the shoulder area to treat a bone abscess or osteomyelitis. The physician makes an incision over the affected area of the shoulder. Dissection is carried down through the soft tissues to expose the bone. The periosteum is split and reflected from the bone overlying the infected area. A curette may be used to scrape away the abscess or infected portion down to healthy bony tissue or drill holes may be made through the cortex into the medullary canal in a window outline around the infected or abscessed bone. The area is drained and debrided of infected bony and soft tissue. The physician irrigates the area with antibiotic solution, the periosteum is closed over the bone, and the soft tissues are sutured closed; or the wound is packed and left open, allowing the area to drain. Secondary closure is performed approximately three weeks later. Dressings are changed daily. A splint may be applied to limit shoulder movement.

Coding Tips

If significant additional time and effort is documented, append modifier 22 and submit a cover letter and operative report. For incision and drainage of a deep abscess or hematoma in the shoulder area, see 23030; of infected bursa, see 23031.

ICD-9-CM Procedural

- 77.11 Other incision of scapula, clavicle, and thorax (ribs and sternum) without division
- 77.12 Other incision of humerus without division

Anesthesia

23035 01630

ICD-9-CM Diagnostic

- 682.3 Cellulitis and abscess of upper arm and forearm — (Use additional code to identify organism, such as 041.1, etc.)
- 730.11 Chronic osteomyelitis, shoulder region — (Use additional code to identify organism: 041.1. Use additional code to identify major osseous defect, if applicable: 731.3)
- 730.21 Unspecified osteomyelitis, shoulder region — (Use additional code to identify organism: 041.1. Use additional code to identify major osseous defect, if applicable: 731.3)
- 730.81 Other infections involving bone diseases classified elsewhere, shoulder region — (Use additional code to identify organism: 041.1. Code first underlying disease: 002.0, 015.0-015.9)
- 731.3 Major osseous defects — (Code first underlying disease: 170.0-170.9, 730.00-730.29, 733.00-733.09, 733.40-733.49, 996.45)
- 998.51 Infected postoperative seroma — (Use additional code to identify organism)
- 998.59 Other postoperative infection — (Use additional code to identify infection)

Terms To Know

abscess. Circumscribed collection of pus resulting from bacteria, frequently associated with swelling and other signs of inflammation.

cellulitis. Sudden, severe, suppurative inflammation and edema in subcutaneous tissue or muscle, most often caused by bacterial infection secondary to a cutaneous lesion.

chronic. Persistent, continuing, or recurring.

infected postoperative seroma. Infection within a tumor-like growth of serum following surgery.

infection. Presence of microorganisms in body tissues that may result in cellular damage.

osteomyelitis. Inflammation of bone that may remain localized or spread to the marrow, cortex, or periosteum, in response to an infecting organism, usually bacterial and pyogenic.

periosteum. Double-layered connective membrane on the outer surface of bone.

soft tissue. Nonepithelial tissues outside of the skeleton that includes subcutaneous adipose tissue, fibrous tissue, fascia, muscles, blood and lymph vessels, and peripheral nervous system tissue.

CCI Version 16.3

01610, 0213T, 0216T, 0228T, 0230T, 10060, 10140, 10160, 11044, 20000-20005, 20103, 20615, 36000, 36400-36410, 36420-36430, 36440, 36600, 36640, 37202, 43752, 51701-51703, 62310-62319, 64400-64435, 64445-64450, 64479, 64483, 64490, 64493, 64505-64530, 69990, 93000-93010, 93040-93042, 93318, 94002, 94200, 94250, 94680-94690, 94770, 95812-95816, 95819, 95822, 95829, 95955, 96360, 96365, 96372, 96374-96376, 97597-97598, 97602-97606, 99148-99149, 99150

Note: These CCI edits are used for Medicare. Other payers may reimburse on codes listed above.

Medicare Edits

	Fac RVU	Non-Fac RVU	FUD	Assist
23035	19.87	19.87	90	80

Medicare References: 100-2,15,260; 100-4,12,30; 100-4,12,90.3; 100-4,14,10

23040-23044

23040 Arthrotomy, glenohumeral joint, including exploration, drainage, or removal of foreign body

23044 Arthrotomy, acromioclavicular, sternoclavicular joint, including exploration, drainage, or removal of foreign body

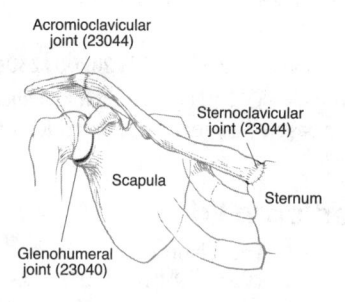

Acromioclavicular joint (23044)
Sternoclavicular joint (23044)
Scapula
Sternum
Glenohumeral joint (23040)

Report 23044 for the acromioclavicular or sternoclavicular joints

A joint of the shoulder area is surgically opened and explored, drained, and debris or foreign bodies removed as needed. Report 23040 for the glenohumeral joint

Explanation
The physician performs an arthrotomy of the glenohumeral joint in 23040 or the acromioclavicular or sternoclavicular joint in 23044 that includes exploration, drainage, or removal of any foreign body. An incision is made over the joint to be exposed. The soft tissues are dissected away and the joint capsule is exposed and incised. The joint space is explored, any necrotic tissue is removed, and infection or abnormal fluid is drained. If a foreign body is present (e.g., bullet, nail, gravel), it is exposed and removed. The wound is irrigated with antibiotic solution. The physician may leave the wound packed open with daily dressing changes to allow for further drainage and secondary healing by granulation. If the incision is repaired, drain tubes may be inserted and the incision is repaired in layers with sutures, staples, and/or Steri-strips. A splint may be applied to limit shoulder motion.

Coding Tips
If significant additional time and effort is documented, append modifier 22 and submit a cover letter and operative report. For simple removal of a superficial foreign body of the subcutaneous tissue of the shoulder area, see 10120; complicated superficial foreign body, see 10121.

ICD-9-CM Procedural
- 80.11 Other arthrotomy of shoulder
- 80.19 Other arthrotomy of other specified site

Anesthesia
01630

ICD-9-CM Diagnostic
- 711.01 Pyogenic arthritis, shoulder region — (Use additional code to identify infectious organism: 041.0-041.8)
- 711.81 Arthropathy associated with other infectious and parasitic diseases, shoulder region — (Code first underlying disease: 080-088, 100-104, 130-136)
- 711.91 Unspecified infective arthritis, shoulder region
- 715.00 Generalized osteoarthrosis, unspecified site
- 715.09 Generalized osteoarthrosis, involving multiple sites
- 715.11 Primary localized osteoarthrosis, shoulder region
- 716.11 Traumatic arthropathy, shoulder region
- 718.01 Articular cartilage disorder, shoulder region
- 718.11 Loose body in shoulder joint
- 718.21 Pathological dislocation of shoulder joint
- 718.41 Contracture of shoulder joint
- 718.51 Ankylosis of joint of shoulder region
- 718.71 Developmental dislocation of joint, shoulder region
- 719.01 Effusion of shoulder joint
- 719.11 Hemarthrosis, shoulder region
- 719.41 Pain in joint, shoulder region
- 719.81 Other specified disorders of shoulder joint
- 729.6 Residual foreign body in soft tissue — (Use additional code to identify foreign body (V90.01-V90.9))
- 998.51 Infected postoperative seroma — (Use additional code to identify organism)
- 998.59 Other postoperative infection — (Use additional code to identify infection)

Terms To Know
ankylosis. Abnormal union or fusion of bones in a joint, which is normally moveable.

contracture. Shortening of muscle or connective tissue.

effusion. Escape of fluid from within a body cavity.

hemarthrosis. Occurrence of blood within a joint space.

infected postoperative seroma. Infection within a tumor-like growth of serum following surgery.

CCI Version 16.3
01610, 0213T, 0216T, 0228T, 0230T, 10060, 10140, 10160, 11040-11043, 20103, 23030-23035, 29819, 29822-29823, 29825, 36000, 36400-36410, 36420-36430, 36440, 36600, 36640, 37202, 43752, 51701-51703, 62310-62319, 64400-64435, 64445-64450, 64479, 64483, 64490, 64493, 64505-64530, 69990, 93000-93010, 93040-93042, 93318, 94002, 94200, 94250, 94680-94690, 94770, 95812-95816, 95819, 95822, 95829, 95955, 96360, 96365, 96372, 96374-96376, 99148-99149, 99150

Also not with 23040: 23100, 23105, 23107, 23700, 24332

Also not with 23044: 11012❖, 21750, 23101, 23106

Note: These CCI edits are used for Medicare. Other payers may reimburse on codes listed above.

Medicare Edits

	Fac RVU	Non-Fac RVU	FUD	Assist
23040	20.94	20.94	90	80
23044	16.6	16.6	90	N/A

Medicare References: 100-2,15,260; 100-4,12,30; 100-4,12,90.3; 100-4,14,10

23065-23066

23065 Biopsy, soft tissue of shoulder area; superficial
23066 deep

Soft tissues of the shoulder area, such as muscle and fascia, are biopsied. Report 23065 for superficial biopsy and 23066 when deep tissues are accessed

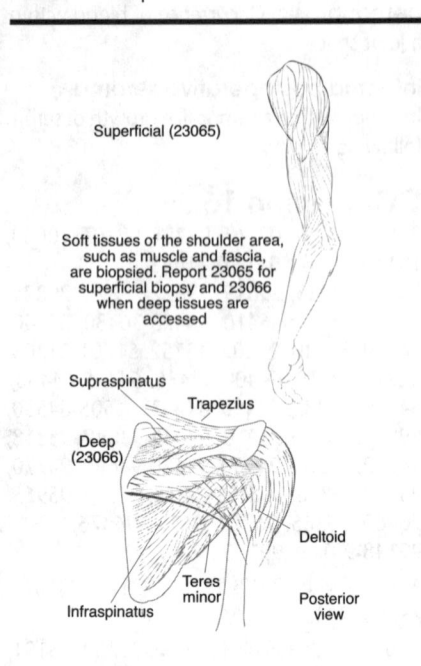

Explanation

The physician performs a biopsy of the soft tissues of the shoulder area. With proper anesthesia administered, an incision is made over the biopsy area. Dissection is carried down within the superficial soft tissue layers in 23065, usually the subcutaneous fat to the uppermost fascial layer. In 23066, dissection is taken down deep within the soft tissue, such as into the fascial layer or within the muscle. A portion of the tissue is excised and submitted for pathology. The area is irrigated and the incision is closed with layered sutures, staples, or Steri-strips.

Coding Tips

If multiple areas are biopsied, report 23065 or 23066 for each site taken and append modifier 51 to additional codes. An excisional biopsy is not reported separately when a therapeutic excision is performed during the same surgical session. For needle biopsy of muscle, see 20206. Surgical trays, A4550, are not separately reimbursed by Medicare; however, other third-party payers may cover them. Check with the specific payer to determine coverage.

ICD-9-CM Procedural

83.21 Open biopsy of soft tissue

Anesthesia

23065 00300, 00400
23066 01610

ICD-9-CM Diagnostic

171.2	Malignant neoplasm of connective and other soft tissue of upper limb, including shoulder
195.4	Malignant neoplasm of upper limb
198.89	Secondary malignant neoplasm of other specified sites
214.1	Lipoma of other skin and subcutaneous tissue
215.2	Other benign neoplasm of connective and other soft tissue of upper limb, including shoulder
238.1	Neoplasm of uncertain behavior of connective and other soft tissue
239.2	Neoplasms of unspecified nature of bone, soft tissue, and skin
728.82	Foreign body granuloma of muscle — (Use additional code to identify foreign body (V90.01-V90.9))
782.2	Localized superficial swelling, mass, or lump

Terms To Know

benign. Mild or nonmalignant in nature.

foreign body. Any object or substance found in an organ and tissue that does not belong under normal circumstances.

granuloma. Abnormal, dense collections or cells forming a mass or nodule of chronically inflamed tissue with granulations that is usually associated with an infective process.

lipoma. Benign tumor containing fat cells and the most common of soft tissue lesions, which are usually painless and asymptomatic, with the exception of an angiolipoma.

malignant. Any condition tending to progress toward death, specifically an invasive tumor with a loss of cellular differentiation that has the ability to spread or metastasize to other areas in the body.

neoplasm. New abnormal growth, tumor.

secondary. Second in order of occurrence or importance, or appearing during the course of another disease or condition.

soft tissue. Nonepithelial tissues outside of the skeleton that includes subcutaneous adipose tissue, fibrous tissue, fascia, muscles, blood and lymph vessels, and peripheral nervous system tissue.

subcutaneous tissue. Sheet or wide band of adipose (fat) and areolar connective tissue in two layers attached to the dermis.

superficial. On the skin surface or near the surface of any involved structure or field of interest.

CCI Version 16.3

01610, 0213T, 0216T, 0228T, 0230T, 10021-10022, 10060, 10140, 10160, 11010-11012❖, 20103, 29805, 36000, 36400-36410, 36420-36430, 36440, 36600, 36640, 37202, 43752, 51701-51703, 62310-62319, 64400-64435, 64445-64450, 64479, 64483, 64490, 64493, 64505-64530, 69990, 93000-93010, 93040-93042, 93318, 94002, 94200, 94250, 94680-94690, 94770, 95812-95816, 95819, 95822, 95829, 95955, 96360, 96365, 96372, 96374-96376, 99148-99149, 99150, J0670, J2001

Also not with 23065: 11900-11901, 13121, 38500

Also not with 23066: 12031, 20200, 23065

Note: These CCI edits are used for Medicare. Other payers may reimburse on codes listed above.

Medicare Edits

	Fac RVU	Non-Fac RVU	FUD	Assist
23065	4.92	6.27	10	N/A
23066	10.01	15.12	90	N/A

Medicare References: 100-2,15,260; 100-4,12,30; 100-4,12,90.3; 100-4,14,10

23075-23076 (23071, 23073)

23075 Excision, tumor, soft tissue of shoulder area, subcutaneous; less than 3 cm
23071 3 cm or greater
23076 Excision, tumor, soft tissue of shoulder area, subfascial (eg, intramuscular); less than 5 cm
23073 5 cm or greater

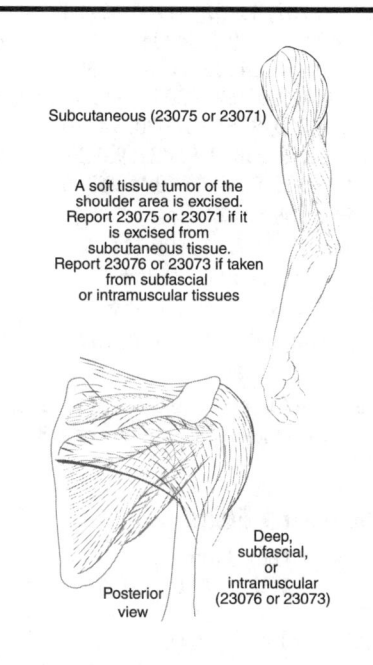

A soft tissue tumor of the shoulder area is excised. Report 23075 or 23071 if it is excised from subcutaneous tissue. Report 23076 or 23073 if taken from subfascial or intramuscular tissues

Subcutaneous (23075 or 23071)

Deep, subfascial, or intramuscular (23076 or 23073)

Posterior view

Explanation

The physician removes a tumor from the soft tissue of the shoulder area that is located in the subcutaneous tissue in 23071 and 23075 and in the deep soft tissue, below the fascial plane or within the muscle, in 23073 and 23076. With the proper anesthesia administered, the physician makes an incision in the skin overlying the mass and dissects down to the tumor. The extent of the tumor is identified and a dissection is undertaken all the way around the tumor. A portion of neighboring soft tissue may also be removed to ensure adequate removal of all tumor tissue. A drain may be inserted and the incision is repaired with layers of sutures, staples, or Steri-strips. Report 23075 for excision of subcutaneous tumors less than 3 cm and 23071 for excision of subcutaneous tumors 3 cm or greater. Report 23076 for excision of subfascial or intramuscular tumors less than 5 cm and 23073 for excision of subfascial or intramuscular tumors 5 cm or greater.

Coding Tips

Codes 23071 and 23073 are resequenced codes and will not display in numeric order. When these codes are performed with another separately identifiable procedure, the highest dollar value code is listed as the primary procedure and subsequent procedures are appended with modifier 51. For radical resection of a tumor of the soft tissue of the shoulder area, see 23077. When medically necessary, report moderate (conscious) sedation provided by the performing physician with 99143–99145. When provided by another physician, report 99148–99150.

ICD-9-CM Procedural

83.32	Excision of lesion of muscle
83.39	Excision of lesion of other soft tissue
83.49	Other excision of soft tissue
86.3	Other local excision or destruction of lesion or tissue of skin and subcutaneous tissue
86.4	Radical excision of skin lesion

Anesthesia

23071	00300, 00400
23073	01610
23075	00300, 00400
23076	01610

ICD-9-CM Diagnostic

171.2	Malignant neoplasm of connective and other soft tissue of upper limb, including shoulder
172.6	Malignant melanoma of skin of upper limb, including shoulder
173.6	Other malignant neoplasm of skin of upper limb, including shoulder
195.4	Malignant neoplasm of upper limb
198.89	Secondary malignant neoplasm of other specified sites
209.33	Merkel cell carcinoma of the upper limb
209.35	Merkel cell carcinoma of the trunk
209.75	Secondary Merkel cell carcinoma
214.1	Lipoma of other skin and subcutaneous tissue
215.2	Other benign neoplasm of connective and other soft tissue of upper limb, including shoulder
228.01	Hemangioma of skin and subcutaneous tissue
238.1	Neoplasm of uncertain behavior of connective and other soft tissue
239.2	Neoplasms of unspecified nature of bone, soft tissue, and skin
728.82	Foreign body granuloma of muscle — (Use additional code to identify foreign body (V90.01-V90.9))
782.2	Localized superficial swelling, mass, or lump

Terms To Know

benign. Mild or nonmalignant in nature.

lipoma. Benign tumor containing fat cells and the most common of soft tissue lesions, which are usually painless and asymptomatic, with the exception of an angiolipoma.

malignant. Any condition tending to progress toward death, specifically an invasive tumor with a loss of cellular differentiation that has the ability to spread or metastasize to other areas in the body.

subcutaneous tissue. Sheet or wide band of adipose (fat) and areolar connective tissue in two layers attached to the dermis.

subfascial. Beneath the band of fibrous tissue that lies deep to the skin, encloses muscles, and separates their layers.

CCI Version 16.3

01610, 0228T, 0230T, 10060, 10140, 10160, 11010-11012❖, 11040-11044, 12001-12007, 12020-12037, 13100-13101, 13120-13121, 23030-23031, 24300, 36000, 36400-36410, 36420-36430, 36440, 36600, 36640, 37202, 38525❖, 38550-38555❖, 38740-38745❖, 43752, 51701-51703, 62310-62319, 64400-64435, 64445-64450, 64479, 64483, 64505-64530, 69990, 93000-93010, 93040-93042, 93318, 94002, 94200, 94250, 94680-94690, 94770, 95812-95816, 95819, 95822, 95829, 95955, 96360, 96365, 96372, 96374-96376, 99148-99149, 99150

Also not with 23071: 0213T, 0216T, 13132, 23000, 23065-23066, 23075, 38500-38505, 64490, 64493, J2001

Also not with 23073: 0213T, 0216T, 23000, 23065-23071, 23075-23076, 38505, 64490, 64493, 64718

Also not with 23075: 13132, 23065-23066, 38500-38505, J0670, J2001

Also not with 23076: 11400, 11406, 11600-11606, 23000, 23065-23071, 23075, 38505, 64718

Note: These CCI edits are used for Medicare. Other payers may reimburse on codes listed above.

Medicare Edits

	Fac RVU	Non-Fac RVU	FUD	Assist
23071	12.48	12.48	90	80
23073	20.68	20.68	90	80
23075	8.44	11.6	90	N/A
23076	15.77	15.77	90	N/A

Medicare References: 100-2,15,260; 100-4,12,30; 100-4,12,90.3; 100-4,14,10

23077-23078

23077 Radical resection of tumor (eg, malignant neoplasm), soft tissue of shoulder area; less than 5 cm
23078 5 cm or greater

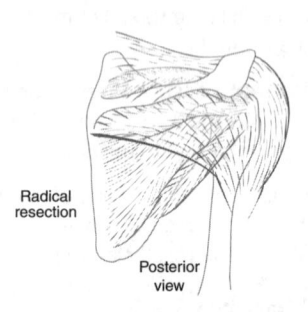

Radical resection of soft tissue tumor of the shoulder area is reported with 23077 if less than 5 cm and with 23078 if 5 cm or greater

Explanation

The physician performs a radical resection of a malignant soft tissue tumor from the shoulder area, not involving bone. An incision is made over the tumor and dissection exposes it. The tumor and any adjacent tissue that may be affected by the spread of the neoplasm are excised. Large resections may be needed. The type and stage of the lesion determines the extent of the tumor margin resection area. Muscle or fascia may need to be repaired and drains may be placed. The surgical wound is repaired by intermediate or complex closure, adjacent tissue transfer, or graft. Report 23077 for excision of tumors less than 5 cm and 23078 for excision of tumors 5 cm or greater.

Coding Tips

Report any grafts or flaps separately. If significant additional time and effort is documented, append modifier 22 and submit a cover letter and operative report. For excision of a subcutaneous soft tissue tumor of the shoulder area, see 23075. For excision of a deep, a subfascial, or an intramuscular tumor of the shoulder area, see 23076.

ICD-9-CM Procedural

83.32	Excision of lesion of muscle
83.39	Excision of lesion of other soft tissue
83.49	Other excision of soft tissue
86.3	Other local excision or destruction of lesion or tissue of skin and subcutaneous tissue
86.4	Radical excision of skin lesion

Anesthesia

01610

ICD-9-CM Diagnostic

171.2	Malignant neoplasm of connective and other soft tissue of upper limb, including shoulder
172.6	Malignant melanoma of skin of upper limb, including shoulder
173.6	Other malignant neoplasm of skin of upper limb, including shoulder
195.4	Malignant neoplasm of upper limb
198.89	Secondary malignant neoplasm of other specified sites
209.33	Merkel cell carcinoma of the upper limb
209.35	Merkel cell carcinoma of the trunk
209.75	Secondary Merkel cell carcinoma
214.1	Lipoma of other skin and subcutaneous tissue
215.2	Other benign neoplasm of connective and other soft tissue of upper limb, including shoulder
228.01	Hemangioma of skin and subcutaneous tissue
238.1	Neoplasm of uncertain behavior of connective and other soft tissue
239.2	Neoplasms of unspecified nature of bone, soft tissue, and skin
728.82	Foreign body granuloma of muscle — (Use additional code to identify foreign body (V90.01-V90.9))
782.2	Localized superficial swelling, mass, or lump

Terms To Know

lesion. Area of damaged tissue that has lost continuity or function, due to disease or trauma. Lesions may be located on internal structures such as the brain, nerves, or kidneys, or visible on the skin.

malignant. Any condition tending to progress toward death, specifically an invasive tumor with a loss of cellular differentiation that has the ability to spread or metastasize to other areas in the body.

secondary. Second in order of occurrence or importance, or appearing during the course of another disease or condition.

soft tissue. Nonepithelial tissues outside of the skeleton that includes subcutaneous adipose tissue, fibrous tissue, fascia, muscles, blood and lymph vessels, and peripheral nervous system tissue.

CCI Version 16.3

01610, 0228T, 0230T, 10060, 10140, 10160, 11010-11012❖, 11040-11044, 12001-12007, 12020-12037, 13100-13101, 13120-13121, 23000, 23030-23031, 24300, 36000, 36400-36410, 36420-36430, 36440, 36600, 36640, 37202, 43752, 51701-51703, 62310-62319, 64400-64435, 64445-64450, 64479, 64483, 64505-64530, 69990, 93000-93010, 93040-93042, 93318, 94002, 94200, 94250, 94680-94690, 94770, 95812-95816, 95819, 95822, 95829, 95955, 96360, 96365, 96372, 96374-96376, 99148-99149, 99150

Also not with 23077: 11600-11606, 23065-23076, 38505, 38525❖, 38550-38555❖, 38740-38745❖

Also not with 23078: 0213T, 0216T, 23065-23077, 64490, 64493

Note: These CCI edits are used for Medicare. Other payers may reimburse on codes listed above.

Medicare Edits

	Fac RVU	Non-Fac RVU	FUD	Assist
23077	33.96	33.96	90	80
23078	41.46	41.46	90	80

Medicare References: 100-2,15,260; 100-4,12,30; 100-4,12,90.3; 100-4,14,10

23100

23100 Arthrotomy, glenohumeral joint, including biopsy

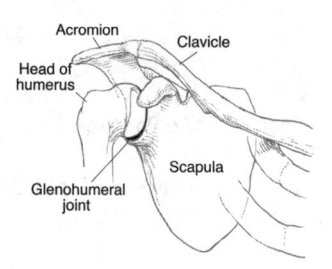

The glenohumeral joint is the shoulder joint and is located between the head of the humerus and the concave neck of the scapula

The glenohumeral joint is surgically accessed and a biopsy is performed

Explanation
The physician performs an arthrotomy and biopsy of the glenohumeral joint. An incision is made over the shoulder joint and carried down through the soft tissues to gain access into the glenohumeral joint. A biopsy sample of the joint tissue is removed and saved for testing. The wound is repaired in layered sutures.

Coding Tips
If a biopsy is performed in addition to the arthrotomy, it should not be reported separately; it is included in the description of the code. For arthrotomy, glenohumeral joint, with synovectomy, with or without biopsy, see 23105. For arthrotomy, glenohumeral joint, with joint exploration, with or without removal of loose or foreign body, see 23107.

ICD-9-CM Procedural
- 80.11 Other arthrotomy of shoulder
- 80.31 Biopsy of joint structure of shoulder

Anesthesia
23100 01630

ICD-9-CM Diagnostic
- 170.4 Malignant neoplasm of scapula and long bones of upper limb
- 171.2 Malignant neoplasm of connective and other soft tissue of upper limb, including shoulder
- 198.5 Secondary malignant neoplasm of bone and bone marrow
- 198.89 Secondary malignant neoplasm of other specified sites
- 213.4 Benign neoplasm of scapula and long bones of upper limb
- 215.2 Other benign neoplasm of connective and other soft tissue of upper limb, including shoulder
- 238.0 Neoplasm of uncertain behavior of bone and articular cartilage
- 238.1 Neoplasm of uncertain behavior of connective and other soft tissue
- 239.2 Neoplasms of unspecified nature of bone, soft tissue, and skin
- 275.40 Unspecified disorder of calcium metabolism — (Use additional code to identify any associated mental retardation)
- 275.42 Hypercalcemia — (Use additional code to identify any associated mental retardation)
- 275.49 Other disorders of calcium metabolism — (Use additional code to identify any associated mental retardation)
- 275.5 Hungry bone syndrome
- 357.1 Polyneuropathy in collagen vascular disease — (Code first underlying disease: 446.0, 710.0, 714.0)
- 359.6 Symptomatic inflammatory myopathy in diseases classified elsewhere — (Code first underlying disease: 135, 140.0-208.9, 277.30-277.39, 446.0, 710.0, 710.1, 710.2, 714.0)
- 446.0 Polyarteritis nodosa
- 710.0 Systemic lupus erythematosus — (Use additional code to identify manifestation: 424.91, 581.81, 582.81, 583.81)
- 714.0 Rheumatoid arthritis — (Use additional code to identify manifestation: 357.1, 359.6)
- 998.51 Infected postoperative seroma — (Use additional code to identify organism)
- 998.59 Other postoperative infection — (Use additional code to identify infection)
- V64.43 Arthroscopic surgical procedure converted to open procedure

Terms To Know
infected postoperative seroma. Infection within a tumor-like growth of serum following surgery.

malignant. Any condition tending to progress toward death, specifically an invasive tumor with a loss of cellular differentiation that has the ability to spread or metastasize to other areas in the body.

CCI Version 16.3
01610, 0213T, 0216T, 0228T, 0230T, 10060, 10140, 10160, 11012❖, 23700, 24332, 29805, 29822-29823, 29825, 36000, 36400-36410, 36420-36430, 36440, 36600, 36640, 37202, 43752, 51701-51703, 62310-62319, 64400-64435, 64445-64450, 64479, 64483, 64490, 64493, 64505-64530, 69990, 93000-93010, 93040-93042, 93318, 94002, 94200, 94250, 94680-94690, 94770, 95812-95816, 95819, 95822, 95829, 95955, 96360, 96365, 96372, 96374-96376, 99148-99149, 99150

Note: These CCI edits are used for Medicare. Other payers may reimburse on codes listed above.

Medicare Edits

	Fac RVU	Non-Fac RVU	FUD	Assist
23100	14.36	14.36	90	80

Medicare References: 100-2,15,260; 100-4,12,30; 100-4,12,90.3; 100-4,14,10

23101

23101 Arthrotomy, acromioclavicular joint or sternoclavicular joint, including biopsy and/or excision of torn cartilage

The acromioclavicular joint or the sternoclavicular joint is surgically accessed. A biopsy is performed and/or torn cartilage is excised

Explanation
The physician makes an incision into the acromioclavicular or sternoclavicular joint to remove torn cartilage and take a tissue sample. An incision is made through the skin and the underlying muscle is divided to gain access to the joint capsule. Once the capsule is penetrated, any torn cartilage is identified and removed. A tissue specimen is removed for biopsy. The joint is irrigated, the capsule is closed, and the soft tissues are sutured in layers. A soft dressing is applied.

Coding Tips
If a biopsy is performed in addition to the arthrotomy, it should not be reported separately; it is included in the description of the code. For arthrotomy, sternoclavicular joint, with synovectomy, with or without biopsy, see 23106.

ICD-9-CM Procedural
- 80.31 Biopsy of joint structure of shoulder
- 80.91 Other excision of shoulder joint

Anesthesia
23101 01630

ICD-9-CM Diagnostic
- 170.4 Malignant neoplasm of scapula and long bones of upper limb
- 171.2 Malignant neoplasm of connective and other soft tissue of upper limb, including shoulder
- 195.4 Malignant neoplasm of upper limb
- 198.89 Secondary malignant neoplasm of other specified sites
- 213.4 Benign neoplasm of scapula and long bones of upper limb
- 215.2 Other benign neoplasm of connective and other soft tissue of upper limb, including shoulder
- 239.2 Neoplasms of unspecified nature of bone, soft tissue, and skin
- 275.40 Unspecified disorder of calcium metabolism — (Use additional code to identify any associated mental retardation)
- 275.42 Hypercalcemia — (Use additional code to identify any associated mental retardation)
- 275.49 Other disorders of calcium metabolism — (Use additional code to identify any associated mental retardation)
- 275.5 Hungry bone syndrome
- 357.1 Polyneuropathy in collagen vascular disease — (Code first underlying disease: 446.0, 710.0, 714.0)
- 359.6 Symptomatic inflammatory myopathy in diseases classified elsewhere — (Code first underlying disease: 135, 140.0-208.9, 277.30-277.39, 446.0, 710.0, 710.1, 710.2, 714.0)
- 446.0 Polyarteritis nodosa
- 710.0 Systemic lupus erythematosus — (Use additional code to identify manifestation: 424.91, 581.81, 582.81, 583.81)
- 714.0 Rheumatoid arthritis — (Use additional code to identify manifestation: 357.1, 359.6)
- 718.01 Articular cartilage disorder, shoulder region
- 719.41 Pain in joint, shoulder region
- V64.43 Arthroscopic surgical procedure converted to open procedure

Terms To Know
polyarteritis nodosa. Systemic necrotizing vasculitis of small and medium arteries that results in the infarction and scarring within the affected organs.

polyneuropathy. Disease process of severe inflammation of multiple nerves.

CCI Version 16.3
01610, 0213T, 0216T, 0228T, 0230T, 10060, 10140, 10160, 11012❖, 11040-11043, 20103, 21750, 23700, 29240, 29805, 29822-29823, 29825, 36000, 36400-36410, 36420-36430, 36440, 36600, 36640, 37202, 43752, 51701-51703, 62310-62319, 64400-64435, 64445-64450, 64479, 64483, 64490, 64493, 64505-64530, 69990, 93000-93010, 93040-93042, 93318, 94002, 94200, 94250, 94680-94690, 94770, 95812-95816, 95819, 95822, 95829, 95955, 96360, 96365, 96372, 96374-96376, 99148-99149, 99150

Note: These CCI edits are used for Medicare. Other payers may reimburse on codes listed above.

Medicare Edits

	Fac RVU	Non-Fac RVU	FUD	Assist
23101	13.04	13.04	90	N/A

Medicare References: 100-2,15,260; 100-4,12,30; 100-4,12,90.3; 100-4,14,10

23105-23106

23105 Arthrotomy; glenohumeral joint, with synovectomy, with or without biopsy
23106 sternoclavicular joint, with synovectomy, with or without biopsy

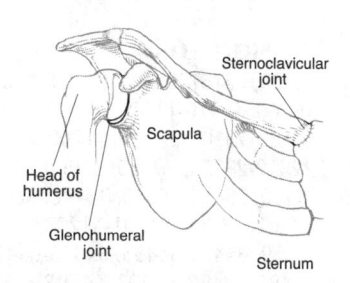

The sternoclavicular joint is surgically accessed and synovial matter removed. Biopsy tissues may be collected (23106)

The glenohumeral joint is surgically accessed and synovial matter removed. Biopsy tissues may be collected (23105)

Explanation
The physician performs an arthrotomy and synovectomy of the glenohumeral joint, with or without biopsy. With the patient lying on one side and the arm suspended in traction, the physician makes an incision overlying the shoulder. The joint capsule is exposed by dissecting down through the soft tissues and freeing and reflecting the muscles. The joint capsule is incised to expose the synovium. Motorized resectors are used to remove the synovium, the inner membrane of the articular capsule that lines the joint cavity. A sample of the tissue for biopsy may also be removed. Following completion of the synovectomy, the shoulder is irrigated, a drain tube may be placed, and the incision is closed in layers with sutures, staples, or Steri-strips. Report 23106 if the procedure is done on the sternoclavicular joint.

Coding Tips
For arthrotomy, glenohumeral joint, see 23100. For arthrotomy, acromioclavicular joint or sternoclavicular joint, including biopsy and/or excision of torn cartilage, see 23101. For arthrotomy, glenohumeral joint, with joint exploration, with or without removal of a loose or foreign body, see 23107. For arthroscopic synovectomy of the shoulder, see 29820–29821.

ICD-9-CM Procedural
80.11 Other arthrotomy of shoulder
80.19 Other arthrotomy of other specified site
80.31 Biopsy of joint structure of shoulder
80.71 Synovectomy of shoulder

Anesthesia
01630

ICD-9-CM Diagnostic
357.1 Polyneuropathy in collagen vascular disease — (Code first underlying disease: 446.0, 710.0, 714.0)
359.6 Symptomatic inflammatory myopathy in diseases classified elsewhere — (Code first underlying disease: 135, 140.0-208.9, 277.30-277.39, 446.0, 710.0, 710.1, 710.2, 714.0)
446.0 Polyarteritis nodosa
710.0 Systemic lupus erythematosus — (Use additional code to identify manifestation: 424.91, 581.81, 582.81, 583.81)
714.0 Rheumatoid arthritis — (Use additional code to identify manifestation: 357.1, 359.6)
715.91 Osteoarthrosis, unspecified whether generalized or localized, shoulder region
716.61 Unspecified monoarthritis, shoulder region
719.21 Villonodular synovitis, shoulder region
719.41 Pain in joint, shoulder region
727.00 Unspecified synovitis and tenosynovitis
727.01 Synovitis and tenosynovitis in diseases classified elsewhere — (Code first underlying disease: 015.0-015.9)
727.02 Giant cell tumor of tendon sheath
V64.43 Arthroscopic surgical procedure converted to open procedure

Terms To Know
osteoarthrosis. Most common form of a noninflammatory degenerative joint disease with degenerating articular cartilage, bone enlargement, and synovial membrane changes.

CCI Version 16.3
01610, 0213T, 0216T, 0228T, 0230T, 10060, 10140, 10160, 11040-11043, 20103, 23700, 24332, 29820-29823, 29825, 36000, 36400-36410, 36420-36430, 36440, 36600, 36640, 37202, 43752, 51701-51703, 62310-62319, 64400-64435, 64445-64450, 64479, 64483, 64490, 64493, 64505-64530, 69990, 93000-93010, 93040-93042, 93318, 94002, 94200, 94250, 94680-94690, 94770, 95812-95816, 95819, 95822, 95829, 95955, 96360, 96365, 96372, 96374-96376, 99148-99149, 99150

Also not with 23105: 23100, 29805
Also not with 23106: 11012❖, 23101

Note: These CCI edits are used for Medicare. Other payers may reimburse on codes listed above.

Medicare Edits

	Fac RVU	Non-Fac RVU	FUD	Assist
23105	18.53	18.53	90	80
23106	14.14	14.14	90	N/A

Medicare References: 100-2,15,260; 100-4,12,30; 100-4,12,90.3; 100-4,14,10

23107

23107 Arthrotomy, glenohumeral joint, with joint exploration, with or without removal of loose or foreign body

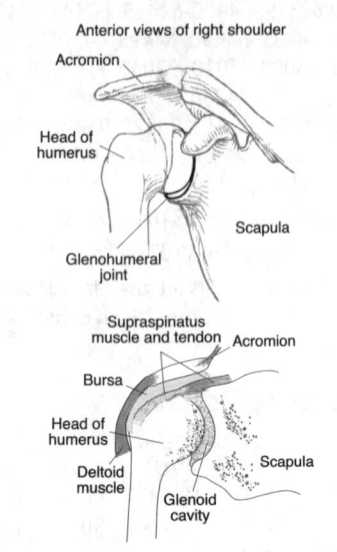

Anterior views of right shoulder

The glenohumeral joint is surgically accessed and explored. Loose or foreign bodies may or may not be removed during the surgery.

Explanation

The physician performs an arthrotomy of the glenohumeral joint with joint exploration and removal of any loose or foreign bodies. An incision is made over the glenohumeral joint. The soft tissues are dissected away and the joint capsule is exposed and incised. The joint space is explored and any loose or foreign body (e.g., free cartilage, bone fragments, gravel) is exposed and removed. The wound is irrigated with antibiotic solution. The physician may leave the wound packed open with daily dressing changes to allow for further drainage and secondary healing by granulation. If the incision is repaired, drain tubes may be inserted and the incision is repaired in layers with sutures, staples, and/or Steri-strips. A splint may be applied to limit shoulder motion.

Coding Tips

For exploration of a penetrating wound, see 20103. For arthroscopic removal of a loose or foreign body from the shoulder, see 29819.

ICD-9-CM Procedural

80.11 Other arthrotomy of shoulder

Anesthesia

23107   01630

ICD-9-CM Diagnostic

- 275.40 Unspecified disorder of calcium metabolism — (Use additional code to identify any associated mental retardation)
- 275.41 Hypocalcemia — (Use additional code to identify any associated mental retardation)
- 275.42 Hypercalcemia — (Use additional code to identify any associated mental retardation)
- 275.49 Other disorders of calcium metabolism — (Use additional code to identify any associated mental retardation)
- 275.5 Hungry bone syndrome
- 357.1 Polyneuropathy in collagen vascular disease — (Code first underlying disease: 446.0, 710.0, 714.0)
- 359.6 Symptomatic inflammatory myopathy in diseases classified elsewhere — (Code first underlying disease: 135, 140.0-208.9, 277.30-277.39, 446.0, 710.0, 710.1, 710.2, 714.0)
- 446.0 Polyarteritis nodosa
- 710.0 Systemic lupus erythematosus — (Use additional code to identify manifestation: 424.91, 581.81, 582.81, 583.81)
- 712.11 Chondrocalcinosis due to dicalcium phosphate crystals, shoulder region — (Code first underlying disease: 275.4)
- 712.21 Chondrocalcinosis due to pyrophosphate crystals, shoulder region — (Code first underlying disease: 275.4)
- 714.0 Rheumatoid arthritis — (Use additional code to identify manifestation: 357.1, 359.6)
- 715.91 Osteoarthrosis, unspecified whether generalized or localized, shoulder region
- 716.61 Unspecified monoarthritis, shoulder region
- 718.11 Loose body in shoulder joint
- 719.41 Pain in joint, shoulder region
- 727.02 Giant cell tumor of tendon sheath
- V64.43 Arthroscopic surgical procedure converted to open procedure

Terms To Know

chondrocalcinosis. Presence of calcium salt deposits within joint cartilage.

foreign body. Any object or substance found in an organ and tissue that does not belong under normal circumstances.

hypercalcemia. Abnormally high levels of calcium in the blood, resulting in symptoms of muscle weakness, fatigue, nausea, depression, and constipation.

polyarteritis nodosa. Systemic necrotizing vasculitis of small and medium arteries that results in the infarction and scarring within the affected organs.

polyneuropathy. Disease process of severe inflammation of multiple nerves.

CCI Version 16.3

01610, 0213T, 0216T, 0228T, 0230T, 10060, 10140, 10160, 11010-11012, 11040-11043, 12034, 20103, 23100, 23105, 23700, 24332, 29805, 29819-29823, 29825, 36000, 36400-36410, 36420-36430, 36440, 36600, 36640, 37202, 43752, 51701-51703, 62310-62319, 64400-64435, 64445-64450, 64479, 64483, 64490, 64493, 64505-64530, 69990, 93000-93010, 93040-93042, 93318, 94002, 94200, 94250, 94680-94690, 94770, 95812-95816, 95819, 95822, 95829, 95955, 96360, 96365, 96372, 96374-96376, 99148-99149, 99150

Note: These CCI edits are used for Medicare. Other payers may reimburse on codes listed above.

Medicare Edits

	Fac RVU	Non-Fac RVU	FUD	Assist
23107	19.2	19.2	90	80

Medicare References: 100-2,15,260; 100-4,12,30; 100-4,12,90.3; 100-4,14,10

23120-23125

23120 Claviculectomy; partial
23125 total

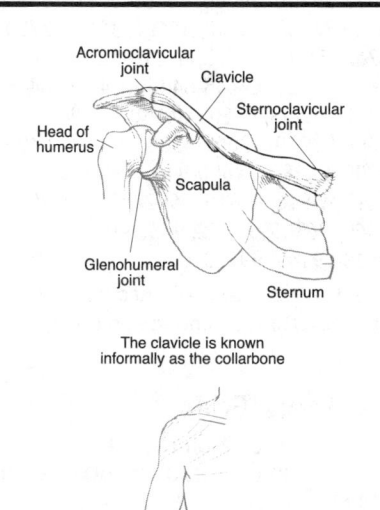

Explanation
Removal of the clavicle (collar bone) is successfully performed without significant loss of function to the upper extremity for such problems as old, chronic, or acute unreduced dislocations. An incision is made horizontally along the portion of the bone to be removed. The skin is reflected, the bone is cleared of soft tissue attachments, and divided with an osteotome or bone-cutting rongeurs. For a partial resection, the remaining end of the clavicle is rounded and smoothed to eliminate the rough edge. If the medial end of the clavicle is removed, the clavicle may be stabilized to the first rib and the sternocleidomastoid may be detached. The periosteum and soft tissues are plicated and sutured over the raw end of the clavicle. The wound is closed and a soft dressing is applied. Report 23120 for a partial claviculectomy and 23125 for total claviculectomy.

Coding Tips
For partial excision involving craterization, saucerization, or diaphysectomy of the clavicle to treat conditions such as osteomyelitis, see 23180. For excision or curettage of a bone cyst or benign tumor of the clavicle, see 23140–23146. For sequestrectomy, clavicle, see 23170. For radical resection of a clavicular tumor, see 23200.

ICD-9-CM Procedural
- 77.81 Other partial ostectomy of scapula, clavicle, and thorax (ribs and sternum)
- 77.91 Total ostectomy of scapula, clavicle, and thorax (ribs and sternum)

Anesthesia
23120 00450
23125 00452

ICD-9-CM Diagnostic
- 170.3 Malignant neoplasm of ribs, sternum, and clavicle
- 196.3 Secondary and unspecified malignant neoplasm of lymph nodes of axilla and upper limb
- 198.5 Secondary malignant neoplasm of bone and bone marrow
- 198.89 Secondary malignant neoplasm of other specified sites
- 209.73 Secondary neuroendocrine tumor of bone
- 213.3 Benign neoplasm of ribs, sternum, and clavicle
- 238.0 Neoplasm of uncertain behavior of bone and articular cartilage
- 239.2 Neoplasms of unspecified nature of bone, soft tissue, and skin
- 715.11 Primary localized osteoarthrosis, shoulder region
- 715.21 Secondary localized osteoarthrosis, shoulder region
- 716.11 Traumatic arthropathy, shoulder region
- 716.61 Unspecified monoarthritis, shoulder region
- 718.01 Articular cartilage disorder, shoulder region
- 718.31 Recurrent dislocation of shoulder joint
- 719.01 Effusion of shoulder joint
- 728.86 Necrotizing fasciitis — (Use additional code to identify infectious organism, 041.00-041.89, 785.4, if applicable)
- 730.11 Chronic osteomyelitis, shoulder region — (Use additional code to identify organism: 041.1. Use additional code to identify major osseous defect, if applicable: 731.3)
- 731.3 Major osseous defects — (Code first underlying disease: 170.0-170.9, 730.00-730.29, 733.00-733.09, 733.40-733.49, 996.45)
- 733.49 Aseptic necrosis of other bone site — (Use additional code to identify major osseous defect, if applicable: 731.3)
- 733.90 Disorder of bone and cartilage, unspecified
- 738.8 Acquired musculoskeletal deformity of other specified site
- 785.4 Gangrene — (Code first any associated underlying condition)
- 831.04 Closed dislocation of acromioclavicular (joint)

Terms To Know
aseptic necrosis. Death of bone tissue resulting from a disruption in the vascular supply, caused by a noninfectious disease process, such as a fracture or the administration of immunosuppressive drugs.

gangrene. Death of tissue, usually resulting from a loss of vascular supply, followed by a bacterial attack or onset of disease.

osteomyelitis. Inflammation of bone that may remain localized or spread to the marrow, cortex, or periosteum, in response to an infecting organism, usually bacterial and pyogenic.

CCI Version 16.3
01610, 0213T, 0216T, 0228T, 0230T, 14020-14021, 23044, 23101, 23106, 23140-23146, 23480❖, 23700, 24301, 24320, 36000, 36400-36410, 36420-36430, 36440, 36600, 36640, 37202, 43752, 51701-51703, 62310-62319, 64400-64435, 64445-64450, 64479, 64483, 64490, 64493, 64505-64530, 69990, 93000-93010, 93040-93042, 93318, 94002, 94200, 94250, 94680-94690, 94770, 95812-95816, 95819, 95822, 95829, 95955, 96360, 96365, 96372, 96374-96376, 99148-99149, 99150

Also not with 23120: 11012❖, 12020, 29805, 29819-29822, 29824-29825

Also not with 23125: 23120, 23415, 29819-29826

Note: These CCI edits are used for Medicare. Other payers may reimburse on codes listed above.

Medicare Edits

	Fac RVU	Non-Fac RVU	FUD	Assist
23120	16.86	16.86	90	80
23125	20.55	20.55	90	80

Medicare References: 100-2,15,260; 100-4,12,30; 100-4,12,90.3; 100-4,14,10

23130

23130 Acromioplasty or acromionectomy, partial, with or without coracoacromial ligament release

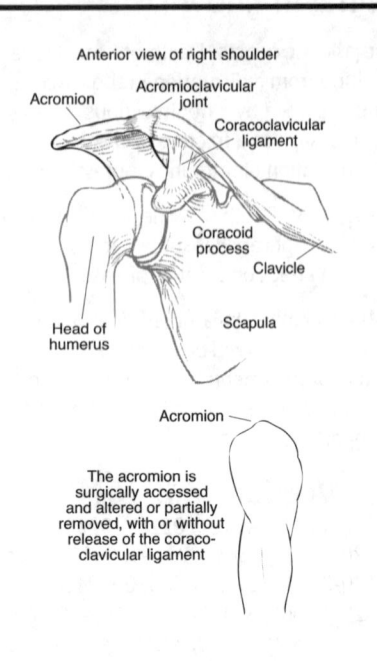

Anterior view of right shoulder

Acromion, Acromioclavicular joint, Coracoclavicular ligament, Coracoid process, Clavicle, Head of humerus, Scapula, Acromion

The acromion is surgically accessed and altered or partially removed, with or without release of the coracoclavicular ligament

Explanation
A partial acromioplasty or acromionectomy, with or without coracoacromial ligament release, is done. This procedure is also commonly performed during repair to the rotator cuff in an effort to increase the space below the acromion where the cuff tendons traverse toward their insertion on the humerus. An incision is made overlying the area. Dissection is carried down to the acromion. Acromioplasty involves the division of the acromioclavicular ligament followed by the use of a burr to cut away the under surface of the acromion. During acromionectomy, the distal portion of the acromion is removed. The coracoacromial ligament, a wide, strong band spanning between the acromion and the coracoid process of the scapula, may also be released. The joint is irrigated and the incisions are closed with sutures or Steri-strips.

Coding Tips
Release of the acromial ligament should not be reported separately. For arthroscopic partial acromioplasty with decompression of the subacromial space, see 29826.

ICD-9-CM Procedural
- 77.81 Other partial ostectomy of scapula, clavicle, and thorax (ribs and sternum)
- 81.81 Partial shoulder replacement
- 81.82 Repair of recurrent dislocation of shoulder
- 81.83 Other repair of shoulder

Anesthesia
23130   01630

ICD-9-CM Diagnostic
- 715.11 Primary localized osteoarthrosis, shoulder region
- 715.21 Secondary localized osteoarthrosis, shoulder region
- 716.11 Traumatic arthropathy, shoulder region
- 716.61 Unspecified monoarthritis, shoulder region
- 716.91 Unspecified arthropathy, shoulder region
- 718.01 Articular cartilage disorder, shoulder region
- 719.41 Pain in joint, shoulder region
- 726.10 Unspecified disorders of bursae and tendons in shoulder region
- 726.2 Other affections of shoulder region, not elsewhere classified
- 727.61 Complete rupture of rotator cuff
- 811.01 Closed fracture of acromial process of scapula
- 811.11 Open fracture of acromial process of scapula
- 831.14 Open dislocation of acromioclavicular (joint)

Terms To Know

closed fracture. Break in a bone without a concomitant opening in the skin. A closed fracture is coded when the type of fracture is not specified.

open fracture. Exposed break in a bone, always considered compound due to its high risk of infection from the open wound leading to the fracture. Broken bone ends may protrude through the skin and contaminants or foreign bodies are often embedded in the tissues.

osteoarthrosis. Most common form of a noninflammatory degenerative joint disease with degenerating articular cartilage, bone enlargement, and synovial membrane changes.

primary. Principal or first in the order of occurrence or importance.

secondary. Second in order of occurrence or importance, or appearing during the course of another disease or condition.

CCI Version 16.3
01610, 0213T, 0216T, 0228T, 0230T, 14020-14021, 23000, 23075, 23140, 23700, 24301, 24320, 29805, 29819-29823, 29825-29826, 36000, 36400-36410, 36420-36430, 36440, 36600, 36640, 37202, 43752, 51701-51703, 62310-62319, 64400-64435, 64445-64450, 64479, 64483, 64490, 64493, 64505-64530, 69990, 93000-93010, 93040-93042, 93318, 94002, 94200, 94250, 94680-94690, 94770, 95812-95816, 95819, 95822, 95829, 95955, 96360, 96365, 96372, 96374-96376, 99148-99149, 99150

Note: These CCI edits are used for Medicare. Other payers may reimburse on codes listed above.

Medicare Edits

	Fac RVU	Non-Fac RVU	FUD	Assist
23130	17.64	17.64	90	N/A

Medicare References: 100-2,15,260; 100-4,12,30; 100-4,12,90.3; 100-4,14,10

23140-23146

23140 Excision or curettage of bone cyst or benign tumor of clavicle or scapula;
23145 with autograft (includes obtaining graft)
23146 with allograft

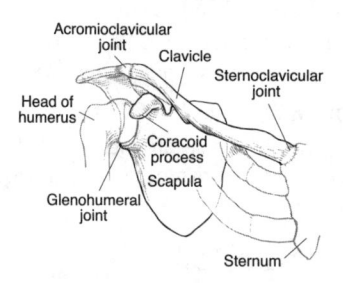

A cyst or benign tumor of the clavicle or scapula is excised or removed by curettage. Report 23145 when an autograft (from the patient) is harvested for the repair. Report 23146 when an allograft (from another human) is used

Explanation
A bone cyst or benign tumor of the clavicle or scapula is removed. The physician makes an incision overlying the cyst or tumor. The skin and underlying soft tissues are reflected to expose the periosteum, which is separated from the bone. Curettes or osteotomes are used to scrape or cut the lesion from the bone. Once the benign tumor or cyst is removed and healthy bone tissue is present, the periosteum is repositioned and the incision is repaired in layers. If the bone defect created requires a graft for repair, the physician obtains the necessary size bone graft from a separate donor site on the patient and packs it into the site where the tumor or bone cyst was removed or uses a bone bank allograft. Report 23145 if an autograft is obtained and 23146 if an allograft is used.

Coding Tips
Grafts are included in the description of 23145 and 23146 and should not be reported separately. For partial excision of the clavicle or scapula, see 23180–23182. For radical resection for a tumor of the clavicle or scapula, see 23200–23210.

ICD-9-CM Procedural
- **77.61** Local excision of lesion or tissue of scapula, clavicle, and thorax (ribs and sternum)
- **77.77** Excision of tibia and fibula for graft
- **77.79** Excision of other bone for graft, except facial bones
- **78.01** Bone graft of scapula, clavicle, and thorax (ribs and sternum)

Anesthesia
00450

ICD-9-CM Diagnostic
- **213.3** Benign neoplasm of ribs, sternum, and clavicle
- **213.4** Benign neoplasm of scapula and long bones of upper limb
- **238.0** Neoplasm of uncertain behavior of bone and articular cartilage
- **239.2** Neoplasms of unspecified nature of bone, soft tissue, and skin
- **733.21** Solitary bone cyst
- **733.22** Aneurysmal bone cyst
- **733.29** Other cyst of bone

Terms To Know
aneurysmal bone cyst. Solitary bone lesion that bulges into the periosteum, marked by a calcified rim.

benign. Mild or nonmalignant in nature.

cyst. Elevated encapsulated mass containing fluid, semisolid, or solid material with a membranous lining.

neoplasm. New abnormal growth, tumor.

soft tissue. Nonepithelial tissues outside of the skeleton that includes subcutaneous adipose tissue, fibrous tissue, fascia, muscles, blood and lymph vessels, and peripheral nervous system tissue.

CCI Version 16.3
01610, 0213T, 0216T, 0228T, 0230T, 10060, 10140, 10160, 20000-20005, 20615, 23700, 24332, 36000, 36400-36410, 36420-36430, 36440, 36600, 36640, 37202, 43752, 51701-51703, 62310-62319, 64400-64435, 64445-64450, 64479, 64483, 64490, 64493, 64505-64530, 69990, 93000-93010, 93040-93042, 93318, 94002, 94200, 94250, 94680-94690, 94770, 95812-95816, 95819, 95822, 95829, 95955, 96360, 96365, 96372, 96374-96376, 99148-99149, 99150

Also not with 23140: 11012❖, 23180❖, 23182❖, 23190❖

Also not with 23145: 20900-20902, 23140, 23515, 23585

Also not with 23146: 23140-23145❖, 23180❖, 23182❖, 23515, 23585

Note: These CCI edits are used for Medicare. Other payers may reimburse on codes listed above.

Medicare Edits

	Fac RVU	Non-Fac RVU	FUD	Assist
23140	15.11	15.11	90	N/A
23145	20.2	20.2	90	80
23146	17.77	17.77	90	80

Medicare References: 100-2,15,260; 100-4,12,30; 100-4,12,90.3; 100-4,14,10

23150-23156

23150 Excision or curettage of bone cyst or benign tumor of proximal humerus;
23155 with autograft (includes obtaining graft)
23156 with allograft

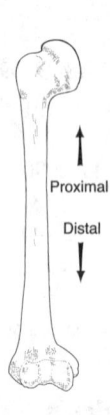

A bone cyst or benign tumor of the proximal humerus is excised or removed by curettage. Report 23155 when an autograft (same patient) is harvested and used to treat the site. Report 23156 when an allograft (another human donor) is used

Explanation

A bone cyst or benign tumor of the proximal humerus is removed. The physician makes an incision in the upper arm overlying the cyst or tumor. The skin and underlying soft tissues are reflected to expose the periosteum, which is separated from the bone. Curettes or osteotomes are used to scrape or cut the lesion from the bone. Once the benign tumor or cyst is removed and healthy bone tissue is present, the periosteum is repositioned and the incision is repaired in layers. If the bone defect created requires a graft for repair, the physician obtains the necessary size bone graft from a separate donor site on the patient and packs it into the site where the tumor or bone cyst was removed or uses a bone bank allograft. Report 23155 if the procedure is done with an autograft and 23156 if an allograft is used.

Coding Tips

Grafts are included in the description of 23155 and 23156 and should not be reported separately. For partial excision of the proximal humerus, see 23184; for radical resection for a tumor of the proximal humerus, see 23220.

ICD-9-CM Procedural

- 77.62 Local excision of lesion or tissue of humerus
- 77.77 Excision of tibia and fibula for graft
- 77.79 Excision of other bone for graft, except facial bones
- 78.02 Bone graft of humerus

Anesthesia
01630

ICD-9-CM Diagnostic

- 213.4 Benign neoplasm of scapula and long bones of upper limb
- 238.0 Neoplasm of uncertain behavior of bone and articular cartilage
- 239.2 Neoplasms of unspecified nature of bone, soft tissue, and skin
- 733.21 Solitary bone cyst
- 733.22 Aneurysmal bone cyst
- 733.29 Other cyst of bone

Terms To Know

allograft. Graft from one individual to another of the same species.

aneurysmal bone cyst. Solitary bone lesion that bulges into the periosteum, marked by a calcified rim.

autograft. Any tissue harvested from one anatomical site of a person and grafted to another anatomical site of the same person. Most commonly, blood vessels, skin, tendons, fascia, and bone are used as autografts.

benign. Mild or nonmalignant in nature.

cyst. Elevated encapsulated mass containing fluid, semisolid, or solid material with a membranous lining.

distal. Located farther away from a specified reference point.

neoplasm. New abnormal growth, tumor.

proximal. Located closest to a specified reference point, usually the midline.

soft tissue. Nonepithelial tissues outside of the skeleton that includes subcutaneous adipose tissue, fibrous tissue, fascia, muscles, blood and lymph vessels, and peripheral nervous system tissue.

CCI Version 16.3

01610, 0213T, 0216T, 0228T, 0230T, 10060, 10140, 10160, 20000-20005, 20615, 23100, 23700, 24332, 36000, 36400-36410, 36420-36430, 36440, 36600, 36640, 37202, 43752, 51701-51703, 62310-62319, 64400-64435, 64445-64450, 64479, 64483, 64490, 64493, 64505-64530, 69990, 93000-93010, 93040-93042, 93318, 94002, 94200, 94250, 94680-94690, 94770, 95812-95816, 95819, 95822, 95829, 95955, 96360, 96365, 96372, 96374-96376, 99148-99149, 99150

Also not with 23150: 23184❖

Also not with 23155: 20900-20902, 23150

Also not with 23156: 23150-23155❖, 23184❖

Note: These CCI edits are used for Medicare. Other payers may reimburse on codes listed above.

Medicare Edits

	Fac RVU	Non-Fac RVU	FUD	Assist
23150	19.11	19.11	90	80
23155	23.07	23.07	90	80
23156	19.67	19.67	90	80

Medicare References: 100-2,15,260; 100-4,12,30; 100-4,12,90.3; 100-4,14,10

23170-23174

23170 Sequestrectomy (eg, for osteomyelitis or bone abscess), clavicle

23172 Sequestrectomy (eg, for osteomyelitis or bone abscess), scapula

23174 Sequestrectomy (eg, for osteomyelitis or bone abscess), humeral head to surgical neck

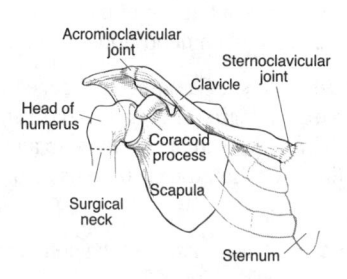

Sequestrum is dead bone tissue and these codes report its removal or removal of an associated bone abscess. Report 23170 for sequestrectomy of the clavicle. Report 23172 for sequestrectomy of the scapula. And report 23174 for sequestrectomy of the humeral head above the surgical neck

Explanation

The physician removes infected portions of the clavicle in 23170 due to a bone abscess or osteomyelitis. This infection often leaves open sinus tracts in the bone that require removal. The physician makes an incision overlying the sequestered area of bone in the clavicle. Once the skin and soft tissues are reflected, a small window is cut into the bone to gain access to the sequestrum, or necrosed piece of bone that has become separated from sound bone. All purulent material and scarred or necrotic tissue are removed. The remaining space is filled with surrounding soft tissues or free tissue transfer. The area is irrigated and an antibiotic solution is used to prevent further infection. The wound is closed loosely over drains if possible. The arm is positioned in a sling or splint and protected to prevent fracture of the clavicle. Report 23172 if the sequestrectomy is performed on the scapula and 23174 if this procedure is performed on the humeral head to the surgical neck.

Coding Tips

For partial excision of the clavicle, scapula, or humeral head, see 23180–23184. For radical resection of the clavicle, scapula, or humeral head for a bone tumor, see 23200–23222. If significant additional time and effort is documented, append modifier 22 and submit a cover letter and operative report.

ICD-9-CM Procedural

77.01 Sequestrectomy of scapula, clavicle, and thorax (ribs and sternum)
77.02 Sequestrectomy of humerus

Anesthesia

23170 00450
23172 00450
23174 01630

ICD-9-CM Diagnostic

730.01 Acute osteomyelitis, shoulder region — (Use additional code to identify organism: 041.1. Use additional code to identify major osseous defect, if applicable: 731.3)

730.02 Acute osteomyelitis, upper arm — (Use additional code to identify organism: 041.1. Use additional code to identify major osseous defect, if applicable: 731.3)

730.11 Chronic osteomyelitis, shoulder region — (Use additional code to identify organism: 041.1. Use additional code to identify major osseous defect, if applicable: 731.3)

730.12 Chronic osteomyelitis, upper arm — (Use additional code to identify organism: 041.1. Use additional code to identify major osseous defect, if applicable: 731.3)

730.21 Unspecified osteomyelitis, shoulder region — (Use additional code to identify organism: 041.1. Use additional code to identify major osseous defect, if applicable: 731.3)

730.22 Unspecified osteomyelitis, upper arm — (Use additional code to identify organism: 041.1. Use additional code to identify major osseous defect, if applicable: 731.3)

730.31 Periostitis, without mention of osteomyelitis, shoulder region — (Use additional code to identify organism: 041.1)

730.32 Periostitis, without mention of osteomyelitis, upper arm — (Use additional code to identify organism: 041.1)

730.82 Other infections involving bone diseases classified elsewhere, upper arm — (Use additional code to identify organism: 041.1. Code first underlying disease: 002.0, 015.0-015.9)

730.88 Other infections involving bone diseases classified elsewhere, other specified sites — (Use additional code to identify organism: 041.1. Code first underlying disease: 002.0, 015.0-015.9)

731.3 Major osseous defects — (Code first underlying disease: 170.0-170.9, 730.00-730.29, 733.00-733.09, 733.40-733.49, 996.45)

733.41 Aseptic necrosis of head of humerus — (Use additional code to identify major osseous defect, if applicable: 731.3)

733.49 Aseptic necrosis of other bone site — (Use additional code to identify major osseous defect, if applicable: 731.3)

Terms To Know

abscess. Circumscribed collection of pus resulting from bacteria, frequently associated with swelling and other signs of inflammation.

osteomyelitis. Inflammation of bone that may remain localized or spread to the marrow, cortex, or periosteum, in response to an infecting organism, usually bacterial and pyogenic.

periostitis. Inflammation of the outer layers of bone.

CCI Version 16.3

01610, 0213T, 0216T, 0228T, 0230T, 10060, 10140, 10160, 20000-20005, 20500, 23030-23035, 23700, 36000, 36400-36410, 36420-36430, 36440, 36600, 36640, 37202, 43752, 51701-51703, 62310-62319, 64400-64435, 64445-64450, 64479, 64483, 64490, 64493, 64505-64530, 69990, 93000-93010, 93040-93042, 93318, 94002, 94200, 94250, 94680-94690, 94770, 95812-95816, 95819, 95822, 95829, 95955, 96360, 96365, 96372, 96374-96376, 99148-99149, 99150

Also not with 23170: 11012❖, 23120-23125❖, 23140-23146❖, 23180

Also not with 23172: 11012❖, 23040, 23140-23146❖, 23182, 23190❖

Also not with 23174: 23040, 23184, 23195❖

Note: These CCI edits are used for Medicare. Other payers may reimburse on codes listed above.

Medicare Edits

	Fac RVU	Non-Fac RVU	FUD	Assist
23170	15.86	15.86	90	N/A
23172	16.22	16.22	90	80
23174	22.01	22.01	90	80

Medicare References: 100-2,15,260; 100-4,12,30; 100-4,12,90.3; 100-4,14,10

23180-23184

23180 Partial excision (craterization, saucerization, or diaphysectomy) bone (eg, osteomyelitis), clavicle

23182 Partial excision (craterization, saucerization, or diaphysectomy) bone (eg, osteomyelitis), scapula

23184 Partial excision (craterization, saucerization, or diaphysectomy) bone (eg, osteomyelitis), proximal humerus

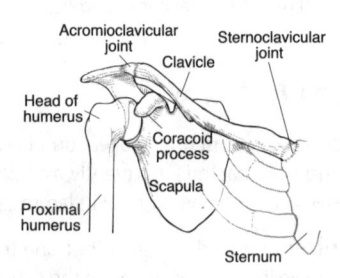

Bone is partially excised. Report 23180 for partial excision of the clavicle. Report 23182 for the scapula. And report 23184 for partial excision of the proximal humerus

Explanation

The physician performs a partial excision of the clavicle in 23180 to remove infected bone. An incision is made over the infected part of the clavicle and the underlying soft tissues are divided to expose the bone. The periosteum is reflected and the infected portion of bone is removed and irrigated. The excavation of bone may excise a crater-like piece, leave a small saucer-like shelf depression in the bone, or may remove a portion of the shaft (diaphysis) of a long bone. If a significant portion of bone is removed, the physician may use bone graft material to fill the cavity left in the bone. The periosteum is closed over the bone, the soft tissues are sutured closed, and a soft dressing is applied. Report 23182 for partial excision of the scapula and 23184 for partial excision of the proximal humerus.

Coding Tips

If a bone graft/graft material is used, it may be reported separately; see 20900–20902. For sequestrectomy of the clavicle, scapula, or humeral head to surgical neck, see 23170–23174. If significant additional time and effort is documented, append modifier 22 and submit a cover letter and operative report.

ICD-9-CM Procedural

77.81 Other partial ostectomy of scapula, clavicle, and thorax (ribs and sternum)
77.82 Other partial ostectomy of humerus

Anesthesia

23180 00450
23182 00450
23184 01630

ICD-9-CM Diagnostic

730.11 Chronic osteomyelitis, shoulder region — (Use additional code to identify organism: 041.1. Use additional code to identify major osseous defect, if applicable: 731.3)
730.12 Chronic osteomyelitis, upper arm — (Use additional code to identify organism: 041.1. Use additional code to identify major osseous defect, if applicable: 731.3)
730.21 Unspecified osteomyelitis, shoulder region — (Use additional code to identify organism: 041.1. Use additional code to identify major osseous defect, if applicable: 731.3)
730.22 Unspecified osteomyelitis, upper arm — (Use additional code to identify organism: 041.1. Use additional code to identify major osseous defect, if applicable: 731.3)
730.31 Periostitis, without mention of osteomyelitis, shoulder region — (Use additional code to identify organism: 041.1)
730.32 Periostitis, without mention of osteomyelitis, upper arm — (Use additional code to identify organism: 041.1)
730.81 Other infections involving bone diseases classified elsewhere, shoulder region — (Use additional code to identify organism: 041.1. Code first underlying disease: 002.0, 015.0-015.9)
730.82 Other infections involving bone diseases classified elsewhere, upper arm — (Use additional code to identify organism: 041.1. Code first underlying disease: 002.0, 015.0-015.9)
731.3 Major osseous defects — (Code first underlying disease: 170.0-170.9, 730.00-730.29, 733.00-733.09, 733.40-733.49, 996.45)
733.41 Aseptic necrosis of head of humerus — (Use additional code to identify major osseous defect, if applicable: 731.3)
733.49 Aseptic necrosis of other bone site — (Use additional code to identify major osseous defect, if applicable: 731.3)

Terms To Know

aseptic necrosis. Death of bone tissue resulting from a disruption in the vascular supply, caused by a noninfectious disease process, such as a fracture or the administration of immunosuppressive drugs.

osteomyelitis. Inflammation of bone that may remain localized or spread to the marrow, cortex, or periosteum, in response to an infecting organism, usually bacterial and pyogenic.

periostitis. Inflammation of the outer layers of bone.

CCI Version 16.3

01610, 0213T, 0216T, 0228T, 0230T, 10060, 10140, 10160, 20000-20005, 20500, 23030-23035, 23700, 36000, 36400-36410, 36420-36430, 36440, 36600, 36640, 37202, 43752, 51701-51703, 62310-62319, 64400-64435, 64445-64450, 64479, 64483, 64490, 64493, 64505-64530, 69990, 93000-93010, 93040-93042, 93318, 94002, 94200, 94250, 94680-94690, 94770, 95812-95816, 95819, 95822, 95829, 95955, 96360, 96365, 96372, 96374-96376, 99148-99149, 99150

Also not with 23180: 23044, 23101, 23106, 23120-23125❖, 23145❖

Also not with 23182: 23040, 23145❖, 24332

Also not with 23184: 23040, 23155❖, 24332

Note: These CCI edits are used for Medicare. Other payers may reimburse on codes listed above.

Medicare Edits

	Fac RVU	Non-Fac RVU	FUD	Assist
23180	19.78	19.78	90	N/A
23182	19.31	19.31	90	80
23184	21.52	21.52	90	80

Medicare References: 100-2,15,260; 100-4,12,30; 100-4,12,90.3; 100-4,14,10

23190

23190 Ostectomy of scapula, partial (eg, superior medial angle)

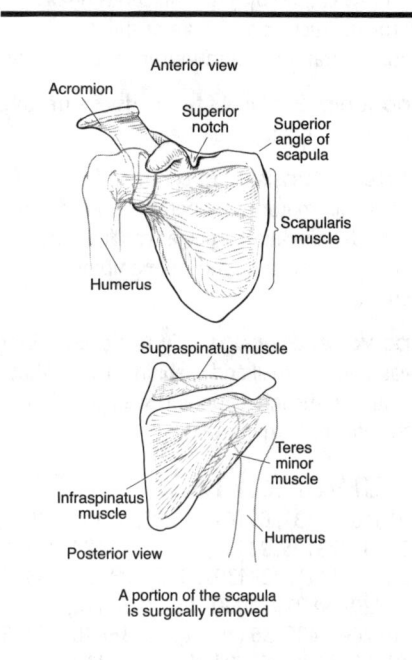

Explanation
The physician removes a portion of the scapula (shoulder blade). An oblique skin incision is made across the scapula and the underlying trapezius muscle is reflected to expose the superior medial angle. The portion of the scapula is removed and the remaining border is smoothed to prevent trauma to the surrounding tissues. A portion of the supraspinatus and levator scapulae tendons are resected and sutured to the trapezius muscle and remaining border of the scapula. The wound is irrigated and the incision is sutured. A soft dressing is applied.

Coding Tips
For radical resection of the scapula for a tumor, see 23210. If significant additional time and effort is documented, append modifier 22 and submit a cover letter and operative report.

ICD-9-CM Procedural
- **77.81** Other partial ostectomy of scapula, clavicle, and thorax (ribs and sternum)

Anesthesia
23190 00450

ICD-9-CM Diagnostic
- **170.4** Malignant neoplasm of scapula and long bones of upper limb
- **171.4** Malignant neoplasm of connective and other soft tissue of thorax
- **195.1** Malignant neoplasm of thorax
- **198.5** Secondary malignant neoplasm of bone and bone marrow
- **213.4** Benign neoplasm of scapula and long bones of upper limb
- **238.0** Neoplasm of uncertain behavior of bone and articular cartilage
- **239.2** Neoplasms of unspecified nature of bone, soft tissue, and skin
- **731.3** Major osseous defects — (Code first underlying disease: 170.0-170.9, 730.00-730.29, 733.00-733.09, 733.40-733.49, 996.45)
- **733.90** Disorder of bone and cartilage, unspecified
- **736.89** Other acquired deformity of other parts of limb

Terms To Know
benign. Mild or nonmalignant in nature.

malignant. Any condition tending to progress toward death, specifically an invasive tumor with a loss of cellular differentiation that has the ability to spread or metastasize to other areas in the body.

neoplasm. New abnormal growth, tumor.

osteomyelitis. Inflammation of bone that may remain localized or spread to the marrow, cortex, or periosteum, in response to an infecting organism, usually bacterial and pyogenic.

secondary. Second in order of occurrence or importance, or appearing during the course of another disease or condition.

soft tissue. Nonepithelial tissues outside of the skeleton that includes subcutaneous adipose tissue, fibrous tissue, fascia, muscles, blood and lymph vessels, and peripheral nervous system tissue.

CCI Version 16.3
01610, 0213T, 0216T, 0228T, 0230T, 11012❖, 23040, 23145-23146❖, 23182❖, 23700, 24332, 36000, 36400-36410, 36420-36430, 36440, 36600, 36640, 37202, 43752, 51701-51703, 62310-62319, 64400-64435, 64445-64450, 64479, 64483, 64490, 64493, 64505-64530, 69990, 93000-93010, 93040-93042, 93318, 94002, 94200, 94250, 94680-94690, 94770, 95812-95816, 95819, 95822, 95829, 95955, 96360, 96365, 96372, 96374-96376, 99148-99149, 99150

Note: These CCI edits are used for Medicare. Other payers may reimburse on codes listed above.

Medicare Edits

	Fac RVU	Non-Fac RVU	FUD	Assist
23190	16.44	16.44	90	80

Medicare References: 100-2,15,260; 100-4,12,30; 100-4,12,90.3; 100-4,14,10

23195

23195 Resection, humeral head

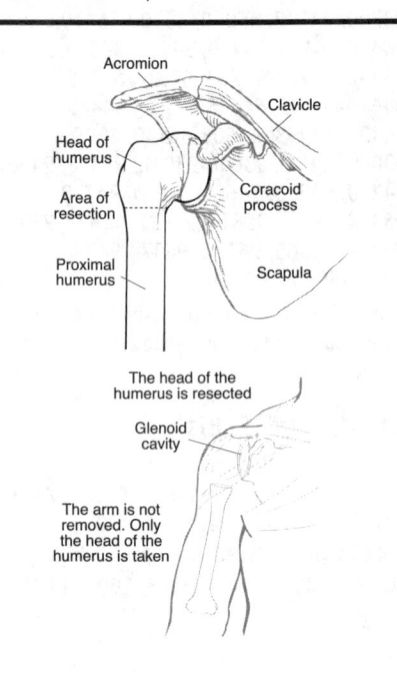

Explanation
The physician performs a resection of the humeral head. An incision is made over the joint in the upper arm and the underlying muscles are divided to expose the bone. The joint capsule is incised and tendons are removed from the bone. The physician makes a horizontal cut through the humerus just distal to the head and removes the bone. Separately reportable hemiarthroplasty to replace the proximal humeral bone with an implant for attaching the tendons and reconstructing the joint usually follows.

Coding Tips
When 23195 is performed with another separately identifiable procedure, the highest dollar value code is listed as the primary procedure and subsequent procedures are appended with modifier 51. If significant additional time and effort is documented, append modifier 22 and submit a cover letter and operative report. For radical resection of the proximal humerus for a tumor, see 23220–23222. For arthroplasty of the glenohumeral joint, see 23470–23472; for arthrodesis of the glenohumeral joint, see 23800–23802.

ICD-9-CM Procedural
77.82 Other partial ostectomy of humerus

Anesthesia
23195 01630

ICD-9-CM Diagnostic
- 170.4 Malignant neoplasm of scapula and long bones of upper limb
- 195.4 Malignant neoplasm of upper limb
- 213.4 Benign neoplasm of scapula and long bones of upper limb
- 357.1 Polyneuropathy in collagen vascular disease — (Code first underlying disease: 446.0, 710.0, 714.0)
- 359.6 Symptomatic inflammatory myopathy in diseases classified elsewhere — (Code first underlying disease: 135, 140.0-208.9, 277.30-277.39, 446.0, 710.0, 710.1, 710.2, 714.0)
- 446.0 Polyarteritis nodosa
- 710.0 Systemic lupus erythematosus — (Use additional code to identify manifestation: 424.91, 581.81, 582.81, 583.81)
- 714.0 Rheumatoid arthritis — (Use additional code to identify manifestation: 357.1, 359.6)
- 715.11 Primary localized osteoarthrosis, shoulder region
- 715.12 Primary localized osteoarthrosis, upper arm
- 715.31 Localized osteoarthrosis not specified whether primary or secondary, shoulder region
- 715.32 Localized osteoarthrosis not specified whether primary or secondary, upper arm
- 716.11 Traumatic arthropathy, shoulder region
- 716.12 Traumatic arthropathy, upper arm
- 716.61 Unspecified monoarthritis, shoulder region
- 716.62 Unspecified monoarthritis, upper arm
- 718.81 Other joint derangement, not elsewhere classified, shoulder region
- 718.82 Other joint derangement, not elsewhere classified, upper arm
- 731.3 Major osseous defects — (Code first underlying disease: 170.0-170.9, 730.00-730.29, 733.00-733.09, 733.40-733.49, 996.45)
- 733.41 Aseptic necrosis of head of humerus — (Use additional code to identify major osseous defect, if applicable: 731.3)
- 733.82 Nonunion of fracture
- 812.03 Closed fracture of greater tuberosity of humerus
- 812.09 Other closed fractures of upper end of humerus

Terms To Know
aseptic necrosis. Death of bone tissue resulting from a disruption in the vascular supply, caused by a noninfectious disease process, such as a fracture or the administration of immunosuppressive drugs.

nonunion. Failure of two ends of a fracture to mend or completely heal.

osteoarthrosis. Most common form of a noninflammatory degenerative joint disease with degenerating articular cartilage, bone enlargement, and synovial membrane changes.

polyarteritis nodosa. Systemic necrotizing vasculitis of small and medium arteries that results in the infarction and scarring within the affected organs.

CCI Version 16.3
01610, 0213T, 0216T, 0228T, 0230T, 23000, 23040, 23105, 23130, 23150, 23184, 23405, 23410-23412, 23430, 23450, 23700, 24332, 29820-29821, 36000, 36400-36410, 36420-36430, 36440, 36600, 36640, 37202, 43752, 51701-51703, 62310-62319, 64400-64435, 64445-64450, 64479, 64483, 64490, 64493, 64505-64530, 69990, 93000-93010, 93040-93042, 93318, 94002, 94200, 94250, 94680-94690, 94770, 95812-95816, 95819, 95822, 95829, 95955, 96360, 96365, 96372, 96374-96376, 99148-99149, 99150

Note: These CCI edits are used for Medicare. Other payers may reimburse on codes listed above.

Medicare Edits

	Fac RVU	Non-Fac RVU	FUD	Assist
23195	21.95	21.95	90	80

Medicare References: 100-2,15,260; 100-4,12,30; 100-4,12,90.3; 100-4,14,10

23200-23210

23200 Radical resection of tumor; clavicle
23210 scapula

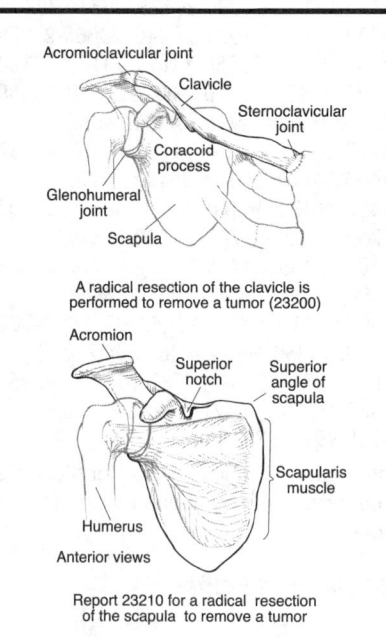

Explanation
The physician performs a radical resection of a tumor of the clavicle bone in 23200. Either end may be resected or the bone may be excised. An incision is made horizontally along the portion of the bone with the tumor to be removed. The skin and soft tissues are reflected. The acromioclavicular and/or sternoclavicular ligaments may need to be divided to free the bone from the joint at either respective end. The bone is cleared of soft tissue attachments, such as the platysma and pectoral muscles, and the diseased bone is resected with an osteotome or bone-cutting rongeurs, along with any soft tissues involved with the tumor. If the tumor is removed from one end, the remaining end of the clavicle is rounded and smoothed to eliminate the rough edge. The periosteum and soft tissues are plicated and sutured over the raw end of the clavicle. The wound is closed and a soft dressing is applied. Report 23210 if a similar procedure is performed on the scapula.

Coding Tips
For partial excision of the clavicle, see 23120 and 23180. For a total claviculectomy, see 23125. For partial excision of the scapula, see 23182 and 23190. For excision or curettage of a bone cyst of the clavicle or scapula, see 23140–23146.

ICD-9-CM Procedural
77.81 Other partial ostectomy of scapula, clavicle, and thorax (ribs and sternum)

Anesthesia
00452

ICD-9-CM Diagnostic
170.3 Malignant neoplasm of ribs, sternum, and clavicle
170.4 Malignant neoplasm of scapula and long bones of upper limb
171.0 Malignant neoplasm of connective and other soft tissue of head, face, and neck
171.4 Malignant neoplasm of connective and other soft tissue of thorax
171.7 Malignant neoplasm of connective and other soft tissue of trunk, unspecified site
198.5 Secondary malignant neoplasm of bone and bone marrow
199.0 Disseminated malignant neoplasm
209.73 Secondary neuroendocrine tumor of bone
213.3 Benign neoplasm of ribs, sternum, and clavicle
213.4 Benign neoplasm of scapula and long bones of upper limb
238.0 Neoplasm of uncertain behavior of bone and articular cartilage
239.2 Neoplasms of unspecified nature of bone, soft tissue, and skin
731.3 Major osseous defects — (Code first underlying disease: 170.0-170.9, 730.00-730.29, 733.00-733.09, 733.40-733.49, 996.45)

Terms To Know
benign. Mild or nonmalignant in nature.

disseminated. Spread over an extensive area.

malignant. Any condition tending to progress toward death, specifically an invasive tumor with a loss of cellular differentiation that has the ability to spread or metastasize to other areas in the body.

neoplasm. New abnormal growth, tumor.

osteotome. Tool used for cutting bone.

resect. Cutting out or removing a portion or all of a bone, organ, or other structure.

rongeur. Sharp-edged instrument with a scoop-tip used to cut through tissue and bone.

secondary. Second in order of occurrence or importance, or appearing during the course of another disease or condition.

soft tissue. Nonepithelial tissues outside of the skeleton that includes subcutaneous adipose tissue, fibrous tissue, fascia, muscles, blood and lymph vessels, and peripheral nervous system tissue.

CCI Version 16.3
01610, 0213T, 0216T, 0228T, 0230T, 10060, 10140, 10160, 11010-11012❖, 11040-11044, 12001-12007, 12020-12037, 13100-13101, 13120-13121, 20220-20225, 20240-20245, 23000, 23030-23035, 23065-23078, 23700, 24300, 36000, 36400-36410, 36420-36430, 36440, 36600, 36640, 37202, 43752, 51701-51703, 62310-62319, 64400-64435, 64445-64450, 64479, 64483, 64490, 64493, 64505-64530, 69990, 93000-93010, 93040-93042, 93318, 94002, 94200, 94250, 94680-94690, 94770, 95812-95816, 95819, 95822, 95829, 95955, 96360, 96365, 96372, 96374-96376, 99148-99149, 99150

Also not with 23200: 23101, 23106, 23120-23125, 23140-23146, 23170, 23180, 23480-23485

Also not with 23210: 23040, 23130-23146, 23172, 23182, 23190, 24332

Note: These CCI edits are used for Medicare. Other payers may reimburse on codes listed above.

Medicare Edits

	Fac RVU	Non-Fac RVU	FUD	Assist
23200	41.43	41.43	90	80
23210	48.48	48.48	90	80

Medicare References: None

23220

23220 Radical resection of tumor, proximal humerus

Section of right shoulder (anterior view)
Supraspinatus muscle and tendon
Acromion
Bursa
Deltoid muscle
Head of humerus
Scapula
Glenoid cavity

A radical resection of the proximal humerus is performed for a bone tumor.

Explanation

The physician performs a radical resection of a tumor of the proximal humerus. Removal of the proximal portion of the humerus is often performed for aggressive benign lesions and low-grade malignancies. A longitudinal incision is made from the acromioclavicular joint to the lateral border of the biceps tendon. The underlying muscles are divided to expose the bone. The joint capsule is incised and tendons are removed from the bone at the level of the proximal joint. The humerus is divided by a horizontal cut a few centimeters distal to the tumor site. A portion of the remaining medullary bone is taken for testing. The proximal portion of the bone is removed, along with any soft tissues involved with the tumor. Reconstructive alternatives following resection include reconstruction with flail shoulder, with passive spacer, with arthrodesis, and with arthroplasty.

Coding Tips

Grafts and prosthetic implants are included in 23221–23222 and should not be reported separately. For excision or curettage of a bone cyst or benign tumor of the proximal humerus, see 23150–23156. For partial excision of the proximal humerus, see 23184.

ICD-9-CM Procedural

77.82 Other partial ostectomy of humerus

Anesthesia

23220 01630

ICD-9-CM Diagnostic

170.4	Malignant neoplasm of scapula and long bones of upper limb
171.2	Malignant neoplasm of connective and other soft tissue of upper limb, including shoulder
198.5	Secondary malignant neoplasm of bone and bone marrow
199.0	Disseminated malignant neoplasm
209.73	Secondary neuroendocrine tumor of bone
213.4	Benign neoplasm of scapula and long bones of upper limb
238.0	Neoplasm of uncertain behavior of bone and articular cartilage
239.2	Neoplasms of unspecified nature of bone, soft tissue, and skin
731.3	Major osseous defects — (Code first underlying disease: 170.0-170.9, 730.00-730.29, 733.00-733.09, 733.40-733.49, 996.45)

Terms To Know

benign. Mild or nonmalignant in nature.

disseminated. Spread over an extensive area.

distal. Located farther away from a specified reference point.

lesion. Area of damaged tissue that has lost continuity or function, due to disease or trauma. Lesions may be located on internal structures such as the brain, nerves, or kidneys, or visible on the skin.

malignant. Any condition tending to progress toward death, specifically an invasive tumor with a loss of cellular differentiation that has the ability to spread or metastasize to other areas in the body.

proximal. Located closest to a specified reference point, usually the midline.

secondary. Second in order of occurrence or importance, or appearing during the course of another disease or condition.

soft tissue. Nonepithelial tissues outside of the skeleton that includes subcutaneous adipose tissue, fibrous tissue, fascia, muscles, blood and lymph vessels, and peripheral nervous system tissue.

CCI Version 16.3

01610, 0213T, 0216T, 0228T, 0230T, 10060, 10140, 10160, 11010-11012❖, 11040-11044, 12001-12007, 12020-12037, 13100-13101, 13120-13121, 20220-20225, 20240-20245, 23000, 23030-23035, 23040, 23065-23078, 23105, 23130, 23150-23156, 23174, 23184, 23195, 23405, 23410-23412, 23430, 23450, 23700, 23930-23935, 24065-24066, 24110-24116, 24134, 24140, 24300, 24332, 24400-24410, 36000, 36400-36410, 36420-36430, 36440, 36600, 36640, 37202, 43752, 51701-51703, 62310-62319, 64400-64435, 64445-64450, 64479, 64483, 64490, 64493, 64505-64530, 69990, 93000-93010, 93040-93042, 93318, 94002, 94200, 94250, 94680-94690, 94770, 95812-95816, 95819, 95822, 95829, 95955, 96360, 96365, 96372, 96374-96376, 99148-99149, 99150

Note: These CCI edits are used for Medicare. Other payers may reimburse on codes listed above.

Medicare Edits

	Fac RVU	Non-Fac RVU	FUD	Assist
23220	53.52	53.52	90	80

Medicare References: None

23330

23330 Removal of foreign body, shoulder; subcutaneous

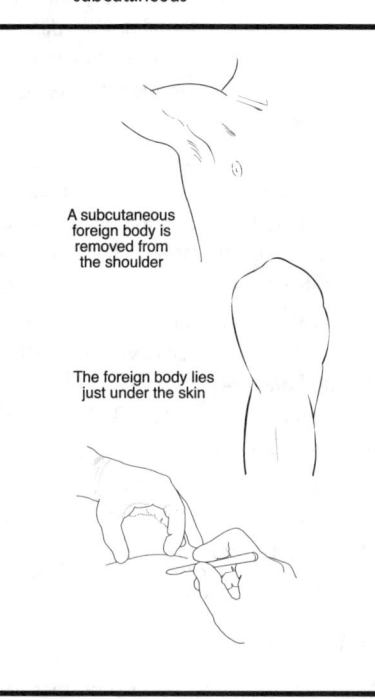

A subcutaneous foreign body is removed from the shoulder

The foreign body lies just under the skin

Explanation

The physician removes a foreign body of the shoulder. The physician makes a small incision over the foreign body and reflects the skin to expose the foreign body. It is removed and the wound is irrigated and the skin is closed with sutures or Steri-strips.

Coding Tips

For K-wire or pin insertion or removal, see 20650, 20670, and 20680. For removal of a foreign body, deep, see 23331; for complicated removal of a foreign body, see 23332.

ICD-9-CM Procedural

- 86.05 Incision with removal of foreign body or device from skin and subcutaneous tissue
- 98.27 Removal of foreign body without incision from upper limb, except hand

Anesthesia

23330 00400

ICD-9-CM Diagnostic

- 709.4 Foreign body granuloma of skin and subcutaneous tissue — (Use additional code to identify foreign body (V90.01-V90.9))
- 729.6 Residual foreign body in soft tissue — (Use additional code to identify foreign body (V90.01-V90.9))
- 880.10 Open wound of shoulder region, complicated
- 912.6 Shoulder and upper arm, superficial foreign body (splinter), without major open wound and without mention of infection
- 912.7 Shoulder and upper arm, superficial foreign body (splinter), without major open wound, infected

Terms To Know

foreign body. Any object or substance found in an organ and tissue that does not belong under normal circumstances.

granuloma. Abnormal, dense collections or cells forming a mass or nodule of chronically inflamed tissue with granulations that is usually associated with an infective process.

infection. Presence of microorganisms in body tissues that may result in cellular damage.

open wound. Opening or break of the skin.

soft tissue. Nonepithelial tissues outside of the skeleton that includes subcutaneous adipose tissue, fibrous tissue, fascia, muscles, blood and lymph vessels, and peripheral nervous system tissue.

subcutaneous tissue. Sheet or wide band of adipose (fat) and areolar connective tissue in two layers attached to the dermis.

CCI Version 16.3

01610, 0213T, 0216T, 0228T, 0230T, 11010-11012❖, 20103, 20650, 20670, 29240, 36000, 36400-36410, 36420-36430, 36440, 36600, 36640, 37202, 43752, 51701-51703, 62310-62319, 64400-64435, 64445-64450, 64479, 64483, 64490, 64493, 64505-64530, 69990, 93000-93010, 93040-93042, 93318, 94002, 94200, 94250, 94680-94690, 94770, 95812-95816, 95819, 95822, 95829, 95955, 96360, 96365, 96372, 96374-96376, 99148-99149, 99150, J0670, J2001

Note: These CCI edits are used for Medicare. Other payers may reimburse on codes listed above.

Medicare Edits

	Fac RVU	Non-Fac RVU	FUD	Assist
23330	4.35	6.63	10	80

Medicare References: 100-2,15,260; 100-4,12,30; 100-4,12,90.3; 100-4,14,10

23331-23332

23331 Removal of foreign body, shoulder; deep (eg, Neer hemiarthroplasty removal)
23332 complicated (eg, total shoulder)

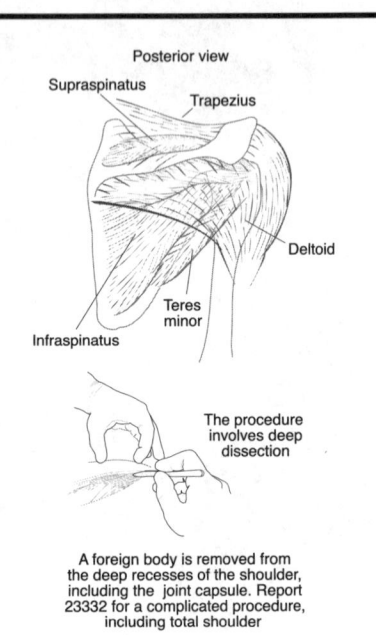

A foreign body is removed from the deep recesses of the shoulder, including the joint capsule. Report 23332 for a complicated procedure, including total shoulder

Explanation

The physician removes a foreign body from deep within the shoulder, such as an artificial shoulder joint. A long incision is made overlying the shoulder. The physician dissects through each layer of tissue down to the bones in the shoulder. The shoulder joint is exposed. The physician may debride any inflamed synovial or other scar tissues. The foreign body is removed from within the joint and from inside the humerus bone. The physician irrigates the joint with antibiotic solution. The wound is closed in layers unless there is infection present. If infection is present, the wound is left open to drain. Report 23332 if complicated, including "total shoulder."

Coding Tips

These codes should be used for removal of prosthetic implants (e.g., Neer hemiarthroplasty, total shoulder). For subcutaneous removal of a foreign body, see 23330.

ICD-9-CM Procedural

- 80.01 Arthrotomy for removal of prosthesis without replacement, shoulder
- 84.57 Removal of (cement) spacer

Anesthesia

23331 01630
23332 01638

ICD-9-CM Diagnostic

- 719.41 Pain in joint, shoulder region
- 728.82 Foreign body granuloma of muscle — (Use additional code to identify foreign body (V90.01-V90.9))
- 729.6 Residual foreign body in soft tissue — (Use additional code to identify foreign body (V90.01-V90.9))
- 731.3 Major osseous defects — (Code first underlying disease: 170.0-170.9, 730.00-730.29, 733.00-733.09, 733.40-733.49, 996.45)
- 880.10 Open wound of shoulder region, complicated
- 996.40 Unspecified mechanical complication of internal orthopedic device, implant, and graft — (Use additional code to identify prosthetic joint with mechanical complication, V43.60-V43.69)
- 996.41 Mechanical loosening of prosthetic joint — (Use additional code to identify prosthetic joint with mechanical complication, V43.60-V43.69)
- 996.42 Dislocation of prosthetic joint — (Use additional code to identify prosthetic joint with mechanical complication, V43.60-V43.69)
- 996.43 Broken prosthetic joint implant — (Use additional code to identify prosthetic joint with mechanical complication, V43.60-V43.69)
- 996.44 Peri-prosthetic fracture around prosthetic joint — (Use additional code to identify prosthetic joint with mechanical complication, V43.60-V43.69)
- 996.45 Peri-prosthetic osteolysis — (Use additional code to identify prosthetic joint with mechanical complication, V43.60-V43.69. Use additional code to identify major osseous defect, if applicable: 731.3)
- 996.47 Other mechanical complication of prosthetic joint implant — (Use additional code to identify prosthetic joint with mechanical complication, V43.60-V43.69)
- 996.49 Other mechanical complication of other internal orthopedic device, implant, and graft — (Use additional code to identify prosthetic joint with mechanical complication, V43.60-V43.69)
- 996.66 Infection and inflammatory reaction due to internal joint prosthesis — (Use additional code to identify specified infections. Use additional code to identify infected prosthetic joint: V43.60-V43.69)
- 996.67 Infection and inflammatory reaction due to other internal orthopedic device, implant, and graft — (Use additional code to identify specified infections)
- 996.78 Other complications due to other internal orthopedic device, implant, and graft — (Use additional code to identify complication: 338.18-338.19, 338.28-338.29)
- 996.79 Other complications due to other internal prosthetic device, implant, and graft — (Use additional code to identify complication: 338.18-338.19, 338.28-338.29)
- 998.59 Other postoperative infection — (Use additional code to identify infection)
- V43.61 Shoulder joint replacement by other means

Terms To Know

foreign body. Any object or substance found in an organ and tissue that does not belong under normal circumstances.

infection. Presence of microorganisms in body tissues that may result in cellular damage.

CCI Version 16.3

01610, 0213T, 0216T, 0228T, 0230T, 20103, 20670, 23000, 23100, 23105, 23405, 23450, 23700, 29820-29821, 36000, 36400-36410, 36420-36430, 36440, 36600, 36640, 37202, 43752, 51701-51703, 62310-62319, 64400-64435, 64445-64450, 64479, 64483, 64490, 64493, 64505-64530, 69990, 93000-93010, 93040-93042, 93318, 94002, 94200, 94250, 94680-94690, 94770, 95812-95816, 95819, 95822, 95829, 95955, 96360, 96365, 96372, 96374-96376, 99148-99149, 99150

Also not with 23331: 10120-10121, 23330
Also not with 23332: 10121, 23330-23331

Note: These CCI edits are used for Medicare. Other payers may reimburse on codes listed above.

Medicare Edits

	Fac RVU	Non-Fac RVU	FUD	Assist
23331	17.14	17.14	90	80
23332	25.77	25.77	90	80

Medicare References: 100-2,15,260; 100-4,12,30; 100-4,12,90.3; 100-4,14,10

23350

23350 Injection procedure for shoulder arthrography or enhanced CT/MRI shoulder arthrography

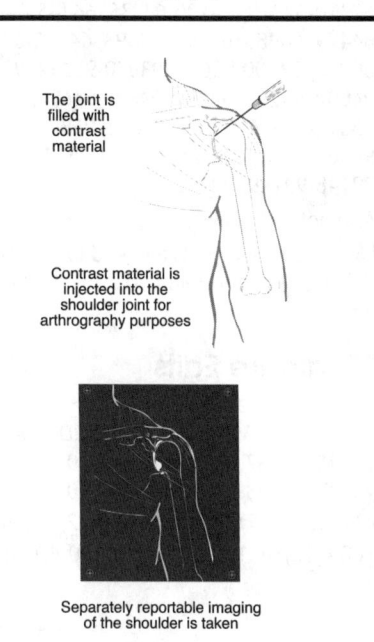

The joint is filled with contrast material

Contrast material is injected into the shoulder joint for arthrography purposes

Separately reportable imaging of the shoulder is taken

Explanation

This procedure is commonly used in the diagnosis of a rotator cuff tear. The patient is positioned supine on the x-ray table. The skin and deep tissues lateral to the coracoid process are injected with a local anesthetic. A number 20 spinal needle, 7.5 cm long, is inserted into the joint at the same location and the position is checked by separately reportable x-ray. From 15.0 ml to 20.0 ml of a suitable contrast medium is injected; resistance is felt when the joint is full. The shoulder is taken through a full range of motion and x-rays are taken to see if there is leakage of the substance to other parts of the joint and a proper diagnosis is made.

Coding Tips

For radiological supervision and interpretation of the arthrography, see 73040. When fluoroscopic-guided injection is performed for enhanced CT arthrogram, use 23350, 77002, and 73201 or 73202. When fluoroscopic-guided injection is performed for enhanced MRI arthrogram, use 23350, 77002, and 73222 or 73223. For enhanced CT or enhanced MRI arthrogram, use 77002 and 73201, 73202, 73222, or 73223.

ICD-9-CM Procedural

- 81.92 Injection of therapeutic substance into joint or ligament
- 88.32 Contrast arthrogram

Anesthesia

23350   01620

ICD-9-CM Diagnostic

- 275.40 Unspecified disorder of calcium metabolism — (Use additional code to identify any associated mental retardation)
- 275.42 Hypercalcemia — (Use additional code to identify any associated mental retardation)
- 275.49 Other disorders of calcium metabolism — (Use additional code to identify any associated mental retardation)
- 275.5 Hungry bone syndrome
- 715.11 Primary localized osteoarthrosis, shoulder region
- 715.21 Secondary localized osteoarthrosis, shoulder region
- 715.31 Localized osteoarthrosis not specified whether primary or secondary, shoulder region
- 715.91 Osteoarthrosis, unspecified whether generalized or localized, shoulder region
- 716.11 Traumatic arthropathy, shoulder region
- 716.41 Transient arthropathy, shoulder region
- 716.61 Unspecified monoarthritis, shoulder region
- 716.81 Other specified arthropathy, shoulder region
- 716.91 Unspecified arthropathy, shoulder region
- 718.01 Articular cartilage disorder, shoulder region
- 718.11 Loose body in shoulder joint
- 718.21 Pathological dislocation of shoulder joint
- 718.31 Recurrent dislocation of shoulder joint
- 718.41 Contracture of shoulder joint
- 718.71 Developmental dislocation of joint, shoulder region
- 719.01 Effusion of shoulder joint
- 719.41 Pain in joint, shoulder region
- 719.42 Pain in joint, upper arm
- 726.90 Enthesopathy of unspecified site
- 727.61 Complete rupture of rotator cuff
- 831.00 Closed dislocation of shoulder, unspecified site
- 831.01 Closed anterior dislocation of humerus
- 831.02 Closed posterior dislocation of humerus
- 831.03 Closed inferior dislocation of humerus
- 831.04 Closed dislocation of acromioclavicular (joint)
- 831.09 Closed dislocation of other site of shoulder
- 831.10 Open unspecified dislocation of shoulder
- 831.11 Open anterior dislocation of humerus
- 831.12 Open posterior dislocation of humerus
- 831.13 Open inferior dislocation of humerus
- 831.14 Open dislocation of acromioclavicular (joint)
- 831.19 Open dislocation of other site of shoulder
- 840.0 Acromioclavicular (joint) (ligament) sprain and strain
- 840.1 Coracoclavicular (ligament) sprain and strain
- 840.2 Coracohumeral (ligament) sprain and strain
- 840.3 Infraspinatus (muscle) (tendon) sprain and strain
- 840.4 Rotator cuff (capsule) sprain and strain
- 923.00 Contusion of shoulder region

CCI Version 16.3

01610, 0213T, 0216T, 0228T, 0230T, 11010-11012❖, 36000, 36400-36410, 36420-36430, 36440, 36600, 36640, 37202, 43752, 51701-51703, 62310-62319, 64400-64435, 64445-64450, 64479, 64483, 64490, 64493, 64505-64530, 69990, 72265, 76000-76001, 93000-93010, 93040-93042, 93318, 94002, 94200, 94250, 94680-94690, 94770, 95812-95816, 95819, 95822, 95829, 95955, 96360, 96365, 96372, 96374-96376, 99148-99149, 99150

Note: These CCI edits are used for Medicare. Other payers may reimburse on codes listed above.

Medicare Edits

	Fac RVU	Non-Fac RVU	FUD	Assist
23350	1.53	4.37	0	N/A

Medicare References: None

23395-23397

23395 Muscle transfer, any type, shoulder or upper arm; single
23397 multiple

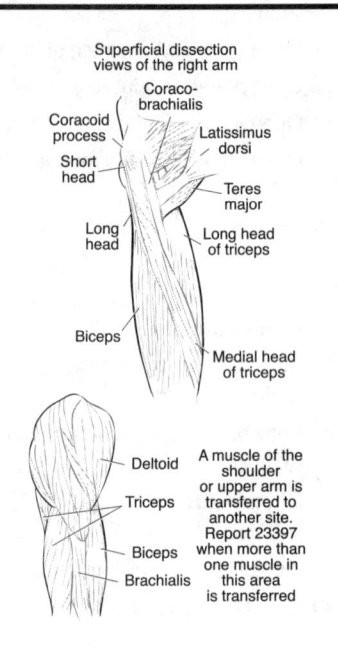

Explanation

In the case of a bicipital syndrome with rotator cuff pathology, the biceps tendon has become detached from the shoulder. The physician makes an anterior superior approach to the shoulder and splits and reflects the deltoid muscle. An acromioplasty is performed and the coracoacromial ligament is excised. The long head of the biceps tendon is identified and reattached to the humerus by tenodesis procedure. The rotator cuff is repaired prior to closure of the incisions. A soft dressing and sling are applied for two weeks. If the rotator cuff was repaired, an abduction pillow is used for four to six weeks. Report 23397 if multiple transfers are performed during the procedure.

Coding Tips

Acromioplasty and excision of coracoacromial ligament is included in this procedure and should not be reported separately.

ICD-9-CM Procedural

83.77 Muscle transfer or transplantation

Anesthesia

01610

ICD-9-CM Diagnostic

880.10 Open wound of shoulder region, complicated
880.11 Open wound of scapular region, complicated
880.12 Open wound of axillary region, complicated
880.13 Open wound of upper arm, complicated
880.19 Open wound of multiple sites of shoulder and upper arm, complicated
880.20 Open wound of shoulder region, with tendon involvement
880.21 Open wound of scapular region, with tendon involvement
880.22 Open wound of axillary region, with tendon involvement
880.23 Open wound of upper arm, with tendon involvement
880.29 Open wound of multiple sites of shoulder and upper arm, with tendon involvement
906.1 Late effect of open wound of extremities without mention of tendon injury
906.7 Late effect of burn of other extremities
927.00 Crushing injury of shoulder region — (Use additional code to identify any associated injuries: 800-829, 850.0-854.1, 860.0-869.1)
927.01 Crushing injury of scapular region — (Use additional code to identify any associated injuries: 800-829, 850.0-854.1, 860.0-869.1)
927.02 Crushing injury of axillary region — (Use additional code to identify any associated injuries: 800-829, 850.0-854.1, 860.0-869.1)
927.03 Crushing injury of upper arm — (Use additional code to identify any associated injuries: 800-829, 850.0-854.1, 860.0-869.1)
927.09 Crushing injury of multiple sites of upper arm — (Use additional code to identify any associated injuries: 800-829, 850.0-854.1, 860.0-869.1)
953.4 Injury to brachial plexus
V10.89 Personal history of malignant neoplasm of other site

Terms To Know

abduction. Pulling away from a central reference line, such as moving away from the midline of the body.

late effect. Abnormality, dysfunction, or other residual condition produced after the acute phase of an illness, injury, or disease is over. There is no time limit on when late effects can appear.

tendon. Fibrous tissue that connects muscle to bone, consisting primarily of collagen and containing little vasculature.

CCI Version 16.3

01610, 0213T, 0216T, 0228T, 0230T, 23405, 23430, 29035, 29055-29058, 29240, 36000, 36400-36410, 36420-36430, 36440, 36600, 36640, 37202, 43752, 51701-51703, 62310-62319, 64400-64435, 64445-64450, 64479, 64483, 64490, 64493, 64505-64530, 69990, 93000-93010, 93040-93042, 93318, 94002, 94200, 94250, 94680-94690, 94770, 95812-95816, 95819, 95822, 95829, 95955, 96360, 96365, 96372, 96374-96376, 99148-99149, 99150

Also not with 23397: 23395

Note: These CCI edits are used for Medicare. Other payers may reimburse on codes listed above.

Medicare Edits

	Fac RVU	Non-Fac RVU	FUD	Assist
23395	37.64	37.64	90	80
23397	33.54	33.54	90	80

Medicare References: 100-2,15,260; 100-4,12,30; 100-4,12,90.3; 100-4,14,10

23400

23400 Scapulopexy (eg, Sprengels deformity or for paralysis)

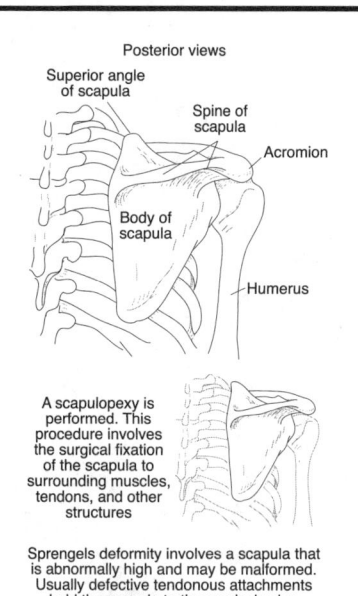

A scapulopexy is performed. This procedure involves the surgical fixation of the scapula to surrounding muscles, tendons, and other structures

Sprengels deformity involves a scapula that is abnormally high and may be malformed. Usually defective tendonous attachments hold the scapula to the cervical spine or other structures

Explanation

Sprengel's deformity is a congenital deformity where the scapula is positioned higher in the thoracic region than normal. The physician makes an incision beginning 1.0 cm superior to the middle of the scapular spine continuing medially along the spine to the medial portion of the bone and inferiorly the inferior angle of the scapula. The deep fascia is reflected back to expose the insertion of the trapezius on the scapular spine. It is reflected back along with the supraspinatus muscle. The rhomboid major and minor and levator scapula muscles are also reflected back to release the scapula from its abnormal position. If the upper portion of the bone is abnormally shaped, a portion of it may be removed. Once the scapula is normally positioned to match the opposite side, the muscles are reattached to the bone in their new orientation. A portion of the trapezius may now form a flap or may require a portion to be excised in order to take up slack in the muscle. The incision is closed with sutures and a Velpeau bandage is applied for two weeks.

Coding Tips

When this procedure is performed with another separately identifiable procedure, the highest dollar value code is listed as the primary procedure and subsequent procedures are appended with modifier 51. If significant additional time and effort is documented, append modifier 22 and submit a cover letter and operative report. For capsular contracture release, see 23020.

ICD-9-CM Procedural

78.41 Other repair or plastic operations on scapula, clavicle, and thorax (ribs and sternum)

Anesthesia

23400 00450

ICD-9-CM Diagnostic

342.10 Spastic hemiplegia affecting unspecified side
342.11 Spastic hemiplegia affecting dominant side
342.12 Spastic hemiplegia affecting nondominant side
353.0 Brachial plexus lesions
718.41 Contracture of shoulder joint
755.52 Congenital elevation of scapula

Terms To Know

congenital. Present at birth, occurring through heredity or an influence during gestation up to the moment of birth.

contracture. Shortening of muscle or connective tissue.

fascia. Fibrous sheet or band of tissue that envelops organs, muscles, and groupings of muscles.

lesion. Area of damaged tissue that has lost continuity or function, due to disease or trauma. Lesions may be located on internal structures such as the brain, nerves, or kidneys, or visible on the skin.

spastic hemiplegia. Paralytic condition affecting one side of the body marked by spasticity of the impaired muscles and an increase in tendon reflexes.

CCI Version 16.3

01610, 0213T, 0216T, 0228T, 0230T, 23190, 23395-23397, 23405, 29035, 29055-29058, 29240, 36000, 36400-36410, 36420-36430, 36440, 36600, 36640, 37202, 43752, 51701-51703, 62310-62319, 64400-64435, 64445-64450, 64479, 64483, 64490, 64493, 64505-64530, 69990, 93000-93010, 93040-93042, 93318, 94002, 94200, 94250, 94680-94690, 94770, 95812-95816, 95819, 95822, 95829, 95955, 96360, 96365, 96372, 96374-96376, 99148-99149, 99150

Note: These CCI edits are used for Medicare. Other payers may reimburse on codes listed above.

Medicare Edits

	Fac RVU	Non-Fac RVU	FUD	Assist
23400	28.47	28.47	90	80

Medicare References: 100-2,15,260; 100-4,12,30; 100-4,12,90.3; 100-4,14,10

23405-23406

23405 Tenotomy, shoulder area; single tendon
23406 multiple tendons through same incision

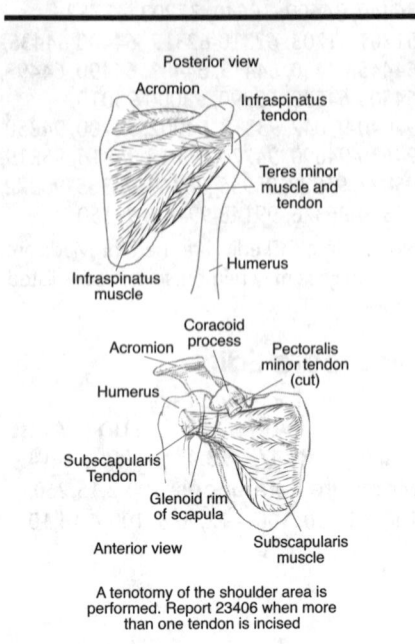

A tenotomy of the shoulder area is performed. Report 23406 when more than one tendon is incised

Explanation

These procedures may be performed if closed manipulation under anesthesia is unsuccessful to gain adequate motion of the shoulder. An incision along the anterior deltoid and pectoral region is made and the skin is reflected back to expose the underlying muscles. The subscapularis tendon is removed from the glenoid rim of the scapula. The physician may also release portions of the pectoral muscle fibers to gain further motion of the shoulder. The incision is closed with sutures and the arm is passively placed in abduction. Report 23406 if multiple tendons are released through the same incision.

Coding Tips

For tenodesis of the long tendon of biceps, see 23430; for resection or transplantation of the long tendon of biceps, see 23440. For capsular contracture release (Sever type), see 23020. For muscle transfer, any type, shoulder or upper arm, see 23395 and 23397. According to CPT guidelines, cast application or strapping (including removal) is only reported as a replacement procedure or when the cast application or strapping is an initial service performed without a restorative treatment or procedure. See "Application of Casts and Strapping" in the CPT book in the Surgery Section, under the Musculoskeletal system.

ICD-9-CM Procedural

83.13 Other tenotomy

Anesthesia
01610

ICD-9-CM Diagnostic

342.10 Spastic hemiplegia affecting unspecified side
342.11 Spastic hemiplegia affecting dominant side
342.12 Spastic hemiplegia affecting nondominant side
718.41 Contracture of shoulder joint
727.02 Giant cell tumor of tendon sheath
755.52 Congenital elevation of scapula
756.89 Other specified congenital anomaly of muscle, tendon, fascia, and connective tissue

Terms To Know

congenital. Present at birth, occurring through heredity or an influence during gestation up to the moment of birth.

contracture. Shortening of muscle or connective tissue.

fascia. Fibrous sheet or band of tissue that envelops organs, muscles, and groupings of muscles.

spastic hemiplegia. Paralytic condition affecting one side of the body marked by spasticity of the impaired muscles and an increase in tendon reflexes.

tendon. Fibrous tissue that connects muscle to bone, consisting primarily of collagen and containing little vasculature.

CCI Version 16.3

01610, 0213T, 0216T, 0228T, 0230T, 24332, 29035, 29055-29058, 29240, 36000, 36400-36410, 36420-36430, 36440, 36600, 36640, 37202, 43752, 51701-51703, 62310-62319, 64400-64435, 64445-64450, 64479, 64483, 64490, 64493, 64505-64530, 69990, 93000-93010, 93040-93042, 93318, 94002, 94200, 94250, 94680-94690, 94770, 95812-95816, 95819, 95822, 95829, 95955, 96360, 96365, 96372, 96374-96376, 99148-99149, 99150

Also not with 23406: 23405

Note: These CCI edits are used for Medicare. Other payers may reimburse on codes listed above.

Medicare Edits

	Fac RVU	Non-Fac RVU	FUD	Assist
23405	18.29	18.29	90	80
23406	22.79	22.79	90	80

Medicare References: 100-2,15,260; 100-4,12,30; 100-4,12,90.3; 100-4,14,10

23410-23412

23410 Repair of ruptured musculotendinous cuff (eg, rotator cuff) open; acute
23412 chronic

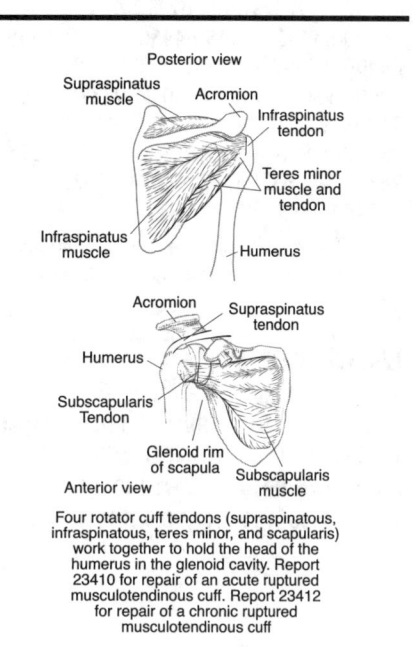

Four rotator cuff tendons (supraspinatus, infraspinatus, teres minor, and scapularis) work together to hold the head of the humerus in the glenoid cavity. Report 23410 for repair of an acute ruptured musculotendinous cuff. Report 23412 for repair of a chronic ruptured musculotendinous cuff

Explanation
The physician repairs a ruptured rotator cuff. A longitudinal incision is made along the anterior portion of the shoulder and the skin is reflected. The deltoid fibers and the underlying tissues are divided. The coracoacromial ligament is divided and the supraspinatus tendon is detached by a transverse incision along the greater tuberosity. The distal frayed edges of the tendon are removed. A trench is chiseled into the humeral bone along the level of the anatomical neck of the humerus. The supraspinatus tendon flap is buried in it. The flap is fixed with sutures tied to the tendon and passed through holes drilled in the bone. The repair is completed with side-to-side sutures of the supraspinatus to the adjacent subscapularis and infraspinatus tendons. The incision is closed and a soft dressing is applied. Protected motion in a specific progression of exercises is followed. Report 23410 if the repair is done for an acute rupture of the musculotendinous cuff and 23412 if chronic.

Coding Tips
These procedures are sometimes referred to as "mini open." For muscle transfer of the shoulder or upper arm, see 23395. For reconstruction of complete shoulder cuff avulsion, see 23420. For surgical arthroscopy with rotator cuff repair, see 29827. According to CPT guidelines, cast application or strapping (including removal) is only reported as a replacement procedure or when the cast application or strapping is an initial service performed without a restorative treatment or procedure. See "Application of Casts and Strapping" in the CPT book in the Surgery Section, under the Musculoskeletal system.

ICD-9-CM Procedural
83.63 Rotator cuff repair

Anesthesia
01610

ICD-9-CM Diagnostic
715.10 Primary localized osteoarthrosis, specified site
715.11 Primary localized osteoarthrosis, shoulder region
715.21 Secondary localized osteoarthrosis, shoulder region
715.31 Localized osteoarthrosis not specified whether primary or secondary, shoulder region
716.11 Traumatic arthropathy, shoulder region
716.61 Unspecified monoarthritis, shoulder region
719.41 Pain in joint, shoulder region
726.10 Unspecified disorders of bursae and tendons in shoulder region
727.61 Complete rupture of rotator cuff
831.00 Closed dislocation of shoulder, unspecified site
831.01 Closed anterior dislocation of humerus
831.02 Closed posterior dislocation of humerus
831.03 Closed inferior dislocation of humerus
831.10 Open unspecified dislocation of shoulder
831.11 Open anterior dislocation of humerus
831.12 Open posterior dislocation of humerus
831.13 Open inferior dislocation of humerus
840.4   Rotator cuff (capsule) sprain and strain
880.20 Open wound of shoulder region, with tendon involvement
927.00 Crushing injury of shoulder region — (Use additional code to identify any associated injuries: 800-829, 850.0-854.1, 860.0-869.1)
959.2   Injury, other and unspecified, shoulder and upper arm

Terms To Know
rotator cuff. Four muscles that originate on the scapula and form a single tendon that inserts on the head of the humerus. The supraspinatus, infraspinatus, subscapulari, and teres minor are the four muscles that come together to help lift and rotate the arm.

CCI Version 16.3
01610, 0213T, 0216T, 0228T, 0230T, 14020-14021, 23000, 23040, 23075-23076, 23130-23140, 23700, 24332, 29035, 29055-29058, 29240, 29805, 29825-29827, 36000, 36400-36410, 36420-36430, 36440, 36600, 36640, 37202, 43752, 51701-51703, 62310-62319, 64400-64435, 64445-64450, 64479, 64483, 64490, 64493, 64505-64530, 69990, 93000-93010, 93040-93042, 93318, 94002, 94200, 94250, 94680-94690, 94770, 95812-95816, 95819, 95822, 95829, 95955, 96360, 96365, 96372, 96374-96376, 99148-99149, 99150

Also not with 23410: 12034, 20103, 23412-23415, 29819-29823

Also not with 23412: 23415, 29819

Note: These CCI edits are used for Medicare. Other payers may reimburse on codes listed above.

Medicare Edits

	Fac RVU	Non-Fac RVU	FUD	Assist
23410	24.06	24.06	90	80
23412	25.04	25.04	90	80

Medicare References: 100-2,15,260; 100-4,12,30; 100-4,12,90.3; 100-4,14,10

23415

23415 Coracoacromial ligament release, with or without acromioplasty

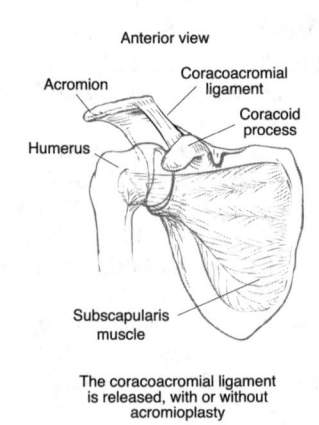

Anterior view
- Acromion
- Coracoacromial ligament
- Coracoid process
- Humerus
- Subscapularis muscle

The coracoacromial ligament is released, with or without acromioplasty

Explanation
The physician performs a coracoacromial ligament release, with or without acromioplasty. The patient is positioned on the side with the affected side up. The physician makes an incision centered over the acromioclavicular joint. The soft tissues are reflected and the ligament between the coracoid and the acromion is released. The physician may perform an acromioplasty where the underside of the acromion is reduced to allow more room for the rotator cuff tendons. Acromioplasty involves the division of the acromioclavicular ligament followed by the use of a burr to cut away the under surface of the acromion. During acromionectomy, the distal portion of the acromion is removed. Following completion, the joint is irrigated and the incisions are closed with sutures or Steri-strips.

Coding Tips
Any manipulation of the shoulder joint is included in the procedure. For arthroscopic decompression of the subacromial space with partial acromioplasty, with or without coracoacromial release, see 29826. According to CPT guidelines, cast application or strapping (including removal) is only reported as a replacement procedure or when the cast application or strapping is an initial service performed without a restorative treatment or procedure. See "Application of Casts and Strapping" in the CPT book in the Surgery Section, under the Musculoskeletal system.

ICD-9-CM Procedural
- 80.41 Division of joint capsule, ligament, or cartilage of shoulder
- 81.83 Other repair of shoulder

Anesthesia
23415 01630

ICD-9-CM Diagnostic
- 715.11 Primary localized osteoarthrosis, shoulder region
- 715.31 Localized osteoarthrosis not specified whether primary or secondary, shoulder region
- 716.11 Traumatic arthropathy, shoulder region
- 716.91 Unspecified arthropathy, shoulder region
- 719.41 Pain in joint, shoulder region
- 726.10 Unspecified disorders of bursae and tendons in shoulder region
- 726.11 Calcifying tendinitis of shoulder
- 726.2 Other affections of shoulder region, not elsewhere classified
- 727.61 Complete rupture of rotator cuff
- 840.4 Rotator cuff (capsule) sprain and strain

Terms To Know
osteoarthrosis. Most common form of a noninflammatory degenerative joint disease with degenerating articular cartilage, bone enlargement, and synovial membrane changes.

primary. Principal or first in the order of occurrence or importance.

secondary. Second in order of occurrence or importance, or appearing during the course of another disease or condition.

soft tissue. Nonepithelial tissues outside of the skeleton that includes subcutaneous adipose tissue, fibrous tissue, fascia, muscles, blood and lymph vessels, and peripheral nervous system tissue.

CCI Version 16.3
01610, 0213T, 0216T, 0228T, 0230T, 23000, 23120, 23130, 23700, 29035, 29055-29058, 29240, 29805, 29826, 36000, 36400-36410, 36420-36430, 36440, 36600, 36640, 37202, 43752, 51701-51703, 62310-62319, 64400-64435, 64445-64450, 64479, 64483, 64490, 64493, 64505-64530, 69990, 93000-93010, 93040-93042, 93318, 94002, 94200, 94250, 94680-94690, 94770, 95812-95816, 95819, 95822, 95829, 95955, 96360, 96365, 96372, 96374-96376, 99148-99149, 99150

Note: These CCI edits are used for Medicare. Other payers may reimburse on codes listed above.

Medicare Edits

	Fac RVU	Non-Fac RVU	FUD	Assist
23415	20.25	20.25	90	N/A

Medicare References: 100-2,15,260; 100-4,12,30; 100-4,12,90.3; 100-4,14,10

23420

23420 Reconstruction of complete shoulder (rotator) cuff avulsion, chronic (includes acromioplasty)

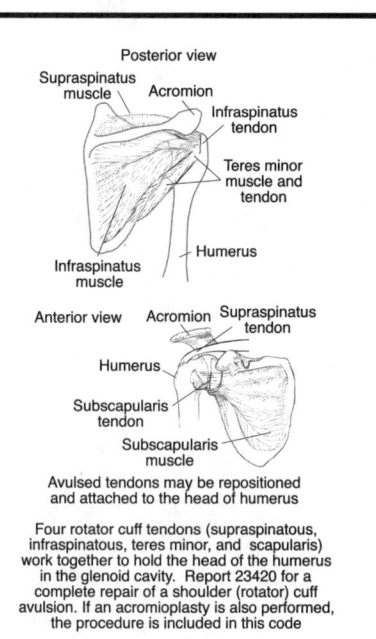

Avulsed tendons may be repositioned and attached to the head of humerus

Four rotator cuff tendons (supraspinatous, infraspinatous, teres minor, and scapularis) work together to hold the head of the humerus in the glenoid cavity. Report 23420 for a complete repair of a shoulder (rotator) cuff avulsion. If an acromioplasty is also performed, the procedure is included in this code

Explanation

The most common approach to reconstruct a massive avulsion tear of the rotator cuff is an anterior approach through an incision over the acromioclavicular joint. If the infraspinatus is to be shifted, a second incision is made along the scapular spine posteriorly. Detaching a portion of the posterior deltoid is necessary. The margins of the tear are freshened and a non-absorbable suture closes the longitudinal portion of the tear. A portion of the articular cartilage on the under side of the humeral head is removed. The raw edges of the torn tendon are brought into contact with raw bone and the ends of the sutures are passed through holes drilled through the greater tuberosity and tied over its lateral aspect. The physician performs an acromioplasty. Acromioplasty involves the division of the acromioclavicular ligament followed by a burr that is used to cut away the under surface of the acromion. During acromionectomy, the entire distal portion of the acromion is removed. Once the reconstruction is complete, the incision is closed and the arm may be positioned in an abduction splint or pillow to protect the reconstruction.

Coding Tips

Any manipulation of the shoulder joint is included in the procedure. For repair of acute ruptured musculotendinous (rotator) cuff, see 23410; for repair of chronic ruptured musculotendinous (rotator) cuff, see 23412.

For arthroscopic decompression of the subacromial space with partial acromioplasty, with or without coracoacromial release, see 29826. According to CPT guidelines, cast application or strapping (including removal) is only reported as a replacement procedure or when the cast application or strapping is an initial service performed without a restorative treatment or procedure. See "Application of Casts and Strapping" in the CPT book in the Surgery Section, under the Musculoskeletal system.

ICD-9-CM Procedural

81.82 Repair of recurrent dislocation of shoulder
83.63 Rotator cuff repair

Anesthesia

23420   01630

ICD-9-CM Diagnostic

715.11 Primary localized osteoarthrosis, shoulder region
715.21 Secondary localized osteoarthrosis, shoulder region
715.31 Localized osteoarthrosis not specified whether primary or secondary, shoulder region
716.61 Unspecified monoarthritis, shoulder region
719.41 Pain in joint, shoulder region
726.10 Unspecified disorders of bursae and tendons in shoulder region
727.61 Complete rupture of rotator cuff
840.4 Rotator cuff (capsule) sprain and strain
V64.43 Arthroscopic surgical procedure converted to open procedure

Terms To Know

bursa. Cavity or sac containing fluid that occurs between articulating surfaces and serves to reduce friction from moving parts. An anatomical structure frequently referenced in orthopedic notes as it may become diseased or need removal.

ligament. Band or sheet of fibrous tissue that connects the articular surfaces of bones or supports visceral organs.

tendon. Fibrous tissue that connects muscle to bone, consisting primarily of collagen and containing little vasculature.

CCI Version 16.3

01610, 0213T, 0216T, 0228T, 0230T, 12020, 14020-14021, 23000, 23040, 23075-23076, 23130-23140, 23180, 23410-23415, 23430-23440, 23480, 23615, 23700, 29035, 29055-29058, 29240, 29805, 29819, 29825-29827, 36000, 36400-36410, 36420-36430, 36440, 36600, 36640, 37202, 43752, 51701-51703, 62310-62319, 64400-64435, 64445-64450, 64479, 64483, 64490, 64493, 64505-64530, 64722, 69990, 93000-93010, 93040-93042, 93318, 94002, 94200, 94250, 94680-94690, 94770, 95812-95816, 95819, 95822, 95829, 95955, 96360, 96365, 96372, 96374-96376, 99148-99149, 99150

Note: These CCI edits are used for Medicare. Other payers may reimburse on codes listed above.

Medicare Edits

	Fac RVU	Non-Fac RVU	FUD	Assist
23420	28.42	28.42	90	80

Medicare References: 100-2,15,260; 100-4,12,30; 100-4,12,90.3; 100-4,14,10

23430

23430 Tenodesis of long tendon of biceps

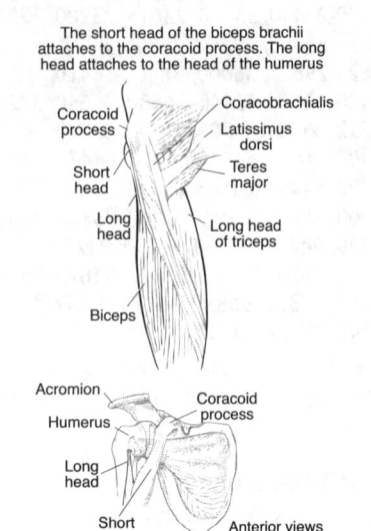

The short head of the biceps brachii attaches to the coracoid process. The long head attaches to the head of the humerus

A tenodesis of the long head of the biceps brachii is performed. The tendon may be repositioned and is reattached to the bone

Explanation
Tenodesis is performed on the long tendon of the biceps. The long head of the biceps tendon may become frayed and ruptured in chronic impingement syndrome, bicipital tenosynovitis, or degenerative conditions of the shoulder. Complete ruptures may leave a frayed proximal segment attached to the supraglenoid tubercle, which may become trapped between the humeral head and glenoid. In this case, the remaining stump of the tendon can be removed by a motorized shaver. A simultaneous subacromial decompression may be performed. Debridement of the frayed portion of the tendon may be performed.

Coding Tips
Subacromial decompression and debridement of the tendon are included in 23430 and should not be reported separately. For resection or transplantation of the long tendon of biceps, see 23440. For tenodesis of the biceps tendon at the elbow, see 24340. According to CPT guidelines, cast application or strapping (including removal) is only reported as a replacement procedure or when the cast application or strapping is an initial service performed without a restorative treatment or procedure. See "Application of Casts and Strapping" in the CPT book in the Surgery Section, under the Musculoskeletal system.

ICD-9-CM Procedural
83.88 Other plastic operations on tendon

Anesthesia
23430 01716

ICD-9-CM Diagnostic
- 718.91 Unspecified derangement, shoulder region
- 719.42 Pain in joint, upper arm
- 719.61 Other symptoms referable to shoulder joint
- 726.12 Bicipital tenosynovitis
- 727.62 Nontraumatic rupture of tendons of biceps (long head)
- 840.8 Sprain and strain of other specified sites of shoulder and upper arm
- 880.20 Open wound of shoulder region, with tendon involvement
- 927.03 Crushing injury of upper arm — (Use additional code to identify any associated injuries: 800-829, 850.0-854.1, 860.0-869.1)

Terms To Know
bicipital tenosynovitis. Inflammatory condition affecting the bicipital tendon.

open wound. Opening or break of the skin.

sprain and strain. Injuries to a joint, in which the fibers of supporting ligaments or muscles are overstretched or slightly ruptured, with the ligaments and muscles maintaining continuity.

tendon. Fibrous tissue that connects muscle to bone, consisting primarily of collagen and containing little vasculature.

CCI Version 16.3
01610, 0213T, 0216T, 0228T, 0230T, 12034, 13121, 23107, 23405, 23700, 29035, 29055-29058, 29240, 29828, 36000, 36400-36410, 36420-36430, 36440, 36600, 36640, 37202, 43752, 51701-51703, 62310-62319, 64400-64435, 64445-64450, 64479, 64483, 64490, 64493, 64505-64530, 69990, 93000-93010, 93040-93042, 93318, 94002, 94200, 94250, 94680-94690, 94770, 95812-95816, 95819, 95822, 95829, 95955, 96360, 96365, 96372, 96374-96376, 99148-99149, 99150

Note: These CCI edits are used for Medicare. Other payers may reimburse on codes listed above.

Medicare Edits

	Fac RVU	Non-Fac RVU	FUD	Assist
23430	21.65	21.65	90	80

Medicare References: 100-2,15,260; 100-4,12,30; 100-4,12,90.3; 100-4,14,10

23440

23440 Resection or transplantation of long tendon of biceps

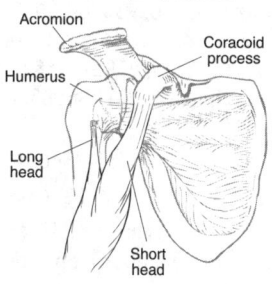

Anterior view, deep dissection

The short head of the biceps brachii attaches to the coracoid process. The long head attaches to the head of the humerus.

The long tendon of the biceps brachii is resected or transplanted

Explanation

The long tendon of the biceps is resected or transplanted. The long head of the biceps tendon is an important stabilizer of the humeral head. When the proximal end of the tendon is detached from the glenoid, it is rolled or knotted, sutured, and inserted through a keyhole-shaped opening in the cortex of the humerus in the floor of the bicipital groove. This is performed through a longitudinal incision at the anterior aspect of the shoulder. Once proper fixation is obtained, the incision is closed and the arm is supported in a sling. Active elbow flexion and shoulder elevation are limited until proper fixation and healing are complete.

Coding Tips

According to CPT guidelines, cast application or strapping (including removal) is only reported as a replacement procedure or when the cast application or strapping is an initial service performed without a restorative treatment or procedure. See "Application of Casts and Strapping" in the CPT book in the Surgery Section, under the Musculoskeletal system. For tenodesis of the long tendon of biceps, see 23430. For reinsertion of ruptured biceps tendon, distal, with or without tendon graft, see 24342.

ICD-9-CM Procedural

- 83.42 Other tenonectomy
- 83.75 Tendon transfer or transplantation

Anesthesia

23440 01610

ICD-9-CM Diagnostic

- 726.12 Bicipital tenosynovitis
- 727.62 Nontraumatic rupture of tendons of biceps (long head)
- 880.20 Open wound of shoulder region, with tendon involvement
- 880.23 Open wound of upper arm, with tendon involvement
- 927.03 Crushing injury of upper arm — (Use additional code to identify any associated injuries: 800-829, 850.0-854.1, 860.0-869.1)

Terms To Know

bicipital tenosynovitis. Inflammatory condition affecting the bicipital tendon.

open wound. Opening or break of the skin.

proximal. Located closest to a specified reference point, usually the midline.

tendon. Fibrous tissue that connects muscle to bone, consisting primarily of collagen and containing little vasculature.

CCI Version 16.3

01610, 0213T, 0216T, 0228T, 0230T, 23107, 23405, 23472❖, 23700, 29035, 29055-29058, 29240, 36000, 36400-36410, 36420-36430, 36440, 36600, 36640, 37202, 43752, 51701-51703, 62310-62319, 64400-64435, 64445-64450, 64479, 64483, 64490, 64493, 64505-64530, 69990, 93000-93010, 93040-93042, 93318, 94002, 94200, 94250, 94680-94690, 94770, 95812-95816, 95819, 95822, 95829, 95955, 96360, 96365, 96372, 96374-96376, 99148-99149, 99150

Note: These CCI edits are used for Medicare. Other payers may reimburse on codes listed above.

Medicare Edits

	Fac RVU	Non-Fac RVU	FUD	Assist
23440	22.09	22.09	90	80

Medicare References: 100-2,15,260; 100-4,12,30; 100-4,12,90.3; 100-4,14,10

23450-23455

23450 Capsulorrhaphy, anterior; Putti-Platt procedure or Magnuson type operation
23455 with labral repair (eg, Bankart procedure)

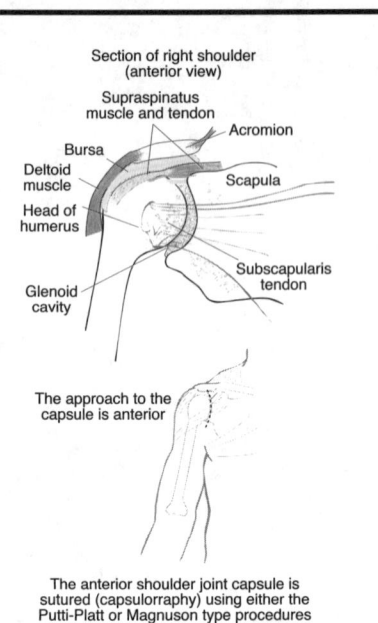

Explanation

An anterior capsulorrhaphy is performed on the shoulder in a Putti-Platt or Magnuson type operation. An anterior incision is made at the deltopectoral-pectoral interval. The coracoid process is identified and the tendon of the biceps (short head) is at times incised distal to the coracoid for exposure. The anterior capsule is visualized through a small transverse incision of the subscapularis tendon, which is tagged for identification and removed from its attachment on the capsule. The quality and laxity of the capsule are assessed and the joint is explored for damage to the labrum or glenoid. The joint is irrigated to remove any loose bodies. If there is no other abnormal laxity, the capsule is advanced superiorly and attached to the labrum with sutures. An appropriate amount of slack is taken up to provide stability within the joint. Once the capsule is reattached, the subscapularis tendon is reapproximated but not tightened and repaired. A subcutaneous drain is placed and the wound is closed. Report 23455 if a Bankart type operation with labral repair is done.

Coding Tips

According to CPT guidelines, cast application or strapping (including removal) is only reported as a replacement procedure or when the cast application or strapping is an initial service performed without a restorative treatment or procedure. See "Application of Casts and Strapping" in the CPT book in the Surgery Section, under the Musculoskeletal system. For anterior capsulorrhaphy with bone block, see code 23460; with coracoid process transfer, see code 23462. For posterior capsulorrhaphy (glenohumeral joint), see 23465 or 23466. For arthroscopic capsulorrhaphy, see 29806. For open thermal capsulorrhaphy, use unlisted procedure code 23929. For arthroscopic thermal capsulorrhaphy, use unlisted procedure code 29999.

ICD-9-CM Procedural

- 81.82 Repair of recurrent dislocation of shoulder
- 81.83 Other repair of shoulder
- 81.93 Suture of capsule or ligament of upper extremity

Anesthesia
01630

ICD-9-CM Diagnostic

- 718.21 Pathological dislocation of shoulder joint
- 718.31 Recurrent dislocation of shoulder joint
- 831.01 Closed anterior dislocation of humerus
- 831.11 Open anterior dislocation of humerus
- 840.5 Subscapularis (muscle) sprain and strain
- 840.7 Superior glenoid labrum lesions (SLAP)
- V64.43 Arthroscopic surgical procedure converted to open procedure

Terms To Know

anterior. Situated in the front area or toward the belly surface of the body; an anatomical reference point used to show the position and relationship of one body structure to another.

distal. Located farther away from a specified reference point.

pathological dislocation. Displacement of a bone or joint caused by a disease process, such as infection, lesions, or muscle weakness, and not traumatic injury.

tendon. Fibrous tissue that connects muscle to bone, consisting primarily of collagen and containing little vasculature.

CCI Version 16.3

01610, 0213T, 0216T, 0228T, 0230T, 14020-14021, 23040, 23100, 23105, 23107, 23415, 23650-23655, 23660, 23700, 29035, 29055-29058, 29240, 29805-29806, 36000, 36400-36410, 36420-36430, 36440, 36600, 36640, 37202, 43752, 51701-51703, 62310-62319, 64400-64435, 64445-64450, 64479, 64483, 64490, 64493, 64505-64530, 69990, 93000-93010, 93040-93042, 93318, 94002, 94200, 94250, 94680-94690, 94770, 95812-95816, 95819, 95822, 95829, 95955, 96360, 96365, 96372, 96374-96376, 99148-99149, 99150

Also not with 23450: 23455-23466❖

Also not with 23455: 23460-23465❖

Note: These CCI edits are used for Medicare. Other payers may reimburse on codes listed above.

Medicare Edits

	Fac RVU	Non-Fac RVU	FUD	Assist
23450	27.77	27.77	90	80
23455	29.5	29.5	90	80

Medicare References: 100-2,15,260; 100-4,12,30; 100-4,12,90.3; 100-4,14,10

23460-23462

23460 Capsulorrhaphy, anterior, any type; with bone block
23462 with coracoid process transfer

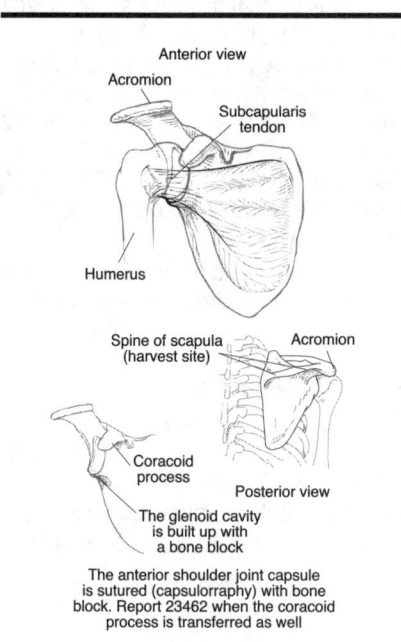

Anterior view
Acromion
Subcapularis tendon
Humerus

Spine of scapula (harvest site)
Acromion
Coracoid process
Posterior view
The glenoid cavity is built up with a bone block

The anterior shoulder joint capsule is sutured (capsulorrhaphy) with bone block. Report 23462 when the coracoid process is transferred as well

Explanation

An anterior capsulorrhaphy of any type with bone block is performed on the shoulder. If there is significant damage to the glenoid where more than one third of the glenoid is deficient, a bone block procedure is performed to increase the surface area of the glenoid. The patient is placed in a lateral position or modified beach chair position. A horizontal or vertical incision is placed inferior to the scapular spine, allowing a bone graft to be taken from the scapular spine if necessary. An additional incision is made at the lateral border of the acromion and carried posteriorly to the axillary crease. The deltoid is split to expose the infraspinatus and teres minor tendons. The capsule is exposed and incised with a T-shaped cut. The capsule is reattached to the glenoid through drill holes or by means of suture anchors taking up slack on the inferior portion of the capsule. The capsular repair may be reinforced using the infraspinatus tendon if the local tissue is felt to be insufficient. The bone block is placed on the posterior inferior portion of the glenoid fossa and fixated with a screw. This bone fragment is usually obtained from the spine of the scapula through a posterior incision. Report 23462 if the procedure is performed with coracoid process transfer.

Coding Tips

According to CPT guidelines, cast application or strapping (including removal) is only reported as a replacement procedure or when the cast application or strapping is an initial service performed without a restorative treatment or procedure. See "Application of Casts and Strapping" in the CPT book in the Surgery Section, under the Musculoskeletal system. For an anterior capsulorrhaphy, Putti-Platt procedure or Magnuson type, see 23450; for Bankhart procedure, see 23455. For capsulorrhaphy of the glenohumeral joint, see 23465 and 23466. For arthroscopic capsulorrhaphy, see 29806. For open thermal capsulorrhaphy, use unlisted procedure code 23929. For arthroscopic thermal capsulorrhaphy, use unlisted procedure code 29999.

ICD-9-CM Procedural

- 81.82 Repair of recurrent dislocation of shoulder
- 81.83 Other repair of shoulder
- 81.93 Suture of capsule or ligament of upper extremity

Anesthesia

01630

ICD-9-CM Diagnostic

- 718.21 Pathological dislocation of shoulder joint
- 718.31 Recurrent dislocation of shoulder joint
- 831.01 Closed anterior dislocation of humerus
- 831.11 Open anterior dislocation of humerus
- 840.2 Coracohumeral (ligament) sprain and strain
- 840.5 Subscapularis (muscle) sprain and strain
- 840.7 Superior glenoid labrum lesions (SLAP)
- V64.43 Arthroscopic surgical procedure converted to open procedure

Terms To Know

anterior. Situated in the front area or toward the belly surface of the body; an anatomical reference point used to show the position and relationship of one body structure to another.

joint capsule. Sac-like enclosure enveloping the synovial joint cavity with a fibrous membrane attached to the articular ends of the bones in the joint.

pathological dislocation. Displacement of a bone or joint caused by a disease process, such as infection, lesions, or muscle weakness, and not traumatic injury.

posterior. Located in the back part or caudal end of the body.

tendon. Fibrous tissue that connects muscle to bone, consisting primarily of collagen and containing little vasculature.

CCI Version 16.3

01610, 0213T, 0216T, 0228T, 0230T, 14020-14021, 23040, 23100, 23105, 23107, 23415, 23465❖, 23650-23655, 23660, 23700, 29035, 29055-29058, 29240, 29805-29806, 36000, 36400-36410, 36420-36430, 36440, 36600, 36640, 37202, 43752, 51701-51703, 62310-62319, 64400-64435, 64445-64450, 64479, 64483, 64490, 64493, 64505-64530, 69990, 93000-93010, 93040-93042, 93318, 94002, 94200, 94250, 94680-94690, 94770, 95812-95816, 95819, 95822, 95829, 95955, 96360, 96365, 96372, 96374-96376, 99148-99149, 99150

Also not with 23460: 20900-20902
Also not with 23462: 20690, 20692

Note: These CCI edits are used for Medicare. Other payers may reimburse on codes listed above.

Medicare Edits

	Fac RVU	Non-Fac RVU	FUD	Assist
23460	32.04	32.04	90	80
23462	31.49	31.49	90	80

Medicare References: 100-2,15,260; 100-4,12,30; 100-4,12,90.3; 100-4,14,10

23465

23465 Capsulorrhaphy, glenohumeral joint, posterior, with or without bone block

Posterior views
Supraspinatus muscle, Acromion, Supraspinatus tendon, Capsule of shoulder joint, Scapula, Humerus, Deep dissection

Spine of scapula, Supraspinatus muscle, Acromion, Teres minor muscle, Infraspinatus muscle, Humerus

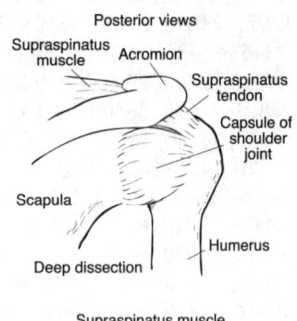

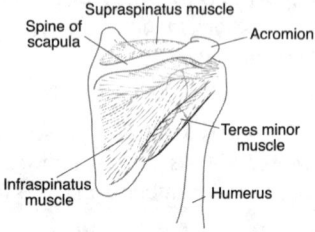

The posterior glenohumeral joint is sutured, with or without bone block graft

Explanation

A posterior capsulorrhaphy of the glenohumeral joint is done with or without bone block. The patient is placed in a lateral position or modified beach chair position. A horizontal or vertical incision is placed inferior to the scapular spine, allowing a bone graft to be taken from the scapular spine if necessary. An additional incision is made at the lateral border of the acromion and carried posteriorly to the axillary crease. The deltoid is split to expose the infraspinatus and teres minor tendons. The capsule is exposed and incised with a T-shaped cut. The capsule is reattached to the glenohumeral joint through drill holes or by means of suture anchors taking up slack on the inferior portion of the capsule. The capsular repair may be reinforced using the infraspinatus tendon if the local tissue is felt to be insufficient. When a bone block is used, it is placed at the posterior inferior quadrant of the glenohumeral joint to increase the articulation surface of the glenoid. This technique is rarely used. Once the incision is closed, the arm is placed in an Orthoplast splint with the arm in external rotation for the first six weeks. Motion is protected.

Coding Tips

According to CPT guidelines, cast application or strapping (including removal) is only reported as a replacement procedure or when the cast application or strapping is an initial service performed without a restorative treatment or procedure. See "Application of Casts and Strapping" in the CPT book in the Surgery section, under the musculoskeletal system. For a capsulorrhaphy of the glenohumeral joint for any type of multi-directional instability, see 23466. For an anterior capsulorrhaphy, Putti-Platt procedure or Magnuson type, see 23450; for Bankhart procedure, see 23455. For arthroscopic capsulorrhaphy, see 29806. For open thermal capsulorrhaphy, use unlisted procedure code 23929. For arthroscopic thermal capsulorrhaphy, use unlisted procedure code 29999. For sternoclavicular reconstruction, see 23530. For acromioclavicular reconstruction, see 23550.

ICD-9-CM Procedural

- 81.82 Repair of recurrent dislocation of shoulder
- 81.83 Other repair of shoulder
- 81.93 Suture of capsule or ligament of upper extremity

Anesthesia
23465 01630

ICD-9-CM Diagnostic

- 718.21 Pathological dislocation of shoulder joint
- 718.31 Recurrent dislocation of shoulder joint
- 831.00 Closed dislocation of shoulder, unspecified site
- 831.02 Closed posterior dislocation of humerus
- 831.10 Open unspecified dislocation of shoulder
- 831.12 Open posterior dislocation of humerus
- 840.4 Rotator cuff (capsule) sprain and strain
- V64.43 Arthroscopic surgical procedure converted to open procedure

Terms To Know

joint capsule. Sac-like enclosure enveloping the synovial joint cavity with a fibrous membrane attached to the articular ends of the bones in the joint.

pathological dislocation. Displacement of a bone or joint caused by a disease process, such as infection, lesions, or muscle weakness, and not traumatic injury.

posterior. Located in the back part or caudal end of the body.

tendon. Fibrous tissue that connects muscle to bone, consisting primarily of collagen and containing little vasculature.

CCI Version 16.3

01610, 0213T, 0216T, 0228T, 0230T, 23040, 23100, 23105, 23107, 23415, 23650-23655, 23660, 23700, 24332, 29035, 29055-29058, 29240, 29805-29806, 36000, 36400-36410, 36420-36430, 36440, 36600, 36640, 37202, 43752, 51701-51703, 62310-62319, 64400-64435, 64445-64450, 64479, 64483, 64490, 64493, 64505-64530, 69990, 93000-93010, 93040-93042, 93318, 94002, 94200, 94250, 94680-94690, 94770, 95812-95816, 95819, 95822, 95829, 95955, 96360, 96365, 96372, 96374-96376, 99148-99149, 99150

Note: These CCI edits are used for Medicare. Other payers may reimburse on codes listed above.

Medicare Edits

	Fac RVU	Non-Fac RVU	FUD	Assist
23465	32.77	32.77	90	80

Medicare References: 100-2,15,260; 100-4,12,30; 100-4,12,90.3; 100-4,14,10

23466

23466 Capsulorrhaphy, glenohumeral joint, any type multi-directional instability

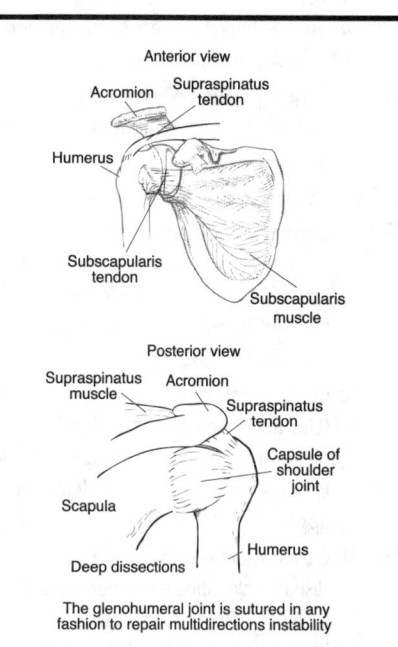

Anterior view
Acromion, Supraspinatus tendon, Humerus, Subscapularis tendon, Subscapularis muscle

Posterior view
Supraspinatus muscle, Acromion, Supraspinatus tendon, Capsule of shoulder joint, Scapula, Humerus, Deep dissections

The glenohumeral joint is sutured in any fashion to repair multidirections instability

Explanation
A capsulorrhaphy of the glenohumeral joint for any type multidirectional instability is done. The surgical approach may differ from patient to patient depending upon the patient's history. The incision is determined by the side of most significant instability. A separately reportable arthroscopic examination of the shoulder should be performed first to fully determine the extent of damage to the joint and the appropriate surgical approach. An anterior H-plasty is commonly used to tighten the capsule. In some cases, both medial and lateral capsular incisions may be required to provide sufficient capsular tension.

Coding Tips
According to CPT guidelines, cast application or strapping (including removal) is only reported as a replacement procedure or when the cast application or strapping is an initial service performed without a restorative treatment or procedure. See "Application of Casts and Strapping" in the CPT book in the Surgery section, under the musculoskeletal system. For capsulorrhaphy of the posterior glenohumeral joint, with or without bone block, see 23465. For arthroscopic capsulorrhaphy, see 29806. For open thermal capsulorrhaphy, use unlisted procedure code 23929. For arthroscopic thermal capsulorrhaphy, use unlisted procedure code 29999.

ICD-9-CM Procedural
81.82 Repair of recurrent dislocation of shoulder
81.83 Other repair of shoulder
81.93 Suture of capsule or ligament of upper extremity

Anesthesia
23466 01630

ICD-9-CM Diagnostic
718.21 Pathological dislocation of shoulder joint
718.31 Recurrent dislocation of shoulder joint
831.00 Closed dislocation of shoulder, unspecified site
831.01 Closed anterior dislocation of humerus
831.02 Closed posterior dislocation of humerus
831.03 Closed inferior dislocation of humerus
831.10 Open unspecified dislocation of shoulder
831.11 Open anterior dislocation of humerus
831.12 Open posterior dislocation of humerus
831.13 Open inferior dislocation of humerus
840.4 Rotator cuff (capsule) sprain and strain
V64.43 Arthroscopic surgical procedure converted to open procedure

Terms To Know
anterior. Situated in the front area or toward the belly surface of the body; an anatomical reference point used to show the position and relationship of one body structure to another.

lateral. To/on the side.

medial. Middle or midline.

pathological dislocation. Displacement of a bone or joint caused by a disease process, such as infection, lesions, or muscle weakness, and not traumatic injury.

posterior. Located in the back part or caudal end of the body.

CCI Version 16.3
01610, 0213T, 0216T, 0228T, 0230T, 14020-14021, 20690, 20692, 23040, 23100, 23105, 23107, 23415, 23455-23465❖, 23650-23655, 23660, 23700, 24332, 29035, 29055-29058, 29240, 29805-29806, 36000, 36400-36410, 36420-36430, 36440, 36600, 36640, 37202, 43752, 51701-51703, 62310-62319, 64400-64435, 64445-64450, 64479, 64483, 64490, 64493, 64505-64530, 69990, 93000-93010, 93040-93042, 93318, 94002, 94200, 94250, 94680-94690, 94770, 95812-95816, 95819, 95822, 95829, 95955, 96360, 96365, 96372, 96374-96376, 99148-99149, 99150

Note: These CCI edits are used for Medicare. Other payers may reimburse on codes listed above.

Medicare Edits

	Fac RVU	Non-Fac RVU	FUD	Assist
23466	32.73	32.73	90	80

Medicare References: 100-2,15,260; 100-4,12,30; 100-4,12,90.3; 100-4,14,10

23470

23470 Arthroplasty, glenohumeral joint; hemiarthroplasty

Explanation
Hemiarthroplasty is performed on the glenohumeral joint. A long curved incision is made from the superior aspect of the acromion along the deltopectoral interval to the deltoid insertion. The deltoid is retracted laterally and the pectoralis medially. The fascia between the pectoralis and the clavicle is divided and the subacromial space is freed with a gloved finger or periosteal elevator. The coracoacromial ligament is freed and often an acromioplasty is performed to allow for freedom of movement after surgery. The subscapularis tendon is tagged and removed from the capsule. The anterior joint capsule is divided and the glenohumeral joint is dislocated by further external rotation and extension of the arm. The joint is explored and all loose bodies are removed. The humeral head is removed with a reciprocating saw or osteotome. A trial prosthesis is placed along the proximal humerus as a guide for proper inclination of the osteotomy. A horizontal cut (osteotomy) is made as previously determined and a large curette is used to open the medullary canal for placement of the stem of the prosthesis. The canal is enlarged with a reamer to the appropriate size. The prosthesis is positioned in proper rotational alignment to articulate with the glenoid. Any remaining osteophytes (bone spurs) are removed. The joint is irrigated. The prosthesis is reduced into the glenoid and the subscapularis tendon is sutured in place with multiple interrupted non-absorbable sutures with the shoulder in neutral position. The deltopectoral interval is closed loosely over drainage tubes. The arm is placed in a sling and swathe bandage.

Coding Tips
If significant additional time and effort is documented, append modifier 22 and submit a cover letter and operative report.

ICD-9-CM Procedural
- 81.81 Partial shoulder replacement
- 81.97 Revision of joint replacement of upper extremity

Anesthesia
23470 01630

ICD-9-CM Diagnostic
- 170.4 Malignant neoplasm of scapula and long bones of upper limb
- 171.2 Malignant neoplasm of connective and other soft tissue of upper limb, including shoulder
- 198.5 Secondary malignant neoplasm of bone and bone marrow
- 238.0 Neoplasm of uncertain behavior of bone and articular cartilage
- 239.2 Neoplasms of unspecified nature of bone, soft tissue, and skin
- 357.1 Polyneuropathy in collagen vascular disease — (Code first underlying disease: 446.0, 710.0, 714.0)
- 359.6 Symptomatic inflammatory myopathy in diseases classified elsewhere — (Code first underlying disease: 135, 140.0-208.9, 277.30-277.39, 446.0, 710.0, 710.1, 710.2, 714.0)
- 446.0 Polyarteritis nodosa
- 710.0 Systemic lupus erythematosus — (Use additional code to identify manifestation: 424.91, 581.81, 582.81, 583.81)
- 714.0 Rheumatoid arthritis — (Use additional code to identify manifestation: 357.1, 359.6)
- 715.11 Primary localized osteoarthrosis, shoulder region
- 715.21 Secondary localized osteoarthrosis, shoulder region
- 715.31 Localized osteoarthrosis not specified whether primary or secondary, shoulder region
- 715.91 Osteoarthrosis, unspecified whether generalized or localized, shoulder region
- 716.11 Traumatic arthropathy, shoulder region
- 716.81 Other specified arthropathy, shoulder region
- 718.01 Articular cartilage disorder, shoulder region
- 726.10 Unspecified disorders of bursae and tendons in shoulder region
- 726.19 Other specified disorders of rotator cuff syndrome of shoulder and allied disorders
- 727.61 Complete rupture of rotator cuff
- 730.11 Chronic osteomyelitis, shoulder region — (Use additional code to identify organism: 041.1. Use additional code to identify major osseous defect, if applicable: 731.3)
- 730.12 Chronic osteomyelitis, upper arm — (Use additional code to identify organism: 041.1. Use additional code to identify major osseous defect, if applicable: 731.3)
- 730.81 Other infections involving bone diseases classified elsewhere, shoulder region — (Use additional code to identify organism: 041.1. Code first underlying disease: 002.0, 015.0-015.9)
- 731.3 Major osseous defects — (Code first underlying disease: 170.0-170.9, 730.00-730.29, 733.00-733.09, 733.40-733.49, 996.45)
- 733.41 Aseptic necrosis of head of humerus — (Use additional code to identify major osseous defect, if applicable: 731.3)

CCI Version 16.3
01610, 0213T, 0216T, 0228T, 0230T, 23040, 23100, 23105, 23107, 23130, 23150-23156, 23182, 23184, 23410-23450, 23616❖, 24332, 24515, 29035, 29055-29058, 29240, 29820-29823, 29825, 36000, 36400-36410, 36420-36430, 36440, 36600, 36640, 37202, 43752, 51701-51703, 62310-62319, 64400-64435, 64445-64450, 64479, 64483, 64490, 64493, 64505-64530, 69990, 93000-93010, 93040-93042, 93318, 94002, 94200, 94250, 94680-94690, 94770, 95812-95816, 95819, 95822, 95829, 95955, 96360, 96365, 96372, 96374-96376, 99148-99149, 99150

Note: These CCI edits are used for Medicare. Other payers may reimburse on codes listed above.

Medicare Edits

	Fac RVU	Non-Fac RVU	FUD	Assist
23470	35.57	35.57	90	80

Medicare References: None

23472

23472 Arthroplasty, glenohumeral joint; total shoulder (glenoid and proximal humeral replacement (eg, total shoulder))

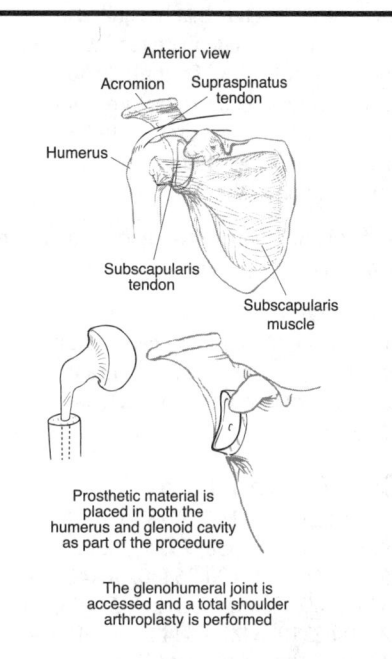

Explanation

A total shoulder replacement is done for the glenohumeral joint. A long curved incision is made from the superior aspect of the acromion along the deltopectoral interval to the deltoid insertion. The deltoid is retracted laterally and pectoralis medially. The fascia between the pectoralis and the clavicle is divided and the subacromial space is freed with a gloved finger or periosteal elevator. The coracoacromial ligament is freed and often an acromioplasty is performed to allow for freedom of movement after surgery. The subscapularis tendon is tagged and removed from the capsule. The anterior joint capsule is divided and the glenohumeral joint is dislocated by further external rotation and extension of the arm. The joint is explored and all loose bodies are removed. The humeral head is removed with a reciprocating saw or osteotome. In addition, a prosthetic device is placed proximally at the glenoid to articulate with the prosthetic humeral head. Prior to placement of the humeral prosthesis, the joint is opened to fully expose the glenoid surface. The surface cartilage of the glenoid is removed. A power drill is used to cut a slot into the glenoid the exact size of the holding device of the glenoid component. Small curettes are used to remove cancellous bone from the base of the coracoid bone. With a bur, articular cartilage is removed from the surface of the glenoid. A trial glenoid component is used to properly prepare the bone and fit the prosthesis. Once the glenoid preparation is complete, the glenoid vault is drilled and filled with polymethylmethacrylate (bone cement). The glenoid component is pushed into place and held until the cement is cured. Prior to final insertion of the humeral component, an anterior acromioplasty and acromioclavicular arthroplasty are performed, if necessary. If large rotator cuff tears are found, they are repaired at this time. The joint is brought through a full range of motion and fully irrigated. The subscapularis tendon is repaired to stabilize the joint; however, the joint capsule is not usually resutured. Drains are placed and the deltopectoral interval is sutured closed. The arm is placed in a sling and swathe.

Coding Tips

If significant additional time and effort is documented, append modifier 22 and submit a cover letter and operative report. If a partial hemiplasty is performed, see 23470. Report removal of total shoulder implants, 23331 or 23332, in addition to 23472, when a revision procedure is performed. For an osteotomy of the proximal humerus, see 24400.

ICD-9-CM Procedural

81.80	Other total shoulder replacement
81.88	Reverse total shoulder replacement
81.97	Revision of joint replacement of upper extremity

Anesthesia

23472 01638

ICD-9-CM Diagnostic

170.4	Malignant neoplasm of scapula and long bones of upper limb
171.2	Malignant neoplasm of connective and other soft tissue of upper limb, including shoulder
198.5	Secondary malignant neoplasm of bone and bone marrow
357.1	Polyneuropathy in collagen vascular disease — (Code first underlying disease: 446.0, 710.0, 714.0)
710.1	Systemic sclerosis — (Use additional code to identify manifestation: 359.6, 517.2)
710.2	Sicca syndrome
714.0	Rheumatoid arthritis — (Use additional code to identify manifestation: 357.1, 359.6)
715.11	Primary localized osteoarthrosis, shoulder region
715.21	Secondary localized osteoarthrosis, shoulder region
715.31	Localized osteoarthrosis not specified whether primary or secondary, shoulder region
715.91	Osteoarthrosis, unspecified whether generalized or localized, shoulder region
716.11	Traumatic arthropathy, shoulder region
718.01	Articular cartilage disorder, shoulder region
730.11	Chronic osteomyelitis, shoulder region — (Use additional code to identify organism: 041.1. Use additional code to identify major osseous defect, if applicable: 731.3)
733.41	Aseptic necrosis of head of humerus — (Use additional code to identify major osseous defect, if applicable: 731.3)
733.81	Malunion of fracture
733.82	Nonunion of fracture
927.00	Crushing injury of shoulder region — (Use additional code to identify any associated injuries: 800-829, 850.0-854.1, 860.0-869.1)

CCI Version 16.3

01610, 0213T, 0216T, 0228T, 0230T, 23040, 23100, 23105, 23107, 23130, 23150-23156, 23184, 23410-23430, 23450, 23470, 24332, 29035, 29055-29058, 29240, 29820-29823, 29825, 36000, 36400-36410, 36420-36430, 36440, 36600, 36640, 37202, 43752, 51701-51703, 62310-62319, 64400-64435, 64445-64450, 64479, 64483, 64490, 64493, 64505-64530, 69990, 93000-93010, 93040-93042, 93318, 94002, 94200, 94250, 94680-94690, 94770, 95812-95816, 95819, 95822, 95829, 95955, 96360, 96365, 96372, 96374-96376, 99148-99149, 99150

Note: These CCI edits are used for Medicare. Other payers may reimburse on codes listed above.

Medicare Edits

	Fac RVU	Non-Fac RVU	FUD	Assist
23472	44.07	44.07	90	80

Medicare References: None

23480-23485

23480 Osteotomy, clavicle, with or without internal fixation;

23485 with bone graft for nonunion or malunion (includes obtaining graft and/or necessary fixation)

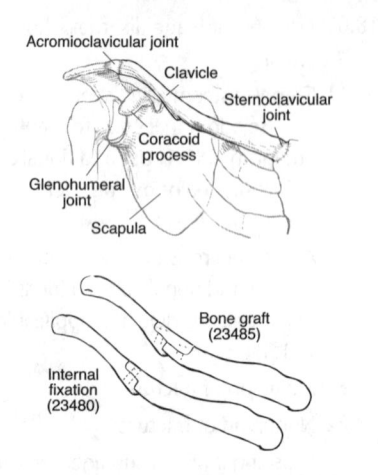

The clavicle is surgically accessed and cut as required (osteotomy). The bone is reapproximated and may be fixed with screws, plates, or wires. Report 23485 when a bone graft is used to repair nonunion or malunion

Explanation

The physician performs an osteotomy of the clavicle. The physician makes an incision in the skin overlying the clavicle. Tissue is dissected down to the bone. Using a surgical saw or other sharp instrument, the physician cuts through the bone. Surgical screws, a metal plate, or wires may secure the cut bone in the correct position. The wound is irrigated with antibiotic solution and the skin is closed in layers. In 23485, the physician performs an osteotomy of the clavicle that is not healing or has healed in an unacceptable position. The physician harvests a bone graft from the patient through a separate incision and places it, with the help of implants, onto the clavicle.

Coding Tips

According to CPT guidelines, cast application or strapping (including removal) is only reported as a replacement procedure or when the cast application or strapping is an initial service performed without a restorative treatment or procedure. See "Application of Casts and Strapping" in the CPT book in the Surgery Section, under the Musculoskeletal system. Internal fixation (23480) and obtaining the bone graft (23485) is included and should not be reported separately. For removal of internal fixation, see 23330–23332.

ICD-9-CM Procedural

- 77.21 Wedge osteotomy of scapula, clavicle, and thorax (ribs and sternum)
- 77.31 Other division of scapula, clavicle, and thorax (ribs and sternum)
- 77.71 Excision of scapula, clavicle, and thorax (ribs and sternum) for graft
- 77.77 Excision of tibia and fibula for graft
- 77.79 Excision of other bone for graft, except facial bones
- 78.01 Bone graft of scapula, clavicle, and thorax (ribs and sternum)
- 78.41 Other repair or plastic operations on scapula, clavicle, and thorax (ribs and sternum)

Anesthesia
00450

ICD-9-CM Diagnostic

- 170.3 Malignant neoplasm of ribs, sternum, and clavicle
- 213.3 Benign neoplasm of ribs, sternum, and clavicle
- 730.11 Chronic osteomyelitis, shoulder region — (Use additional code to identify organism: 041.1. Use additional code to identify major osseous defect, if applicable: 731.3)
- 731.3 Major osseous defects — (Code first underlying disease: 170.0-170.9, 730.00-730.29, 733.00-733.09, 733.40-733.49, 996.45)
- 733.81 Malunion of fracture
- 733.82 Nonunion of fracture
- 738.8 Acquired musculoskeletal deformity of other specified site
- 755.51 Congenital deformity of clavicle
- 905.1 Late effect of fracture of spine and trunk without mention of spinal cord lesion

Terms To Know

benign. Mild or nonmalignant in nature.

chronic. Persistent, continuing, or recurring.

congenital. Present at birth, occurring through heredity or an influence during gestation up to the moment of birth.

late effect. Abnormality, dysfunction, or other residual condition produced after the acute phase of an illness, injury, or disease is over. There is no time limit on when late effects can appear.

malignant. Any condition tending to progress toward death, specifically an invasive tumor with a loss of cellular differentiation that has the ability to spread or metastasize to other areas in the body.

malunion. Fracture that has united in a faulty position due to inadequate reduction of the original fracture, insufficient holding of a previously well-reduced fracture, contracture of the soft tissues, or comminuted or osteoporotic bone causing a slow disintegration of the fracture.

nonunion. Failure of two ends of a fracture to mend or completely heal.

osteomyelitis. Inflammation of bone that may remain localized or spread to the marrow, cortex, or periosteum, in response to an infecting organism, usually bacterial and pyogenic.

CCI Version 16.3

01610, 0213T, 0216T, 0228T, 0230T, 23180, 29035, 29055-29058, 29240, 36000, 36400-36410, 36420-36430, 36440, 36600, 36640, 37202, 43752, 51701-51703, 62310-62319, 64400-64435, 64445-64450, 64479, 64483, 64490, 64493, 64505-64530, 69990, 93000-93010, 93040-93042, 93318, 94002, 94200, 94250, 94680-94690, 94770, 95812-95816, 95819, 95822, 95829, 95955, 96360, 96365, 96372, 96374-96376, 99148-99149, 99150

Also not with 23485: 20680, 20900-20902, 23480

Note: These CCI edits are used for Medicare. Other payers may reimburse on codes listed above.

Medicare Edits

	Fac RVU	Non-Fac RVU	FUD	Assist
23480	23.97	23.97	90	N/A
23485	28.15	28.15	90	80

Medicare References: 100-2,15,260; 100-4,12,30; 100-4,12,90.3; 100-4,14,10

23490-23491

23490 Prophylactic treatment (nailing, pinning, plating or wiring) with or without methylmethacrylate; clavicle
23491 proximal humerus

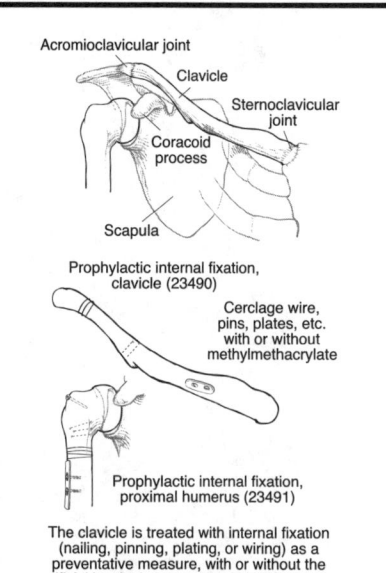

The clavicle is treated with internal fixation (nailing, pinning, plating, or wiring) as a preventative measure, with or without the artificial hardening agent methylmethacrylate. Report 23491 when the proximal humerus is similarly treated

Explanation

The physician performs a preventative nailing, plating, pinning, or wiring of the clavicle to the coracoid process in order to gain better fixation and prevent further dislocation of the acromioclavicular joint. Access to the joint is obtained through a lateral incision over the acromion process. The skin and soft tissues are reflected. The screw or other fixation device of choice is positioned and may be checked by separately reportable x-ray. The procedure may be accomplished with the use of methylmethacrylate, which can be injected into a weak or defective bone area and hardens to act like a bone cement. The incision is closed with sutures and movement is restricted for four to six weeks. The hardware is removed when stability is determined. Report 23491 for similar prophylactic treatment of the proximal humerus.

Coding Tips

According to CPT guidelines, cast application or strapping (including removal) is only reported as a replacement procedure or when the cast application or strapping is an initial service performed without a restorative treatment or procedure. See "Application of Casts and Strapping" in the CPT book in the Surgery Section, under the Musculoskeletal system. For removal of hardware, see 23330–23332. For treatment of a clavicular fracture, see 23500–23515. For prophylactic treatment of the humeral shaft, see 24498. For radiology services, see 73000, 73020, 73030, and 73060.

ICD-9-CM Procedural

78.51 Internal fixation of scapula, clavicle, and thorax (ribs and sternum) without fracture reduction
78.52 Internal fixation of humerus without fracture reduction
84.55 Insertion of bone void filler

Anesthesia

23490 00450
23491 01630

ICD-9-CM Diagnostic

170.4 Malignant neoplasm of scapula and long bones of upper limb
198.5 Secondary malignant neoplasm of bone and bone marrow
238.0 Neoplasm of uncertain behavior of bone and articular cartilage
239.2 Neoplasms of unspecified nature of bone, soft tissue, and skin
731.3 Major osseous defects — (Code first underlying disease: 170.0-170.9, 730.00-730.29, 733.00-733.09, 733.40-733.49, 996.45)
733.00 Unspecified osteoporosis — (Use additional code to identify major osseous defect, if applicable: 731.3) (Use additional code to identify personal history of pathologic (healed) fracture: V13.51)
733.01 Senile osteoporosis — (Use additional code to identify major osseous defect, if applicable: 731.3) (Use additional code to identify personal history of pathologic (healed) fracture: V13.51)
733.02 Idiopathic osteoporosis — (Use additional code to identify major osseous defect, if applicable: 731.3) (Use additional code to identify personal history of pathologic (healed) fracture: V13.51)
733.7 Algoneurodystrophy
831.00 Closed dislocation of shoulder, unspecified site
831.01 Closed anterior dislocation of humerus
831.02 Closed posterior dislocation of humerus
831.03 Closed inferior dislocation of humerus
831.04 Closed dislocation of acromioclavicular (joint)
831.10 Open unspecified dislocation of shoulder
831.11 Open anterior dislocation of humerus
831.12 Open posterior dislocation of humerus
831.13 Open inferior dislocation of humerus
831.14 Open dislocation of acromioclavicular (joint)

Terms To Know

algoneurodystrophy. Neuropathy of the peripheral nervous system.

malignant. Any condition tending to progress toward death, specifically an invasive tumor with a loss of cellular differentiation that has the ability to spread or metastasize to other areas in the body.

neoplasm. New abnormal growth, tumor.

proximal. Located closest to a specified reference point, usually the midline.

secondary. Second in order of occurrence or importance, or appearing during the course of another disease or condition.

soft tissue. Nonepithelial tissues outside of the skeleton that includes subcutaneous adipose tissue, fibrous tissue, fascia, muscles, blood and lymph vessels, and peripheral nervous system tissue.

CCI Version 16.3

01610, 0213T, 0216T, 0228T, 0230T, 20690, 20692, 20696-20697, 29035, 29055-29058, 29240, 36000, 36400-36410, 36420-36430, 36440, 36600, 36640, 37202, 43752, 51701-51703, 62310-62319, 64400-64435, 64445-64450, 64479, 64483, 64490, 64493, 64505-64530, 69990, 93000-93010, 93040-93042, 93318, 94002, 94200, 94250, 94680-94690, 94770, 95812-95816, 95819, 95822, 95829, 95955, 96360, 96365, 96372, 96374-96376, 99148-99149, 99150

Also not with 23490: 20650

Also not with 23491: 23000, 23040, 23100, 23105, 23107, 23130, 23150, 23184, 23195, 23410-23412, 23430, 23450, 23470-23472❖, 23700, 24332, 29820-29821

Note: These CCI edits are used for Medicare. Other payers may reimburse on codes listed above.

Medicare Edits

	Fac RVU	Non-Fac RVU	FUD	Assist
23490	25.52	25.52	90	80
23491	29.71	29.71	90	80

Medicare References: 100-2,15,260; 100-4,12,30; 100-4,12,90.3; 100-4,14,10

23500-23505

23500 Closed treatment of clavicular fracture; without manipulation
23505 with manipulation

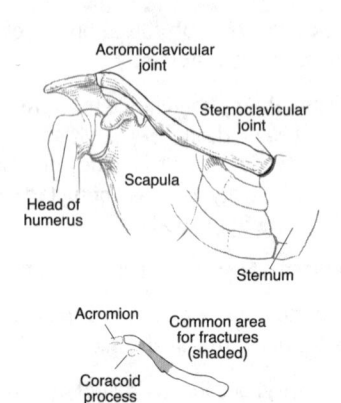

A fracture of the clavicle is treated in a closed fashion without manipulation. Report 23505 when manipulation is required to treat the fracture

Explanation

The physician treats a fracture of the clavicle bone without surgery or manipulation. X-rays confirm the stable position of the fractured pieces. No manipulation is required. The physician may apply a clavicle brace, tape, or splint until the fracture heals. In 23505, the fracture is displaced and manipulation is required. A local anesthetic may be applied. The physician then pushes or pulls on the bony pieces or manipulates the shoulder in such a way to properly align the fracture. The physician may apply a clavicle brace, tape, or splint until the fracture heals.

Coding Tips

According to CPT guidelines, cast application or strapping (including removal) is only reported as a replacement procedure or when the cast application or strapping is an initial service performed without a restorative treatment or procedure. See "Application of Casts and Strapping" in the CPT book in the Surgery Section, under the Musculoskeletal system. When 23500 or 23505 is performed with another separately identifiable procedure, the highest dollar value code is listed as the primary procedure and subsequent procedures are appended with modifier 51. For radiology services, see 73000, and add modifier 26 to identify the professional component only, unless the physician owns the equipment.

ICD-9-CM Procedural

79.09 Closed reduction of fracture of other specified bone, except facial bones, without internal fixation
93.54 Application of splint

Anesthesia
00450

ICD-9-CM Diagnostic

733.19 Pathologic fracture of other specified site
810.00 Unspecified part of closed fracture of clavicle
810.01 Closed fracture of sternal end of clavicle
810.02 Closed fracture of shaft of clavicle
810.03 Closed fracture of acromial end of clavicle

Terms To Know

closed fracture. Break in a bone without a concomitant opening in the skin. A closed fracture is coded when the type of fracture is not specified.

fracture. Break in bone or cartilage.

pathologic fracture. Break in bone due to a disease process that weakens the bone structure, such as osteoporosis, osteomalacia, or neoplasia, and not traumatic injury.

CCI Version 16.3

01610, 0213T, 0216T, 0228T, 0230T, 23700, 29000-29065, 29105, 29240, 29700-29715, 36000, 36400-36410, 36420-36430, 36440, 36600, 36640, 37202, 43752, 51701-51703, 62310-62319, 64400-64435, 64445-64450, 64479, 64483, 64490, 64493, 64505-64530, 69990, 93000-93010, 93040-93042, 93318, 94002, 94200, 94250, 94680-94690, 94770, 95812-95816, 95819, 95822, 95829, 95955, 96360, 96365, 96372, 96374-96376, 97597-97598, 97602-97606, 99148-99149, 99150

Also not with 23500: 12001, 12013-12014, G0168

Also not with 23505: 23500, J0670, J2001

Note: These CCI edits are used for Medicare. Other payers may reimburse on codes listed above.

Medicare Edits

	Fac RVU	Non-Fac RVU	FUD	Assist
23500	6.14	6.11	90	N/A
23505	9.4	9.93	90	N/A

Medicare References: 100-2,15,260; 100-4,12,30; 100-4,12,90.3; 100-4,14,10

23515

23515 Open treatment of clavicular fracture, includes internal fixation, when performed

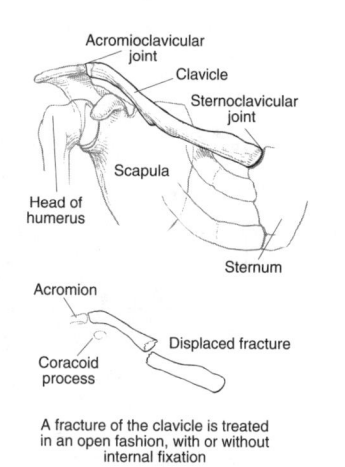

A fracture of the clavicle is treated in an open fashion, with or without internal fixation

Explanation

The physician treats a fracture of the clavicle with open surgery. The physician makes an incision overlying the fractured area of the clavicle. Tissue is dissected down to the bone and the fracture is identified. The physician debrides any nonviable tissues. Any tissue that has become lodged between the fracture pieces is removed. The physician may apply screws, wires, or plates to secure the fracture. The wound is irrigated and the incision is closed. A splint or brace may also be applied on the outside of the clavicle or shoulder.

Coding Tips

When 23515 is performed with another separately identifiable procedure, the highest dollar value code is listed as the primary procedure and subsequent procedures are appended with modifier 51. According to CPT guidelines, cast application or strapping (including removal) is only reported as a replacement procedure or when the cast application or strapping is an initial service performed without a restorative treatment or procedure. See "Application of Casts and Strapping" in the CPT book in the Surgery Section, under the Musculoskeletal system. For radiology services, see 73000. For debridement of an open fracture, see 11010–11012. For removal of internal fixation, see 23330–23332. For closed treatment of a clavicular fracture, see 23500–23505.

ICD-9-CM Procedural

- 79.29 Open reduction of fracture of other specified bone, except facial bones, without internal fixation
- 79.39 Open reduction of fracture of other specified bone, except facial bones, with internal fixation

Anesthesia

23515   00450

ICD-9-CM Diagnostic

- 733.19 Pathologic fracture of other specified site
- 733.81 Malunion of fracture
- 733.82 Nonunion of fracture
- 810.00 Unspecified part of closed fracture of clavicle
- 810.02 Closed fracture of shaft of clavicle
- 810.03 Closed fracture of acromial end of clavicle
- 810.10 Unspecified part of open fracture of clavicle
- 810.11 Open fracture of sternal end of clavicle
- 810.12 Open fracture of shaft of clavicle
- 810.13 Open fracture of acromial end of clavicle

Terms To Know

open fracture. Exposed break in a bone, always considered compound due to its high risk of infection from the open wound leading to the fracture. Broken bone ends may protrude through the skin and contaminants or foreign bodies are often embedded in the tissues.

pathologic fracture. Break in bone due to a disease process that weakens the bone structure, such as osteoporosis, osteomalacia, or neoplasia, and not traumatic injury.

CCI Version 16.3

01610, 0213T, 0216T, 0228T, 0230T, 20650, 23500-23505, 23700, 29000-29065, 29105, 29240, 29700-29715, 36000, 36400-36410, 36420-36430, 36440, 36600, 36640, 37202, 43752, 51701-51703, 62310-62319, 64400-64435, 64445-64450, 64479, 64483, 64490, 64493, 64505-64530, 69990, 93000-93010, 93040-93042, 93318, 94002, 94200, 94250, 94680-94690, 94770, 95812-95816, 95819, 95822, 95829, 95955, 96360, 96365, 96372, 96374-96376, 97597-97598, 97602-97606, 99148-99149, 99150

Note: These CCI edits are used for Medicare. Other payers may reimburse on codes listed above.

Medicare Edits

	Fac RVU	Non-Fac RVU	FUD	Assist
23515	20.98	20.98	90	80

Medicare References: 100-2,15,260; 100-4,12,30; 100-4,12,90.3; 100-4,14,10

23520-23525

23520 Closed treatment of sternoclavicular dislocation; without manipulation
23525 with manipulation

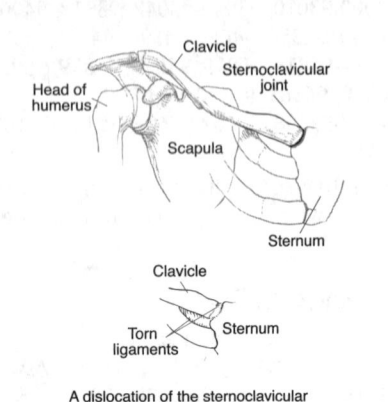

A dislocation of the sternoclavicular joint is treated in a closed fashion without manipulation. Report 23525 when manipulation is required to treat the dislocation

Explanation

The physician treats a dislocation of the joint between the sternum and the clavicle (sternoclavicular) without making incisions and without any manipulation in 23520. The physician applies a splint or brace to hold the joint in place until it has healed. In 23525, manipulation is required. Anesthesia may be necessary. The physician pushes, pulls, or moves the arm and chest to restore the joint to correct position and alignment. After manipulation, the patient is placed in a brace or splint.

Coding Tips

According to CPT guidelines, cast application or strapping (including removal) is only reported as a replacement procedure or when the cast application or strapping is an initial service performed without a restorative treatment or procedure. See "Application of Casts and Strapping" in the CPT book in the Surgery Section, under the Musculoskeletal system. For radiology services, see 71130. For open treatment of an acute or a chronic sternoclavicular dislocation, see 23530 and 23532.

ICD-9-CM Procedural

79.79 Closed reduction of dislocation of other specified site, except temporomandibular
93.54 Application of splint
93.59 Other immobilization, pressure, and attention to wound

Anesthesia
01620

ICD-9-CM Diagnostic

718.21 Pathological dislocation of shoulder joint
718.71 Developmental dislocation of joint, shoulder region
839.61 Closed dislocation, sternum

Terms To Know

closed dislocation. Simple displacement of a body part without an open wound.

pathological dislocation. Displacement of a bone or joint caused by a disease process, such as infection, lesions, or muscle weakness, and not traumatic injury.

CCI Version 16.3

01610, 0213T, 0216T, 0228T, 0230T, 23700, 29000-29065, 29105, 29240, 29700-29715, 36000, 36400-36410, 36420-36430, 36440, 36600, 36640, 37202, 43752, 51701-51703, 62310-62319, 64400-64435, 64445-64450, 64479, 64483, 64490, 64493, 64505-64530, 69990, 93000-93010, 93040-93042, 93318, 94002, 94200, 94250, 94680-94690, 94770, 95812-95816, 95819, 95822, 95829, 95955, 96360, 96365, 96372, 96374-96376, 97597-97598, 97602-97606, 99148-99149, 99150

Also not with 23525: 23520, J0670, J2001

Note: These CCI edits are used for Medicare. Other payers may reimburse on codes listed above.

Medicare Edits

	Fac RVU	Non-Fac RVU	FUD	Assist
23520	6.49	6.42	90	80
23525	9.67	10.53	90	80

Medicare References: 100-2,15,260; 100-4,12,30; 100-4,12,90.3; 100-4,14,10

23530-23532

23530 Open treatment of sternoclavicular dislocation, acute or chronic;

23532 with fascial graft (includes obtaining graft)

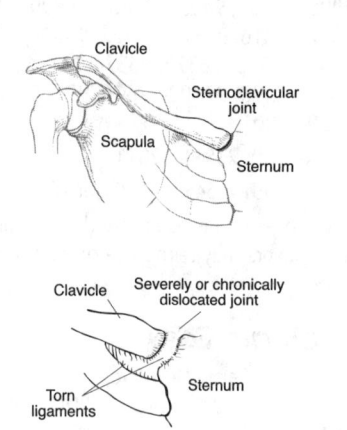

A chronic or acute dislocation of the sternoclavicular joint is treated in an open surgical session. Report code 23532 when a fascial graft is required during repair

Explanation
The physician treats a chronic or acute dislocation of the sternoclavicular joint. The physician makes an incision overlying the joint between the clavicle and sternum where the dislocation has occurred. The tissues are dissected down to the joint and the dislocation is visualized. The physician may debride the area before realigning the joint back to proper position. In 23532, the physician harvests a fascial graft from the patient through a separate incision. The physician repairs the surgically created graft donor site. The fascial graft is attached to the bones in the sternoclavicular joint, preventing recurrent dislocation. Fixation may be applied. The joint is irrigated and the incision is closed in layers. A splint or brace may be applied to the outside of the body.

Coding Tips
When 23530 or 23532 is performed with another separately identifiable procedure, the highest dollar value code is listed as the primary procedure and subsequent procedures are appended with modifier 51. According to CPT guidelines, cast application or strapping (including removal) is only reported as a replacement procedure or when the cast application or strapping is an initial service performed without a restorative treatment or procedure. See "Application of Casts and Strapping" in the CPT book in the Surgery Section, under the Musculoskeletal system. For debridement of an open dislocation, see 11010–11012. For closed treatment of a sternoclavicular dislocation, see 23520–23525.

ICD-9-CM Procedural
- **79.89** Open reduction of dislocation of other specified site, except temporomandibular
- **83.82** Graft of muscle or fascia

Anesthesia
01630

ICD-9-CM Diagnostic
- **718.21** Pathological dislocation of shoulder joint
- **718.31** Recurrent dislocation of shoulder joint
- **718.71** Developmental dislocation of joint, shoulder region
- **718.78** Developmental dislocation of joint, other specified sites
- **839.61** Closed dislocation, sternum
- **839.71** Open dislocation, sternum

Terms To Know
acute. Sudden, severe. Documentation and reporting of an acute condition is important to establishing medical necessity.

chronic. Persistent, continuing, or recurring.

closed dislocation. Simple displacement of a body part without an open wound.

fascia. Fibrous sheet or band of tissue that envelops organs, muscles, and groupings of muscles.

open dislocation. Displacement of a bone or joint with an open wound.

pathological dislocation. Displacement of a bone or joint caused by a disease process, such as infection, lesions, or muscle weakness, and not traumatic injury.

CCI Version 16.3
01610, 0213T, 0216T, 0228T, 0230T, 23044, 23101, 23106, 23700, 29000-29065, 29105, 29240, 29700-29715, 36000, 36400-36410, 36420-36430, 36440, 36600, 36640, 37202, 43752, 51701-51703, 62310-62319, 64400-64435, 64445-64450, 64479, 64483, 64490, 64493, 64505-64530, 69990, 93000-93010, 93040-93042, 93318, 94002, 94200, 94250, 94680-94690, 94770, 95812-95816, 95819, 95822, 95829, 95955, 96360, 96365, 96372, 96374-96376, 97597-97598, 97602-97606, 99148-99149, 99150

Also not with 23530: 23520-23525

Also not with 23532: 20920-20922, 20926, 23520-23530

Note: These CCI edits are used for Medicare. Other payers may reimburse on codes listed above.

Medicare Edits

	Fac RVU	Non-Fac RVU	FUD	Assist
23530	16.18	16.18	90	80
23532	18.08	18.08	90	80

Medicare References: 100-2,15,260; 100-4,12,30; 100-4,12,90.3; 100-4,14,10

23540-23545

23540 Closed treatment of acromioclavicular dislocation; without manipulation
23545 with manipulation

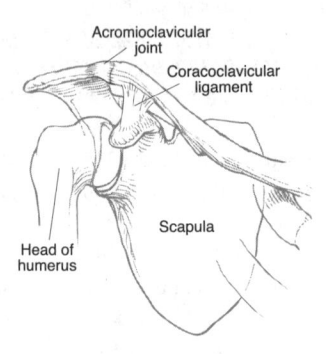

A dislocation of the acromioclavicular joint is treated in a closed fashion without manipulation. Report 23545 when manipulation is required to treat the dislocation.

Explanation

The physician treats a dislocation of the acromioclavicular joint (between the acromion process of the scapula and the clavicle). Neither incisions nor manipulation are necessary. The physician places the affected shoulder and arm in a sling or other brace. In 23545, manipulation is necessary to correct the dislocation. Anesthesia may be necessary. The physician then manipulates the joint by pushing or pulling on the shoulder and arm to align the bones. The physician applies a sling or other brace.

Coding Tips

According to CPT guidelines, cast application or strapping (including removal) is only reported as a replacement procedure or when the cast application or strapping is an initial service performed without a restorative treatment or procedure. See "Application of Casts and Strapping" in the CPT book in the Surgery Section, under the Musculoskeletal system. In 23545, local anesthesia is included in the service. However, this procedure may be performed under general anesthesia, depending on the age and/or condition of the patient. For radiology services, see 73000, 73010, and 73050 and report the appropriate code for the view taken. For open treatment of an acromioclavicular dislocation, see 23550–23552.

ICD-9-CM Procedural

79.79 Closed reduction of dislocation of other specified site, except temporomandibular
93.59 Other immobilization, pressure, and attention to wound

Anesthesia
01620

ICD-9-CM Diagnostic

718.21 Pathological dislocation of shoulder joint
718.31 Recurrent dislocation of shoulder joint
718.71 Developmental dislocation of joint, shoulder region
831.04 Closed dislocation of acromioclavicular (joint)
840.0 Acromioclavicular (joint) (ligament) sprain and strain

Terms To Know

closed dislocation. Simple displacement of a body part without an open wound.

developmental dislocation. Displacement of a body part occurring in the developmental phase of childhood.

pathological dislocation. Displacement of a bone or joint caused by a disease process, such as infection, lesions, or muscle weakness, and not traumatic injury.

sprain and strain. Injuries to a joint, in which the fibers of supporting ligaments or muscles are overstretched or slightly ruptured, with the ligaments and muscles maintaining continuity.

CCI Version 16.3

01610, 0213T, 0216T, 0228T, 0230T, 23700, 29000-29065, 29105, 29240, 29700-29715, 36000, 36400-36410, 36420-36430, 36440, 36600, 36640, 37202, 43752, 51701-51703, 62310-62319, 64400-64435, 64445-64450, 64479, 64483, 64490, 64493, 64505-64530, 69990, 93000-93010, 93040-93042, 93318, 94002, 94200, 94250, 94680-94690, 94770, 95812-95816, 95819, 95822, 95829, 95955, 96360, 96365, 96372, 96374-96376, 97597-97598, 97602-97606, 99148-99149, 99150, J2001

Also not with 23540: 12011
Also not with 23545: 23540, J0670

Note: These CCI edits are used for Medicare. Other payers may reimburse on codes listed above.

Medicare Edits

	Fac RVU	Non-Fac RVU	FUD	Assist
23540	6.24	6.24	90	N/A
23545	8.36	9.13	90	80

Medicare References: 100-2,15,260; 100-4,12,30; 100-4,12,90.3; 100-4,14,10

23550-23552

23550 Open treatment of acromioclavicular dislocation, acute or chronic;
23552 with fascial graft (includes obtaining graft)

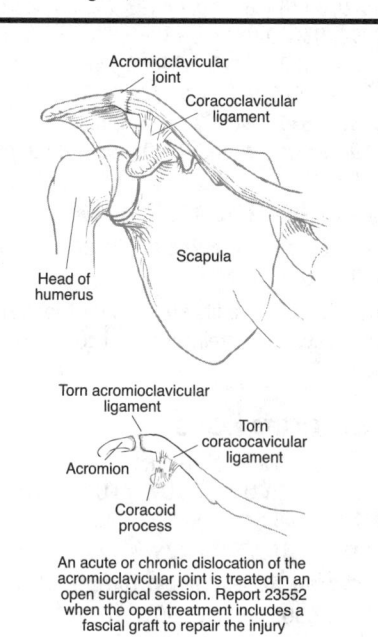

An acute or chronic dislocation of the acromioclavicular joint is treated in an open surgical session. Report 23552 when the open treatment includes a fascial graft to repair the injury

Explanation

The physician treats an acute or chronic dislocation of the acromioclavicular joint (between the acromion process of the scapula and the clavicle). An incision is made overlying the shoulder at the articulation of the acromion of the scapula and the end of the clavicle. Dissection is carried through the tissues to the joint. Any nonviable tissue is removed. The bones are identified and the dislocation visualized. In 23552, the physician harvests a fascial graft from the patient through a separate incision. The physician repairs the surgically created graft donor site. The graft is then connected to the pieces of dislocated joint to restore alignment. In both 23550 and 23552, the physician uses a heavy nonabsorbable suture, a wire, or screws to secure the two bones in their proper joint alignment. When the joint is restored, the wound is irrigated with antibiotic solution. The incision is closed in multiple layers. A sterile dressing is applied. A sling or brace is applied to the shoulder and arm.

Coding Tips

A fascial graft should not be reported separately. When 23550 or 23552 is performed with another separately identifiable procedure, the highest dollar value code is listed as the primary procedure and subsequent procedures are appended with modifier 51. According to CPT guidelines, cast application or strapping (including removal) is only reported as a replacement procedure or when the cast application or strapping is an initial service performed without a restorative treatment or procedure. See "Application of Casts and Strapping" in the CPT book in the Surgery Section, under the Musculoskeletal system. For debridement of an open dislocation, see 11010–11012. For closed treatment of an acromioclavicular dislocation, see 23540–23545.

ICD-9-CM Procedural

79.89 Open reduction of dislocation of other specified site, except temporomandibular
83.82 Graft of muscle or fascia

Anesthesia
01630

ICD-9-CM Diagnostic

718.21 Pathological dislocation of shoulder joint
718.31 Recurrent dislocation of shoulder joint
718.71 Developmental dislocation of joint, shoulder region
831.04 Closed dislocation of acromioclavicular (joint)
831.14 Open dislocation of acromioclavicular (joint)
840.0 Acromioclavicular (joint) (ligament) sprain and strain

Terms To Know

acute. Sudden, severe. Documentation and reporting of an acute condition is important to establishing medical necessity.

chronic. Persistent, continuing, or recurring.

developmental dislocation. Displacement of a body part occurring in the developmental phase of childhood.

fascia. Fibrous sheet or band of tissue that envelops organs, muscles, and groupings of muscles.

pathological dislocation. Displacement of a bone or joint caused by a disease process, such as infection, lesions, or muscle weakness, and not traumatic injury.

sprain and strain. Injuries to a joint, in which the fibers of supporting ligaments or muscles are overstretched or slightly ruptured, with the ligaments and muscles maintaining continuity.

CCI Version 16.3

01610, 0213T, 0216T, 0228T, 0230T, 23044, 23101, 23700, 29000-29065, 29105, 29240, 29700-29715, 36000, 36400-36410, 36420-36430, 36440, 36600, 36640, 37202, 43752, 51701-51703, 62310-62319, 64400-64435, 64445-64450, 64479, 64483, 64490, 64493, 64505-64530, 69990, 93000-93010, 93040-93042, 93318, 94002, 94200, 94250, 94680-94690, 94770, 95812-95816, 95819, 95822, 95829, 95955, 96360, 96365, 96372, 96374-96376, 97597-97598, 97602-97606, 99148-99149, 99150

Also not with 23550: 23540-23545, 29540

Also not with 23552: 20920-20922, 20926, 23540-23550

Note: These CCI edits are used for Medicare. Other payers may reimburse on codes listed above.

Medicare Edits

	Fac RVU	Non-Fac RVU	FUD	Assist
23550	16.61	16.61	90	80
23552	19.14	19.14	90	80

Medicare References: 100-2,15,260; 100-4,12,30; 100-4,12,90.3; 100-4,14,10

23570-23575

23570 Closed treatment of scapular fracture; without manipulation
23575 with manipulation, with or without skeletal traction (with or without shoulder joint involvement)

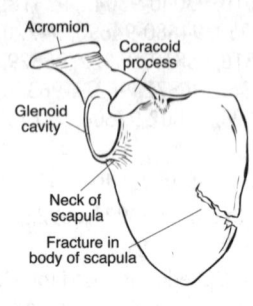

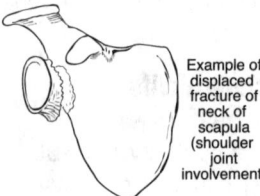

A fracture of the scapula is treated in a closed fashion without manipulation. Report 23575 if manipulation is required, with or without skeletal traction or shoulder joint involvement

Explanation

In 23570, the physician treats a fracture of the scapula bone without surgery or any type of manipulation. X-rays confirm the stable position of the fractured pieces. The physician then places the shoulder in a sling or other brace until the fracture heals. In 23575, with the patient under anesthesia, the physician manipulates (pushes, pulls, or moves) the scapula and arm to align the fractured pieces. Serial x-rays may be necessary while the manipulation is performed to confirm alignment. The physician may apply traction devices to the body to maintain satisfactory fracture position. A brace, splint, or cast may be applied to hold the bones in the correct position until they are healed.

Coding Tips

According to CPT guidelines, cast application or strapping (including removal) is only reported as a replacement procedure or when the cast application or strapping is an initial service performed without a restorative treatment or procedure. See "Application of Casts and Strapping" in the CPT book in the Surgery Section, under the Musculoskeletal system. In 23575, local anesthesia is included in the service. However, this procedure may be performed under general anesthesia, depending on the age and/or condition of the patient. For radiology services, see 73010.

Check with individual payers to determine additional payment for x-rays. For open treatment of a scapular fracture, see 23585.

ICD-9-CM Procedural

- 79.09 Closed reduction of fracture of other specified bone, except facial bones, without internal fixation
- 79.19 Closed reduction of fracture of other specified bone, except facial bones, with internal fixation
- 93.44 Other skeletal traction
- 93.54 Application of splint
- 93.59 Other immobilization, pressure, and attention to wound

Anesthesia
00450

ICD-9-CM Diagnostic

- 733.19 Pathologic fracture of other specified site
- 811.01 Closed fracture of acromial process of scapula
- 811.02 Closed fracture of coracoid process of scapula
- 811.03 Closed fracture of glenoid cavity and neck of scapula
- 811.09 Closed fracture of other part of scapula

Terms To Know

closed fracture. Break in a bone without a concomitant opening in the skin. A closed fracture is coded when the type of fracture is not specified.

pathologic fracture. Break in bone due to a disease process that weakens the bone structure, such as osteoporosis, osteomalacia, or neoplasia, and not traumatic injury.

CCI Version 16.3

01610, 0213T, 0216T, 0228T, 0230T, 23700, 29000-29065, 29105, 29240, 29700-29715, 36000, 36400-36410, 36420-36430, 36440, 36600, 36640, 37202, 43752, 51701-51703, 62310-62319, 64400-64435, 64445-64450, 64479, 64483, 64490, 64493, 64505-64530, 69990, 93000-93010, 93040-93042, 93318, 94002, 94200, 94250, 94680-94690, 94770, 95812-95816, 95819, 95822, 95829, 95955, 96360, 96365, 96372, 96374-96376, 97597-97598, 97602-97606, 99148-99149, 99150

Also not with 23570: 12002, 12054

Also not with 23575: 20650, 20690, 23570, J0670, J2001

Note: These CCI edits are used for Medicare. Other payers may reimburse on codes listed above.

Medicare Edits

	Fac RVU	Non-Fac RVU	FUD	Assist
23570	6.64	6.5	90	N/A
23575	10.59	11.25	90	80

Medicare References: 100-2,15,260; 100-4,12,30; 100-4,12,90.3; 100-4,14,10

23585

23585 Open treatment of scapular fracture (body, glenoid or acromion) includes internal fixation, when performed

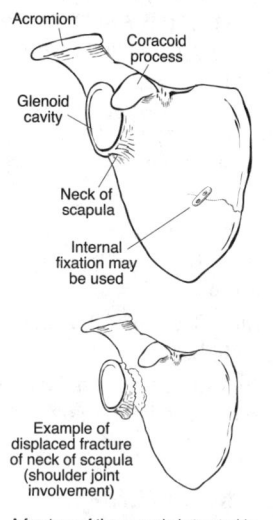

A fracture of the scapula is treated in an open surgical session. Report this code for fractures to the scapular body, glenoid, or acromion, with or without internal fixation

Explanation

The physician treats a fracture of the scapula with open surgery. The physician makes an incision overlying the area of the fractured scapula and dissects the tissues down to the bone to visualize the fracture. Nonviable tissues or those between the fragments are debrided. The physician places the fragments back together in their correct anatomic position manually or with instruments. Internal fixation devices such as screws, metal plates, sutures, or wire may be applied to secure the bones. The wound is irrigated and the incisions are closed in layers with sutures.

Coding Tips

According to CPT guidelines, cast application or strapping (including removal) is only reported as a replacement procedure or when the cast application or strapping is an initial service performed without a restorative treatment or procedure. See "Application of Casts and Strapping" in the CPT book in the Surgery Section, under the Musculoskeletal system. When 23585 is performed with another separately identifiable procedure, the highest dollar value code is listed as the primary procedure and subsequent procedures are appended with modifier 51. For debridement of an open fracture, see 11010–11012. For closed treatment of a scapular fracture, see 23570–23575.

ICD-9-CM Procedural

- 79.29 Open reduction of fracture of other specified bone, except facial bones, without internal fixation
- 79.39 Open reduction of fracture of other specified bone, except facial bones, with internal fixation

Anesthesia

23585 00450

ICD-9-CM Diagnostic

- 733.19 Pathologic fracture of other specified site
- 733.81 Malunion of fracture
- 733.82 Nonunion of fracture
- 811.01 Closed fracture of acromial process of scapula
- 811.03 Closed fracture of glenoid cavity and neck of scapula
- 811.09 Closed fracture of other part of scapula
- 811.11 Open fracture of acromial process of scapula
- 811.13 Open fracture of glenoid cavity and neck of scapula
- 811.19 Open fracture of other part of scapula

Terms To Know

malunion. Fracture that has united in a faulty position due to inadequate reduction of the original fracture, insufficient holding of a previously well-reduced fracture, contracture of the soft tissues, or comminuted or osteoporotic bone causing a slow disintegration of the fracture.

nonunion. Failure of two ends of a fracture to mend or completely heal.

nonviable. Unable to live.

pathologic fracture. Break in bone due to a disease process that weakens the bone structure, such as osteoporosis, osteomalacia, or neoplasia, and not traumatic injury.

CCI Version 16.3

01610, 0213T, 0216T, 0228T, 0230T, 20650, 23040, 23100, 23105, 23107, 23570-23575, 23700, 24332, 29000-29065, 29105, 29240, 29700-29715, 36000, 36400-36410, 36420-36430, 36440, 36600, 36640, 37202, 43752, 51701-51703, 62310-62319, 64400-64435, 64445-64450, 64479, 64483, 64490, 64493, 64505-64530, 69990, 93000-93010, 93040-93042, 93318, 94002, 94200, 94250, 94680-94690, 94770, 95812-95816, 95819, 95822, 95829, 95955, 96360, 96365, 96372, 96374-96376, 97597-97598, 97602-97606, 99148-99149, 99150

Note: These CCI edits are used for Medicare. Other payers may reimburse on codes listed above.

Medicare Edits

	Fac RVU	Non-Fac RVU	FUD	Assist
23585	28.47	28.47	90	80

Medicare References: 100-2,15,260; 100-4,12,30; 100-4,12,90.3; 100-4,14,10

23600-23605

23600 Closed treatment of proximal humeral (surgical or anatomical neck) fracture; without manipulation
23605 with manipulation, with or without skeletal traction

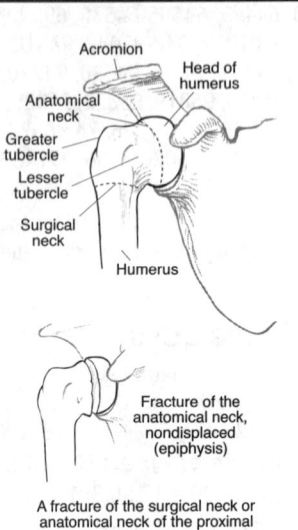

A fracture of the surgical neck or anatomical neck of the proximal humerus is treated in a closed fashion without manipulation. Report 23605 if manipulation is required, with or without skeletal traction

Explanation

Separately reportable x-rays confirm a stable, non-displaced proximal humeral fracture. No manipulation or open reduction is required in 23600. The arm is positioned in a sling and protected from movement to allow adequate healing. In 23605, the physician manipulates (pushes, pulls, or moves) the upper arm in the shoulder area to align the fractured pieces. Separately reportable serial x-rays may be necessary while the manipulation is performed to confirm alignment. The physician may apply traction devices to the body to maintain satisfactory fracture reduction. A brace, splint, or cast may be applied to hold the bones in the correct position until they are healed.

Coding Tips

According to CPT guidelines, cast application or strapping (including removal) is only reported as a replacement procedure or when the cast application or strapping is an initial service performed without a restorative treatment or procedure. See "Application of Casts and Strapping" in the CPT book in the Surgery Section, under the Musculoskeletal system. In 23605, local anesthesia is included in the service. However, this procedure may be performed under general anesthesia, depending on the age and/or condition of the patient. For radiology services, see 73020 and 73030. For treatment of a surgical or an anatomical humeral neck fracture in conjunction with closed treatment of a shoulder dislocation, see 23675. For open treatment of a proximal humerus fracture, see 23615–23616.

ICD-9-CM Procedural

- 79.01 Closed reduction of fracture of humerus without internal fixation
- 79.11 Closed reduction of fracture of humerus with internal fixation
- 93.54 Application of splint

Anesthesia
01620

ICD-9-CM Diagnostic

- 733.11 Pathologic fracture of humerus
- 812.01 Closed fracture of surgical neck of humerus
- 812.02 Closed fracture of anatomical neck of humerus

Terms To Know

closed fracture. Break in a bone without a concomitant opening in the skin. A closed fracture is coded when the type of fracture is not specified.

pathologic fracture. Break in bone due to a disease process that weakens the bone structure, such as osteoporosis, osteomalacia, or neoplasia, and not traumatic injury.

proximal. Located closest to a specified reference point, usually the midline.

CCI Version 16.3

01610, 0213T, 0216T, 0228T, 0230T, 23470-23472❖, 23700, 29000-29065, 29105-29125, 29240, 29700-29715, 36000, 36400-36410, 36420-36430, 36440, 36600, 36640, 37202, 43752, 51701-51703, 62310-62319, 64400-64435, 64445-64450, 64479, 64483, 64490, 64493, 64505-64530, 69990, 93000-93010, 93040-93042, 93318, 94002, 94200, 94250, 94680-94690, 94770, 95812-95816, 95819, 95822, 95829, 95955, 96360, 96365, 96372, 96374-96376, 97597-97598, 97602-97606, 99148-99149, 99150

Also not with 23600: 12001-12002, 12011-12013, 12032, 12051, 13132, 23620, 29085, G0168

Also not with 23605: 20650, 20690, 23600, 23625, J0670, J2001

Note: These CCI edits are used for Medicare. Other payers may reimburse on codes listed above.

Medicare Edits

	Fac RVU	Non-Fac RVU	FUD	Assist
23600	8.5	9.13	90	N/A
23605	12.23	13.27	90	N/A

Medicare References: 100-2,15,260; 100-4,12,30; 100-4,12,90.3; 100-4,14,10

23615-23616

23615 Open treatment of proximal humeral (surgical or anatomical neck) fracture, includes internal fixation, when performed, includes repair of tuberosity(s), when performed;

23616 with proximal humeral prosthetic replacement

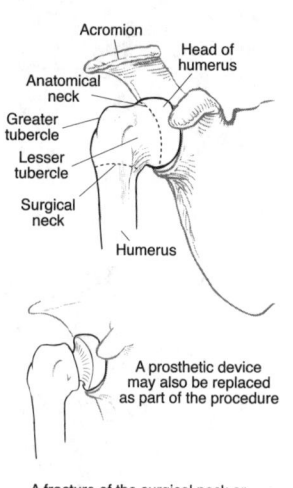

A fracture of the surgical neck or anatomical neck of the proximal humerus is treated in an open surgical session. A repair to the tubercles may be included. Report 23616 when a humeral prosthetic is also replaced

Explanation

The physician performs open treatment of a proximal humeral (surgical or anatomical neck) fracture. An incision is made anteromedially extending posteriorly along the acromion to the lateral half of the spine of the scapula. The deltoid is detached from the exposed portion of the spine of the scapula. The deltoid is reflected down to expose the joint capsule and the humerus. The fractured portion of the proximal humerus (surgical or anatomical neck) is identified and the fracture is aligned. If the tuberosity is involved, it may also be repaired. Internal fixation may be used to stabilize the fracture site. Once the fracture is stabilized, the wound is irrigated. The deltoid is repositioned and sutured in place. The skin is sutured and the wound is covered with a soft dressing. The arm is positioned in a sling and movement is restricted to allow for proper healing. Report 23616 when the fracture cannot be repaired and a prosthetic proximal humeral replacement is necessary.

Coding Tips

When 23615 or 23616 is performed with another separately identifiable procedure, the highest dollar value code is listed as the primary procedure and subsequent procedures are appended with modifier 51. According to CPT guidelines, cast application or strapping (including removal) is only reported as a replacement procedure or when the cast application or strapping is an initial service performed without a restorative treatment or procedure. See "Application of Casts and Strapping" in the CPT book in the Surgery Section, under the Musculoskeletal system. For treatment of a surgical or an anatomical humeral neck fracture in conjunction with open treatment of a shoulder dislocation, see 23680. For debridement of an open fracture, see 11010–11012. For closed treatment of a proximal humeral fracture, see 23600–23605.

ICD-9-CM Procedural

79.21	Open reduction of fracture of humerus without internal fixation
79.31	Open reduction of fracture of humerus with internal fixation
81.81	Partial shoulder replacement

Anesthesia
01630

ICD-9-CM Diagnostic

733.11	Pathologic fracture of humerus
733.81	Malunion of fracture
733.82	Nonunion of fracture
812.01	Closed fracture of surgical neck of humerus
812.02	Closed fracture of anatomical neck of humerus
812.03	Closed fracture of greater tuberosity of humerus
812.09	Other closed fractures of upper end of humerus
812.11	Open fracture of surgical neck of humerus
812.12	Open fracture of anatomical neck of humerus
812.13	Open fracture of greater tuberosity of humerus
812.19	Other open fracture of upper end of humerus

CCI Version 16.3

01610, 0213T, 0216T, 0228T, 0230T, 20650, 23040, 23100, 23105, 23107, 23410-23412, 23600-23605, 23620-23630, 23700, 24332, 29000-29065, 29105, 29240, 29700-29715, 36000, 36400-36410, 36420-36430, 36440, 36600, 36640, 37202, 43752, 51701-51703, 62310-62319, 64400-64435, 64445-64450, 64479, 64483, 64490, 64493, 64505-64530, 69990, 93000-93010, 93040-93042, 93318, 94002, 94200, 94250, 94680-94690, 94770, 95812-95816, 95819, 95822, 95829, 95955, 96360, 96365, 96372, 96374-96376, 97597-97598, 97602-97606, 99148-99149, 99150

Also not with 23615: 23470-23472❖, 29820-29821

Also not with 23616: 23000, 23195, 23420-23430, 23450, 23615

Note: These CCI edits are used for Medicare. Other payers may reimburse on codes listed above.

Medicare Edits

	Fac RVU	Non-Fac RVU	FUD	Assist
23615	25.76	25.76	90	80
23616	36.81	36.81	90	80

Medicare References: 100-2,15,260; 100-4,12,30; 100-4,12,90.3; 100-4,14,10

23620-23625

23620 Closed treatment of greater humeral tuberosity fracture; without manipulation
23625 with manipulation

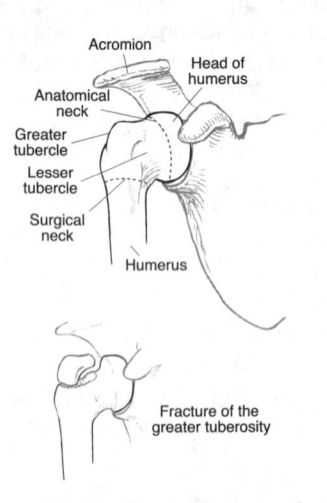

A fracture of the greater humeral tuberosity is treated in a closed fashion without manipulation. Report 23625 when manipulation is required to treat the fracture

Explanation

Separately reportable x-rays determine a stable, non-displaced greater humeral tuberosity fracture. The arm is positioned in a sling and motion of the shoulder is protected to prevent pull of the muscles that attach to the bone of the upper arm. Report 23625 if the fracture is displaced and manipulation is required. A local anesthetic may be given. The physician pushes or pulls on the bony pieces or manipulates them in such a way to properly align the fracture.

Coding Tips

According to CPT guidelines, cast application or strapping (including removal) is only reported as a replacement procedure or when the cast application or strapping is an initial service performed without a restorative treatment or procedure. See "Application of Casts and Strapping" in the CPT book in the Surgery Section, under the Musculoskeletal system. In 23625, local anesthesia is included in the service. However, this procedure may be performed under general anesthesia, depending on the age and/or condition of the patient. For radiology services, see 73020 and 73030. For open treatment of a greater humeral tuberosity fracture, see 23630.

ICD-9-CM Procedural

79.01 Closed reduction of fracture of humerus without internal fixation
93.54 Application of splint

Anesthesia
01620

ICD-9-CM Diagnostic

733.11 Pathologic fracture of humerus
812.03 Closed fracture of greater tuberosity of humerus

Terms To Know

closed fracture. Break in a bone without a concomitant opening in the skin. A closed fracture is coded when the type of fracture is not specified.

pathologic fracture. Break in bone due to a disease process that weakens the bone structure, such as osteoporosis, osteomalacia, or neoplasia, and not traumatic injury.

CCI Version 16.3

01610, 0213T, 0216T, 0228T, 0230T, 23700, 29000-29065, 29105, 29240, 29700-29715, 36000, 36400-36410, 36420-36430, 36440, 36600, 36640, 37202, 43752, 51701-51703, 62310-62319, 64400-64435, 64445-64450, 64479, 64483, 64490, 64493, 64505-64530, 69990, 93000-93010, 93040-93042, 93318, 94002, 94200, 94250, 94680-94690, 94770, 95812-95816, 95819, 95822, 95829, 95955, 96360, 96365, 96372, 96374-96376, 97597-97598, 97602-97606, 99148-99149, 99150

Also not with 23625: 23620, J0670, J2001

Note: These CCI edits are used for Medicare. Other payers may reimburse on codes listed above.

Medicare Edits

	Fac RVU	Non-Fac RVU	FUD	Assist
23620	7.16	7.55	90	N/A
23625	10.1	10.79	90	N/A

Medicare References: 100-2,15,260; 100-4,12,30; 100-4,12,90.3; 100-4,14,10

23630

23630 Open treatment of greater humeral tuberosity fracture, includes internal fixation, when performed

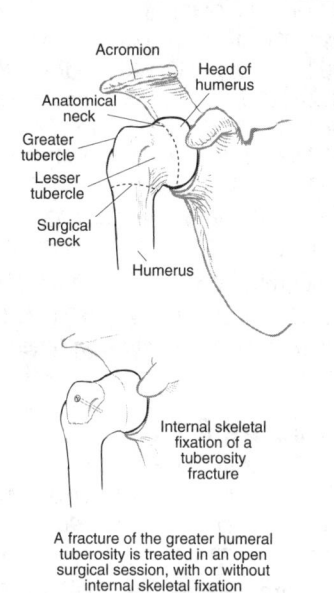

A fracture of the greater humeral tuberosity is treated in an open surgical session, with or without internal skeletal fixation

Explanation
The physician performs open treatment of a greater humeral tuberosity fracture. An anterior longitudinal incision is made and the underlying deltoid fibers are divided to expose the fracture site. Often this injury will include damage to the rotator cuff tendons requiring repair of the soft tissues in addition to the fracture site. The soft tissues are reflected to expose the bone and any loose bodies are removed. The fracture may be stabilized by internal fixation and the soft tissues are reattached by suture. The skin incision is closed and a soft dressing is applied. The arm is placed in a sling and movement is restricted to allow for adequate healing.

Coding Tips
When 23630 is performed with another separately identifiable procedure, the highest dollar value code is listed as the primary procedure and subsequent procedures are appended with modifier 51. According to CPT guidelines, cast application or strapping (including removal) is only reported as a replacement procedure or when the cast application or strapping is an initial service performed without a restorative treatment or procedure. See "Application of Casts and Strapping" in the CPT book in the Surgery Section, under the Musculoskeletal system. For debridement of an open fracture, see 11010–11012. For treatment of a greater humeral tuberosity with closed treatment of a shoulder dislocation, see 23665. For closed treatment of a greater humeral tuberosity fracture, see 23620–23625.

ICD-9-CM Procedural
- 79.21 Open reduction of fracture of humerus without internal fixation
- 79.31 Open reduction of fracture of humerus with internal fixation

Anesthesia
23630 01630

ICD-9-CM Diagnostic
- 733.19 Pathologic fracture of other specified site
- 733.81 Malunion of fracture
- 733.82 Nonunion of fracture
- 812.03 Closed fracture of greater tuberosity of humerus
- 812.13 Open fracture of greater tuberosity of humerus

Terms To Know

closed fracture. Break in a bone without a concomitant opening in the skin. A closed fracture is coded when the type of fracture is not specified.

malunion. Fracture that has united in a faulty position due to inadequate reduction of the original fracture, insufficient holding of a previously well-reduced fracture, contracture of the soft tissues, or comminuted or osteoporotic bone causing a slow disintegration of the fracture.

nonunion. Failure of two ends of a fracture to mend or completely heal.

open fracture. Exposed break in a bone, always considered compound due to its high risk of infection from the open wound leading to the fracture. Broken bone ends may protrude through the skin and contaminants or foreign bodies are often embedded in the tissues.

pathologic fracture. Break in bone due to a disease process that weakens the bone structure, such as osteoporosis, osteomalacia, or neoplasia, and not traumatic injury.

CCI Version 16.3
01610, 0213T, 0216T, 0228T, 0230T, 12020, 20650, 23040, 23100, 23105, 23107, 23410-23412, 23420, 23450, 23620-23625, 23700, 24332, 29000-29065, 29105, 29240, 29700-29715, 36000, 36400-36410, 36420-36430, 36440, 36600, 36640, 37202, 43752, 51701-51703, 62310-62319, 64400-64435, 64445-64450, 64479, 64483, 64490, 64493, 64505-64530, 69990, 93000-93010, 93040-93042, 93318, 94002, 94200, 94250, 94680-94690, 94770, 95812-95816, 95819, 95822, 95829, 95955, 96360, 96365, 96372, 96374-96376, 97597-97598, 97602-97606, 99148-99149, 99150

Note: These CCI edits are used for Medicare. Other payers may reimburse on codes listed above.

Medicare Edits

	Fac RVU	Non-Fac RVU	FUD	Assist
23630	22.51	22.51	90	80

Medicare References: 100-2,15,260; 100-4,12,30; 100-4,12,90.3; 100-4,14,10

23650-23655

23650 Closed treatment of shoulder dislocation, with manipulation; without anesthesia
23655 requiring anesthesia

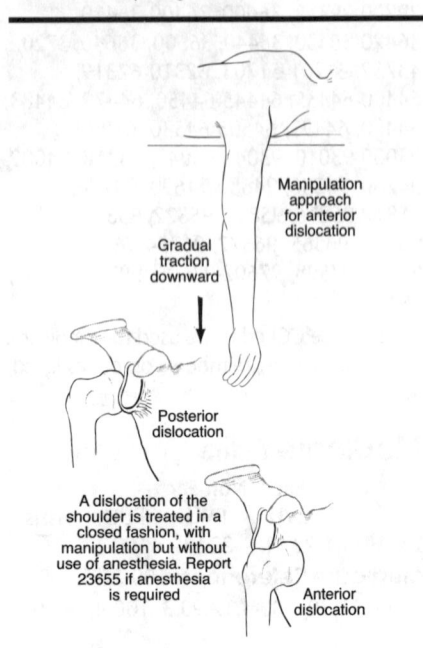

Explanation
The physician performs closed treatment of a shoulder dislocation by manipulation. The most common form of shoulder dislocation is the traumatic anterior inferior dislocation. A closed manipulation requires the patient to be positioned to allow the arm to hang forward. The physician applies gentle traction to distract the joint and manually relocates the glenohumeral joint back into position. Report 23655 if the manipulation treatment requires anesthesia.

Coding Tips
According to CPT guidelines, cast application or strapping (including removal) is only reported as a replacement procedure or when the cast application or strapping is an initial service performed without a restorative treatment or procedure. See "Application of Casts and Strapping" in the CPT book in the Surgery Section, under the Musculoskeletal system. For radiology services, see 73020 and 73030. For open treatment of an acute shoulder dislocation, see 23660.

ICD-9-CM Procedural
79.71 Closed reduction of dislocation of shoulder

Anesthesia
23650 N/A
23655 01620

ICD-9-CM Diagnostic
718.21 Pathological dislocation of shoulder joint
718.31 Recurrent dislocation of shoulder joint
718.71 Developmental dislocation of joint, shoulder region
831.00 Closed dislocation of shoulder, unspecified site
831.01 Closed anterior dislocation of humerus
831.02 Closed posterior dislocation of humerus
831.03 Closed inferior dislocation of humerus
831.09 Closed dislocation of other site of shoulder

Terms To Know
anterior. Situated in the front area or toward the belly surface of the body; an anatomical reference point used to show the position and relationship of one body structure to another.

developmental dislocation. Displacement of a body part occurring in the developmental phase of childhood.

dislocation. Displacement of a bone in relation to its neighboring tissue, especially a joint.

pathological dislocation. Displacement of a bone or joint caused by a disease process, such as infection, lesions, or muscle weakness, and not traumatic injury.

posterior. Located in the back part or caudal end of the body.

CCI Version 16.3
01610, 0213T, 0216T, 0228T, 0230T, 29000-29065, 29105, 29240, 29700-29715, 36000, 36400-36410, 36420-36430, 36440, 36600, 36640, 37202, 43752, 51701-51703, 62310-62319, 64400-64435, 64445-64450, 64479, 64483, 64490, 64493, 64505-64530, 69990, 93000-93010, 93040-93042, 93318, 94002, 94200, 94250, 94680-94690, 94770, 95812-95816, 95819, 95822, 95829, 95955, 96360, 96365, 96372, 96374-96376, 97597-97598, 97602-97606, 99148-99149, 99150, G0168

Also not with 23650: 12001-12002, 12011-12013, 12052, 29505, J0670, J2001
Also not with 23655: 12001, 12032, 23650
Note: These CCI edits are used for Medicare. Other payers may reimburse on codes listed above.

Medicare Edits

	Fac RVU	Non-Fac RVU	FUD	Assist
23650	7.81	8.49	90	N/A
23655	11.23	11.23	90	N/A

Medicare References: 100-2,15,260; 100-4,12,30; 100-4,12,90.3; 100-4,14,10

23660

23660 Open treatment of acute shoulder dislocation

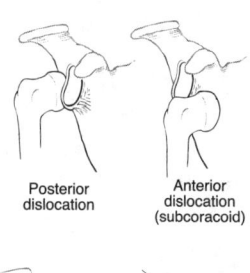

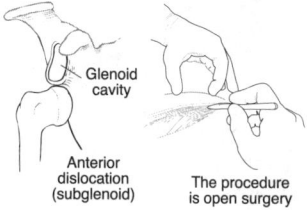

Posterior dislocation
Anterior dislocation (subcoracoid)
Glenoid cavity
Anterior dislocation (subglenoid)
The procedure is open surgery

An acute dislocation of the shoulder is treated in an open surgical session

Explanation
The physician performs open treatment of an acute shoulder dislocation. A posterior dislocation would be more likely to require an open reduction procedure than an anterior dislocation. The shoulder is approached through a deltopectoral incision. The joint is inspected and the head of the humerus is reduced into its proper position. The subscapularis tendon is attached to the head of the humerus with sutures or screws. If there is significant posterior translation, the posterior capsule is tightened. The incision is closed and the arm is immobilized in 20 degrees of external rotation.

Coding Tips
According to CPT guidelines, cast application or strapping (including removal) is only reported as a replacement procedure or when the cast application or strapping is an initial service performed without a restorative treatment or procedure. See "Application of Casts and Strapping" in the CPT book in the Surgery Section, under the Musculoskeletal system. For closed treatment of a shoulder dislocation, see 23650–23655. For surgical repair for recurrent shoulder dislocations, see 23450–23466.

ICD-9-CM Procedural
79.81 Open reduction of dislocation of shoulder

Anesthesia
23660 01630

ICD-9-CM Diagnostic
718.21 Pathological dislocation of shoulder joint
718.71 Developmental dislocation of joint, shoulder region
831.00 Closed dislocation of shoulder, unspecified site
831.01 Closed anterior dislocation of humerus
831.02 Closed posterior dislocation of humerus
831.03 Closed inferior dislocation of humerus
831.04 Closed dislocation of acromioclavicular (joint)
831.09 Closed dislocation of other site of shoulder
831.10 Open unspecified dislocation of shoulder
831.11 Open anterior dislocation of humerus
831.12 Open posterior dislocation of humerus
831.13 Open inferior dislocation of humerus
831.14 Open dislocation of acromioclavicular (joint)
831.19 Open dislocation of other site of shoulder

Terms To Know

anterior. Situated in the front area or toward the belly surface of the body; an anatomical reference point used to show the position and relationship of one body structure to another.

developmental dislocation. Displacement of a body part occurring in the developmental phase of childhood.

dislocation. Displacement of a bone in relation to its neighboring tissue, especially a joint.

pathological dislocation. Displacement of a bone or joint caused by a disease process, such as infection, lesions, or muscle weakness, and not traumatic injury.

posterior. Located in the back part or caudal end of the body.

tendon. Fibrous tissue that connects muscle to bone, consisting primarily of collagen and containing little vasculature.

CCI Version 16.3
01610, 0213T, 0216T, 0228T, 0230T, 12034, 23040, 23100, 23105, 23107, 23650-23655, 23700, 24332, 29000-29065, 29105, 29240, 29700-29715, 36000, 36400-36410, 36420-36430, 36440, 36600, 36640, 37202, 43752, 51701-51703, 62310-62319, 64400-64435, 64445-64450, 64479, 64483, 64490, 64493, 64505-64530, 69990, 93000-93010, 93040-93042, 93318, 94002, 94200, 94250, 94680-94690, 94770, 95812-95816, 95819, 95822, 95829, 95955, 96360, 96365, 96372, 96374-96376, 97597-97598, 97602-97606, 99148-99149, 99150

Note: These CCI edits are used for Medicare. Other payers may reimburse on codes listed above.

Medicare Edits

	Fac RVU	Non-Fac RVU	FUD	Assist
23660	16.9	16.9	90	80

Medicare References: 100-2,15,260; 100-4,12,30; 100-4,12,90.3; 100-4,14,10

23665

23665 Closed treatment of shoulder dislocation, with fracture of greater humeral tuberosity, with manipulation

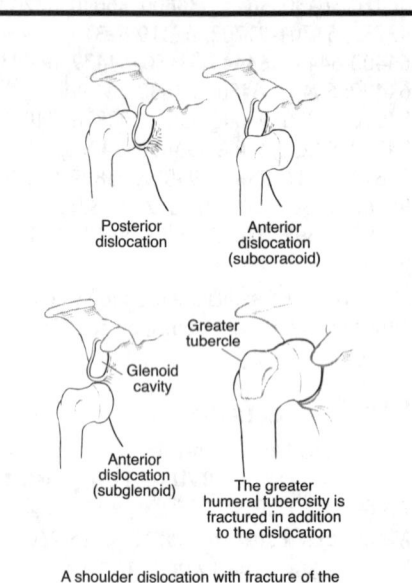

Posterior dislocation
Anterior dislocation (subcoracoid)
Glenoid cavity
Greater tubercle
Anterior dislocation (subglenoid)
The greater humeral tuberosity is fractured in addition to the dislocation

A shoulder dislocation with fracture of the greater humeral tuberosity is treated in a closed fashion with manipulation

Explanation
The physician performs closed reduction of a shoulder dislocation with greater humeral tuberosity fracture. With the patient positioned prone and the arm hanging toward the floor, manual distraction is attempted. If not successful, the physician may hang a five-pound weight from the arm in an attempt to reduce the shoulder into place. Once shoulder reduction is obtained, a neurovascular examination is performed and treatment of the humeral tuberosity fracture is addressed. The arm is immobilized for three to six weeks.

Coding Tips
According to CPT guidelines, cast application or strapping (including removal) is only reported as a replacement procedure or when the cast application or strapping is an initial service performed without a restorative treatment or procedure. See "Application of Casts and Strapping" in the CPT book in the Surgery Section, under the Musculoskeletal system. Local anesthesia is included in this service. However, this procedure may be performed under general anesthesia, depending on the age and/or condition of the patient. For open treatment of a shoulder dislocation with a greater humeral tuberosity fracture, see 23670. For closed treatment of a shoulder dislocation alone, see 23650 and 23655. For open treatment of a shoulder dislocation alone, see 23660.

ICD-9-CM Procedural
- 79.01 Closed reduction of fracture of humerus without internal fixation
- 79.71 Closed reduction of dislocation of shoulder

Anesthesia
23665 01620

ICD-9-CM Diagnostic
- 733.11 Pathologic fracture of humerus
- 812.03 Closed fracture of greater tuberosity of humerus
- 831.00 Closed dislocation of shoulder, unspecified site

Terms To Know

closed fracture. Break in a bone without a concomitant opening in the skin. A closed fracture is coded when the type of fracture is not specified.

developmental dislocation. Displacement of a body part occurring in the developmental phase of childhood.

dislocation. Displacement of a bone in relation to its neighboring tissue, especially a joint.

pathologic fracture. Break in bone due to a disease process that weakens the bone structure, such as osteoporosis, osteomalacia, or neoplasia, and not traumatic injury.

prone. Lying face downward.

CCI Version 16.3
01610, 0213T, 0216T, 0228T, 0230T, 23700, 29000-29065, 29105, 29240, 29700-29715, 36000, 36400-36410, 36420-36430, 36440, 36600, 36640, 37202, 43752, 51701-51703, 62310-62319, 64400-64435, 64445-64450, 64479, 64483, 64490, 64493, 64505-64530, 69990, 93000-93010, 93040-93042, 93318, 94002, 94200, 94250, 94680-94690, 94770, 95812-95816, 95819, 95822, 95829, 95955, 96360, 96365, 96372, 96374-96376, 97597-97598, 97602-97606, 99148-99149, 99150, J0670, J2001

Note: These CCI edits are used for Medicare. Other payers may reimburse on codes listed above.

Medicare Edits

	Fac RVU	Non-Fac RVU	FUD	Assist
23665	11.28	12.03	90	N/A

Medicare References: 100-2,15,260; 100-4,12,30; 100-4,12,90.3; 100-4,14,10

23670

23670 Open treatment of shoulder dislocation, with fracture of greater humeral tuberosity, includes internal fixation, when performed

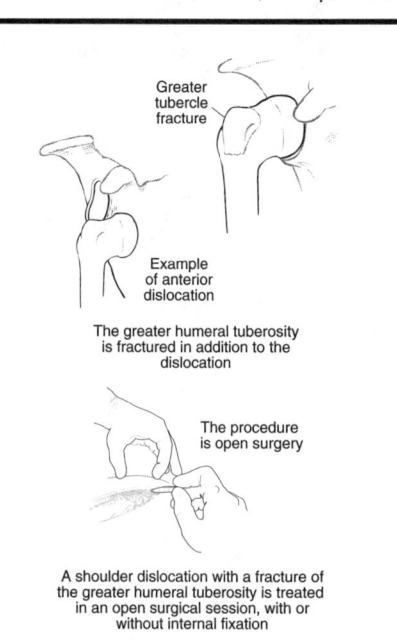

Greater tubercle fracture

Example of anterior dislocation

The greater humeral tuberosity is fractured in addition to the dislocation

The procedure is open surgery

A shoulder dislocation with a fracture of the greater humeral tuberosity is treated in an open surgical session, with or without internal fixation

Explanation

The physician performs open reduction of a shoulder dislocation with greater humeral tuberosity fracture. The physician may enter the shoulder anteriorly through a deltopectoral approach or superiorly through a deltoid splitting approach. The soft tissues are reflected and the fracture is observed. Once the dislocated joint is reduced into proper position, the repair of the humeral tuberosity fracture is addressed. Larger fragments may be stabilized with screws, wire sutures, staples, or other internal fixation measures. These fragments usually require later removal of the fixation device to allow full motion of the shoulder. If the fragment is small, it can be removed and the tendons of the rotator cuff advanced and attached to the defect in the bone. Once the fracture is stable, the incision is closed and the arm is protected in a sling for four to six weeks.

Coding Tips

According to CPT guidelines, cast application or strapping (including removal) is only reported as a replacement procedure or when the cast application or strapping is an initial service performed without a restorative treatment or procedure. See "Application of Casts and Strapping" in the CPT book in the Surgery Section, under the Musculoskeletal system. For debridement of an open fracture, see 11010–11012. For closed treatment of a shoulder dislocation with a greater humeral tuberosity fracture, see 23665. For closed treatment of a shoulder dislocation alone, see 23650 and 23655. For open treatment of a shoulder dislocation alone, see 23660.

ICD-9-CM Procedural

- 79.21 Open reduction of fracture of humerus without internal fixation
- 79.31 Open reduction of fracture of humerus with internal fixation
- 79.81 Open reduction of dislocation of shoulder

Anesthesia

23670 01630

ICD-9-CM Diagnostic

- 733.11 Pathologic fracture of humerus
- 812.03 Closed fracture of greater tuberosity of humerus
- 812.13 Open fracture of greater tuberosity of humerus
- 831.00 Closed dislocation of shoulder, unspecified site
- 831.10 Open unspecified dislocation of shoulder
- 831.19 Open dislocation of other site of shoulder

Terms To Know

closed fracture. Break in a bone without a concomitant opening in the skin. A closed fracture is coded when the type of fracture is not specified.

developmental dislocation. Displacement of a body part occurring in the developmental phase of childhood.

dislocation. Displacement of a bone in relation to its neighboring tissue, especially a joint.

open fracture. Exposed break in a bone, always considered compound due to its high risk of infection from the open wound leading to the fracture. Broken bone ends may protrude through the skin and contaminants or foreign bodies are often embedded in the tissues.

pathologic fracture. Break in bone due to a disease process that weakens the bone structure, such as osteoporosis, osteomalacia, or neoplasia, and not traumatic injury.

soft tissue. Nonepithelial tissues outside of the skeleton that includes subcutaneous adipose tissue, fibrous tissue, fascia, muscles, blood and lymph vessels, and peripheral nervous system tissue.

CCI Version 16.3

01610, 0213T, 0216T, 0228T, 0230T, 20650, 23040, 23100, 23105, 23107, 23410-23412, 23420, 23450, 23625, 23650-23655, 23660-23665, 23700, 24332, 29000-29065, 29105, 29240, 29700-29715, 36000, 36400-36410, 36420-36430, 36440, 36600, 36640, 37202, 43752, 51701-51703, 62310-62319, 64400-64435, 64445-64450, 64479, 64483, 64490, 64493, 64505-64530, 69990, 93000-93010, 93040-93042, 93318, 94002, 94200, 94250, 94680-94690, 94770, 95812-95816, 95819, 95822, 95829, 95955, 96360, 96365, 96372, 96374-96376, 97597-97598, 97602-97606, 99148-99149, 99150

Note: These CCI edits are used for Medicare. Other payers may reimburse on codes listed above.

Medicare Edits

	Fac RVU	Non-Fac RVU	FUD	Assist
23670	25.24	25.24	90	80

Medicare References: 100-2,15,260; 100-4,12,30; 100-4,12,90.3; 100-4,14,10

23675

23675 Closed treatment of shoulder dislocation, with surgical or anatomical neck fracture, with manipulation

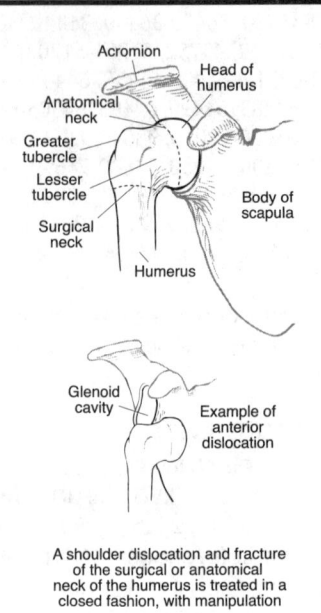

A shoulder dislocation and fracture of the surgical or anatomical neck of the humerus is treated in a closed fashion, with manipulation

Explanation
The physician performs closed reduction of a shoulder dislocation with surgical or anatomical neck fracture. With the patient positioned prone and the arm hanging toward the floor, manual distraction is attempted. If not successful, the physician may hang a five-pound weight from the arm in an attempt to reduce the shoulder into place. Once shoulder reduction is obtained, a neurovascular examination is performed and treatment of the humeral surgical or anatomical neck fracture is addressed. The arm is immobilized for three to six weeks.

Coding Tips
According to CPT guidelines, cast application or strapping (including removal) is only reported as a replacement procedure or when the cast application or strapping is an initial service performed without a restorative treatment or procedure. See "Application of Casts and Strapping" in the CPT book in the Surgery Section, under the Musculoskeletal system. Local anesthesia is included in this service. However, this procedure may be performed under general anesthesia, depending on the age and/or condition of the patient. For radiology services, see 73020 and 73030. For open treatment of a dislocation with a surgical or an anatomical neck fracture, see 23680. For closed treatment of a shoulder dislocation alone, see 23650 and 23655.

ICD-9-CM Procedural
- 79.01 Closed reduction of fracture of humerus without internal fixation
- 79.71 Closed reduction of dislocation of shoulder

Anesthesia
23675 01620

ICD-9-CM Diagnostic
- 733.11 Pathologic fracture of humerus
- 812.01 Closed fracture of surgical neck of humerus
- 812.02 Closed fracture of anatomical neck of humerus
- 831.00 Closed dislocation of shoulder, unspecified site

Terms To Know
closed fracture. Break in a bone without a concomitant opening in the skin. A closed fracture is coded when the type of fracture is not specified.

developmental dislocation. Displacement of a body part occurring in the developmental phase of childhood.

dislocation. Displacement of a bone in relation to its neighboring tissue, especially a joint.

pathologic fracture. Break in bone due to a disease process that weakens the bone structure, such as osteoporosis, osteomalacia, or neoplasia, and not traumatic injury.

prone. Lying face downward.

CCI Version 16.3
01610, 0213T, 0216T, 0228T, 0230T, 23700, 29000-29065, 29105, 29240, 29700-29715, 36000, 36400-36410, 36420-36430, 36440, 36600, 36640, 37202, 43752, 51701-51703, 62310-62319, 64400-64435, 64445-64450, 64479, 64483, 64490, 64493, 64505-64530, 69990, 93000-93010, 93040-93042, 93318, 94002, 94200, 94250, 94680-94690, 94770, 95812-95816, 95819, 95822, 95829, 95955, 96360, 96365, 96372, 96374-96376, 97597-97598, 97602-97606, 99148-99149, 99150, J0670, J2001

Note: These CCI edits are used for Medicare. Other payers may reimburse on codes listed above.

Medicare Edits

	Fac RVU	Non-Fac RVU	FUD	Assist
23675	14.41	15.67	90	N/A

Medicare References: 100-2,15,260; 100-4,12,30; 100-4,12,90.3; 100-4,14,10

23680

23680 Open treatment of shoulder dislocation, with surgical or anatomical neck fracture, includes internal fixation, when performed

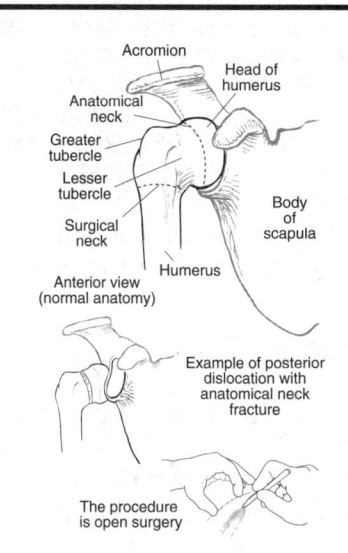

Upper shoulder dislocation with fracture of the surgical or anatomical neck of the humerus is treated in an open surgical session, with or without internal fixation

Explanation

The physician performs open reduction of a shoulder dislocation with surgical or anatomical neck fracture. The physician may enter the shoulder anteriorly through a deltopectoral approach or superiorly through a deltoid splitting approach. The soft tissues are reflected and the fracture is observed. Once the dislocated joint is reduced into proper position, the repair of the humeral surgical or anatomical neck fracture is addressed. Larger fragments may be stabilized with screws, wire sutures, staples, or other internal fixation measures. These fragments usually require later removal of the fixation device to allow full motion of the shoulder. An intramedullary rod may be placed through the shaft of the bone as well. Once the fracture is stable, the incision is closed and the arm is protected in a sling for four to six weeks.

Coding Tips

According to CPT guidelines, cast application or strapping (including removal) is only reported as a replacement procedure or when the cast application or strapping is an initial service performed without a restorative treatment or procedure. See "Application of Casts and Strapping" in the CPT book in the Surgery Section, under the Musculoskeletal system. For closed treatment of a dislocation with a surgical or an anatomical neck fracture, see 23675. For closed treatment of a shoulder dislocation alone, see 23650 and 23655.

ICD-9-CM Procedural

- 79.21 Open reduction of fracture of humerus without internal fixation
- 79.31 Open reduction of fracture of humerus with internal fixation
- 79.81 Open reduction of dislocation of shoulder

Anesthesia

23680 01630

ICD-9-CM Diagnostic

- 733.11 Pathologic fracture of humerus
- 812.01 Closed fracture of surgical neck of humerus
- 812.02 Closed fracture of anatomical neck of humerus
- 812.11 Open fracture of surgical neck of humerus
- 812.12 Open fracture of anatomical neck of humerus
- 831.00 Closed dislocation of shoulder, unspecified site
- 831.10 Open unspecified dislocation of shoulder
- 831.19 Open dislocation of other site of shoulder

Terms To Know

closed fracture. Break in a bone without a concomitant opening in the skin. A closed fracture is coded when the type of fracture is not specified.

developmental dislocation. Displacement of a body part occurring in the developmental phase of childhood.

dislocation. Displacement of a bone in relation to its neighboring tissue, especially a joint.

open fracture. Exposed break in a bone, always considered compound due to its high risk of infection from the open wound leading to the fracture. Broken bone ends may protrude through the skin and contaminants or foreign bodies are often embedded in the tissues.

pathologic fracture. Break in bone due to a disease process that weakens the bone structure, such as osteoporosis, osteomalacia, or neoplasia, and not traumatic injury.

CCI Version 16.3

01610, 0213T, 0216T, 0228T, 0230T, 20650, 23040, 23100, 23105, 23107, 23410-23412, 23420, 23450, 23600-23605, 23615, 23650-23655, 23660, 23675, 23700, 24332, 29000-29065, 29105, 29240, 29700-29715, 29820-29821, 36000, 36400-36410, 36420-36430, 36440, 36600, 36640, 37202, 43752, 51701-51703, 62310-62319, 64400-64435, 64445-64450, 64479, 64483, 64490, 64493, 64505-64530, 69990, 93000-93010, 93040-93042, 93318, 94002, 94200, 94250, 94680-94690, 94770, 95812-95816, 95819, 95822, 95829, 95955, 96360, 96365, 96372, 96374-96376, 97597-97598, 97602-97606, 99148-99149, 99150

Note: These CCI edits are used for Medicare. Other payers may reimburse on codes listed above.

Medicare Edits

	Fac RVU	Non-Fac RVU	FUD	Assist
23680	26.94	26.94	90	80

Medicare References: 100-2,15,260; 100-4,12,30; 100-4,12,90.3; 100-4,14,10

23700

23700 Manipulation under anesthesia, shoulder joint, including application of fixation apparatus (dislocation excluded)

The patient is under anesthesia

Dislocation is excluded

A shoulder joint is manipulated while the patient is under anesthesia. Application of fixation apparatus is included

Explanation

Manipulation of the shoulder under anesthesia may be necessary to regain the loss of motion that occurs in the case of frozen shoulder or following a surgical procedure. The patient is positioned supine and given general anesthesia. Following full evaluation, the physician manipulates the shoulder to achieve the appropriate range of motion. A fixation apparatus may also be applied.

Coding Tips

For closed treatment of a shoulder dislocation with manipulation, see 23655.

ICD-9-CM Procedural

- 78.11 Application of external fixator device, scapula, clavicle, and thorax [ribs and sternum]
- 78.12 Application of external fixator device, humerus
- 78.19 Application of external fixator device, other
- 84.71 Application of external fixator device, monoplanar system
- 84.72 Application of external fixator device, ring system
- 84.73 Application of hybrid external fixator device
- 93.25 Forced extension of limb
- 93.26 Manual rupture of joint adhesions

Anesthesia
23700 01620

ICD-9-CM Diagnostic

- 354.4 Causalgia of upper limb
- 719.41 Pain in joint, shoulder region
- 723.4 Brachial neuritis or radiculitis nos.
- 726.0 Adhesive capsulitis of shoulder
- 726.10 Unspecified disorders of bursae and tendons in shoulder region
- 726.11 Calcifying tendinitis of shoulder
- 726.2 Other affections of shoulder region, not elsewhere classified
- 727.82 Calcium deposits in tendon and bursa
- 728.85 Spasm of muscle
- 729.1 Unspecified myalgia and myositis
- 729.2 Unspecified neuralgia, neuritis, and radiculitis
- 739.7 Nonallopathic lesion of upper extremities, not elsewhere classified

Terms To Know

adhesive capsulitis. Excessive scar tissue in the shoulder, causing stiffness and pain.

calcifying tendinitis. Inflammation and hardening of tissue due to calcium salt deposits, occurring in the tendons and areas of tendonomuscular attachment.

causalgia. Condition due to an injury of a peripheral nerve causing burning pain and possible trophic skin changes.

lesion. Area of damaged tissue that has lost continuity or function, due to disease or trauma. Lesions may be located on internal structures such as the brain, nerves, or kidneys, or visible on the skin.

myalgia. Pain in the muscles.

spasm. Involuntary muscle contraction.

tendon. Fibrous tissue that connects muscle to bone, consisting primarily of collagen and containing little vasculature.

CCI Version 16.3

01610, 0213T, 0216T, 0228T, 0230T, 11010-11012❖, 20650, 20690, 20692, 20696-20697, 23650-23655❖, 36000, 36400-36410, 36420-36430, 36440, 36600, 36640, 37202, 43752, 51701-51703, 62310-62319, 64400-64435, 64445-64450, 64479, 64483, 64490, 64493, 64505-64530, 64713, 69990, 93000-93010, 93040-93042, 93318, 94002, 94200, 94250, 94680-94690, 94770, 95812-95816, 95819, 95822, 95829, 95955, 96360, 96365, 96372, 96374-96376, 99148-99149, 99150

Note: These CCI edits are used for Medicare. Other payers may reimburse on codes listed above.

Medicare Edits

	Fac RVU	Non-Fac RVU	FUD	Assist
23700	5.64	5.64	10	N/A

Medicare References: 100-2,15,260; 100-4,12,30; 100-4,12,90.3; 100-4,14,10

23800-23802

23800 Arthrodesis, glenohumeral joint;
23802 with autogenous graft (includes obtaining graft)

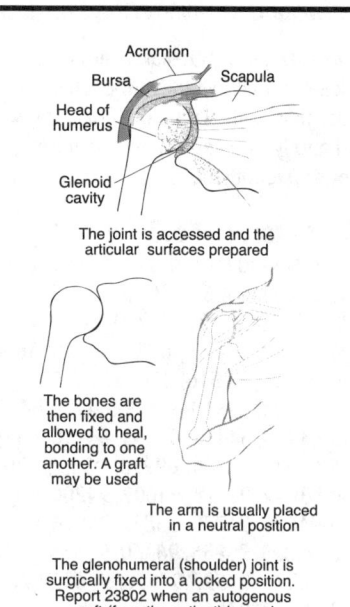

The joint is accessed and the articular surfaces prepared

The bones are then fixed and allowed to heal, bonding to one another. A graft may be used

The arm is usually placed in a neutral position

The glenohumeral (shoulder) joint is surgically fixed into a locked position. Report 23802 when an autogenous graft (from the patient) is used

Explanation
The physician performs arthrodesis of the glenohumeral joint. The shoulder is positioned in what is considered the most functional position, slightly abducted to the side with forward elevation. A dorsolateral semicircular incision is made across the glenohumeral joint and carried distally at the midpoint. The articular cartilage is removed from the head of the humerus (ball) and the glenoid cavity (socket). The head is split and a wedge of bone is removed. This wedge is where the acromion will rest when the arm is positioned in abduction. At this point, bone grafting or plate fixation may be added to the procedure to stabilize the glenohumeral joint. If a plate is used, a second procedure will be needed to remove the hardware. Cast application or external fixation may be used in a number of ways. Report 23802 if an autogenous graft is used.

Coding Tips
A graft is included in 23802 and should not be reported separately. For removal of an internal fixation, see 23330–23332. According to CPT guidelines, cast application or strapping (including removal) is only reported as a replacement procedure or when the cast application or strapping is an initial service performed without a restorative treatment or procedure. See "Application of Casts and Strapping" in the CPT book in the Surgery Section, under the Musculoskeletal system.

ICD-9-CM Procedural
77.71	Excision of scapula, clavicle, and thorax (ribs and sternum) for graft
77.77	Excision of tibia and fibula for graft
77.79	Excision of other bone for graft, except facial bones
78.02	Bone graft of humerus
81.23	Arthrodesis of shoulder

Anesthesia
01630

ICD-9-CM Diagnostic
171.2	Malignant neoplasm of connective and other soft tissue of upper limb, including shoulder
198.5	Secondary malignant neoplasm of bone and bone marrow
238.0	Neoplasm of uncertain behavior of bone and articular cartilage
239.2	Neoplasms of unspecified nature of bone, soft tissue, and skin
357.1	Polyneuropathy in collagen vascular disease — (Code first underlying disease: 446.0, 710.0, 714.0)
359.6	Symptomatic inflammatory myopathy in diseases classified elsewhere — (Code first underlying disease: 135, 140.0-208.9, 277.30-277.39, 446.0, 710.0, 710.1, 710.2, 714.0)
711.01	Pyogenic arthritis, shoulder region — (Use additional code to identify infectious organism: 041.0-041.8)
714.0	Rheumatoid arthritis — (Use additional code to identify manifestation: 357.1, 359.6)
715.11	Primary localized osteoarthrosis, shoulder region
715.21	Secondary localized osteoarthrosis, shoulder region
715.31	Localized osteoarthrosis not specified whether primary or secondary, shoulder region
715.91	Osteoarthrosis, unspecified whether generalized or localized, shoulder region
716.11	Traumatic arthropathy, shoulder region
718.01	Articular cartilage disorder, shoulder region
718.31	Recurrent dislocation of shoulder joint
730.11	Chronic osteomyelitis, shoulder region — (Use additional code to identify organism: 041.1. Use additional code to identify major osseous defect, if applicable: 731.3)
731.3	Major osseous defects — (Code first underlying disease: 170.0-170.9, 730.00-730.29, 733.00-733.09, 733.40-733.49, 996.45)

Terms To Know
myopathy. Any disease process within muscle tissue.

osteoarthrosis. Most common form of a noninflammatory degenerative joint disease with degenerating articular cartilage, bone enlargement, and synovial membrane changes.

osteomyelitis. Inflammation of bone that may remain localized or spread to the marrow, cortex, or periosteum, in response to an infecting organism, usually bacterial and pyogenic.

CCI Version 16.3
01610, 0213T, 0216T, 0228T, 0230T, 20690, 20692, 23000, 23040, 23100, 23105, 23107, 23130-23140, 23415, 23700, 24332, 29822-29823, 36000, 36400-36410, 36420-36430, 36440, 36600, 36640, 37202, 43752, 51701-51703, 62310-62319, 64400-64435, 64445-64450, 64479, 64483, 64490, 64493, 64505-64530, 69990, 93000-93010, 93040-93042, 93318, 94002, 94200, 94250, 94680-94690, 94770, 95812-95816, 95819, 95822, 95829, 95955, 96360, 96365, 96372, 96374-96376, 99148-99149, 99150

Also not with 23802: 20900-20902

Note: These CCI edits are used for Medicare. Other payers may reimburse on codes listed above.

Medicare Edits
	Fac RVU	Non-Fac RVU	FUD	Assist
23800	30.06	30.06	90	80
23802	37.17	37.17	90	80

Medicare References: 100-2,15,260; 100-4,12,30; 100-4,12,90.3; 100-4,14,10

23900

23900 Interthoracoscapular amputation (forequarter)

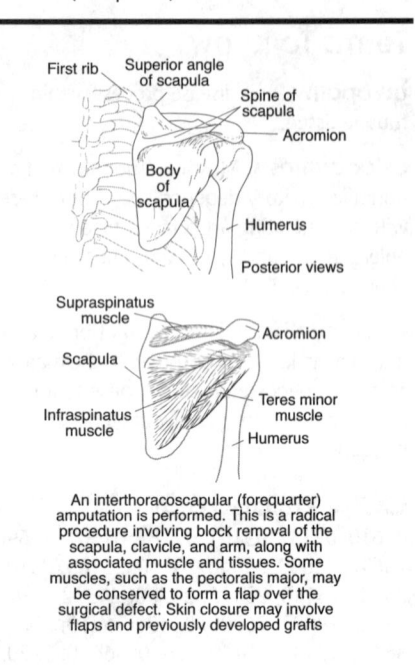

An interthoracoscapular (forequarter) amputation is performed. This is a radical procedure involving block removal of the scapula, clavicle, and arm, along with associated muscle and tissues. Some muscles, such as the pectoralis major, may be conserved to form a flap over the surgical defect. Skin closure may involve flaps and previously developed grafts

Explanation

The physician preforms a forequarter amputation (interthoracoscapular). The physician incises the skin overlying the shoulder and dissects the disease-free soft tissue away from the bone to create a skin flap to cover the wound. The clavicle is disarticulated from the sternum and the chest wall is freed from muscular attachments to the arm. The quarter section is removed and the wound is closed in sutured layers. If enough disease-free tissue is not available for primary closure, the wound is packed closed with gauze.

Coding Tips

If significant additional time and effort is documented, append modifier 22 and submit a cover letter and operative report. For disarticulation of the shoulder, see 23920–23921.

ICD-9-CM Procedural

84.09 Interthoracoscapular amputation

Anesthesia

23900 01636

ICD-9-CM Diagnostic

- 170.4 Malignant neoplasm of scapula and long bones of upper limb
- 171.2 Malignant neoplasm of connective and other soft tissue of upper limb, including shoulder
- 199.0 Disseminated malignant neoplasm
- 238.0 Neoplasm of uncertain behavior of bone and articular cartilage
- 728.86 Necrotizing fasciitis — (Use additional code to identify infectious organism, 041.00-041.89, 785.4, if applicable)
- 785.4 Gangrene — (Code first any associated underlying condition)
- 880.10 Open wound of shoulder region, complicated
- 880.11 Open wound of scapular region, complicated
- 880.12 Open wound of axillary region, complicated
- 880.13 Open wound of upper arm, complicated
- 880.20 Open wound of shoulder region, with tendon involvement
- 880.21 Open wound of scapular region, with tendon involvement
- 880.22 Open wound of axillary region, with tendon involvement
- 880.23 Open wound of upper arm, with tendon involvement
- 887.2 Traumatic amputation of arm and hand (complete) (partial), unilateral, at or above elbow, without mention of complication
- 887.3 Traumatic amputation of arm and hand (complete) (partial), unilateral, at or above elbow, complicated
- 906.7 Late effect of burn of other extremities
- 927.00 Crushing injury of shoulder region — (Use additional code to identify any associated injuries: 800-829, 850.0-854.1, 860.0-869.1)
- 927.01 Crushing injury of scapular region — (Use additional code to identify any associated injuries: 800-829, 850.0-854.1, 860.0-869.1)
- 927.02 Crushing injury of axillary region — (Use additional code to identify any associated injuries: 800-829, 850.0-854.1, 860.0-869.1)

Terms To Know

gangrene. Death of tissue, usually resulting from a loss of vascular supply, followed by a bacterial attack or onset of disease.

late effect. Abnormality, dysfunction, or other residual condition produced after the acute phase of an illness, injury, or disease is over. There is no time limit on when late effects can appear.

malignant. Any condition tending to progress toward death, specifically an invasive tumor with a loss of cellular differentiation that has the ability to spread or metastasize to other areas in the body.

open wound. Opening or break of the skin.

soft tissue. Nonepithelial tissues outside of the skeleton that includes subcutaneous adipose tissue, fibrous tissue, fascia, muscles, blood and lymph vessels, and peripheral nervous system tissue.

CCI Version 16.3

01610, 0213T, 0216T, 0228T, 0230T, 20103, 20200-20205, 23065-23066, 23075-23077, 23125, 23140, 23182, 23210, 36000, 36400-36410, 36420-36430, 36440, 36600, 36640, 37202, 37616, 37618, 43752, 51701-51703, 62310-62319, 64400-64435, 64445-64450, 64479, 64483, 64490, 64493, 64505-64530, 64784, 69990, 93000-93010, 93040-93042, 93318, 94002, 94200, 94250, 94680-94690, 94770, 95812-95816, 95819, 95822, 95829, 95955, 96360, 96365, 96372, 96374-96376, 97597-97598, 97602-97606, 99148-99149, 99150

Note: These CCI edits are used for Medicare. Other payers may reimburse on codes listed above.

Medicare Edits

	Fac RVU	Non-Fac RVU	FUD	Assist
23900	39.83	39.83	90	80

Medicare References: None

23920-23921

23920 Disarticulation of shoulder;
23921 secondary closure or scar revision

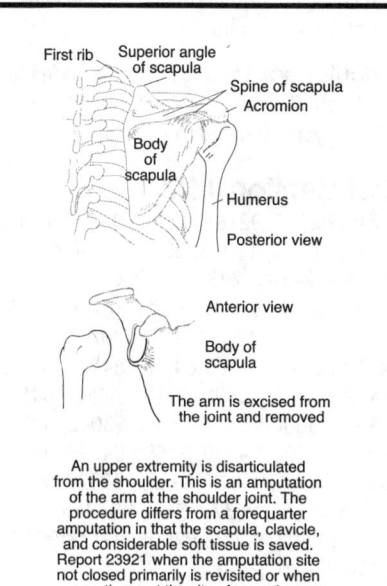

An upper extremity is disarticulated from the shoulder. This is an amputation of the arm at the shoulder joint. The procedure differs from a forequarter amputation in that the scapula, clavicle, and considerable soft tissue is saved. Report 23921 when the amputation site not closed primarily is revisited or when scar tissue at the site of a previous disarticulation requires revision

Explanation

The physician disarticulates the shoulder. The physician incises the skin overlying the shoulder. The rotator cuff is incised freeing the arm of ligamentous and muscular attachments. The arm is removed and the wound is closed in sutured layers. Report 23920 for the initial amputation. Report 23921 for a secondary closure of the wound or scar revision.

Coding Tips

If significant additional time and effort is documented, append modifier 22 and submit a cover letter and operative report. For interthoracoscapular amputation, see 23900.

ICD-9-CM Procedural

84.08 Disarticulation of shoulder
84.3 Revision of amputation stump

Anesthesia

23920 01634
23921 00300, 00400

ICD-9-CM Diagnostic

170.4 Malignant neoplasm of scapula and long bones of upper limb
171.2 Malignant neoplasm of connective and other soft tissue of upper limb, including shoulder
199.0 Disseminated malignant neoplasm
238.0 Neoplasm of uncertain behavior of bone and articular cartilage
728.86 Necrotizing fasciitis — (Use additional code to identify infectious organism, 041.00-041.89, 785.4, if applicable)
785.4 Gangrene — (Code first any associated underlying condition)
880.10 Open wound of shoulder region, complicated
880.12 Open wound of axillary region, complicated
880.13 Open wound of upper arm, complicated
880.19 Open wound of multiple sites of shoulder and upper arm, complicated
880.20 Open wound of shoulder region, with tendon involvement
880.22 Open wound of axillary region, with tendon involvement
880.23 Open wound of upper arm, with tendon involvement
880.29 Open wound of multiple sites of shoulder and upper arm, with tendon involvement
887.2 Traumatic amputation of arm and hand (complete) (partial), unilateral, at or above elbow, without mention of complication
887.3 Traumatic amputation of arm and hand (complete) (partial), unilateral, at or above elbow, complicated
906.7 Late effect of burn of other extremities
908.6 Late effect of certain complications of trauma
927.00 Crushing injury of shoulder region — (Use additional code to identify any associated injuries: 800-829, 850.0-854.1, 860.0-869.1)
927.01 Crushing injury of scapular region — (Use additional code to identify any associated injuries: 800-829, 850.0-854.1, 860.0-869.1)
927.02 Crushing injury of axillary region — (Use additional code to identify any associated injuries: 800-829, 850.0-854.1, 860.0-869.1)
927.03 Crushing injury of upper arm — (Use additional code to identify any associated injuries: 800-829, 850.0-854.1, 860.0-869.1)
927.09 Crushing injury of multiple sites of upper arm — (Use additional code to identify any associated injuries: 800-829, 850.0-854.1, 860.0-869.1)
997.69 Other late amputation stump complication — (Use additional code to identify complications)
V49.67 Upper limb amputation, shoulder
V51.8 Other aftercare involving the use of plastic surgery

CCI Version 16.3

01610, 0213T, 0216T, 0228T, 0230T, 36000, 36400-36410, 36420-36430, 36440, 36600, 36640, 37202, 43752, 51701-51703, 62310-62319, 64400-64435, 64445-64450, 64479, 64483, 64490, 64493, 64505-64530, 69990, 93000-93010, 93040-93042, 93318, 94002, 94200, 94250, 94680-94690, 94770, 95812-95816, 95819, 95822, 95829, 95955, 96360, 96365, 96372, 96374-96376, 97597-97598, 97602-97606, 99148-99149, 99150

Also not with 23920: 20103, 23040, 23075-23077, 23100, 23105, 23107, 23220, 37618, 64784

Also not with 23921: 11012❖, 23920, J2001

Note: These CCI edits are used for Medicare. Other payers may reimburse on codes listed above.

Medicare Edits

	Fac RVU	Non-Fac RVU	FUD	Assist
23920	32.34	32.34	90	80
23921	12.83	12.83	90	N/A

Medicare References: 100-2,15,260; 100-4,12,30; 100-4,12,90.3; 100-4,14,10

23930-23931

23930 Incision and drainage, upper arm or elbow area; deep abscess or hematoma
23931 bursa

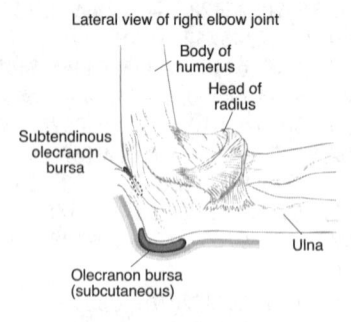

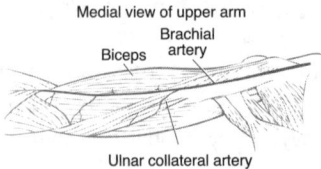

Lateral view of right elbow joint
- Body of humerus
- Head of radius
- Subtendinous olecranon bursa
- Ulna
- Olecranon bursa (subcutaneous)

Medial view of upper arm
- Biceps
- Brachial artery
- Ulnar collateral artery

A deep abscess or hematoma of the upper arm or elbow area is incised and drained. Report 23931 when a bursa of the area is incised and drained

Explanation
The physician drains a deep abscess or hematoma in 23930 or an infected bursa in 23931 from within the upper arm or elbow area. With proper anesthesia administered, the physician makes an incision in the upper arm or elbow overlying the site of the abscess, hematoma, or bursa to be incised. Dissection is carried down through the deep subcutaneous tissues and may be continued into the fascia or muscle to expose the abscess or hematoma. The incision may be extended if the mass is larger than expected. When the infected bursa, abscess, or hematoma is identified, it is incised and the contents are drained. The area is irrigated and the incision is repaired in layers with sutures, staples, and/or Steri-strips; closed with drains in place; or simply left open to further facilitate drainage of infection.

Coding Tips
For deep incision with opening of bone cortex for osteomyelitis or bone abscess, see 23935.

ICD-9-CM Procedural
- 83.03 Bursotomy
- 83.09 Other incision of soft tissue

Anesthesia
- **23930** 01740
- **23931** 01710

ICD-9-CM Diagnostic
- 682.3 Cellulitis and abscess of upper arm and forearm — (Use additional code to identify organism, such as 041.1, etc.)
- 711.02 Pyogenic arthritis, upper arm — (Use additional code to identify infectious organism: 041.0-041.8)
- 719.02 Effusion of upper arm joint
- 719.12 Hemarthrosis, upper arm
- 719.82 Other specified disorders of upper arm joint
- 726.33 Olecranon bursitis
- 727.89 Other disorders of synovium, tendon, and bursa
- 728.0 Infective myositis
- 729.4 Unspecified fasciitis
- 729.5 Pain in soft tissues of limb
- 730.02 Acute osteomyelitis, upper arm — (Use additional code to identify organism: 041.1. Use additional code to identify major osseous defect, if applicable: 731.3)
- 730.12 Chronic osteomyelitis, upper arm — (Use additional code to identify organism: 041.1. Use additional code to identify major osseous defect, if applicable: 731.3)
- 780.62 Postprocedural fever
- 903.1 Brachial blood vessels injury
- 923.03 Contusion of upper arm
- 923.11 Contusion of elbow
- 958.8 Other early complications of trauma
- 996.1 Mechanical complication of other vascular device, implant, and graft
- 998.59 Other postoperative infection — (Use additional code to identify infection)

Terms To Know
abscess. Circumscribed collection of pus resulting from bacteria, frequently associated with swelling and other signs of inflammation.

bursa. Cavity or sac containing fluid that occurs between articulating surfaces and serves to reduce friction from moving parts. An anatomical structure frequently referenced in orthopedic notes as it may become diseased or need removal.

cellulitis. Sudden, severe, suppurative inflammation and edema in subcutaneous tissue or muscle, most often caused by bacterial infection secondary to a cutaneous lesion.

effusion. Escape of fluid from within a body cavity.

hematoma. Tumor-like collection of blood in some part of the body caused by a break in a blood vessel wall, usually as a result of trauma.

myositis. Inflammation of a muscle with voluntary movement.

subcutaneous tissue. Sheet or wide band of adipose (fat) and areolar connective tissue in two layers attached to the dermis.

CCI Version 16.3
01710, 0213T, 0216T, 0228T, 0230T, 10060, 10140, 10160, 11043, 20103, 20500, 23935❖, 24149, 24300, 36000, 36400-36410, 36420-36430, 36440, 36600, 36640, 37202, 43752, 51701-51703, 62310-62319, 64400-64435, 64445-64450, 64479, 64483, 64490, 64493, 64505-64530, 69990, 93000-93010, 93040-93042, 93318, 94002, 94200, 94250, 94680-94690, 94770, 95812-95816, 95819, 95822, 95829, 95955, 96360, 96365, 96372, 96374-96376, 97597-97598, 97602-97606, 99148-99149, 99150, J0670, J2001

Also not with 23930: 29075, 35761

Also not with 23931: 23930❖, 24332, 29105

Note: These CCI edits are used for Medicare. Other payers may reimburse on codes listed above.

Medicare Edits

	Fac RVU	Non-Fac RVU	FUD	Assist
23930	6.31	10.22	10	N/A
23931	4.59	8.08	10	N/A

Medicare References: 100-2,15,260; 100-4,12,30; 100-4,12,90.3; 100-4,14,10

23935

23935 Incision, deep, with opening of bone cortex (eg, for osteomyelitis or bone abscess), humerus or elbow

Anterior view of right arm and elbow

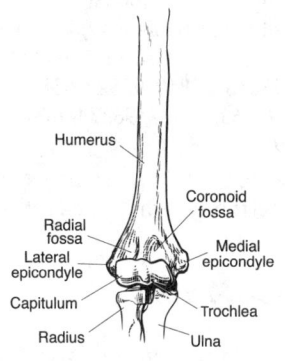

Humerus
Radial fossa
Lateral epicondyle
Capitulum
Radius
Coronoid fossa
Medial epicondyle
Trochlea
Ulna

An incision is made into the bone cortex of the humerus or into the proximal ulna and/or radius of the elbow. Typically a bone abscess is treated or dead bone tissue removed

Explanation

The physician incises the bone cortex of infected bone in the humerus or elbow to treat an abscess or osteomyelitis. The physician makes an incision over the affected area. Dissection is carried down through the soft tissues to expose the bone. The periosteum is split and reflected from the bone overlying the infected area. A curette may be used to scrape away the abscess or infected portion down to healthy bony tissue or drill holes may be made through the cortex into the medullary canal in a window outline around the infected or abscessed bone. The area is drained and debrided of infected bony and soft tissue. The physician irrigates the area with antibiotic solution, the periosteum is closed over the bone, and the soft tissues are sutured closed; or the wound is packed and left open, allowing the area to drain. Secondary closure is performed approximately three weeks later. Dressings are changed daily. A splint may be applied to limit elbow movement.

Coding Tips

For incision and drainage of an upper arm or elbow deep abscess, hematoma, see 23930. For incision and drainage of an elbow bursa, see 23931. According to CPT guidelines, cast application or strapping (including removal) is only reported as a replacement procedure or when the cast application or strapping is an initial service performed without a restorative treatment or procedure. See "Application of Casts and Strapping" in the CPT book in the Surgery Section, under the Musculoskeletal system.

ICD-9-CM Procedural

77.12 Other incision of humerus without division
77.19 Other incision of other bone, except facial bones, without division

Anesthesia

23935 01740

ICD-9-CM Diagnostic

682.3 Cellulitis and abscess of upper arm and forearm — (Use additional code to identify organism, such as 041.1, etc.)
730.12 Chronic osteomyelitis, upper arm — (Use additional code to identify organism: 041.1. Use additional code to identify major osseous defect, if applicable: 731.3)
730.22 Unspecified osteomyelitis, upper arm — (Use additional code to identify organism: 041.1. Use additional code to identify major osseous defect, if applicable: 731.3)
730.28 Unspecified osteomyelitis, other specified sites — (Use additional code to identify organism: 041.1. Use additional code to identify major osseous defect, if applicable: 731.3)
730.29 Unspecified osteomyelitis, multiple sites — (Use additional code to identify organism: 041.1. Use additional code to identify major osseous defect, if applicable: 731.3)
730.30 Periostitis, without mention of osteomyelitis, unspecified site — (Use additional code to identify organism: 041.1)
730.32 Periostitis, without mention of osteomyelitis, upper arm — (Use additional code to identify organism: 041.1)
730.80 Other infections involving bone in diseases classified elsewhere, site unspecified — (Use additional code to identify organism: 041.1. Code first underlying disease: 002.0, 015.0-015.9)
730.82 Other infections involving bone diseases classified elsewhere, upper arm — (Use additional code to identify organism: 041.1. Code first underlying disease: 002.0, 015.0-015.9)
730.88 Other infections involving bone diseases classified elsewhere, other specified sites — (Use additional code to identify organism: 041.1. Code first underlying disease: 002.0, 015.0-015.9)
730.92 Unspecified infection of bone, upper arm — (Use additional code to identify organism: 041.1)
731.3 Major osseous defects — (Code first underlying disease: 170.0-170.9, 730.00-730.29, 733.00-733.09, 733.40-733.49, 996.45)

Terms To Know

abscess. Circumscribed collection of pus resulting from bacteria, frequently associated with swelling and other signs of inflammation.

cellulitis. Sudden, severe, suppurative inflammation and edema in subcutaneous tissue or muscle, most often caused by bacterial infection secondary to a cutaneous lesion.

osteomyelitis. Inflammation of bone that may remain localized or spread to the marrow, cortex, or periosteum, in response to an infecting organism, usually bacterial and pyogenic.

periostitis. Inflammation of the outer layers of bone.

CCI Version 16.3

01710, 0213T, 0216T, 0228T, 0230T, 10060, 10140, 10160, 11010-11011, 20000-20005, 20103, 20500, 20615, 24071, 24075, 24149, 24300, 24332, 36000, 36400-36410, 36420-36430, 36440, 36600, 36640, 37202, 43752, 51701-51703, 62310-62319, 64400-64435, 64445-64450, 64479, 64483, 64490, 64493, 64505-64530, 69990, 93000-93010, 93040-93042, 93318, 94002, 94200, 94250, 94680-94690, 94770, 95812-95816, 95819, 95822, 95829, 95955, 96360, 96365, 96372, 96374-96376, 97597-97598, 97602-97606, 99148-99149, 99150

Note: These CCI edits are used for Medicare. Other payers may reimburse on codes listed above.

Medicare Edits

	Fac RVU	Non-Fac RVU	FUD	Assist
23935	14.59	14.59	90	80

Medicare References: 100-2,15,260; 100-4,12,30; 100-4,12,90.3; 100-4,14,10

24000

24000 Arthrotomy, elbow, including exploration, drainage, or removal of foreign body

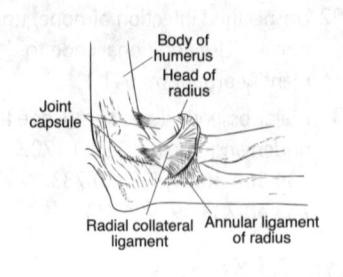

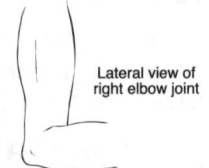

An elbow joint is surgically accessed, explored, drained, and any foreign bodies removed

Explanation

The physician performs an arthrotomy on the elbow that includes exploration, drainage, or removal of any foreign body. A longitudinal incision over the part of the elbow to be exposed (e.g., the anterior, posterior, medial, or lateral aspect) is made. The soft tissues are dissected away and the joint capsule is exposed and incised. The joint is explored, any necrotic tissue is removed, and infection or abnormal fluid is drained. If a foreign body is present (e.g., bullet, nail, gravel), it is exposed and removed. The wound is irrigated with antibiotic solution. The physician may leave the wound packed open with daily dressing changes to allow for further drainage and secondary healing by granulation. If the incision is repaired, drain tubes may be inserted and the incision is repaired in layers with sutures, staples, and/or Steri-strips. A splint may be applied to limit elbow motion.

Coding Tips

For needle biopsy of soft tissue, see 20206.

ICD-9-CM Procedural

80.12 Other arthrotomy of elbow

Anesthesia

24000 01740

ICD-9-CM Diagnostic

711.02 Pyogenic arthritis, upper arm — (Use additional code to identify infectious organism: 041.0-041.8)
711.92 Unspecified infective arthritis, upper arm
711.98 Unspecified infective arthritis, other specified sites
715.92 Osteoarthrosis, unspecified whether generalized or localized, upper arm
718.12 Loose body in upper arm joint
719.02 Effusion of upper arm joint
719.12 Hemarthrosis, upper arm
726.33 Olecranon bursitis
729.6 Residual foreign body in soft tissue — (Use additional code to identify foreign body (V90.01-V90.9))
881.01 Open wound of elbow, without mention of complication
881.11 Open wound of elbow, complicated
998.51 Infected postoperative seroma — (Use additional code to identify organism)
998.59 Other postoperative infection — (Use additional code to identify infection)
V64.43 Arthroscopic surgical procedure converted to open procedure

Terms To Know

anterior. Situated in the front area or toward the belly surface of the body; an anatomical reference point used to show the position and relationship of one body structure to another.

effusion. Escape of fluid from within a body cavity.

foreign body. Any object or substance found in an organ and tissue that does not belong under normal circumstances.

hemarthrosis. Occurrence of blood within a joint space.

infected postoperative seroma. Infection within a tumor-like growth of serum following surgery.

lateral. To/on the side.

medial. Middle or midline.

necrosis. Death of cells or tissue within a living organ or structure.

open wound. Opening or break of the skin.

posterior. Located in the back part or caudal end of the body.

CCI Version 16.3

01710, 0213T, 0216T, 0228T, 0230T, 10060, 10140, 10160, 11010-11011, 11040-11044, 20500, 23100, 24006, 24076, 24101-24102, 24110, 24149, 24300, 24332, 29834-29835, 29837-29838, 36000, 36400-36410, 36420-36430, 36440, 36600, 36640, 37202, 43752, 51701-51703, 62310-62319, 64400-64435, 64445-64450, 64479, 64483, 64490, 64493, 64505-64530, 69990, 93000-93010, 93040-93042, 93318, 94002, 94200, 94250, 94680-94690, 94770, 95812-95816, 95819, 95822, 95829, 95955, 96360, 96365, 96372, 96374-96376, 99148-99149, 99150

Note: These CCI edits are used for Medicare. Other payers may reimburse on codes listed above.

Medicare Edits

	Fac RVU	Non-Fac RVU	FUD	Assist
24000	13.8	13.8	90	80

Medicare References: 100-2,15,260; 100-4,12,30; 100-4,12,90.3; 100-4,14,10

24006

24006 Arthrotomy of the elbow, with capsular excision for capsular release (separate procedure)

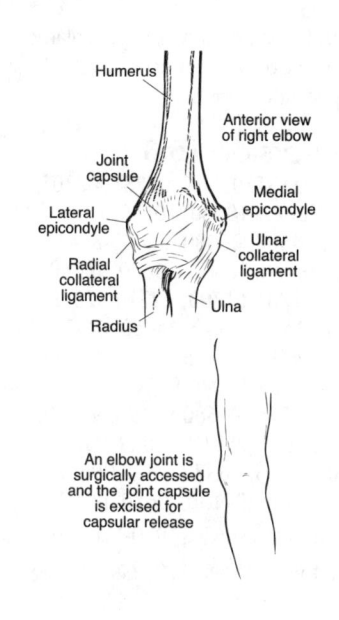

Explanation
The physician performs an arthrotomy of the elbow with capsular excision for release. The physician makes an incision over the anterior part of the elbow. Dissection exposes the joint capsule. The radial nerve is identified and protected. The anterior elbow joint capsule is incised and portions of it are removed. By excising the capsule, any scarring limiting elbow motion is minimal. Additional incisions (e.g., medial elbow incision) are made if other parts of the capsule are also to be excised. The physician repairs the incision in layers with sutures, staples, and/or Steri-strips. The elbow is placed in a posterior splint.

Coding Tips
This separate procedure by definition is usually a component of a more complex service and is not identified separately. When performed alone or with other unrelated procedures/services, it may be reported. If performed alone, list the code; if performed with other procedures/services, list the code and append modifier 59. According to CPT guidelines, cast application or strapping (including removal) is only reported as a replacement procedure or when the cast application or strapping is an initial service performed without a restorative treatment or procedure. See "Application of Casts and Strapping" in the CPT book in the Surgery Section, under the Musculoskeletal system. For arthrotomy with a synovial biopsy, see 24100; for synovectomy, see 24102; or for joint exploration with or without a biopsy, with or without removal of a loose or foreign body, see 24101.

ICD-9-CM Procedural
80.92 Other excision of elbow joint

Anesthesia
24006 01740

ICD-9-CM Diagnostic
711.02 Pyogenic arthritis, upper arm — (Use additional code to identify infectious organism: 041.0-041.8)
711.92 Unspecified infective arthritis, upper arm
715.12 Primary localized osteoarthrosis, upper arm
715.92 Osteoarthrosis, unspecified whether generalized or localized, upper arm
716.12 Traumatic arthropathy, upper arm
718.42 Contracture of upper arm joint
718.52 Ankylosis of upper arm joint
726.30 Unspecified enthesopathy of elbow
726.31 Medial epicondylitis of elbow
726.32 Lateral epicondylitis of elbow
726.33 Olecranon bursitis
726.39 Other enthesopathy of elbow region
V64.43 Arthroscopic surgical procedure converted to open procedure

Terms To Know
ankylosis. Abnormal union or fusion of bones in a joint, which is normally moveable.

anterior. Situated in the front area or toward the belly surface of the body; an anatomical reference point used to show the position and relationship of one body structure to another.

contracture. Shortening of muscle or connective tissue.

epicondylitis. Inflammation of the humeral epicondyle and the tissues adjoining it.

joint capsule. Sac-like enclosure enveloping the synovial joint cavity with a fibrous membrane attached to the articular ends of the bones in the joint.

posterior. Located in the back part or caudal end of the body.

CCI Version 16.3
01710, 0213T, 0216T, 0228T, 0230T, 11010-11012, 20500, 24300, 24332, 24357, 36000, 36400-36410, 36420-36430, 36440, 36600, 36640, 37202, 43752, 51701-51703, 62310-62319, 64400-64435, 64445-64450, 64479, 64483, 64490, 64493, 64505-64530, 69990, 93000-93010, 93040-93042, 93318, 94002, 94200, 94250, 94680-94690, 94770, 95812-95816, 95819, 95822, 95829, 95955, 96360, 96365, 96372, 96374-96376, 99148-99149, 99150

Note: These CCI edits are used for Medicare. Other payers may reimburse on codes listed above.

Medicare Edits

	Fac RVU	Non-Fac RVU	FUD	Assist
24006	20.72	20.72	90	80

Medicare References: 100-2,15,260; 100-4,12,30; 100-4,12,90.3; 100-4,14,10

24065-24066

24065 Biopsy, soft tissue of upper arm or elbow area; superficial
24066 deep (subfascial or intramuscular)

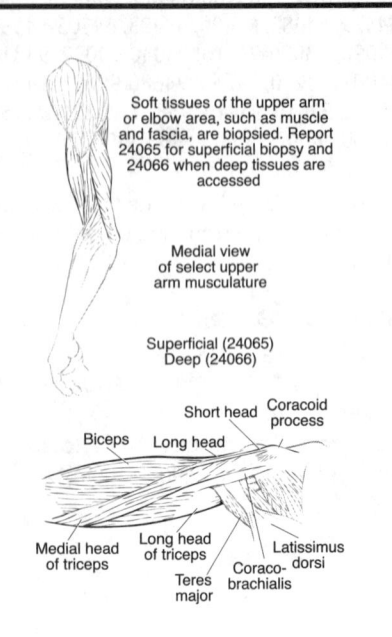

Soft tissues of the upper arm or elbow area, such as muscle and fascia, are biopsied. Report 24065 for superficial biopsy and 24066 when deep tissues are accessed

Medial view of select upper arm musculature

Superficial (24065)
Deep (24066)

Short head — Coracoid process
Biceps — Long head
Medial head of triceps — Long head of triceps — Teres major — Coraco-brachialis — Latissimus dorsi

Explanation
The physician performs a biopsy of the soft tissues of the upper arm or elbow area. With proper anesthesia administered, an incision is made over the biopsy area. Dissection is carried down within the superficial soft tissue layers in 24065, usually the subcutaneous fat to the uppermost fascial layer. In 24066, dissection is taken down deep within the soft tissue, such as into the fascial layer or within the muscle. A portion of the tissue is excised and submitted for pathology. The area is irrigated and the incision is closed with layered sutures, staples, or Steri-strips.

Coding Tips
Local anesthesia is included in these procedures. However, these procedures may be performed under general anesthesia, depending on the age and/or condition of the patient. For needle biopsy of soft tissue, see 20206.

ICD-9-CM Procedural
83.21 Open biopsy of soft tissue

Anesthesia
24065 00400
24066 01710

ICD-9-CM Diagnostic
171.2 Malignant neoplasm of connective and other soft tissue of upper limb, including shoulder
195.4 Malignant neoplasm of upper limb
198.89 Secondary malignant neoplasm of other specified sites
214.1 Lipoma of other skin and subcutaneous tissue
215.2 Other benign neoplasm of connective and other soft tissue of upper limb, including shoulder
238.1 Neoplasm of uncertain behavior of connective and other soft tissue
239.2 Neoplasms of unspecified nature of bone, soft tissue, and skin
682.3 Cellulitis and abscess of upper arm and forearm — (Use additional code to identify organism, such as 041.1, etc.)
686.8 Other specified local infections of skin and subcutaneous tissue — (Use additional code to identify any infectious organism: 041.0-041.8)
709.9 Unspecified disorder of skin and subcutaneous tissue
728.82 Foreign body granuloma of muscle — (Use additional code to identify foreign body (V90.01-V90.9))

Terms To Know

abscess. Circumscribed collection of pus resulting from bacteria, frequently associated with swelling and other signs of inflammation.

benign. Mild or nonmalignant in nature.

cyst. Elevated encapsulated mass containing fluid, semisolid, or solid material with a membranous lining.

lipoma. Benign tumor containing fat cells and the most common of soft tissue lesions, which are usually painless and asymptomatic, with the exception of an angiolipoma.

malignant. Any condition tending to progress toward death, specifically an invasive tumor with a loss of cellular differentiation that has the ability to spread or metastasize to other areas in the body.

soft tissue. Nonepithelial tissues outside of the skeleton that includes subcutaneous adipose tissue, fibrous tissue, fascia, muscles, blood and lymph vessels, and peripheral nervous system tissue.

subcutaneous tissue. Sheet or wide band of adipose (fat) and areolar connective tissue in two layers attached to the dermis.

subfascial. Beneath the band of fibrous tissue that lies deep to the skin, encloses muscles, and separates their layers.

superficial. On the skin surface or near the surface of any involved structure or field of interest.

tumor. Pathological swelling or enlargement; a neoplastic growth of uncontrolled, abnormal multiplication of cells.

CCI Version 16.3
01710, 0213T, 0216T, 0228T, 0230T, 10021-10022, 10060, 10140, 10160, 20103, 24149, 24300, 36000, 36400-36410, 36420-36430, 36440, 36600, 36640, 37202, 43752, 51701-51703, 62310-62319, 64400-64435, 64445-64450, 64479, 64483, 64490, 64493, 64505-64530, 69990, 93000-93010, 93040-93042, 93318, 94002, 94200, 94250, 94680-94690, 94770, 95812-95816, 95819, 95822, 95829, 95955, 96360, 96365, 96372, 96374-96376, 99148-99149, 99150, J0670, J2001

Also not with 24065: 11010-11012❖, 38500

Also not with 24066: 11012❖, 23065, 24006-24065, 24075

Note: These CCI edits are used for Medicare. Other payers may reimburse on codes listed above.

Medicare Edits

	Fac RVU	Non-Fac RVU	FUD	Assist
24065	4.92	7.4	10	N/A
24066	11.77	17.33	90	N/A

Medicare References: 100-2,15,260; 100-4,12,30; 100-4,12,90.3; 100-4,14,10

24075-24076 (24071, 24073)

24075 Excision, tumor, soft tissue of upper arm or elbow area, subcutaneous; less than 3 cm
24071 3 cm or greater
24076 Excision, tumor, soft tissue of upper arm or elbow area, subfascial (eg, intramuscular); less than 5 cm
24073 5 cm or greater

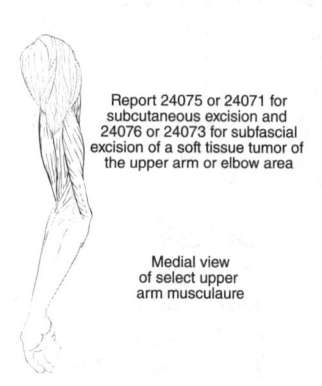

Report 24075 or 24071 for subcutaneous excision and 24076 or 24073 for subfascial excision of a soft tissue tumor of the upper arm or elbow area

Medial view of select upper arm musculaure

Explanation

The physician removes a tumor from the soft tissue of the upper arm or elbow area that is located in the subcutaneous tissue in 24071 and 24075 and in the deep soft tissue, below the fascial plane or within the muscle, in 24073 and 24076. With the proper anesthesia administered, the physician makes an incision in the skin overlying the mass and dissects down to the tumor. The extent of the tumor is identified and a dissection is undertaken all the way around the tumor. A portion of neighboring soft tissue may also be removed to ensure adequate removal of all tumor tissue. A drain may be inserted and the incision is repaired with layers of sutures, staples, or Steri-strips. Report 24075 for excision of subcutaneous tumors less than 3 cm and 24071 for excision of subcutaneous tumors 3 cm or greater. Report 24076 for excision of subfascial or intramuscular tumors less than 5 cm and 24073 for excision of subfascial or intramuscular tumors 5 cm or greater.

Coding Tips

Codes 24071 and 24073 are resequenced codes and will not display in numeric order. For an excision of soft tissues of other sites, see the specific anatomical section. An excisional biopsy is not reported separately when a therapeutic excision is performed during the same surgical session. Report any free grafts or flaps separately. When medically necessary, report moderate (conscious) sedation provided by the performing physician with 99143–99145. When provided by another physician, report 99148–99150.

ICD-9-CM Procedural

83.32	Excision of lesion of muscle
83.39	Excision of lesion of other soft tissue
83.49	Other excision of soft tissue
86.3	Other local excision or destruction of lesion or tissue of skin and subcutaneous tissue
86.4	Radical excision of skin lesion

Anesthesia

24071	00400
24073	01710
24075	00400
24076	01710

ICD-9-CM Diagnostic

171.2	Malignant neoplasm of connective and other soft tissue of upper limb, including shoulder
172.6	Malignant melanoma of skin of upper limb, including shoulder
173.6	Other malignant neoplasm of skin of upper limb, including shoulder
195.4	Malignant neoplasm of upper limb
209.33	Merkel cell carcinoma of the upper limb
209.75	Secondary Merkel cell carcinoma
214.1	Lipoma of other skin and subcutaneous tissue
214.8	Lipoma of other specified sites
215.2	Other benign neoplasm of connective and other soft tissue of upper limb, including shoulder
238.1	Neoplasm of uncertain behavior of connective and other soft tissue
239.2	Neoplasms of unspecified nature of bone, soft tissue, and skin
782.2	Localized superficial swelling, mass, or lump

Terms To Know

benign. Mild or nonmalignant in nature.

fascia. Fibrous sheet or band of tissue that envelops organs, muscles, and groupings of muscles.

malignant. Any condition tending to progress toward death, specifically an invasive tumor with a loss of cellular differentiation that has the ability to spread or metastasize to other areas in the body.

neoplasm. New abnormal growth, tumor.

soft tissue. Nonepithelial tissues outside of the skeleton that includes subcutaneous adipose tissue, fibrous tissue, fascia, muscles, blood and lymph vessels, and peripheral nervous system tissue.

CCI Version 16.3

01710, 0228T, 0230T, 10060, 10140, 10160, 11010-11012❖, 11040-11044, 12001-12007, 12020-12037, 13120-13121, 24105, 24149, 24300, 36000, 36400-36410, 36420-36430, 36440, 36600, 36640, 37202, 43752, 51701-51703, 62310-62319, 64400-64435, 64445-64450, 64479, 64483, 64505-64530, 64718, 69990, 93000-93010, 93040-93042, 93318, 94002, 94200, 94250, 94680-94690, 94770, 95812-95816, 95819, 95822, 95829, 95955, 96360, 96365, 96372, 96374-96376, 99148-99149, 99150

Also not with 24071: 0213T, 0216T, 23930-23931, 24065-24066, 24075, 38500, 64490, 64493, J2001

Also not with 24073: 0213T, 0216T, 11403, 23930-23935, 24006-24071, 24075-24076, 24101, 24341, 64490, 64493

Also not with 24075: 23930-23931, 24065, 38500, J0670, J2001

Also not with 24076: 11400-11406, 11600-11606, 23075, 23930-23935, 24006-24071, 24075, 24101

Note: These CCI edits are used for Medicare. Other payers may reimburse on codes listed above.

Medicare Edits

	Fac RVU	Non-Fac RVU	FUD	Assist
24071	12.16	12.16	90	80
24073	20.74	20.74	90	80
24075	9.47	14.07	90	N/A
24076	15.39	15.39	90	N/A

Medicare References: 100-2,15,260; 100-4,12,30; 100-4,12,90.3; 100-4,14,10

24077-24079

24077 Radical resection of tumor (eg, malignant neoplasm), soft tissue of upper arm or elbow area; less than 5 cm
24079 5 cm or greater

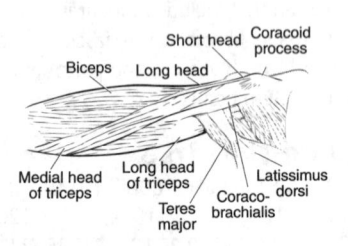

Radical resection of soft tissue tumor of the upper arm or elbow area is reported with 24077 if less than 5 cm and with 24079 if 5 cm or greater

Explanation

The physician performs a radical resection of a malignant soft tissue tumor from the upper arm or elbow area, not involving bone. An incision is made over the tumor and dissection exposes it. The tumor and any adjacent tissue that may be affected by the spread of the neoplasm are excised. Large resections may be needed. The type and stage of the lesion determines the extent of the tumor margin resection area. Muscle or fascia may need to be repaired and drains may be placed. The surgical wound is repaired by intermediate or complex closure, adjacent tissue transfer, or graft. The arm may be placed in a posterior splint. Report 24077 for excision of tumors less than 5 cm and 24079 for excision of tumors 5 cm or greater.

Coding Tips

For radical tumor resection of the soft tissue of the forearm or wrist area, see 25077–25078. For radical tumor resection of the soft tissue of the shoulder area, see 23077–23078. For resection of soft tissues of other sites, see the specific anatomical section.

ICD-9-CM Procedural

83.32	Excision of lesion of muscle
83.39	Excision of lesion of other soft tissue
83.49	Other excision of soft tissue
86.3	Other local excision or destruction of lesion or tissue of skin and subcutaneous tissue
86.4	Radical excision of skin lesion

Anesthesia

24077 00400, 01756
24079 01756

ICD-9-CM Diagnostic

171.2	Malignant neoplasm of connective and other soft tissue of upper limb, including shoulder
172.6	Malignant melanoma of skin of upper limb, including shoulder
173.6	Other malignant neoplasm of skin of upper limb, including shoulder
195.4	Malignant neoplasm of upper limb
209.33	Merkel cell carcinoma of the upper limb
209.75	Secondary Merkel cell carcinoma
214.1	Lipoma of other skin and subcutaneous tissue
214.8	Lipoma of other specified sites
215.2	Other benign neoplasm of connective and other soft tissue of upper limb, including shoulder
238.1	Neoplasm of uncertain behavior of connective and other soft tissue
239.2	Neoplasms of unspecified nature of bone, soft tissue, and skin
782.2	Localized superficial swelling, mass, or lump

Terms To Know

benign. Mild or nonmalignant in nature.

fascia. Fibrous sheet or band of tissue that envelops organs, muscles, and groupings of muscles.

malignant. Any condition tending to progress toward death, specifically an invasive tumor with a loss of cellular differentiation that has the ability to spread or metastasize to other areas in the body.

Merkel cell carcinoma. Malignant cutaneous cancer predominantly found in immunocompromised and elderly patients with a history of sun exposure.

neoplasm. New abnormal growth, tumor.

radical resection. Removal of an entire tumor (e.g., malignant neoplasm) along with a large area of surrounding tissue, including adjacent lymph nodes that may have been infiltrated.

soft tissue. Nonepithelial tissues outside of the skeleton.

subfascial. Beneath the band of fibrous tissue that lies deep to the skin, encloses muscles, and separates their layers.

CCI Version 16.3

01710, 0228T, 0230T, 10060, 10140, 10160, 11010-11012❖, 11040-11044, 12001-12007, 12020-12037, 13120-13121, 23930-23935, 24105, 24149, 24300, 36000, 36400-36410, 36420-36430, 36440, 36600, 36640, 37202, 43752, 51701-51703, 62310-62319, 64400-64435, 64445-64450, 64479, 64483, 64505-64530, 69990, 93000-93010, 93040-93042, 93318, 94002, 94200, 94250, 94680-94690, 94770, 95812-95816, 95819, 95822, 95829, 95955, 96360, 96365, 96372, 96374-96376, 99148-99149, 99150

Also not with 24077: 24000, 24065-24076

Also not with 24079: 0213T, 0216T, 24065-24077, 24152, 24155, 24341, 64490, 64493

Note: These CCI edits are used for Medicare. Other payers may reimburse on codes listed above.

Medicare Edits

	Fac RVU	Non-Fac RVU	FUD	Assist
24077	29.41	29.41	90	N/A
24079	38.23	38.23	90	80

Medicare References: 100-2,15,260; 100-4,12,30; 100-4,12,90.3; 100-4,14,10

24100-24102

24100 Arthrotomy, elbow; with synovial biopsy only
24101 with joint exploration, with or without biopsy, with or without removal of loose or foreign body
24102 with synovectomy

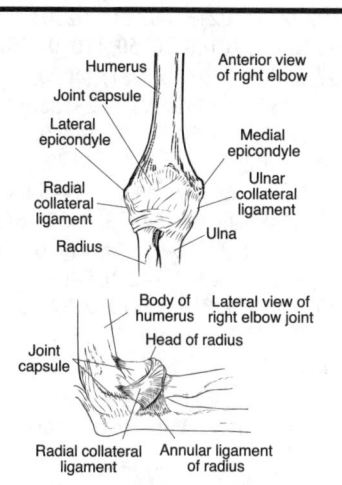

An elbow joint is surgically accessed and synovial fluids are collected for biopsy. Report 24101 when the joint is explored, with or without biopsy and with or without removal of loose or foreign body. Report 24102 when synovial tissues are removed

Explanation

The physician makes a straight, 10 cm, lateral, longitudinal incision to access the elbow joint. The physician may also use a medial, anterior, or posterior approach. The synovium lies within the joint capsule. The elbow joint is exposed by freeing and reflecting the common origin of the extensor muscles. The physician incises the joint capsule to expose the synovium. A small portion of the synovium is excised for biopsy. In 24101, additional dissection is carried out to further explore the joint and soft tissues. Any loose or foreign bodies are then removed. The physician thoroughly irrigates the joint. A drain tube may be inserted. The capsule is closed with sutures. In 24102, the physician makes a straight, longitudinal, lateral incision beginning 5 cm above the lateral epicondyle, and extending 5 cm along the anterolateral surface of the forearm. The physician may also make a medial incision if significant ulnar nerve symptoms coexist. The elbow joint is exposed by freeing and reflecting the common origin of the extensor muscles. Inflamed and enlarged synovium is removed from all aspects of the joint. A drain is then inserted. For all three procedures, the physician repairs the incision in multiple layers with sutures, staples, and/or Steri-strips. A posterior, plaster, long arm splint is applied.

Coding Tips

For arthrotomy for capsular excision or release, see 24006. For arthroscopy of the elbow, diagnostic or with synovial biopsy, see 29830. For arthroscopy of the elbow for removal of a loose or foreign body, see 29834. For arthroscopy of the elbow for synovectomy partial, see 29835; for complete synovectomy, see 29836.

ICD-9-CM Procedural

80.32 Biopsy of joint structure of elbow
80.72 Synovectomy of elbow
80.92 Other excision of elbow joint

Anesthesia
01740

ICD-9-CM Diagnostic

171.2 Malignant neoplasm of connective and other soft tissue of upper limb, including shoulder
215.2 Other benign neoplasm of connective and other soft tissue of upper limb, including shoulder
238.1 Neoplasm of uncertain behavior of connective and other soft tissue
239.2 Neoplasms of unspecified nature of bone, soft tissue, and skin
357.1 Polyneuropathy in collagen vascular disease — (Code first underlying disease: 446.0, 710.0, 714.0)
359.6 Symptomatic inflammatory myopathy in diseases classified elsewhere — (Code first underlying disease: 135, 140.0-208.9, 277.30-277.39, 446.0, 710.0, 710.1, 710.2, 714.0)
446.0 Polyarteritis nodosa
710.0 Systemic lupus erythematosus — (Use additional code to identify manifestation: 424.91, 581.81, 582.81, 583.81)
710.1 Systemic sclerosis — (Use additional code to identify manifestation: 359.6, 517.2)
710.2 Sicca syndrome
711.02 Pyogenic arthritis, upper arm — (Use additional code to identify infectious organism: 041.0-041.8)
711.32 Postdysenteric arthropathy, upper arm — (Code first underlying disease: 002.0-002.9, 008.0-009.3)
711.42 Arthropathy associated with other bacterial diseases, upper arm — (Code first underlying disease, such as diseases classifiable to 010-040 (except 036.82), 090-099 (except 098.50))
711.52 Arthropathy associated with other viral diseases, upper arm — (Code first underlying disease: 045-049, 050-079, 480, 487)
711.62 Arthropathy associated with mycoses, upper arm — (Code first underlying disease: 110.0-118)
711.82 Arthropathy associated with other infectious and parasitic diseases, upper arm — (Code first underlying disease: 080-088, 100-104, 130-136)
714.0 Rheumatoid arthritis — (Use additional code to identify manifestation: 357.1, 359.6)
714.1 Felty's syndrome
718.12 Loose body in upper arm joint
719.02 Effusion of upper arm joint
719.22 Villonodular synovitis, upper arm
732.7 Osteochondritis dissecans
V64.43 Arthroscopic surgical procedure converted to open procedure

CCI Version 16.3

01710, 0213T, 0216T, 0228T, 0230T, 10060, 10140, 10160, 24006, 24149, 24300, 24332, 36000, 36400-36410, 36420-36430, 36440, 36600, 36640, 37202, 43752, 51701-51703, 62310-62319, 64400-64435, 64445-64450, 64479, 64483, 64490, 64493, 64505-64530, 69990, 93000-93010, 93040-93042, 93318, 94002, 94200, 94250, 94680-94690, 94770, 95812-95816, 95819, 95822, 95829, 95955, 96360, 96365, 96372, 96374-96376, 99148-99149, 99150

Also not with 24100: 11011-11012❖, 29830-29835, 29837-29838

Also not with 24101: 11012❖, 20103, 24100, 29830-29835, 29837-29838, 64718

Also not with 24102: 24101, 24341, 29830-29838

Note: These CCI edits are used for Medicare. Other payers may reimburse on codes listed above.

Medicare Edits

	Fac RVU	Non-Fac RVU	FUD	Assist
24100	11.91	11.91	90	80
24101	14.48	14.48	90	80
24102	17.85	17.85	90	80

Medicare References: 100-2,15,260; 100-4,12,30; 100-4,12,90.3; 100-4,14,10

24105

24105 Excision, olecranon bursa

Explanation
The physician excises the olecranon bursa by making a longitudinal incision along the posteromedial border of the elbow and dissecting down to expose the bursa, the fluid filled sac that lubricates the joint against friction. The bursa is excised. The surrounding tissue is examined for any sign of infection. The wound is irrigated and the incision is repaired in layers with sutures, staples, and/or Steri-strips.

Coding Tips
According to CPT guidelines, cast application or strapping (including removal) is only reported as a replacement procedure or when the cast application or strapping is an initial service performed without a restorative treatment or procedure. See "Application of Casts and Strapping" in the CPT book in the Surgery Section, under the Musculoskeletal system. For excision and drainage of olecranon bursa, see 23931.

ICD-9-CM Procedural
83.5 Bursectomy

Anesthesia
24105   01710

ICD-9-CM Diagnostic
357.1 Polyneuropathy in collagen vascular disease — (Code first underlying disease: 446.0, 710.0, 714.0)
359.6 Symptomatic inflammatory myopathy in diseases classified elsewhere — (Code first underlying disease: 135, 140.0-208.9, 277.30-277.39, 446.0, 710.0, 710.1, 710.2, 714.0)
446.0 Polyarteritis nodosa
710.0 Systemic lupus erythematosus — (Use additional code to identify manifestation: 424.91, 581.81, 582.81, 583.81)
710.1 Systemic sclerosis — (Use additional code to identify manifestation: 359.6, 517.2)
710.2 Sicca syndrome
714.0 Rheumatoid arthritis — (Use additional code to identify manifestation: 357.1, 359.6)
719.42 Pain in joint, upper arm
719.43 Pain in joint, forearm
719.62 Other symptoms referable to upper arm joint
726.33 Olecranon bursitis
727.2 Specific bursitides often of occupational origin
727.3 Other bursitis disorders
727.49 Other ganglion and cyst of synovium, tendon, and bursa

Terms To Know
bursa. Cavity or sac containing fluid that occurs between articulating surfaces and serves to reduce friction from moving parts. An anatomical structure frequently referenced in orthopedic notes as it may become diseased or need removal.

cyst. Elevated encapsulated mass containing fluid, semisolid, or solid material with a membranous lining.

ganglion. Fluid-filled, benign cyst appearing on a tendon sheath or aponeurosis, frequently found in the hand, wrist, or foot and connecting to an underlying joint.

infection. Presence of microorganisms in body tissues that may result in cellular damage.

polyarteritis nodosa. Systemic necrotizing vasculitis of small and medium arteries that results in the infarction and scarring within the affected organs.

polyneuropathy. Disease process of severe inflammation of multiple nerves.

sicca syndrome. Complex of symptoms of unknown source in middle-aged women in which the following triad exists: keratoconjunctivitis sicca, zerostomia, and connective tissue disease (usually rheumatoid arthritis but sometimes systemic lupus erythematosus).

CCI Version 16.3
01710, 0213T, 0216T, 0228T, 0230T, 10060-10061, 10140, 10160, 11010-11012❖, 12032, 20605, 23930-23931, 24000, 24101, 24300, 24332, 29065, 29105-29125, 36000, 36400-36410, 36420-36430, 36440, 36600, 36640, 37202, 43752, 51701-51703, 62310-62319, 64400-64435, 64445-64450, 64479, 64483, 64490, 64493, 64505-64530, 64718, 69990, 93000-93010, 93040-93042, 93318, 94002, 94200, 94250, 94680-94690, 94770, 95812-95816, 95819, 95822, 95829, 95955, 96360, 96365, 96372, 96374-96376, 99148-99149, 99150

Note: These CCI edits are used for Medicare. Other payers may reimburse on codes listed above.

Medicare Edits

	Fac RVU	Non-Fac RVU	FUD	Assist
24105	9.94	9.94	90	N/A

Medicare References: 100-2,15,260; 100-4,12,30; 100-4,12,90.3; 100-4,14,10

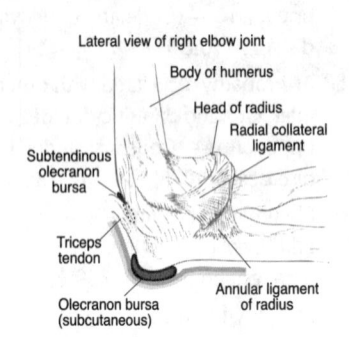

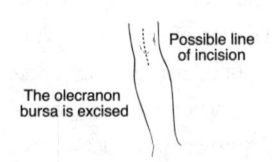

24110-24116

24110	Excision or curettage of bone cyst or benign tumor, humerus;
24115	with autograft (includes obtaining graft)
24116	with allograft

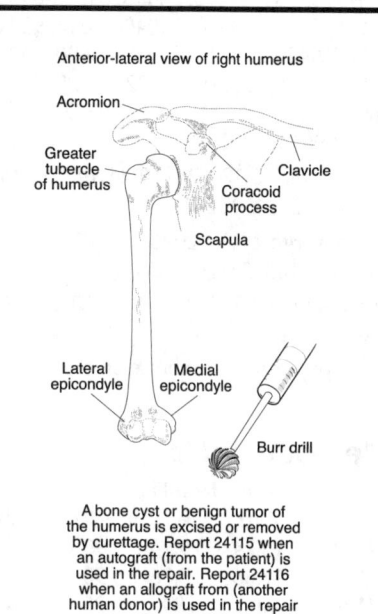

Explanation
A bone cyst or benign tumor of the humerus is removed. The physician makes an incision in the upper arm overlying the cyst or tumor. The skin and underlying soft tissues are reflected to expose the periosteum, which is separated from the bone. Curettes or osteotomes are used to scrape or cut the lesion from the bone. Once the benign tumor or cyst is removed and healthy bone tissue is present, the periosteum is repositioned and the incision is repaired in layers. If the bone defect created requires a graft for repair, the physician obtains the necessary size bone graft from a separate donor site on the patient and packs it into the site where the tumor or bone cyst was removed, or uses a bone bank allograft. Report 24115 if the procedure is done with an autograft and 24116 if an allograft is used.

Coding Tips
Any bone graft harvest is not reported separately. For radical resection of a tumor of the distal or shaft of the humerus, see 24150–24151.

ICD-9-CM Procedural
77.62	Local excision of lesion or tissue of humerus
77.77	Excision of tibia and fibula for graft
77.79	Excision of other bone for graft, except facial bones
78.02	Bone graft of humerus

Anesthesia
01758

ICD-9-CM Diagnostic
213.4	Benign neoplasm of scapula and long bones of upper limb
238.0	Neoplasm of uncertain behavior of bone and articular cartilage
239.2	Neoplasms of unspecified nature of bone, soft tissue, and skin
726.91	Exostosis of unspecified site
733.21	Solitary bone cyst
733.22	Aneurysmal bone cyst
733.29	Other cyst of bone

Terms To Know

allograft. Graft from one individual to another of the same species.

aneurysmal bone cyst. Solitary bone lesion that bulges into the periosteum, marked by a calcified rim.

autograft. Any tissue harvested from one anatomical site of a person and grafted to another anatomical site of the same person. Most commonly, blood vessels, skin, tendons, fascia, and bone are used as autografts.

benign. Mild or nonmalignant in nature.

curettage. Removal of tissue by scraping.

cyst. Elevated encapsulated mass containing fluid, semisolid, or solid material with a membranous lining.

exostosis. Abnormal formation of a benign bony growth.

neoplasm. New abnormal growth, tumor.

CCI Version 16.3
01710, 0213T, 0216T, 0228T, 0230T, 10060, 10140, 10160, 20000-20005, 20615, 24300, 24332, 24343-24346, 29834-29838, 36000, 36400-36410, 36420-36430, 36440, 36600, 36640, 37202, 43752, 51701-51703, 62310-62319, 64400-64435, 64445-64450, 64479, 64483, 64490, 64493, 64505-64530, 69990, 93000-93010, 93040-93042, 93318, 94002, 94200, 94250, 94680-94690, 94770, 95812-95816, 95819, 95822, 95829, 95955, 96360, 96365, 96372, 96374-96376, 99148-99149, 99150

Also not with 24110: 24100-24105, 24134❖, 24140❖

Also not with 24115: 20900-20902, 24100-24110, 24134❖, 24341

Also not with 24116: 24100-24110, 24341

Note: These CCI edits are used for Medicare. Other payers may reimburse on codes listed above.

Medicare Edits

	Fac RVU	Non-Fac RVU	FUD	Assist
24110	16.98	16.98	90	N/A
24115	21.38	21.38	90	80
24116	25.18	25.18	90	80

Medicare References: 100-2,15,260; 100-4,12,30; 100-4,12,90.3; 100-4,14,10

24120-24126

24120 Excision or curettage of bone cyst or benign tumor of head or neck of radius or olecranon process;
24125 with autograft (includes obtaining graft)
24126 with allograft

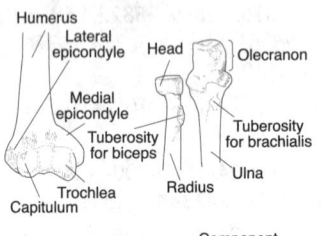

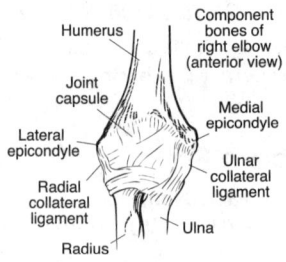

A bone cyst or benign tumor of the head or neck of the radius or olecranon process is excised or removed by curettage. Report 24125 when an autograft is required in the repair. And report 24126 when an allograft is used in the repair

Explanation

The physician uses excision or curettage to remove a bone cyst or benign tumor of the head or neck of the radius or olecranon process in 24120. The physician makes a longitudinal incision along the lateral aspect of the elbow. A posterior incision may also be made to access the olecranon process. To expose the radial head and/or neck, the common origin of the extensor muscles is reflected and the joint capsule is incised. The bone cyst or tumor is identified and the periosteum is separated from the bone. Curettes or osteotomes are used to scrape or cut the lesion from the bone. Once the benign tumor or cyst is removed and healthy bone tissue is present, the periosteum is repositioned and the incision is repaired in layers, including the joint capsule, if incised. If the bone defect created requires a graft for repair, the physician obtains the necessary size bone graft from a separate donor site on the patient and packs it into the site where the tumor or bone cyst was removed or uses a bone bank allograft. Report 24125 if an autograft is obtained and 24126 if an allograft is used.

Coding Tips

Any bone graft harvest is not reported separately. According to CPT guidelines, cast application or strapping (including removal) is only reported as a replacement procedure or when the cast application or strapping is an initial service performed without a restorative treatment or procedure. See "Application of Casts and Strapping" in the CPT book in the Surgery Section, under the Musculoskeletal system. For radical resection of a tumor, radial head or neck, see 24152–24153.

ICD-9-CM Procedural

77.63 Local excision of lesion or tissue of radius and ulna
77.77 Excision of tibia and fibula for graft
77.79 Excision of other bone for graft, except facial bones
78.03 Bone graft of radius and ulna

Anesthesia
01740

ICD-9-CM Diagnostic

213.4 Benign neoplasm of scapula and long bones of upper limb
229.8 Benign neoplasm of other specified sites
238.0 Neoplasm of uncertain behavior of bone and articular cartilage
239.2 Neoplasms of unspecified nature of bone, soft tissue, and skin
726.91 Exostosis of unspecified site
733.21 Solitary bone cyst
733.22 Aneurysmal bone cyst
733.29 Other cyst of bone

Terms To Know

cyst. Elevated encapsulated mass containing fluid, semisolid, or solid material with a membranous lining.

exostosis. Abnormal formation of a benign bony growth.

CCI Version 16.3

01710, 0213T, 0216T, 0228T, 0230T, 10060, 10140, 10160, 20000-20005, 20615, 24149, 24300, 24332, 24343-24346, 29834-29838, 36000, 36400-36410, 36420-36430, 36440, 36600, 36640, 37202, 43752, 51701-51703, 62310-62319, 64400-64435, 64445-64450, 64479, 64483, 64490, 64493, 64505-64530, 69990, 93000-93010, 93040-93042, 93318, 94002, 94200, 94250, 94680-94690, 94770, 95812-95816, 95819, 95822, 95829, 95955, 96360, 96365, 96372, 96374-96376, 99148-99149, 99150

Also not with 24120: 24100-24105, 24136❖, 24138❖, 24145❖, 24147❖

Also not with 24125: 20900-20902, 24100-24105, 24120

Also not with 24126: 24100-24110, 24120

Note: These CCI edits are used for Medicare. Other payers may reimburse on codes listed above.

Medicare Edits

	Fac RVU	Non-Fac RVU	FUD	Assist
24120	15.24	15.24	90	80
24125	17.86	17.86	90	80
24126	18.8	18.8	90	80

Medicare References: 100-2,15,260; 100-4,12,30; 100-4,12,90.3; 100-4,14,10

24130

24130 Excision, radial head

Explanation
The radial head is excised in this procedure. The physician makes a longitudinal incision along the lateral aspect of the elbow. The elbow joint is exposed by freeing and reflecting the common origin of the extensor muscles. The joint capsule is incised and the radial head is exposed. The physician uses a bone-cutting saw to excise the radial head. The capsule is closed with sutures and the incision is repaired in layers with sutures, staples, and/or Steri-strips.

Coding Tips
According to CPT guidelines, cast application or strapping (including removal) is only reported as a replacement procedure or when the cast application or strapping is an initial service performed without a restorative treatment or procedure. See "Application of Casts and Strapping" in the CPT book in the Surgery Section, under the Musculoskeletal system. For replacement of the radial head with an implant, see 24366.

ICD-9-CM Procedural
77.83 Other partial ostectomy of radius and ulna

Anesthesia
24130 01740

ICD-9-CM Diagnostic
170.4 Malignant neoplasm of scapula and long bones of upper limb
171.2 Malignant neoplasm of connective and other soft tissue of upper limb, including shoulder
195.4 Malignant neoplasm of upper limb
213.4 Benign neoplasm of scapula and long bones of upper limb
238.0 Neoplasm of uncertain behavior of bone and articular cartilage
239.2 Neoplasms of unspecified nature of bone, soft tissue, and skin
277.30 Amyloidosis, unspecified — (Use additional code to identify any associated mental retardation)
277.31 Familial Mediterranean fever — (Use additional code to identify any associated mental retardation)
277.39 Other amyloidosis — (Use additional code to identify any associated mental retardation)
357.1 Polyneuropathy in collagen vascular disease — (Code first underlying disease: 446.0, 710.0, 714.0)
359.6 Symptomatic inflammatory myopathy in diseases classified elsewhere — (Code first underlying disease: 135, 140.0-208.9, 277.30-277.39, 446.0, 710.0, 710.1, 710.2, 714.0)
446.0 Polyarteritis nodosa
710.0 Systemic lupus erythematosus — (Use additional code to identify manifestation: 424.91, 581.81, 582.81, 583.81)
710.1 Systemic sclerosis — (Use additional code to identify manifestation: 359.6, 517.2)
710.2 Sicca syndrome
714.0 Rheumatoid arthritis — (Use additional code to identify manifestation: 357.1, 359.6)
715.13 Primary localized osteoarthrosis, forearm
718.93 Unspecified derangement, forearm joint
719.43 Pain in joint, forearm
733.81 Malunion of fracture
754.89 Other specified nonteratogenic anomalies

Terms To Know
amyloidosis. Condition in which insoluble, fibril-like proteins (amyloid) build up in one or more organs and tissues within the body.

osteoarthrosis. Most common form of a noninflammatory degenerative joint disease with degenerating articular cartilage, bone enlargement, and synovial membrane changes.

polyarteritis nodosa. Systemic necrotizing vasculitis of small and medium arteries that results in the infarction and scarring within the affected organs.

CCI Version 16.3
01710, 0213T, 0216T, 0228T, 0230T, 24000, 24100-24105, 24120-24126, 24145, 24149, 24300, 24332, 24343-24346, 25355, 29105, 36000, 36400-36410, 36420-36430, 36440, 36600, 36640, 37202, 43752, 51701-51703, 62310-62319, 64400-64435, 64445-64450, 64479, 64483, 64490, 64493, 64505-64530, 69990, 93000-93010, 93040-93042, 93318, 94002, 94200, 94250, 94680-94690, 94770, 95812-95816, 95819, 95822, 95829, 95955, 96360, 96365, 96372, 96374-96376, 99148-99149, 99150

Note: These CCI edits are used for Medicare. Other payers may reimburse on codes listed above.

Medicare Edits

	Fac RVU	Non-Fac RVU	FUD	Assist
24130	14.67	14.67	90	N/A

Medicare References: 100-2,15,260; 100-4,12,30; 100-4,12,90.3; 100-4,14,10

24134

24134 Sequestrectomy (eg, for osteomyelitis or bone abscess), shaft or distal humerus

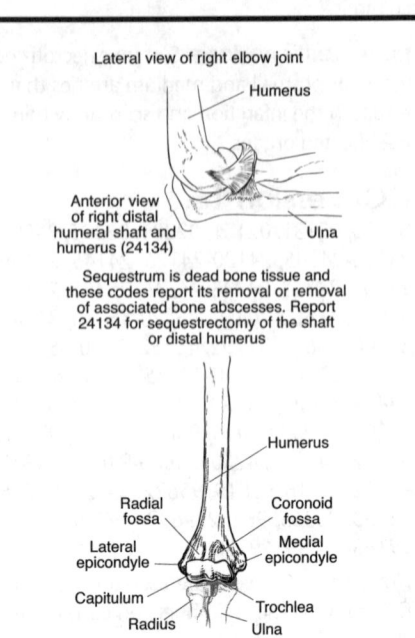

Lateral view of right elbow joint

Anterior view of right distal humeral shaft and humerus (24134)

Sequestrum is dead bone tissue and these codes report its removal or removal of associated bone abscesses. Report 24134 for sequestrectomy of the shaft or distal humerus.

Explanation

The physician removes infected portions of bone, due to a bone abscess or osteomyelitis, from the shaft or distal humerus in 24134, from the radial head or neck in 24136, and from the olecranon process in 24138. This infection often leaves open sinus tracts in the bone that require removal. The physician makes an incision overlying the sequestered area of bone, which includes incising the capsule if the elbow joint is involved. Once the skin and soft tissues are reflected, a small window is cut into the bone to gain access to the sequestrum, or necrosed piece of bone that has become separated from sound bone. All purulent material and scarred or necrotic tissue are removed. The remaining space is filled with surrounding soft tissues or free tissue transfer. The area is irrigated and an antibiotic solution is used to prevent further infection. The wound is closed loosely over drains if possible or may be packed open with dressings. The patient may be placed in a splint to limit elbow motion.

Coding Tips

For craterization, saucerization, or diaphysectomy (partial excision of bone) for osteomyelitis of the humerus, see 24140. For sequestrectomy for osteomyelitis or bone abscess of the radial head or neck, see 24136; for the olecranon process, see 24138.

ICD-9-CM Procedural

77.02 Sequestrectomy of humerus

Anesthesia

24134   01740

ICD-9-CM Diagnostic

715.12 Primary localized osteoarthrosis, upper arm
715.32 Localized osteoarthrosis not specified whether primary or secondary, upper arm
715.92 Osteoarthrosis, unspecified whether generalized or localized, upper arm
716.62 Unspecified monoarthritis, upper arm
730.12 Chronic osteomyelitis, upper arm — (Use additional code to identify organism: 041.1. Use additional code to identify major osseous defect, if applicable: 731.3)
730.22 Unspecified osteomyelitis, upper arm — (Use additional code to identify organism: 041.1. Use additional code to identify major osseous defect, if applicable: 731.3)
730.32 Periostitis, without mention of osteomyelitis, upper arm — (Use additional code to identify organism: 041.1)
730.72 Osteopathy resulting from poliomyelitis, upper arm — (Use additional code to identify organism: 041.1. Code first underlying disease: 045.0-045.9)
730.82 Other infections involving bone diseases classified elsewhere, upper arm — (Use additional code to identify organism: 041.1. Code first underlying disease: 002.0, 015.0-015.9)
731.3 Major osseous defects — (Code first underlying disease: 170.0-170.9, 730.00-730.29, 733.00-733.09, 733.40-733.49, 996.45)
733.49 Aseptic necrosis of other bone site — (Use additional code to identify major osseous defect, if applicable: 731.3)
905.2 Late effect of fracture of upper extremities

Terms To Know

abscess. Circumscribed collection of pus resulting from bacteria, frequently associated with swelling and other signs of inflammation.

late effect. Abnormality, dysfunction, or other residual condition produced after the acute phase of an illness, injury, or disease is over. There is no time limit on when late effects can appear.

necrosis. Death of cells or tissue within a living organ or structure.

osteomyelitis. Inflammation of bone that may remain localized or spread to the marrow, cortex, or periosteum, in response to an infecting organism, usually bacterial and pyogenic.

periostitis. Inflammation of the outer layers of bone.

CCI Version 16.3

01710, 0213T, 0216T, 0228T, 0230T, 10060, 10140, 10160, 20500, 23930-23935, 24116❖, 24140, 24149, 24300, 24332, 24343-24346, 36000, 36400-36410, 36420-36430, 36440, 36600, 36640, 37202, 43752, 51701-51703, 62310-62319, 64400-64435, 64445-64450, 64479, 64483, 64490, 64493, 64505-64530, 69990, 93000-93010, 93040-93042, 93318, 94002, 94200, 94250, 94680-94690, 94770, 95812-95816, 95819, 95822, 95829, 95955, 96360, 96365, 96372, 96374-96376, 99148-99149, 99150

Note: These CCI edits are used for Medicare. Other payers may reimburse on codes listed above.

Medicare Edits

	Fac RVU	Non-Fac RVU	FUD	Assist
24134	21.86	21.86	90	80

Medicare References: 100-2,15,260; 100-4,12,30; 100-4,12,90.3; 100-4,14,10

24136-24138

24136 Sequestrectomy (eg, for osteomyelitis or bone abscess), radial head or neck
24138 Sequestrectomy (eg, for osteomyelitis or bone abscess), olecranon process

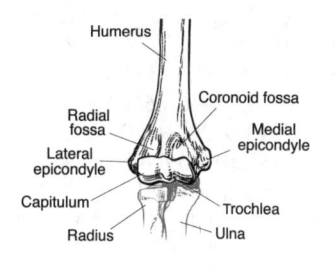

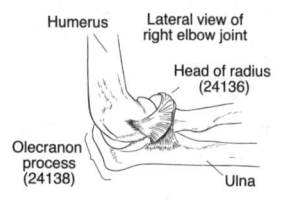

Sequestrum is dead bone tissue and these codes report its removal or removal of associated bone abscesses. Report 24136 for sequestrectomy of the radial head or neck. And report 24138 for sequestrectomy of the olecranon process.

Explanation

The physician removes infected portions of bone, due to a bone abscess or osteomyelitis, from the shaft or distal humerus in 24134, from the radial head or neck in 24136, and from the olecranon process in 24138. This infection often leaves open sinus tracts in the bone that require removal. The physician makes an incision overlying the sequestered area of bone, which includes incising the capsule if the elbow joint is involved. Once the skin and soft tissues are reflected, a small window is cut into the bone to gain access to the sequestrum, or necrosed piece of bone that has become separated from sound bone. All purulent material and scarred or necrotic tissue are removed. The remaining space is filled with surrounding soft tissues or free tissue transfer. The area is irrigated and an antibiotic solution is used to prevent further infection. The wound is closed loosely over drains if possible or may be packed open with dressings. The patient may be placed in a splint to limit elbow motion.

Coding Tips

If significant additional time and effort is documented, append modifier 22 and submit a cover letter and operative report. For sequestrectomy for osteomyelitis or a bone abscess of the shaft or distal humerus, see 24134. For craterization, saucerization, or diaphysectomy (partial excision of bone) for osteomyelitis of the radial head or neck, see 24145; olecranon process, see 24147.

ICD-9-CM Procedural

77.03 Sequestrectomy of radius and ulna
77.09 Sequestrectomy of other bone, except facial bones

Anesthesia
01740

ICD-9-CM Diagnostic

715.12 Primary localized osteoarthrosis, upper arm
715.32 Localized osteoarthrosis not specified whether primary or secondary, upper arm
715.92 Osteoarthrosis, unspecified whether generalized or localized, upper arm
716.62 Unspecified monoarthritis, upper arm
730.12 Chronic osteomyelitis, upper arm — (Use additional code to identify organism: 041.1. Use additional code to identify major osseous defect, if applicable: 731.3)
730.22 Unspecified osteomyelitis, upper arm — (Use additional code to identify organism: 041.1. Use additional code to identify major osseous defect, if applicable: 731.3)
730.32 Periostitis, without mention of osteomyelitis, upper arm — (Use additional code to identify organism: 041.1)
730.72 Osteopathy resulting from poliomyelitis, upper arm — (Use additional code to identify organism: 041.1. Code first underlying disease: 045.0-045.9)
730.82 Other infections involving bone diseases classified elsewhere, upper arm — (Use additional code to identify organism: 041.1. Code first underlying disease: 002.0, 015.0-015.9)
730.92 Unspecified infection of bone, upper arm — (Use additional code to identify organism: 041.1)
731.3 Major osseous defects — (Code first underlying disease: 170.0-170.9, 730.00-730.29, 733.00-733.09, 733.40-733.49, 996.45)
733.49 Aseptic necrosis of other bone site — (Use additional code to identify major osseous defect, if applicable: 731.3)
905.2 Late effect of fracture of upper extremities

Terms To Know

abscess. Circumscribed collection of pus resulting from bacteria, frequently associated with swelling and other signs of inflammation.

late effect. Abnormality, dysfunction, or other residual condition produced after the acute phase of an illness, injury, or disease is over. There is no time limit on when late effects can appear.

lateral. To/on the side.

necrosis. Death of cells or tissue within a living organ or structure.

osteomyelitis. Inflammation of bone that may remain localized or spread to the marrow, cortex, or periosteum, in response to an infecting organism, usually bacterial and pyogenic.

periostitis. Inflammation of the outer layers of bone.

CCI Version 16.3

01710, 0213T, 0216T, 0228T, 0230T, 10060, 10140, 10160, 20500, 23930-23935, 24125-24126✦, 24149, 24300, 24332, 24341, 24343-24346, 36000, 36400-36410, 36420-36430, 36440, 36600, 36640, 37202, 43752, 51701-51703, 62310-62319, 64400-64435, 64445-64450, 64479, 64483, 64490, 64493, 64505-64530, 69990, 93000-93010, 93040-93042, 93318, 94002, 94200, 94250, 94680-94690, 94770, 95812-95816, 95819, 95822, 95829, 95955, 96360, 96365, 96372, 96374-96376, 99148-99149, 99150

Also not with 24136: 24145
Also not with 24138: 24105, 24147

Note: These CCI edits are used for Medicare. Other payers may reimburse on codes listed above.

Medicare Edits

	Fac RVU	Non-Fac RVU	FUD	Assist
24136	17.83	17.83	90	N/A
24138	19.45	19.45	90	80

Medicare References: 100-2,15,260; 100-4,12,30; 100-4,12,90.3; 100-4,14,10

24140

24140 Partial excision (craterization, saucerization, or diaphysectomy) bone (eg, osteomyelitis), humerus

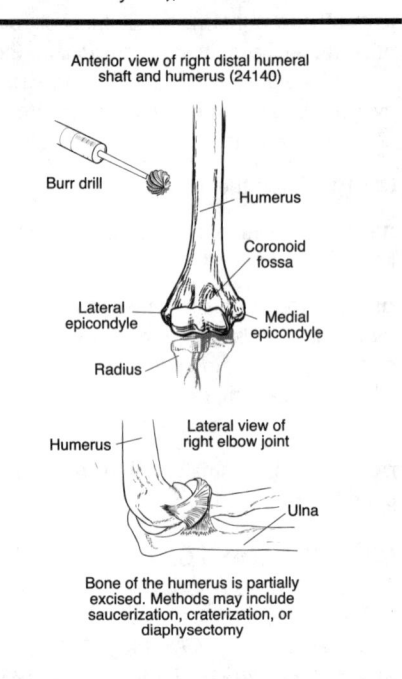

Anterior view of right distal humeral shaft and humerus (24140)

Burr drill — Humerus — Coronoid fossa — Lateral epicondyle — Medial epicondyle — Radius

Lateral view of right elbow joint

Humerus — Ulna

Bone of the humerus is partially excised. Methods may include saucerization, craterization, or diaphysectomy

Explanation
The physician performs a partial excision of the humerus in 24140, to remove infected bone. An incision is made over the infected part of the bone and the underlying soft tissues are divided to expose the bone. The elbow joint capsule may be incised if necessary. The periosteum is reflected and the infected portion of bone is removed and irrigated. The excavation of bone may excise a crater-like piece, leave a small saucer-like shelf depression in the bone, or may remove a portion of the shaft (diaphysis) of a long bone. If a significant portion of bone is removed, the physician may use bone graft material to fill the cavity left in the bone. The periosteum is closed over the bone, the soft tissues are sutured closed, and a soft dressing is applied. A long splint may be applied to limit elbow motion.

Coding Tips
If significant additional time and effort is documented, append modifier 22 and submit a cover letter and operative report. For sequestrectomy for osteomyelitis or a bone abscess, shaft or distal humerus, see 24134. For craterization, saucerization, or diaphysectomy (partial excision of bone) for osteomyelitis of the radial head or neck, see 24145; olecranon process, see 24147.

ICD-9-CM Procedural
77.82 Other partial ostectomy of humerus

Anesthesia
24140 01740

ICD-9-CM Diagnostic
729.5 Pain in soft tissues of limb
730.12 Chronic osteomyelitis, upper arm — (Use additional code to identify organism: 041.1. Use additional code to identify major osseous defect, if applicable: 731.3)
730.22 Unspecified osteomyelitis, upper arm — (Use additional code to identify organism: 041.1. Use additional code to identify major osseous defect, if applicable: 731.3)
730.32 Periostitis, without mention of osteomyelitis, upper arm — (Use additional code to identify organism: 041.1)
730.72 Osteopathy resulting from poliomyelitis, upper arm — (Use additional code to identify organism: 041.1. Code first underlying disease: 045.0-045.9)
730.82 Other infections involving bone diseases classified elsewhere, upper arm — (Use additional code to identify organism: 041.1. Code first underlying disease: 002.0, 015.0-015.9)
730.92 Unspecified infection of bone, upper arm — (Use additional code to identify organism: 041.1)
731.3 Major osseous defects — (Code first underlying disease: 170.0-170.9, 730.00-730.29, 733.00-733.09, 733.40-733.49, 996.45)
733.49 Aseptic necrosis of other bone site — (Use additional code to identify major osseous defect, if applicable: 731.3)

Terms To Know
abscess. Circumscribed collection of pus resulting from bacteria, frequently associated with swelling and other signs of inflammation.

chronic. Persistent, continuing, or recurring.

necrosis. Death of cells or tissue within a living organ or structure.

osteomyelitis. Inflammation of bone that may remain localized or spread to the marrow, cortex, or periosteum, in response to an infecting organism, usually bacterial and pyogenic.

periostitis. Inflammation of the outer layers of bone.

soft tissue. Nonepithelial tissues outside of the skeleton that includes subcutaneous adipose tissue, fibrous tissue, fascia, muscles, blood and lymph vessels, and peripheral nervous system tissue.

CCI Version 16.3
01710, 0213T, 0216T, 0228T, 0230T, 10060, 10140, 10160, 20500, 23930-23935, 24115-24116❖, 24300, 24332, 24341, 24357, 24359, 36000, 36400-36410, 36420-36430, 36440, 36600, 36640, 37202, 43752, 51701-51703, 62310-62319, 64400-64435, 64445-64450, 64479, 64483, 64490, 64493, 64505-64530, 64718, 69990, 93000-93010, 93040-93042, 93318, 94002, 94200, 94250, 94680-94690, 94770, 95812-95816, 95819, 95822, 95829, 95955, 96360, 96365, 96372, 96374-96376, 99148-99149, 99150

Note: These CCI edits are used for Medicare. Other payers may reimburse on codes listed above.

Medicare Edits

	Fac RVU	Non-Fac RVU	FUD	Assist
24140	20.69	20.69	90	80

Medicare References: 100-2,15,260; 100-4,12,30; 100-4,12,90.3; 100-4,14,10

24145-24147

24145 Partial excision (craterization, saucerization, or diaphysectomy) bone (eg, osteomyelitis), radial head or neck

24147 Partial excision (craterization, saucerization, or diaphysectomy) bone (eg, osteomyelitis), olecranon process

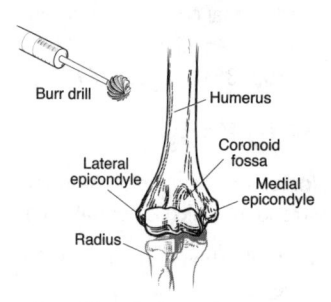

Bone of the radius is partially excised. Methods may include saucerization, craterization, or diaphysectomy. Report 24145 when the radial head or neck is treated. Report 24147 when the olecranon process is treated

Lateral view of right elbow joint

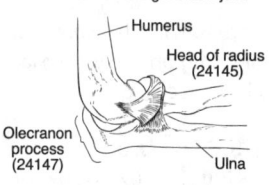

Explanation

The physician performs a partial excision of the radial head or neck in 24145, or the olecranon process in 24147 to remove infected bone. An incision is made over the infected part of the bone and the underlying soft tissues are divided to expose the bone. The elbow joint capsule may be incised if necessary. The periosteum is reflected and the infected portion of bone is removed and irrigated. The excavation of bone may excise a crater-like piece, leave a small saucer-like shelf depression in the bone, or may remove a portion of the shaft (diaphysis) of a long bone. If a significant portion of bone is removed, the physician may use bone graft material to fill the cavity left in the bone. The periosteum is closed over the bone, the soft tissues are sutured closed, and a soft dressing is applied. A long splint may be applied to limit elbow motion.

Coding Tips

If significant additional time and effort are documented, append modifier 22 and submit a cover letter and operative report. For craterization, saucerization, or diaphysectomy (partial excision of bone) for osteomyelitis of the humerus, see 24140. For sequestrectomy for osteomyelitis or a bone abscess of the radial head or neck, see 24136; olecranon process, see 24138.

ICD-9-CM Procedural

77.83 Other partial ostectomy of radius and ulna

77.89 Other partial ostectomy of other bone, except facial bones

Anesthesia
01740

ICD-9-CM Diagnostic

729.5 Pain in soft tissues of limb

730.12 Chronic osteomyelitis, upper arm — (Use additional code to identify organism: 041.1. Use additional code to identify major osseous defect, if applicable: 731.3)

730.13 Chronic osteomyelitis, forearm — (Use additional code to identify organism: 041.1. Use additional code to identify major osseous defect, if applicable: 731.3)

730.22 Unspecified osteomyelitis, upper arm — (Use additional code to identify organism: 041.1. Use additional code to identify major osseous defect, if applicable: 731.3)

730.23 Unspecified osteomyelitis, forearm — (Use additional code to identify organism: 041.1. Use additional code to identify major osseous defect, if applicable: 731.3)

730.32 Periostitis, without mention of osteomyelitis, upper arm — (Use additional code to identify organism: 041.1)

730.33 Periostitis, without mention of osteomyelitis, forearm — (Use additional code to identify organism: 041.1)

730.73 Osteopathy resulting from poliomyelitis, forearm — (Use additional code to identify organism: 041.1. Code first underlying disease: 045.0-045.9)

730.82 Other infections involving bone diseases classified elsewhere, upper arm — (Use additional code to identify organism: 041.1. Code first underlying disease: 002.0, 015.0-015.9)

730.83 Other infections involving bone in diseases classified elsewhere, forearm — (Use additional code to identify organism: 041.1. Code first underlying disease: 002.0, 015.0-015.9)

730.92 Unspecified infection of bone, upper arm — (Use additional code to identify organism: 041.1)

730.93 Unspecified infection of bone, forearm — (Use additional code to identify organism: 041.1)

731.3 Major osseous defects — (Code first underlying disease: 170.0-170.9, 730.00-730.29, 733.00-733.09, 733.40-733.49, 996.45)

733.49 Aseptic necrosis of other bone site — (Use additional code to identify major osseous defect, if applicable: 731.3)

Terms To Know

necrosis. Death of cells or tissue within a living organ or structure.

osteomyelitis. Inflammation of bone that may remain localized or spread to the marrow, cortex, or periosteum, in response to an infecting organism, usually bacterial and pyogenic.

periostitis. Inflammation of the outer layers of bone.

posterolateral. Located in the back and off to the side.

CCI Version 16.3

01710, 0213T, 0216T, 0228T, 0230T, 10060, 10140, 10160, 20500, 23930-23935, 24125-24126❖, 24149, 24300, 24332, 24343-24346, 36000, 36400-36410, 36420-36430, 36440, 36600, 36640, 37202, 43752, 51701-51703, 62310-62319, 64400-64435, 64445-64450, 64479, 64483, 64490, 64493, 64505-64530, 69990, 93000-93010, 93040-93042, 93318, 94002, 94200, 94250, 94680-94690, 94770, 95812-95816, 95819, 95822, 95829, 95955, 96360, 96365, 96372, 96374-96376, 99148-99149, 99150

Also not with 24145: 64718

Also not with 24147: 24105

Note: These CCI edits are used for Medicare. Other payers may reimburse on codes listed above.

Medicare Edits

	Fac RVU	Non-Fac RVU	FUD	Assist
24145	17.39	17.39	90	N/A
24147	18.2	18.2	90	N/A

Medicare References: 100-2,15,260; 100-4,12,30; 100-4,12,90.3; 100-4,14,10

24149

24149 Radical resection of capsule, soft tissue, and heterotopic bone, elbow, with contracture release (separate procedure)

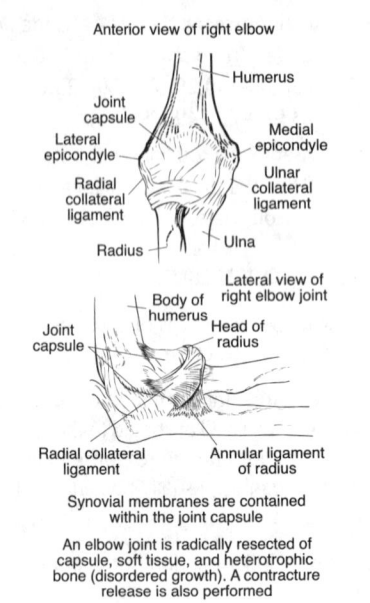

Anterior view of right elbow
Lateral view of right elbow joint
Synovial membranes are contained within the joint capsule
An elbow joint is radically resected of capsule, soft tissue, and heterotrophic bone (disordered growth). A contracture release is also performed

Explanation
The physician radically resects the elbow joint capsule, undesirable soft tissue and bone, and releases a contracture of a muscle or tendon. With the patient under anesthesia, the physician makes a long longitudinal incision overlying the elbow. Depending on the extent of the excess bone to be removed or the severity of the contracture, additional incisions may be required. The incision is continued deep to the elbow joint capsule itself. Nerves, vessels, and tendons are retracted. The capsule is fully exposed. A thorough debridement is undertaken to excise unwanted soft tissue. The overgrown and excess bone is isolated and excised. The capsule is resected. The contracture of the elbow involving muscle, tendon, scar tissue, or soft tissue is identified and explored. The physician releases the offending tissue to allow full elbow range of motion. The wound or wounds are irrigated and closed in layers. A dressing is applied.

Coding Tips
This separate procedure by definition is usually a component of a more complex service and is not identified separately. When performed alone or with other unrelated procedures/services it may be reported. If performed alone, list the code; if performed with other procedures/services, list the code and append modifier 59. For capsular and soft tissue release only, see 24006.

ICD-9-CM Procedural
- 77.62 Local excision of lesion or tissue of humerus
- 80.42 Division of joint capsule, ligament, or cartilage of elbow
- 83.49 Other excision of soft tissue

Anesthesia
24149 01756

ICD-9-CM Diagnostic
- 357.1 Polyneuropathy in collagen vascular disease — (Code first underlying disease: 446.0, 710.0, 714.0)
- 359.6 Symptomatic inflammatory myopathy in diseases classified elsewhere — (Code first underlying disease: 135, 140.0-208.9, 277.30-277.39, 446.0, 710.0, 710.1, 710.2, 714.0)
- 446.0 Polyarteritis nodosa
- 710.0 Systemic lupus erythematosus — (Use additional code to identify manifestation: 424.91, 581.81, 582.81, 583.81)
- 710.1 Systemic sclerosis — (Use additional code to identify manifestation: 359.6, 517.2)
- 710.2 Sicca syndrome
- 711.02 Pyogenic arthritis, upper arm — (Use additional code to identify infectious organism: 041.0-041.8)
- 711.92 Unspecified infective arthritis, upper arm
- 714.0 Rheumatoid arthritis — (Use additional code to identify manifestation: 357.1, 359.6)
- 718.52 Ankylosis of upper arm joint
- 719.22 Villonodular synovitis, upper arm
- 719.42 Pain in joint, upper arm
- 730.12 Chronic osteomyelitis, upper arm — (Use additional code to identify organism: 041.1. Use additional code to identify major osseous defect, if applicable: 731.3)
- 730.22 Unspecified osteomyelitis, upper arm — (Use additional code to identify organism: 041.1. Use additional code to identify major osseous defect, if applicable: 731.3)
- 730.92 Unspecified infection of bone, upper arm — (Use additional code to identify organism: 041.1)
- 731.3 Major osseous defects — (Code first underlying disease: 170.0-170.9, 730.00-730.29, 733.00-733.09, 733.40-733.49, 996.45)
- 733.49 Aseptic necrosis of other bone site — (Use additional code to identify major osseous defect, if applicable: 731.3)
- 905.2 Late effect of fracture of upper extremities
- 905.6 Late effect of dislocation
- 906.4 Late effect of crushing
- 927.11 Crushing injury of elbow — (Use additional code to identify any associated injuries: 800-829, 850.0-854.1, 860.0-869.1)

Terms To Know
ankylosis. Abnormal union or fusion of bones in a joint, which is normally moveable.

contracture. Shortening of muscle or connective tissue.

scar tissue. Fibrous connective tissue that forms around a wounded area or injury, composed mainly of fibroblasts or collagenous fibers.

tendon. Fibrous tissue that connects muscle to bone, consisting primarily of collagen and containing little vasculature.

CCI Version 16.3
01710, 0213T, 0216T, 0228T, 0230T, 11900-11901, 12001-12007, 12011-12057, 13100-13101, 13120-13121, 13131-13132, 13150-13152, 15851-15860, 20500-20501, 24006, 24300, 24332, 24343-24346, 29049-29085, 29105-29126, 29240-29280, 29705-29715, 29730, 29834, 35761, 36000, 36400-36410, 36420-36430, 36440, 36600, 36640, 37202, 37618, 43752, 51701-51703, 62310-62319, 64400-64435, 64445-64450, 64479, 64483, 64490, 64493, 64505-64560, 64565, 64573-64580, 64585-64595, 64702-64713, 64716-64726, 69990, 76000-76001, 76080, 77002, 87070, 87076-87077, 87102, 93000-93010, 93040-93042, 93318, 94002, 94200, 94250, 94680-94690, 94770, 95812-95816, 95819, 95822, 95829, 95860, 95900, 95955, 96360, 96365, 96372, 96374-96376, 99148-99149, 99150, G0168

Note: These CCI edits are used for Medicare. Other payers may reimburse on codes listed above.

Medicare Edits

	Fac RVU	Non-Fac RVU	FUD	Assist
24149	34.09	34.09	90	80

Medicare References: None

24150

24150 Radical resection of tumor, shaft or distal humerus

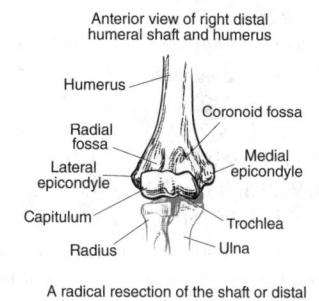

Anterior view of right distal humeral shaft and humerus

A radical resection of the shaft or distal humerus is performed to remove a tumor.

Explanation
The physician performs a radical resection of a tumor of the shaft or distal humerus. The physician makes an incision overlying the involved area of bone, dissecting down to expose the tumor site. The involved vessels and nerves are protected. Proximate muscles are detached extraperiosteally by sharp dissection, and the tumor is excised, including the immediately surrounding bone and any involved soft tissue. The wound is closed with layered sutures.

Coding Tips
Any bone graft harvest is not reported separately. According to CPT guidelines, cast application or strapping (including removal) is only reported as a replacement procedure or when the cast application or strapping is an initial service performed without a restorative treatment or procedure. See "Application of Casts and Strapping" in the CPT book in the Surgery Section, under the Musculoskeletal system.

ICD-9-CM Procedural
77.82 Other partial ostectomy of humerus

Anesthesia
24150 01756

ICD-9-CM Diagnostic
170.4 Malignant neoplasm of scapula and long bones of upper limb
198.5 Secondary malignant neoplasm of bone and bone marrow
209.73 Secondary neuroendocrine tumor of bone
238.0 Neoplasm of uncertain behavior of bone and articular cartilage
239.2 Neoplasms of unspecified nature of bone, soft tissue, and skin

Terms To Know
distal. Located farther away from a specified reference point.

malignant. Any condition tending to progress toward death, specifically an invasive tumor with a loss of cellular differentiation that has the ability to spread or metastasize to other areas in the body.

neoplasm. New abnormal growth, tumor.

radical. Extensive surgery.

resection. Surgical removal of a part or all of an organ or body part.

soft tissue. Nonepithelial tissues outside of the skeleton that includes subcutaneous adipose tissue, fibrous tissue, fascia, muscles, blood and lymph vessels, and peripheral nervous system tissue.

strapping. Application of overlapping strips of tape or bandaging to put pressure on the affected area.

tumor. Pathological swelling or enlargement; a neoplastic growth of uncontrolled, abnormal multiplication of cells.

CCI Version 16.3
01710, 0213T, 0216T, 0228T, 0230T, 10060, 10140, 10160, 11010-11012❖, 11040-11044, 12001-12007, 12020-12037, 13120-13121, 20220-20225, 20240-20245, 23930-23935, 24000, 24006-24116, 24134, 24140, 24149, 24300, 24332, 24341, 24343-24346, 24400-24410, 24495, 29835-29836, 36000, 36400-36410, 36420-36430, 36440, 36600, 36640, 37202, 43752, 51701-51703, 62310-62319, 64400-64435, 64445-64450, 64479, 64483, 64490, 64493, 64505-64530, 69990, 93000-93010, 93040-93042, 93318, 94002, 94200, 94250, 94680-94690, 94770, 95812-95816, 95819, 95822, 95829, 95955, 96360, 96365, 96372, 96374-96376, 99148-99149, 99150

Note: These CCI edits are used for Medicare. Other payers may reimburse on codes listed above.

Medicare Edits

	Fac RVU	Non-Fac RVU	FUD	Assist
24150	43.11	43.11	90	80

Medicare References: None

24152

24152 Radical resection of tumor, radial head or neck

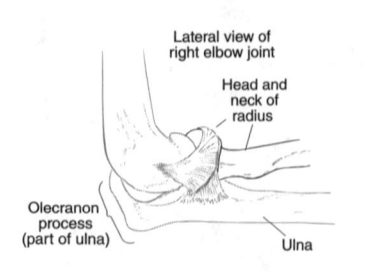

Lateral view of right elbow joint
Head and neck of radius
Olecranon process (part of ulna)
Ulna

A radical resection of the radial head or neck is performed to remove a tumor.

Explanation
The physician performs a radical resection of a tumor of the radial head or neck. The physician makes an anterolateral incision overlying the elbow or forearm. Dissection exposes the radial head or neck. The radial vessels and nerve are protected. The tumor is excised, including the radial head or neck. The physician selects the level of the radius to be divided. The physician uses a bone saw to divide the bone at the appropriate level. The muscles are detached by sharp dissection. Radical resection may also include removal of surrounding soft tissues such as muscles, fascia, and vessels. The wound is closed with layered sutures.

Coding Tips
Any bone graft harvest is not reported separately. According to CPT guidelines, cast application or strapping (including removal) is only reported as a replacement procedure or when the cast application or strapping is an initial service performed without a restorative treatment or procedure. See "Application of Casts and Strapping" in the CPT book in the Surgery Section, under the Musculoskeletal system.

ICD-9-CM Procedural
77.83   Other partial ostectomy of radius and ulna

Anesthesia
24152   01756

ICD-9-CM Diagnostic
170.4   Malignant neoplasm of scapula and long bones of upper limb
198.5   Secondary malignant neoplasm of bone and bone marrow
209.73 Secondary neuroendocrine tumor of bone
238.0   Neoplasm of uncertain behavior of bone and articular cartilage
239.2   Neoplasms of unspecified nature of bone, soft tissue, and skin

Terms To Know
anterolateral. Situated in the front and off to one side.

fascia. Fibrous sheet or band of tissue that envelops organs, muscles, and groupings of muscles.

malignant. Any condition tending to progress toward death, specifically an invasive tumor with a loss of cellular differentiation that has the ability to spread or metastasize to other areas in the body.

neoplasm. New abnormal growth, tumor.

posterior. Located in the back part or caudal end of the body.

secondary. Second in order of occurrence or importance, or appearing during the course of another disease or condition.

soft tissue. Nonepithelial tissues outside of the skeleton that includes subcutaneous adipose tissue, fibrous tissue, fascia, muscles, blood and lymph vessels, and peripheral nervous system tissue.

CCI Version 16.3
01710, 0213T, 0216T, 0228T, 0230T, 10060, 10140, 10160, 11010-11012✦, 11040-11044, 12001-12007, 12020-12037, 13120-13121, 20220-20225, 20240-20245, 23930-23935, 24000, 24006-24077, 24100-24105, 24120-24130, 24136, 24138, 24145, 24147, 24149, 24155✦, 24300, 24332, 24341, 24343-24346, 24495, 29835-29836, 36000, 36400-36410, 36420-36430, 36440, 36600, 36640, 37202, 43752, 51701-51703, 62310-62319, 64400-64435, 64445-64450, 64479, 64483, 64490, 64493, 64505-64530, 69990, 93000-93010, 93040-93042, 93318, 94002, 94200, 94250, 94680-94690, 94770, 95812-95816, 95819, 95822, 95829, 95955, 96360, 96365, 96372, 96374-96376, 99148-99149, 99150

Note: These CCI edits are used for Medicare. Other payers may reimburse on codes listed above.

Medicare Edits

	Fac RVU	Non-Fac RVU	FUD	Assist
24152	36.67	36.67	90	80

Medicare References: None

24155

24155 Resection of elbow joint (arthrectomy)

Explanation
An elbow joint arthrectomy is performed to remove the joint by resection of the distal humerus and the proximal radius and ulna. The physician makes a longitudinal incision along the lateral elbow. Dissection is carried down through the joint capsule to expose the distal humerus and the proximal radius and ulna. The physician selects the level at which the bones are to be resected. The physician uses a bone saw to divide the bones at the appropriate level. The physician preserves the surrounding muscle attachments to maintain some support and function for moving the elbow. However, gross instability of the elbow is present. The incision is repaired in layers using staples, sutures, and/or Steri-strips.

Coding Tips
According to CPT guidelines, cast application or strapping (including removal) is only reported as a replacement procedure or when the cast application or strapping is an initial service performed without a restorative treatment or procedure. See "Application of Casts and Strapping" in the CPT book in the Surgery Section, under the Musculoskeletal system.

ICD-9-CM Procedural
80.92   Other excision of elbow joint

Anesthesia
24155   01740

ICD-9-CM Diagnostic
170.4   Malignant neoplasm of scapula and long bones of upper limb
195.4   Malignant neoplasm of upper limb
238.0   Neoplasm of uncertain behavior of bone and articular cartilage
357.1   Polyneuropathy in collagen vascular disease — (Code first underlying disease: 446.0, 710.0, 714.0)
359.6   Symptomatic inflammatory myopathy in diseases classified elsewhere — (Code first underlying disease: 135, 140.0-208.9, 277.30-277.39, 446.0, 710.0, 710.1, 710.2, 714.0)
710.2   Sicca syndrome
714.0   Rheumatoid arthritis — (Use additional code to identify manifestation: 357.1, 359.6)
718.52 Ankylosis of upper arm joint
718.72 Developmental dislocation of joint, upper arm
719.22 Villonodular synovitis, upper arm
730.12 Chronic osteomyelitis, upper arm — (Use additional code to identify organism: 041.1. Use additional code to identify major osseous defect, if applicable: 731.3)
733.49 Aseptic necrosis of other bone site — (Use additional code to identify major osseous defect, if applicable: 731.3)
812.41 Closed fracture of supracondylar humerus
812.42 Closed fracture of lateral condyle of humerus
812.43 Closed fracture of medial condyle of humerus
812.44 Closed fracture of unspecified condyle(s) of humerus
812.49 Other closed fracture of lower end of humerus
812.51 Open fracture of supracondylar humerus
812.52 Open fracture of lateral condyle of humerus
812.53 Open fracture of medial condyle of humerus
812.59 Other open fracture of lower end of humerus
813.01 Closed fracture of olecranon process of ulna
813.02 Closed fracture of coronoid process of ulna
813.05 Closed fracture of head of radius
813.06 Closed fracture of neck of radius
813.08 Closed fracture of radius with ulna, upper end (any part)
813.11 Open fracture of olecranon process of ulna
813.12 Open fracture of coronoid process of ulna
813.15 Open fracture of head of radius
813.16 Open fracture of neck of radius
813.17 Other and unspecified open fractures of proximal end of radius (alone)
813.18 Open fracture of radius with ulna, upper end (any part)
832.01 Closed anterior dislocation of elbow
832.02 Closed posterior dislocation of elbow
832.10 Open unspecified dislocation of elbow
832.11 Open anterior dislocation of elbow
832.12 Open posterior dislocation of elbow
832.13 Open medial dislocation of elbow
832.14 Open lateral dislocation of elbow
832.19 Open dislocation of other site of elbow

CCI Version 16.3
01710, 0213T, 0216T, 0228T, 0230T, 23930-23935, 24000, 24006-24077, 24100-24134, 24136, 24138, 24140, 24145, 24147, 24149-24150❖, 24300, 24332, 24341, 24343-24346, 24495, 29835-29836, 36000, 36400-36410, 36420-36430, 36440, 36600, 36640, 37202, 43752, 51701-51703, 62310-62319, 64400-64435, 64445-64450, 64479, 64483, 64490, 64493, 64505-64530, 69990, 93000-93010, 93040-93042, 93318, 94002, 94200, 94250, 94680-94690, 94770, 95812-95816, 95819, 95822, 95829, 95955, 96360, 96365, 96372, 96374-96376, 99148-99149, 99150

Note: These CCI edits are used for Medicare. Other payers may reimburse on codes listed above.

Medicare Edits

	Fac RVU	Non-Fac RVU	FUD	Assist
24155	24.88	24.88	90	80

Medicare References: 100-2,15,260; 100-4,12,30; 100-4,12,90.3; 100-4,14,10

24160-24164

24160 Implant removal; elbow joint
24164 radial head

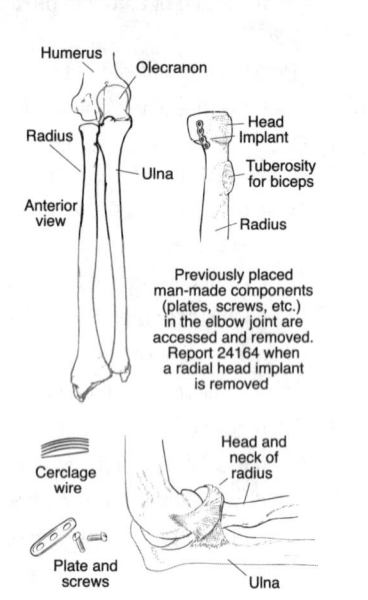

Explanation

The physician makes an incision overlying the area of the implant of the elbow joint. The incision may be made on the medial, lateral, or posterior portion of the elbow. In 24164, the incision may be made along the lateral elbow to expose the radial head. Dissection is carried down to expose the implant (e.g., pin, wire, screw). The physician uses instruments to remove the implant from the bone. The incision is then repaired with sutures and/or Steri-strips.

Coding Tips

For removal of a K-wire or pin, see 20670 or 20680.

ICD-9-CM Procedural

78.63 Removal of implanted device from radius and ulna
78.69 Removal of implanted device from other bone

Anesthesia

01740

ICD-9-CM Diagnostic

731.3 Major osseous defects — (Code first underlying disease: 170.0-170.9, 730.00-730.29, 733.00-733.09, 733.40-733.49, 996.45)
996.40 Unspecified mechanical complication of internal orthopedic device, implant, and graft — (Use additional code to identify prosthetic joint with mechanical complication, V43.60-V43.69)
996.41 Mechanical loosening of prosthetic joint — (Use additional code to identify prosthetic joint with mechanical complication, V43.60-V43.69)
996.42 Dislocation of prosthetic joint — (Use additional code to identify prosthetic joint with mechanical complication, V43.60-V43.69)
996.43 Broken prosthetic joint implant — (Use additional code to identify prosthetic joint with mechanical complication, V43.60-V43.69)
996.44 Peri-prosthetic fracture around prosthetic joint — (Use additional code to identify prosthetic joint with mechanical complication, V43.60-V43.69.
996.45 Peri-prosthetic osteolysis — (Use additional code to identify prosthetic joint with mechanical complication, V43.60-V43.69. Use additional code to identify major osseous defect, if applicable: 731.3)
996.47 Other mechanical complication of prosthetic joint implant — (Use additional code to identify prosthetic joint with mechanical complication, V43.60-V43.69)
996.49 Other mechanical complication of other internal orthopedic device, implant, and graft — (Use additional code to identify prosthetic joint with mechanical complication, V43.60-V43.69)
996.66 Infection and inflammatory reaction due to internal joint prosthesis — (Use additional code to identify specified infections. Use additional code to identify infected prosthetic joint: V43.60-V43.69)
996.67 Infection and inflammatory reaction due to other internal orthopedic device, implant, and graft — (Use additional code to identify specified infections)
996.77 Other complications due to internal joint prosthesis — (Use additional code to identify complication: 338.18-338.19, 338.28-338.29)
996.78 Other complications due to other internal orthopedic device, implant, and graft — (Use additional code to identify complication: 338.18-338.19, 338.28-338.29)
996.79 Other complications due to other internal prosthetic device, implant, and graft — (Use additional code to identify complication: 338.18-338.19, 338.28-338.29)
998.59 Other postoperative infection — (Use additional code to identify infection)
V43.62 Elbow joint replacement by other means

Terms To Know

complication. Condition arising after the beginning of observation and treatment that modifies the course of the patient's illness or the medical care required, or an undesired result or misadventure in medical care.

infection. Presence of microorganisms in body tissues that may result in cellular damage.

lateral. To/on the side.

posterior. Located in the back part or caudal end of the body.

CCI Version 16.3

01710, 0213T, 0216T, 0228T, 0230T, 20670, 24000, 24006, 24100-24102, 24300, 24332, 29835-29836, 36000, 36400-36410, 36420-36430, 36440, 36600, 36640, 37202, 43752, 51701-51703, 62310-62319, 64400-64435, 64445-64450, 64479, 64483, 64490, 64493, 64505-64530, 69990, 93000-93010, 93040-93042, 93318, 94002, 94200, 94250, 94680-94690, 94770, 95812-95816, 95819, 95822, 95829, 95955, 96360, 96365, 96372, 96374-96376, 99148-99149, 99150

Also not with 24160: 24341, 24343-24346
Also not with 24164: 24160❖

Note: These CCI edits are used for Medicare. Other payers may reimburse on codes listed above.

Medicare Edits

	Fac RVU	Non-Fac RVU	FUD	Assist
24160	17.6	17.6	90	N/A
24164	14.42	14.42	90	N/A

Medicare References: 100-2,15,260; 100-4,12,30; 100-4,12,90.3; 100-4,14,10

24200-24201

24200 Removal of foreign body, upper arm or elbow area; subcutaneous
24201 deep (subfascial or intramuscular)

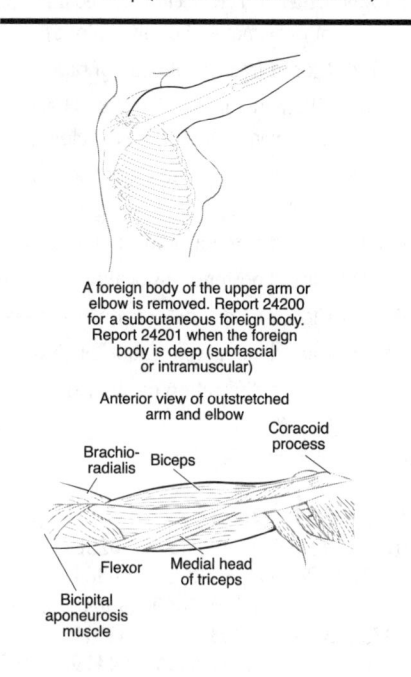

A foreign body of the upper arm or elbow is removed. Report 24200 for a subcutaneous foreign body. Report 24201 when the foreign body is deep (subfascial or intramuscular).

Anterior view of outstretched arm and elbow

Explanation

The physician removes a foreign body of the upper arm or elbow area. If the foreign body is a result of trauma, an open wound may already exist. The physician may make a separate incision or access the foreign body through the open wound. Location of the foreign body may be determined prior to surgery by separately reportable x-rays. A subcutaneous foreign body is located between the skin and muscle layer in 24200. The foreign body is deep and may be within muscle in 24201. More extensive dissection and a larger incision may be necessary for a deep foreign body. Once the foreign body is visualized, it is removed. The physician may also debride any surrounding damaged soft tissue. The wound is thoroughly irrigated. Drains may be placed in the wound and the incision repaired in multiple layers with sutures, staples, and/or Steri-strips. A splint may be applied to limit elbow motion.

Coding Tips

According to CPT guidelines, cast application or strapping (including removal) is only reported as a replacement procedure or when the cast application or strapping is an initial service performed without a restorative treatment or procedure. See "Application of Casts and Strapping" in the CPT book in the Surgery Section, under the Musculoskeletal system. Local anesthesia is included in these services. However, these procedures may be performed under general anesthesia, depending on the age and/or condition of the patient.

ICD-9-CM Procedural

- 83.02 Myotomy
- 83.09 Other incision of soft tissue
- 86.05 Incision with removal of foreign body or device from skin and subcutaneous tissue
- 98.27 Removal of foreign body without incision from upper limb, except hand

Anesthesia

- **24200** 00400
- **24201** 01710

ICD-9-CM Diagnostic

- 709.4 Foreign body granuloma of skin and subcutaneous tissue — (Use additional code to identify foreign body (V90.01-V90.9))
- 728.82 Foreign body granuloma of muscle — (Use additional code to identify foreign body (V90.01-V90.9))
- 729.6 Residual foreign body in soft tissue — (Use additional code to identify foreign body (V90.01-V90.9))
- 733.99 Other disorders of bone and cartilage
- 880.13 Open wound of upper arm, complicated
- 881.11 Open wound of elbow, complicated
- 906.1 Late effect of open wound of extremities without mention of tendon injury
- 913.6 Elbow, forearm, and wrist, superficial foreign body (splinter), without major open wound and without mention of infection
- 913.7 Elbow, forearm, and wrist, superficial foreign body (splinter), without major open wound, infected
- 998.4 Foreign body accidentally left during procedure, not elsewhere classified

Terms To Know

foreign body. Any object or substance found in an organ and tissue that does not belong under normal circumstances.

soft tissue. Nonepithelial tissues outside of the skeleton that includes subcutaneous adipose tissue, fibrous tissue, fascia, muscles, blood and lymph vessels, and peripheral nervous system tissue.

subfascial. Beneath the band of fibrous tissue that lies deep to the skin, encloses muscles, and separates their layers.

CCI Version 16.3

01710, 0213T, 0216T, 0228T, 0230T, 20103, 24300, 36000, 36400-36410, 36420-36430, 36440, 36600, 36640, 37202, 43752, 51701-51703, 62310-62319, 64400-64435, 64445-64450, 64479, 64483, 64490, 64493, 64505-64530, 69990, 93000-93010, 93040-93042, 93318, 94002, 94200, 94250, 94680-94690, 94770, 95812-95816, 95819, 95822, 95829, 95955, 96360, 96365, 96372, 96374-96376, 99148-99149, 99150, J0670, J2001

Also not with 24200: 11010❖

Also not with 24201: 24200

Note: These CCI edits are used for Medicare. Other payers may reimburse on codes listed above.

Medicare Edits

	Fac RVU	Non-Fac RVU	FUD	Assist
24200	4.01	5.81	10	80
24201	10.6	15.96	90	N/A

Medicare References: 100-2,15,260; 100-4,12,30; 100-4,12,90.3; 100-4,14,10

24220

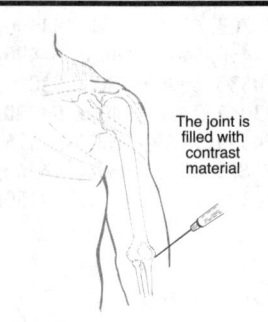

24220 Injection procedure for elbow arthrography

The joint is filled with contrast material

Contrast material is injected into the elbow joint for arthrography purposes

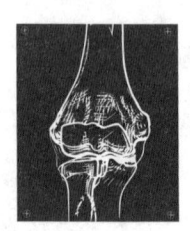

Separately reportable imaging of the elbow is taken

Explanation
Elbow arthrography provides information about the capsule size, the synovial lining, the articular surfaces of the joints, and detects loose bodies and capsular leaks. The patient is positioned sitting or supine (lying face up) with the elbow flexed at 90 degrees. One of two injection sites may be used, a lateral or posterior approach. The contrast medium is injected. A fluoroscope is used to study the elbow. No incisions are made. This code reports the injection only. The radiological exam is reported separately.

Coding Tips
For radiology supervision and interpretation, see 73085. For injection for tennis elbow, see 20550.

ICD-9-CM Procedural
- 81.92 Injection of therapeutic substance into joint or ligament
- 88.32 Contrast arthrogram

Anesthesia
24220 01730

ICD-9-CM Diagnostic
- 229.8 Benign neoplasm of other specified sites
- 275.40 Unspecified disorder of calcium metabolism — (Use additional code to identify any associated mental retardation)
- 275.42 Hypercalcemia — (Use additional code to identify any associated mental retardation)
- 275.49 Other disorders of calcium metabolism — (Use additional code to identify any associated mental retardation)
- 275.5 Hungry bone syndrome
- 357.1 Polyneuropathy in collagen vascular disease — (Code first underlying disease: 446.0, 710.0, 714.0)
- 359.6 Symptomatic inflammatory myopathy in diseases classified elsewhere — (Code first underlying disease: 135, 140.0-208.9, 277.30-277.39, 446.0, 710.0, 710.1, 710.2, 714.0)
- 446.0 Polyarteritis nodosa
- 710.0 Systemic lupus erythematosus — (Use additional code to identify manifestation: 424.91, 581.81, 582.81, 583.81)
- 710.1 Systemic sclerosis — (Use additional code to identify manifestation: 359.6, 517.2)
- 710.2 Sicca syndrome
- 714.0 Rheumatoid arthritis — (Use additional code to identify manifestation: 357.1, 359.6)
- 715.12 Primary localized osteoarthrosis, upper arm
- 715.92 Osteoarthrosis, unspecified whether generalized or localized, upper arm
- 716.12 Traumatic arthropathy, upper arm
- 718.12 Loose body in upper arm joint
- 718.72 Developmental dislocation of joint, upper arm
- 718.82 Other joint derangement, not elsewhere classified, upper arm
- 719.42 Pain in joint, upper arm
- 719.52 Stiffness of joint, not elsewhere classified, upper arm
- 719.82 Other specified disorders of upper arm joint
- 812.40 Closed fracture of unspecified part of lower end of humerus
- 812.41 Closed fracture of supracondylar humerus
- 812.42 Closed fracture of lateral condyle of humerus
- 812.43 Closed fracture of medial condyle of humerus
- 812.44 Closed fracture of unspecified condyle(s) of humerus
- 812.49 Other closed fracture of lower end of humerus
- 813.01 Closed fracture of olecranon process of ulna
- 813.02 Closed fracture of coronoid process of ulna
- 813.04 Other and unspecified closed fractures of proximal end of ulna (alone)
- 813.05 Closed fracture of head of radius
- 813.07 Other and unspecified closed fractures of proximal end of radius (alone)
- 832.00 Closed unspecified dislocation of elbow
- 832.01 Closed anterior dislocation of elbow
- 832.02 Closed posterior dislocation of elbow
- 832.03 Closed medial dislocation of elbow
- 832.04 Closed lateral dislocation of elbow
- 832.09 Closed dislocation of other site of elbow
- 832.2 Nursemaid's elbow

CCI Version 16.3
01710, 0213T, 0216T, 0228T, 0230T, 11010❖, 24300, 36000, 36400-36410, 36420-36430, 36440, 36600, 36640, 37202, 43752, 51701-51703, 62310-62319, 64400-64435, 64445-64450, 64479, 64483, 64490, 64493, 64505-64530, 69990, 76000-76001, 93000-93010, 93040-93042, 93318, 94002, 94200, 94250, 94680-94690, 94770, 95812-95816, 95819, 95822, 95829, 95955, 96360, 96365, 96372, 96374-96376, 99148-99149, 99150, J1644, J2001

Note: These CCI edits are used for Medicare. Other payers may reimburse on codes listed above.

Medicare Edits

	Fac RVU	Non-Fac RVU	FUD	Assist
24220	2.02	4.75	0	80

Medicare References: None

24300

24300 Manipulation, elbow, under anesthesia

Lateral view of right elbow joint
- Body of humerus
- Head of radius
- Joint capsule
- Radial collateral ligament
- Annular ligament of radius

Explanation

Manipulation of the elbow under anesthesia may be necessary to gain the loss of motion following a surgical procedure or due to scar tissue. Following the induction of general anesthesia, the physician evaluates the elbow. The elbow is manipulated by stretching, rotation, and other maneuvers to gain the appropriate range of motion.

Coding Tips

This is a unilateral procedure. If performed bilaterally, some payers require that the service be reported twice with modifier 50 appended to the second code while others require identification of the service only once with modifier 50 appended. Check with individual payers. Modifier 50 identifies a procedure performed identically on the opposite side of the body (mirror image). Local anesthesia is included in this service. For application of external fixation, see 20690 or 29692.

ICD-9-CM Procedural

- 93.25 Forced extension of limb
- 93.26 Manual rupture of joint adhesions
- 93.29 Other forcible correction of musculoskeletal deformity

Anesthesia

24300 01730

ICD-9-CM Diagnostic

- 357.1 Polyneuropathy in collagen vascular disease — (Code first underlying disease: 446.0, 710.0, 714.0)
- 359.6 Symptomatic inflammatory myopathy in diseases classified elsewhere — (Code first underlying disease: 135, 140.0-208.9, 277.30-277.39, 446.0, 710.0, 710.1, 710.2, 714.0)
- 446.0 Polyarteritis nodosa
- 710.0 Systemic lupus erythematosus — (Use additional code to identify manifestation: 424.91, 581.81, 582.81, 583.81)
- 710.1 Systemic sclerosis — (Use additional code to identify manifestation: 359.6, 517.2)
- 710.2 Sicca syndrome
- 714.0 Rheumatoid arthritis — (Use additional code to identify manifestation: 357.1, 359.6)
- 715.12 Primary localized osteoarthrosis, upper arm
- 715.92 Osteoarthrosis, unspecified whether generalized or localized, upper arm
- 718.42 Contracture of upper arm joint
- 718.52 Ankylosis of upper arm joint
- 719.22 Villonodular synovitis, upper arm
- 719.52 Stiffness of joint, not elsewhere classified, upper arm
- 726.30 Unspecified enthesopathy of elbow
- 726.31 Medial epicondylitis of elbow
- 726.32 Lateral epicondylitis of elbow
- 726.33 Olecranon bursitis
- 726.39 Other enthesopathy of elbow region

Terms To Know

adhesion. Abnormal fibrous connection between two structures, soft tissue or bony structures, that may occur as the result of surgery, infection, or trauma.

ankylosis. Abnormal union or fusion of bones in a joint, which is normally moveable.

contracture. Shortening of muscle or connective tissue.

polyneuropathy. Disease process of severe inflammation of multiple nerves.

sicca syndrome. Complex of symptoms of unknown source in middle-aged women in which the following triad exists: keratoconjunctivitis sicca, zerostomia, and connective tissue disease (usually rheumatoid arthritis but sometimes systemic lupus erythematosus).

synovitis. Inflammation of the synovial membrane that lines a synovial joint, resulting in pain and swelling.

CCI Version 16.3

01710, 0213T, 0216T, 0228T, 0230T, 29058-29075, 29105, 29260, 36000, 36400-36410, 36420-36430, 36440, 36600, 36640, 37202, 43752, 51701-51703, 62310-62319, 64400-64435, 64445-64450, 64479, 64483, 64490, 64493, 64505-64530, 93000-93010, 93040-93042, 93318, 94002, 94200, 94250, 94680-94690, 94770, 95812-95816, 95819, 95822, 95829, 95955, 96360, 96365, 96372, 96374-96376, 99148-99149, 99150

Note: These CCI edits are used for Medicare. Other payers may reimburse on codes listed above.

Medicare Edits

	Fac RVU	Non-Fac RVU	FUD	Assist
24300	11.63	11.63	90	N/A

Medicare References: None

24301

24301 Muscle or tendon transfer, any type, upper arm or elbow, single (excluding 24320-24331)

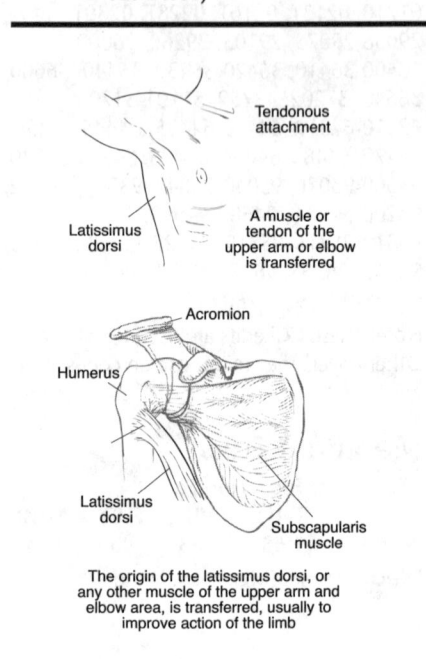

Explanation

The physician performs a muscle or tendon transfer of the upper arm or elbow. An example is transfer of the latissimus dorsi muscle. This transfer restores active elbow flexion by transferring the origin and belly of the latissimus dorsi to the arm and anchoring the origin near the radial head. The patient is placed side-lying with the affected side up. An incision is made starting at the loin and extending up to the axilla and then distally along the medial aspect of the arm to the anterior elbow. The physician cuts free the origin of the latissimus dorsi. The muscle itself is cut free from the underlying abdominal muscles. The origin of the latissimus dorsi muscle is sutured to the biceps tendon and the periosteal tissues about the radial tuberosity. The incision is repaired in multiple layers with sutures, staples, and/or Steri-strips.

Coding Tips

Tenoplasty with muscle transfer from the elbow to the shoulder should not be reported with 24301, instead see 24320. Flexor-plasty, elbow, also has more specific procedure codes and should be reported with 24330 or 24331. According to CPT guidelines, cast application or strapping (including removal) is only reported as a replacement procedure or when the cast application or strapping is an initial service performed without a restorative treatment or procedure. See "Application of Casts and Strapping" in the CPT book in the Surgery Section, under the Musculoskeletal system.

ICD-9-CM Procedural

83.75	Tendon transfer or transplantation
83.77	Muscle transfer or transplantation

Anesthesia

24301   01710

ICD-9-CM Diagnostic

342.10	Spastic hemiplegia affecting unspecified side
342.11	Spastic hemiplegia affecting dominant side
342.12	Spastic hemiplegia affecting nondominant side
343.0	Diplegic infantile cerebral palsy
343.1	Hemiplegic infantile cerebral palsy
343.2	Quadriplegic infantile cerebral palsy
343.3	Monoplegic infantile cerebral palsy
718.32	Recurrent dislocation of upper arm joint
726.30	Unspecified enthesopathy of elbow
726.39	Other enthesopathy of elbow region
727.62	Nontraumatic rupture of tendons of biceps (long head)
727.63	Nontraumatic rupture of extensor tendons of hand and wrist
727.64	Nontraumatic rupture of flexor tendons of hand and wrist
728.4	Laxity of ligament
728.5	Hypermobility syndrome
841.0	Radial collateral ligament sprain and strain
841.1	Ulnar collateral ligament sprain and strain
841.2	Radiohumeral (joint) sprain and strain
841.3	Ulnohumeral (joint) sprain and strain
841.8	Sprain and strain of other specified sites of elbow and forearm
841.9	Sprain and strain of unspecified site of elbow and forearm
881.11	Open wound of elbow, complicated
881.21	Open wound of elbow, with tendon involvement
884.1	Multiple and unspecified open wound of upper limb, complicated
884.2	Multiple and unspecified open wound of upper limb, with tendon involvement

Terms To Know

diplegic infantile cerebral palsy. Bilateral paralysis and delayed or abnormal motor development caused by trauma at birth or intrauterine pathology.

ligament. Band or sheet of fibrous tissue that connects the articular surfaces of bones or supports visceral organs.

tendon. Fibrous tissue that connects muscle to bone, consisting primarily of collagen and containing little vasculature.

CCI Version 16.3

01710, 0213T, 0216T, 0228T, 0230T, 24300, 24310, 24332-24341, 29055-29065, 29105, 29260, 36000, 36400-36410, 36420-36430, 36440, 36600, 36640, 37202, 43752, 51701-51703, 62310-62319, 64400-64435, 64445-64450, 64479, 64483, 64490, 64493, 64505-64530, 69990, 93000-93010, 93040-93042, 93318, 94002, 94200, 94250, 94680-94690, 94770, 95812-95816, 95819, 95822, 95829, 95955, 96360, 96365, 96372, 96374-96376, 99148-99149, 99150

Note: These CCI edits are used for Medicare. Other payers may reimburse on codes listed above.

Medicare Edits

	Fac RVU	Non-Fac RVU	FUD	Assist
24301	21.91	21.91	90	80

Medicare References: 100-2,15,260; 100-4,12,30; 100-4,12,90.3; 100-4,14,10

24305

24305 Tendon lengthening, upper arm or elbow, each tendon

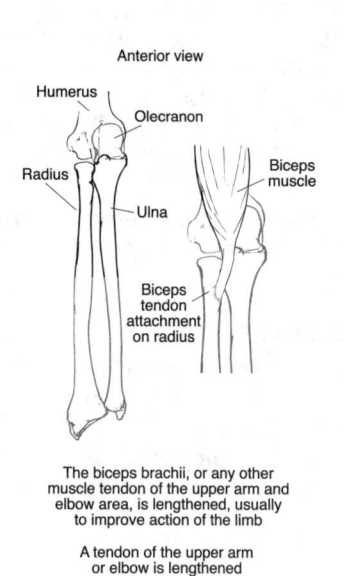

Anterior view

The biceps brachii, or any other muscle tendon of the upper arm and elbow area, is lengthened, usually to improve action of the limb

A tendon of the upper arm or elbow is lengthened

Explanation

The physician lengthens a tendon of the upper arm or elbow. An anterior curvilinear incision is made, for example, over the anterior elbow to lengthen the biceps tendon. Dissection is carried down to expose the distal biceps tendon. The biceps tendon is divided by Z-plasty and then stretched into extension, causing it to stretch and release to a lengthened position. If the elbow joint capsule is thickened, the physician may elect to excise this part of the capsule and any fibrous bands or bone spurs in the anterior part of the elbow joint. A drain is inserted into the wound and the incision is repaired in multiple layers using sutures, staples, and/or Steri-strips. The elbow is placed in a splint or cast in an extended position.

Coding Tips

Code 24305 should be reported for each tendon lengthening performed. When multiple tendon lengthening is performed, report one tendon as the primary procedure and append modifier 51 to subsequent procedures. According to CPT guidelines, cast application or strapping (including removal) is only reported as a replacement procedure or when the cast application or strapping is an initial service performed without a restorative treatment or procedure. See "Application of Casts and Strapping" in the CPT book in the Surgery Section, under the Musculoskeletal system.

ICD-9-CM Procedural

83.85 Other change in muscle or tendon length

Anesthesia

24305 01710

ICD-9-CM Diagnostic

- 343.0 Diplegic infantile cerebral palsy
- 715.31 Localized osteoarthrosis not specified whether primary or secondary, shoulder region
- 718.41 Contracture of shoulder joint
- 718.42 Contracture of upper arm joint
- 728.3 Other specific muscle disorders
- 840.8 Sprain and strain of other specified sites of shoulder and upper arm
- 840.9 Sprain and strain of unspecified site of shoulder and upper arm
- 841.0 Radial collateral ligament sprain and strain
- 841.1 Ulnar collateral ligament sprain and strain
- 841.2 Radiohumeral (joint) sprain and strain
- 841.3 Ulnohumeral (joint) sprain and strain
- 841.8 Sprain and strain of other specified sites of elbow and forearm
- 841.9 Sprain and strain of unspecified site of elbow and forearm

Terms To Know

anterior. Situated in the front area or toward the belly surface of the body; an anatomical reference point used to show the position and relationship of one body structure to another.

contracture. Shortening of muscle or connective tissue.

diplegic infantile cerebral palsy. Bilateral paralysis and delayed or abnormal motor development caused by trauma at birth or intrauterine pathology.

osteoarthrosis. Most common form of a noninflammatory degenerative joint disease with degenerating articular cartilage, bone enlargement, and synovial membrane changes.

sprain and strain. Injuries to a joint, in which the fibers of supporting ligaments or muscles are overstretched or slightly ruptured, with the ligaments and muscles maintaining continuity.

tendon. Fibrous tissue that connects muscle to bone, consisting primarily of collagen and containing little vasculature.

CCI Version 16.3

01710, 0213T, 0216T, 0228T, 0230T, 24300, 24310, 24332-24340, 29055-29065, 29105, 29260, 36000, 36400-36410, 36420-36430, 36440, 36600, 36640, 37202, 43752, 51701-51703, 62310-62319, 64400-64435, 64445-64450, 64479, 64483, 64490, 64493, 64505-64530, 64718, 69990, 93000-93010, 93040-93042, 93318, 94002, 94200, 94250, 94680-94690, 94770, 95812-95816, 95819, 95822, 95829, 95955, 96360, 96365, 96372, 96374-96376, 99148-99149, 99150

Note: These CCI edits are used for Medicare. Other payers may reimburse on codes listed above.

Medicare Edits

	Fac RVU	Non-Fac RVU	FUD	Assist
24305	16.83	16.83	90	80

Medicare References: 100-2,15,260; 100-4,12,30; 100-4,12,90.3; 100-4,14,10

24310

24310 Tenotomy, open, elbow to shoulder, each tendon

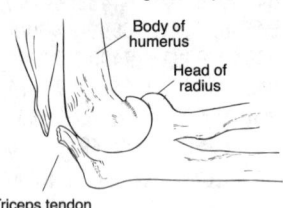

Lateral view of right elbow joint
Body of humerus
Head of radius
Triceps tendon at attachment on olecranon

Anterior view of right elbow joint
Biceps muscle
The biceps brachii, or any other muscle tendon of the upper arm and elbow area, is incised, usually to release a locked arm position
Biceps tendon attachment on radius

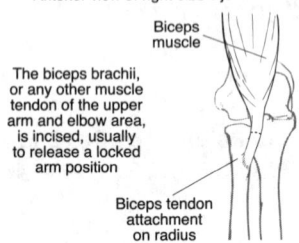

A tendon of the upper arm or elbow is cut

Explanation

For tenotomy of distal biceps tendon, an incision is made over the anterior elbow to expose the biceps tendon. The tendon is cut all the way through so as to release the flexion contracture. No repair of the tendon is made. The incision is repaired with sutures. The elbow may be placed in a splint to keep it in as much extension as possible.

Coding Tips

Code 24310 should be reported for each tenotomy performed. When multiple tenotomies are performed, report one tendon as the primary procedure and append modifier 51 to subsequent procedures. According to CPT guidelines, cast application or strapping (including removal) is only reported as a replacement procedure or when the cast application or strapping is an initial service performed without a restorative treatment or procedure. See "Application of Casts and Strapping" in the CPT book in the Surgery Section, under the Musculoskeletal system.

ICD-9-CM Procedural

83.13 Other tenotomy

Anesthesia

24310 01712

ICD-9-CM Diagnostic

716.51 Unspecified polyarthropathy or polyarthritis, shoulder region
716.52 Unspecified polyarthropathy or polyarthritis, upper arm
718.41 Contracture of shoulder joint
718.42 Contracture of upper arm joint
718.51 Ankylosis of joint of shoulder region
718.52 Ankylosis of upper arm joint
718.81 Other joint derangement, not elsewhere classified, shoulder region
718.82 Other joint derangement, not elsewhere classified, upper arm
718.91 Unspecified derangement, shoulder region
718.92 Unspecified derangement, upper arm joint
728.3 Other specific muscle disorders
840.8 Sprain and strain of other specified sites of shoulder and upper arm

Terms To Know

ankylosis. Abnormal union or fusion of bones in a joint, which is normally moveable.

anterior. Situated in the front area or toward the belly surface of the body; an anatomical reference point used to show the position and relationship of one body structure to another.

contracture. Shortening of muscle or connective tissue.

distal. Located farther away from a specified reference point.

flexion. Act of bending or being bent.

sprain and strain. Injuries to a joint, in which the fibers of supporting ligaments or muscles are overstretched or slightly ruptured, with the ligaments and muscles maintaining continuity.

tendon. Fibrous tissue that connects muscle to bone, consisting primarily of collagen and containing little vasculature.

CCI Version 16.3

01710, 0213T, 0216T, 0228T, 0230T, 24300, 24332-24340, 29055-29065, 29105, 29260, 36000, 36400-36410, 36420-36430, 36440, 36600, 36640, 37202, 43752, 51701-51703, 62310-62319, 64400-64435, 64445-64450, 64479, 64483, 64490, 64493, 64505-64530, 69990, 93000-93010, 93040-93042, 93318, 94002, 94200, 94250, 94680-94690, 94770, 95812-95816, 95819, 95822, 95829, 95955, 96360, 96365, 96372, 96374-96376, 99148-99149, 99150

Note: These CCI edits are used for Medicare. Other payers may reimburse on codes listed above.

Medicare Edits

	Fac RVU	Non-Fac RVU	FUD	Assist
24310	13.82	13.82	90	80

Medicare References: 100-2,15,260; 100-4,12,30; 100-4,12,90.3; 100-4,14,10

24320

24320 Tenoplasty, with muscle transfer, with or without free graft, elbow to shoulder, single (Seddon-Brookes type procedure)

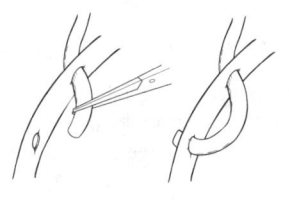

Typical tenoplasty approach to link tendons, as in a free graft procedure

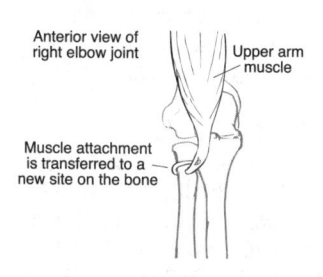

Anterior view of right elbow joint — Upper arm muscle — Muscle attachment is transferred to a new site on the bone

A tenoplasty is performed in the elbow to shoulder region, with muscle transfer, with or without free graft

Explanation

A Seddon-Brookes type upper arm tenoplasty with muscle transfer restores elbow flexion by prolonging the tendon of the pectoralis major muscle with the long head of the biceps brachii. The physician makes an incision from the deltopectoral groove to the midportion of the upper arm. The pectoralis major tendon is exposed through dissection, detached from its insertion, and mobilized from the chest wall toward the clavicle. The tendon of the long head of the biceps is exposed and severed from its origin and withdrawn into the wound. The long head of the biceps is dissected from the short head. An L-shaped incision is made over the anterior aspect of the elbow. The long head of the biceps is divided and freed distally to its attachment on the radius. The biceps tendon and muscle are withdrawn through the distal L-shaped incision. Through the proximal incision, the tendon and muscle belly of the long head of the biceps is passed through two slits in the tendon of the pectoralis major and looped on itself so that its proximal tendon is brought into the distal L-shaped incision. The end of the proximal tendon is sutured through a slit in the distal tendon and the tendon of the pectoralis major is sutured to the long head of the biceps at their junction. The incisions are repaired in layers using sutures, staples, and/or Steri-strips. A posterior plaster splint is applied with the elbow in flexion.

Coding Tips

Any tendon graft harvest is not reported separately. Code 24320 should be reported for each tenoplasty performed. When multiple tenoplasties are performed, report one tendon as the primary procedure and append modifier 51 to subsequent procedures. According to CPT guidelines, cast application or strapping (including removal) is only reported as a replacement procedure or when the cast application or strapping is an initial service performed without a restorative treatment or procedure. See "Application of Casts and Strapping" in the CPT book in the Surgery Section, under the Musculoskeletal system.

ICD-9-CM Procedural

- 83.77 Muscle transfer or transplantation
- 83.81 Tendon graft
- 83.88 Other plastic operations on tendon

Anesthesia

24320 01714

ICD-9-CM Diagnostic

- 343.0 Diplegic infantile cerebral palsy
- 718.41 Contracture of shoulder joint
- 718.42 Contracture of upper arm joint
- 718.81 Other joint derangement, not elsewhere classified, shoulder region
- 718.82 Other joint derangement, not elsewhere classified, upper arm
- 718.91 Unspecified derangement, shoulder region
- 718.92 Unspecified derangement, upper arm joint
- 718.98 Unspecified derangement of joint, other specified sites
- 727.62 Nontraumatic rupture of tendons of biceps (long head)
- 880.23 Open wound of upper arm, with tendon involvement
- 881.21 Open wound of elbow, with tendon involvement

Terms To Know

contracture. Shortening of muscle or connective tissue.

diplegic infantile cerebral palsy. Bilateral paralysis and delayed or abnormal motor development caused by trauma at birth or intrauterine pathology.

distal. Located farther away from a specified reference point.

open wound. Opening or break of the skin.

posterior. Located in the back part or caudal end of the body.

proximal. Located closest to a specified reference point, usually the midline.

tendon. Fibrous tissue that connects muscle to bone, consisting primarily of collagen and containing little vasculature.

CCI Version 16.3

01710, 0213T, 0216T, 0228T, 0230T, 20920-20924, 24300-24301, 24310, 24332-24341, 29055-29065, 29105, 29260, 36000, 36400-36410, 36420-36430, 36440, 36600, 36640, 37202, 43752, 51701-51703, 62310-62319, 64400-64435, 64445-64450, 64479, 64483, 64490, 64493, 64505-64530, 69990, 93000-93010, 93040-93042, 93318, 94002, 94200, 94250, 94680-94690, 94770, 95812-95816, 95819, 95822, 95829, 95955, 96360, 96365, 96372, 96374-96376, 99148-99149, 99150

Note: These CCI edits are used for Medicare. Other payers may reimburse on codes listed above.

Medicare Edits

	Fac RVU	Non-Fac RVU	FUD	Assist
24320	22.7	22.7	90	80

Medicare References: 100-2,15,260; 100-4,12,30; 100-4,12,90.3; 100-4,14,10

24330-24331

24330 Flexor-plasty, elbow (eg, Steindler type advancement);
24331 with extensor advancement

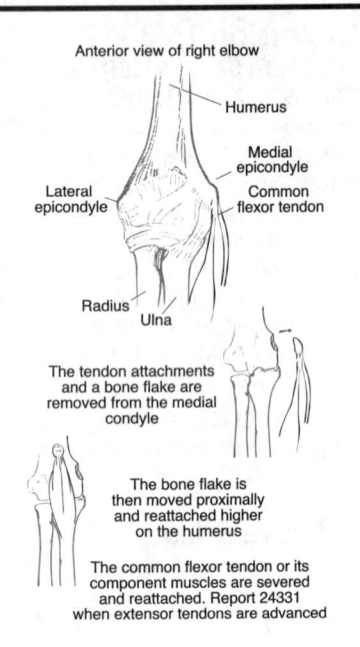

Anterior view of right elbow
- Humerus
- Medial epicondyle
- Lateral epicondyle
- Common flexor tendon
- Radius
- Ulna

The tendon attachments and a bone flake are removed from the medial condyle

The bone flake is then moved proximally and reattached higher on the humerus

The common flexor tendon or its component muscles are severed and reattached. Report 24331 when extensor tendons are advanced

Explanation

To perform a Steindler-type advancement for flexor-plasty of the elbow, the physician transfers the common origin of the pronator teres, flexor carpi radialis, palmaris longus, flexor digitorum sublimis, and flexor carpi ulnaris from the medial epicondyle of the humerus proximally and laterally onto the anterior surface of the humerus so that it performs elbow flexion rather than forearm pronation. This is done when the biceps brachii and brachialis are paralyzed. The physician makes a curved longitudinal incision over the medial side of the elbow extending over the medial condyle area and along the pronator teres. The ulnar nerve is identified and retracted for protection. The common origin of the pronator teres, flexor carpi radialis, palmaris longus, flexor digitorum sublimis, and flexor carpi ulnaris is detached as a whole from the medial epicondyle. These muscles are freed up for about 4 cm. A fascia lata graft is taken from the lateral thigh and one end is sutured to the common origin to extend it, while the other end is advanced and attached 5 cm up the lateral side of the humerus. A cast is applied with the elbow in flexion. In 24331, an anterior transfer of the triceps (extensor advancement) is performed in conjunction with elbow flexor-plasty. A posterolateral incision is made over the lower upper arm. The triceps tendon is exposed and divided at its insertion, dissected from the back of the lower humerus, and brought around to the lateral side. An anterolateral curvilinear incision is made to expose the radial tuberosity. Another 4 cm long fascia lata graft is harvested and attached to the triceps tendon to extend it for advancement. The other end of the fascia lata graft is attached to the tuberosity of the radius. This creates added elbow flexibility. A cast is applied with the elbow in flexion.

Coding Tips

For other muscle or tendon transfer procedures of the upper arm or elbow, see 24301 or 24320. According to CPT guidelines, cast application or strapping (including removal) is only reported as a replacement procedure or when the cast application or strapping is an initial service performed without a restorative treatment or procedure. See "Application of Casts and Strapping" in the CPT book in the Surgery Section, under the Musculoskeletal system.

ICD-9-CM Procedural

- 83.71 Advancement of tendon
- 83.77 Muscle transfer or transplantation
- 83.81 Tendon graft

Anesthesia
01710, 01714

ICD-9-CM Diagnostic

- 343.0 Diplegic infantile cerebral palsy
- 344.2 Diplegia of upper limbs
- 344.40 Monoplegia of upper limb affecting unspecified side
- 344.41 Monoplegia of upper limb affecting dominant side
- 344.42 Monoplegia of upper limb affecting nondominant side
- 718.32 Recurrent dislocation of upper arm joint
- 718.42 Contracture of upper arm joint
- 718.82 Other joint derangement, not elsewhere classified, upper arm
- 718.92 Unspecified derangement, upper arm joint
- 719.42 Pain in joint, upper arm
- 767.6 Injury to brachial plexus, birth trauma — (Use additional code(s) to further specify condition)
- 953.4 Injury to brachial plexus

Terms To Know

anterior. Situated in the front area or toward the belly surface of the body; an anatomical reference point used to show the position and relationship of one body structure to another.

contracture. Shortening of muscle or connective tissue.

diplegic infantile cerebral palsy. Bilateral paralysis and delayed or abnormal motor development caused by trauma at birth or intrauterine pathology.

dislocation. Displacement of a bone in relation to its neighboring tissue, especially a joint.

flexion. Act of bending or being bent.

pronation. Lying on the stomach or in a face down position; turning the palm toward the back or downward; lowering of the medial margin of the foot by an everting and abducting movement.

tendon. Fibrous tissue that connects muscle to bone, consisting primarily of collagen and containing little vasculature.

CCI Version 16.3

01710, 0213T, 0216T, 0228T, 0230T, 24300-24301, 24310, 24332-24341, 29055-29065, 29105, 29260, 36000, 36400-36410, 36420-36430, 36440, 36600, 36640, 37202, 43752, 51701-51703, 62310-62319, 64400-64435, 64445-64450, 64479, 64483, 64490, 64493, 64505-64530, 69990, 93000-93010, 93040-93042, 93318, 94002, 94200, 94250, 94680-94690, 94770, 95812-95816, 95819, 95822, 95829, 95955, 96360, 96365, 96372, 96374-96376, 99148-99149, 99150

Also not with 24330: 64718
Also not with 24331: 24330

Note: These CCI edits are used for Medicare. Other payers may reimburse on codes listed above.

Medicare Edits

	Fac RVU	Non-Fac RVU	FUD	Assist
24330	20.89	20.89	90	80
24331	23.48	23.48	90	80

Medicare References: 100-2,15,260; 100-4,12,30; 100-4,12,90.3; 100-4,14,10

24332

24332 Tenolysis, triceps

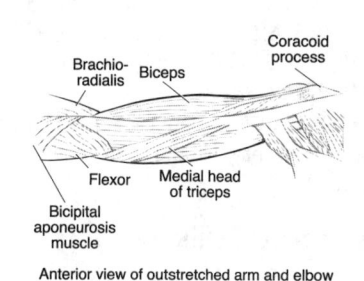

Anterior view of outstretched arm and elbow — Brachioradialis, Biceps, Coracoid process, Flexor, Medial head of triceps, Bicipital aponeurosis muscle

Explanation
Tenolysis involves transection of adhesions that have formed between the tendon and its surrounding tissues. Beginning proximally along the supracondylar ridge and ending near the subcutaneous border of the ulna, the physician makes a deep dissection to the anterior aspect of the capsule. The triceps tendon is retracted posteriorly to expose the olecranon fossa and tenolysis of the triceps and posterior capsulectomy is performed. Tenolysis should be performed under a local anesthetic so that full release can be confirmed. If, however, general or regional anesthesia is used, the physician may check the adequacy of the removal of all adhesions by manually pulling the tendons.

Coding Tips
This is a unilateral procedure. If performed bilaterally, some payers require that the service be reported twice with modifier 50 appended to the second code, while others require identification of the service only once with modifier 50 appended. Check with individual payers. Modifier 50 identifies a procedure performed identically on the opposite side of the body (mirror image). Local anesthesia is included in this service.

ICD-9-CM Procedural
83.91 Lysis of adhesions of muscle, tendon, fascia, and bursa

Anesthesia
24332 01710

ICD-9-CM Diagnostic
- 357.1 Polyneuropathy in collagen vascular disease — (Code first underlying disease: 446.0, 710.0, 714.0)
- 359.6 Symptomatic inflammatory myopathy in diseases classified elsewhere — (Code first underlying disease: 135, 140.0-208.9, 277.30-277.39, 446.0, 710.0, 710.1, 710.2, 714.0)
- 446.0 Polyarteritis nodosa
- 710.0 Systemic lupus erythematosus — (Use additional code to identify manifestation: 424.91, 581.81, 582.81, 583.81)
- 710.1 Systemic sclerosis — (Use additional code to identify manifestation: 359.6, 517.2)
- 710.2 Sicca syndrome
- 714.0 Rheumatoid arthritis — (Use additional code to identify manifestation: 357.1, 359.6)
- 718.52 Ankylosis of upper arm joint
- 719.52 Stiffness of joint, not elsewhere classified, upper arm
- 727.00 Unspecified synovitis and tenosynovitis
- 727.01 Synovitis and tenosynovitis in diseases classified elsewhere — (Code first underlying disease: 015.0-015.9)
- 727.09 Other synovitis and tenosynovitis
- 727.81 Contracture of tendon (sheath)
- 727.82 Calcium deposits in tendon and bursa
- 727.89 Other disorders of synovium, tendon, and bursa
- 727.9 Unspecified disorder of synovium, tendon, and bursa

Terms To Know
adhesion. Abnormal fibrous connection between two structures, soft tissue or bony structures, that may occur as the result of surgery, infection, or trauma.

polyneuropathy. Disease process of severe inflammation of multiple nerves.

sheath. Covering enclosing an organ or part.

subcutaneous tissue. Sheet or wide band of adipose (fat) and areolar connective tissue in two layers attached to the dermis.

tendon. Fibrous tissue that connects muscle to bone, consisting primarily of collagen and containing little vasculature.

CCI Version 16.3
01710, 0213T, 0216T, 0228T, 0230T, 24300, 24357, 29049-29075, 29105, 29240-29260, 36000, 36400-36410, 36420-36430, 36440, 36600, 36640, 37202, 43752, 51701-51703, 62310-62319, 64400-64435, 64445-64450, 64479, 64483, 64490, 64493, 64505-64530, 69990, 93000-93010, 93040-93042, 93318, 94002, 94200, 94250, 94680-94690, 94770, 95812-95816, 95819, 95822, 95829, 95955, 96360, 96365, 96372, 96374-96376, 99148-99149, 99150

Note: These CCI edits are used for Medicare. Other payers may reimburse on codes listed above.

Medicare Edits

	Fac RVU	Non-Fac RVU	FUD	Assist
24332	17.71	17.71	90	N/A

Medicare References: None

24340

24340 Tenodesis of biceps tendon at elbow (separate procedure)

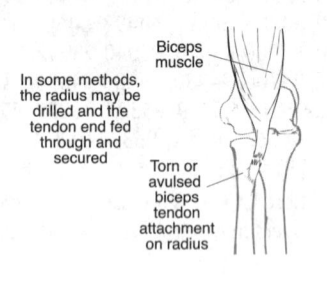

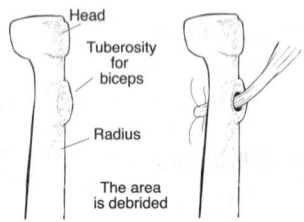

Explanation

The physician treats a rupture of a distal biceps tendon by reattachment of the biceps tendon to the radius, direct reimplantation, or inserting a loop of fascia lata graft around the proximal radius. Reattachment of the biceps tendon to the radius is described. The patient is placed supine. The physician makes an anterior lateral incision on the lower upper arm and extending transversely across the antecubital fossa. The torn biceps tendon is identified and the tear is minimally debrided. Two Bunnell sutures are placed in the torn end. A second incision is made over the dorsal aspect of the proximal forearm to expose the radial tuberosity. The physician uses a high speed burr to evacuate a 5.0 mm to 7.0 mm defect in the radial tuberosity. Three holes are drilled through this window to the opposite side of the tuberosity. The physician places sutures through the holes and places the tendon into the window in the tuberosity. The sutures are pulled tight and secured. The incisions are repaired in multiple layers with drains inserted. The elbow is placed in a splint in 90 degrees of flexion and full supination.

Coding Tips

This separate procedure by definition is usually a component of a more complex service and is not identified separately. When performed alone or with other unrelated procedures/services it may be reported. If performed alone, list the code; if performed with other procedures/services, list the code and append modifier 59. According to CPT guidelines, cast application or strapping (including removal) is only reported as a replacement procedure or when the cast application or strapping is an initial service performed without a restorative treatment or procedure. See "Application of Casts and Strapping" in the CPT book in the Surgery Section, under the Musculoskeletal system.

ICD-9-CM Procedural

83.88 Other plastic operations on tendon

Anesthesia

24340 01710

ICD-9-CM Diagnostic

727.62 Nontraumatic rupture of tendons of biceps (long head)

728.83 Rupture of muscle, nontraumatic

841.8 Sprain and strain of other specified sites of elbow and forearm

Terms To Know

anterior. Situated in the front area or toward the belly surface of the body; an anatomical reference point used to show the position and relationship of one body structure to another.

distal. Located farther away from a specified reference point.

dorsal. Pertaining to the back or posterior aspect.

flexion. Act of bending or being bent.

proximal. Located closest to a specified reference point, usually the midline.

supination. Lying on the back; turning the palm toward the front or upward; raising the medial margin of the foot by an inverting and adducting movement.

tendon. Fibrous tissue that connects muscle to bone, consisting primarily of collagen and containing little vasculature.

CCI Version 16.3

01710, 0213T, 0216T, 0228T, 0230T, 24000, 24006, 24100-24102, 24300, 24341, 29055-29075, 29105, 29260, 36000, 36400-36410, 36420-36430, 36440, 36600, 36640, 37202, 43752, 51701-51703, 62310-62319, 64400-64435, 64445-64450, 64479, 64483, 64490, 64493, 64505-64530, 69990, 93000-93010, 93040-93042, 93318, 94002, 94200, 94250, 94680-94690, 94770, 95812-95816, 95819, 95822, 95829, 95955, 96360, 96365, 96372, 96374-96376, 99148-99149, 99150

Note: These CCI edits are used for Medicare. Other payers may reimburse on codes listed above.

Medicare Edits

	Fac RVU	Non-Fac RVU	FUD	Assist
24340	17.83	17.83	90	80

Medicare References: 100-2,15,260; 100-4,12,30; 100-4,12,90.3; 100-4,14,10

24341

24341 Repair, tendon or muscle, upper arm or elbow, each tendon or muscle, primary or secondary (excludes rotator cuff)

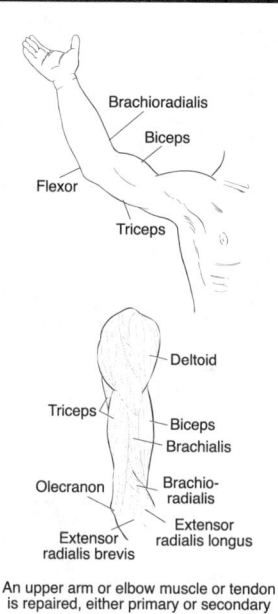

An upper arm or elbow muscle or tendon is repaired, either primary or secondary

Explanation

The physician repairs one of the muscles or tendons in the upper arm or elbow, not including those of the rotator cuff. With the patient under general anesthesia, the physician makes an incision directly overlying the torn muscles or tendon. The incision is carried deep through the subcutaneous tissue. The extent of the tear is ascertained through debridement and exploration. The physician repairs the tissue using appropriate fixation devices such as sutures, wires, or screws. Additional incisions are often required when a tendon is completely ruptured. When the repair is complete, the incision is closed in layers. Use this code to report both the initial, primary repair done near the time of injury or a secondary repair, done sometime after the incident of injury or following a previous surgical repair.

Coding Tips

For repair of the rotator cuff, see 23410–23412. According to CPT guidelines, cast application or strapping (including removal) is only reported as a replacement procedure or when the cast application or strapping is an initial service performed without a restorative treatment or procedure. See "Application of Casts and Strapping" in the CPT book in the Surgery Section, under the Musculoskeletal system.

ICD-9-CM Procedural

83.64	Other suture of tendon
83.65	Other suture of muscle or fascia
83.87	Other plastic operations on muscle
83.88	Other plastic operations on tendon

Anesthesia

24341   01710

ICD-9-CM Diagnostic

727.62	Nontraumatic rupture of tendons of biceps (long head)
727.69	Nontraumatic rupture of other tendon
831.00	Closed dislocation of shoulder, unspecified site
831.02	Closed posterior dislocation of humerus
831.03	Closed inferior dislocation of humerus
831.04	Closed dislocation of acromioclavicular (joint)
831.09	Closed dislocation of other site of shoulder
831.11	Open anterior dislocation of humerus
831.12	Open posterior dislocation of humerus
831.13	Open inferior dislocation of humerus
831.14	Open dislocation of acromioclavicular (joint)
831.19	Open dislocation of other site of shoulder
832.01	Closed anterior dislocation of elbow
832.02	Closed posterior dislocation of elbow
832.03	Closed medial dislocation of elbow
832.04	Closed lateral dislocation of elbow
832.09	Closed dislocation of other site of elbow
832.11	Open anterior dislocation of elbow
832.12	Open posterior dislocation of elbow
832.13	Open medial dislocation of elbow
832.14	Open lateral dislocation of elbow
832.19	Open dislocation of other site of elbow
841.8	Sprain and strain of other specified sites of elbow and forearm
880.03	Open wound of upper arm, without mention of complication
880.23	Open wound of upper arm, with tendon involvement
884.1	Multiple and unspecified open wound of upper limb, complicated
884.2	Multiple and unspecified open wound of upper limb, with tendon involvement
927.00	Crushing injury of shoulder region — (Use additional code to identify any associated injuries: 800-829, 850.0-854.1, 860.0-869.1)
927.01	Crushing injury of scapular region — (Use additional code to identify any associated injuries: 800-829, 850.0-854.1, 860.0-869.1)
927.03	Crushing injury of upper arm — (Use additional code to identify any associated injuries: 800-829, 850.0-854.1, 860.0-869.1)
927.11	Crushing injury of elbow — (Use additional code to identify any associated injuries: 800-829, 850.0-854.1, 860.0-869.1)
998.2	Accidental puncture or laceration during procedure

CCI Version 16.3

01710, 0213T, 0216T, 0228T, 0230T, 11900-11901, 12001-12007, 12011-12057, 13100-13101, 13120-13121, 13132, 13150-13152, 15851-15860, 20500-20501, 24000, 24006-24071, 24101, 24110, 24130, 24145, 24147, 24201, 24300, 24305-24310, 24332, 24357-24359, 29049-29085, 29105-29126, 29240-29280, 35761, 36000, 36400-36410, 36420-36430, 36440, 36600, 36640, 37202, 37618, 43752, 51701-51703, 62310-62319, 64400-64435, 64445-64450, 64479, 64483, 64490, 64493, 64505-64560, 64565, 64573-64580, 64585-64595, 64702-64708, 64713, 64718-64726, 69990, 87070, 87076-87077, 87102, 93000-93010, 93040-93042, 93318, 94002, 94200, 94250, 94680-94690, 94770, 95812-95816, 95819, 95822, 95829, 95860, 95900, 95955, 96360, 96365, 96372, 96374-96376, 99148-99149, 99150, G0168

Note: These CCI edits are used for Medicare. Other payers may reimburse on codes listed above.

Medicare Edits

	Fac RVU	Non-Fac RVU	FUD	Assist
24341	21.51	21.51	90	80

Medicare References: 100-2,15,260; 100-4,12,30; 100-4,12,90.3; 100-4,14,10

24342

24342 Reinsertion of ruptured biceps or triceps tendon, distal, with or without tendon graft

The biceps brachii tendon or the triceps brachii tendon at the elbow is reinserted to a bone attachment, with or without a tendon graft

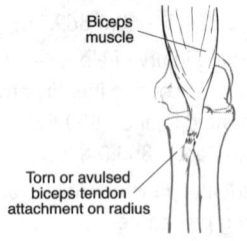

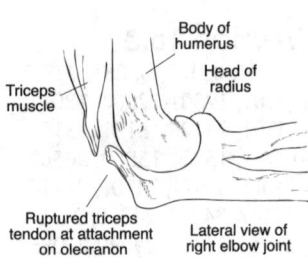

- Biceps muscle
- Torn or avulsed biceps tendon attachment on radius
- Body of humerus
- Head of radius
- Triceps muscle
- Ruptured triceps tendon at attachment on olecranon
- Lateral view of right elbow joint

Explanation

The physician performs reinsertion of a distal ruptured biceps or triceps tendon. For the triceps tendon, a posterior longitudinal incision is made to expose the tendinous portion of the triceps. Drill holes are made in the olecranon. Sutures from the triceps tendon are passed through the drill holes, pulled tight, and secured. The physician may harvest a fascia graft from the forearm. The proximal attachment of the fascia graft is left attached to the epicondyle. The distal part is detached, raised, and sutured to the distal triceps for reinforcement. The incision is repaired in layers with sutures, staples, and/or Steri-strips. The arm is immobilized in less than 90 degrees of flexion.

Coding Tips

According to CPT guidelines, cast application or strapping (including removal) is only reported as a replacement procedure or when the cast application or strapping is an initial service performed without a restorative treatment or procedure. See "Application of Casts and Strapping" in the CPT book in the Surgery Section, under the Musculoskeletal system.

ICD-9-CM Procedural

- 83.75 Tendon transfer or transplantation
- 83.82 Graft of muscle or fascia

Anesthesia

24342 01710

ICD-9-CM Diagnostic

- 727.62 Nontraumatic rupture of tendons of biceps (long head)
- 841.8 Sprain and strain of other specified sites of elbow and forearm
- 880.23 Open wound of upper arm, with tendon involvement

Terms To Know

distal. Located farther away from a specified reference point.

fascia. Fibrous sheet or band of tissue that envelops organs, muscles, and groupings of muscles.

flexion. Act of bending or being bent.

posterior. Located in the back part or caudal end of the body.

proximal. Located closest to a specified reference point, usually the midline.

rupture. Tearing or breaking open of tissue.

sprain and strain. Injuries to a joint, in which the fibers of supporting ligaments or muscles are overstretched or slightly ruptured, with the ligaments and muscles maintaining continuity.

tendon. Fibrous tissue that connects muscle to bone, consisting primarily of collagen and containing little vasculature.

CCI Version 16.3

01710, 0213T, 0216T, 0228T, 0230T, 24000, 24006, 24100-24102, 24300-24310, 24332-24341, 29055-29075, 29105, 29260, 36000, 36400-36410, 36420-36430, 36440, 36600, 36640, 37202, 43752, 51701-51703, 62310-62319, 64400-64435, 64445-64450, 64479, 64483, 64490, 64493, 64505-64530, 69990, 93000-93010, 93040-93042, 93318, 94002, 94200, 94250, 94680-94690, 94770, 95812-95816, 95819, 95822, 95829, 95955, 96360, 96365, 96372, 96374-96376, 99148-99149, 99150

Note: These CCI edits are used for Medicare. Other payers may reimburse on codes listed above.

Medicare Edits

	Fac RVU	Non-Fac RVU	FUD	Assist
24342	22.75	22.75	90	80

Medicare References: 100-2,15,260; 100-4,12,30; 100-4,12,90.3; 100-4,14,10

24343

24343 Repair lateral collateral ligament, elbow, with local tissue

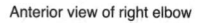

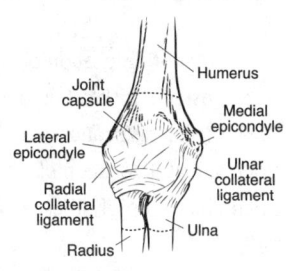

Explanation

The lateral collateral ligament (LCL) is the ligament of the elbow along the outer aspect that connects the distal end of the humerus to the proximal end of the ulna. It provides lateral stability to the joint and injury to the LCL can lead to elbow dislocation. Anterior-posterior and lateral x-rays of the elbow are taken and reported separately. The physician administers a local anesthetic block and makes an incision and dissects the lateral ligament to the head and neck of the humerus to expose the anterior surface of the lateral epicondyle. Repair of a freshly torn collateral ligament usually requires the surgeon to make an incision through the skin over the area where the tear in the ligament has occurred. If the ligament has been pulled from its attachment on the bone, the ligament is reattached to the bone with either large sutures or a special metal bone staple. The ends of the ligament are sewn together to repair mid-ligament tears.

Coding Tips

Local anesthesia is included in this service.

ICD-9-CM Procedural

81.96 Other repair of joint

Anesthesia

24343 01710

ICD-9-CM Diagnostic

- 716.12 Traumatic arthropathy, upper arm
- 718.02 Articular cartilage disorder, upper arm
- 718.32 Recurrent dislocation of upper arm joint
- 718.82 Other joint derangement, not elsewhere classified, upper arm
- 728.89 Other disorder of muscle, ligament, and fascia — (Use additional E code to identify drug, if drug-induced)
- 728.9 Unspecified disorder of muscle, ligament, and fascia
- 812.40 Closed fracture of unspecified part of lower end of humerus
- 812.41 Closed fracture of supracondylar humerus
- 812.42 Closed fracture of lateral condyle of humerus
- 812.43 Closed fracture of medial condyle of humerus
- 812.49 Other closed fracture of lower end of humerus
- 812.51 Open fracture of supracondylar humerus
- 812.52 Open fracture of lateral condyle of humerus
- 812.53 Open fracture of medial condyle of humerus
- 812.59 Other open fracture of lower end of humerus
- 813.01 Closed fracture of olecranon process of ulna
- 813.02 Closed fracture of coronoid process of ulna
- 813.03 Closed Monteggia's fracture
- 813.04 Other and unspecified closed fractures of proximal end of ulna (alone)
- 813.07 Other and unspecified closed fractures of proximal end of radius (alone)
- 813.08 Closed fracture of radius with ulna, upper end (any part)
- 813.11 Open fracture of olecranon process of ulna
- 813.12 Open fracture of coronoid process of ulna
- 813.13 Open Monteggia's fracture
- 813.14 Other and unspecified open fractures of proximal end of ulna (alone)
- 813.15 Open fracture of head of radius
- 813.16 Open fracture of neck of radius
- 813.17 Other and unspecified open fractures of proximal end of radius (alone)
- 832.00 Closed unspecified dislocation of elbow
- 832.01 Closed anterior dislocation of elbow
- 832.02 Closed posterior dislocation of elbow
- 832.03 Closed medial dislocation of elbow
- 832.04 Closed lateral dislocation of elbow
- 832.11 Open anterior dislocation of elbow
- 832.12 Open posterior dislocation of elbow
- 832.13 Open medial dislocation of elbow
- 832.14 Open lateral dislocation of elbow
- 832.19 Open dislocation of other site of elbow
- 841.0 Radial collateral ligament sprain and strain
- 841.1 Ulnar collateral ligament sprain and strain
- 841.2 Radiohumeral (joint) sprain and strain
- 841.3 Ulnohumeral (joint) sprain and strain
- 841.8 Sprain and strain of other specified sites of elbow and forearm
- 841.9 Sprain and strain of unspecified site of elbow and forearm
- 881.21 Open wound of elbow, with tendon involvement
- 927.11 Crushing injury of elbow — (Use additional code to identify any associated injuries: 800-829, 850.0-854.1, 860.0-869.1)

CCI Version 16.3

01710, 0213T, 0216T, 0228T, 0230T, 20605, 24000, 24006, 24100-24102, 24300, 24332, 24341, 24357-24359, 29049-29075, 29105-29126, 29260, 36000, 36400-36410, 36420-36430, 36440, 36600, 36640, 37202, 43752, 51701-51703, 62310-62319, 64400-64435, 64445-64450, 64479, 64483, 64490, 64493, 64505-64530, 69990, 93000-93010, 93040-93042, 93318, 94002, 94200, 94250, 94680-94690, 94770, 95812-95816, 95819, 95822, 95829, 95955, 96360, 96365, 96372, 96374-96376, 99148-99149, 99150

Note: These CCI edits are used for Medicare. Other payers may reimburse on codes listed above.

Medicare Edits

	Fac RVU	Non-Fac RVU	FUD	Assist
24343	20.45	20.45	90	80

Medicare References: None

24344

24344 Reconstruction lateral collateral ligament, elbow, with tendon graft (includes harvesting of graft)

Anterior view of right elbow

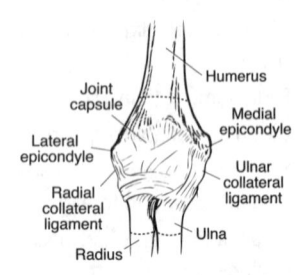

Explanation

The lateral collateral ligament (LCL) is the ligament of the elbow along the outer aspect that connects the distal end of the humerus to the proximal end of the ulna. It provides lateral stability to the joint and injury to the LCL can lead to elbow dislocation. Anterior-posterior and lateral x-rays of the elbow are taken and reported separately. The physician administers a local anesthetic block and makes an incision and dissects the lateral ligament to the head and neck of the humerus to expose the anterior surface of the lateral epicondyle. The palmaris longus tendon is usually used for the graft. The physician makes transverse wrist incision and spreads the areolar tissue to identify the tendon. A second transverse incision is made about eight centimeters above the first incision to again identify the tendon. The physician pulls on the tendon from both incisions to ensure that the same tendon has been isolated and makes a third transverse incision proximally. Alternatively, tendon stripper can be used. The tendon is cut and reattached in a new position, either by stitching it to another tendon or through a hole drilled into the bone. The wound is closed and a dressing applied. The hand and wrist may be put in a plaster cast, splint, or bandage, depending on which tendons have been moved.

Coding Tips

According to CPT guidelines, cast application or strapping (including removal) is only reported as a replacement procedure or when the cast application or strapping is an initial service performed without a restorative treatment or procedure. See "Application of Casts and Strapping" in the CPT book in the Surgery Section, under the Musculoskeletal system.

ICD-9-CM Procedural

81.96	Other repair of joint
83.81	Tendon graft

Anesthesia

24344 01710

ICD-9-CM Diagnostic

716.12	Traumatic arthropathy, upper arm
718.02	Articular cartilage disorder, upper arm
718.32	Recurrent dislocation of upper arm joint
718.82	Other joint derangement, not elsewhere classified, upper arm
728.89	Other disorder of muscle, ligament, and fascia — (Use additional E code to identify drug, if drug-induced)
728.9	Unspecified disorder of muscle, ligament, and fascia
812.41	Closed fracture of supracondylar humerus
812.42	Closed fracture of lateral condyle of humerus
812.49	Other closed fracture of lower end of humerus
812.51	Open fracture of supracondylar humerus
812.52	Open fracture of lateral condyle of humerus
812.53	Open fracture of medial condyle of humerus
812.59	Other open fracture of lower end of humerus
813.01	Closed fracture of olecranon process of ulna
813.02	Closed fracture of coronoid process of ulna
813.03	Closed Monteggia's fracture
813.05	Closed fracture of head of radius
813.06	Closed fracture of neck of radius
813.08	Closed fracture of radius with ulna, upper end (any part)
813.11	Open fracture of olecranon process of ulna
813.12	Open fracture of coronoid process of ulna
813.13	Open Monteggia's fracture
813.15	Open fracture of head of radius
813.16	Open fracture of neck of radius
813.18	Open fracture of radius with ulna, upper end (any part)
832.01	Closed anterior dislocation of elbow
832.02	Closed posterior dislocation of elbow
832.03	Closed medial dislocation of elbow
832.04	Closed lateral dislocation of elbow
832.09	Closed dislocation of other site of elbow
832.11	Open anterior dislocation of elbow
832.12	Open posterior dislocation of elbow
832.13	Open medial dislocation of elbow
832.14	Open lateral dislocation of elbow
832.19	Open dislocation of other site of elbow
841.2	Radiohumeral (joint) sprain and strain
841.3	Ulnohumeral (joint) sprain and strain
880.23	Open wound of upper arm, with tendon involvement
881.21	Open wound of elbow, with tendon involvement
927.11	Crushing injury of elbow — (Use additional code to identify any associated injuries: 800-829, 850.0-854.1, 860.0-869.1)

CCI Version 16.3

01710, 0213T, 0216T, 0228T, 0230T, 20605, 20924, 24000, 24006, 24100-24102, 24300, 24332, 24341, 24343, 24357-24359, 29049-29075, 29105-29126, 29260, 36000, 36400-36410, 36420-36430, 36440, 36600, 36640, 37202, 43752, 51701-51703, 62310-62319, 64400-64435, 64445-64450, 64479, 64483, 64490, 64493, 64505-64530, 69990, 93000-93010, 93040-93042, 93318, 94002, 94200, 94250, 94680-94690, 94770, 95812-95816, 95819, 95822, 95829, 95955, 96360, 96365, 96372, 96374-96376, 99148-99149, 99150

Note: These CCI edits are used for Medicare. Other payers may reimburse on codes listed above.

Medicare Edits

	Fac RVU	Non-Fac RVU	FUD	Assist
24344	32.0	32.0	90	80

Medicare References: None

24345

24345 Repair medial collateral ligament, elbow, with local tissue

Anterior view of right elbow

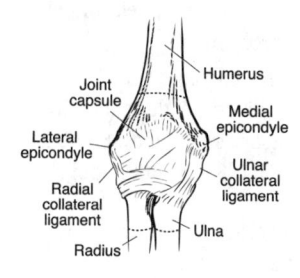

Explanation
The medial collateral ligament (MCL) is posterior to the axis of elbow flexion and primarily serves as the medial stabilizer of the flexed elbow joint. X-rays (reported separately) are taken to identify abnormally wide joint space on the medial side. An MRI (reported separately) may be taken to show focal discontinuity of the ligament and joint fluid extravasation. Repair of a freshly torn medial collateral ligament usually requires the surgeon to make an incision through the skin over the area where the tear in the ligament has occurred. If the ligament has been pulled from its attachment on the bone, the ligament is reattached with large sutures or a metal bone staple. More than one incision may be necessary. The damaged ligament is repaired with local tissue that can be used to restore its functionality. For mid-ligament tears, the ends of the ligament are sewed together to repair ligament continuity. The procedure is normally performed under general anesthesia or with a local block.

Coding Tips
Local anesthesia is included in this service.

ICD-9-CM Procedural
81.96 Other repair of joint

Anesthesia
24345 01710

ICD-9-CM Diagnostic
- 716.12 Traumatic arthropathy, upper arm
- 718.02 Articular cartilage disorder, upper arm
- 718.32 Recurrent dislocation of upper arm joint
- 718.82 Other joint derangement, not elsewhere classified, upper arm
- 728.89 Other disorder of muscle, ligament, and fascia — (Use additional E code to identify drug, if drug-induced)
- 812.40 Closed fracture of unspecified part of lower end of humerus
- 812.41 Closed fracture of supracondylar humerus
- 812.43 Closed fracture of medial condyle of humerus
- 812.49 Other closed fracture of lower end of humerus
- 812.50 Open fracture of unspecified part of lower end of humerus
- 812.51 Open fracture of supracondylar humerus
- 812.52 Open fracture of lateral condyle of humerus
- 812.53 Open fracture of medial condyle of humerus
- 812.54 Open fracture of unspecified condyle(s) of humerus
- 812.59 Other open fracture of lower end of humerus
- 813.01 Closed fracture of olecranon process of ulna
- 813.02 Closed fracture of coronoid process of ulna
- 813.03 Closed Monteggia's fracture
- 813.05 Closed fracture of head of radius
- 813.06 Closed fracture of neck of radius
- 813.08 Closed fracture of radius with ulna, upper end (any part)
- 813.11 Open fracture of olecranon process of ulna
- 813.12 Open fracture of coronoid process of ulna
- 813.13 Open Monteggia's fracture
- 813.15 Open fracture of head of radius
- 813.16 Open fracture of neck of radius
- 813.18 Open fracture of radius with ulna, upper end (any part)
- 832.00 Closed unspecified dislocation of elbow
- 832.01 Closed anterior dislocation of elbow
- 832.02 Closed posterior dislocation of elbow
- 832.03 Closed medial dislocation of elbow
- 832.04 Closed lateral dislocation of elbow
- 832.09 Closed dislocation of other site of elbow
- 832.11 Open anterior dislocation of elbow
- 832.12 Open posterior dislocation of elbow
- 832.13 Open medial dislocation of elbow
- 832.14 Open lateral dislocation of elbow
- 841.0 Radial collateral ligament sprain and strain
- 841.1 Ulnar collateral ligament sprain and strain
- 841.2 Radiohumeral (joint) sprain and strain
- 841.3 Ulnohumeral (joint) sprain and strain
- 880.23 Open wound of upper arm, with tendon involvement
- 881.21 Open wound of elbow, with tendon involvement
- 927.11 Crushing injury of elbow — (Use additional code to identify any associated injuries: 800-829, 850.0-854.1, 860.0-869.1)

CCI Version 16.3
01710, 0213T, 0216T, 0228T, 0230T, 20605, 24000, 24006, 24100-24102, 24300, 24332, 24357-24359, 29049-29075, 29105-29126, 29260, 36000, 36400-36410, 36420-36430, 36440, 36600, 36640, 37202, 43752, 51701-51703, 62310-62319, 64400-64435, 64445-64450, 64479, 64483, 64490, 64493, 64505-64530, 69990, 93000-93010, 93040-93042, 93318, 94002, 94200, 94250, 94680-94690, 94770, 95812-95816, 95819, 95822, 95829, 95955, 96360, 96365, 96372, 96374-96376, 99148-99149, 99150

Note: These CCI edits are used for Medicare. Other payers may reimburse on codes listed above.

Medicare Edits

	Fac RVU	Non-Fac RVU	FUD	Assist
24345	20.32	20.32	90	80

Medicare References: 100-2,15,260; 100-4,12,30; 100-4,12,90.3; 100-4,14,10

24346

24346 Reconstruction medial collateral ligament, elbow, with tendon graft (includes harvesting of graft)

Anterior view of right elbow

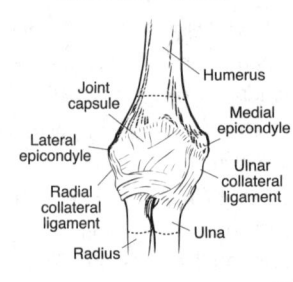

Explanation
The medial collateral ligament (MCL) is posterior to the axis of elbow flexion and primarily serves as the medial stabilizer of the flexed elbow joint. X-rays (reported separately) are taken to identify abnormally wide joint space on the medial side. An MRI (reported separately) may be taken to show focal discontinuity of the ligament and joint fluid extravasation. The palmaris longus tendon is the most commonly used tendon graft for the elbow. The procedure is normally performed under general anesthesia. The physician makes a transverse proximal wrist crease incision directly over the tendon, divides it, and holds it taut. A second transverse incision is made about 8 cm above the first incision on the forearm to again identify the tendon. The graft segment is divided and withdrawn. Alternatively, a tendon stripper can be used. The tendon is grafted to the medial collateral ligament to restore functionality. The wound is closed and a dressing applied. The hand and wrist may be put in a plaster cast, splint, or bandage, depending on which tendons were involved.

Coding Tips
According to CPT guidelines, cast application or strapping (including removal) is only reported as a replacement procedure or when the cast application or strapping is an initial service performed without a restorative treatment or procedure. See "Application of Casts and Strapping" in the CPT book in the Surgery Section, under the Musculoskeletal system.

ICD-9-CM Procedural
81.96 Other repair of joint
83.81 Tendon graft

Anesthesia
24346 01710

ICD-9-CM Diagnostic
716.12 Traumatic arthropathy, upper arm
718.02 Articular cartilage disorder, upper arm
718.32 Recurrent dislocation of upper arm joint
812.40 Closed fracture of unspecified part of lower end of humerus
812.41 Closed fracture of supracondylar humerus
812.42 Closed fracture of lateral condyle of humerus
812.43 Closed fracture of medial condyle of humerus
812.51 Open fracture of supracondylar humerus
812.53 Open fracture of medial condyle of humerus
813.01 Closed fracture of olecranon process of ulna
813.02 Closed fracture of coronoid process of ulna
813.03 Closed Monteggia's fracture
813.05 Closed fracture of head of radius
813.06 Closed fracture of neck of radius
813.08 Closed fracture of radius with ulna, upper end (any part)
813.11 Open fracture of olecranon process of ulna
813.12 Open fracture of coronoid process of ulna
813.13 Open Monteggia's fracture
813.15 Open fracture of head of radius
813.16 Open fracture of neck of radius
813.18 Open fracture of radius with ulna, upper end (any part)
832.01 Closed anterior dislocation of elbow
832.02 Closed posterior dislocation of elbow
832.03 Closed medial dislocation of elbow
832.04 Closed lateral dislocation of elbow
832.09 Closed dislocation of other site of elbow
832.11 Open anterior dislocation of elbow
832.12 Open posterior dislocation of elbow
832.13 Open medial dislocation of elbow
832.14 Open lateral dislocation of elbow
832.19 Open dislocation of other site of elbow
841.0 Radial collateral ligament sprain and strain
841.1 Ulnar collateral ligament sprain and strain
841.2 Radiohumeral (joint) sprain and strain
841.3 Ulnohumeral (joint) sprain and strain
880.23 Open wound of upper arm, with tendon involvement
881.21 Open wound of elbow, with tendon involvement
927.11 Crushing injury of elbow — (Use additional code to identify any associated injuries: 800-829, 850.0-854.1, 860.0-869.1)

CCI Version 16.3
01710, 0213T, 0216T, 0228T, 0230T, 20605, 20924, 24000, 24006, 24100-24102, 24300, 24332, 24345, 24357-24359, 29049-29075, 29105-29126, 29260, 36000, 36400-36410, 36420-36430, 36440, 36600, 36640, 37202, 43752, 51701-51703, 62310-62319, 64400-64435, 64445-64450, 64479, 64483, 64490, 64493, 64505-64530, 69990, 93000-93010, 93040-93042, 93318, 94002, 94200, 94250, 94680-94690, 94770, 95812-95816, 95819, 95822, 95829, 95955, 96360, 96365, 96372, 96374-96376, 99148-99149, 99150

Note: These CCI edits are used for Medicare. Other payers may reimburse on codes listed above.

Medicare Edits

	Fac RVU	Non-Fac RVU	FUD	Assist
24346	32.04	32.04	90	80

Medicare References: None

24357

24357 Tenotomy, elbow, lateral or medial (eg, epicondylitis, tennis elbow, golfer's elbow); percutaneous

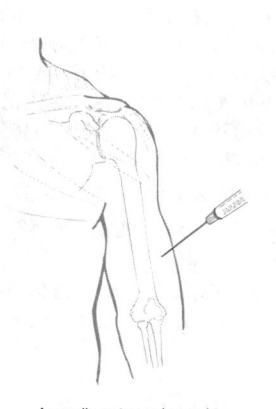

A needle or trocar is used to percutaneously treat the infection

Explanation
The physician performs a percutaneous (through the skin) lateral or medial tenotomy for tennis elbow, golfer's elbow, or epicondylitis. Following administration of a local anesthetic, the physician advances an 18- or 20-guage needle through the abnormal region of the tendon. The tip of the needle is drawn back and forth to repeatedly perforate (fenestrate) the tendinotic tissue in multiple locations. Any calcifications or spurs are mechanically fragmented and the bony surface of the apex and epicondylar face are abraded to stimulate new blood vessels. The fenestrated tendon is then infiltrated with a corticosteroid/bupivacaine solution.

Coding Tips
Code 24357 should not be reported with 29837 and 29838.

ICD-9-CM Procedural
- 77.89 Other partial ostectomy of other bone, except facial bones
- 80.99 Other excision of joint of other specified site
- 83.14 Fasciotomy
- 83.82 Graft of muscle or fascia

Anesthesia
24357   01710

ICD-9-CM Diagnostic
- 719.42 Pain in joint, upper arm
- 726.31 Medial epicondylitis of elbow
- 726.32 Lateral epicondylitis of elbow
- 726.39 Other enthesopathy of elbow region
- 726.90 Enthesopathy of unspecified site
- 727.09 Other synovitis and tenosynovitis
- 729.71 Nontraumatic compartment syndrome of upper extremity — (Code first, if applicable, postprocedural complication: 998.89)
- 958.91 Traumatic compartment syndrome of upper extremity

Terms To Know
anterior. Situated in the front area or toward the belly surface of the body; an anatomical reference point used to show the position and relationship of one body structure to another.

epicondylitis. Inflammation of the humeral epicondyle and the tissues adjoining it.

extensor. Any muscle that extends a joint.

flexor. Muscle/tendon that bends or flexes a limb or part as opposed to extending it.

lateral. To/on the side.

medial. Middle or midline.

percutaneous. Through the skin.

synovitis. Inflammation of the synovial membrane that lines a synovial joint, resulting in pain and swelling.

tendon. Fibrous tissue that connects muscle to bone, consisting primarily of collagen and containing little vasculature.

CCI Version 16.3
01710-01712, 0213T, 0216T, 0228T, 0230T, 11010-11012, 11040-11044, 24100-24102, 24300, 24340, 25270-25275, 29058-29075, 29105, 29260, 36000, 36400-36410, 36420-36430, 36440, 36600, 36640, 37202, 43752, 62310-62319, 64400-64435, 64445-64450, 64479, 64483, 64490, 64493, 64505-64530, 69990, 93000-93010, 93040-93042, 93318, 94002, 94200, 94250, 94680-94690, 94770, 95812-95816, 95819, 95822, 95829, 95955, 96360, 96365, 96372, 96374-96376, 99148-99149, 99150

Note: These CCI edits are used for Medicare. Other payers may reimburse on codes listed above.

Medicare Edits

	Fac RVU	Non-Fac RVU	FUD	Assist
24357	12.89	12.89	90	80

Medicare References: None

24358-24359

24358 Tenotomy, elbow, lateral or medial (eg, epicondylitis, tennis elbow, golfer's elbow); debridement, soft tissue and/or bone, open

24359 debridement, soft tissue and/or bone, open with tendon repair or reattachment

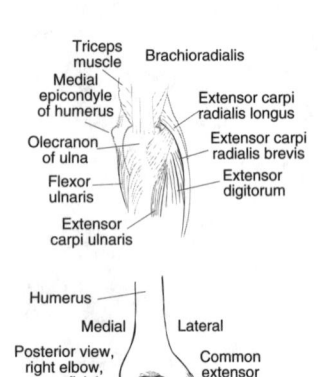

Tenotomy of the lateral or medial tendons is performed.

Explanation

The physician performs open tenotomy (cutting or release) to treat lateral epicondylitis (tennis elbow) or medial epicondylitis (golfer's elbow). An incision is made over the lateral epicondyle of the humerus. In 24358, the physician removes (debrides) damaged soft tissue or bone. In 24359, the physician also repairs or reattaches the affected tendon. The incision is repaired in layers with sutures, staples, and/or Steri-strips. The arm is placed in a sling.

Coding Tips

These codes should not be reported with 29837 and 29838.

ICD-9-CM Procedural

- 77.89 Other partial ostectomy of other bone, except facial bones
- 80.99 Other excision of joint of other specified site
- 83.14 Fasciotomy
- 83.82 Graft of muscle or fascia

Anesthesia

01710, 01712

ICD-9-CM Diagnostic

- 719.42 Pain in joint, upper arm
- 726.31 Medial epicondylitis of elbow
- 726.32 Lateral epicondylitis of elbow
- 726.39 Other enthesopathy of elbow region
- 726.90 Enthesopathy of unspecified site
- 727.09 Other synovitis and tenosynovitis
- 729.71 Nontraumatic compartment syndrome of upper extremity — (Code first, if applicable, postprocedural complication: 998.89)
- 958.91 Traumatic compartment syndrome of upper extremity

Terms To Know

anterior. Situated in the front area or toward the belly surface of the body; an anatomical reference point used to show the position and relationship of one body structure to another.

debridement. Removal of dead or contaminated tissue and foreign matter from a wound.

epicondylitis. Inflammation of the humeral epicondyle and the tissues adjoining it.

extensor. Any muscle that extends a joint.

flexor. Muscle/tendon that bends or flexes a limb or part as opposed to extending it.

lateral. To/on the side.

medial. Middle or midline.

synovitis. Inflammation of the synovial membrane that lines a synovial joint, resulting in pain and swelling.

tendon. Fibrous tissue that connects muscle to bone, consisting primarily of collagen and containing little vasculature.

CCI Version 16.3

01710-01712, 0213T, 0216T, 0228T, 0230T, 11010-11012, 11040-11044, 24000, 24006, 24100-24102, 24110, 24300, 24332-24340, 25270-25275, 29058-29075, 29105, 29240-29260, 36000, 36400-36410, 36420-36430, 36440, 36600, 36640, 37202, 43752, 62310-62319, 64400-64435, 64445-64450, 64479, 64483, 64490, 64493, 64505-64530, 69990, 93000-93010, 93040-93042, 93318, 94002, 94200, 94250, 94680-94690, 94770, 95812-95816, 95819, 95822, 95829, 95955, 96360, 96365, 96372, 96374-96376, 99148-99149, 99150

Also not with 24358: 24140, 24357

Also not with 24359: 24357-24358, 29837-29838, 64718

Note: These CCI edits are used for Medicare. Other payers may reimburse on codes listed above.

Medicare Edits

	Fac RVU	Non-Fac RVU	FUD	Assist
24358	15.18	15.18	90	80
24359	19.1	19.1	90	80

Medicare References: None

24360

24360 Arthroplasty, elbow; with membrane (eg, fascial)

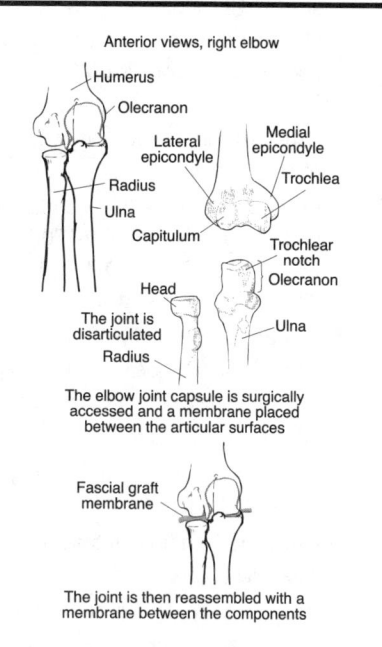

Explanation
The physician performs a membrane arthroplasty of the elbow. A longitudinal incision is made over the lateral elbow. All soft tissue is dissected from the distal humerus. The elbow is dislocated. Osteophytes and articular cartilage are removed from the distal humerus so that a smooth, rounded surface remains. Articular cartilage is left intact on the proximal ulna and radius. The physician uses a motorized dermatome to remove a thin split-thickness skin graft from the patient's lower abdomen. Small drill holes are made in the distal end of the humerus. The graft is sutured into place over the distal end of the humerus with the dermal surface placed against the bone and the fat facing the new joint space. The elbow joint is reduced (realigned). The physician repairs the incision in layers using sutures, staples, and/or Steri-strips. The elbow is placed in a posterior splint in 90 degrees of flexion.

Coding Tips
According to CPT guidelines, cast application or strapping (including removal) is only reported as a replacement procedure or when the cast application or strapping is an initial service performed without a restorative treatment or procedure. See "Application of Casts and Strapping" in the CPT book in the Surgery Section, under the Musculoskeletal system.

ICD-9-CM Procedural
81.85   Other repair of elbow

Anesthesia
24360   01740

ICD-9-CM Diagnostic
357.1   Polyneuropathy in collagen vascular disease — (Code first underlying disease: 446.0, 710.0, 714.0)
359.6   Symptomatic inflammatory myopathy in diseases classified elsewhere — (Code first underlying disease: 135, 140.0-208.9, 277.30-277.39, 446.0, 710.0, 710.1, 710.2, 714.0)
446.0   Polyarteritis nodosa
710.0   Systemic lupus erythematosus — (Use additional code to identify manifestation: 424.91, 581.81, 582.81, 583.81)
710.1   Systemic sclerosis — (Use additional code to identify manifestation: 359.6, 517.2)
710.2   Sicca syndrome
711.02 Pyogenic arthritis, upper arm — (Use additional code to identify infectious organism: 041.0-041.8)
714.0   Rheumatoid arthritis — (Use additional code to identify manifestation: 357.1, 359.6)
715.12 Primary localized osteoarthrosis, upper arm
715.32 Localized osteoarthrosis not specified whether primary or secondary, upper arm
716.12 Traumatic arthropathy, upper arm
716.22 Allergic arthritis, upper arm
730.12 Chronic osteomyelitis, upper arm — (Use additional code to identify organism: 041.1. Use additional code to identify major osseous defect, if applicable: 731.3)
730.32 Periostitis, without mention of osteomyelitis, upper arm — (Use additional code to identify organism: 041.1)
731.0   Osteitis deformans without mention of bone tumor
733.49 Aseptic necrosis of other bone site — (Use additional code to identify major osseous defect, if applicable: 731.3)
733.82 Nonunion of fracture
756.51 Osteogenesis imperfecta
812.41 Closed fracture of supracondylar humerus
812.42 Closed fracture of lateral condyle of humerus
812.43 Closed fracture of medial condyle of humerus
812.44 Closed fracture of unspecified condyle(s) of humerus
812.49 Other closed fracture of lower end of humerus
812.51 Open fracture of supracondylar humerus
812.52 Open fracture of lateral condyle of humerus
812.53 Open fracture of medial condyle of humerus
813.02 Closed fracture of coronoid process of ulna
813.03 Closed Monteggia's fracture
813.05 Closed fracture of head of radius
813.06 Closed fracture of neck of radius
813.08 Closed fracture of radius with ulna, upper end (any part)
813.11 Open fracture of olecranon process of ulna
813.12 Open fracture of coronoid process of ulna
813.13 Open Monteggia's fracture
813.15 Open fracture of head of radius
813.16 Open fracture of neck of radius
813.18 Open fracture of radius with ulna, upper end (any part)

CCI Version 16.3
01710, 0213T, 0216T, 0228T, 0230T, 24000, 24006, 24100-24102, 24110-24126, 24149, 24300, 24332-24346, 24365-24400, 24495, 29058-29075, 29105, 29260, 29835-29836, 36000, 36400-36410, 36420-36430, 36440, 36600, 36640, 37202, 43752, 51701-51703, 62310-62319, 64400-64435, 64445-64450, 64479, 64483, 64490, 64493, 64505-64530, 64708, 64718, 69990, 93000-93010, 93040-93042, 93318, 94002, 94200, 94250, 94680-94690, 94770, 95812-95816, 95819, 95822, 95829, 95955, 96360, 96365, 96372, 96374-96376, 99148-99149, 99150

Note: These CCI edits are used for Medicare. Other payers may reimburse on codes listed above.

Medicare Edits

	Fac RVU	Non-Fac RVU	FUD	Assist
24360	26.29	26.29	90	80

Medicare References: 100-2,15,260; 100-4,12,30; 100-4,12,90.3; 100-4,14,10

24361

24361 Arthroplasty, elbow; with distal humeral prosthetic replacement

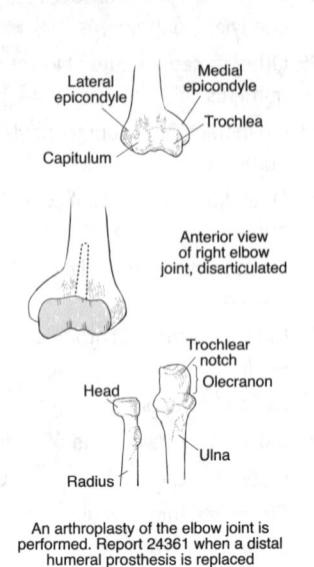

An arthroplasty of the elbow joint is performed. Report 24361 when a distal humeral prosthesis is replaced.

Explanation

The physician performs an arthroplasty of the elbow with distal humeral prosthetic replacement. The physician makes a 10 cm longitudinal incision over the medial aspect of the elbow. The ulnar nerve is identified and retracted to protect it from injury. The joint capsule is excised and the radius and ulna are separated from the humerus. A Kirschner wire is drilled into the trochlea (distal humerus) along the axis of the joint. Using an osteotome, high speed burr, or saw, the physician trims and remodels the distal end of the humerus. A prosthesis is fitted to the distal humerus and hammered into place. The ulna and radius are reduced to the prosthesis. If the radial head is severely deformed or arthritic, the physician may resect (remove) it. Other adjustments may be made, such as sculpting the semilunar notch or olecranon. Sculpting allows better articulation with the prosthesis and better elbow motion. The flexor origins are reattached to the epicondyle. The physician repairs the incision in layers with sutures, staples, and/or Steri-strips. A long arm cast or splint is applied with the elbow in 90 degrees of flexion.

Coding Tips

According to CPT guidelines, cast application or strapping (including removal) is only reported as a replacement procedure or when the cast application or strapping is an initial service performed without a restorative treatment or procedure. See "Application of Casts and Strapping" in the CPT book in the Surgery Section, under the Musculoskeletal system.

ICD-9-CM Procedural

81.85   Other repair of elbow

Anesthesia

24361   01740

ICD-9-CM Diagnostic

- 357.1 Polyneuropathy in collagen vascular disease — (Code first underlying disease: 446.0, 710.0, 714.0)
- 359.6 Symptomatic inflammatory myopathy in diseases classified elsewhere — (Code first underlying disease: 135, 140.0-208.9, 277.30-277.39, 446.0, 710.0, 710.1, 710.2, 714.0)
- 446.0 Polyarteritis nodosa
- 710.0 Systemic lupus erythematosus — (Use additional code to identify manifestation: 424.91, 581.81, 582.81, 583.81)
- 710.1 Systemic sclerosis — (Use additional code to identify manifestation: 359.6, 517.2)
- 710.2 Sicca syndrome
- 711.02 Pyogenic arthritis, upper arm — (Use additional code to identify infectious organism: 041.0-041.8)
- 711.92 Unspecified infective arthritis, upper arm
- 714.0 Rheumatoid arthritis — (Use additional code to identify manifestation: 357.1, 359.6)
- 715.12 Primary localized osteoarthrosis, upper arm
- 715.32 Localized osteoarthrosis not specified whether primary or secondary, upper arm
- 716.12 Traumatic arthropathy, upper arm
- 716.22 Allergic arthritis, upper arm
- 716.62 Unspecified monoarthritis, upper arm
- 719.22 Villonodular synovitis, upper arm
- 719.42 Pain in joint, upper arm
- 730.12 Chronic osteomyelitis, upper arm — (Use additional code to identify organism: 041.1. Use additional code to identify major osseous defect, if applicable: 731.3)
- 730.22 Unspecified osteomyelitis, upper arm — (Use additional code to identify organism: 041.1. Use additional code to identify major osseous defect, if applicable: 731.3)
- 730.32 Periostitis, without mention of osteomyelitis, upper arm — (Use additional code to identify organism: 041.1)
- 730.82 Other infections involving bone diseases classified elsewhere, upper arm — (Use additional code to identify organism: 041.1. Code first underlying disease: 002.0, 015.0-015.9)
- 731.0 Osteitis deformans without mention of bone tumor
- 731.3 Major osseous defects — (Code first underlying disease: 170.0-170.9, 730.00-730.29, 733.00-733.09, 733.40-733.49, 996.45)
- 733.49 Aseptic necrosis of other bone site — (Use additional code to identify major osseous defect, if applicable: 731.3)
- 733.82 Nonunion of fracture
- 736.00 Unspecified deformity of forearm, excluding fingers
- 754.89 Other specified nonteratogenic anomalies
- 755.50 Unspecified congenital anomaly of upper limb
- 756.51 Osteogenesis imperfecta

Terms To Know

distal. Located farther away from a specified reference point.

flexion. Act of bending or being bent.

CCI Version 16.3

01710, 0213T, 0216T, 0228T, 0230T, 24000, 24006, 24100-24102, 24110-24126, 24140, 24149, 24300, 24332-24346, 24360❖, 24365-24400, 24495, 29065, 29105, 29260, 36000, 36400-36410, 36420-36430, 36440, 36600, 36640, 37202, 43752, 51701-51703, 62310-62319, 64400-64435, 64445-64450, 64479, 64483, 64490, 64493, 64505-64530, 64708, 64718, 69990, 93000-93010, 93040-93042, 93318, 94002, 94200, 94250, 94680-94690, 94770, 95812-95816, 95819, 95822, 95829, 95955, 96360, 96365, 96372, 96374-96376, 99148-99149, 99150

Note: These CCI edits are used for Medicare. Other payers may reimburse on codes listed above.

Medicare Edits

	Fac RVU	Non-Fac RVU	FUD	Assist
24361	29.54	29.54	90	80

Medicare References: 100-2,15,260; 100-4,12,30; 100-4,12,90.3; 100-4,14,10

24362

24362 Arthroplasty, elbow; with implant and fascia lata ligament reconstruction

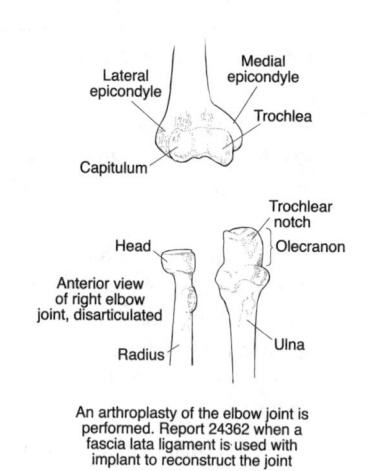

An arthroplasty of the elbow joint is performed. Report 24362 when a fascia lata ligament is used with implant to reconstruct the joint

Explanation

The physician performs an arthroplasty of the elbow with an implant and fascia lata ligament reconstruction. The physician makes a 10 cm longitudinal incision over the medial aspect of the elbow. The ulnar nerve is identified and retracted to protect it from injury. The joint capsule is excised and the radius and ulna are separated from the humerus. A Kirschner wire is drilled into the trochlea (distal humerus) along the axis of the joint. Using an osteotome, high speed burr, or saw, the physician trims and remodels the distal end of the humerus. A prosthesis is fitted to the distal humerus and hammered into place. The ulna and radius are reduced to the prosthesis. If the radial head is severely deformed or arthritic, the physician may resect (remove) it. Other adjustments may be made, such as sculpting the semilunar notch or olecranon. Sculpting allows better articulation with the prosthesis and better elbow motion. The flexor origins are reattached to the epicondyle. For the fascia lata ligament reconstruction, an additional incision may be necessary on the posterior aspect of the elbow and forearm. The radial head and olecranon are exposed. Through an incision on the lateral side of the thigh, a long rectangle of fascia lata is removed. The fascia is folded in half crosswise and the folded edge is anchored to the anterior part of the capsule with sutures. The distal half is sutured in place over the trochlear notch. A fold of the same fascia is inserted between the radial head and ulna and fixed with sutures. The capsule is sutured closed. The incisions are repaired in layers with sutures, staples, and/or Steri-strips. A long arm cast or splint immobilizes the elbow at 90 degrees of flexion.

Coding Tips

According to CPT guidelines, cast application or strapping (including removal) is only reported as a replacement procedure or when the cast application or strapping is an initial service performed without a restorative treatment or procedure. See "Application of Casts and Strapping" in the CPT book in the Surgery Section, under the Musculoskeletal system. For arthroplasty with membrane (e.g., fascial), see 24360; for distal humeral prosthetic replacement, see 24361.

ICD-9-CM Procedural

81.85 Other repair of elbow

Anesthesia

24362 01740

ICD-9-CM Diagnostic

- 357.1 Polyneuropathy in collagen vascular disease — (Code first underlying disease: 446.0, 710.0, 714.0)
- 359.6 Symptomatic inflammatory myopathy in diseases classified elsewhere — (Code first underlying disease: 135, 140.0-208.9, 277.30-277.39, 446.0, 710.0, 710.1, 710.2, 714.0)
- 446.0 Polyarteritis nodosa
- 710.0 Systemic lupus erythematosus — (Use additional code to identify manifestation: 424.91, 581.81, 582.81, 583.81)
- 710.1 Systemic sclerosis — (Use additional code to identify manifestation: 359.6, 517.2)
- 710.2 Sicca syndrome
- 711.02 Pyogenic arthritis, upper arm — (Use additional code to identify infectious organism: 041.0-041.8)
- 711.92 Unspecified infective arthritis, upper arm
- 714.0 Rheumatoid arthritis — (Use additional code to identify manifestation: 357.1, 359.6)
- 715.12 Primary localized osteoarthrosis, upper arm
- 715.32 Localized osteoarthrosis not specified whether primary or secondary, upper arm
- 716.12 Traumatic arthropathy, upper arm
- 716.22 Allergic arthritis, upper arm
- 716.62 Unspecified monoarthritis, upper arm
- 719.22 Villonodular synovitis, upper arm
- 730.12 Chronic osteomyelitis, upper arm — (Use additional code to identify organism: 041.1. Use additional code to identify major osseous defect, if applicable: 731.3)
- 730.22 Unspecified osteomyelitis, upper arm — (Use additional code to identify organism: 041.1. Use additional code to identify major osseous defect, if applicable: 731.3)
- 730.32 Periostitis, without mention of osteomyelitis, upper arm — (Use additional code to identify organism: 041.1)
- 730.82 Other infections involving bone diseases classified elsewhere, upper arm — (Use additional code to identify organism: 041.1. Code first underlying disease: 002.0, 015.0-015.9)
- 731.0 Osteitis deformans without mention of bone tumor
- 731.3 Major osseous defects — (Code first underlying disease: 170.0-170.9, 730.00-730.29, 733.00-733.09, 733.40-733.49, 996.45)
- 733.49 Aseptic necrosis of other bone site — (Use additional code to identify major osseous defect, if applicable: 731.3)
- 733.82 Nonunion of fracture
- 736.00 Unspecified deformity of forearm, excluding fingers
- 756.51 Osteogenesis imperfecta

CCI Version 16.3

01710, 0213T, 0216T, 0228T, 0230T, 24000, 24006, 24100-24102, 24110-24126, 24149, 24300, 24332-24346, 24360-24361❖, 24365-24400, 24495, 29835-29836, 36000, 36400-36410, 36420-36430, 36440, 36600, 36640, 37202, 43752, 51701-51703, 62310-62319, 64400-64435, 64445-64450, 64479, 64483, 64490, 64493, 64505-64530, 64708, 64718, 69990, 93000-93010, 93040-93042, 93318, 94002, 94200, 94250, 94680-94690, 94770, 95812-95816, 95819, 95822, 95829, 95955, 96360, 96365, 96372, 96374-96376, 99148-99149, 99150

Note: These CCI edits are used for Medicare. Other payers may reimburse on codes listed above.

Medicare Edits

	Fac RVU	Non-Fac RVU	FUD	Assist
24362	31.08	31.08	90	80

Medicare References: 100-2,15,260; 100-4,12,30; 100-4,12,90.3; 100-4,14,10

24363

24363 Arthroplasty, elbow; with distal humerus and proximal ulnar prosthetic replacement (eg, total elbow)

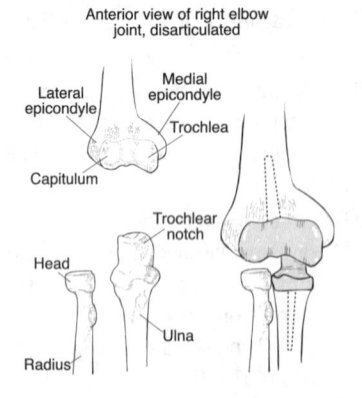

Anterior view of right elbow joint, disarticulated

Lateral epicondyle, Medial epicondyle, Trochlea, Capitulum, Trochlear notch, Head, Ulna, Radius

An arthroplasty of the elbow is performed. During the surgical session, a prosthetic replacement is fitted for the distal humerus and the proximal ulna (total elbow)

Explanation

The physician performs a total elbow arthroplasty with distal humerus and proximal ulnar prosthetic replacement. The patient is placed supine with the affected arm on the chest and a sandbag beneath the shoulder. Different types of prosthetic implants are available. Selection depends on capsuloligamentous structures, muscular integrity, and the amount of bone remaining at the elbow joint. A technique for a semiconstrained (two to three part) hinged prosthesis is described. The physician makes a straight, midline, posterior incision. The ulnar nerve is identified and retracted for protection. The triceps mechanism is elevated from the olecranon. The collateral ligaments are preserved. A portion of the olecranon is cut and removed to allow implantation of the ulnar stem. The distal humerus is prepared by removing cancellous bone with a curette. The physician uses a rasp to open and contour the humeral and ulnar medullary canals for insertion of the prosthetic stems. Cement is inserted into the ulnar and humeral medullary canals with a cement gun or syringe. The elbow is flexed and the prosthesis is inserted into the humeral and ulnar medullary canals at the same time. The elbow joint is fully extended while the cement hardens. The triceps mechanism is sutured back to fascia. The ulnar nerve is positioned anterior to the elbow. The physician inserts drain tubes. The incision is repaired in layers with sutures, staples, and/or Steri-strips. A posterior splint is applied to the elbow in 90 degrees of flexion.

Coding Tips

For arthroplasty, distal humeral replacement only, see 24361. This code should be used also for revision of total elbow replacement. For total elbow arthroplasty when performed during open treatment of a fracture, see 24587. For implant removal, elbow joint, see 24160. According to CPT guidelines, cast application or strapping (including removal) is only reported as a replacement procedure or when the cast application or strapping is an initial service performed without a restorative treatment or procedure. See "Application of Casts and Strapping" in the CPT book in the Surgery Section, under the Musculoskeletal system.

ICD-9-CM Procedural

81.84 Total elbow replacement

Anesthesia

24363 01760

ICD-9-CM Diagnostic

357.1 Polyneuropathy in collagen vascular disease — (Code first underlying disease: 446.0, 710.0, 714.0)
359.6 Symptomatic inflammatory myopathy in diseases classified elsewhere — (Code first underlying disease: 135, 140.0-208.9, 277.30-277.39, 446.0, 710.0, 710.1, 710.2, 714.0)
446.0 Polyarteritis nodosa
710.0 Systemic lupus erythematosus — (Use additional code to identify manifestation: 424.91, 581.81, 582.81, 583.81)
710.1 Systemic sclerosis — (Use additional code to identify manifestation: 359.6, 517.2)
710.2 Sicca syndrome
711.02 Pyogenic arthritis, upper arm — (Use additional code to identify infectious organism: 041.0-041.8)
714.0 Rheumatoid arthritis — (Use additional code to identify manifestation: 357.1, 359.6)
715.12 Primary localized osteoarthrosis, upper arm
715.32 Localized osteoarthrosis not specified whether primary or secondary, upper arm
716.12 Traumatic arthropathy, upper arm
716.22 Allergic arthritis, upper arm
719.22 Villonodular synovitis, upper arm
730.12 Chronic osteomyelitis, upper arm — (Use additional code to identify organism: 041.1. Use additional code to identify major osseous defect, if applicable: 731.3)
730.22 Unspecified osteomyelitis, upper arm — (Use additional code to identify organism: 041.1. Use additional code to identify major osseous defect, if applicable: 731.3)
730.32 Periostitis, without mention of osteomyelitis, upper arm — (Use additional code to identify organism: 041.1)
730.82 Other infections involving bone diseases classified elsewhere, upper arm — (Use additional code to identify organism: 041.1. Code first underlying disease: 002.0, 015.0-015.9)
731.0 Osteitis deformans without mention of bone tumor
731.3 Major osseous defects — (Code first underlying disease: 170.0-170.9, 730.00-730.29, 733.00-733.09, 733.40-733.49, 996.45)
733.49 Aseptic necrosis of other bone site — (Use additional code to identify major osseous defect, if applicable: 731.3)
733.82 Nonunion of fracture
756.51 Osteogenesis imperfecta

CCI Version 16.3

01710, 0213T, 0216T, 0228T, 0230T, 24000, 24006, 24100-24102, 24110-24126, 24149, 24300, 24332-24346, 24360-24362❖, 24365-24400, 24495, 29065, 29105, 29260, 29835-29836, 36000, 36400-36410, 36420-36430, 36440, 36600, 36640, 37202, 43752, 51701-51703, 62310-62319, 64400-64435, 64445-64450, 64479, 64483, 64490, 64493, 64505-64530, 64708, 64718, 64722, 69990, 93000-93010, 93040-93042, 93318, 94002, 94200, 94250, 94680-94690, 94770, 95812-95816, 95819, 95822, 95829, 95955, 96360, 96365, 96372, 96374-96376, 99148-99149, 99150

Note: These CCI edits are used for Medicare. Other payers may reimburse on codes listed above.

Medicare Edits

	Fac RVU	Non-Fac RVU	FUD	Assist
24363	43.95	43.95	90	80

Medicare References: 100-2,15,260; 100-4,12,30; 100-4,12,90.3; 100-4,14,10

24365

24365 Arthroplasty, radial head;

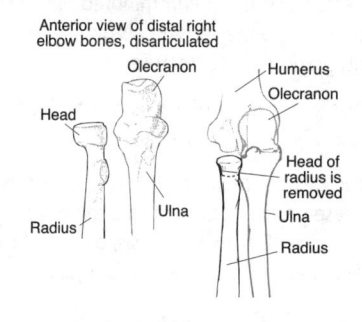

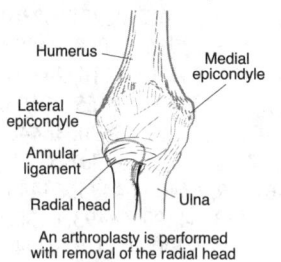

Explanation
The physician performs an arthroplasty on the radial head by making a 5 cm to 6 cm longitudinal incision along the lateral aspect of the elbow. The elbow joint is exposed by freeing and reflecting the common origin of the extensor muscles. The joint capsule is incised and the radial head is exposed. The physician uses a bone cutting saw to excise the radial head. The capsule is closed with sutures and the incision is repaired in layers with sutures, staples, and/or Steri-strips.

Coding Tips
For arthroplasty, radial head with implant, see 24366. For removal of radial head implant, see 24164. According to CPT guidelines, cast application or strapping (including removal) is only reported as a replacement procedure or when the cast application or strapping is an initial service performed without a restorative treatment or procedure. See "Application of Casts and Strapping" in the CPT book in the Surgery Section, under the Musculoskeletal system.

ICD-9-CM Procedural
81.85   Other repair of elbow

Anesthesia
24365   01740

ICD-9-CM Diagnostic
357.1   Polyneuropathy in collagen vascular disease — (Code first underlying disease: 446.0, 710.0, 714.0)
359.6   Symptomatic inflammatory myopathy in diseases classified elsewhere — (Code first underlying disease: 135, 140.0-208.9, 277.30-277.39, 446.0, 710.0, 710.1, 710.2, 714.0)
446.0   Polyarteritis nodosa
710.0   Systemic lupus erythematosus — (Use additional code to identify manifestation: 424.91, 581.81, 582.81, 583.81)
710.1   Systemic sclerosis — (Use additional code to identify manifestation: 359.6, 517.2)
710.2   Sicca syndrome
711.02 Pyogenic arthritis, upper arm — (Use additional code to identify infectious organism: 041.0-041.8)
711.92 Unspecified infective arthritis, upper arm
714.0   Rheumatoid arthritis — (Use additional code to identify manifestation: 357.1, 359.6)
715.00 Generalized osteoarthrosis, unspecified site
715.12 Primary localized osteoarthrosis, upper arm
715.32 Localized osteoarthrosis not specified whether primary or secondary, upper arm
716.12 Traumatic arthropathy, upper arm
716.22 Allergic arthritis, upper arm
716.62 Unspecified monoarthritis, upper arm
718.82 Other joint derangement, not elsewhere classified, upper arm
719.22 Villonodular synovitis, upper arm
719.42 Pain in joint, upper arm
719.52 Stiffness of joint, not elsewhere classified, upper arm
730.12 Chronic osteomyelitis, upper arm — (Use additional code to identify organism: 041.1. Use additional code to identify major osseous defect, if applicable: 731.3)
730.22 Unspecified osteomyelitis, upper arm — (Use additional code to identify organism: 041.1. Use additional code to identify major osseous defect, if applicable: 731.3)
730.32 Periostitis, without mention of osteomyelitis, upper arm — (Use additional code to identify organism: 041.1)
730.82 Other infections involving bone diseases classified elsewhere, upper arm — (Use additional code to identify organism: 041.1. Code first underlying disease: 002.0, 015.0-015.9)
731.0   Osteitis deformans without mention of bone tumor
731.3   Major osseous defects — (Code first underlying disease: 170.0-170.9, 730.00-730.29, 733.00-733.09, 733.40-733.49, 996.45)
733.49 Aseptic necrosis of other bone site — (Use additional code to identify major osseous defect, if applicable: 731.3)
733.82 Nonunion of fracture
736.00 Unspecified deformity of forearm, excluding fingers
756.51 Osteogenesis imperfecta

CCI Version 16.3
01710, 0213T, 0216T, 0228T, 0230T, 24000, 24006, 24100-24102, 24110-24130, 24300, 24332, 24341, 24400, 24495, 29065, 29105, 29260, 29834, 36000, 36400-36410, 36420-36430, 36440, 36600, 36640, 37202, 43752, 51701-51703, 62310-62319, 64400-64435, 64445-64450, 64479, 64483, 64490, 64493, 64505-64530, 64708, 64718, 69990, 93000-93010, 93040-93042, 93318, 94002, 94200, 94250, 94680-94690, 94770, 95812-95816, 95819, 95822, 95829, 95955, 96360, 96365, 96372, 96374-96376, 99148-99149, 99150

Note: These CCI edits are used for Medicare. Other payers may reimburse on codes listed above.

Medicare Edits

	Fac RVU	Non-Fac RVU	FUD	Assist
24365	18.61	18.61	90	80

Medicare References: 100-2,15,260; 100-4,12,30; 100-4,12,90.3; 100-4,14,10

24400

24400 Osteotomy, humerus, with or without internal fixation

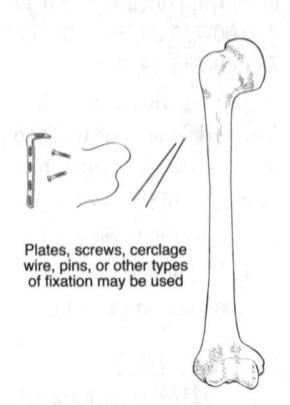

Plates, screws, cerclage wire, pins, or other types of fixation may be used

An osteotomy (surgical cutting of bone) is performed on the humerus, with or without internal fixation

The osteotomy may occur anywhere along the humeral shaft or distal portions

Explanation

The physician performs an osteotomy of the humerus with or without internal fixation. The physician makes a longitudinal incision overlying the involved portion of the shaft of the humerus to expose the affected part of the bone. An osteotomy is made through the humerus, usually in a wedge shape. This allows the bone to be realigned. The physician may apply plates and screws to hold the bone together in the correct position (internal fixation). The incision is repaired in multiple layers with sutures, staples, and/or Steri-strips. The arm may be placed in a cast or splint for immobilization.

Coding Tips

According to CPT guidelines, cast application or strapping (including removal) is only reported as a replacement procedure or when the cast application or strapping is an initial service performed without a restorative treatment or procedure. See "Application of Casts and Strapping" in the CPT book in the Surgery Section, under the Musculoskeletal system.

ICD-9-CM Procedural

- 77.22 Wedge osteotomy of humerus
- 77.32 Other division of humerus

Anesthesia

24400 01742

ICD-9-CM Diagnostic

- 170.4 Malignant neoplasm of scapula and long bones of upper limb
- 213.4 Benign neoplasm of scapula and long bones of upper limb
- 715.10 Primary localized osteoarthrosis, specified site
- 715.22 Secondary localized osteoarthrosis, upper arm
- 715.32 Localized osteoarthrosis not specified whether primary or secondary, upper arm
- 730.12 Chronic osteomyelitis, upper arm — (Use additional code to identify organism: 041.1. Use additional code to identify major osseous defect, if applicable: 731.3)
- 731.3 Major osseous defects — (Code first underlying disease: 170.0-170.9, 730.00-730.29, 733.00-733.09, 733.40-733.49, 996.45)
- 733.11 Pathologic fracture of humerus
- 733.41 Aseptic necrosis of head of humerus — (Use additional code to identify major osseous defect, if applicable: 731.3)
- 733.81 Malunion of fracture
- 733.82 Nonunion of fracture
- 736.89 Other acquired deformity of other parts of limb
- 756.4 Chondrodystrophy
- 756.51 Osteogenesis imperfecta
- 812.21 Closed fracture of shaft of humerus
- 812.31 Open fracture of shaft of humerus
- 812.49 Other closed fracture of lower end of humerus

Terms To Know

aseptic necrosis. Death of bone tissue resulting from a disruption in the vascular supply, caused by a noninfectious disease process, such as a fracture or the administration of immunosuppressive drugs.

benign. Mild or nonmalignant in nature.

distal. Located farther away from a specified reference point.

malignant. Any condition tending to progress toward death, specifically an invasive tumor with a loss of cellular differentiation that has the ability to spread or metastasize to other areas in the body.

malunion. Fracture that has united in a faulty position due to inadequate reduction of the original fracture, insufficient holding of a previously well-reduced fracture, contracture of the soft tissues, or comminuted or osteoporotic bone causing a slow disintegration of the fracture.

nonunion. Failure of two ends of a fracture to mend or completely heal.

pathologic fracture. Break in bone due to a disease process that weakens the bone structure, such as osteoporosis, osteomalacia, or neoplasia, and not traumatic injury.

CCI Version 16.3

01710, 0213T, 0216T, 0228T, 0230T, 23155-23156, 23935, 24000, 24006-24066, 24100-24101, 24110-24116, 24160, 24300, 24332, 24341, 24495, 29065, 29105, 36000, 36400-36410, 36420-36430, 36440, 36600, 36640, 37202, 43752, 51701-51703, 62310-62319, 64400-64435, 64445-64450, 64479, 64483, 64490, 64493, 64505-64530, 64718, 69990, 93000-93010, 93040-93042, 93318, 94002, 94200, 94250, 94680-94690, 94770, 95812-95816, 95819, 95822, 95829, 95955, 96360, 96365, 96372, 96374-96376, 99148-99149, 99150

Note: These CCI edits are used for Medicare. Other payers may reimburse on codes listed above.

Medicare Edits

	Fac RVU	Non-Fac RVU	FUD	Assist
24400	23.93	23.93	90	80

Medicare References: 100-2,15,260; 100-4,12,30; 100-4,12,90.3; 100-4,14,10

24410

24410 Multiple osteotomies with realignment on intramedullary rod, humeral shaft (Sofield type procedure)

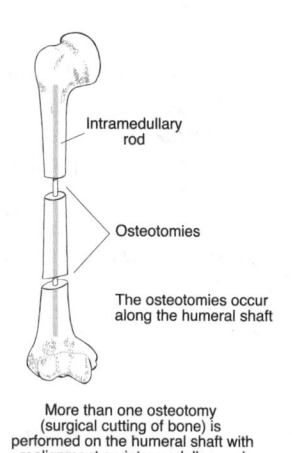

Intramedullary rod

Osteotomies

The osteotomies occur along the humeral shaft

More than one osteotomy (surgical cutting of bone) is performed on the humeral shaft with realignment on intramedullary rod

Explanation
The physician performs multiple osteotomies with realignment on an intramedullary rod of the humeral shaft. This is done to treat the deformities of osteogenesis imperfecta. The physician makes a longitudinal incision through the skin, fascia, and muscle to expose the shaft of the bone subperiosteally. Osteotomies are made through the proximal and distal metaphyses; the shaft is removed and studied to determine how many osteotomies must be made to thread the segments onto the intramedullary rod. Additional osteotomies, usually three or four, are performed to correct the alignment. The fragments are shifted and rotated to facilitate aligning them end to end on the straight nail. Autografts may be added if the cortex is thin. The intramedullary nail is inserted so that the ends extend into the canals at the distal and proximal ends. The periosteum is sutured over the bone and the wound is closed and dressed.

Coding Tips
According to CPT guidelines, cast application or strapping (including removal) is only reported as a replacement procedure or when the cast application or strapping is an initial service performed without a restorative treatment or procedure. See "Application of Casts and Strapping" in the CPT book in the Surgery Section, under the Musculoskeletal system.

ICD-9-CM Procedural
77.32 Other division of humerus

Anesthesia
24410 01742

ICD-9-CM Diagnostic
- 170.4 Malignant neoplasm of scapula and long bones of upper limb
- 213.4 Benign neoplasm of scapula and long bones of upper limb
- 715.12 Primary localized osteoarthrosis, upper arm
- 715.22 Secondary localized osteoarthrosis, upper arm
- 715.32 Localized osteoarthrosis not specified whether primary or secondary, upper arm
- 730.12 Chronic osteomyelitis, upper arm — (Use additional code to identify organism: 041.1. Use additional code to identify major osseous defect, if applicable: 731.3)
- 731.3 Major osseous defects — (Code first underlying disease: 170.0-170.9, 730.00-730.29, 733.00-733.09, 733.40-733.49, 996.45)
- 733.11 Pathologic fracture of humerus
- 733.41 Aseptic necrosis of head of humerus — (Use additional code to identify major osseous defect, if applicable: 731.3)
- 733.81 Malunion of fracture
- 733.82 Nonunion of fracture
- 736.89 Other acquired deformity of other parts of limb
- 756.4 Chondrodystrophy
- 756.51 Osteogenesis imperfecta
- V54.02 Encounter for lengthening/adjustment of growth rod

Terms To Know
aseptic necrosis. Death of bone tissue resulting from a disruption in the vascular supply, caused by a noninfectious disease process, such as a fracture or the administration of immunosuppressive drugs.

benign. Mild or nonmalignant in nature.

distal. Located farther away from a specified reference point.

fascia. Fibrous sheet or band of tissue that envelops organs, muscles, and groupings of muscles.

malignant. Any condition tending to progress toward death, specifically an invasive tumor with a loss of cellular differentiation that has the ability to spread or metastasize to other areas in the body.

malunion. Fracture that has united in a faulty position due to inadequate reduction of the original fracture, insufficient holding of a previously well-reduced fracture, contracture of the soft tissues, or comminuted or osteoporotic bone causing a slow disintegration of the fracture.

nonunion. Failure of two ends of a fracture to mend or completely heal.

proximal. Located closest to a specified reference point, usually the midline.

CCI Version 16.3
01710, 0213T, 0216T, 0228T, 0230T, 23935, 24000, 24006-24066, 24100-24101, 24110-24116, 24140, 24300, 24332, 24341, 24495, 29065, 29105, 36000, 36400-36410, 36420-36430, 36440, 36600, 36640, 37202, 43752, 51701-51703, 62310-62319, 64400-64435, 64445-64450, 64479, 64483, 64490, 64493, 64505-64530, 69990, 93000-93010, 93040-93042, 93318, 94002, 94200, 94250, 94680-94690, 94770, 95812-95816, 95819, 95822, 95829, 95955, 96360, 96365, 96372, 96374-96376, 99148-99149, 99150

Note: These CCI edits are used for Medicare. Other payers may reimburse on codes listed above.

Medicare Edits

	Fac RVU	Non-Fac RVU	FUD	Assist
24410	30.77	30.77	90	80

Medicare References: 100-2,15,260; 100-4,12,30; 100-4,12,90.3; 100-4,14,10

24420

24420 Osteoplasty, humerus (eg, shortening or lengthening) (excluding 64876)

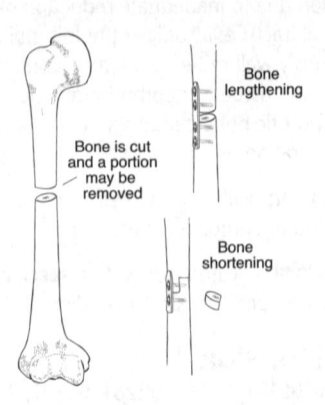

An osteoplasty (surgical manipulation of bone) is performed on the humerus to shorten or lengthen the humerus

The osteoplasty may occur anywhere along the humerus

Explanation
The physician performs osteoplasty of the humerus for shortening or lengthening. An incision is made through the skin, fascia, and muscle in the upper arm over the humeral shaft. Vessels and nerves are exposed and retracted. Dissection continues to expose the shaft of the humerus. An osteotomy is made at the determined point on the humerus. The physician removes a wedge of bone. To shorten the humeral shaft, a plate is attached to the distal segment with screws. Reduction forceps are used to hold and compress the osteotomy while the plate is attached to the proximal fragment with screws. To lengthen the bone, the segments are retracted, usually 2 mm to 3 mm, and fixed at that distance with plates and screws. X-rays (reported separately) are used to check rotational alignment of the segments. Drain tubes are inserted, the incision is repaired in layers with sutures, staples, and/or Steri-strips, and the arm is immobilized.

Coding Tips
According to CPT guidelines, cast application or strapping (including removal) is only reported as a replacement procedure or when the cast application or strapping is an initial service performed without a restorative treatment or procedure. See "Application of Casts and Strapping" in the CPT book in the Surgery Section, under the Musculoskeletal system. Do not report 24420 when shortening of humerus is performed to facilitate nerve repair. For suture of nerve requiring shortening of bone, see 64876.

ICD-9-CM Procedural
- 77.32 Other division of humerus
- 78.12 Application of external fixator device, humerus
- 78.22 Limb shortening procedures, humerus
- 78.32 Limb lengthening procedures, humerus
- 84.53 Implantation of internal limb lengthening device with kinetic distraction
- 84.54 Implantation of other internal limb lengthening device
- 84.71 Application of external fixator device, monoplanar system
- 84.72 Application of external fixator device, ring system
- 84.73 Application of hybrid external fixator device

Anesthesia
24420 01742

ICD-9-CM Diagnostic
- 170.4 Malignant neoplasm of scapula and long bones of upper limb
- 198.5 Secondary malignant neoplasm of bone and bone marrow
- 213.4 Benign neoplasm of scapula and long bones of upper limb
- 715.10 Primary localized osteoarthrosis, specified site
- 715.22 Secondary localized osteoarthrosis, upper arm
- 715.31 Localized osteoarthrosis not specified whether primary or secondary, shoulder region
- 715.32 Localized osteoarthrosis not specified whether primary or secondary, upper arm
- 730.12 Chronic osteomyelitis, upper arm — (Use additional code to identify organism: 041.1. Use additional code to identify major osseous defect, if applicable: 731.3)
- 731.3 Major osseous defects — (Code first underlying disease: 170.0-170.9, 730.00-730.29, 733.00-733.09, 733.40-733.49, 996.45)
- 733.41 Aseptic necrosis of head of humerus — (Use additional code to identify major osseous defect, if applicable: 731.3)
- 733.81 Malunion of fracture
- 733.82 Nonunion of fracture
- 733.91 Arrest of bone development or growth
- 736.89 Other acquired deformity of other parts of limb
- 756.4 Chondrodystrophy
- 756.51 Osteogenesis imperfecta

Terms To Know
aseptic necrosis. Death of bone tissue resulting from a disruption in the vascular supply, caused by a noninfectious disease process, such as a fracture or the administration of immunosuppressive drugs.

benign. Mild or nonmalignant in nature.

distal. Located farther away from a specified reference point.

fascia. Fibrous sheet or band of tissue that envelops organs, muscles, and groupings of muscles.

malignant. Any condition tending to progress toward death, specifically an invasive tumor with a loss of cellular differentiation that has the ability to spread or metastasize to other areas in the body.

malunion. Fracture that has united in a faulty position due to inadequate reduction of the original fracture, insufficient holding of a previously well-reduced fracture, contracture of the soft tissues, or comminuted or osteoporotic bone causing a slow disintegration of the fracture.

CCI Version 16.3
01710, 0213T, 0216T, 0228T, 0230T, 23935, 24000, 24006-24066, 24100-24101, 24110-24116, 24140, 24300, 24332, 24341, 24400-24410, 24495, 24515-24516, 29065, 29105, 36000, 36400-36410, 36420-36430, 36440, 36600, 36640, 37202, 43752, 51701-51703, 62310-62319, 64400-64435, 64445-64450, 64479, 64483, 64490, 64493, 64505-64530, 69990, 93000-93010, 93040-93042, 93318, 94002, 94200, 94250, 94680-94690, 94770, 95812-95816, 95819, 95822, 95829, 95955, 96360, 96365, 96372, 96374-96376, 99148-99149, 99150

Note: These CCI edits are used for Medicare. Other payers may reimburse on codes listed above.

Medicare Edits

	Fac RVU	Non-Fac RVU	FUD	Assist
24420	28.93	28.93	90	80

Medicare References: 100-2,15,260; 100-4,12,30; 100-4,12,90.3; 100-4,14,10

24430-24435

24430 Repair of nonunion or malunion, humerus; without graft (eg, compression technique)
24435 with iliac or other autograft (includes obtaining graft)

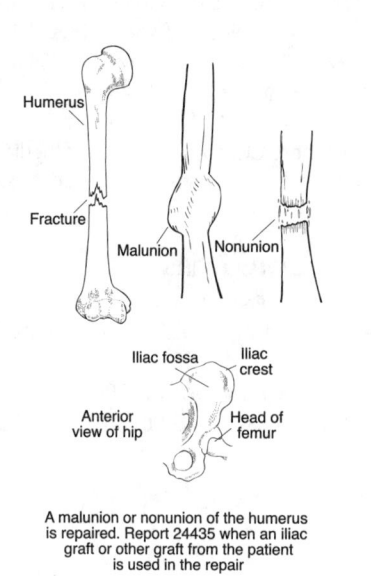

A malunion or nonunion of the humerus is repaired. Report 24435 when an iliac graft or other graft from the patient is used in the repair

Explanation
The physician repairs a nonunion or malunion of the humerus without using a graft in 24430 and with an iliac or other autograft in 24435. The physician exposes the nonunion or malunion of the humerus by making a 10 cm to 15 cm longitudinal incision through the skin, fascia, and muscle over the fracture site. With a reciprocating saw, the bone is divided through the nonunion. The fragments are aligned. A compression plate is centered over the fracture and screws are inserted. In 24435, a bone graft is needed to help heal the fracture due to bone loss. Autogenous iliac bone is typically used, but proximal tibia grafts may also be used. Both require a separate incision and wound closure of the harvest site. The physician uses an osteotome to harvest strips of bone, which are placed around the ends of the humeral fracture in addition to the compression plate for internal fixation. The incision is repaired in layers with sutures, staples, and/or Steri-strips. The limb is immobilized.

Coding Tips
In 24435, the bone graft harvest is not reported separately. According to CPT guidelines, cast application or strapping (including removal) is only reported as a replacement procedure or when the cast application or strapping is an initial service performed without a restorative treatment or procedure. See "Application of Casts and Strapping" in the CPT book in the Surgery Section, under the Musculoskeletal system. For repair of malunion of proximal radius and/or ulna, see 25400–25420.

ICD-9-CM Procedural
77.79 Excision of other bone for graft, except facial bones
78.02 Bone graft of humerus
78.42 Other repair or plastic operation on humerus

Anesthesia
01744

ICD-9-CM Diagnostic
733.81 Malunion of fracture
733.82 Nonunion of fracture

Terms To Know
fascia. Fibrous sheet or band of tissue that envelops organs, muscles, and groupings of muscles.

fracture. Break in bone or cartilage.

malunion. Fracture that has united in a faulty position due to inadequate reduction of the original fracture, insufficient holding of a previously well-reduced fracture, contracture of the soft tissues, or comminuted or osteoporotic bone causing a slow disintegration of the fracture.

nonunion. Failure of two ends of a fracture to mend or completely heal.

proximal. Located closest to a specified reference point, usually the midline.

CCI Version 16.3
01710, 0213T, 0216T, 0228T, 0230T, 20680, 24140, 24300, 24332, 24400-24410, 24495, 24515-24516, 25020, 25024-25025, 29065, 29105, 36000, 36400-36410, 36420-36430, 36440, 36600, 36640, 37202, 43752, 51701-51703, 62310-62319, 64400-64435, 64445-64450, 64479, 64483, 64490, 64493, 64505-64530, 64708, 69990, 93000-93010, 93040-93042, 93318, 94002, 94200, 94250, 94680-94690, 94770, 95812-95816, 95819, 95822, 95829, 95955, 96360, 96365, 96372, 96374-96376, 99148-99149, 99150

Also not with 24435: 20900-20902, 24430, 76000-76001

Note: These CCI edits are used for Medicare. Other payers may reimburse on codes listed above.

Medicare Edits

	Fac RVU	Non-Fac RVU	FUD	Assist
24430	30.91	30.91	90	80
24435	31.43	31.43	90	80

Medicare References: 100-2,15,260; 100-4,12,30; 100-4,12,90.3; 100-4,14,10

24470

24470 Hemiepiphyseal arrest (eg, cubitus varus or valgus, distal humerus)

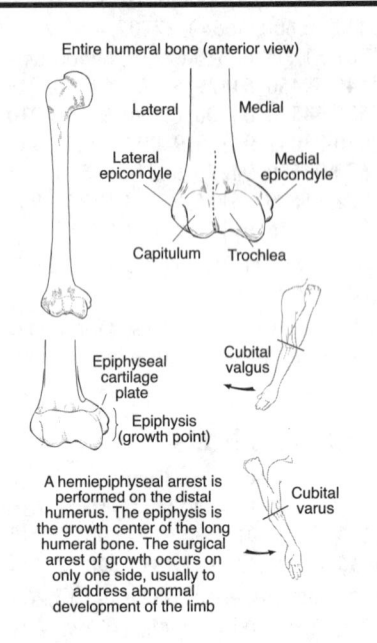

Entire humeral bone (anterior view)

Lateral — Medial
Lateral epicondyle — Medial epicondyle
Capitulum — Trochlea
Epiphyseal cartilage plate
Epiphysis (growth point)
Cubital valgus
Cubital varus

A hemiepiphyseal arrest is performed on the distal humerus. The epiphysis is the growth center of the long humeral bone. The surgical arrest of growth occurs on only one side, usually to address abnormal development of the limb

Explanation

The physician performs a hemiepiphyseal arrest. Angular deformities are typically a complication of fractures of the lateral condylar physis. The most common deformity is cubitus valgus. To treat cubitus valgus, the physician makes a longitudinal posterior incision along the distal humerus. The humerus is then exposed. If a nonunion exists from a previous condylar physeal fracture, it may be approached from the same incision. If a nonunion is present, the ends are denuded and a local bone graft is applied. The physician applies a cancellous screw to provide fixation and compression across the nonunion. An osteotomy is then performed across the distal humerus, correcting both the angulation and realigning the longitudinal axis of the humerus with that of the forearm. The osteotomy is secured with screws. The physician repairs the incision in layers with sutures, staples, and/or Steri-strips. The elbow is immobilized in a splint or brace.

Coding Tips

According to CPT guidelines, cast application or strapping (including removal) is only reported as a replacement procedure or when the cast application or strapping is an initial service performed without a restorative treatment or procedure. See "Application of Casts and Strapping" in the CPT book in the Surgery Section, under the Musculoskeletal system.

ICD-9-CM Procedural

78.42 Other repair or plastic operation on humerus

Anesthesia

24470 01740

ICD-9-CM Diagnostic

268.1 Rickets, late effect — (Use additional code to identify the nature of late effect)
736.01 Cubitus valgus (acquired)
736.02 Cubitus varus (acquired)
755.59 Other congenital anomaly of upper limb, including shoulder girdle

Terms To Know

complication. Condition arising after the beginning of observation and treatment that modifies the course of the patient's illness or the medical care required, or an undesired result or misadventure in medical care.

cubitus valgus. Congenital or acquired condition in which the forearm deviates away from the midline on extension.

cubitus varus. Congenital or acquired condition in which the forearm deviates inward toward the midline when extended.

distal. Located farther away from a specified reference point.

late effect. Abnormality, dysfunction, or other residual condition produced after the acute phase of an illness, injury, or disease is over. There is no time limit on when late effects can appear.

nonunion. Failure of two ends of a fracture to mend or completely heal.

posterior. Located in the back part or caudal end of the body.

CCI Version 16.3

01710, 0213T, 0216T, 0228T, 0230T, 24300, 24332, 24575, 24579, 29065, 29105, 29260, 36000, 36400-36410, 36420-36430, 36440, 36600, 36640, 37202, 43752, 51701-51703, 62310-62319, 64400-64435, 64445-64450, 64479, 64483, 64490, 64493, 64505-64530, 69990, 93000-93010, 93040-93042, 93318, 94002, 94200, 94250, 94680-94690, 94770, 95812-95816, 95819, 95822, 95829, 95955, 96360, 96365, 96372, 96374-96376, 99148-99149, 99150

Note: These CCI edits are used for Medicare. Other payers may reimburse on codes listed above.

Medicare Edits

	Fac RVU	Non-Fac RVU	FUD	Assist
24470	18.94	18.94	90	80

Medicare References: 100-2,15,260; 100-4,12,30; 100-4,12,90.3; 100-4,14,10

24495

24495 Decompression fasciotomy, forearm, with brachial artery exploration

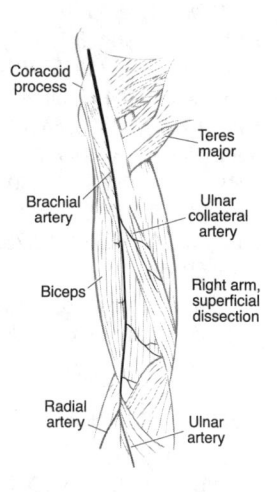

A decompression fasciotomy of the forearm is performed, with exploration of the brachial artery

Explanation

The physician performs a decompression fasciotomy in the forearm with exploration of the brachial artery. The physician makes a longitudinal incision on the anterior forearm, from just lateral and proximal to the biceps tendon distal toward the radial styloid, excising the deep fascia, exposing brachioradialis laterally and biceps and brachialis medially, decompressing the compartment. The brachial artery is explored proximally to identify the origin of decreased circulation. The fascial incision remains open. The skin incision may be left open or closed.

Coding Tips

For tenotomy, lateral or medial, for tennis or golfer's elbow, see 24357; with debridement, see 24358; with tendon repair or reattachment, see 24359.

ICD-9-CM Procedural

83.14   Fasciotomy

Anesthesia

24495   01810

ICD-9-CM Diagnostic

682.3   Cellulitis and abscess of upper arm and forearm — (Use additional code to identify organism, such as 041.1, etc.)
728.88 Rhabdomyolysis
729.71 Nontraumatic compartment syndrome of upper extremity — (Code first, if applicable, postprocedural complication: 998.89)
813.21 Closed fracture of shaft of radius (alone)
813.22 Closed fracture of shaft of ulna (alone)
813.23 Closed fracture of shaft of radius with ulna
813.31 Open fracture of shaft of radius (alone)
813.32 Open fracture of shaft of ulna (alone)
813.33 Open fracture of shaft of radius with ulna
813.80 Closed fracture of unspecified part of forearm
813.90 Open fracture of unspecified part of forearm
832.00 Closed unspecified dislocation of elbow
832.10 Open unspecified dislocation of elbow
881.01 Open wound of elbow, without mention of complication
881.10 Open wound of forearm, complicated
881.11 Open wound of elbow, complicated
881.20 Open wound of forearm, with tendon involvement
903.1   Brachial blood vessels injury
923.10 Contusion of forearm
923.11 Contusion of elbow
927.10 Crushing injury of forearm — (Use additional code to identify any associated injuries: 800-829, 850.0-854.1, 860.0-869.1)
927.11 Crushing injury of elbow — (Use additional code to identify any associated injuries: 800-829, 850.0-854.1, 860.0-869.1)
958.8   Other early complications of trauma
958.91 Traumatic compartment syndrome of upper extremity

Terms To Know

anterior. Situated in the front area or toward the belly surface of the body; an anatomical reference point used to show the position and relationship of one body structure to another.

cellulitis. Sudden, severe, suppurative inflammation and edema in subcutaneous tissue or muscle, most often caused by bacterial infection secondary to a cutaneous lesion.

contusion. Superficial injury (bruising) produced by impact without a break in the skin.

distal. Located farther away from a specified reference point.

fascia. Fibrous sheet or band of tissue that envelops organs, muscles, and groupings of muscles.

open wound. Opening or break of the skin.

proximal. Located closest to a specified reference point, usually the midline.

tendon. Fibrous tissue that connects muscle to bone, consisting primarily of collagen and containing little vasculature.

CCI Version 16.3

01710, 0213T, 0216T, 0228T, 0230T, 11040, 11043, 20103, 24300, 29105-29126, 35860, 36000, 36400-36410, 36420-36430, 36440, 36600, 36640, 37202, 43752, 51701-51703, 62310-62319, 64400-64435, 64445-64450, 64479, 64483, 64490, 64493, 64505-64530, 69990, 93000-93010, 93040-93042, 93318, 94002, 94200, 94250, 94680-94690, 94770, 95812-95816, 95819, 95822, 95829, 95955, 96360, 96365, 96372, 96374-96376, 99148-99149, 99150

Note: These CCI edits are used for Medicare. Other payers may reimburse on codes listed above.

Medicare Edits

	Fac RVU	Non-Fac RVU	FUD	Assist
24495	19.18	19.18	90	80

Medicare References: 100-2,15,260; 100-4,12,30; 100-4,12,90.3; 100-4,14,10

24498

24498 Prophylactic treatment (nailing, pinning, plating or wiring), with or without methylmethacrylate, humeral shaft

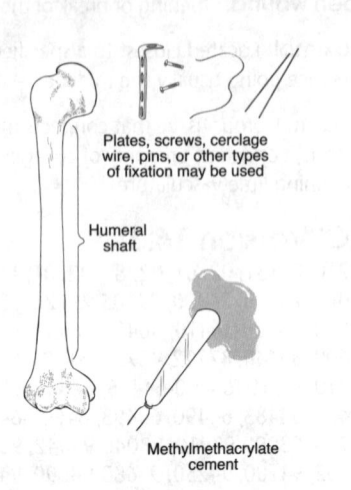

Plates, screws, cerclage wire, pins, or other types of fixation may be used

Humeral shaft

Methylmethacrylate cement

The humeral shaft is surgically treated with internal fixation as a preventive measure against fractures, with or without the use of the artificial bone compound, methylmethacrylate

Explanation
The physician applies prophylactic treatment to prevent fracture. A longitudinal incision is made through the skin, fascia, and muscle along the humerus to expose the worrisome area. Pins or a plate and screws are used to stabilize the bone. If defects in the bone do not allow for good internal fixation, methylmethacrylate, a bone cementing substance when hard, may be used to fill in the gaps. Wiring may also be wrapped around the bone to provide additional fixation. An intramedullary nail may also be inserted through the canal of the humerus to provide internal stabilization. The incisions are repaired in layers with sutures, staples, and/or Steri-strips.

Coding Tips
For prophylactic treatment (nailing, pinning, plating, or wiring) of proximal humerus, see 23491. For radiology services, see 73060.

ICD-9-CM Procedural
- 78.52 Internal fixation of humerus without fracture reduction
- 84.55 Insertion of bone void filler

Anesthesia
24498 01740

ICD-9-CM Diagnostic
- 170.4 Malignant neoplasm of scapula and long bones of upper limb
- 198.5 Secondary malignant neoplasm of bone and bone marrow
- 213.4 Benign neoplasm of scapula and long bones of upper limb
- 238.0 Neoplasm of uncertain behavior of bone and articular cartilage
- 239.2 Neoplasms of unspecified nature of bone, soft tissue, and skin
- 732.3 Juvenile osteochondrosis of upper extremity
- 733.11 Pathologic fracture of humerus
- 756.4 Chondrodystrophy
- 756.51 Osteogenesis imperfecta

Terms To Know
benign. Mild or nonmalignant in nature.

chondrodystrophy. Abnormal development of cartilage, the primary cause of short limb dwarfism.

fascia. Fibrous sheet or band of tissue that envelops organs, muscles, and groupings of muscles.

malignant. Any condition tending to progress toward death, specifically an invasive tumor with a loss of cellular differentiation that has the ability to spread or metastasize to other areas in the body.

neoplasm. New abnormal growth, tumor.

pathologic fracture. Break in bone due to a disease process that weakens the bone structure, such as osteoporosis, osteomalacia, or neoplasia, and not traumatic injury.

CCI Version 16.3
01710, 0213T, 0216T, 0228T, 0230T, 20650, 23000, 23040, 23100, 23105, 23107, 23130, 23150, 23184, 23195, 23410-23412, 23430, 23450, 23700, 24000, 24006, 24100-24110, 24140, 24300, 24332-24340, 24410, 29065, 29105, 29819-29821, 29834-29835, 29837, 36000, 36400-36410, 36420-36430, 36440, 36600, 36640, 37202, 43752, 51701-51703, 62310-62319, 64400-64435, 64445-64450, 64479, 64483, 64490, 64493, 64505-64530, 69990, 93000-93010, 93040-93042, 93318, 94002, 94200, 94250, 94680-94690, 94770, 95812-95816, 95819, 95822, 95829, 95955, 96360, 96365, 96372, 96374-96376, 99148-99149, 99150

Note: These CCI edits are used for Medicare. Other payers may reimburse on codes listed above.

Medicare Edits

	Fac RVU	Non-Fac RVU	FUD	Assist
24498	25.39	25.39	90	80

Medicare References: 100-2,15,260; 100-4,12,30; 100-4,12,90.3; 100-4,14,10

24500-24505

24500 Closed treatment of humeral shaft fracture; without manipulation
24505 with manipulation, with or without skeletal traction

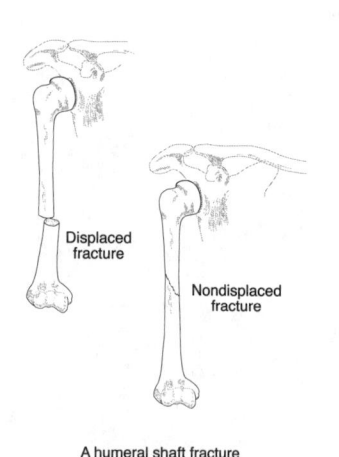

A humeral shaft fracture is treated in a closed fashion without manipulation in 24500. Report 24505 when manipulation is required to treat the fracture, with or without skeletal traction

Explanation
The physician performs closed treatment of a humeral shaft fracture. In 24500, the segments are determined to be aligned and stable and no manipulation of the bone fragments is necessary. Treatment involves immobilization, using one of several methods, of the elbow and possibly of the glenohumeral joint for several weeks until union is established. In 24505, the physician must first manually coerce the fractured bone into alignment. Skeletal traction may also be applied in 24505.

Coding Tips
According to CPT guidelines, cast application or strapping (including removal) is only reported as a replacement procedure or when the cast application or strapping is an initial service performed without a restorative treatment or procedure. See "Application of Casts and Strapping" in the CPT book in the Surgery Section, under the Musculoskeletal system. In 24505, local anesthesia is included in this service. However, this procedure may be performed under general anesthesia, depending on the age and/or condition of the patient. For radiology services, see 73060. For open treatment of a humeral shaft fracture with plate/screws, with or without cerclage, see 24515; with insertion of an intramedullary implant, see 24516. For humeral supracondylar or transcondylar fracture treatments, see 24530–24546. For humeral epicondylar fracture treatments, see 24560–24575. For a humeral condylar fracture, medial or lateral, see 24576–24582.

ICD-9-CM Procedural
79.01 Closed reduction of fracture of humerus without internal fixation
93.43 Intermittent skeletal traction
93.44 Other skeletal traction
93.53 Application of other cast
93.54 Application of splint

Anesthesia
01730

ICD-9-CM Diagnostic
733.11 Pathologic fracture of humerus
812.21 Closed fracture of shaft of humerus

Terms To Know
closed fracture. Break in a bone without a concomitant opening in the skin. A closed fracture is coded when the type of fracture is not specified.

pathologic fracture. Break in bone due to a disease process that weakens the bone structure, such as osteoporosis, osteomalacia, or neoplasia, and not traumatic injury.

CCI Version 16.3
01710, 0213T, 0216T, 0228T, 0230T, 24300, 29049-29075, 29105-29125, 29240-29260, 29700-29715, 36000, 36400-36410, 36420-36430, 36440, 36600, 36640, 37202, 43752, 51701-51703, 62310-62319, 64400-64435, 64445-64450, 64479, 64483, 64490, 64493, 64505-64530, 69990, 93000-93010, 93040-93042, 93318, 94002, 94200, 94250, 94680-94690, 94770, 95812-95816, 95819, 95822, 95829, 95955, 96360, 96365, 96372, 96374-96376, 97597-97598, 97602-97606, 99148-99149, 99150
Also not with 24500: 12011, 76000-76001
Also not with 24505: 12001, 12032, 24500, 29130, G0168, J0670, J2001
Note: These CCI edits are used for Medicare. Other payers may reimburse on codes listed above.

Medicare Edits

	Fac RVU	Non-Fac RVU	FUD	Assist
24500	9.07	9.97	90	N/A
24505	12.98	14.25	90	N/A

Medicare References: 100-2,15,260; 100-4,12,30; 100-4,12,90.3; 100-4,14,10

24515

24515 Open treatment of humeral shaft fracture with plate/screws, with or without cerclage

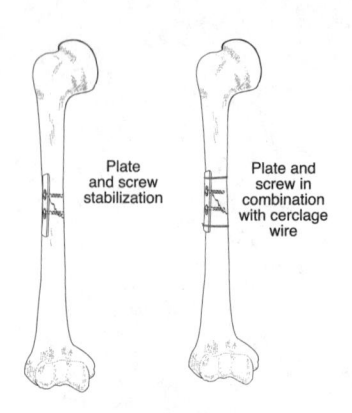

A humeral shaft fracture is treated in an open surgical session and fixed with plates/screws. Cerclage wire may also be used to stabilize the fracture

Explanation

The physician repairs a humeral shaft fracture with a plate or screws, with or without cerclage. A lateral or anterolateral incision is made overlying a fracture site. The fracture is reduced by manipulation and bone reduction forceps. A compression plate with screws secures and compresses the fragments. Cerclage wiring might be used to facilitate fixation of the fracture. One or more wires may be placed around the humerus, over the fracture site. The incision is closed with sutures, staples, and/or Steri-strips.

Coding Tips

According to CPT guidelines, cast application or strapping (including removal) is only reported as a replacement procedure or when the cast application or strapping is an initial service performed without a restorative treatment or procedure. See "Application of Casts and Strapping" in the CPT book in the Surgery Section, under the Musculoskeletal system. For closed treatment of a humeral shaft fracture, without manipulation, see 24500; with manipulation, with or without skeletal traction, see 24505. For open treatment of a humeral shaft fracture, with insertion of an intramedullary implant, see 24516. For a humeral supracondylar or transcondylar fracture treatments, see 24530–24546. For humeral epicondylar fracture treatments, see 24560–24575. For humeral condylar fracture, medial or lateral, see 24576–24582.

ICD-9-CM Procedural

79.31 Open reduction of fracture of humerus with internal fixation

Anesthesia

24515 01740

ICD-9-CM Diagnostic

733.11 Pathologic fracture of humerus
812.21 Closed fracture of shaft of humerus
812.31 Open fracture of shaft of humerus

Terms To Know

anterolateral. Situated in the front and off to one side.

closed fracture. Break in a bone without a concomitant opening in the skin. A closed fracture is coded when the type of fracture is not specified.

lateral. To/on the side.

open fracture. Exposed break in a bone, always considered compound due to its high risk of infection from the open wound leading to the fracture. Broken bone ends may protrude through the skin and contaminants or foreign bodies are often embedded in the tissues.

pathologic fracture. Break in bone due to a disease process that weakens the bone structure, such as osteoporosis, osteomalacia, or neoplasia, and not traumatic injury.

CCI Version 16.3

01710, 0213T, 0216T, 0228T, 0230T, 20680, 24300, 24332, 24495, 24500-24505, 25020, 29049-29075, 29105, 29240-29260, 29700-29715, 36000, 36400-36410, 36420-36430, 36440, 36600, 36640, 37202, 43752, 51701-51703, 62310-62319, 64400-64435, 64445-64450, 64479, 64483, 64490, 64493, 64505-64530, 64708, 64718, 69990, 93000-93010, 93040-93042, 93318, 94002, 94200, 94250, 94680-94690, 94770, 95812-95816, 95819, 95822, 95829, 95955, 96360, 96365, 96372, 96374-96376, 97597-97598, 97602-97606, 99148-99149, 99150

Note: These CCI edits are used for Medicare. Other payers may reimburse on codes listed above.

Medicare Edits

	Fac RVU	Non-Fac RVU	FUD	Assist
24515	25.57	25.57	90	80

Medicare References: 100-2,15,260; 100-4,12,30; 100-4,12,90.3; 100-4,14,10

24516

24516 Treatment of humeral shaft fracture, with insertion of intramedullary implant, with or without cerclage and/or locking screws

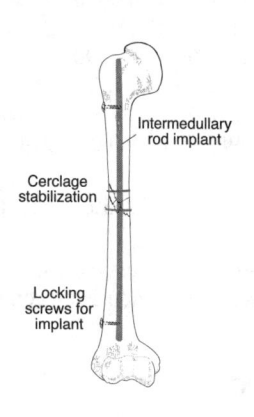

A humeral shaft fracture is treated in an open surgical session with insertion of an intermedullary implant. Locking screws and/or cerclage wire may be used in the procedure as well

Explanation

The physician repairs a humeral shaft fracture with insertion of an intramedullary implant, with or without cerclage and/or locking screws. A straight lateral incision is made through skin, fascia, and muscles to expose the fracture site. If there are multiple fragments or if there is a long spiral fracture, cerclage wires may be wrapped around the bone to hold the fragments in place. Using a guide rod to direct a reamer and rod, an intermedullary nail is placed within the humeral shaft. The nail may be locked in place proximally and distally with locking screws. The wound is irrigated, a drain may be inserted, and the wound is closed in layers.

Coding Tips

According to CPT guidelines, cast application or strapping (including removal) is only reported as a replacement procedure or when the cast application or strapping is an initial service performed without a restorative treatment or procedure. See "Application of Casts and Strapping" in the CPT book in the Surgery Section, under the Musculoskeletal system. For closed treatment of a humeral shaft fracture, without manipulation, see 24500; with manipulation, with or without skeletal traction, see 24505. For open treatment of a humeral shaft fracture, with plate/screws, with or without cerclage, see 24515. For humeral supracondylar or transcondylar fracture treatments, see 24530–24546. For humeral epicondylar fracture treatments, see 24560–24575. For a humeral condylar fracture, medial or lateral, see 24576–24582.

ICD-9-CM Procedural

79.21 Open reduction of fracture of humerus without internal fixation
79.31 Open reduction of fracture of humerus with internal fixation

Anesthesia

24516 01740

ICD-9-CM Diagnostic

733.11 Pathologic fracture of humerus
812.21 Closed fracture of shaft of humerus
812.31 Open fracture of shaft of humerus

Terms To Know

closed fracture. Break in a bone without a concomitant opening in the skin. A closed fracture is coded when the type of fracture is not specified.

distal. Located farther away from a specified reference point.

fascia. Fibrous sheet or band of tissue that envelops organs, muscles, and groupings of muscles.

lateral. To/on the side.

open fracture. Exposed break in a bone, always considered compound due to its high risk of infection from the open wound leading to the fracture. Broken bone ends may protrude through the skin and contaminants or foreign bodies are often embedded in the tissues.

pathologic fracture. Break in bone due to a disease process that weakens the bone structure, such as osteoporosis, osteomalacia, or neoplasia, and not traumatic injury.

proximal. Located closest to a specified reference point, usually the midline.

CCI Version 16.3

01710, 0213T, 0216T, 0228T, 0230T, 20680, 24300, 24332, 24495, 24500-24505, 24515❖, 25020, 29049-29075, 29105, 29240-29260, 29700-29715, 36000, 36400-36410, 36420-36430, 36440, 36600, 36640, 37202, 43752, 51701-51703, 62310-62319, 64400-64435, 64445-64450, 64479, 64483, 64490, 64493, 64505-64530, 64708, 64722, 69990, 76000-76001, 93000-93010, 93040-93042, 93318, 94002, 94200, 94250, 94680-94690, 94770, 95812-95816, 95819, 95822, 95829, 95955, 96360, 96365, 96372, 96374-96376, 97597-97598, 97602-97606, 99148-99149, 99150

Note: These CCI edits are used for Medicare. Other payers may reimburse on codes listed above.

Medicare Edits

	Fac RVU	Non-Fac RVU	FUD	Assist
24516	25.2	25.2	90	80

Medicare References: 100-2,15,260; 100-4,12,30; 100-4,12,90.3; 100-4,14,10

24530-24535

24530 Closed treatment of supracondylar or transcondylar humeral fracture, with or without intercondylar extension; without manipulation

24535 with manipulation, with or without skin or skeletal traction

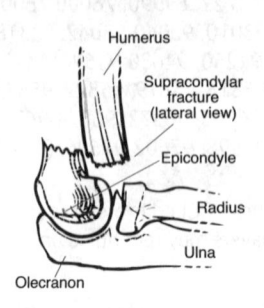

Humerus
Supracondylar fracture (lateral view)
Epicondyle
Radius
Ulna
Olecranon

A supracondylar or transcondylar humeral fracture is treated in a closed fashion, with or without condylar extension. Report 24530 when the procedure does not require manipulation or skin or skeletal traction. Report 24535 when manipulation is required, with or without skin or skeletal traction

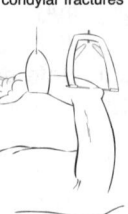

One type of skeletal traction for condylar fractures

Explanation

Closed treatment of a supracondylar or transcondylar fracture, which may have an extending fracture line between the condyles, is indicated when the fragments are not separated and appear stable. No manipulation is required in 24530. Supracondylar fractures in the adult are usually treated with a caption splint or hanging arm cast. Transcondylar fractures may be treated conservatively with a hanging arm cast and elbow immobilization. In 24535, manipulation is necessary to realign the fracture into proper reduction. Skin or skeletal traction may also be applied. Pins, wires, or tongs are inserted into the bone for skeletal traction through a small incision without opening the fracture. A weight and pulley system is attached to exert a constant force of traction and keep the fractured bones in alignment.

Coding Tips

According to CPT guidelines, cast application or strapping (including removal) is only reported as a replacement procedure or when the cast application or strapping is an initial service performed without a restorative treatment or procedure. See "Application of Casts and Strapping" in the CPT book in the Surgery Section, under the Musculoskeletal system. In 24535, local anesthesia is included in the service. However, this procedure may be performed under general anesthesia, depending on the age and/or condition of the patient. For radiology services, see 73060–73080. Distal humeral fractures are site specific. For percutaneous skeletal fixation of supracondylar or transcondylar humeral fractures, see 24538. For open treatment, see 24545 and 24546. For humeral shaft fractures, see 24500–24516. For humeral epicondylar fractures, see 24560–24575. For humeral condylar fractures, medial or lateral, see 24576–24582.

ICD-9-CM Procedural

- 79.01 Closed reduction of fracture of humerus without internal fixation
- 79.11 Closed reduction of fracture of humerus with internal fixation
- 93.43 Intermittent skeletal traction
- 93.44 Other skeletal traction
- 93.46 Other skin traction of limbs
- 93.53 Application of other cast
- 93.54 Application of splint

Anesthesia
01730

ICD-9-CM Diagnostic

- 733.11 Pathologic fracture of humerus
- 812.40 Closed fracture of unspecified part of lower end of humerus
- 812.41 Closed fracture of supracondylar humerus
- 812.42 Closed fracture of lateral condyle of humerus
- 812.43 Closed fracture of medial condyle of humerus
- 812.44 Closed fracture of unspecified condyle(s) of humerus
- 812.49 Other closed fracture of lower end of humerus

CCI Version 16.3

01710, 0213T, 0216T, 0228T, 0230T, 24300, 29049-29075, 29105, 29240-29260, 29700-29715, 36000, 36400-36410, 36420-36430, 36440, 36600, 36640, 37202, 43752, 51701-51703, 62310-62319, 64400-64435, 64445-64450, 64479, 64483, 64490, 64493, 64505-64530, 69990, 93000-93010, 93040-93042, 93318, 94002, 94200, 94250, 94680-94690, 94770, 95812-95816, 95819, 95822, 95829, 95955, 96360, 96365, 96372, 96374-96376, 97597-97598, 97602-97606, 99148-99149, 99150

Also not with 24535: 20650, 24530, J0670, J2001

Note: These CCI edits are used for Medicare. Other payers may reimburse on codes listed above.

Medicare Edits

	Fac RVU	Non-Fac RVU	FUD	Assist
24530	9.69	10.68	90	N/A
24535	16.42	17.68	90	N/A

Medicare References: 100-2,15,260; 100-4,12,30; 100-4,12,90.3; 100-4,14,10

24538

24538 Percutaneous skeletal fixation of supracondylar or transcondylar humeral fracture, with or without intercondylar extension

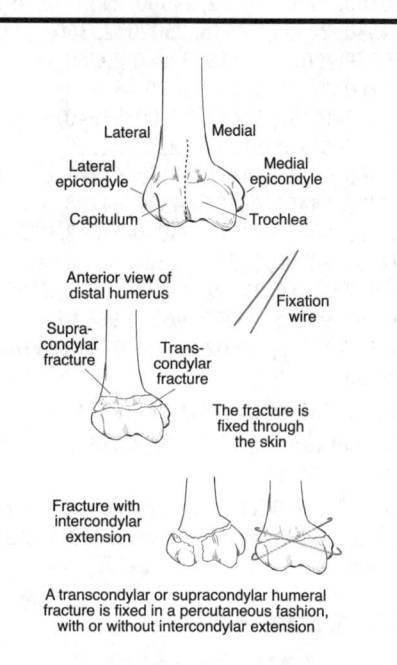

Explanation
The physician performs percutaneous skeletal fixation of a supracondylar or transcondylar humeral fracture, which may have an extending fracture line between the condyles. The elbow is prepared and draped. The fracture is reduced by applying longitudinal traction and manipulating the fracture into alignment. Pins are inserted through the condyles and metaphysis diagonally, avoiding the ulnar nerve to hold the fractured pieces stable. The pins are clipped and bent beneath the skin. The incision is closed with layered sutures and the arm is immobilized.

Coding Tips
According to CPT guidelines, cast application or strapping (including removal) is only reported as a replacement procedure or when the cast application or strapping is an initial service performed without a restorative treatment or procedure. See "Application of Casts and Strapping" in the CPT book in the Surgery Section, under the Musculoskeletal system. For radiology services, see 73060–73080. Distal humeral fractures are site specific. For closed treatment of supracondylar or transcondylar humeral fractures, see 24530 and 24535. For open treatment, see 24545 and 24546. For humeral shaft fractures, see 24500–24516. For humeral epicondylar fractures, see 24560–24575. For humeral condylar fractures, medial or lateral, see 24576–24582.

ICD-9-CM Procedural
79.31 Open reduction of fracture of humerus with internal fixation

Anesthesia
24538 01730

ICD-9-CM Diagnostic
733.11 Pathologic fracture of humerus
812.20 Closed fracture of unspecified part of humerus
812.40 Closed fracture of unspecified part of lower end of humerus
812.41 Closed fracture of supracondylar humerus
812.42 Closed fracture of lateral condyle of humerus
812.43 Closed fracture of medial condyle of humerus
812.49 Other closed fracture of lower end of humerus
812.50 Open fracture of unspecified part of lower end of humerus
812.51 Open fracture of supracondylar humerus
812.52 Open fracture of lateral condyle of humerus
812.53 Open fracture of medial condyle of humerus
812.54 Open fracture of unspecified condyle(s) of humerus
812.59 Other open fracture of lower end of humerus

Terms To Know

closed fracture. Break in a bone without a concomitant opening in the skin. A closed fracture is coded when the type of fracture is not specified.

open fracture. Exposed break in a bone, always considered compound due to its high risk of infection from the open wound leading to the fracture. Broken bone ends may protrude through the skin and contaminants or foreign bodies are often embedded in the tissues.

pathologic fracture. Break in bone due to a disease process that weakens the bone structure, such as osteoporosis, osteomalacia, or neoplasia, and not traumatic injury.

CCI Version 16.3
01710, 0213T, 0216T, 0228T, 0230T, 20650, 24300, 24530, 24535, 29049-29075, 29105, 29240-29260, 36000, 36400-36410, 36420-36430, 36440, 36600, 36640, 37202, 43752, 51701-51703, 62310-62319, 64400-64435, 64445-64450, 64479, 64483, 64490, 64493, 64505-64530, 69990, 93000-93010, 93040-93042, 93318, 94002, 94200, 94250, 94680-94690, 94770, 95812-95816, 95819, 95822, 95829, 95955, 96360, 96365, 96372, 96374-96376, 97597-97598, 97602-97606, 99148-99149, 99150

Note: These CCI edits are used for Medicare. Other payers may reimburse on codes listed above.

Medicare Edits

	Fac RVU	Non-Fac RVU	FUD	Assist
24538	21.64	21.64	90	N/A

Medicare References: 100-2,15,260; 100-4,12,30; 100-4,12,90.3; 100-4,14,10

24545-24546

24545 Open treatment of humeral supracondylar or transcondylar fracture, includes internal fixation, when performed; without intercondylar extension

24546 with intercondylar extension

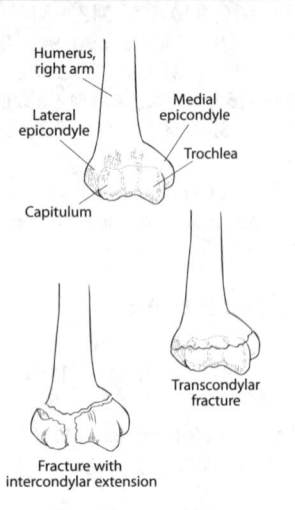

A humeral supracondylar or transcondylar fracture is treated in an open surgical session, with or without internal fixation. Report 24546 when intercondylar extension is present

Explanation
In 24545, the physician performs open treatment of a supracondylar or transcondylar humeral fracture that does not have an extending fracture line present between the condyles. In 24546, the humeral condylar fracture has an extending fracture line between the condyles that may create a third fracture piece. The physician makes a posterior incision from midline of the arm to just distal to the olecranon, exposing the olecranon, triceps tendon, and distal humerus. The ulnar nerve is isolated and retracted. Preserving as much soft tissue attachment as possible, the physician exposes and assembles the fragments, reducing the condyles and fixing the fragments with screws, pins, or plates as may be needed to hold the condyles firmly reduced to the metaphysis. The joint is irrigated and the wounds are closed with drain placement if needed.

Coding Tips
According to CPT guidelines, cast application or strapping (including removal) is only reported as a replacement procedure or when the cast application or strapping is an initial service performed without a restorative treatment or procedure. See "Application of Casts and Strapping" in the CPT book in the Surgery Section, under the Musculoskeletal system. Distal humeral fractures are site specific. For percutaneous skeletal fixation of supracondylar or transcondylar humeral fractures, see 24538. For closed treatment of supracondylar or transcondylar humeral fractures, see 24530 and 24535. For humeral shaft fractures, see 24500–24516. For humeral epicondylar fractures, see 24560–24575. For humeral condylar fractures, medial or lateral, see 24576–24582.

ICD-9-CM Procedural
79.21 Open reduction of fracture of humerus without internal fixation
79.31 Open reduction of fracture of humerus with internal fixation

Anesthesia
01740

ICD-9-CM Diagnostic
733.11 Pathologic fracture of humerus
812.40 Closed fracture of unspecified part of lower end of humerus
812.41 Closed fracture of supracondylar humerus
812.42 Closed fracture of lateral condyle of humerus
812.43 Closed fracture of medial condyle of humerus
812.49 Other closed fracture of lower end of humerus
812.50 Open fracture of unspecified part of lower end of humerus
812.51 Open fracture of supracondylar humerus
812.52 Open fracture of lateral condyle of humerus
812.53 Open fracture of medial condyle of humerus
812.54 Open fracture of unspecified condyle(s) of humerus
812.59 Other open fracture of lower end of humerus

Terms To Know
closed fracture. Break in a bone without a concomitant opening in the skin. A closed fracture is coded when the type of fracture is not specified.

distal. Located farther away from a specified reference point.

soft tissue. Nonepithelial tissues outside of the skeleton that includes subcutaneous adipose tissue, fibrous tissue, fascia, muscles, blood and lymph vessels, and peripheral nervous system tissue.

tendon. Fibrous tissue that connects muscle to bone, consisting primarily of collagen and containing little vasculature.

CCI Version 16.3
01710, 0213T, 0216T, 0228T, 0230T, 20650, 20680, 24100-24102, 24300, 24332, 24495, 24530, 24535, 24538, 25020, 25360, 29049-29075, 29105, 29240-29260, 29700-29715, 36000, 36400-36410, 36420-36430, 36440, 36600, 36640, 37202, 43752, 51701-51703, 62310-62319, 64400-64435, 64445-64450, 64479, 64483, 64490, 64493, 64505-64530, 64708, 64718, 69990, 93000-93010, 93040-93042, 93318, 94002, 94200, 94250, 94680-94690, 94770, 95812-95816, 95819, 95822, 95829, 95955, 96360, 96365, 96372, 96374-96376, 97597-97598, 97602-97606, 99148-99149, 99150

Also not with 24545: 12004, 29834

Also not with 24546: 24400, 24545, 25024-25025

Note: These CCI edits are used for Medicare. Other payers may reimburse on codes listed above.

Medicare Edits

	Fac RVU	Non-Fac RVU	FUD	Assist
24545	27.02	27.02	90	80
24546	30.57	30.57	90	80

Medicare References: 100-2,15,260; 100-4,12,30; 100-4,12,90.3; 100-4,14,10

24560-24565

24560 Closed treatment of humeral epicondylar fracture, medial or lateral; without manipulation
24565 with manipulation

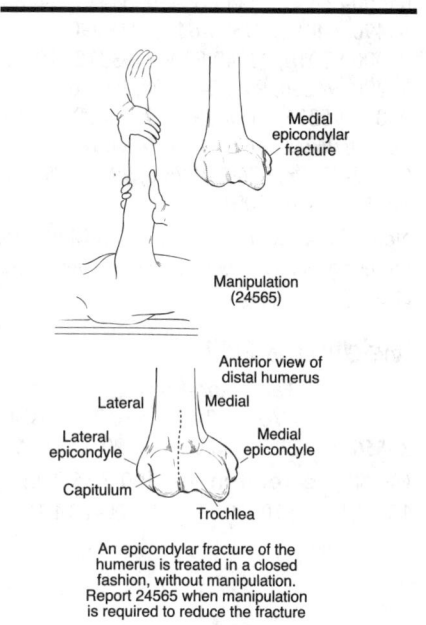

Explanation
The physician repairs a humeral medial or lateral epicondylar fracture without incision or manipulation in 24560. Closed treatment of a humeral epicondylar fracture is indicated when the fragments are not separated and appear stable. No manipulation is required. No incisions are made. The arm is placed in a posterior elbow splint at 90 degrees of flexion. Report 24565 if manipulation is required to reduce the fracture into position.

Coding Tips
According to CPT guidelines, cast application or strapping (including removal) is only reported as a replacement procedure or when the cast application or strapping is an initial service performed without a restorative treatment or procedure. See "Application of Casts and Strapping" in the CPT book in the Surgery Section, under the Musculoskeletal system. In 24565, local anesthesia is included in the service. However, this procedure may be performed under general anesthesia, depending on the age and/or condition of the patient. For radiology services, see 73060–73080. Distal humeral fractures are site specific. For percutaneous skeletal fixation of humeral epicondylar fractures, see 24566. For open treatment of humeral epicondylar fractures, see 24575. For supracondylar or transcondylar humeral fracture treatments, see 24530–24546. For humeral shaft fractures, see 24500–24516. For humeral condylar fractures, medial or lateral, see 24576–24582.

ICD-9-CM Procedural
79.01 Closed reduction of fracture of humerus without internal fixation
93.54 Application of splint

Anesthesia
01730

ICD-9-CM Diagnostic
733.11 Pathologic fracture of humerus
812.40 Closed fracture of unspecified part of lower end of humerus
812.42 Closed fracture of lateral condyle of humerus
812.43 Closed fracture of medial condyle of humerus
812.44 Closed fracture of unspecified condyle(s) of humerus
812.49 Other closed fracture of lower end of humerus

Terms To Know
closed fracture. Break in a bone without a concomitant opening in the skin. A closed fracture is coded when the type of fracture is not specified.

flexion. Act of bending or being bent.

lateral. To/on the side.

medial. Middle or midline.

posterior. Located in the back part or caudal end of the body.

CCI Version 16.3
01710, 0213T, 0216T, 0228T, 0230T, 24300, 29049-29075, 29105, 29240-29260, 29700-29715, 36000, 36400-36410, 36420-36430, 36440, 36600, 36640, 37202, 43752, 51701-51703, 62310-62319, 64400-64435, 64445-64450, 64479, 64483, 64490, 64493, 64505-64530, 69990, 93000-93010, 93040-93042, 93318, 94002, 94200, 94250, 94680-94690, 94770, 95812-95816, 95819, 95822, 95829, 95955, 96360, 96365, 96372, 96374-96376, 97597-97598, 97602-97606, 99148-99149, 99150

Also not with 24565: 24560, J0670, J2001

Note: These CCI edits are used for Medicare. Other payers may reimburse on codes listed above.

Medicare Edits

	Fac RVU	Non-Fac RVU	FUD	Assist
24560	8.0	8.95	90	N/A
24565	13.78	14.94	90	N/A

Medicare References: 100-2,15,260; 100-4,12,30; 100-4,12,90.3; 100-4,14,10

24566

24566 Percutaneous skeletal fixation of humeral epicondylar fracture, medial or lateral, with manipulation

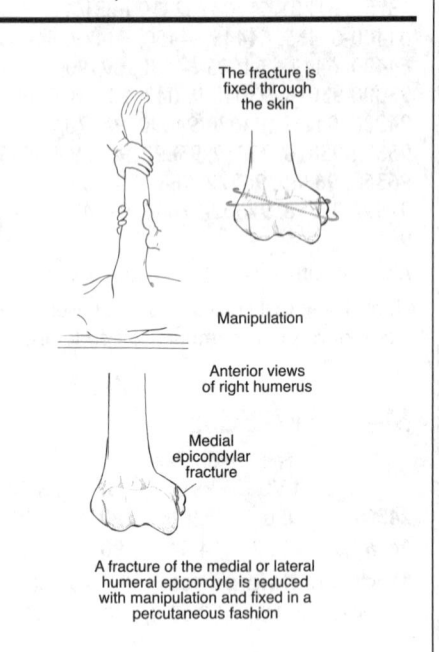

The fracture is fixed through the skin

Manipulation

Anterior views of right humerus

Medial epicondylar fracture

A fracture of the medial or lateral humeral epicondyle is reduced with manipulation and fixed in a percutaneous fashion

Explanation
The physician fixates a humeral medial or lateral epicondylar fracture percutaneously. The physician uses separately reportable fluoroscopy to realign the fracture by manipulation first. Once the bone is realigned, the physician fixates the pieces to the humeral shaft by driving percutaneous wires through the pieces and into the shaft.

Coding Tips
According to CPT guidelines, cast application or strapping (including removal) is only reported as a replacement procedure or when the cast application or strapping is an initial service performed without a restorative treatment or procedure. See "Application of Casts and Strapping" in the CPT book in the Surgery Section, under the Musculoskeletal system. Distal humeral fractures are site specific. For closed treatment of humeral epicondylar fractures, see 24560 and 24565. For open treatment of humeral epicondylar fractures, see 24575. For supracondylar or transcondylar humeral fracture treatments, see 24530–24546. For humeral shaft fractures, see 24500–24516. For humeral condylar fractures, medial or lateral, see 24576–24582.

ICD-9-CM Procedural
79.11 Closed reduction of fracture of humerus with internal fixation

Anesthesia
24566 01730

ICD-9-CM Diagnostic
733.11 Pathologic fracture of humerus
812.40 Closed fracture of unspecified part of lower end of humerus
812.42 Closed fracture of lateral condyle of humerus
812.43 Closed fracture of medial condyle of humerus
812.44 Closed fracture of unspecified condyle(s) of humerus
812.49 Other closed fracture of lower end of humerus
812.50 Open fracture of unspecified part of lower end of humerus
812.52 Open fracture of lateral condyle of humerus
812.53 Open fracture of medial condyle of humerus
812.54 Open fracture of unspecified condyle(s) of humerus
812.59 Other open fracture of lower end of humerus

Terms To Know

closed fracture. Break in a bone without a concomitant opening in the skin. A closed fracture is coded when the type of fracture is not specified.

lateral. To/on the side.

medial. Middle or midline.

open fracture. Exposed break in a bone, always considered compound due to its high risk of infection from the open wound leading to the fracture. Broken bone ends may protrude through the skin and contaminants or foreign bodies are often embedded in the tissues.

CCI Version 16.3
01710, 0213T, 0216T, 0228T, 0230T, 20650, 24300, 24560-24565, 29049-29075, 29105, 29240-29260, 36000, 36400-36410, 36420-36430, 36440, 36600, 36640, 37202, 43752, 51701-51703, 62310-62319, 64400-64435, 64445-64450, 64479, 64483, 64490, 64493, 64505-64530, 69990, 93000-93010, 93040-93042, 93318, 94002, 94200, 94250, 94680-94690, 94770, 95812-95816, 95819, 95822, 95829, 95955, 96360, 96365, 96372, 96374-96376, 97597-97598, 97602-97606, 99148-99149, 99150, J0670, J2001

Note: These CCI edits are used for Medicare. Other payers may reimburse on codes listed above.

Medicare Edits

	Fac RVU	Non-Fac RVU	FUD	Assist
24566	20.7	20.7	90	N/A

Medicare References: 100-2,15,260; 100-4,12,30; 100-4,12,90.3; 100-4,14,10

24575

24575 Open treatment of humeral epicondylar fracture, medial or lateral, includes internal fixation, when performed

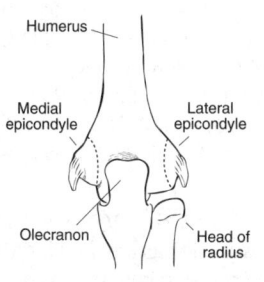

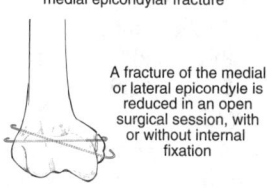

Explanation

The physician openly treats a fracture of the medial or lateral epicondyle of the humerus. The physician makes an incision in the skin overlying the fractured epicondyle. This is carried deep through the fascia to the bone. Fracture fragments are identified and manipulated into the appropriate anatomic position. The epicondyle may be immobilized in place using internal fixation devices such as plates, screws, or wires if needed. The wound is irrigated and closed in layers.

Coding Tips

According to CPT guidelines, cast application or strapping (including removal) is only reported as a replacement procedure or when the cast application or strapping is an initial service performed without a restorative treatment or procedure. See "Application of Casts and Strapping" in the CPT book in the Surgery Section, under the Musculoskeletal system. Distal humeral fractures are site specific. For closed treatment of humeral epicondylar fractures, see 24560 and 24565. For percutaneous skeletal fixation of humeral epicondylar fractures, see 24566. For supracondylar or transcondylar humeral fracture treatments, see 24530–24546. For humeral shaft fractures, see 24500–24516. For humeral condylar fractures, medial or lateral, see 24576–24582.

ICD-9-CM Procedural

- 79.21 Open reduction of fracture of humerus without internal fixation
- 79.31 Open reduction of fracture of humerus with internal fixation

Anesthesia

24575 01740

ICD-9-CM Diagnostic

- 733.11 Pathologic fracture of humerus
- 812.40 Closed fracture of unspecified part of lower end of humerus
- 812.42 Closed fracture of lateral condyle of humerus
- 812.43 Closed fracture of medial condyle of humerus
- 812.49 Other closed fracture of lower end of humerus
- 812.50 Open fracture of unspecified part of lower end of humerus
- 812.52 Open fracture of lateral condyle of humerus
- 812.53 Open fracture of medial condyle of humerus
- 812.54 Open fracture of unspecified condyle(s) of humerus
- 812.59 Other open fracture of lower end of humerus

Terms To Know

closed fracture. Break in a bone without a concomitant opening in the skin. A closed fracture is coded when the type of fracture is not specified.

fascia. Fibrous sheet or band of tissue that envelops organs, muscles, and groupings of muscles.

medial. Middle or midline.

open fracture. Exposed break in a bone, always considered compound due to its high risk of infection from the open wound leading to the fracture. Broken bone ends may protrude through the skin and contaminants or foreign bodies are often embedded in the tissues.

CCI Version 16.3

01710, 0213T, 0216T, 0228T, 0230T, 20650, 20680, 24000, 24006, 24100-24102, 24300, 24332, 24495, 24560-24566, 25020, 25024-25025, 29049-29075, 29105, 29240-29260, 29700-29715, 36000, 36400-36410, 36420-36430, 36440, 36600, 36640, 37202, 43752, 51701-51703, 62310-62319, 64400-64435, 64445-64450, 64479, 64483, 64490, 64493, 64505-64530, 64708, 69990, 93000-93010, 93040-93042, 93318, 94002, 94200, 94250, 94680-94690, 94770, 95812-95816, 95819, 95822, 95829, 95955, 96360, 96365, 96372, 96374-96376, 97597-97598, 97602-97606, 99148-99149, 99150

Note: These CCI edits are used for Medicare. Other payers may reimburse on codes listed above.

Medicare Edits

	Fac RVU	Non-Fac RVU	FUD	Assist
24575	21.32	21.32	90	80

Medicare References: 100-2,15,260; 100-4,12,30; 100-4,12,90.3; 100-4,14,10

24576-24577

24576 Closed treatment of humeral condylar fracture, medial or lateral; without manipulation
24577 with manipulation

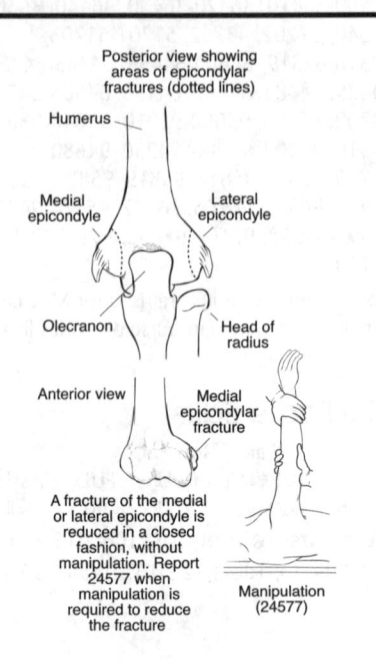

Posterior view showing areas of epicondylar fractures (dotted lines)

A fracture of the medial or lateral epicondyle is reduced in a closed fashion, without manipulation. Report 24577 when manipulation is required to reduce the fracture

Explanation

The physician repairs a humeral medial or lateral condylar fracture without incision or manipulation in 24576. Closed treatment of a humeral condylar fracture is indicated when the fragments are not separated and appear stable. No manipulation is required. No incisions are made. The arm is placed in a posterior elbow splint at 90 degrees of flexion. Report 24577 if manipulation is required to reduce the fracture into position.

Coding Tips

According to CPT guidelines, cast application or strapping (including removal) is only reported as a replacement procedure or when the cast application or strapping is an initial service performed without a restorative treatment or procedure. See "Application of Casts and Strapping" in the CPT book in the Surgery Section, under the Musculoskeletal system. In 24577, local anesthesia is included in the service. However, this procedure may be performed under general anesthesia, depending on the age and/or condition of the patient. For radiology services, see 73060–73080. Distal humeral fractures are site specific. For open treatment of humeral condylar fractures, medial or lateral, see 24579. For percutaneous skeletal fixation of condylar fractures, see 24582. For closed treatment of humeral epicondylar fractures, see 24560 and 24565. For percutaneous skeletal fixation of humeral epicondylar fractures, see 24566. For supracondylar or transcondylar humeral fracture treatments, see 24530–24546. For humeral shaft fractures, see 24500–24516.

ICD-9-CM Procedural

- 79.01 Closed reduction of fracture of humerus without internal fixation
- 93.54 Application of splint

Anesthesia
01730

ICD-9-CM Diagnostic

- 733.11 Pathologic fracture of humerus
- 812.40 Closed fracture of unspecified part of lower end of humerus
- 812.41 Closed fracture of supracondylar humerus
- 812.42 Closed fracture of lateral condyle of humerus
- 812.43 Closed fracture of medial condyle of humerus
- 812.44 Closed fracture of unspecified condyle(s) of humerus
- 812.49 Other closed fracture of lower end of humerus

Terms To Know

closed fracture. Break in a bone without a concomitant opening in the skin. A closed fracture is coded when the type of fracture is not specified.

condyle. Rounded end of a bone that forms an articulation.

flexion. Act of bending or being bent.

manipulation. Skillful treatment by hand to reduce fractures and dislocations, or provide therapy through forceful passive movement of a joint beyond its active limit of motion.

posterior. Located in the back part or caudal end of the body.

CCI Version 16.3

01710, 0213T, 0216T, 0228T, 0230T, 24300, 29049-29075, 29105, 29240-29260, 29700-29715, 36000, 36400-36410, 36420-36430, 36440, 36600, 36640, 37202, 43752, 51701-51703, 62310-62319, 64400-64435, 64445-64450, 64479, 64483, 64490, 64493, 64505-64530, 69990, 93000-93010, 93040-93042, 93318, 94002, 94200, 94250, 94680-94690, 94770, 95812-95816, 95819, 95822, 95829, 95955, 96360, 96365, 96372, 96374-96376, 97597-97598, 97602-97606, 99148-99149, 99150

Also not with 24577: 24576, J0670, J2001

Note: These CCI edits are used for Medicare. Other payers may reimburse on codes listed above.

Medicare Edits

	Fac RVU	Non-Fac RVU	FUD	Assist
24576	8.54	9.49	90	N/A
24577	14.23	15.46	90	N/A

Medicare References: 100-2,15,260; 100-4,12,30; 100-4,12,90.3; 100-4,14,10

24579

24579 Open treatment of humeral condylar fracture, medial or lateral, includes internal fixation, when performed

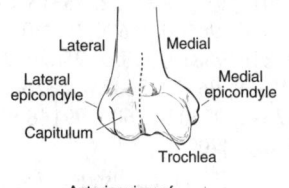

Lateral
Medial
Lateral epicondyle
Medial epicondyle
Capitulum
Trochlea
Anterior view of distal humerus

Lateral condylar fracture
Medial condylar fracture
Several types of condylar fractures are described in current literature

A medial or lateral humeral condylar fracture is treated in an open surgical session, with or without internal fixation

Explanation

The physician openly repairs a humeral condylar fracture, medial or lateral. The physician makes an incision exposing the posterior elbow. Skin and subcutaneous tissue are reflected to expose the olecranon and triceps tendon. The ulnar nerve is retracted. The condyles are reduced and may be temporarily fixed with internal fixation devices such as wires, or screws may be placed across the major fragments. Small fragments may require excision. The incision is closed with sutures and the elbow is immobilized in a posterior elbow splint.

Coding Tips

According to CPT guidelines, cast application or strapping (including removal) is only reported as a replacement procedure or when the cast application or strapping is an initial service performed without a restorative treatment or procedure. See "Application of Casts and Strapping" in the CPT book in the Surgery Section, under the Musculoskeletal system. Distal humeral fractures are site specific. For closed treatment of humeral condylar fractures, medial or lateral, see 24576 and 24577. For percutaneous skeletal fixation of condylar fractures, see 24582. For closed treatment of humeral epicondylar fractures, see 24560 and 24565. For percutaneous skeletal fixation of humeral epicondylar fractures, see 24566. For supracondylar or transcondylar humeral fracture treatments, see 24530–24546. For humeral shaft fractures, see 24500–24516.

ICD-9-CM Procedural

- 79.21 Open reduction of fracture of humerus without internal fixation
- 79.31 Open reduction of fracture of humerus with internal fixation

Anesthesia
24579   01740

ICD-9-CM Diagnostic

- 733.11 Pathologic fracture of humerus
- 812.40 Closed fracture of unspecified part of lower end of humerus
- 812.42 Closed fracture of lateral condyle of humerus
- 812.43 Closed fracture of medial condyle of humerus
- 812.44 Closed fracture of unspecified condyle(s) of humerus
- 812.49 Other closed fracture of lower end of humerus
- 812.50 Open fracture of unspecified part of lower end of humerus
- 812.52 Open fracture of lateral condyle of humerus
- 812.53 Open fracture of medial condyle of humerus
- 812.54 Open fracture of unspecified condyle(s) of humerus
- 812.59 Other open fracture of lower end of humerus

Terms To Know

closed fracture. Break in a bone without a concomitant opening in the skin. A closed fracture is coded when the type of fracture is not specified.

condyle. Rounded end of a bone that forms an articulation.

medial. Middle or midline.

open fracture. Exposed break in a bone, always considered compound due to its high risk of infection from the open wound leading to the fracture. Broken bone ends may protrude through the skin and contaminants or foreign bodies are often embedded in the tissues.

posterior. Located in the back part or caudal end of the body.

tendon. Fibrous tissue that connects muscle to bone, consisting primarily of collagen and containing little vasculature.

CCI Version 16.3

01710, 0213T, 0216T, 0228T, 0230T, 20650, 20680, 24000, 24006, 24100-24102, 24300, 24332, 24495, 24576-24577, 24582, 25020, 25024-25025, 29049-29075, 29105, 29240-29260, 29700-29715, 36000, 36400-36410, 36420-36430, 36440, 36600, 36640, 37202, 43752, 51701-51703, 62310-62319, 64400-64435, 64445-64450, 64479, 64483, 64490, 64493, 64505-64530, 64708, 64718, 69990, 93000-93010, 93040-93042, 93318, 94002, 94200, 94250, 94680-94690, 94770, 95812-95816, 95819, 95822, 95829, 95955, 96360, 96365, 96372, 96374-96376, 97597-97598, 97602-97606, 99148-99149, 99150

Note: These CCI edits are used for Medicare. Other payers may reimburse on codes listed above.

Medicare Edits

	Fac RVU	Non-Fac RVU	FUD	Assist
24579	24.32	24.32	90	80

Medicare References: 100-2,15,260; 100-4,12,30; 100-4,12,90.3; 100-4,14,10

24582

24582 Percutaneous skeletal fixation of humeral condylar fracture, medial or lateral, with manipulation

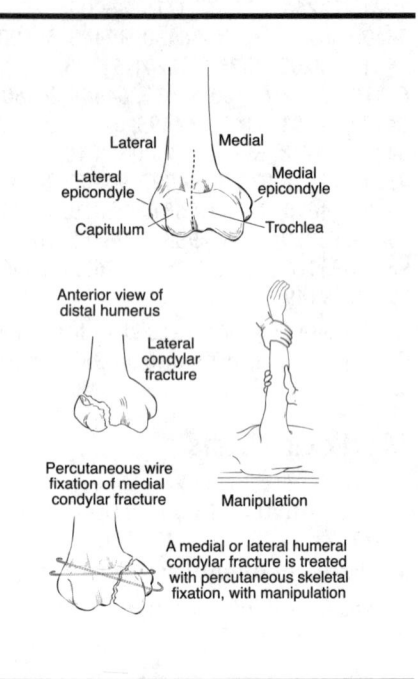

Explanation
The physician fixates a humeral medial or lateral condylar fracture percutaneously by manipulating the fracture in a closed fashion and inserting pins through the skin and bones to maintain appropriate position. Separately reportable x-rays, including fluoroscopic views, are obtained to ascertain the extent of the fracture. The physician manipulates the arm, elbow, and forearm in such a way to restore the fractured pieces to the acceptable position. The physician places pins through the skin and into the bones to immobilize the reduction until healing is complete.

Coding Tips
According to CPT guidelines, cast application or strapping (including removal) is only reported as a replacement procedure or when the cast application or strapping is an initial service performed without a restorative treatment or procedure. See "Application of Casts and Strapping" in the CPT book in the Surgery Section, under the Musculoskeletal system. Distal humeral fractures are site specific. For closed treatment of humeral condylar fractures, medial or lateral, see 24576 and 24577. For open treatment of condylar fractures, see 24579. For closed treatment of humeral epicondylar fractures, see 24560 and 24565. For percutaneous skeletal fixation of humeral epicondylar fractures, see 24566. For supracondylar or transcondylar humeral fracture treatments, see 24530–24546. For humeral shaft fractures, see 24500–24516.

ICD-9-CM Procedural
79.11 Closed reduction of fracture of humerus with internal fixation

Anesthesia
24582 01730

ICD-9-CM Diagnostic
733.11 Pathologic fracture of humerus
812.40 Closed fracture of unspecified part of lower end of humerus
812.42 Closed fracture of lateral condyle of humerus
812.43 Closed fracture of medial condyle of humerus
812.44 Closed fracture of unspecified condyle(s) of humerus
812.49 Other closed fracture of lower end of humerus
812.50 Open fracture of unspecified part of lower end of humerus
812.52 Open fracture of lateral condyle of humerus
812.53 Open fracture of medial condyle of humerus
812.54 Open fracture of unspecified condyle(s) of humerus
812.59 Other open fracture of lower end of humerus

Terms To Know
closed fracture. Break in a bone without a concomitant opening in the skin. A closed fracture is coded when the type of fracture is not specified.

lateral. To/on the side.

medial. Middle or midline.

open fracture. Exposed break in a bone, always considered compound due to its high risk of infection from the open wound leading to the fracture. Broken bone ends may protrude through the skin and contaminants or foreign bodies are often embedded in the tissues.

CCI Version 16.3
01710, 0213T, 0216T, 0228T, 0230T, 20650, 24300, 24577, 29049-29075, 29105, 29240-29260, 36000, 36400-36410, 36420-36430, 36440, 36600, 36640, 37202, 43752, 51701-51703, 62310-62319, 64400-64435, 64445-64450, 64479, 64483, 64490, 64493, 64505-64530, 69990, 93000-93010, 93040-93042, 93318, 94002, 94200, 94250, 94680-94690, 94770, 95812-95816, 95819, 95822, 95829, 95955, 96360, 96365, 96372, 96374-96376, 97597-97598, 97602-97606, 99148-99149, 99150, J0670, J2001

Note: These CCI edits are used for Medicare. Other payers may reimburse on codes listed above.

Medicare Edits

	Fac RVU	Non-Fac RVU	FUD	Assist
24582	23.2	23.2	90	N/A

Medicare References: 100-2,15,260; 100-4,12,30; 100-4,12,90.3; 100-4,14,10

24586-24587

24586 Open treatment of periarticular fracture and/or dislocation of the elbow (fracture distal humerus and proximal ulna and/or proximal radius);

24587 with implant arthroplasty

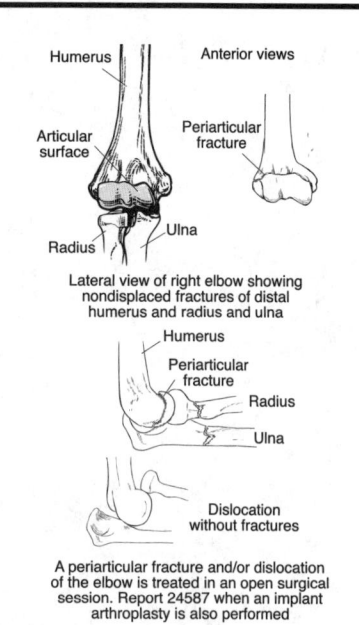

A periarticular fracture and/or dislocation of the elbow is treated in an open surgical session. Report 24587 when an implant arthroplasty is also performed.

Explanation

The physician openly treats a periarticular fracture (distal humerus and proximal ulna and/or proximal radius) and/or dislocation of the elbow. The physician may make more than one incision depending on the extent of the fractures and/or dislocation. If there is a dislocation, it is reduced (realigned) first. The fractures are reduced and secured with plates, screws, pins, wires, or a combination of these. The physician may place a pin through the olecranon for skeletal traction in a patient with multiple injuries to temporarily stabilize the fracture and/or dislocation. In 24587, if joint surface congruity cannot be restored, the physician performs a total elbow arthroplasty. For elbow arthroplasty, the physician makes a straight, midline, posterior incision. The ulnar nerve is identified and retracted for protection. The triceps mechanism is elevated from the olecranon. The collateral ligaments are preserved. A portion of the olecranon is cut and removed to allow implantation of the ulnar stem. The distal humerus is prepared by removing cancellous bone with a curette. The physician uses a rasp to open and contour the humeral and ulnar medullary canals for insertion of the prosthetic stems. Cement is inserted into the ulnar and humeral medullary canals with a cement gun or syringe. The elbow is flexed and the prosthesis is inserted into the humeral and ulnar medullary canals at the same time. The elbow joint is fully extended while the cement hardens. The triceps mechanism is sutured back to fascia. The ulnar nerve is positioned anterior to the elbow. Arthroplasty may be performed in conjunction with some internal fixation for fracture reduction and stabilization.

Coding Tips

According to CPT guidelines, cast application or strapping (including removal) is only reported as a replacement procedure or when the cast application or strapping is an initial service performed without a restorative treatment or procedure. See "Application of Casts and Strapping" in the CPT book in the Surgery Section, under the Musculoskeletal system. For arthroplasty of elbow with distal humeral prosthetic replacement without fracture, see 24361.

ICD-9-CM Procedural

- 79.21 Open reduction of fracture of humerus without internal fixation
- 79.32 Open reduction of fracture of radius and ulna with internal fixation
- 79.82 Open reduction of dislocation of elbow
- 81.84 Total elbow replacement

Anesthesia
01740

ICD-9-CM Diagnostic

- 718.72 Developmental dislocation of joint, upper arm
- 733.11 Pathologic fracture of humerus
- 733.19 Pathologic fracture of other specified site
- 812.41 Closed fracture of supracondylar humerus
- 812.42 Closed fracture of lateral condyle of humerus
- 812.43 Closed fracture of medial condyle of humerus
- 812.49 Other closed fracture of lower end of humerus
- 812.51 Open fracture of supracondylar humerus
- 812.52 Open fracture of lateral condyle of humerus
- 812.53 Open fracture of medial condyle of humerus
- 812.59 Other open fracture of lower end of humerus
- 813.01 Closed fracture of olecranon process of ulna
- 813.02 Closed fracture of coronoid process of ulna
- 813.05 Closed fracture of head of radius
- 813.06 Closed fracture of neck of radius
- 813.08 Closed fracture of radius with ulna, upper end (any part)
- 813.11 Open fracture of olecranon process of ulna
- 813.12 Open fracture of coronoid process of ulna
- 813.14 Other and unspecified open fractures of proximal end of ulna (alone)
- 813.15 Open fracture of head of radius
- 813.17 Other and unspecified open fractures of proximal end of radius (alone)
- 832.01 Closed anterior dislocation of elbow
- 832.10 Open unspecified dislocation of elbow
- 832.11 Open anterior dislocation of elbow
- 832.12 Open posterior dislocation of elbow
- 832.13 Open medial dislocation of elbow
- 832.14 Open lateral dislocation of elbow
- 832.19 Open dislocation of other site of elbow

CCI Version 16.3

01710, 0213T, 0216T, 0228T, 0230T, 20680, 24006, 24100-24102, 24130, 24300, 24332, 24495, 24600-24605, 25020, 25024-25025, 25360-25365, 29049-29075, 29105, 29240-29260, 29700-29715, 36000, 36400-36410, 36420-36430, 36440, 36600, 36640, 37202, 43752, 51701-51703, 62310-62319, 64400-64435, 64445-64450, 64479, 64483, 64490, 64493, 64505-64530, 64708, 64718, 69990, 93000-93010, 93040-93042, 93318, 94002, 94200, 94250, 94680-94690, 94770, 95812-95816, 95819, 95822, 95829, 95955, 96360, 96365, 96372, 96374-96376, 97597-97598, 97602-97606, 99148-99149, 99150

Also not with 24586: 24343-24346, 29425, 29834

Also not with 24587: 24000, 24400-24410, 24586, 29834-29836

Note: These CCI edits are used for Medicare. Other payers may reimburse on codes listed above.

Medicare Edits

	Fac RVU	Non-Fac RVU	FUD	Assist
24586	31.9	31.9	90	80
24587	31.83	31.83	90	80

Medicare References: 100-2,15,260; 100-4,12,30; 100-4,12,90.3; 100-4,14,10

24600-24605

24600 Treatment of closed elbow dislocation; without anesthesia
24605 requiring anesthesia

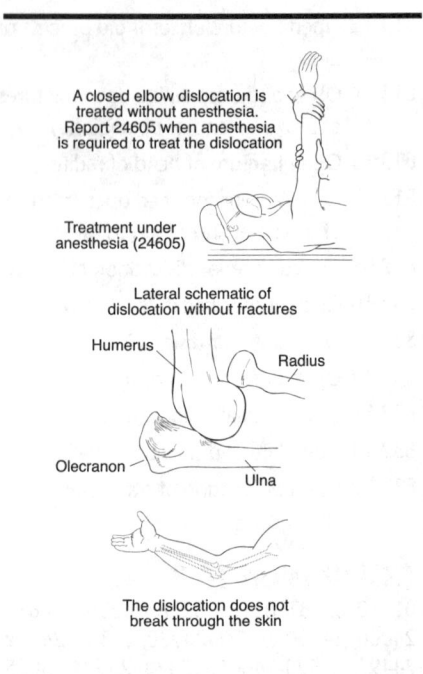

A closed elbow dislocation is treated without anesthesia. Report 24605 when anesthesia is required to treat the dislocation

Treatment under anesthesia (24605)

Lateral schematic of dislocation without fractures

Humerus
Radius
Olecranon
Ulna

The dislocation does not break through the skin

Explanation

The physician performs closed treatment of elbow dislocation when there are no fractures. The forearm typically dislocates posteriorly. The physician manually reduces (realigns) the dislocation with pressure to the area. The elbow is then placed in a posterior elbow splint or elbow brace at 90 degrees of flexion with the forearm supinated. The procedure is performed without anesthesia in 24600 or with anesthesia in 24605.

Coding Tips

According to CPT guidelines, cast application or strapping (including removal) is only reported as a replacement procedure or when the cast application or strapping is an initial service performed without a restorative treatment or procedure. See "Application of Casts and Strapping" in the CPT book in the Surgery Section, under the Musculoskeletal system. For radiology services, see 73070–73085. For open treatment of an elbow dislocation, see 24615. For a periarticular fracture dislocation of the elbow, see 24586 or 24587. For a Monteggia type fracture dislocation, see 24620 or 24635. For treatment of a radial head subluxation (nursemaid elbow), see 24640.

ICD-9-CM Procedural

79.72 Closed reduction of dislocation of elbow

Anesthesia
24600 N/A
24605 01730

ICD-9-CM Diagnostic

718.72 Developmental dislocation of joint, upper arm
832.00 Closed unspecified dislocation of elbow
832.01 Closed anterior dislocation of elbow
832.02 Closed posterior dislocation of elbow
832.03 Closed medial dislocation of elbow
832.04 Closed lateral dislocation of elbow
832.09 Closed dislocation of other site of elbow
832.2 Nursemaid's elbow

Terms To Know

anterior. Situated in the front area or toward the belly surface of the body; an anatomical reference point used to show the position and relationship of one body structure to another.

developmental dislocation. Displacement of a body part occurring in the developmental phase of childhood.

flexion. Act of bending or being bent.

lateral. To/on the side.

medial. Middle or midline.

posterior. Located in the back part or caudal end of the body.

CCI Version 16.3

01710, 0213T, 0216T, 0228T, 0230T, 24300, 24640, 29049-29075, 29105, 29240-29260, 36000, 36400-36410, 36420-36430, 36440, 36600, 36640, 37202, 43752, 51701-51703, 62310-62319, 64400-64435, 64445-64450, 64479, 64483, 64490, 64493, 64505-64530, 69990, 93000-93010, 93040-93042, 93318, 94002, 94200, 94250, 94680-94690, 94770, 95812-95816, 95819, 95822, 95829, 95955, 96360, 96365, 96372, 96374-96376, 97597-97598, 97602-97606, 99148-99149, 99150

Also not with 24605: 24600

Note: These CCI edits are used for Medicare. Other payers may reimburse on codes listed above.

Medicare Edits

	Fac RVU	Non-Fac RVU	FUD	Assist
24600	9.37	10.23	90	N/A
24605	13.39	13.39	90	N/A

Medicare References: 100-2,15,260; 100-4,12,30; 100-4,12,90.3; 100-4,14,10

24615

24615 Open treatment of acute or chronic elbow dislocation

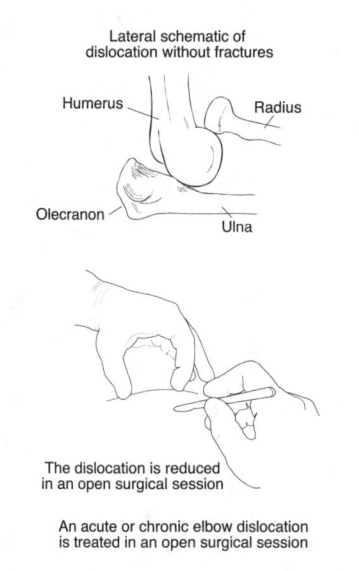

Lateral schematic of dislocation without fractures

The dislocation is reduced in an open surgical session

An acute or chronic elbow dislocation is treated in an open surgical session

Explanation

To openly treat an acute or chronic elbow dislocation, the physician may use the Osborne-Cotterill technique of dislocation treatment. The physician makes a longitudinal incision over the lateral aspect of the elbow. The physician dissects the elbow posterior to the lateral collateral ligament. Any bone fragments are removed. The physician roughens the bone at the lateral epicondyle and lateral side of the capitellum. The physician uses an awl to make one or two transverse holes through the lateral condyle close to the articular surface of the humerus. Sutures are passed through these holes and through the posterolateral part of the capsule. The capsule is fixed to the bone as tightly as possible. The incision is repaired in layers. A long arm cast or splint is applied with the elbow in 40 degrees of flexion for approximately four weeks.

Coding Tips

According to CPT guidelines, cast application or strapping (including removal) is only reported as a replacement procedure or when the cast application or strapping is an initial service performed without a restorative treatment or procedure. See "Application of Casts and Strapping" in the CPT book in the Surgery Section, under the Musculoskeletal system. For closed treatment of an elbow dislocation, see 24600–24605. For a periarticular fracture dislocation of the elbow, see 24586 or 24587. For a Monteggia type fracture dislocation, see 24620 or 24635. For treatment of a radial head subluxation (nursemaid elbow), see 24640.

ICD-9-CM Procedural

79.82 Open reduction of dislocation of elbow

Anesthesia

24615 01740

ICD-9-CM Diagnostic

718.32 Recurrent dislocation of upper arm joint
718.72 Developmental dislocation of joint, upper arm
754.89 Other specified nonteratogenic anomalies
832.01 Closed anterior dislocation of elbow
832.02 Closed posterior dislocation of elbow
832.03 Closed medial dislocation of elbow
832.04 Closed lateral dislocation of elbow
832.09 Closed dislocation of other site of elbow
832.10 Open unspecified dislocation of elbow
832.11 Open anterior dislocation of elbow
832.12 Open posterior dislocation of elbow
832.13 Open medial dislocation of elbow
832.14 Open lateral dislocation of elbow
832.19 Open dislocation of other site of elbow

Terms To Know

acute. Sudden, severe. Documentation and reporting of an acute condition is important to establishing medical necessity.

anterior. Situated in the front area or toward the belly surface of the body; an anatomical reference point used to show the position and relationship of one body structure to another.

chronic. Persistent, continuing, or recurring.

flexion. Act of bending or being bent.

lateral. To/on the side.

medial. Middle or midline.

posterior. Located in the back part or caudal end of the body.

CCI Version 16.3

01710, 0213T, 0216T, 0228T, 0230T, 24000, 24006, 24100-24102, 24300, 24332, 24343-24346, 24357, 24600-24605, 25360, 29049-29075, 29105, 29240-29260, 29834, 36000, 36400-36410, 36420-36430, 36440, 36600, 36640, 37202, 43752, 51701-51703, 62310-62319, 64400-64435, 64445-64450, 64479, 64483, 64490, 64493, 64505-64530, 64718, 69990, 93000-93010, 93040-93042, 93318, 94002, 94200, 94250, 94680-94690, 94770, 95812-95816, 95819, 95822, 95829, 95955, 96360, 96365, 96372, 96374-96376, 97597-97598, 97602-97606, 99148-99149, 99150

Note: These CCI edits are used for Medicare. Other payers may reimburse on codes listed above.

Medicare Edits

	Fac RVU	Non-Fac RVU	FUD	Assist
24615	20.76	20.76	90	80

Medicare References: 100-2,15,260; 100-4,12,30; 100-4,12,90.3; 100-4,14,10

24620

24620 Closed treatment of Monteggia type of fracture dislocation at elbow (fracture proximal end of ulna with dislocation of radial head), with manipulation

Explanation
The physician treats a Monteggia type fracture dislocation at the elbow (fracture of the proximal end of the ulna with dislocation of the radial head) by manipulation. No incisions are made. The physician manually realigns the radial head back into position. If alignment of the ulnar fracture is not adequate, the physician may also manually align this fracture. Once satisfactory and stable reduction (realignment) is achieved, the elbow is placed in a posterior splint or cast. The elbow is immobilized at 120 degrees of flexion to prevent recurrent dislocation of the radial head.

Coding Tips
According to CPT guidelines, cast application or strapping (including removal) is only reported as a replacement procedure or when the cast application or strapping is an initial service performed without a restorative treatment or procedure. See "Application of Casts and Strapping" in the CPT book in the Surgery Section, under the Musculoskeletal system. Local anesthesia is included in this service. However, this procedure may be performed under general anesthesia, depending on the age and/or condition of the patient. For open treatment of a Monteggia type fracture dislocation, see 24635. For treatment of a radial head subluxation (nursemaid elbow), see 24640. For closed treatment of an elbow dislocation, see 24600–24605. For a periarticular fracture dislocation of the elbow, see 24586 or 24587.

ICD-9-CM Procedural
79.02 Closed reduction of fracture of radius and ulna without internal fixation
79.72 Closed reduction of dislocation of elbow

Anesthesia
24620 01730

ICD-9-CM Diagnostic
733.19 Pathologic fracture of other specified site
813.03 Closed Monteggia's fracture
813.13 Open Monteggia's fracture

Terms To Know
flexion. Act of bending or being bent.

Monteggia's fracture. Break in the proximal half of the ulnar shaft accompanied by a dislocation of the radial head.

posterior. Located in the back part or caudal end of the body.

proximal. Located closest to a specified reference point, usually the midline.

CCI Version 16.3
01710, 0213T, 0216T, 0228T, 0230T, 24300, 29049-29075, 29105, 29240-29260, 29700-29715, 36000, 36400-36410, 36420-36430, 36440, 36600, 36640, 37202, 43752, 51701-51703, 62310-62319, 64400-64435, 64445-64450, 64479, 64483, 64490, 64493, 64505-64530, 69990, 93000-93010, 93040-93042, 93318, 94002, 94200, 94250, 94680-94690, 94770, 95812-95816, 95819, 95822, 95829, 95955, 96360, 96365, 96372, 96374-96376, 97597-97598, 97602-97606, 99148-99149, 99150

Note: These CCI edits are used for Medicare. Other payers may reimburse on codes listed above.

Medicare Edits

	Fac RVU	Non-Fac RVU	FUD	Assist
24620	16.0	16.0	90	80

Medicare References: 100-2,15,260; 100-4,12,30; 100-4,12,90.3; 100-4,14,10

24635

24635 Open treatment of Monteggia type of fracture dislocation at elbow (fracture proximal end of ulna with dislocation of radial head), includes internal fixation, when performed

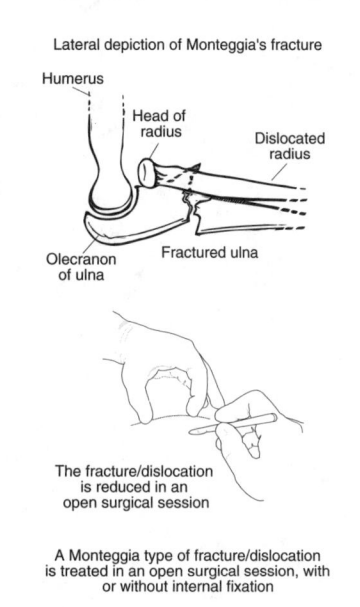

Lateral depiction of Monteggia's fracture

The fracture/dislocation is reduced in an open surgical session

A Monteggia type of fracture/dislocation is treated in an open surgical session, with or without internal fixation

Explanation

The physician openly treats a Monteggia type fracture dislocation at the elbow (fracture of the proximal end of the ulna with dislocation of the radial head), with or without internal fixation. The physician makes a longitudinal incision along the lateral aspect of the elbow. Dissection exposes the radial head and proximal ulna. The physician determines the status of the annular ligament. If the ligament is intact, the physician incises it so the radial head can be reduced. The ligament is repaired with nonabsorbable sutures. More commonly, the ligament is torn or avulsed, requiring reconstruction. If so, a strip of fascia 1.3 cm wide and 11 cm long is dissected from the muscles of the forearm. If the ulnar fracture is stable, no internal fixation is required. If the fracture is unstable, internal fixation is typically applied. A compression plate or an intramedullary nail may be utilized for internal fixation. The new annular ligament (fascial strip) is sutured about the radial neck. The incision is repaired in layers with sutures, staples, and/or Steri-strips. The elbow is placed in a posterior splint or cast at 120 degrees of flexion, preventing redislocation of the radial head.

Coding Tips

According to CPT guidelines, cast application or strapping (including removal) is only reported as a replacement procedure or when the cast application or strapping is an initial service performed without a restorative treatment or procedure. See "Application of Casts and Strapping" in the CPT book in the Surgery Section, under the Musculoskeletal system. For closed treatment of a Monteggia type fracture dislocation, see 24620. For treatment of a radial head subluxation (nursemaid elbow), see 24640. For closed treatment of an elbow dislocation, see 24600–24605. For a periarticular fracture dislocation of the elbow, see 24586 or 24587.

ICD-9-CM Procedural

- 79.22 Open reduction of fracture of radius and ulna without internal fixation
- 79.32 Open reduction of fracture of radius and ulna with internal fixation
- 79.82 Open reduction of dislocation of elbow
- 81.85 Other repair of elbow

Anesthesia

24635 01740

ICD-9-CM Diagnostic

- 813.03 Closed Monteggia's fracture
- 813.13 Open Monteggia's fracture

Terms To Know

dislocation. Displacement of a bone in relation to its neighboring tissue, especially a joint.

fascia. Fibrous sheet or band of tissue that envelops organs, muscles, and groupings of muscles.

internal fixation. Wires, pins, screws, and plates placed through or within the fractured area to stabilize and immobilize the injury.

ligament. Band or sheet of fibrous tissue that connects the articular surfaces of bones or supports visceral organs.

Monteggia's fracture. Break in the proximal half of the ulnar shaft accompanied by a dislocation of the radial head.

open wound. Opening or break of the skin.

reconstruction. Recreating, restoring, or rebuilding a body part or organ.

CCI Version 16.3

01710, 0213T, 0216T, 0228T, 0230T, 20650, 20680, 24000, 24006, 24100-24102, 24130, 24300, 24332, 24343-24346, 24495, 24600-24605, 24620, 25020, 25024-25025, 25360-25365, 29049-29075, 29105, 29240-29260, 29700-29715, 36000, 36400-36410, 36420-36430, 36440, 36600, 36640, 37202, 43752, 51701-51703, 62310-62319, 64400-64435, 64445-64450, 64479, 64483, 64490, 64493, 64505-64530, 64708, 64718, 69990, 93000-93010, 93040-93042, 93318, 94002, 94200, 94250, 94680-94690, 94770, 95812-95816, 95819, 95822, 95829, 95955, 96360, 96365, 96372, 96374-96376, 97597-97598, 97602-97606, 99148-99149, 99150

Note: These CCI edits are used for Medicare. Other payers may reimburse on codes listed above.

Medicare Edits

	Fac RVU	Non-Fac RVU	FUD	Assist
24635	20.49	20.49	90	80

Medicare References: 100-2,15,260; 100-4,12,30; 100-4,12,90.3; 100-4,14,10

24640

24640 Closed treatment of radial head subluxation in child, nursemaid elbow, with manipulation

Medial view of right elbow joint
Annular ligament on head of radius
Body of humerus
Medial epicondyle
Ulnar collateral ligaments
Ulna
Tubercle of coronoid process
Olecranon

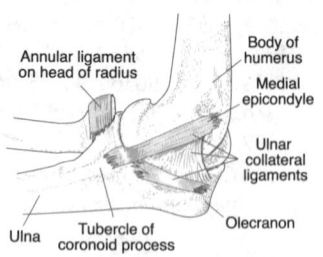

A subluxation (partial dislocation) of the radial head in a child is treated in a closed fashion with manipulation

Explanation

The physician performs closed treatment of nursemaid elbow in a child with manipulation. To realign a subluxated (partially dislocated) radial head, the physician supinates the forearm (palm upward) while flexing the elbow. No incisions are made. If stability of the radial head is questionable, a cast or splint is applied with the elbow in 90 degrees of flexion.

Coding Tips

According to CPT guidelines, cast application or strapping (including removal) is only reported as a replacement procedure or when the cast application or strapping is an initial service performed without a restorative treatment or procedure. See "Application of Casts and Strapping" in the CPT book in the Surgery Section, under the Musculoskeletal system. For radiology services, see 73060–73080. For treatment of a Monteggia type fracture dislocation, see 24620 and 24635. For a periarticular fracture dislocation of the elbow, see 24586 or 24587. For closed treatment of an elbow dislocation, see 24600–24605.

ICD-9-CM Procedural

79.72 Closed reduction of dislocation of elbow

Anesthesia

24640 01730

ICD-9-CM Diagnostic

832.2 Nursemaid's elbow

Terms To Know

closed reduction. Treatment of a fracture by manipulating it into proper alignment without opening the skin.

developmental dislocation. Displacement of a body part occurring in the developmental phase of childhood.

flexion. Act of bending or being bent.

incision. Act of cutting into tissue or an organ.

lateral. To/on the side.

medial. Middle or midline.

Monteggia's fracture. Break in the proximal half of the ulnar shaft accompanied by a dislocation of the radial head.

strapping. Application of overlapping strips of tape or bandaging to put pressure on the affected area.

subluxation. Partial or complete dislocation.

CCI Version 16.3

01710, 0213T, 0216T, 0228T, 0230T, 24300, 29049-29075, 29105, 29240-29260, 29700-29715, 36000, 36400-36410, 36420-36430, 36440, 36600, 36640, 37202, 43752, 51701-51703, 62310-62319, 64400-64435, 64445-64450, 64479, 64483, 64490, 64493, 64505-64530, 69990, 93000-93010, 93040-93042, 93318, 94002, 94200, 94250, 94680-94690, 94770, 95812-95816, 95819, 95822, 95829, 95955, 96360, 96365, 96372, 96374-96376, 97597-97598, 97602-97606, 99148-99149, 99150, J2001

Note: These CCI edits are used for Medicare. Other payers may reimburse on codes listed above.

Medicare Edits

	Fac RVU	Non-Fac RVU	FUD	Assist
24640	2.56	3.62	10	80

Medicare References: None

24650-24655

24650 Closed treatment of radial head or neck fracture; without manipulation
24655 with manipulation

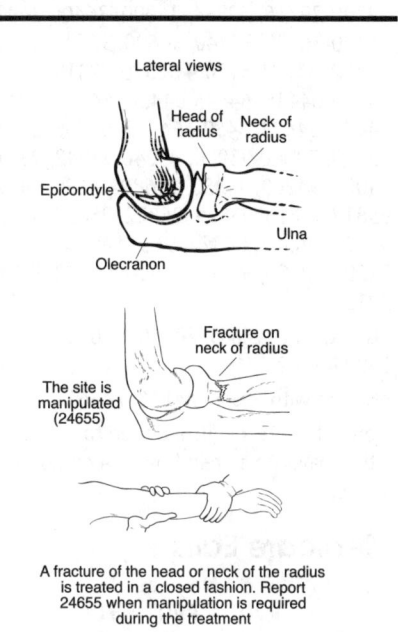

A fracture of the head or neck of the radius is treated in a closed fashion. Report 24655 when manipulation is required during the treatment

Explanation

The physician performs closed treatment of a radial head or neck fracture without manipulation in 24650 and with manipulation in 24655. In 24650, the radial fracture is determined to be stable and nondisplaced and can be splinted or braced without requiring manipulation. In 24655, the physician performs manual manipulation to realign the fractured bone by applying pressure. No incisions are made. The arm is placed in a posterior elbow splint or brace.

Coding Tips

According to CPT guidelines, cast application or strapping (including removal) is only reported as a replacement procedure or when the cast application or strapping is an initial service performed without a restorative treatment or procedure. See "Application of Casts and Strapping" in the CPT book in the Surgery Section, under the Musculoskeletal system. In 24655, local anesthesia is included in the service. However, this procedure may be performed under general anesthesia, depending on the age and/or condition of the patient. For radiology services, see 73070–73085. For open treatment of a radial head or neck fracture see 24665; with radial head prosthetic replacement, see 24666.

ICD-9-CM Procedural

79.02 Closed reduction of fracture of radius and ulna without internal fixation

93.54 Application of splint

Anesthesia

01730

ICD-9-CM Diagnostic

733.19 Pathologic fracture of other specified site
813.05 Closed fracture of head of radius
813.06 Closed fracture of neck of radius
813.07 Other and unspecified closed fractures of proximal end of radius (alone)

Terms To Know

closed fracture. Break in a bone without a concomitant opening in the skin. A closed fracture is coded when the type of fracture is not specified.

fracture types. There are three basic degrees of fracture: type I: a small crack in the bone without displacement; type II: a fracture in which the bone is slightly displaced; type III: a fracture in which there are more than three broken pieces of bone that cannot fit together.

lateral. To/on the side.

manipulation. Skillful treatment by hand to reduce fractures and dislocations, or provide therapy through forceful passive movement of a joint beyond its active limit of motion.

posterior. Located in the back part or caudal end of the body.

splint. Brace or support for an anatomical structure after surgery or injury.

CCI Version 16.3

01710, 0213T, 0216T, 0228T, 0230T, 20605, 24300, 29049-29075, 29240-29260, 29700-29715, 36000, 36400-36410, 36420-36430, 36440, 36600, 36640, 37202, 43752, 51701-51703, 62310-62319, 64400-64435, 64445-64450, 64479, 64483, 64490, 64493, 64505-64530, 69990, 93000-93010, 93040-93042, 93318, 94002, 94200, 94250, 94680-94690, 94770, 95812-95816, 95819, 95822, 95829, 95955, 96360, 96365, 96372, 96374-96376, 97597-97598, 97602-97606, 99148-99149, 99150

Also not with 24650: 12005, 12011-12014, 15851, 29105-29125

Also not with 24655: 24650, 29105, J0670, J2001

Note: These CCI edits are used for Medicare. Other payers may reimburse on codes listed above.

Medicare Edits

	Fac RVU	Non-Fac RVU	FUD	Assist
24650	6.64	7.28	90	N/A
24655	11.31	12.34	90	N/A

Medicare References: 100-2,15,260; 100-4,12,30; 100-4,12,90.3; 100-4,14,10

24665-24666

24665 Open treatment of radial head or neck fracture, includes internal fixation or radial head excision, when performed;

24666 with radial head prosthetic replacement

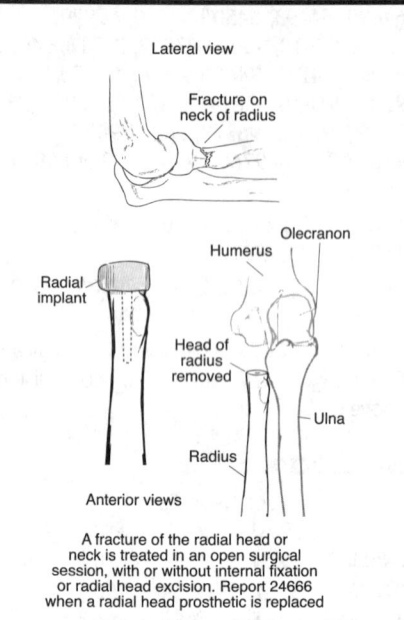

A fracture of the radial head or neck is treated in an open surgical session, with or without internal fixation or radial head excision. Report 24666 when a radial head prosthetic is replaced

Explanation

The physician performs open treatment of a radial head or neck fracture, with or without internal fixation or radial head excision in 24665 and with radial head prosthetic replacement in 24666. The physician makes an incision along the posterolateral aspect of the elbow. The common origin of the extensor muscles is reflected and the joint capsule is incised, exposing the radial head and neck. All loose particles of bone are removed, the elbow joint is irrigated, and the fractured fragments are reduced. In 24665, the physician may need to remove the radial head to achieve good reduction and screws or other internal fixation devices may be employed to stabilize the fracture. In 24666, the physician uses a bone cutting saw to excise the radial head and replaces it with a prosthesis before repairing the capsule and the incision in layers with sutures, staples, and/or Steri-strips. A posterior elbow splint is applied with the elbow at 90 degrees of flexion.

Coding Tips

According to CPT guidelines, cast application or strapping (including removal) is only reported as a replacement procedure or when the cast application or strapping is an initial service performed without a restorative treatment or procedure. See "Application of Casts and Strapping" in the CPT book in the Surgery Section, under the Musculoskeletal system. For radiology services, see 73070–73085. For closed treatment of a radial head or neck fracture, see 24650–24655.

ICD-9-CM Procedural

- 77.83 Other partial ostectomy of radius and ulna
- 79.22 Open reduction of fracture of radius and ulna without internal fixation
- 79.32 Open reduction of fracture of radius and ulna with internal fixation
- 81.85 Other repair of elbow

Anesthesia
01830

ICD-9-CM Diagnostic

- 733.19 Pathologic fracture of other specified site
- 733.81 Malunion of fracture
- 813.05 Closed fracture of head of radius
- 813.06 Closed fracture of neck of radius
- 813.07 Other and unspecified closed fractures of proximal end of radius (alone)
- 813.15 Open fracture of head of radius
- 813.16 Open fracture of neck of radius
- 813.17 Other and unspecified open fractures of proximal end of radius (alone)

Terms To Know

closed fracture. Break in a bone without a concomitant opening in the skin. A closed fracture is coded when the type of fracture is not specified.

comminuted fracture. Any type of fracture in which the bone is splintered or crushed, resulting in multiple bone fragments.

flexion. Act of bending or being bent.

fracture types. There are three basic degrees of fracture: type I: a small crack in the bone without displacement; type II: a fracture in which the bone is slightly displaced; type III: a fracture in which there are more than three broken pieces of bone that cannot fit together.

open fracture. Exposed break in a bone, always considered compound due to its high risk of infection from the open wound leading to the fracture. Broken bone ends may protrude through the skin and contaminants or foreign bodies are often embedded in the tissues.

posterior. Located in the back part or caudal end of the body.

CCI Version 16.3

01710, 0213T, 0216T, 0228T, 0230T, 20680, 24000, 24006, 24100-24102, 24130, 24300, 24332, 24495, 24640-24655, 25360-25365, 29049-29075, 29105, 29240-29260, 29700-29715, 29834, 36000, 36400-36410, 36420-36430, 36440, 36600, 36640, 37202, 43752, 51701-51703, 62310-62319, 64400-64435, 64445-64450, 64479, 64483, 64490, 64493, 64505-64530, 64708, 64718, 69990, 93000-93010, 93040-93042, 93318, 94002, 94200, 94250, 94680-94690, 94770, 95812-95816, 95819, 95822, 95829, 95955, 96360, 96365, 96372, 96374-96376, 97597-97598, 97602-97606, 99148-99149, 99150

Also not with 24665: 20650, 25020, 25024-25025

Also not with 24666: 24145, 24665

Note: These CCI edits are used for Medicare. Other payers may reimburse on codes listed above.

Medicare Edits

	Fac RVU	Non-Fac RVU	FUD	Assist
24665	18.89	18.89	90	80
24666	21.32	21.32	90	80

Medicare References: 100-2,15,260; 100-4,12,30; 100-4,12,90.3; 100-4,14,10

24670-24675

24670 Closed treatment of ulnar fracture, proximal end (eg, olecranon or coronoid process[es]); without manipulation
24675 with manipulation

A fracture of the olecranon process is treated in a closed fashion, without manipulation. Report 24675 when manipulation is required for the treatment

Explanation

The physician performs closed treatment of an olecranon or coronoid process fracture. No manipulation is required in 24670. In 24675, mild or slight separation of the fragments requires manipulation. The physician manually manipulates the area, reducing the proximal end ulnar fracture. No incisions are made. The arm may be placed in a posterior elbow splint at 90 degrees of flexion.

Coding Tips

According to CPT guidelines, cast application or strapping (including removal) is only reported as a replacement procedure or when the cast application or strapping is an initial service performed without a restorative treatment or procedure. See "Application of Casts and Strapping" in the CPT book in the Surgery Section, under the Musculoskeletal system. In 24675, local anesthesia is included in this service. However, this procedure may be performed under general anesthesia, depending on the age and/or condition of the patient. For radiology services, see 73070–73085. For open treatment of the olecranon process, see 24685.

ICD-9-CM Procedural

79.02 Closed reduction of fracture of radius and ulna without internal fixation
93.54 Application of splint

Anesthesia
01820

ICD-9-CM Diagnostic

733.19 Pathologic fracture of other specified site
813.01 Closed fracture of olecranon process of ulna
813.02 Closed fracture of coronoid process of ulna
813.04 Other and unspecified closed fractures of proximal end of ulna (alone)

Terms To Know

closed fracture. Break in a bone without a concomitant opening in the skin. A closed fracture is coded when the type of fracture is not specified.

closed reduction. Treatment of a fracture by manipulating it into proper alignment without opening the skin.

flexion. Act of bending or being bent.

fracture types. There are three basic degrees of fracture: type I: a small crack in the bone without displacement; type II: a fracture in which the bone is slightly displaced; type III: a fracture in which there are more than three broken pieces of bone that cannot fit together.

posterior. Located in the back part or caudal end of the body.

proximal. Located closest to a specified reference point, usually the midline.

strapping. Application of overlapping strips of tape or bandaging to put pressure on the affected area.

CCI Version 16.3

01710, 0213T, 0216T, 0228T, 0230T, 24300, 29049-29075, 29105, 29240-29260, 29700-29715, 36000, 36400-36410, 36420-36430, 36440, 36600, 36640, 37202, 43752, 51701-51703, 62310-62319, 64400-64435, 64445-64450, 64479, 64483, 64490, 64493, 64505-64530, 69990, 93000-93010, 93040-93042, 93318, 94002, 94200, 94250, 94680-94690, 94770, 95812-95816, 95819, 95822, 95829, 95955, 96360, 96365, 96372, 96374-96376, 97597-97598, 97602-97606, 99148-99149, 99150

Also not with 24670: 12001, G0168
Also not with 24675: 24670, J0670, J2001

Note: These CCI edits are used for Medicare. Other payers may reimburse on codes listed above.

Medicare Edits

	Fac RVU	Non-Fac RVU	FUD	Assist
24670	7.34	8.14	90	N/A
24675	11.94	12.99	90	N/A

Medicare References: 100-2,15,260; 100-4,12,30; 100-4,12,90.3; 100-4,14,10

24685

24685 Open treatment of ulnar fracture, proximal end (eg, olecranon or coronoid process[es]), includes internal fixation, when performed

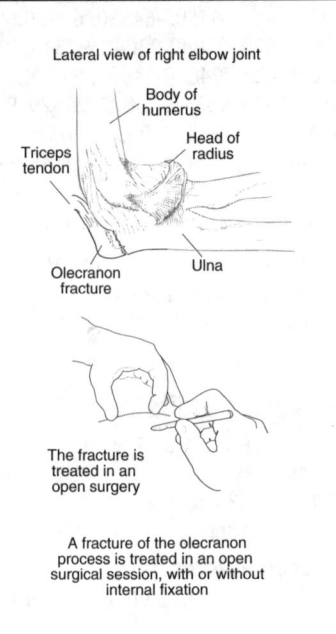

Explanation
The physician openly treats a fracture of the olecranon or coronoid process (proximal end of the ulna). The physician makes a 10 cm incision along the posterolateral border of the elbow. Dissection exposes the fracture. If the fracture is not comminuted, a figure-of-eight wire loop stabilizes the fracture. The physician drills a hole from side to side in the distal fragment. Wire is passed through the drill hole in the distal fragment and through the triceps aponeurosis. This creates a figure-of-eight loop. The wire is pulled tight and twisted. If the fracture is more distal, a medullary pin or screw may be used as well. If medullary fixation is used, the pin or screw is inserted through the olecranon and into the medullary canal of the ulna. The physician repairs the incision in layers with sutures, staples, and/or Steri-strips.

Coding Tips
According to CPT guidelines, cast application or strapping (including removal) is only reported as a replacement procedure or when the cast application or strapping is an initial service performed without a restorative treatment or procedure. See "Application of Casts and Strapping" in the CPT book in the Surgery Section, under the Musculoskeletal system. For radiology services, see 73070-73085. For closed treatment of a proximal ulnar fracture (olecranon process), see 24670-24675.

ICD-9-CM Procedural
- 79.22 Open reduction of fracture of radius and ulna without internal fixation
- 79.32 Open reduction of fracture of radius and ulna with internal fixation

Anesthesia
24685 01830

ICD-9-CM Diagnostic
- 733.19 Pathologic fracture of other specified site
- 733.82 Nonunion of fracture
- 813.01 Closed fracture of olecranon process of ulna
- 813.02 Closed fracture of coronoid process of ulna
- 813.04 Other and unspecified closed fractures of proximal end of ulna (alone)
- 813.11 Open fracture of olecranon process of ulna
- 813.12 Open fracture of coronoid process of ulna
- 813.14 Other and unspecified open fractures of proximal end of ulna (alone)

Terms To Know
aponeurosis. Flat expansion of white, ribbon-like tendinous tissue that functions as the connection of a muscle to its moving part.

closed fracture. Break in a bone without a concomitant opening in the skin. A closed fracture is coded when the type of fracture is not specified.

comminuted fracture. Any type of fracture in which the bone is splintered or crushed, resulting in multiple bone fragments.

open fracture. Exposed break in a bone, always considered compound due to its high risk of infection from the open wound leading to the fracture. Broken bone ends may protrude through the skin and contaminants or foreign bodies are often embedded in the tissues.

posterolateral. Located in the back and off to the side.

CCI Version 16.3
01710, 0213T, 0216T, 0228T, 0230T, 20650, 20680, 24000, 24006, 24100-24102, 24300, 24332, 24495, 24670-24675, 25020, 25024-25025, 29049-29075, 29105, 29240-29260, 29700-29715, 29834, 36000, 36400-36410, 36420-36430, 36440, 36600, 36640, 37202, 43752, 51701-51703, 62310-62319, 64400-64435, 64445-64450, 64479, 64483, 64490, 64493, 64505-64530, 64708, 64718, 69990, 76000-76001, 93000-93010, 93040-93042, 93318, 94002, 94200, 94250, 94680-94690, 94770, 95812-95816, 95819, 95822, 95829, 95955, 96360, 96365, 96372, 96374-96376, 97597-97598, 97602-97606, 99148-99149, 99150

Note: These CCI edits are used for Medicare. Other payers may reimburse on codes listed above.

Medicare Edits

	Fac RVU	Non-Fac RVU	FUD	Assist
24685	18.93	18.93	90	80

Medicare References: 100-2,15,260; 100-4,12,30; 100-4,12,90.3; 100-4,14,10

24800-24802

24800 Arthrodesis, elbow joint; local
24802 with autogenous graft (includes obtaining graft)

Lateral view of right elbow joint
Body of humerus
Head of radius
Olecranon

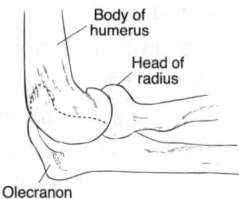

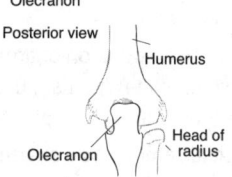

Posterior view
Humerus
Olecranon
Head of radius

The olecranon is shaped and fitted into a locked position into the humerus. A local bone graft may be used in the procedure

The elbow joint is surgically fixed (arthrodesis) into a locked position using bone graft from surrounding bone if necessary. Report 24802 when an autogenous graft (from another incision) is required to perform the arthrodesis

Explanation

The physician performs an arthrodesis of the elbow joint and makes a posterior longitudinal or posterolateral incision. If the physician does not use a bone graft, the triceps tendon is split and released from the olecranon. The joint capsule is incised to expose the radial head and neck and the radial head is excised. A posterior and anterior synovectomy is performed. The physician trims the olecranon into a triangular shape with a saw. A triangular hole is created through the lower end of the humerus and the olecranon is inserted through this triangular hole. The physician places a bone screw obliquely through the humerus and into the ulna. The triceps tendon is repaired with sutures. The physician repairs the incision in layers and the elbow is immobilized in a long arm cast. If a bone graft is used, the physician prepares a bed for the graft in the posterior surface of the lower humerus. A cleft is formed in the upper part of the tip of the olecranon. If local autograft bone is used, it is harvested from the surrounding healthy bone and no separate incision is required. The autograft is fitted into the olecranon cleft and humeral bed. If allograft (donor) bone is used, it is fitted in the same manner. In 24802, an autogenous graft is harvested from the patient's upper tibia or iliac crest with an osteotome. The physician repairs the surgically created graft donor site. One or two screws are inserted through the graft and into the humerus to make it secure. Bone chips are packed into the humeral-ulnar joint. The physician repairs the incision in layers with sutures. A long arm cast is applied with the elbow in approximately 90 degrees of flexion.

Coding Tips

In 24802, any bone graft is not reported separately. According to CPT guidelines, cast application or strapping (including removal) is only reported as a replacement procedure or when the cast application or strapping is an initial service performed without a restorative treatment or procedure. See "Application of Casts and Strapping" in the CPT book in the Surgery Section, under the Musculoskeletal system.

ICD-9-CM Procedural

81.24 Arthrodesis of elbow

Anesthesia

24800 01756
24802 01740

ICD-9-CM Diagnostic

171.2 Malignant neoplasm of connective and other soft tissue of upper limb, including shoulder
198.5 Secondary malignant neoplasm of bone and bone marrow
238.0 Neoplasm of uncertain behavior of bone and articular cartilage
357.1 Polyneuropathy in collagen vascular disease — (Code first underlying disease: 446.0, 710.0, 714.0)
359.6 Symptomatic inflammatory myopathy in diseases classified elsewhere — (Code first underlying disease: 135, 140.0-208.9, 277.30-277.39, 446.0, 710.0, 710.1, 710.2, 714.0)
446.0 Polyarteritis nodosa
710.0 Systemic lupus erythematosus — (Use additional code to identify manifestation: 424.91, 581.81, 582.81, 583.81)
710.1 Systemic sclerosis — (Use additional code to identify manifestation: 359.6, 517.2)
710.2 Sicca syndrome
711.02 Pyogenic arthritis, upper arm — (Use additional code to identify infectious organism: 041.0-041.8)
714.0 Rheumatoid arthritis — (Use additional code to identify manifestation: 357.1, 359.6)
714.1 Felty's syndrome
714.2 Other rheumatoid arthritis with visceral or systemic involvement
714.4 Chronic postrheumatic arthropathy
715.12 Primary localized osteoarthrosis, upper arm
715.32 Localized osteoarthrosis not specified whether primary or secondary, upper arm
716.12 Traumatic arthropathy, upper arm
716.82 Other specified arthropathy, upper arm
716.92 Unspecified arthropathy, upper arm
719.42 Pain in joint, upper arm
728.0 Infective myositis
728.10 Unspecified calcification and ossification
728.11 Progressive myositis ossificans
728.12 Traumatic myositis ossificans
728.13 Postoperative heterotopic calcification
728.19 Other muscular calcification and ossification
728.3 Other specific muscle disorders
728.81 Interstitial myositis
730.12 Chronic osteomyelitis, upper arm — (Use additional code to identify organism: 041.1. Use additional code to identify major osseous defect, if applicable: 731.3)
731.3 Major osseous defects — (Code first underlying disease: 170.0-170.9, 730.00-730.29, 733.00-733.09, 733.40-733.49, 996.45)

CCI Version 16.3

01710, 0213T, 0216T, 0228T, 0230T, 20690, 20692, 24000, 24006, 24100-24102, 24300, 24332, 24400, 24579, 25365, 29834-29838, 36000, 36400-36410, 36420-36430, 36440, 36600, 36640, 37202, 43752, 51701-51703, 62310-62319, 64400-64435, 64445-64450, 64479, 64483, 64490, 64493, 64505-64530, 69990, 93000-93010, 93040-93042, 93318, 94002, 94200, 94250, 94680-94690, 94770, 95812-95816, 95819, 95822, 95829, 95955, 96360, 96365, 96372, 96374-96376, 99148-99149, 99150

Also not with 24802: 20900-20902

Note: These CCI edits are used for Medicare. Other payers may reimburse on codes listed above.

Medicare Edits

	Fac RVU	Non-Fac RVU	FUD	Assist
24800	23.76	23.76	90	80
24802	29.27	29.27	90	80

Medicare References: 100-2,15,260; 100-4,12,30; 100-4,12,90.3; 100-4,14,10

24900

24900 Amputation, arm through humerus; with primary closure

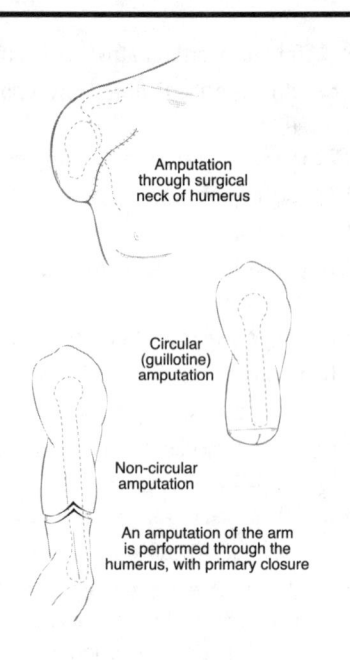

Amputation through surgical neck of humerus

Circular (guillotine) amputation

Non-circular amputation

An amputation of the arm is performed through the humerus, with primary closure

Explanation

The physician amputates the arm through the humerus. An incision is made distal to the intended level of bone section. Anterior and posterior skin flaps are fashioned. The brachial artery and vein are identified, double ligated, and divided just proximal to the level of bone section. Nerves are divided proximally to the site to ensure retraction proximal to the end of the stump. Muscles are sectioned slightly distal to the stump. The humerus is divided and the end is smoothed. The triceps muscle is flapped over the end of the bone and sutured into the anterior fascia. The wound is closed over a drain tube with suction and the fascia and skin flaps are closed.

Coding Tips

Adjacent tissue transfer is included in this procedure. However, report any free grafts separately. For amputation through the humerus, open, circular method, see 24920. For amputation, arm through humerus, secondary closure or scar revision, see 24925. For re-amputation of the upper arm, see 24930. For amputation with implant placement, see 24931.

ICD-9-CM Procedural

84.07   Amputation through humerus

Anesthesia

24900   01756

ICD-9-CM Diagnostic

- 170.4 Malignant neoplasm of scapula and long bones of upper limb
- 171.2 Malignant neoplasm of connective and other soft tissue of upper limb, including shoulder
- 198.5 Secondary malignant neoplasm of bone and bone marrow
- 249.70 Secondary diabetes mellitus with peripheral circulatory disorders, not stated as uncontrolled, or unspecified — (Use additional code to identify manifestation: 443.81, 785.4) (Use additional code to identify any associated insulin use: V58.67)
- 249.71 Secondary diabetes mellitus with peripheral circulatory disorders, uncontrolled — (Use additional code to identify manifestation: 443.81, 785.4) (Use additional code to identify any associated insulin use: V58.67)
- 250.70 Diabetes with peripheral circulatory disorders, type II or unspecified type, not stated as uncontrolled — (Use additional code to identify manifestation: 443.81, 785.4)
- 250.71 Diabetes with peripheral circulatory disorders, type I [juvenile type], not stated as uncontrolled — (Use additional code to identify manifestation: 443.81, 785.4)
- 440.24 Atherosclerosis of native arteries of the extremities with gangrene — (Use additional code for any associated ulceration: 707.10-707.9)
- 443.81 Peripheral angiopathy in diseases classified elsewhere — (Code first underlying disease: 249.7, 250.7)
- 443.9 Unspecified peripheral vascular disease
- 444.21 Embolism and thrombosis of arteries of upper extremity
- 445.01 Atheroembolism of upper extremity
- 446.0 Polyarteritis nodosa
- 728.86 Necrotizing fasciitis — (Use additional code to identify infectious organism, 041.00-041.89, 785.4, if applicable)
- 730.12 Chronic osteomyelitis, upper arm — (Use additional code to identify organism: 041.1. Use additional code to identify major osseous defect, if applicable: 731.3)
- 731.1 Osteitis deformans in diseases classified elsewhere — (Code first underlying disease: 170.0-170.9)
- 731.3 Major osseous defects — (Code first underlying disease: 170.0-170.9, 730.00-730.29, 733.00-733.09, 733.40-733.49, 996.45)
- 785.4 Gangrene — (Code first any associated underlying condition)
- 812.59 Other open fracture of lower end of humerus
- 880.13 Open wound of upper arm, complicated
- 880.23 Open wound of upper arm, with tendon involvement
- 887.2 Traumatic amputation of arm and hand (complete) (partial), unilateral, at or above elbow, without mention of complication
- 887.3 Traumatic amputation of arm and hand (complete) (partial), unilateral, at or above elbow, complicated
- 887.6 Traumatic amputation of arm and hand (complete) (partial), bilateral (any level), without mention of complication
- 887.7 Traumatic amputation of arm and hand (complete) (partial), bilateral (any level), complicated
- 927.03 Crushing injury of upper arm — (Use additional code to identify any associated injuries: 800-829, 850.0-854.1, 860.0-869.1)
- 943.52 Deep necrosis of underlying tissues due to burn (deep third degree) of elbow, with loss of a body part
- 943.53 Deep necrosis of underlying tissues due to burn (deep third degree) of upper arm, with loss of upper a body part

CCI Version 16.3

01710, 0213T, 0216T, 0228T, 0230T, 20103, 24300, 24332, 24400, 24420, 36000, 36400-36410, 36420-36430, 36440, 36600, 36640, 37202, 37618, 43752, 51701-51703, 62310-62319, 64400-64435, 64445-64450, 64479, 64483, 64490, 64493, 64505-64530, 69990, 93000-93010, 93040-93042, 93318, 94002, 94200, 94250, 94680-94690, 94770, 95812-95816, 95819, 95822, 95829, 95955, 96360, 96365, 96372, 96374-96376, 97597-97598, 97602-97606, 99148-99149, 99150

Note: These CCI edits are used for Medicare. Other payers may reimburse on codes listed above.

Medicare Edits

	Fac RVU	Non-Fac RVU	FUD	Assist
24900	21.2	21.2	90	80

Medicare References: None

24920

24920 Amputation, arm through humerus; open, circular (guillotine)

Amputation through surgical neck of humerus

Circular (guillotine) amputation

Non-circular amputation

An amputation of the arm is performed through the humerus. Report 24920 for an open, circular (guillotine) procedure.

Explanation

The physician amputates the arm through the humerus using an open, circular technique. The physician makes an incision distal to the intended level of bone section in a circular manner to the fascia and fashions anterior and posterior skin flaps. The brachial artery and vein are identified, double ligated, and divided just proximal to the level of bone section. Nerves are also divided proximal to the site to ensure retraction to the end of the stump. Muscles are sectioned slightly distal to the stump. The humerus is divided and the end is smoothed. The triceps muscle is flapped over the end of the bone and sutured into the anterior fascia. The wound is closed over a drain tube with suction and the fascia and skin flaps are closed.

Coding Tips

Adjacent tissue transfer is included in these procedures. However, report any free grafts separately. For amputation, arm through humerus, see 24900. For amputation, arm through humerus, secondary closure or scar revision, see 24925. For re-amputation of the upper arm, see 24930. For amputation with implant placement, see 24931.

ICD-9-CM Procedural

84.07 Amputation through humerus

Anesthesia

24920 01756

ICD-9-CM Diagnostic

- 170.4 Malignant neoplasm of scapula and long bones of upper limb
- 171.2 Malignant neoplasm of connective and other soft tissue of upper limb, including shoulder
- 198.5 Secondary malignant neoplasm of bone and bone marrow
- 249.70 Secondary diabetes mellitus with peripheral circulatory disorders, not stated as uncontrolled, or unspecified — (Use additional code to identify manifestation: 443.81, 785.4) (Use additional code to identify any associated insulin use: V58.67)
- 249.71 Secondary diabetes mellitus with peripheral circulatory disorders, uncontrolled — (Use additional code to identify manifestation: 443.81, 785.4) (Use additional code to identify any associated insulin use: V58.67)
- 250.70 Diabetes with peripheral circulatory disorders, type II or unspecified type, not stated as uncontrolled — (Use additional code to identify manifestation: 443.81, 785.4)
- 250.71 Diabetes with peripheral circulatory disorders, type I [juvenile type], not stated as uncontrolled — (Use additional code to identify manifestation: 443.81, 785.4)
- 440.24 Atherosclerosis of native arteries of the extremities with gangrene — (Use additional code for any associated ulceration: 707.10-707.9)
- 443.81 Peripheral angiopathy in diseases classified elsewhere — (Code first underlying disease: 249.7, 250.7)
- 444.21 Embolism and thrombosis of arteries of upper extremity
- 445.01 Atheroembolism of upper extremity
- 446.0 Polyarteritis nodosa
- 728.86 Necrotizing fasciitis — (Use additional code to identify infectious organism, 041.00-041.89, 785.4, if applicable)
- 730.12 Chronic osteomyelitis, upper arm — (Use additional code to identify organism: 041.1. Use additional code to identify major osseous defect, if applicable: 731.3)
- 731.1 Osteitis deformans in diseases classified elsewhere — (Code first underlying disease: 170.0-170.9)
- 731.3 Major osseous defects — (Code first underlying disease: 170.0-170.9, 730.00-730.29, 733.00-733.09, 733.40-733.49, 996.45)
- 785.4 Gangrene — (Code first any associated underlying condition)
- 880.13 Open wound of upper arm, complicated
- 880.23 Open wound of upper arm, with tendon involvement
- 887.2 Traumatic amputation of arm and hand (complete) (partial), unilateral, at or above elbow, without mention of complication
- 887.3 Traumatic amputation of arm and hand (complete) (partial), unilateral, at or above elbow, complicated
- 927.03 Crushing injury of upper arm — (Use additional code to identify any associated injuries: 800-829, 850.0-854.1, 860.0-869.1)
- 943.52 Deep necrosis of underlying tissues due to burn (deep third degree) of elbow, with loss of a body part
- 943.53 Deep necrosis of underlying tissues due to burn (deep third degree) of upper arm, with loss of upper a body part
- 996.94 Complications of reattached upper extremity, other and unspecified

CCI Version 16.3

01710, 0213T, 0216T, 0228T, 0230T, 20103, 24300, 24332, 24400, 24420, 36000, 36400-36410, 36420-36430, 36440, 36600, 36640, 37202, 37618, 43752, 51701-51703, 62310-62319, 64400-64435, 64445-64450, 64479, 64483, 64490, 64493, 64505-64530, 69990, 93000-93010, 93040-93042, 93318, 94002, 94200, 94250, 94680-94690, 94770, 95812-95816, 95819, 95822, 95829, 95955, 96360, 96365, 96372, 96374-96376, 97597-97598, 97602-97606, 99148-99149, 99150

Note: These CCI edits are used for Medicare. Other payers may reimburse on codes listed above.

Medicare Edits

	Fac RVU	Non-Fac RVU	FUD	Assist
24920	21.07	21.07	90	80

Medicare References: None

24925

24925 Amputation, arm through humerus; secondary closure or scar revision

Secondary closure or scar revision

A secondary closure or scar revision is performed at the site of an amputation of the humerus

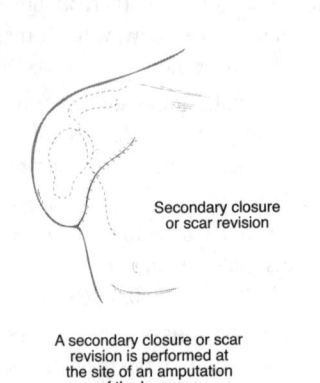

Explanation
The physician performs a secondary closure or scar revision of an existing amputation. The physician excises the granulation and scar tissues and remodels the soft tissues to close over the amputation again. Arteries and veins are identified, ligated, and divided, as necessary, as well as nerves. The wound is closed over a drain tube with suction and the fascia and skin flaps are closed.

Coding Tips
Adjacent tissue transfer is included in this procedure. However, report any free grafts separately. For initial amputation, arm through humerus, see 24900 and 24920. For re-amputation of the upper arm, see 24930. For amputation with implant placement, see 24931.

ICD-9-CM Procedural
84.3   Revision of amputation stump

Anesthesia
24925   00400

ICD-9-CM Diagnostic
- 249.70 Secondary diabetes mellitus with peripheral circulatory disorders, not stated as uncontrolled, or unspecified — (Use additional code to identify manifestation: 443.81, 785.4) (Use additional code to identify any associated insulin use: V58.67)
- 249.71 Secondary diabetes mellitus with peripheral circulatory disorders, uncontrolled — (Use additional code to identify manifestation: 443.81, 785.4) (Use additional code to identify any associated insulin use: V58.67)
- 250.70 Diabetes with peripheral circulatory disorders, type II or unspecified type, not stated as uncontrolled — (Use additional code to identify manifestation: 443.81, 785.4)
- 250.71 Diabetes with peripheral circulatory disorders, type I [juvenile type], not stated as uncontrolled — (Use additional code to identify manifestation: 443.81, 785.4)
- 440.24 Atherosclerosis of native arteries of the extremities with gangrene — (Use additional code for any associated ulceration: 707.10-707.9)
- 443.81 Peripheral angiopathy in diseases classified elsewhere — (Code first underlying disease: 249.7, 250.7)
- 443.9   Unspecified peripheral vascular disease
- 446.0   Polyarteritis nodosa
- 682.3   Cellulitis and abscess of upper arm and forearm — (Use additional code to identify organism, such as 041.1, etc.)
- 707.00 Pressure ulcer, unspecified site — (Use additional code to identify pressure ulcer stage: 707.20-707.25)
- 707.01 Pressure ulcer, elbow — (Use additional code to identify pressure ulcer stage: 707.20-707.25)
- 707.09 Pressure ulcer, other site — (Use additional code to identify pressure ulcer stage: 707.20-707.25)
- 707.20 Pressure ulcer, unspecified stage — (Code first site of pressure ulcer: 707.00-707.09)
- 707.21 Pressure ulcer, stage I — (Code first site of pressure ulcer: 707.00-707.09)
- 707.22 Pressure ulcer stage II — (Code first site of pressure ulcer: 707.00-707.09)
- 707.23 Pressure ulcer stage III — (Code first site of pressure ulcer: 707.00-707.09)
- 707.24 Pressure ulcer stage IV — (Code first site of pressure ulcer: 707.00-707.09)
- 707.25 Pressure ulcer, unstageable — (Code first site of pressure ulcer: 707.00-707.09)
- 707.8   Chronic ulcer of other specified site
- 709.2   Scar condition and fibrosis of skin
- 728.86 Necrotizing fasciitis — (Use additional code to identify infectious organism, 041.00-041.89, 785.4, if applicable)
- 730.12 Chronic osteomyelitis, upper arm — (Use additional code to identify organism: 041.1. Use additional code to identify major osseous defect, if applicable: 731.3)
- 731.3   Major osseous defects — (Code first underlying disease: 170.0-170.9, 730.00-730.29, 733.00-733.09, 733.40-733.49, 996.45)
- 785.4   Gangrene — (Code first any associated underlying condition)
- 880.23 Open wound of upper arm, with tendon involvement
- 997.60 Late complications of amputation stump, unspecified — (Use additional code to identify complications)
- 997.61 Neuroma of amputation stump — (Use additional code to identify complications)
- 997.62 Infection (chronic) of amputation stump — (Use additional code to identify complications)
- 997.69 Other late amputation stump complication — (Use additional code to identify complications)
- 998.83 Non-healing surgical wound
- V51.8   Other aftercare involving the use of plastic surgery
- V58.41 Planned postoperative wound closure — (This code should be used in conjunction with other aftercare codes to fully identify the reason for the aftercare encounter)

CCI Version 16.3
01710, 0213T, 0216T, 0228T, 0230T, 20103, 24300, 24332, 24400, 24420, 36000, 36400-36410, 36420-36430, 36440, 36600, 36640, 37202, 37618, 43752, 51701-51703, 62310-62319, 64400-64435, 64445-64450, 64479, 64483, 64490, 64493, 64505-64530, 69990, 93000-93010, 93040-93042, 93318, 94002, 94200, 94250, 94680-94690, 94770, 95812-95816, 95819, 95822, 95829, 95955, 96360, 96365, 96372, 96374-96376, 97597-97598, 97602-97606, 99148-99149, 99150

Note: These CCI edits are used for Medicare. Other payers may reimburse on codes listed above.

Medicare Edits

	Fac RVU	Non-Fac RVU	FUD	Assist
24925	16.34	16.34	90	80

Medicare References: 100-2,15,260; 100-4,12,30; 100-4,12,90.3; 100-4,14,10

24930

24930 Amputation, arm through humerus; re-amputation

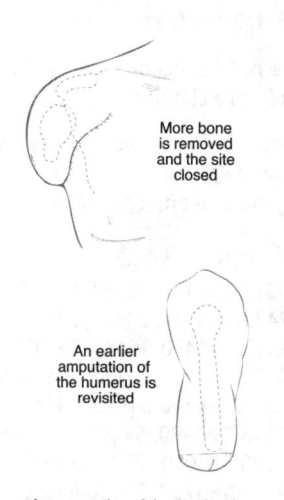

An amputation of the arm has been performed through the humerus. The site must be revisited and a re-amputation performed. Conditions such as infection or non-healing may necessitate removal of more of the humerus

Explanation

The physician re-amputates the arm through the humerus. The physician makes an incision distal to the intended level of bone section and fashions anterior and posterior skin flaps. The brachial artery and vein are identified, double ligated, and divided just proximal to the level of bone section. Nerves are divided proximally to the site to ensure retraction proximal to the end of the stump. Muscles are sectioned slightly distal to the stump. The humerus is divided and the end is smoothed. The triceps muscle is flapped over the end of the bone and sutured into the anterior fascia. The wound is closed over a drain tube with suction and the fascia and skin flaps are closed.

Coding Tips

Adjacent tissue transfer is included in this procedure. However, report any free grafts separately. For initial amputation, arm through humerus, see 24900 and 24920. For amputation, arm through humerus, secondary closure or scar revision, see 24925. For amputation with implant placement, see 24931.

ICD-9-CM Procedural

- 84.07 Amputation through humerus
- 84.3 Revision of amputation stump

Anesthesia

24930 01756

ICD-9-CM Diagnostic

- 170.4 Malignant neoplasm of scapula and long bones of upper limb
- 171.2 Malignant neoplasm of connective and other soft tissue of upper limb, including shoulder
- 198.5 Secondary malignant neoplasm of bone and bone marrow
- 249.70 Secondary diabetes mellitus with peripheral circulatory disorders, not stated as uncontrolled, or unspecified — (Use additional code to identify manifestation: 443.81, 785.4) (Use additional code to identify any associated insulin use: V58.67)
- 249.71 Secondary diabetes mellitus with peripheral circulatory disorders, uncontrolled — (Use additional code to identify manifestation: 443.81, 785.4) (Use additional code to identify any associated insulin use: V58.67)
- 250.70 Diabetes with peripheral circulatory disorders, type II or unspecified type, not stated as uncontrolled — (Use additional code to identify manifestation: 443.81, 785.4)
- 250.71 Diabetes with peripheral circulatory disorders, type I [juvenile type], not stated as uncontrolled — (Use additional code to identify manifestation: 443.81, 785.4)
- 730.12 Chronic osteomyelitis, upper arm — (Use additional code to identify organism: 041.1. Use additional code to identify major osseous defect, if applicable: 731.3)
- 731.8 Other bone involvement in diseases classified elsewhere — (Code first underlying disease: 249.8, 250.8. Use additional code to specify bone condition: 730.00-730.09)
- 785.4 Gangrene — (Code first any associated underlying condition)
- 997.60 Late complications of amputation stump, unspecified — (Use additional code to identify complications)
- 997.61 Neuroma of amputation stump — (Use additional code to identify complications)
- 997.62 Infection (chronic) of amputation stump — (Use additional code to identify complications)
- 997.69 Other late amputation stump complication — (Use additional code to identify complications)
- V49.66 Upper limb amputation, above elbow

Terms To Know

anterior. Situated in the front area or toward the belly surface of the body; an anatomical reference point used to show the position and relationship of one body structure to another.

complication. Condition arising after the beginning of observation and treatment that modifies the course of the patient's illness or the medical care required, or an undesired result or misadventure in medical care.

distal. Located farther away from a specified reference point.

fascia. Fibrous sheet or band of tissue that envelops organs, muscles, and groupings of muscles.

fistula. Abnormal tube-like passage between two body cavities or organs or from an organ to the outside surface.

gangrene. Death of tissue, usually resulting from a loss of vascular supply, followed by a bacterial attack or onset of disease.

neuroma. Any type of tumor growing from a nerve or comprised of nerve cells and fibers.

proximal. Located closest to a specified reference point, usually the midline.

CCI Version 16.3

01710, 0213T, 0216T, 0228T, 0230T, 20103, 24300, 24332, 24341, 24400, 24420, 36000, 36400-36410, 36420-36430, 36440, 36600, 36640, 37202, 37618, 43752, 51701-51703, 62310-62319, 64400-64435, 64445-64450, 64479, 64483, 64490, 64493, 64505-64530, 69990, 93000-93010, 93040-93042, 93318, 94002, 94200, 94250, 94680-94690, 94770, 95812-95816, 95819, 95822, 95829, 95955, 96360, 96365, 96372, 96374-96376, 97597-97598, 97602-97606, 99148-99149, 99150

Note: These CCI edits are used for Medicare. Other payers may reimburse on codes listed above.

Medicare Edits

	Fac RVU	Non-Fac RVU	FUD	Assist
24930	22.34	22.34	90	80

Medicare References: None

24931

24931 Amputation, arm through humerus; with implant

A rod implanted into the medullary cavity at time of amputation

An amputation of the arm is performed through the humerus. An implant, such as a rod, is inserted into the humerus at the time of the amputation. The implant may serve to maintain length or to replace a portion of the amputated arm. The use of a rod in this procedure may allow better function of the remaining arm or offer better fit and function of a prosthesis

Explanation

The physician amputates the arm through the humerus bone and places a surgical implant in the arm. The physician makes an incision in a circular fashion around the entire arm distal to the level of the planned amputation of the humerus. The vessels and nerves are identified, divided, and ligated. The humerus bone is divided in two, completing the amputation. The physician spares the skin, soft tissue, and muscle needed to close the amputation incision. Any of a variety of implants, such as rods, are utilized to maintain the length of the arm or to replace a portion of the amputated humerus. Fixation devices are used. The entire incision is thoroughly irrigated. Retained muscle flaps are closed over exposed bone. The wound is closed in layers and a soft dressing is applied.

Coding Tips

Adjacent tissue transfer is included in this procedure. However, report any free grafts separately. For amputation without implant, see 24900 and 24920. For amputation, arm through humerus, secondary closure or scar revision, see 24925. For re-amputation of the upper arm, see 24930.

ICD-9-CM Procedural

- 81.96 Other repair of joint
- 84.07 Amputation through humerus
- 84.44 Implantation of prosthetic device of arm

Anesthesia

24931 01756

ICD-9-CM Diagnostic

- 170.4 Malignant neoplasm of scapula and long bones of upper limb
- 171.2 Malignant neoplasm of connective and other soft tissue of upper limb, including shoulder
- 198.5 Secondary malignant neoplasm of bone and bone marrow
- 440.24 Atherosclerosis of native arteries of the extremities with gangrene — (Use additional code for any associated ulceration: 707.10-707.9)
- 443.9 Unspecified peripheral vascular disease
- 444.21 Embolism and thrombosis of arteries of upper extremity
- 445.01 Atheroembolism of upper extremity
- 728.86 Necrotizing fasciitis — (Use additional code to identify infectious organism, 041.00-041.89, 785.4, if applicable)
- 785.4 Gangrene — (Code first any associated underlying condition)
- 812.49 Other closed fracture of lower end of humerus
- 812.59 Other open fracture of lower end of humerus
- 880.13 Open wound of upper arm, complicated
- 880.23 Open wound of upper arm, with tendon involvement
- 887.2 Traumatic amputation of arm and hand (complete) (partial), unilateral, at or above elbow, without mention of complication
- 887.3 Traumatic amputation of arm and hand (complete) (partial), unilateral, at or above elbow, complicated
- 887.6 Traumatic amputation of arm and hand (complete) (partial), bilateral (any level), without mention of complication
- 887.7 Traumatic amputation of arm and hand (complete) (partial), bilateral (any level), complicated
- 927.03 Crushing injury of upper arm — (Use additional code to identify any associated injuries: 800-829, 850.0-854.1, 860.0-869.1)
- 943.52 Deep necrosis of underlying tissues due to burn (deep third degree) of elbow, with loss of a body part
- 943.53 Deep necrosis of underlying tissues due to burn (deep third degree) of upper arm, with loss of upper a body part
- 996.94 Complications of reattached upper extremity, other and unspecified

Terms To Know

embolism. Obstruction of a blood vessel resulting from a clot or foreign substance.

gangrene. Death of tissue, usually resulting from a loss of vascular supply, followed by a bacterial attack or onset of disease.

CCI Version 16.3

01710, 0213T, 0216T, 0228T, 0230T, 20103, 24300, 24332, 24341, 24400, 24420, 36000, 36400-36410, 36420-36430, 36440, 36600, 36640, 37202, 37618, 43752, 51701-51703, 62310-62319, 64400-64435, 64445-64450, 64479, 64483, 64490, 64493, 64505-64530, 69990, 93000-93010, 93040-93042, 93318, 94002, 94200, 94250, 94680-94690, 94770, 95812-95816, 95819, 95822, 95829, 95955, 96360, 96365, 96372, 96374-96376, 97597-97598, 97602-97606, 99148-99149, 99150

Note: These CCI edits are used for Medicare. Other payers may reimburse on codes listed above.

Medicare Edits

	Fac RVU	Non-Fac RVU	FUD	Assist
24931	22.57	22.57	90	80

Medicare References: None

24935

24935 Stump elongation, upper extremity

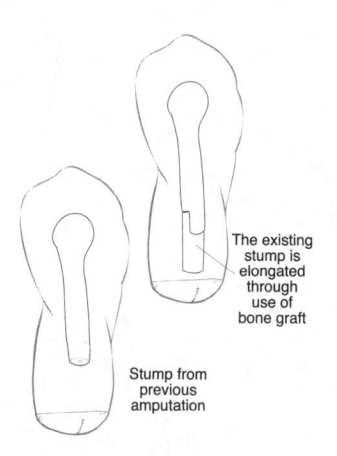

The existing stump is elongated through use of bone graft

Stump from previous amputation

An amputation of the arm has been performed through the humerus. The remaining stump is elongated in this procedure, usually through use of bone grafts. The longer stump may allow better function of the remaining arm or offer better fit and function of a prosthesis

Explanation

The physician elongates a stump of an upper extremity. First, the physician obtains the bone graft. The physician incises the skin over the area where the bone graft is to be obtained (usually the iliac crest). The tissue is dissected away from the bone and the graft is harvested. The wound is closed in sutured layers. The skin overlying the stump is incised to expose the bony stump. The graft is pinned or plated to the existing bone. The tissues are replaced around the bone and the wound is closed in sutured layers.

Coding Tips

If significant additional time and effort is documented, append modifier 22 and submit a cover letter and operative report. Bone graft harvest is not reported separately.

ICD-9-CM Procedural

77.77	Excision of tibia and fibula for graft
77.79	Excision of other bone for graft, except facial bones
78.02	Bone graft of humerus
78.03	Bone graft of radius and ulna
78.32	Limb lengthening procedures, humerus
78.33	Limb lengthening procedures, radius and ulna

Anesthesia

24935 00400, 01710, 01740, 01756, 01810

ICD-9-CM Diagnostic

V51.8	Other aftercare involving the use of plastic surgery
V58.49	Other specified aftercare following surgery — (This code should be used in conjunction with other aftercare codes to fully identify the reason for the aftercare encounter)

Terms To Know

bone graft. Bone that is removed from one part of the body and placed into another bone site without direct re-establishment of blood supply.

graft. Tissue implant from another part of the body or another person.

harvest. Removal of cells or tissue from their native site to be used as a graft or transplant to another part of the donor's body or placed into another person.

CCI Version 16.3

01710, 0213T, 0216T, 0228T, 0230T, 24300, 24332, 24341, 24400, 24420, 36000, 36400-36410, 36420-36430, 36440, 36600, 36640, 37202, 37618, 43752, 51701-51703, 62310-62319, 64400-64435, 64445-64450, 64479, 64483, 64490, 64493, 64505-64530, 69990, 93000-93010, 93040-93042, 93318, 94002, 94200, 94250, 94680-94690, 94770, 95812-95816, 95819, 95822, 95829, 95955, 96360, 96365, 96372, 96374-96376, 97597-97598, 97602-97606, 99148-99149, 99150

Note: These CCI edits are used for Medicare. Other payers may reimburse on codes listed above.

Medicare Edits

	Fac RVU	Non-Fac RVU	FUD	Assist
24935	28.24	28.24	90	80

Medicare References: None

25000

25000 Incision, extensor tendon sheath, wrist (eg, deQuervains disease)

Abductor pollicis longus
Extensor pollicis brevis
Common extensor tendon sheath
Retinaculum
Extensor tendon sheaths (dark)

An extensor tendon sheath is incised

DeQuervain's disease involves the irritation and stenosis of the synovial lining of the common extensor tendon sheath and retinaculum. Symptoms include pain as the tendons move

Explanation

The physician incises the extensor tendon sheath over the wrist. The physician incises the skin just proximal to the anatomic snuffbox. The tissues are dissected and the extensor retinaculum of the first extensor compartment is identified and incised. The incision is closed in sutured layers.

Coding Tips

According to CPT guidelines, cast application or strapping (including removal) is only reported as a replacement procedure or when the cast application or strapping is an initial service performed without a restorative treatment or procedure. See "Application of Casts and Strapping" in the CPT book in the Surgery Section, under the Musculoskeletal system. For decompression of the median nerve (carpel tunnel syndrome), see 64721.

ICD-9-CM Procedural

83.01 Exploration of tendon sheath

Anesthesia

25000 01810

ICD-9-CM Diagnostic

719.23 Villonodular synovitis, forearm
726.4   Enthesopathy of wrist and carpus
727.00 Unspecified synovitis and tenosynovitis
727.04 Radial styloid tenosynovitis
727.05 Other tenosynovitis of hand and wrist
727.2   Specific bursitides often of occupational origin

Terms To Know

extensor. Any muscle that extends a joint.

sheath. Covering enclosing an organ or part.

tendon. Fibrous tissue that connects muscle to bone, consisting primarily of collagen and containing little vasculature.

tenosynovitis. Inflammation of a tendon sheath due to infection or disease.

villonodular synovitis. Inflammation of the synovial membrane due to excessive synovial tissue formation, especially in the knee.

CCI Version 16.3

01810, 0213T, 0216T, 0228T, 0230T, 11010❖, 24300, 25230, 25259, 26500, 29125, 36000, 36400-36410, 36420-36430, 36440, 36600, 36640, 37202, 43752, 51701-51703, 62310-62319, 64400-64435, 64445-64450, 64479, 64483, 64490, 64493, 64505-64530, 69990, 93000-93010, 93040-93042, 93318, 94002, 94200, 94250, 94680-94690, 94770, 95812-95816, 95819, 95822, 95829, 95900, 95955, 96360, 96365, 96372, 96374-96376, 99148-99149, 99150

Note: These CCI edits are used for Medicare. Other payers may reimburse on codes listed above.

Medicare Edits

	Fac RVU	Non-Fac RVU	FUD	Assist
25000	9.94	9.94	90	N/A

Medicare References: 100-2,15,260; 100-4,12,30; 100-4,12,90.3; 100-4,14,10

25001

25001 Incision, flexor tendon sheath, wrist (eg, flexor carpi radialis)

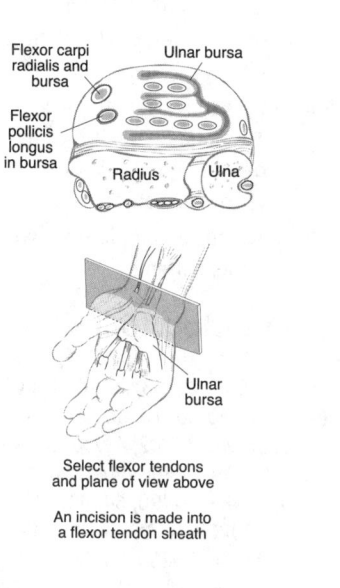

Explanation

The physician incises the flexor tendon sheath over the wrist. The physician makes a radial incision. The tissues are dissected to the tendon sheath. The compartment is identified and incised. When incising the flexor carpi radialis (FCR) the tendon sheath is opened proximal to distal. The fibro-osseous tunnel is released along the ulnar border of the trapezium. The incision is closed with layered suture.

Coding Tips

This is a unilateral procedure. If performed bilaterally, some payers require that the service be reported twice with modifier 50 appended to the second code, while others require identification of the service only once with modifier 50 appended. Check with individual payers. Modifier 50 identifies a procedure performed identically on the opposite side of the body (mirror image).

ICD-9-CM Procedural

83.01 Exploration of tendon sheath

Anesthesia

25001 01810

ICD-9-CM Diagnostic

719.23 Villonodular synovitis, forearm
726.4 Enthesopathy of wrist and carpus
727.00 Unspecified synovitis and tenosynovitis
727.04 Radial styloid tenosynovitis
727.05 Other tenosynovitis of hand and wrist
727.2 Specific bursitides often of occupational origin

Terms To Know

bilateral. Consisting of or affecting two sides.

distal. Located farther away from a specified reference point.

proximal. Located closest to a specified reference point, usually the midline.

sheath. Covering enclosing an organ or part.

tendon. Fibrous tissue that connects muscle to bone, consisting primarily of collagen and containing little vasculature.

tenosynovitis. Inflammation of a tendon sheath due to infection or disease.

unilateral. Located on or affecting one side.

villonodular synovitis. Inflammation of the synovial membrane due to excessive synovial tissue formation, especially in the knee.

CCI Version 16.3

01810, 0213T, 0216T, 0228T, 0230T, 11011-11012❖, 29065-29085, 29105-29126, 29260, 36000, 36400-36410, 36420-36430, 36440, 36600, 36640, 37202, 43752, 51701-51703, 62310-62319, 64400-64435, 64445-64450, 64479, 64483, 64490, 64493, 64505-64530, 69990, 93000-93010, 93040-93042, 93318, 94002, 94200, 94250, 94680-94690, 94770, 95812-95816, 95819, 95822, 95829, 95955, 96360, 96365, 96372, 96374-96376, 99148-99149, 99150

Note: These CCI edits are used for Medicare. Other payers may reimburse on codes listed above.

Medicare Edits

	Fac RVU	Non-Fac RVU	FUD	Assist
25001	9.79	9.79	90	N/A

Medicare References: None

25020-25023

25020 Decompression fasciotomy, forearm and/or wrist, flexor OR extensor compartment; without debridement of nonviable muscle and/or nerve

25023 with debridement of nonviable muscle and/or nerve

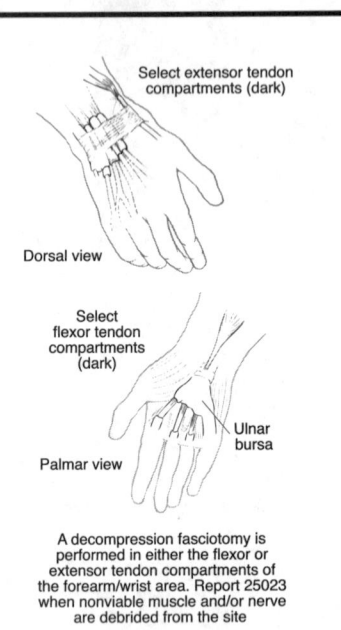

A decompression fasciotomy is performed in either the flexor or extensor tendon compartments of the forearm/wrist area. Report 25023 when nonviable muscle and/or nerve are debrided from the site.

Explanation

The physician performs a decompression fasciotomy of the forearm and/or wrist extensor or flexor compartment without debridement in 25020 and with debridement of any nonviable tissue, including muscles and nerves in 25023. The physician makes an incision over the flexor or extensor compartment of the forearm. This is carried deep to the fascia and the fascia itself is incised and released. In 25020, the skin is sutured closed, if possible. In 25023, the physician explores the compartment and debrides any nonviable tissue that may include muscle, nerve, or fascia. The wound is irrigated and typically left open. Closure is accomplished during a later, separately reportable procedure.

Coding Tips

According to CPT guidelines, cast application or strapping (including removal) is only reported as a replacement procedure or when the cast application or strapping is an initial service performed without a restorative treatment or procedure. See "Application of Casts and Strapping" in the CPT book in the Surgery Section, under the Musculoskeletal system. For decompression fasciotomy with brachial artery exploration, see 24495.

ICD-9-CM Procedural

- 04.07 Other excision or avulsion of cranial and peripheral nerves
- 83.14 Fasciotomy
- 83.45 Other myectomy

Anesthesia

01810

ICD-9-CM Diagnostic

- 682.3 Cellulitis and abscess of upper arm and forearm — (Use additional code to identify organism, such as 041.1, etc.)
- 682.4 Cellulitis and abscess of hand, except fingers and thumb — (Use additional code to identify organism, such as 041.1, etc.)
- 728.86 Necrotizing fasciitis — (Use additional code to identify infectious organism, 041.00-041.89, 785.4, if applicable)
- 728.88 Rhabdomyolysis
- 729.4 Unspecified fasciitis
- 729.71 Nontraumatic compartment syndrome of upper extremity — (Code first, if applicable, postprocedural complication: 998.89)
- 785.4 Gangrene — (Code first any associated underlying condition)
- 813.21 Closed fracture of shaft of radius (alone)
- 813.22 Closed fracture of shaft of ulna (alone)
- 813.23 Closed fracture of shaft of radius with ulna
- 813.31 Open fracture of shaft of radius (alone)
- 813.32 Open fracture of shaft of ulna (alone)
- 813.33 Open fracture of shaft of radius with ulna
- 881.01 Open wound of elbow, without mention of complication
- 881.10 Open wound of forearm, complicated
- 881.12 Open wound of wrist, complicated
- 881.20 Open wound of forearm, with tendon involvement
- 881.22 Open wound of wrist, with tendon involvement
- 927.10 Crushing injury of forearm — (Use additional code to identify any associated injuries: 800-829, 850.0-854.1, 860.0-869.1)
- 927.21 Crushing injury of wrist — (Use additional code to identify any associated injuries: 800-829, 850.0-854.1, 860.0-869.1)
- 943.01 Burn of unspecified degree of forearm
- 943.21 Blisters with epidermal loss due to burn (second degree) of forearm
- 943.31 Full-thickness skin loss due to burn (third degree NOS) of forearm
- 943.41 Deep necrosis of underlying tissues due to burn (deep third degree) of forearm, without mention of loss of a body part
- 948.00 Burn (any degree) involving less than 10% of body surface with third degree burn of less than 10% or unspecified amount
- 958.91 Traumatic compartment syndrome of upper extremity

CCI Version 16.3

01810, 0213T, 0216T, 0228T, 0230T, 11040-11044, 20103, 24300, 25000, 25259, 36000, 36400-36410, 36420-36430, 36440, 36600, 36640, 37202, 43752, 51701-51703, 62310-62319, 64400-64435, 64445-64450, 64479, 64483, 64490, 64493, 64505-64530, 69990, 93000-93010, 93040-93042, 93318, 94002, 94200, 94250, 94680-94690, 94770, 95812-95816, 95819, 95822, 95829, 95955, 96360, 96365, 96372, 96374-96376, 99148-99149, 99150

Also not with 25020: 11010-11011, 25110, 64704, 64718, 64721

Also not with 25023: 11010-11012, 20520-20525, 25020, 25109, 25116, 25248, 64719-64721, 97597-97598, 97602-97606

Note: These CCI edits are used for Medicare. Other payers may reimburse on codes listed above.

Medicare Edits

	Fac RVU	Non-Fac RVU	FUD	Assist
25020	16.72	16.72	90	N/A
25023	32.17	32.17	90	80

Medicare References: 100-2,15,260; 100-4,12,30; 100-4,12,90.3; 100-4,14,10

25024-25025

25024 Decompression fasciotomy, forearm and/or wrist, flexor AND extensor compartment; without debridement of nonviable muscle and/or nerve

25025 with debridement of nonviable muscle and/or nerve

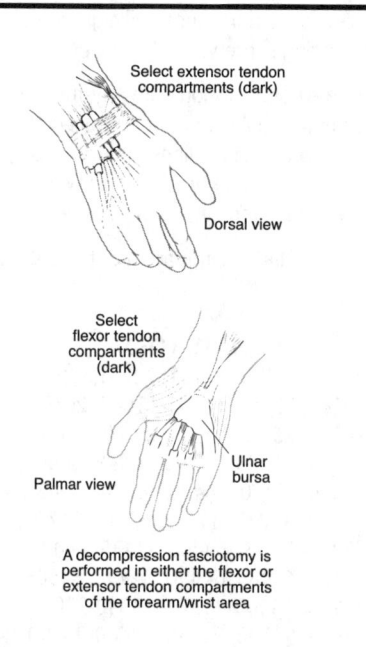

Select extensor tendon compartments (dark)
Dorsal view

Select flexor tendon compartments (dark)
Palmar view
Ulnar bursa

A decompression fasciotomy is performed in either the flexor or extensor tendon compartments of the forearm/wrist area

Explanation

The physician performs a decompression fasciotomy of the forearm and/or wrist extensor and flexor compartment without debridement in 25024 and with debridement of any nonviable tissue, including muscles and nerves in 25025. A decompression fasciotomy of the forearm for compartment syndrome is described here. An anterior curvilinear incision for volar fasciotomy is made beginning on the ulnar side of the forearm, crossing the elbow crease at an angle to reach the radial side, curving back to the ulnar side, and while continuing toward the palm, the incision is centered where it crosses the wrist flexion crease, and extends into the palm medially along the crease. The superficial volar compartment is released along its length, to free the fascia over the compartment muscles. Muscles and nerves are retracted to expose the flexor digitorum profundus in the deep compartment. If its overlying fascia is tight, it too is incised. Report 25025 if any nonviable tissue that may include muscle, nerve, or fascia is found and requires debridement. The dorsal compartments are checked and/or pressure measurements are taken. The volar fasciotomy usually sufficiently decompresses the dorsal musculature also. If the dorsal compartments still require release, an incision is made beginning distal to the lateral epicondyle and extending about 10 cm distally. The subcutaneous tissue is undermined and the fascia is released over the extensor retinaculum. A dressing and a long arm splint are applied to hold the elbow in flexion. The arm is elevated and wound closure is usually done at five days.

Coding Tips

This is a unilateral procedure. If performed bilaterally, some payers require that the service be reported twice with modifier 50 appended to the second code, while others require identification of the service only once with modifier 50 appended. Check with individual payers. Modifier 50 identifies a procedure performed identically on the opposite side of the body (mirror image).

ICD-9-CM Procedural

- 04.07 Other excision or avulsion of cranial and peripheral nerves
- 83.14 Fasciotomy
- 83.45 Other myectomy

Anesthesia
01810

ICD-9-CM Diagnostic

- 682.3 Cellulitis and abscess of upper arm and forearm — (Use additional code to identify organism, such as 041.1, etc.)
- 682.4 Cellulitis and abscess of hand, except fingers and thumb — (Use additional code to identify organism, such as 041.1, etc.)
- 728.86 Necrotizing fasciitis — (Use additional code to identify infectious organism, 041.00-041.89, 785.4, if applicable)
- 728.88 Rhabdomyolysis
- 729.71 Nontraumatic compartment syndrome of upper extremity — (Code first, if applicable, postprocedural complication: 998.89)
- 813.31 Open fracture of shaft of radius (alone)
- 813.32 Open fracture of shaft of ulna (alone)
- 813.33 Open fracture of shaft of radius with ulna
- 881.10 Open wound of forearm, complicated
- 881.12 Open wound of wrist, complicated
- 881.20 Open wound of forearm, with tendon involvement
- 881.22 Open wound of wrist, with tendon involvement
- 923.10 Contusion of forearm
- 923.11 Contusion of elbow
- 927.10 Crushing injury of forearm — (Use additional code to identify any associated injuries: 800-829, 850.0-854.1, 860.0-869.1)
- 927.21 Crushing injury of wrist — (Use additional code to identify any associated injuries: 800-829, 850.0-854.1, 860.0-869.1)
- 943.31 Full-thickness skin loss due to burn (third degree NOS) of forearm
- 943.41 Deep necrosis of underlying tissues due to burn (deep third degree) of forearm, without mention of loss of a body part
- 948.00 Burn (any degree) involving less than 10% of body surface with third degree burn of less than 10% or unspecified amount
- 958.91 Traumatic compartment syndrome of upper extremity

CCI Version 16.3

01810, 0213T, 0216T, 0228T, 0230T, 11010-11012, 11040-11044, 20103, 36000, 36400-36410, 36420-36430, 36440, 36600, 36640, 37202, 43752, 51701-51703, 62310-62319, 64400-64435, 64445-64450, 64479, 64483, 64490, 64493, 64505-64530, 64704, 64718, 64721, 69990, 93000-93010, 93040-93042, 93318, 94002, 94200, 94250, 94680-94690, 94770, 95812-95816, 95819, 95822, 95829, 95955, 96360, 96365, 96372, 96374-96376, 97597-97598, 97602-97606, 99148-99149, 99150

Also not with 25024: 20520-20525, 25020-25023, 25248

Also not with 25025: 25000, 25020-25024, 25109

Note: These CCI edits are used for Medicare. Other payers may reimburse on codes listed above.

Medicare Edits

	Fac RVU	Non-Fac RVU	FUD	Assist
25024	22.67	22.67	90	N/A
25025	35.5	35.5	90	80

Medicare References: 100-2,15,260; 100-4,12,30; 100-4,12,90.3; 100-4,14,10

25028-25031

25028 Incision and drainage, forearm and/or wrist; deep abscess or hematoma
25031 bursa

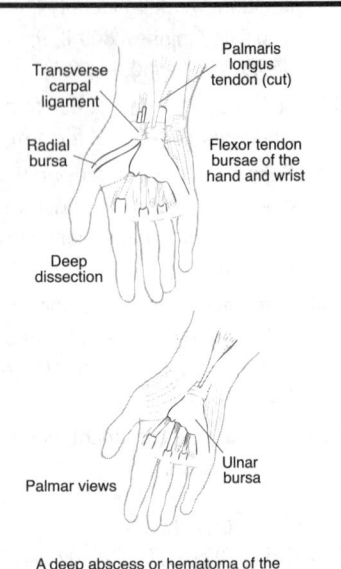

A deep abscess or hematoma of the forearm or wrist area is incised and drained. Report 25031 when a bursa of the same area is incised and drained

Explanation
The physician drains a deep abscess or hematoma in 25028 or an infected bursa in 25031 from the forearm and/or wrist. The physician makes an incision in the forearm or wrist overlying the site of the abscess, hematoma, or bursa. Dissection is carried down through the deep subcutaneous tissues and may be continued into the fascia or muscle to expose the abscess or hematoma. The incision may be extended if the mass is larger than expected. When the infected bursa, abscess, or hematoma is identified, it is incised and the contents are drained. The area is irrigated and the incision is repaired in layers with sutures, staples, and/or Steri-strips; closed with drains in place; or simply left open to further facilitate drainage of infection.

Coding Tips
For superficial incision and drainage of an abscess, see 10060 and 10061. For superficial incision and drainage of a hematoma, seroma, or fluid collection, see 10140. For puncture aspiration of an abscess, a hematoma, a bulla, or a cyst, see 10160. Local anesthesia is included in these services. However, these procedures may be performed under general anesthesia, depending on the age and/or condition of the patient. Surgical trays, A4550, are not separately reimbursed by Medicare; however, other third-party payers may cover them. Check with the specific payer to determine coverage.

ICD-9-CM Procedural
83.02 Myotomy
83.09 Other incision of soft tissue

Anesthesia
01810

ICD-9-CM Diagnostic
682.3 Cellulitis and abscess of upper arm and forearm — (Use additional code to identify organism, such as 041.1, etc.)
682.4 Cellulitis and abscess of hand, except fingers and thumb — (Use additional code to identify organism, such as 041.1, etc.)
727.89 Other disorders of synovium, tendon, and bursa
730.33 Periostitis, without mention of osteomyelitis, forearm — (Use additional code to identify organism: 041.1)
780.62 Postprocedural fever
881.10 Open wound of forearm, complicated
881.12 Open wound of wrist, complicated
923.10 Contusion of forearm
923.21 Contusion of wrist
927.10 Crushing injury of forearm — (Use additional code to identify any associated injuries: 800-829, 850.0-854.1, 860.0-869.1)
927.21 Crushing injury of wrist — (Use additional code to identify any associated injuries: 800-829, 850.0-854.1, 860.0-869.1)
927.8 Crushing injury of multiple sites of upper limb — (Use additional code to identify any associated injuries: 800-829, 850.0-854.1, 860.0-869.1)
998.59 Other postoperative infection — (Use additional code to identify infection)

Terms To Know
abscess. Circumscribed collection of pus resulting from bacteria, frequently associated with swelling and other signs of inflammation.

bursa. Cavity or sac containing fluid that occurs between articulating surfaces and serves to reduce friction from moving parts. An anatomical structure frequently referenced in orthopedic notes as it may become diseased or need removal.

cellulitis. Sudden, severe, suppurative inflammation and edema in subcutaneous tissue or muscle, most often caused by bacterial infection secondary to a cutaneous lesion.

contusion. Superficial injury (bruising) produced by impact without a break in the skin.

hematoma. Tumor-like collection of blood in some part of the body caused by a break in a blood vessel wall, usually as a result of trauma.

infected postoperative seroma. Infection within a tumor-like growth of serum following surgery.

late effect. Abnormality, dysfunction, or other residual condition produced after the acute phase of an illness, injury, or disease is over. There is no time limit on when late effects can appear.

periostitis. Inflammation of the outer layers of bone.

CCI Version 16.3
01810, 0213T, 0216T, 0228T, 0230T, 10060, 10140, 10160, 11041-11043, 20103, 20500, 24300, 25020-25023, 25075, 25115-25118, 25259, 25295, 26445-26449, 36000, 36400-36410, 36420-36430, 36440, 36600, 36640, 37202, 43752, 51701-51703, 62310-62319, 64400-64435, 64445-64450, 64479, 64483, 64490, 64493, 64505-64530, 69990, 93000-93010, 93040-93042, 93318, 94002, 94200, 94250, 94680-94690, 94770, 95812-95816, 95819, 95822, 95829, 95955, 96360, 96365, 96372, 96374-96376, 97597-97598, 97602-97606, 99148-99149, 99150

Also not with 25028: 11010, 25000-25001
Also not with 25031: 25000

Note: These CCI edits are used for Medicare. Other payers may reimburse on codes listed above.

Medicare Edits

	Fac RVU	Non-Fac RVU	FUD	Assist
25028	14.99	14.99	90	N/A
25031	10.53	10.53	90	80

Medicare References: 100-2,15,260; 100-4,12,30; 100-4,12,90.3; 100-4,14,10

25035

25035 Incision, deep, bone cortex, forearm and/or wrist (eg, osteomyelitis or bone abscess)

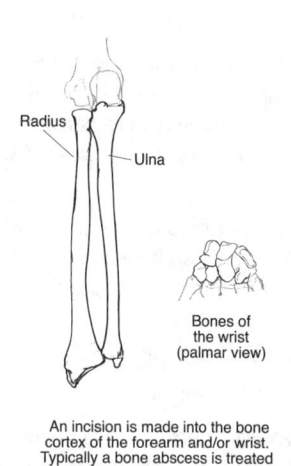

An incision is made into the bone cortex of the forearm and/or wrist. Typically a bone abscess is treated or dead bone tissue (osteomyelitis) is removed

Explanation
The physician incises the bone cortex of infected bone in the forearm and/or wrist to treat an abscess or osteomyelitis. The physician makes an incision over the affected area. Dissection is carried down through the soft tissues to expose the bone. The periosteum is split and reflected from the bone overlying the infected area. A curette may be used to scrape away the abscess or infected portion down to healthy bony tissue or drill holes may be made through the cortex into the medullary canal in a window outline around the infected or abscessed bone. The area is drained and debrided of infected bony and soft tissue. The physician irrigates the area with antibiotic solution, the periosteum is closed over the bone, and the soft tissues are sutured closed; or the wound is packed and left open, allowing the area to drain. Secondary closure is performed approximately three weeks later. Dressings are changed daily. A splint may be applied to limit wrist motion.

Coding Tips
According to CPT guidelines, cast application or strapping (including removal) is only reported as a replacement procedure or when the cast application or strapping is an initial service performed without a restorative treatment or procedure. See "Application of Casts and Strapping" in the CPT book in the Surgery Section, under the Musculoskeletal system. For superficial incision and drainage of an abscess, see 10060 and 10061. For superficial incision and drainage of a hematoma, seroma, or fluid collection, see 10140. For puncture aspiration of an abscess, a hematoma, a bulla, or a cyst, see 10160.

ICD-9-CM Procedural
77.13 Other incision of radius and ulna without division
77.14 Other incision of carpals and metacarpals without division

Anesthesia
25035 01830

ICD-9-CM Diagnostic
730.13 Chronic osteomyelitis, forearm — (Use additional code to identify organism: 041.1. Use additional code to identify major osseous defect, if applicable: 731.3)
730.23 Unspecified osteomyelitis, forearm — (Use additional code to identify organism: 041.1. Use additional code to identify major osseous defect, if applicable: 731.3)
730.83 Other infections involving bone in diseases classified elsewhere, forearm — (Use additional code to identify organism: 041.1. Code first underlying disease: 002.0, 015.0-015.9)
730.88 Other infections involving bone diseases classified elsewhere, other specified sites — (Use additional code to identify organism: 041.1. Code first underlying disease: 002.0, 015.0-015.9)
731.3 Major osseous defects — (Code first underlying disease: 170.0-170.9, 730.00-730.29, 733.00-733.09, 733.40-733.49, 996.45)
998.59 Other postoperative infection — (Use additional code to identify infection)

Terms To Know
abscess. Circumscribed collection of pus resulting from bacteria, frequently associated with swelling and other signs of inflammation.

fascia. Fibrous sheet or band of tissue that envelops organs, muscles, and groupings of muscles.

infection. Presence of microorganisms in body tissues that may result in cellular damage.

osteomyelitis. Inflammation of bone that may remain localized or spread to the marrow, cortex, or periosteum, in response to an infecting organism, usually bacterial and pyogenic.

soft tissue. Nonepithelial tissues outside of the skeleton that includes subcutaneous adipose tissue, fibrous tissue, fascia, muscles, blood and lymph vessels, and peripheral nervous system tissue.

subcutaneous. Below the skin.

CCI Version 16.3
01810, 0213T, 0216T, 0228T, 0230T, 10060-10061, 10140, 10160, 11010-11011, 11041-11043, 20000-20005, 20103, 20500, 20615, 24300, 25000, 25020-25023, 25028-25031, 25115-25118, 25250, 25259, 25295, 26445-26449, 36000, 36400-36410, 36420-36430, 36440, 36600, 36640, 37202, 43752, 51701-51703, 62310-62319, 64400-64435, 64445-64450, 64479, 64483, 64490, 64493, 64505-64530, 69990, 93000-93010, 93040-93042, 93318, 94002, 94200, 94250, 94680-94690, 94770, 95812-95816, 95819, 95822, 95829, 95955, 96360, 96365, 96372, 96374-96376, 97597-97598, 97602-97606, 99148-99149, 99150

Note: These CCI edits are used for Medicare. Other payers may reimburse on codes listed above.

Medicare Edits

	Fac RVU	Non-Fac RVU	FUD	Assist
25035	17.93	17.93	90	80

Medicare References: 100-2,15,260; 100-4,12,30; 100-4,12,90.3; 100-4,14,10

25040

25040 Arthrotomy, radiocarpal or midcarpal joint, with exploration, drainage, or removal of foreign body

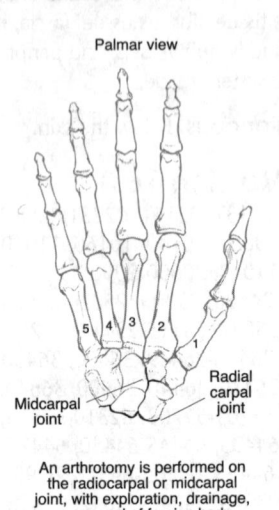

Palmar view

An arthrotomy is performed on the radiocarpal or midcarpal joint, with exploration, drainage, or removal of foreign body

Explanation
The physician performs an arthrotomy of a radiocarpal or midcarpal joint that includes exploration, drainage, or removal of any foreign body. An incision is made over the joint to be exposed. The soft tissues are dissected away and the joint capsule is exposed and incised. The joint space is explored, any necrotic tissue is removed, and infection or abnormal fluid is drained. If a foreign body is present (e.g., bullet, nail, gravel), it is exposed and removed. The wound is irrigated with antibiotic solution. The physician may leave the wound packed open with daily dressing changes to allow for further drainage and secondary healing by granulation. If the incision is repaired, drain tubes may be inserted and the incision is repaired in layers with sutures, staples, and/or Steri-strips.

Coding Tips
According to CPT guidelines, cast application or strapping (including removal) is only reported as a replacement procedure or when the cast application or strapping is an initial service performed without a restorative treatment or procedure. See "Application of Casts and Strapping" in the CPT book in the Surgery Section, under the Musculoskeletal system. For arthroscopy, wrist for lavage and drainage, see 29843.

ICD-9-CM Procedural
80.13   Other arthrotomy of wrist

Anesthesia
25040   01830

ICD-9-CM Diagnostic
- 357.1 Polyneuropathy in collagen vascular disease — (Code first underlying disease: 446.0, 710.0, 714.0)
- 359.6 Symptomatic inflammatory myopathy in diseases classified elsewhere — (Code first underlying disease: 135, 140.0-208.9, 277.30-277.39, 446.0, 710.0, 710.1, 710.2, 714.0)
- 446.0 Polyarteritis nodosa
- 710.0 Systemic lupus erythematosus — (Use additional code to identify manifestation: 424.91, 581.81, 582.81, 583.81)
- 710.1 Systemic sclerosis — (Use additional code to identify manifestation: 359.6, 517.2)
- 710.2 Sicca syndrome
- 711.03 Pyogenic arthritis, forearm — (Use additional code to identify infectious organism: 041.0-041.8)
- 714.0 Rheumatoid arthritis — (Use additional code to identify manifestation: 357.1, 359.6)
- 715.13 Primary localized osteoarthrosis, forearm
- 715.33 Localized osteoarthrosis not specified whether primary or secondary, forearm
- 716.13 Traumatic arthropathy, forearm
- 716.63 Unspecified monoarthritis, forearm
- 718.13 Loose body in forearm joint
- 719.03 Effusion of forearm joint
- 719.23 Villonodular synovitis, forearm
- 719.83 Other specified disorders of forearm joint
- 730.03 Acute osteomyelitis, forearm — (Use additional code to identify organism: 041.1. Use additional code to identify major osseous defect, if applicable: 731.3)
- 730.13 Chronic osteomyelitis, forearm — (Use additional code to identify organism: 041.1. Use additional code to identify major osseous defect, if applicable: 731.3)
- 731.3 Major osseous defects — (Code first underlying disease: 170.0-170.9, 730.00-730.29, 733.00-733.09, 733.40-733.49, 996.45)
- 881.12 Open wound of wrist, complicated

Terms To Know
effusion. Escape of fluid from within a body cavity.

foreign body. Any object or substance found in an organ and tissue that does not belong under normal circumstances.

osteomyelitis. Inflammation of bone that may remain localized or spread to the marrow, cortex, or periosteum, in response to an infecting organism, usually bacterial and pyogenic.

polyarteritis nodosa. Systemic necrotizing vasculitis of small and medium arteries that results in the infarction and scarring within the affected organs.

polyneuropathy. Disease process of severe inflammation of multiple nerves.

villonodular synovitis. Inflammation of the synovial membrane due to excessive synovial tissue formation, especially in the knee.

CCI Version 16.3
01810, 0213T, 0216T, 0228T, 0230T, 11010-11011, 11041-11044, 20103, 20500, 24300, 25000, 25100-25105, 25111, 25115-25118, 25259, 25295, 26449, 29844-29845, 36000, 36400-36410, 36420-36430, 36440, 36600, 36640, 37202, 43752, 51701-51703, 62310-62319, 64400-64435, 64445-64450, 64479, 64483, 64490, 64493, 64505-64530, 69990, 93000-93010, 93040-93042, 93318, 94002, 94200, 94250, 94680-94690, 94770, 95812-95816, 95819, 95822, 95829, 95955, 96360, 96365, 96372, 96374-96376, 99148-99149, 99150

Note: These CCI edits are used for Medicare. Other payers may reimburse on codes listed above.

Medicare Edits

	Fac RVU	Non-Fac RVU	FUD	Assist
25040	16.47	16.47	90	80

Medicare References: 100-2,15,260; 100-4,12,30; 100-4,12,90.3; 100-4,14,10

25065-25066

25065 Biopsy, soft tissue of forearm and/or wrist; superficial
25066 deep (subfascial or intramuscular)

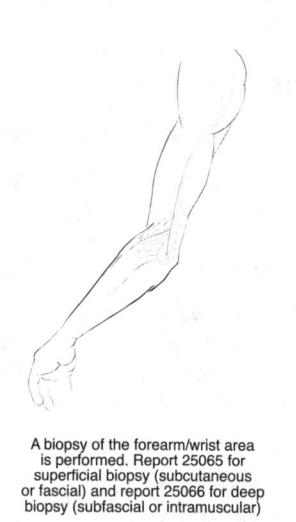

A biopsy of the forearm/wrist area is performed. Report 25065 for superficial biopsy (subcutaneous or fascial) and report 25066 for deep biopsy (subfascial or intramuscular)

Explanation
The physician performs a biopsy of the soft tissues of the forearm and/or wrist. With proper anesthesia administered, an incision is made over the biopsy area. Dissection is carried down within the superficial soft tissue layers in 25065, usually the subcutaneous fat to the uppermost fascial layer. In 25066, dissection is taken down deep within the soft tissue, such as into the fascial layer or within the muscle. A portion of the tissue is excised and submitted for pathology. The area is irrigated and the incision is closed with layered sutures, staples, or Steri-strips. If the wrist is involved, a splint may be applied to limit motion.

Coding Tips
According to CPT guidelines, cast application or strapping (including removal) is only reported as a replacement procedure or when the cast application or strapping is an initial service performed without a restorative treatment or procedure. See "Application of Casts and Strapping" in the CPT book in the Surgery Section, under the Musculoskeletal system. Local anesthesia is included in these services. However, 25066 may be performed under general anesthesia, depending on the age and/or condition of the patient. For needle biopsy of soft tissue, see 20206. Surgical trays, A4550, are not separately reimbursed by Medicare; however, other third-party payers may cover them. Check with the specific payer to determine coverage.

ICD-9-CM Procedural
83.21 Open biopsy of soft tissue

Anesthesia
25065 00400
25066 01810

ICD-9-CM Diagnostic
171.2 Malignant neoplasm of connective and other soft tissue of upper limb, including shoulder
195.4 Malignant neoplasm of upper limb
198.89 Secondary malignant neoplasm of other specified sites
215.2 Other benign neoplasm of connective and other soft tissue of upper limb, including shoulder
238.1 Neoplasm of uncertain behavior of connective and other soft tissue
239.2 Neoplasms of unspecified nature of bone, soft tissue, and skin

Terms To Know
benign. Mild or nonmalignant in nature.

cyst. Elevated encapsulated mass containing fluid, semisolid, or solid material with a membranous lining.

malignant. Any condition tending to progress toward death, specifically an invasive tumor with a loss of cellular differentiation that has the ability to spread or metastasize to other areas in the body.

soft tissue. Nonepithelial tissues outside of the skeleton that includes subcutaneous adipose tissue, fibrous tissue, fascia, muscles, blood and lymph vessels, and peripheral nervous system tissue.

subfascial. Beneath the band of fibrous tissue that lies deep to the skin, encloses muscles, and separates their layers.

superficial. On the skin surface or near the surface of any involved structure or field of interest.

tumor. Pathological swelling or enlargement; a neoplastic growth of uncontrolled, abnormal multiplication of cells.

CCI Version 16.3
01810, 0213T, 0216T, 0228T, 0230T, 10021-10022, 20103, 24300, 25259, 36000, 36400-36410, 36420-36430, 36440, 36600, 36640, 37202, 43752, 51701-51703, 62310-62319, 64400-64435, 64445-64450, 64479, 64483, 64490, 64493, 64505-64530, 69990, 93000-93010, 93040-93042, 93318, 94002, 94200, 94250, 94680-94690, 94770, 95812-95816, 95819, 95822, 95829, 95955, 96360, 96365, 96372, 96374-96376, 99148-99149, 99150

Also not with 25065: 38500, J0670, J2001
Also not with 25066: 11100, 20200-20205, 25001, 25065

Note: These CCI edits are used for Medicare. Other payers may reimburse on codes listed above.

Medicare Edits

	Fac RVU	Non-Fac RVU	FUD	Assist
25065	4.86	7.37	10	N/A
25066	10.69	10.69	90	N/A

Medicare References: 100-2,15,260; 100-4,12,30; 100-4,12,90.3; 100-4,14,10

25075-25076 (25071, 25073)

25075 Excision, tumor, soft tissue of forearm and/or wrist area, subcutaneous; less than 3 cm
25071   3 cm or greater
25076 Excision, tumor, soft tissue of forearm and/or wrist area, subfascial (eg, intramuscular); less than 3 cm
25073   3 cm or greater

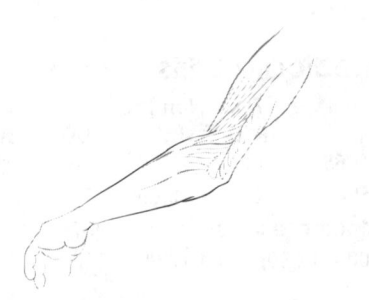

Report 25075 or 25071 for subcutaneous excision and 25076 or 25073 for subfascial excision of a soft tissue tumor of the forearm or wrist area

Explanation
The physician removes a tumor from the soft tissue of the forearm and/or wrist area that is located in the subcutaneous tissue in 25071 and 25075 and in the deep soft tissue, below the fascial plane or within the muscle, in 25073 and 25076. With the proper anesthesia administered, the physician makes an incision in the skin overlying the mass and dissects down to the tumor. The extent of the tumor is identified and a dissection is undertaken all the way around the tumor. A portion of neighboring soft tissue may also be removed to ensure adequate removal of all tumor tissue. A drain may be inserted and the incision is repaired with layers of sutures, staples, or Steri-strips. Report 25075 for excision of subcutaneous tumors less than 3 cm and 25071 for excision of subcutaneous tumors 3 cm or greater. Report 25076 for excision of subfascial or intramuscular tumors less than 3 cm and 25073 for excision of subfascial or intramuscular tumors 3 cm or greater.

Coding Tips
Codes 25071 and 25073 are resequenced codes and will not display in numeric order. According to CPT guidelines, cast application or strapping (including removal) is only reported as a replacement procedure or when the cast application or strapping is an initial service performed without a restorative treatment or procedure. See "Application of Casts and Strapping" in the CPT book in the Surgery Section, under the Musculoskeletal system. These codes include local anesthesia. However, they may be performed under general anesthesia, depending on the age and/or condition of the patient. When medically necessary, report moderate (conscious) sedation provided by the performing physician with 99143–99145. When provided by another physician, report 99148–99150. For needle biopsy of muscle, see 20206.

ICD-9-CM Procedural
83.31 Excision of lesion of tendon sheath
83.32 Excision of lesion of muscle
83.39 Excision of lesion of other soft tissue
83.49 Other excision of soft tissue
86.3 Other local excision or destruction of lesion or tissue of skin and subcutaneous tissue
86.4 Radical excision of skin lesion

Anesthesia
25071 00400
25073 01810
25075 00400
25076 01810

ICD-9-CM Diagnostic
171.2 Malignant neoplasm of connective and other soft tissue of upper limb, including shoulder
172.6 Malignant melanoma of skin of upper limb, including shoulder
173.6 Other malignant neoplasm of skin of upper limb, including shoulder
195.4 Malignant neoplasm of upper limb
198.89 Secondary malignant neoplasm of other specified sites
209.33 Merkel cell carcinoma of the upper limb
209.75 Secondary Merkel cell carcinoma
214.1 Lipoma of other skin and subcutaneous tissue
215.2 Other benign neoplasm of connective and other soft tissue of upper limb, including shoulder
232.6 Carcinoma in situ of skin of upper limb, including shoulder
238.1 Neoplasm of uncertain behavior of connective and other soft tissue
239.2 Neoplasms of unspecified nature of bone, soft tissue, and skin
782.2 Localized superficial swelling, mass, or lump

Terms To Know
benign. Mild or nonmalignant in nature.

lipoma. Benign tumor containing fat cells and the most common of soft tissue lesions, which are usually painless and asymptomatic, with the exception of an angiolipoma.

malignant. Any condition tending to progress toward death, specifically an invasive tumor with a loss of cellular differentiation that has the ability to spread or metastasize to other areas in the body.

CCI Version 16.3
01810, 0228T, 0230T, 10060, 10140, 10160, 11010-11012❖, 11040-11044, 12001-12007, 12020-12047, 13120-13121, 13131-13132, 24300, 25259, 36000, 36400-36410, 36420-36430, 36440, 36600, 36640, 37202, 43752, 51701-51703, 62310-62319, 64400-64435, 64445-64450, 64479, 64483, 64505-64530, 69990, 93000-93010, 93040-93042, 93318, 94002, 94200, 94250, 94680-94690, 94770, 95812-95816, 95819, 95822, 95829, 95955, 96360, 96365, 96372, 96374-96376, 99148-99149, 99150

Also not with 25071: 0213T, 0216T, 11402-11403, 25028-25031, 25065-25066, 25075, 25110-25112, 25118❖, 38500, 64490, 64493

Also not with 25073: 0213T, 0216T, 25001, 25028-25031, 25065-25071, 25075-25076, 25110-25112, 25118❖, 64490, 64493

Also not with 25075: 11400-11401, 11404-11426, 25065-25066, 25111, 38500, J0670, J2001

Also not with 25076: 11400-11406, 11600-11606, 25001, 25028-25031, 25065-25071, 25075, 25110-25115, 25118, 25295

Note: These CCI edits are used for Medicare. Other payers may reimburse on codes listed above.

Medicare Edits

	Fac RVU	Non-Fac RVU	FUD	Assist
25071	12.79	12.79	90	80
25073	15.99	15.99	90	80
25075	9.49	13.92	90	N/A
25076	15.05	15.05	90	N/A

Medicare References: 100-2,15,260; 100-4,12,30; 100-4,12,90.3; 100-4,14,10

25077-25078

25077 Radical resection of tumor (eg, malignant neoplasm), soft tissue of forearm and/or wrist area; less than 3 cm
25078 3 cm or greater

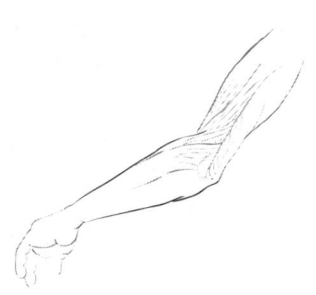

Radical resection of soft tissue tumor of the forearm or wrist area is reported with 25077 if less than 3 cm and with 25078 if 3 cm or greater

Explanation
The physician performs a radical resection of a malignant soft tissue tumor from the forearm and/or wrist area, not involving bone. An incision is made over the tumor and dissection exposes it. The tumor and any adjacent tissue that may be affected by the spread of the neoplasm are excised. Large resections may be needed. The type and stage of the lesion determines the extent of the tumor margin resection area. Muscle or fascia may need to be repaired and drains may be placed. The surgical wound is repaired by intermediate or complex closure, adjacent tissue transfer, or graft. If the wrist is involved, a splint may be applied to limit motion. Report 25077 for excision of tumors less than 3 cm and 25078 for excision of tumors 3 cm or greater.

Coding Tips
If significant additional time and effort is documented, append modifier 22 and submit a cover letter and operative report. For radical tumor resection of the soft tissue of the hand or finger, see 26117.

ICD-9-CM Procedural
- 83.31 Excision of lesion of tendon sheath
- 83.32 Excision of lesion of muscle
- 83.39 Excision of lesion of other soft tissue
- 83.49 Other excision of soft tissue
- 86.3 Other local excision or destruction of lesion or tissue of skin and subcutaneous tissue
- 86.4 Radical excision of skin lesion

Anesthesia
00400, 01810

ICD-9-CM Diagnostic
- 171.2 Malignant neoplasm of connective and other soft tissue of upper limb, including shoulder
- 172.6 Malignant melanoma of skin of upper limb, including shoulder
- 173.6 Other malignant neoplasm of skin of upper limb, including shoulder
- 195.4 Malignant neoplasm of upper limb
- 198.89 Secondary malignant neoplasm of other specified sites
- 209.33 Merkel cell carcinoma of the upper limb
- 209.75 Secondary Merkel cell carcinoma
- 214.1 Lipoma of other skin and subcutaneous tissue
- 215.2 Other benign neoplasm of connective and other soft tissue of upper limb, including shoulder
- 238.1 Neoplasm of uncertain behavior of connective and other soft tissue
- 239.2 Neoplasms of unspecified nature of bone, soft tissue, and skin
- 782.2 Localized superficial swelling, mass, or lump

CCI Version 16.3
01810, 0228T, 0230T, 10060, 10140, 10160, 11010-11012❖, 11040-11044, 12001-12007, 12020-12047, 13120-13121, 13131-13132, 24300, 25001, 25028-25031, 25259, 36000, 36400-36410, 36420-36430, 36440, 36600, 36640, 37202, 43752, 51701-51703, 62310-62319, 64400-64435, 64445-64450, 64479, 64483, 64505-64530, 69990, 93000-93010, 93040-93042, 93318, 94002, 94200, 94250, 94680-94690, 94770, 95812-95816, 95819, 95822, 95829, 95955, 96360, 96365, 96372, 96374-96376, 99148-99149, 99150

Also not with 25077: 11400-11406, 11600-11606, 25065-25076, 25110-25118❖, 25295

Also not with 25078: 0213T, 0216T, 25065-25077, 25110-25116, 64490, 64493

Note: These CCI edits are used for Medicare. Other payers may reimburse on codes listed above.

Medicare Edits

	Fac RVU	Non-Fac RVU	FUD	Assist
25077	25.78	25.78	90	N/A
25078	33.45	33.45	90	80

Medicare References: 100-2,15,260; 100-4,12,30; 100-4,12,90.3; 100-4,14,10

25085

25085 Capsulotomy, wrist (eg, contracture)

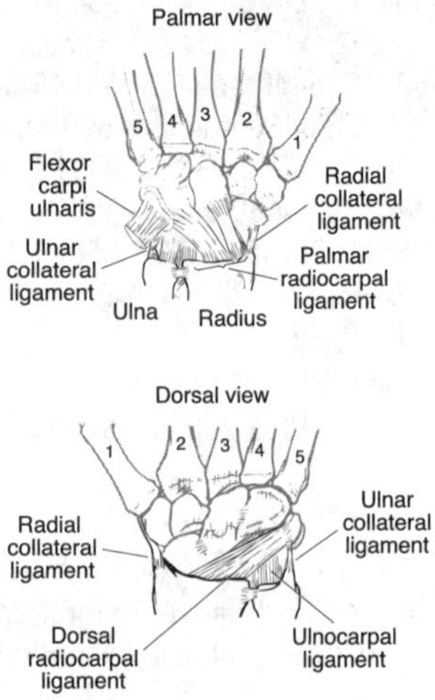

Palmar view

A capsulotomy of the wrist is performed

Explanation

The physician performs a capsulotomy of the wrist. The physician makes an incision overlying the wrist joint. The tissues are dissected to the joint capsule. The physician makes an incision in the capsule, allowing better joint movement. The incision is closed in multiple layers with sutures.

Coding Tips

Capsulotomy is not reported separately when performed as part of a more complex procedure requiring incision into the joint capsule. According to CPT guidelines, cast application or strapping (including removal) is only reported as a replacement procedure or when the cast application or strapping is an initial service performed without a restorative treatment or procedure. See "Application of Casts and Strapping" in the CPT book in the Surgery Section, under the Musculoskeletal system.

ICD-9-CM Procedural

80.43 Division of joint capsule, ligament, or cartilage of wrist

Anesthesia

25085 01810

ICD-9-CM Diagnostic

718.43 Contracture of forearm joint
728.10 Unspecified calcification and ossification

Terms To Know

calcification. Normal process of calcium salts deposition in bone.

contracture. Shortening of muscle or connective tissue.

joint capsule. Sac-like enclosure enveloping the synovial joint cavity with a fibrous membrane attached to the articular ends of the bones in the joint.

ossification. Formation of bony growth or hardening into bone-like substance.

CCI Version 16.3

01810, 0213T, 0216T, 0228T, 0230T, 11012❖, 24300, 25040, 25100-25101, 25259, 36000, 36400-36410, 36420-36430, 36440, 36600, 36640, 37202, 43752, 51701-51703, 62310-62319, 64400-64435, 64445-64450, 64479, 64483, 64490, 64493, 64505-64530, 69990, 93000-93010, 93040-93042, 93318, 94002, 94200, 94250, 94680-94690, 94770, 95812-95816, 95819, 95822, 95829, 95955, 96360, 96365, 96372, 96374-96376, 99148-99149, 99150

Note: These CCI edits are used for Medicare. Other payers may reimburse on codes listed above.

Medicare Edits

	Fac RVU	Non-Fac RVU	FUD	Assist
25085	13.31	13.31	90	80

Medicare References: 100-2,15,260; 100-4,12,30; 100-4,12,90.3; 100-4,14,10

25100-25105

25100	Arthrotomy, wrist joint; with biopsy
25101	with joint exploration, with or without biopsy, with or without removal of loose or foreign body
25105	with synovectomy

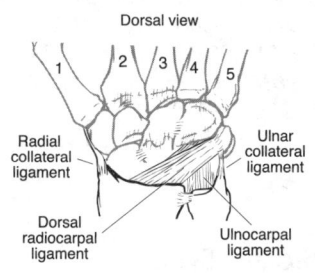

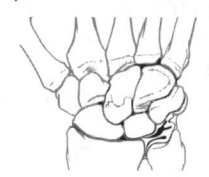

The wrist joint is surgically accessed and a biopsy is collected. Report 25101 when the joint is explored, with or without biopsy and with or without removal of loose or foreign body. Report 25105 when synovial material is removed

Explanation

The physician makes a longitudinal incision over the part of the wrist to be exposed (e.g., anterior, posterior, medial, or lateral aspect) to access the wrist joint and perform an arthrotomy. The soft tissues are dissected away to expose the joint capsule, which is incised to expose the synovium lying within the capsule. A small portion of the synovium is excised for biopsy in 25100. In 25101, additional dissection is carried out to further explore the joint cavity. Any loose or foreign bodies (e.g., free cartilage, bone chips, gravel) are removed and a biopsy may be taken. In 25105, the joint capsule is incised to expose the synovium, the inner membrane of the articular capsule that lines the joint cavity. The inflamed or enlarged synovium is dissected away from the capsule and the bones and removed. A drain tube may be placed. The physician irrigates the joint. The physician may leave the wound packed open with daily dressing changes to allow for further drainage and secondary healing by granulation. The incision is repaired in layers with sutures, staples, and/or Steri-strips. A splint may be applied to limit wrist movement.

Coding Tips

According to CPT guidelines, cast application or strapping (including removal) is only reported as a replacement procedure or when the cast application or strapping is an initial service performed without a restorative treatment or procedure. See "Application of Casts and Strapping" in the CPT book in the Surgery Section, under the Musculoskeletal system. For wrist arthroscopy, diagnostic with or without synovial biopsy, see 29840. For arthroscopy of the wrist with synovectomy, see 29844 and 29845.

ICD-9-CM Procedural

80.13	Other arthrotomy of wrist
80.33	Biopsy of joint structure of wrist
80.73	Synovectomy of wrist

Anesthesia
01830

ICD-9-CM Diagnostic

170.5	Malignant neoplasm of short bones of upper limb
171.2	Malignant neoplasm of connective and other soft tissue of upper limb, including shoulder
195.4	Malignant neoplasm of upper limb
198.5	Secondary malignant neoplasm of bone and bone marrow
198.89	Secondary malignant neoplasm of other specified sites
213.5	Benign neoplasm of short bones of upper limb
215.2	Other benign neoplasm of connective and other soft tissue of upper limb, including shoulder
238.0	Neoplasm of uncertain behavior of bone and articular cartilage
239.2	Neoplasms of unspecified nature of bone, soft tissue, and skin
357.1	Polyneuropathy in collagen vascular disease — (Code first underlying disease: 446.0, 710.0, 714.0)
359.6	Symptomatic inflammatory myopathy in diseases classified elsewhere — (Code first underlying disease: 135, 140.0-208.9, 277.30-277.39, 446.0, 710.0, 710.1, 710.2, 714.0)
446.0	Polyarteritis nodosa
710.0	Systemic lupus erythematosus — (Use additional code to identify manifestation: 424.91, 581.81, 582.81, 583.81)
710.1	Systemic sclerosis — (Use additional code to identify manifestation: 359.6, 517.2)
710.2	Sicca syndrome
711.03	Pyogenic arthritis, forearm — (Use additional code to identify infectious organism: 041.0-041.8)
711.93	Unspecified infective arthritis, forearm
714.0	Rheumatoid arthritis — (Use additional code to identify manifestation: 357.1, 359.6)
715.13	Primary localized osteoarthrosis, forearm
715.33	Localized osteoarthrosis not specified whether primary or secondary, forearm
716.63	Unspecified monoarthritis, forearm
718.13	Loose body in forearm joint
718.93	Unspecified derangement, forearm joint
719.23	Villonodular synovitis, forearm
727.05	Other tenosynovitis of hand and wrist
729.6	Residual foreign body in soft tissue — (Use additional code to identify foreign body (V90.01-V90.9))
906.3	Late effect of contusion
906.4	Late effect of crushing
V64.43	Arthroscopic surgical procedure converted to open procedure

CCI Version 16.3

01810, 0213T, 0216T, 0228T, 0230T, 24300, 25000, 25116-25118, 25259, 25295, 36000, 36400-36410, 36420-36430, 36440, 36600, 36640, 37202, 43752, 51701-51703, 62310-62319, 64400-64435, 64445-64450, 64479, 64483, 64490, 64493, 64505-64530, 64721, 69990, 93000-93010, 93040-93042, 93318, 94002, 94200, 94250, 94680-94690, 94770, 95812-95816, 95819, 95822, 95829, 95955, 96360, 96365, 96372, 96374-96376, 99148-99149, 99150

Also not with 25100: 11010-11012❖, 29843-29848

Also not with 25101: 11010, 20103, 25100, 25250, 29843-29848

Also not with 25105: 11012❖, 25085-25100, 29843-29847, 64718

Note: These CCI edits are used for Medicare. Other payers may reimburse on codes listed above.

Medicare Edits

	Fac RVU	Non-Fac RVU	FUD	Assist
25100	10.02	10.02	90	80
25101	11.76	11.76	90	80
25105	14.17	14.17	90	80

Medicare References: 100-2,15,260; 100-4,12,30; 100-4,12,90.3; 100-4,14,10

25107

25107 Arthrotomy, distal radioulnar joint including repair of triangular cartilage, complex

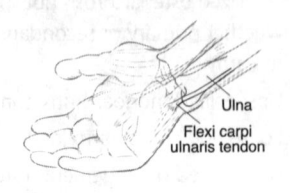

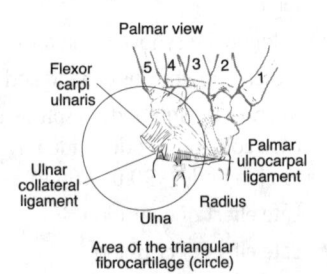

Ulna
Flexi carpi ulnaris tendon

Palmar view
Flexor carpi ulnaris
Ulnar collateral ligament
Palmar ulnocarpal ligament
Ulna
Radius
Area of the triangular fibrocartilage (circle)

The distal radioulnar joint is surgically accessed and repaired along with a complex repair of the triangular cartilage

Explanation
The physician performs a distal radioulnar arthrotomy for repair of a triangular cartilage complex. The physician incises the skin over the wrist and dissects down through the soft tissues to expose the joint and locate the triangular cartilage complex. The defect is identified and debrided or sutured to return to a correct anatomic state. The wound is repaired in layers with sutures, staples, and/or Steri-strips. A splint may be applied to limit wrist movement.

Coding Tips
According to CPT guidelines, cast application or strapping (including removal) is only reported as a replacement procedure or when the cast application or strapping is an initial service performed without a restorative treatment or procedure. See "Application of Casts and Strapping" in the CPT book in the Surgery Section, under the Musculoskeletal system. For arthrotomy of the wrist joint with a biopsy, see 25100. For arthrotomy, wrist joint with synovectomy, see 25105.

ICD-9-CM Procedural
81.96 Other repair of joint

Anesthesia
25107 01830

ICD-9-CM Diagnostic
718.03 Articular cartilage disorder, forearm
718.73 Developmental dislocation of joint, forearm
718.83 Other joint derangement, not elsewhere classified, forearm
718.93 Unspecified derangement, forearm joint
813.40 Unspecified closed fracture of lower end of forearm
813.41 Closed Colles' fracture
813.42 Other closed fractures of distal end of radius (alone)
813.43 Closed fracture of distal end of ulna (alone)
813.44 Closed fracture of lower end of radius with ulna
813.45 Torus fracture of radius (alone)
813.46 Torus fracture of ulna (alone)
813.47 Torus fracture of radius and ulna
813.50 Unspecified open fracture of lower end of forearm
813.51 Open Colles' fracture
813.52 Other open fractures of distal end of radius (alone)
813.53 Open fracture of distal end of ulna (alone)
813.54 Open fracture of lower end of radius with ulna
833.01 Closed dislocation of distal radioulnar (joint)
833.11 Open dislocation of distal radioulnar (joint)
842.09 Other wrist sprain and strain
881.12 Open wound of wrist, complicated
881.22 Open wound of wrist, with tendon involvement

Terms To Know

closed fracture. Break in a bone without a concomitant opening in the skin. A closed fracture is coded when the type of fracture is not specified.

dislocation. Displacement of a bone in relation to its neighboring tissue, especially a joint.

distal. Located farther away from a specified reference point.

open fracture. Exposed break in a bone, always considered compound due to its high risk of infection from the open wound leading to the fracture. Broken bone ends may protrude through the skin and contaminants or foreign bodies are often embedded in the tissues.

open wound. Opening or break of the skin.

CCI Version 16.3
01810, 0213T, 0216T, 0228T, 0230T, 11012❖, 24300, 25040❖, 25100-25105, 25250, 25259, 29846, 36000, 36400-36410, 36420-36430, 36440, 36600, 36640, 37202, 43752, 51701-51703, 62310-62319, 64400-64435, 64445-64450, 64479, 64483, 64490, 64493, 64505-64530, 69990, 93000-93010, 93040-93042, 93318, 94002, 94200, 94250, 94680-94690, 94770, 95812-95816, 95819, 95822, 95829, 95955, 96360, 96365, 96372, 96374-96376, 99148-99149, 99150

Note: These CCI edits are used for Medicare. Other payers may reimburse on codes listed above.

Medicare Edits

	Fac RVU	Non-Fac RVU	FUD	Assist
25107	17.97	17.97	90	80

Medicare References: 100-2,15,260; 100-4,12,30; 100-4,12,90.3; 100-4,14,10

25109

25109 Excision of tendon, forearm and/or wrist, flexor or extensor, each

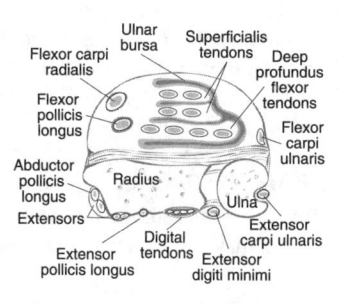

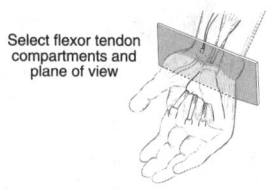

Explanation
The physician excises a flexor or extensor tendon of the wrist or forearm. The physician incises the overlying skin and dissects the tendon. The tendon is freed and resected. The operative incision is closed in sutured layers.

Coding Tips
According to CPT guidelines, cast application or strapping (including removal) is only reported as a replacement procedure or when the cast application or strapping is an initial service performed without a restorative treatment or procedure. See "Application of Casts and Strapping" in the CPT book in the Surgery Section, under the Musculoskeletal system. Local anesthesia is included in this service. For excision of lesion of tendon sheath, forearm/wrist, see 25110.

ICD-9-CM Procedural
- 83.41 Excision of tendon for graft
- 83.42 Other tenonectomy

Anesthesia
25109 01810

ICD-9-CM Diagnostic
- 171.2 Malignant neoplasm of connective and other soft tissue of upper limb, including shoulder
- 215.2 Other benign neoplasm of connective and other soft tissue of upper limb, including shoulder
- 238.1 Neoplasm of uncertain behavior of connective and other soft tissue
- 239.2 Neoplasms of unspecified nature of bone, soft tissue, and skin
- 719.93 Unspecified disorder of forearm joint
- 727.00 Unspecified synovitis and tenosynovitis
- 727.01 Synovitis and tenosynovitis in diseases classified elsewhere — (Code first underlying disease: 015.0-015.9)
- 727.02 Giant cell tumor of tendon sheath
- 727.04 Radial styloid tenosynovitis
- 727.05 Other tenosynovitis of hand and wrist
- 782.2 Localized superficial swelling, mass, or lump

Terms To Know

anterior. Situated in the front area or toward the belly surface of the body; an anatomical reference point used to show the position and relationship of one body structure to another.

flexion. Act of bending or being bent.

lateral. To/on the side.

lesion. Area of damaged tissue that has lost continuity or function, due to disease or trauma. Lesions may be located on internal structures such as the brain, nerves, or kidneys, or visible on the skin.

malignant. Any condition tending to progress toward death, specifically an invasive tumor with a loss of cellular differentiation that has the ability to spread or metastasize to other areas in the body.

proximal. Located closest to a specified reference point, usually the midline.

secondary. Second in order of occurrence or importance, or appearing during the course of another disease or condition.

soft tissue. Nonepithelial tissues outside of the skeleton that includes subcutaneous adipose tissue, fibrous tissue, fascia, muscles, blood and lymph vessels, and peripheral nervous system tissue.

tumor. Pathological swelling or enlargement; a neoplastic growth of uncontrolled, abnormal multiplication of cells.

CCI Version 16.3
01810, 0213T, 0216T, 0228T, 0230T, 11010-11011❖, 24300, 25000-25001, 25110, 25259, 36000, 36400-36410, 36420-36430, 36440, 36600, 36640, 37202, 43752, 51701-51703, 62310-62319, 64400-64435, 64445-64450, 64479, 64483, 64490, 64493, 64505-64530, 69990, 93000-93010, 93040-93042, 93318, 94002, 94200, 94250, 94680-94690, 94770, 95812-95816, 95819, 95822, 95829, 95955, 96360, 96365, 96372, 96374-96376, 99148-99149, 99150

Note: These CCI edits are used for Medicare. Other payers may reimburse on codes listed above.

Medicare Edits

	Fac RVU	Non-Fac RVU	FUD	Assist
25109	15.46	15.46	90	N/A

Medicare References: None

25110

25110 Excision, lesion of tendon sheath, forearm and/or wrist

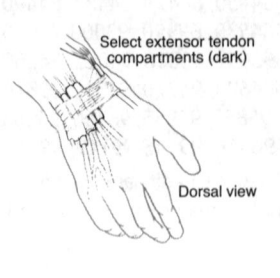

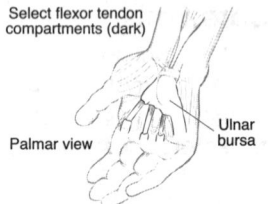

Explanation
The physician makes an incision overlying the affected tendon in the volar or dorsal aspect (flexor or extensor tendons) of the forearm and/or wrist. Dissection exposes the affected tendon. The lesion is excised or shelled out, leaving normal tissue intact. If incised, the tendon sheath is closed. The incision is repaired in layers with sutures, staples, and/or Steri-strips.

Coding Tips
According to CPT guidelines, cast application or strapping (including removal) is only reported as a replacement procedure or when the cast application or strapping is an initial service performed without a restorative treatment or procedure. See "Application of Casts and Strapping" in the CPT book in the Surgery Section, under the Musculoskeletal system. Local anesthesia is included in this service.

ICD-9-CM Procedural
83.31 Excision of lesion of tendon sheath

Anesthesia
25110 01810

ICD-9-CM Diagnostic
171.2 Malignant neoplasm of connective and other soft tissue of upper limb, including shoulder
215.2 Other benign neoplasm of connective and other soft tissue of upper limb, including shoulder
216.6 Benign neoplasm of skin of upper limb, including shoulder
238.1 Neoplasm of uncertain behavior of connective and other soft tissue
239.2 Neoplasms of unspecified nature of bone, soft tissue, and skin
719.93 Unspecified disorder of forearm joint
727.02 Giant cell tumor of tendon sheath
727.05 Other tenosynovitis of hand and wrist
782.2 Localized superficial swelling, mass, or lump

Terms To Know

anterior. Situated in the front area or toward the belly surface of the body; an anatomical reference point used to show the position and relationship of one body structure to another.

benign. Mild or nonmalignant in nature.

lesion. Area of damaged tissue that has lost continuity or function, due to disease or trauma. Lesions may be located on internal structures such as the brain, nerves, or kidneys, or visible on the skin.

malignant. Any condition tending to progress toward death, specifically an invasive tumor with a loss of cellular differentiation that has the ability to spread or metastasize to other areas in the body.

neoplasm. New abnormal growth, tumor.

posterior. Located in the back part or caudal end of the body.

sheath. Covering enclosing an organ or part.

tendon. Fibrous tissue that connects muscle to bone, consisting primarily of collagen and containing little vasculature.

tenosynovitis. Inflammation of a tendon sheath due to infection or disease.

CCI Version 16.3
01810, 0213T, 0216T, 0228T, 0230T, 11010-11012❖, 24300, 25000-25001, 25075, 25100-25105, 25259, 25295, 36000, 36400-36410, 36420-36430, 36440, 36600, 36640, 37202, 43752, 51701-51703, 62310-62319, 64400-64435, 64445-64450, 64479, 64483, 64490, 64493, 64505-64530, 64704-64708, 69990, 93000-93010, 93040-93042, 93318, 94002, 94200, 94250, 94680-94690, 94770, 95812-95816, 95819, 95822, 95829, 95955, 96360, 96365, 96372, 96374-96376, 99148-99149, 99150

Note: These CCI edits are used for Medicare. Other payers may reimburse on codes listed above.

Medicare Edits

	Fac RVU	Non-Fac RVU	FUD	Assist
25110	10.18	10.18	90	N/A

Medicare References: 100-2,15,260; 100-4,12,30; 100-4,12,90.3; 100-4,14,10

25111-25112

25111 Excision of ganglion, wrist (dorsal or volar); primary
25112 recurrent

Ganglia can be found on either the dorsal or volar aspect

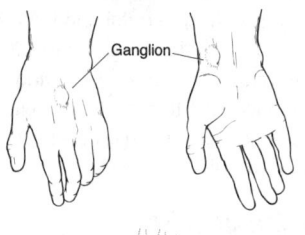

Ganglion

Extensor pollicis longus
Extensor carpi radialis brevis
Extensor retinaculum
Head of ulna

The insertion of the extensor carpi radialis brevis into the base of the metacarpal bones is a common place for ganglia to form

Ganglia are round, often nontender cyst-like growths of nerve cells that often communicate with synovial tendon sheaths. Code 25111 reports the primary removal of ganglia of the wrist. Report 25112 for removal of recurrent ganglia

Explanation

The physician removes a ganglion from the wrist in 25111 or a recurrent ganglion in 25112. An incision is made overlying the ganglion. The tissues are dissected around the ganglion, freeing the ganglion from surrounding tissue. (Scar tissue may be removed in 25112.) The physician may dissect deep within the wrist joint in order to excise all of the ganglion. The ganglion is then removed. The joint or muscle tissue may be repaired in 25112. The physician irrigates the wound with antibiotic solution and closes the wound in layers.

Coding Tips

According to CPT guidelines, cast application or strapping (including removal) is only reported as a replacement procedure or when the cast application or strapping is an initial service performed without a restorative treatment or procedure. See "Application of Casts and Strapping" in the CPT book in the Surgery Section, under the Musculoskeletal system. Local anesthesia is included in these services. For excision of a ganglion, hand or finger, see 26160.

ICD-9-CM Procedural

82.21 Excision of lesion of tendon sheath of hand

Anesthesia

01810

ICD-9-CM Diagnostic

727.41 Ganglion of joint
727.42 Ganglion of tendon sheath

Terms To Know

dorsal. Pertaining to the back or posterior aspect.

ganglion. Fluid-filled, benign cyst appearing on a tendon sheath or aponeurosis, frequently found in the hand, wrist, or foot and connecting to an underlying joint.

muscle tissue. Network of specialized cells for performing contraction to produce voluntary or involuntary movement of body parts, and skeletal, cardiac, or visceral muscles.

primary. Principal or first in the order of occurrence or importance.

volar. Palm of the hand (palmar) or sole of the foot (plantar).

CCI Version 16.3

01810, 0213T, 0216T, 0228T, 0230T, 24300, 25100-25105, 25259, 25295, 29125, 35761, 36000, 36400-36410, 36420-36430, 36440, 36600, 36640, 37202, 43752, 51701-51703, 62310-62319, 64400-64435, 64445-64450, 64479, 64483, 64490, 64493, 64505-64530, 69990, 93000-93010, 93040-93042, 93318, 94002, 94200, 94250, 94680-94690, 94770, 95812-95816, 95819, 95822, 95829, 95955, 96360, 96365, 96372, 96374-96376, 99148-99149, 99150

Also not with 25111: 11010-11012❖, 12001-12007, 12020-12047, 13120-13121, 13131-13132, 25001, 25112❖, 64704-64708

Also not with 25112: 11011-11012❖, 25040, 25075

Note: These CCI edits are used for Medicare. Other payers may reimburse on codes listed above.

Medicare Edits

	Fac RVU	Non-Fac RVU	FUD	Assist
25111	9.21	9.21	90	N/A
25112	11.17	11.17	90	N/A

Medicare References: 100-2,15,260; 100-4,12,30; 100-4,12,90.3; 100-4,14,10

25115-25116

25115 Radical excision of bursa, synovia of wrist, or forearm tendon sheaths (eg, tenosynovitis, fungus, Tbc, or other granulomas, rheumatoid arthritis); flexors

25116 extensors, with or without transposition of dorsal retinaculum

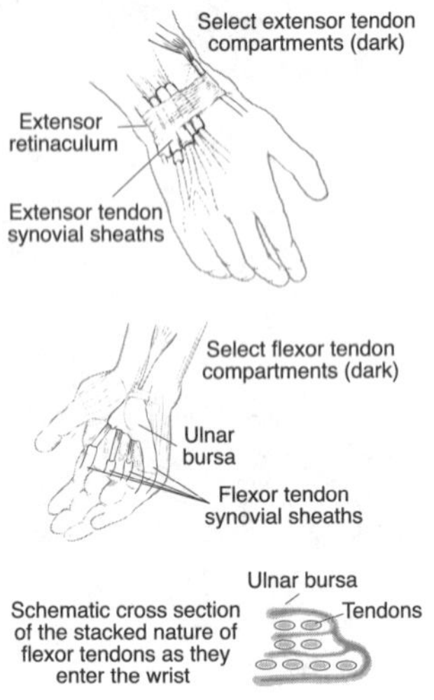

A radical excision of wrist or forearm flexor tendon sheaths is performed, including bursae and synovia. Report 25116 when a radical excision is performed on the extensor tendons, including bursae and synovia.

Explanation

Radical excision is removal of all diseased and/or inflamed tissue and may include removal of a portion of surrounding normal tissue. The physician makes a longitudinal incision over the anterior aspect of the distal forearm and wrist. Dissection is carried down to expose the flexor tendons of the wrist in 25115 or the extensor tendons in 25116. The physician excises the bursa and any inflamed and hypertrophied tissues from around the tendons. The tendons are left intact, allowing them to glide better during wrist movement. The physician may perform a transposition of the dorsal retinaculum if enough tissue is removed from the wrist extensors. A transposition makes a smooth gliding surface no longer present between the extensor tendons and carpal bones of the wrist. The dorsal retinaculum is incised in the mid-line and tucked underneath the extensor tendons and closed with sutures. The incisions are repaired in multiple layers with sutures, staples, and/or Steri-strips. The wrist may be placed in a splint.

Coding Tips

According to CPT guidelines, cast application or strapping (including removal) is only reported as a replacement procedure or when the cast application or strapping is an initial service performed without a restorative treatment or procedure. See "Application of Casts and Strapping" in the CPT book in the Surgery Section, under the Musculoskeletal system. For incision and drainage of a bursa, forearm or wrist, see 25031. For finger synovectomy, see 26145.

ICD-9-CM Procedural

- 83.31 Excision of lesion of tendon sheath
- 83.39 Excision of lesion of other soft tissue
- 83.5 Bursectomy

Anesthesia
01810

ICD-9-CM Diagnostic

- 357.1 Polyneuropathy in collagen vascular disease — (Code first underlying disease: 446.0, 710.0, 714.0)
- 359.6 Symptomatic inflammatory myopathy in diseases classified elsewhere — (Code first underlying disease: 135, 140.0-208.9, 277.30-277.39, 446.0, 710.0, 710.1, 710.2, 714.0)
- 446.0 Polyarteritis nodosa
- 517.8 Lung involvement in other diseases classified elsewhere — (Use additional code to identify infectious organism. Code first underlying disease: 135, 277.30-277.39, 710.0, 710.2, 710.4)
- 710.0 Systemic lupus erythematosus — (Use additional code to identify manifestation: 424.91, 581.81, 582.81, 583.81)
- 710.1 Systemic sclerosis — (Use additional code to identify manifestation: 359.6, 517.2)
- 710.2 Sicca syndrome
- 710.9 Unspecified diffuse connective tissue disease
- 711.03 Pyogenic arthritis, forearm — (Use additional code to identify infectious organism: 041.0-041.8)
- 711.13 Arthropathy associated with Reiter's disease and nonspecific urethritis, forearm — (Code first underlying disease: 099.3, 099.4)
- 711.93 Unspecified infective arthritis, forearm
- 714.0 Rheumatoid arthritis — (Use additional code to identify manifestation: 357.1, 359.6)
- 719.23 Villonodular synovitis, forearm
- 727.00 Unspecified synovitis and tenosynovitis
- 727.01 Synovitis and tenosynovitis in diseases classified elsewhere — (Code first underlying disease: 015.0-015.9)
- 727.02 Giant cell tumor of tendon sheath
- 727.05 Other tenosynovitis of hand and wrist
- 727.42 Ganglion of tendon sheath
- 727.49 Other ganglion and cyst of synovium, tendon, and bursa

Terms To Know

bursa. Cavity or sac containing fluid that occurs between articulating surfaces and serves to reduce friction from moving parts. An anatomical structure frequently referenced in orthopedic notes as it may become diseased or need removal.

CCI Version 16.3

01810, 0213T, 0216T, 0228T, 0230T, 24300, 24495, 25250, 25259, 25295, 29125, 36000, 36400-36410, 36420-36430, 36440, 36600, 36640, 37202, 43752, 51701-51703, 62310-62319, 64400-64435, 64445-64450, 64479, 64483, 64490, 64493, 64505-64530, 64702-64726, 69990, 93000-93010, 93040-93042, 93318, 94002, 94200, 94250, 94680-94690, 94770, 95812-95816, 95819, 95822, 95829, 95955, 96360, 96365, 96372, 96374-96376, 99148-99149, 99150

Also not with 25115: 25000-25001, 25020-25025, 25071-25075, 25100-25105, 25109-25112, 29085

Also not with 25116: 11012❖, 12042, 25000, 25020, 25024-25025, 25071-25076, 25109-25115, 25118-25119, 25275, 26060, 26100-26111, 26115, 26445-26449

Note: These CCI edits are used for Medicare. Other payers may reimburse on codes listed above.

Medicare Edits

	Fac RVU	Non-Fac RVU	FUD	Assist
25115	22.92	22.92	90	N/A
25116	18.27	18.27	90	80

Medicare References: 100-2,15,260; 100-4,12,30; 100-4,12,90.3; 100-4,14,10

25118-25119

25118 Synovectomy, extensor tendon sheath, wrist, single compartment;
25119 with resection of distal ulna

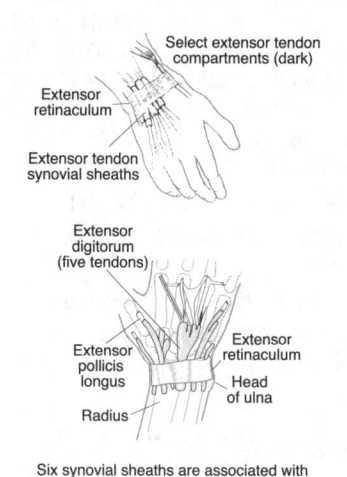

Select extensor tendon compartments (dark)
Extensor retinaculum
Extensor tendon synovial sheaths
Extensor digitorum (five tendons)
Extensor pollicis longus
Extensor retinaculum
Head of ulna
Radius

Six synovial sheaths are associated with the extensor tendons of the dorsal wrist

An excision of synovial material from a single extensor tendon sheath compartment of the wrist is performed. Report 25119 when the distal ulna bone is also resected

Explanation

The physician performs a synovectomy of the extensor tendon sheath in the wrist. The physician makes a curved, longitudinal incision over the back of the wrist, radial to the ulna. A longitudinal incision is made through the deep fascia and the extensor retinaculum, entering the involved compartment. Hypertrophic synovium is removed from each extensor tendon sheath. If an area of a tendon appears frayed to the point of possible rupture, it may be sutured to an adjacent extensor tendon above and below the damaged area. After completing the tenosynovectomy, the physician evaluates the wrist. If synovitis is present, the joint is opened and a wrist synovectomy is performed. The dorsal retinaculum is sutured back into place, deep to the exterior tendons. Closure is performed after a drain is placed. The wrist is held in a neutral position, the fingers in extension. Report 25119 if resection of the distal ulna is performed as part of the procedure.

Coding Tips

According to CPT guidelines, cast application or strapping (including removal) is only reported as a replacement procedure or when the cast application or strapping is an initial service performed without a restorative treatment or procedure. See "Application of Casts and Strapping" in the CPT book in the Surgery Section, under the Musculoskeletal system. For wrist arthroscopy with synovectomy, see 29844 and 29845.

ICD-9-CM Procedural

- 77.83 Other partial ostectomy of radius and ulna
- 80.73 Synovectomy of wrist
- 83.42 Other tenonectomy

Anesthesia

25118 01810
25119 01830

ICD-9-CM Diagnostic

- 171.2 Malignant neoplasm of connective and other soft tissue of upper limb, including shoulder
- 198.89 Secondary malignant neoplasm of other specified sites
- 215.2 Other benign neoplasm of connective and other soft tissue of upper limb, including shoulder
- 238.1 Neoplasm of uncertain behavior of connective and other soft tissue
- 239.2 Neoplasms of unspecified nature of bone, soft tissue, and skin
- 354.5 Mononeuritis multiplex
- 357.1 Polyneuropathy in collagen vascular disease — (Code first underlying disease: 446.0, 710.0, 714.0)
- 359.6 Symptomatic inflammatory myopathy in diseases classified elsewhere — (Code first underlying disease: 135, 140.0-208.9, 277.30-277.39, 446.0, 710.0, 710.1, 710.2, 714.0)
- 446.0 Polyarteritis nodosa
- 710.0 Systemic lupus erythematosus — (Use additional code to identify manifestation: 424.91, 581.81, 582.81, 583.81)
- 710.1 Systemic sclerosis — (Use additional code to identify manifestation: 359.6, 517.2)
- 710.2 Sicca syndrome
- 714.0 Rheumatoid arthritis — (Use additional code to identify manifestation: 357.1, 359.6)
- 715.13 Primary localized osteoarthrosis, forearm
- 716.13 Traumatic arthropathy, forearm
- 719.23 Villonodular synovitis, forearm
- 727.00 Unspecified synovitis and tenosynovitis
- 727.01 Synovitis and tenosynovitis in diseases classified elsewhere — (Code first underlying disease: 015.0-015.9)
- 727.04 Radial styloid tenosynovitis
- 727.05 Other tenosynovitis of hand and wrist
- 727.40 Unspecified synovial cyst
- 727.49 Other ganglion and cyst of synovium, tendon, and bursa
- 881.22 Open wound of wrist, with tendon involvement
- V64.43 Arthroscopic surgical procedure converted to open procedure

Terms To Know

hypertrophy. Overgrowth or enlargement of normal cells in tissue.

sicca syndrome. Complex of symptoms of unknown source in middle-aged women in which the following triad exists: keratoconjunctivitis sicca, zerostomia, and connective tissue disease (usually rheumatoid arthritis but sometimes systemic lupus erythematosus).

systemic sclerosis. Systemic disease characterized by excess fibrotic collagen build-up, turning the skin thickened and hard. Fibrotic changes also occur in various organs and cause vascular abnormalities and affect more women than men.

tendon. Fibrous tissue that connects muscle to bone, consisting primarily of collagen and containing little vasculature.

CCI Version 16.3

01810, 0213T, 0216T, 0228T, 0230T, 24300, 25000, 25020, 25110-25112, 25259, 25275, 36000, 36400-36410, 36420-36430, 36440, 36600, 36640, 37202, 43752, 51701-51703, 62310-62319, 64400-64435, 64445-64450, 64479, 64483, 64490, 64493, 64505-64530, 69990, 93000-93010, 93040-93042, 93318, 94002, 94200, 94250, 94680-94690, 94770, 95812-95816, 95819, 95822, 95829, 95955, 96360, 96365, 96372, 96374-96376, 99148-99149, 99150

Also not with 25118: 11010-11012❖, 25075❖, 29125

Also not with 25119: 11012❖, 25105, 25118, 25150, 25295

Note: These CCI edits are used for Medicare. Other payers may reimburse on codes listed above.

Medicare Edits

	Fac RVU	Non-Fac RVU	FUD	Assist
25118	11.11	11.11	90	N/A
25119	14.63	14.63	90	80

Medicare References: 100-2,15,260; 100-4,12,30; 100-4,12,90.3; 100-4,14,10

25120-25126

25120 Excision or curettage of bone cyst or benign tumor of radius or ulna (excluding head or neck of radius and olecranon process);
25125 with autograft (includes obtaining graft)
25126 with allograft

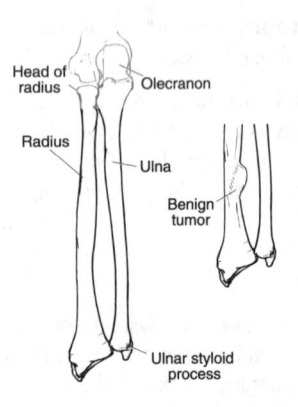

A bone cyst or benign tumor of the radius or ulna (excluding the head of radius and the olecranon of the ulna) is excised or removed by curret. Report 25125 when an autograft (from the patient) is required to repair the surgical defect. Report 25126 when an allograft (another human donor) is used in the repair

Explanation

A bone cyst or benign tumor of the radius or ulna, excluding the head, neck, or olecranon process, is removed. The physician makes an incision in the forearm overlying the cyst or tumor. The skin and underlying soft tissues are reflected to expose the periosteum, which is separated from the bone. Curettes or osteotomes are used to scrape or cut the lesion from the bone. Once the benign tumor or cyst is removed and healthy bone tissue is present, the periosteum is repositioned and the incision is repaired in layers. If the bone defect created requires a graft for repair, the physician obtains the necessary size bone graft from a separate donor site on the patient and packs it into the site where the tumor or bone cyst was removed or uses a bone bank allograft. Report 25125 if the procedure is done with an autograft and 25126 if an allograft is used.

Coding Tips

In 25125, any bone graft harvest is not reported separately. According to CPT guidelines, cast application or strapping (including removal) is only reported as a replacement procedure or when the cast application or strapping is an initial service performed without a restorative treatment or procedure. See "Application of Casts and Strapping" in the CPT book in the Surgery section, under the musculoskeletal system. For excision or curettage of a bone cyst or benign tumor of head or neck of radius or olecranon process, see 24120–24126.

ICD-9-CM Procedural

77.79 Excision of other bone for graft, except facial bones
78.03 Bone graft of radius and ulna
80.83 Other local excision or destruction of lesion of wrist joint

Anesthesia
01830

ICD-9-CM Diagnostic

213.4 Benign neoplasm of scapula and long bones of upper limb
238.0 Neoplasm of uncertain behavior of bone and articular cartilage
239.2 Neoplasms of unspecified nature of bone, soft tissue, and skin
726.91 Exostosis of unspecified site
733.21 Solitary bone cyst
733.22 Aneurysmal bone cyst
733.29 Other cyst of bone

Terms To Know

aneurysmal bone cyst. Solitary bone lesion that bulges into the periosteum, marked by a calcified rim.

benign. Mild or nonmalignant in nature.

cyst. Elevated encapsulated mass containing fluid, semisolid, or solid material with a membranous lining.

exostosis. Abnormal formation of a benign bony growth.

fascia. Fibrous sheet or band of tissue that envelops organs, muscles, and groupings of muscles.

neoplasm. New abnormal growth, tumor.

tumor. Pathological swelling or enlargement; a neoplastic growth of uncontrolled, abnormal multiplication of cells.

CCI Version 16.3

01810, 0213T, 0216T, 0228T, 0230T, 20000-20005, 20615, 24300, 25000, 25020, 25145, 25150-25151, 25259, 25295, 36000, 36400-36410, 36420-36430, 36440, 36600, 36640, 37202, 43752, 51701-51703, 62310-62319, 64400-64435, 64445-64450, 64479, 64483, 64490, 64493, 64505-64530, 69990, 93000-93010, 93040-93042, 93318, 94002, 94200, 94250, 94680-94690, 94770, 95812-95816, 95819, 95822, 95829, 95955, 96360, 96365, 96372, 96374-96376, 99148-99149, 99150

Also not with 25120: 11012❖, 25115-25119

Also not with 25125: 20900-20902, 25115-25120

Also not with 25126: 25115-25120

Note: These CCI edits are used for Medicare. Other payers may reimburse on codes listed above.

Medicare Edits

	Fac RVU	Non-Fac RVU	FUD	Assist
25120	15.35	15.35	90	80
25125	18.13	18.13	90	80
25126	18.2	18.2	90	80

Medicare References: 100-2,15,260; 100-4,12,30; 100-4,12,90.3; 100-4,14,10

25130-25136

25130 Excision or curettage of bone cyst or benign tumor of carpal bones;
25135 with autograft (includes obtaining graft)
25136 with allograft

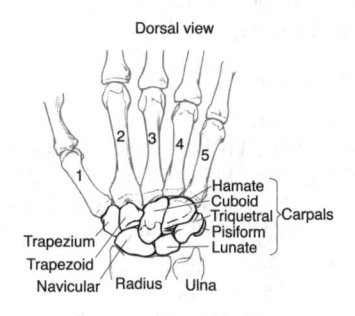

A cyst or benign tumor of the carpal bones is excised or removed by curet. Report 25135 when an autograft (from the patient) is required to repair the surgical defect. Report 25136 when an allograft from (other human donor) is used in the repair

Explanation

A bone cyst or benign tumor of the carpal bones is removed. The physician makes an incision in the wrist overlying the cyst or tumor. The skin and underlying soft tissues are reflected to expose the periosteum, which is separated from the bone. Curettes or osteotomes are used to scrape or cut the lesion from the bone. Once the benign tumor or cyst is removed and healthy bone tissue is present, the periosteum is repositioned and the incision is repaired in layers. If the bone defect created requires a graft for repair, the physician obtains the necessary size bone graft from a separate donor site on the patient and packs it into the site where the tumor or bone cyst was removed or uses a bone bank allograft. Report 25135 if the procedure is done with an autograft and 25136 if an allograft is used.

Coding Tips

In 25135, any bone graft harvest is not reported separately. According to CPT guidelines, cast application or strapping (including removal) is only reported as a replacement procedure or when the cast application or strapping is an initial service performed without a restorative treatment or procedure. See "Application of Casts and Strapping" in the CPT book in the Surgery Section, under the Musculoskeletal system.

ICD-9-CM Procedural

77.77 Excision of tibia and fibula for graft
77.79 Excision of other bone for graft, except facial bones
78.04 Bone graft of carpals and metacarpals
80.83 Other local excision or destruction of lesion of wrist joint

Anesthesia

01830

ICD-9-CM Diagnostic

213.5 Benign neoplasm of short bones of upper limb
238.0 Neoplasm of uncertain behavior of bone and articular cartilage
239.2 Neoplasms of unspecified nature of bone, soft tissue, and skin
726.91 Exostosis of unspecified site
733.21 Solitary bone cyst
733.22 Aneurysmal bone cyst
733.29 Other cyst of bone

Terms To Know

aneurysmal bone cyst. Solitary bone lesion that bulges into the periosteum, marked by a calcified rim.

benign. Mild or nonmalignant in nature.

cyst. Elevated encapsulated mass containing fluid, semisolid, or solid material with a membranous lining.

exostosis. Abnormal formation of a benign bony growth.

neoplasm. New abnormal growth, tumor.

soft tissue. Nonepithelial tissues outside of the skeleton that includes subcutaneous adipose tissue, fibrous tissue, fascia, muscles, blood and lymph vessels, and peripheral nervous system tissue.

CCI Version 16.3

01810, 0213T, 0216T, 0228T, 0230T, 11012❖, 20000-20005, 20615, 24300, 25259, 36000, 36400-36410, 36420-36430, 36440, 36600, 36640, 37202, 43752, 51701-51703, 62310-62319, 64400-64435, 64445-64450, 64479, 64483, 64490, 64493, 64505-64530, 69990, 93000-93010, 93040-93042, 93318, 94002, 94200, 94250, 94680-94690, 94770, 95812-95816, 95819, 95822, 95829, 95955, 96360, 96365, 96372, 96374-96376, 99148-99149, 99150

Also not with 25130: 25000, 25020, 25115-25116, 25295

Also not with 25135: 20900-20902, 25000, 25020, 25115-25116, 25130, 25145, 25295, 25430

Also not with 25136: 25130, 25430

Note: These CCI edits are used for Medicare. Other payers may reimburse on codes listed above.

Medicare Edits

	Fac RVU	Non-Fac RVU	FUD	Assist
25130	13.08	13.08	90	80
25135	16.31	16.31	90	80
25136	14.36	14.36	90	80

Medicare References: 100-2,15,260; 100-4,12,30; 100-4,12,90.3; 100-4,14,10

25145

25145 Sequestrectomy (eg, for osteomyelitis or bone abscess), forearm and/or wrist

Dorsal view

Sequestrum is dead bone tissue and this code reports its removal or removal of an associated bone abscess from the forearm and/or wrist

Explanation
The physician removes infected portions of bone from the forearm and/or wrist. The physician makes an incision overlying the sequestered area of bone, which includes incising the capsule if the wrist joint is involved. Once the skin and soft tissues are reflected, a small window is cut into the bone to gain access to the sequestrum, or necrosed piece of bone that has become separated from sound bone. All purulent material and scarred or necrotic tissue are removed. The remaining space is filled with surrounding soft tissues or free tissue transfer. The area is irrigated and an antibiotic solution is applied. The wound is closed loosely over drains or may be packed open with dressings. The patient may be placed in a posterior elbow splint or wrist splint to limit motion.

Coding Tips
According to CPT guidelines, cast application or strapping (including removal) is only reported as a replacement procedure or when the cast application or strapping is an initial service performed without a restorative treatment or procedure. See "Application of Casts and Strapping" in the CPT book in the Surgery Section, under the Musculoskeletal system. For partial excision of bone, ulna, see 25150; radius, see 25151.

ICD-9-CM Procedural
- 77.03 Sequestrectomy of radius and ulna
- 77.04 Sequestrectomy of carpals and metacarpals
- 77.09 Sequestrectomy of other bone, except facial bones

Anesthesia
25145 01830

ICD-9-CM Diagnostic
- 715.13 Primary localized osteoarthrosis, forearm
- 715.33 Localized osteoarthrosis not specified whether primary or secondary, forearm
- 716.63 Unspecified monoarthritis, forearm
- 730.13 Chronic osteomyelitis, forearm — (Use additional code to identify organism: 041.1. Use additional code to identify major osseous defect, if applicable: 731.3)
- 730.23 Unspecified osteomyelitis, forearm — (Use additional code to identify organism: 041.1. Use additional code to identify major osseous defect, if applicable: 731.3)
- 730.33 Periostitis, without mention of osteomyelitis, forearm — (Use additional code to identify organism: 041.1)
- 730.83 Other infections involving bone in diseases classified elsewhere, forearm — (Use additional code to identify organism: 041.1. Code first underlying disease: 002.0, 015.0-015.9)
- 731.3 Major osseous defects — (Code first underlying disease: 170.0-170.9, 730.00-730.29, 733.00-733.09, 733.40-733.49, 996.45)
- 905.2 Late effect of fracture of upper extremities

Terms To Know
abscess. Circumscribed collection of pus resulting from bacteria, frequently associated with swelling and other signs of inflammation.

chronic. Persistent, continuing, or recurring.

infection. Presence of microorganisms in body tissues that may result in cellular damage.

late effect. Abnormality, dysfunction, or other residual condition produced after the acute phase of an illness, injury, or disease is over. There is no time limit on when late effects can appear.

necrosis. Death of cells or tissue within a living organ or structure.

osteoarthrosis. Most common form of a noninflammatory degenerative joint disease with degenerating articular cartilage, bone enlargement, and synovial membrane changes.

osteomyelitis. Inflammation of bone that may remain localized or spread to the marrow, cortex, or periosteum, in response to an infecting organism, usually bacterial and pyogenic.

posterior. Located in the back part or caudal end of the body.

CCI Version 16.3
01810, 0213T, 0216T, 0228T, 0230T, 10060-10061, 11012❖, 24300, 25000, 25020, 25028, 25115-25116, 25130, 25136, 25250, 25259, 25295, 36000, 36400-36410, 36420-36430, 36440, 36600, 36640, 37202, 43752, 51701-51703, 62310-62319, 64400-64435, 64445-64450, 64479, 64483, 64490, 64493, 64505-64530, 69990, 93000-93010, 93040-93042, 93318, 94002, 94200, 94250, 94680-94690, 94770, 95812-95816, 95819, 95822, 95829, 95955, 96360, 96365, 96372, 96374-96376, 99148-99149, 99150

Note: These CCI edits are used for Medicare. Other payers may reimburse on codes listed above.

Medicare Edits

	Fac RVU	Non-Fac RVU	FUD	Assist
25145	15.86	15.86	90	80

Medicare References: 100-2,15,260; 100-4,12,30; 100-4,12,90.3; 100-4,14,10

25150-25151

25150 Partial excision (craterization, saucerization, or diaphysectomy) of bone (eg, for osteomyelitis); ulna
25151 radius

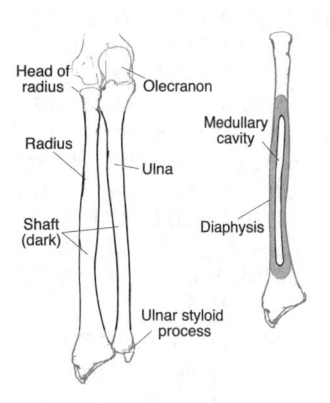

The diaphysis is the bone surrounding the medullary cavity in long bones, such as the radius and ulna. The diaphysis is a growth center in children and teenagers. It is generally associated with the shaft of the bone

A partial excision of bone is performed on the radius. Report 25151 when the excision occurs on the radius

Explanation
The physician performs a partial excision of the ulna in 25150 or the radius in 25151 to remove infected bone. An incision is made over the infected part of the bone and the underlying soft tissues are divided to expose the bone. The periosteum is reflected and the infected portion of bone is removed and irrigated. The excavation of bone may excise a crater-like piece, leave a small saucer-like shelf depression in the bone, or may remove a portion of the shaft (diaphysis) of a long bone. If a significant portion of bone is removed, the physician may fill the cavity in a separately reported grafting procedure The periosteum is closed over the bone, the soft tissues are sutured closed, and a soft dressing is applied to the elbow or a wrist splint may be used to limit elbow and/or wrist motion.

Coding Tips
According to CPT guidelines, cast application or strapping (including removal) is only reported as a replacement procedure or when the cast application or strapping is an initial service performed without a restorative treatment or procedure. See "Application of Casts and Strapping" in the CPT book in the Surgery Section, under the Musculoskeletal system. For sequestrectomy of the forearm and/or wrist, see 25145. For partial excision of bone of the head or neck of radius or olecranon process, see 24145–24147.

ICD-9-CM Procedural
77.83 Other partial ostectomy of radius and ulna

Anesthesia
01830

ICD-9-CM Diagnostic
715.13 Primary localized osteoarthrosis, forearm
715.33 Localized osteoarthrosis not specified whether primary or secondary, forearm
716.63 Unspecified monoarthritis, forearm
730.13 Chronic osteomyelitis, forearm — (Use additional code to identify organism: 041.1. Use additional code to identify major osseous defect, if applicable: 731.3)
730.23 Unspecified osteomyelitis, forearm — (Use additional code to identify organism: 041.1. Use additional code to identify major osseous defect, if applicable: 731.3)
730.33 Periostitis, without mention of osteomyelitis, forearm — (Use additional code to identify organism: 041.1)
730.83 Other infections involving bone in diseases classified elsewhere, forearm — (Use additional code to identify organism: 041.1. Code first underlying disease: 002.0, 015.0-015.9)
731.3 Major osseous defects — (Code first underlying disease: 170.0-170.9, 730.00-730.29, 733.00-733.09, 733.40-733.49, 996.45)
905.2 Late effect of fracture of upper extremities

Terms To Know
anterior. Situated in the front area or toward the belly surface of the body; an anatomical reference point used to show the position and relationship of one body structure to another.

chronic. Persistent, continuing, or recurring.

necrosis. Death of cells or tissue within a living organ or structure.

osteoarthrosis. Most common form of a noninflammatory degenerative joint disease with degenerating articular cartilage, bone enlargement, and synovial membrane changes.

osteomyelitis. Inflammation of bone that may remain localized or spread to the marrow, cortex, or periosteum, in response to an infecting organism, usually bacterial and pyogenic.

periostitis. Inflammation of the outer layers of bone.

posterior. Located in the back part or caudal end of the body.

soft tissue. Nonepithelial tissues outside of the skeleton that includes subcutaneous adipose tissue, fibrous tissue, fascia, muscles, blood and lymph vessels, and peripheral nervous system tissue.

CCI Version 16.3
01810, 0213T, 0216T, 0228T, 0230T, 10060-10061, 11012❖, 24300, 25000, 25020, 25028, 25115-25116, 25145, 25259, 25295, 36000, 36400-36410, 36420-36430, 36440, 36600, 36640, 37202, 43752, 51701-51703, 62310-62319, 64400-64435, 64445-64450, 64479, 64483, 64490, 64493, 64505-64530, 69990, 93000-93010, 93040-93042, 93318, 94002, 94200, 94250, 94680-94690, 94770, 95812-95816, 95819, 95822, 95829, 95955, 96360, 96365, 96372, 96374-96376, 99148-99149, 99150

Note: These CCI edits are used for Medicare. Other payers may reimburse on codes listed above.

Medicare Edits

	Fac RVU	Non-Fac RVU	FUD	Assist
25150	16.65	16.65	90	N/A
25151	17.9	17.9	90	80

Medicare References: 100-2,15,260; 100-4,12,30; 100-4,12,90.3; 100-4,14,10

25170

25170 Radical resection of tumor, radius or ulna

Malignant tumor on radius

Significant hard and soft tissue removal may be required

A radical resection is performed for a tumor of the radius or ulna

Explanation
The physician performs a radical resection of a tumor of the radius or ulna. The physician makes a skin incision along the lateral, anterior, or dorsal aspect of the forearm, depending on the area of resection. Resection of the proximal ulna is described. The physician makes a longitudinal posterior incision, dissecting down to expose the tumor site. The triceps insertion is detached from the ulna. The physician uses a bone saw to make an osteotomy cut in the ulna and the tumor is excised, including the immediate surrounding bone and any involved soft tissue. If much of the proximal ulna is removed, the radius may be dislocated posteriorly so that the radial neck articulates with the trochlea and the triceps tendon is sutured to the radial head. Drains are inserted and the incision is repaired in layers. A posterior splint is applied. No bone graft is used. Similar technique may be used for the radius.

Coding Tips
According to CPT guidelines, cast application or strapping (including removal) is only reported as a replacement procedure or when the cast application or strapping is an initial service performed without a restorative treatment or procedure. See "Application of Casts and Strapping" in the CPT book in the Surgery Section, under the Musculoskeletal system. For partial excision of bone, ulna, see 25150; radius, see 25151.

ICD-9-CM Procedural
77.63 Local excision of lesion or tissue of radius and ulna

Anesthesia
25170 01830

ICD-9-CM Diagnostic
- 170.4 Malignant neoplasm of scapula and long bones of upper limb
- 198.5 Secondary malignant neoplasm of bone and bone marrow
- 209.73 Secondary neuroendocrine tumor of bone
- 238.0 Neoplasm of uncertain behavior of bone and articular cartilage
- 239.2 Neoplasms of unspecified nature of bone, soft tissue, and skin

Terms To Know

anterior. Situated in the front area or toward the belly surface of the body; an anatomical reference point used to show the position and relationship of one body structure to another.

flexion. Act of bending or being bent.

lateral. To/on the side.

lesion. Area of damaged tissue that has lost continuity or function, due to disease or trauma. Lesions may be located on internal structures such as the brain, nerves, or kidneys, or visible on the skin.

malignant. Any condition tending to progress toward death, specifically an invasive tumor with a loss of cellular differentiation that has the ability to spread or metastasize to other areas in the body.

proximal. Located closest to a specified reference point, usually the midline.

secondary. Second in order of occurrence or importance, or appearing during the course of another disease or condition.

soft tissue. Nonepithelial tissues outside of the skeleton that includes subcutaneous adipose tissue, fibrous tissue, fascia, muscles, blood and lymph vessels, and peripheral nervous system tissue.

tumor. Pathological swelling or enlargement; a neoplastic growth of uncontrolled, abnormal multiplication of cells.

CCI Version 16.3
01810, 0213T, 0216T, 0228T, 0230T, 10060, 10140, 10160, 11010-11012❖, 11040-11044, 12001-12007, 12020-12021, 12041-12047, 13120-13121, 13131-13132, 20220-20225, 20240-20245, 24000, 24006, 24100-24102, 24120, 24300, 25000, 25020, 25028-25035, 25040, 25065-25078, 25100-25126, 25145, 25150-25151, 25230-25240, 25248, 25259, 25295, 25350-25375, 36000, 36400-36410, 36420-36430, 36440, 36600, 36640, 37202, 43752, 51701-51703, 62310-62319, 64400-64435, 64445-64450, 64479, 64483, 64490, 64493, 64505-64530, 69990, 93000-93010, 93040-93042, 93318, 94002, 94200, 94250, 94680-94690, 94770, 95812-95816, 95819, 95822, 95829, 95955, 96360, 96365, 96372, 96374-96376, 99148-99149, 99150

Note: These CCI edits are used for Medicare. Other payers may reimburse on codes listed above.

Medicare Edits

	Fac RVU	Non-Fac RVU	FUD	Assist
25170	41.46	41.46	90	80

Medicare References: None

25210-25215

25210 Carpectomy; 1 bone
25215 all bones of proximal row

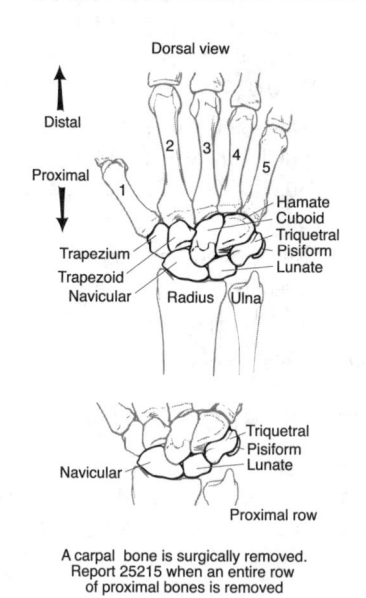

A carpal bone is surgically removed. Report 25215 when an entire row of proximal bones is removed

Explanation

In 25210, the physician removes one of the eight carpal bones of the wrist. An incision is made in the wrist overlying the carpal bone to be removed. The tissues are dissected down to the bone. The physician identifies the bone visually and dissects it free of the surrounding structures. Some ligaments may be reattached to other bones. The carpal bone is excised. In 25215, all four bones in the proximal row of the carpal bones of the wrist are removed. An incision is made overlying the wrist. The physician carries the incision down to the carpal bone. The physician identifies the two rows of carpal bones. The physician removes the bones one by one in the proximal row while preserving tendons, nerves, and blood vessels. Ligaments may need to be reattached to other bones. Each of the bones is dissected free and removed. For both procedures, the wound is irrigated with antibiotic solution and closed in multiple layers.

Coding Tips

According to CPT guidelines, cast application or strapping (including removal) is only reported as a replacement procedure or when the cast application or strapping is an initial service performed without a restorative treatment or procedure. See "Application of Casts and Strapping" in the CPT book in the Surgery Section, under the Musculoskeletal system. For carpectomy with implant, see 25441–25445.

ICD-9-CM Procedural

- **77.84** Other partial ostectomy of carpals and metacarpals
- **77.94** Total ostectomy of carpals and metacarpals

Anesthesia
01830

ICD-9-CM Diagnostic

- **710.1** Systemic sclerosis — (Use additional code to identify manifestation: 359.6, 517.2)
- **710.2** Sicca syndrome
- **715.34** Localized osteoarthrosis not specified whether primary or secondary, hand
- **715.94** Osteoarthrosis, unspecified whether generalized or localized, hand
- **716.14** Traumatic arthropathy, hand
- **727.05** Other tenosynovitis of hand and wrist
- **730.14** Chronic osteomyelitis, hand — (Use additional code to identify organism: 041.1. Use additional code to identify major osseous defect, if applicable: 731.3)
- **730.24** Unspecified osteomyelitis, hand — (Use additional code to identify organism: 041.1. Use additional code to identify major osseous defect, if applicable: 731.3)
- **731.3** Major osseous defects — (Code first underlying disease: 170.0-170.9, 730.00-730.29, 733.00-733.09, 733.40-733.49, 996.45)
- **733.49** Aseptic necrosis of other bone site — (Use additional code to identify major osseous defect, if applicable: 731.3)
- **733.82** Nonunion of fracture
- **814.01** Closed fracture of navicular (scaphoid) bone of wrist
- **814.02** Closed fracture of lunate (semilunar) bone of wrist
- **814.03** Closed fracture of triquetral (cuneiform) bone of wrist
- **814.04** Closed fracture of pisiform bone of wrist
- **814.05** Closed fracture of trapezium bone (larger multangular) of wrist
- **814.06** Closed fracture of trapezoid bone (smaller multangular) of wrist
- **814.07** Closed fracture of capitate bone (os magnum) of wrist
- **814.08** Closed fracture of hamate (unciform) bone of wrist
- **814.09** Closed fracture of other bone of wrist
- **814.11** Open fracture of navicular (scaphoid) bone of wrist
- **814.12** Open fracture of lunate (semilunar) bone of wrist
- **814.13** Open fracture of triquetral (cuneiform) bone of wrist
- **814.14** Open fracture of pisiform bone of wrist
- **814.15** Open fracture of trapezium bone (larger multangular) of wrist
- **814.16** Open fracture of trapezoid bone (smaller multangular) of wrist
- **814.17** Open fracture of capitate bone (os magnum) of wrist
- **814.18** Open fracture of hamate (unciform) bone of wrist
- **814.19** Open fracture of other bone of wrist
- **906.4** Late effect of crushing
- **927.21** Crushing injury of wrist — (Use additional code to identify any associated injuries: 800-829, 850.0-854.1, 860.0-869.1)

CCI Version 16.3

01810, 0213T, 0216T, 0228T, 0230T, 24300, 25020, 25040, 25115-25118, 25130-25145, 25259, 25295, 25320, 36000, 36400-36410, 36420-36430, 36440, 36600, 36640, 37202, 43752, 51701-51703, 62310-62319, 64400-64435, 64445-64450, 64479, 64483, 64490, 64493, 64505-64530, 69990, 93000-93010, 93040-93042, 93318, 94002, 94200, 94250, 94680-94690, 94770, 95812-95816, 95819, 95822, 95829, 95955, 96360, 96365, 96372, 96374-96376, 99148-99149, 99150

Also not with 25210: 11012❖, 25000-25001, 25100, 25105, 64708

Also not with 25215: 25000, 25100-25105, 25210

Note: These CCI edits are used for Medicare. Other payers may reimburse on codes listed above.

Medicare Edits

	Fac RVU	Non-Fac RVU	FUD	Assist
25210	14.27	14.27	90	80
25215	18.18	18.18	90	80

Medicare References: 100-2,15,260; 100-4,12,30; 100-4,12,90.3; 100-4,14,10

25230

25230 Radial styloidectomy (separate procedure)

Explanation
The physician performs a radial styloidectomy by making a bayonet-shaped incision along the radial aspect of the wrist. The radial artery and nerve are exposed. The joint capsule is incised to expose the radial styloid. The physician uses a thin osteotome or thin oscillating saw blade to cut the radial styloid perpendicular to the long axis of the radius. The incision is repaired in layers with sutures, staples, and/or Steri-strips. The wrist is placed in an anterior splint.

Coding Tips
This separate procedure by definition is usually a component of a more complex service and is not identified separately. When performed alone or with other unrelated procedures/services it may be reported. If performed alone, list the code; if performed with other procedures/services, list the code and append modifier 59. According to CPT guidelines, cast application or strapping (including removal) is only reported as a replacement procedure or when the cast application or strapping is an initial service performed without a restorative treatment or procedure. See "Application of Casts and Strapping" in the CPT book in the Surgery Section, under the Musculoskeletal system.

ICD-9-CM Procedural
- 77.83 Other partial ostectomy of radius and ulna

Anesthesia
25230 01830

ICD-9-CM Diagnostic
- 170.5 Malignant neoplasm of short bones of upper limb
- 198.5 Secondary malignant neoplasm of bone and bone marrow
- 213.5 Benign neoplasm of short bones of upper limb
- 238.0 Neoplasm of uncertain behavior of bone and articular cartilage
- 239.2 Neoplasms of unspecified nature of bone, soft tissue, and skin
- 357.1 Polyneuropathy in collagen vascular disease — (Code first underlying disease: 446.0, 710.0, 714.0)
- 359.6 Symptomatic inflammatory myopathy in diseases classified elsewhere — (Code first underlying disease: 135, 140.0-208.9, 277.30-277.39, 446.0, 710.0, 710.1, 710.2, 714.0)
- 446.0 Polyarteritis nodosa
- 710.0 Systemic lupus erythematosus — (Use additional code to identify manifestation: 424.91, 581.81, 582.81, 583.81)
- 710.1 Systemic sclerosis — (Use additional code to identify manifestation: 359.6, 517.2)
- 710.2 Sicca syndrome
- 714.0 Rheumatoid arthritis — (Use additional code to identify manifestation: 357.1, 359.6)
- 715.13 Primary localized osteoarthrosis, forearm
- 715.93 Osteoarthrosis, unspecified whether generalized or localized, forearm
- 716.13 Traumatic arthropathy, forearm
- 716.93 Unspecified arthropathy, forearm
- 718.83 Other joint derangement, not elsewhere classified, forearm
- 727.00 Unspecified synovitis and tenosynovitis
- 727.04 Radial styloid tenosynovitis
- 727.05 Other tenosynovitis of hand and wrist
- 729.5 Pain in soft tissues of limb
- 730.13 Chronic osteomyelitis, forearm — (Use additional code to identify organism: 041.1. Use additional code to identify major osseous defect, if applicable: 731.3)
- 730.23 Unspecified osteomyelitis, forearm — (Use additional code to identify organism: 041.1. Use additional code to identify major osseous defect, if applicable: 731.3)
- 730.83 Other infections involving bone in diseases classified elsewhere, forearm — (Use additional code to identify organism: 041.1. Code first underlying disease: 002.0, 015.0-015.9)
- 731.3 Major osseous defects — (Code first underlying disease: 170.0-170.9, 730.00-730.29, 733.00-733.09, 733.40-733.49, 996.45)
- 732.3 Juvenile osteochondrosis of upper extremity
- 733.81 Malunion of fracture
- 733.82 Nonunion of fracture

Terms To Know
osteomyelitis. Inflammation of bone that may remain localized or spread to the marrow, cortex, or periosteum, in response to an infecting organism, usually bacterial and pyogenic.

sicca syndrome. Complex of symptoms of unknown source in middle-aged women in which the following triad exists: keratoconjunctivitis sicca, zerostomia, and connective tissue disease (usually rheumatoid arthritis but sometimes systemic lupus erythematosus).

systemic sclerosis. Systemic disease characterized by excess fibrotic collagen build-up, turning the skin thickened and hard. Fibrotic changes also occur in various organs and cause vascular abnormalities and affect more women than men.

CCI Version 16.3
01810, 0213T, 0216T, 0228T, 0230T, 11011-11012❖, 24300, 25259, 36000, 36400-36410, 36420-36430, 36440, 36600, 36640, 37202, 43752, 51701-51703, 62310-62319, 64400-64435, 64445-64450, 64479, 64483, 64490, 64493, 64505-64530, 64718, 69990, 93000-93010, 93040-93042, 93318, 94002, 94200, 94250, 94680-94690, 94770, 95812-95816, 95819, 95822, 95829, 95955, 96360, 96365, 96372, 96374-96376, 99148-99149, 99150

Note: These CCI edits are used for Medicare. Other payers may reimburse on codes listed above.

Medicare Edits

	Fac RVU	Non-Fac RVU	FUD	Assist
25230	12.58	12.58	90	N/A

Medicare References: 100-2,15,260; 100-4,12,30; 100-4,12,90.3; 100-4,14,10

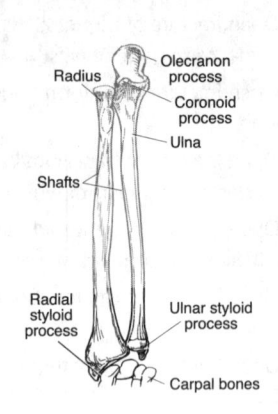

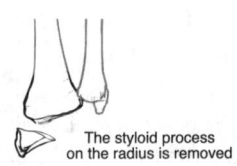

25240

25240 Excision distal ulna partial or complete (eg, Darrach type or matched resection)

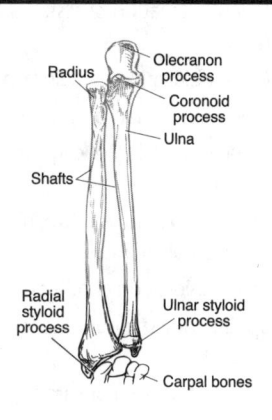

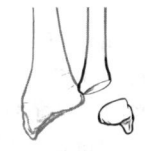

The distal ulna is removed, either partially or completely

Explanation

The distal ulna is partially or completely excised. The physician makes a medial longitudinal incision to expose the distal ulna. The ulna is located subcutaneously and does not require much dissection. The periosteum is incised and reflected to expose the distal ulna. Drill holes are made through the ulna 2.5 cm above the distal head. The physician uses bone-biting forceps to complete the division of the bone and remove the fragment. To stabilize the free end of the ulna, the physician reefs (overlaps) the periosteal envelope and ligament. The incision is repaired in layers with sutures, staples, and/or Steri-strips. Immobilization of the wrist is usually not necessary.

Coding Tips

According to CPT guidelines, cast application or strapping (including removal) is only reported as a replacement procedure or when the cast application or strapping is an initial service performed without a restorative treatment or procedure. See "Application of Casts and Strapping" in the CPT book in the Surgery section, under the musculoskeletal system. For distal ulna implant replacement, see 25442. Report obtaining fascia graft for interposition separately; see 20920 or 20922.

ICD-9-CM Procedural

77.83 Other partial ostectomy of radius and ulna

Anesthesia

25240 01830

ICD-9-CM Diagnostic

- 238.0 Neoplasm of uncertain behavior of bone and articular cartilage
- 239.2 Neoplasms of unspecified nature of bone, soft tissue, and skin
- 357.1 Polyneuropathy in collagen vascular disease — (Code first underlying disease: 446.0, 710.0, 714.0)
- 359.6 Symptomatic inflammatory myopathy in diseases classified elsewhere — (Code first underlying disease: 135, 140.0-208.9, 277.30-277.39, 446.0, 710.0, 710.1, 710.2, 714.0)
- 446.0 Polyarteritis nodosa
- 710.0 Systemic lupus erythematosus — (Use additional code to identify manifestation: 424.91, 581.81, 582.81, 583.81)
- 710.1 Systemic sclerosis — (Use additional code to identify manifestation: 359.6, 517.2)
- 710.2 Sicca syndrome
- 714.0 Rheumatoid arthritis — (Use additional code to identify manifestation: 357.1, 359.6)
- 715.13 Primary localized osteoarthrosis, forearm
- 715.93 Osteoarthrosis, unspecified whether generalized or localized, forearm
- 716.13 Traumatic arthropathy, forearm
- 716.93 Unspecified arthropathy, forearm
- 718.83 Other joint derangement, not elsewhere classified, forearm
- 727.00 Unspecified synovitis and tenosynovitis
- 727.05 Other tenosynovitis of hand and wrist
- 730.13 Chronic osteomyelitis, forearm — (Use additional code to identify organism: 041.1. Use additional code to identify major osseous defect, if applicable: 731.3)
- 730.23 Unspecified osteomyelitis, forearm — (Use additional code to identify organism: 041.1. Use additional code to identify major osseous defect, if applicable: 731.3)
- 730.83 Other infections involving bone in diseases classified elsewhere, forearm — (Use additional code to identify organism: 041.1. Code first underlying disease: 002.0, 015.0-015.9)
- 731.3 Major osseous defects — (Code first underlying disease: 170.0-170.9, 730.00-730.29, 733.00-733.09, 733.40-733.49, 996.45)
- 732.3 Juvenile osteochondrosis of upper extremity
- 733.81 Malunion of fracture
- 733.82 Nonunion of fracture
- 736.09 Other acquired deformities of forearm, excluding fingers

Terms To Know

ligament. Band or sheet of fibrous tissue that connects the articular surfaces of bones or supports visceral organs.

sicca syndrome. Complex of symptoms of unknown source in middle-aged women in which the following triad exists: keratoconjunctivitis sicca, zerostomia, and connective tissue disease (usually rheumatoid arthritis but sometimes systemic lupus erythematosus).

systemic sclerosis. Systemic disease characterized by excess fibrotic collagen build-up, turning the skin thickened and hard. Fibrotic changes also occur in various organs and cause vascular abnormalities and affect more women than men.

CCI Version 16.3

01810, 0213T, 0216T, 0228T, 0230T, 11011-11012✦, 24300, 25040, 25100-25105, 25115-25118, 25259, 25295, 25320, 25350, 25360-25365, 25651-25652✦, 25671✦, 36000, 36400-36410, 36420-36430, 36440, 36600, 36640, 37202, 43752, 51701-51703, 62310-62319, 64400-64435, 64445-64450, 64479, 64483, 64490, 64493, 64505-64530, 64704-64708, 64719, 69990, 93000-93010, 93040-93042, 93318, 94002, 94200, 94250, 94680-94690, 94770, 95812-95816, 95819, 95822, 95829, 95955, 96360, 96365, 96372, 96374-96376, 99148-99149, 99150

Note: These CCI edits are used for Medicare. Other payers may reimburse on codes listed above.

Medicare Edits

	Fac RVU	Non-Fac RVU	FUD	Assist
25240	12.62	12.62	90	80

Medicare References: 100-2,15,260; 100-4,12,30; 100-4,12,90.3; 100-4,14,10

25246

25246 Injection procedure for wrist arthrography

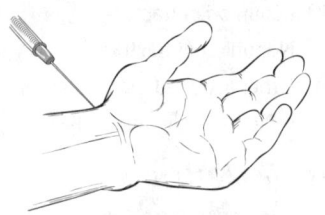

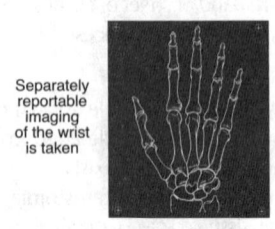

The joint is filled with contrast material

Separately reportable imaging of the wrist is taken

Contrast material is injected into the wrist joint for arthrography purposes

Explanation

The physician injects contrast material into the wrist joint for arthrography. The physician inserts a needle into the wrist and aspirates joint fluid for culture. Contrast material is injected into the wrist and the wrist is manipulated to distribute the dye. As the dye fades, a second injection may be made.

Coding Tips

For radiology supervision and interpretation, see 73115.

ICD-9-CM Procedural

- 81.92 Injection of therapeutic substance into joint or ligament
- 88.32 Contrast arthrogram

Anesthesia

25246 01810, 01820

ICD-9-CM Diagnostic

- 275.40 Unspecified disorder of calcium metabolism — (Use additional code to identify any associated mental retardation)
- 275.42 Hypercalcemia — (Use additional code to identify any associated mental retardation)
- 275.49 Other disorders of calcium metabolism — (Use additional code to identify any associated mental retardation)
- 275.5 Hungry bone syndrome
- 718.03 Articular cartilage disorder, forearm
- 718.13 Loose body in forearm joint
- 718.73 Developmental dislocation of joint, forearm
- 718.93 Unspecified derangement, forearm joint
- 814.00 Unspecified closed fracture of carpal bone
- 814.01 Closed fracture of navicular (scaphoid) bone of wrist
- 814.02 Closed fracture of lunate (semilunar) bone of wrist
- 814.03 Closed fracture of triquetral (cuneiform) bone of wrist
- 814.04 Closed fracture of pisiform bone of wrist
- 814.05 Closed fracture of trapezium bone (larger multangular) of wrist
- 814.06 Closed fracture of trapezoid bone (smaller multangular) of wrist
- 814.07 Closed fracture of capitate bone (os magnum) of wrist
- 814.08 Closed fracture of hamate (unciform) bone of wrist
- 814.09 Closed fracture of other bone of wrist
- 814.10 Unspecified open fracture of carpal bone
- 814.11 Open fracture of navicular (scaphoid) bone of wrist
- 814.12 Open fracture of lunate (semilunar) bone of wrist
- 814.13 Open fracture of triquetral (cuneiform) bone of wrist
- 814.14 Open fracture of pisiform bone of wrist
- 814.15 Open fracture of trapezium bone (larger multangular) of wrist
- 814.16 Open fracture of trapezoid bone (smaller multangular) of wrist
- 814.17 Open fracture of capitate bone (os magnum) of wrist
- 814.18 Open fracture of hamate (unciform) bone of wrist
- 814.19 Open fracture of other bone of wrist
- 833.00 Closed dislocation of wrist, unspecified part
- 833.01 Closed dislocation of distal radioulnar (joint)
- 833.02 Closed dislocation of radiocarpal (joint)
- 833.03 Closed dislocation of midcarpal (joint)
- 833.04 Closed dislocation of carpometacarpal (joint)
- 833.05 Closed dislocation of proximal end of metacarpal (bone)
- 833.09 Closed dislocation of other part of wrist
- 833.10 Open dislocation of wrist, unspecified part
- 833.11 Open dislocation of distal radioulnar (joint)
- 833.12 Open dislocation of radiocarpal (joint)
- 833.13 Open dislocation of midcarpal (joint)
- 833.14 Open dislocation of carpometacarpal (joint)
- 833.15 Open dislocation of proximal end of metacarpal (bone)
- 833.19 Open dislocation of other part of wrist
- 842.00 Sprain and strain of unspecified site of wrist
- 842.01 Sprain and strain of carpal (joint) of wrist
- 842.02 Sprain and strain of radiocarpal (joint) (ligament) of wrist
- 842.09 Other wrist sprain and strain
- 881.12 Open wound of wrist, complicated
- 881.22 Open wound of wrist, with tendon involvement
- 927.21 Crushing injury of wrist — (Use additional code to identify any associated injuries: 800-829, 850.0-854.1, 860.0-869.1)
- 959.3 Injury, other and unspecified, elbow, forearm, and wrist

CCI Version 16.3

01810, 0213T, 0216T, 0228T, 0230T, 11010❖, 24300, 25248-25274❖, 25280-25316❖, 25320❖, 25332-25375❖, 36000, 36400-36410, 36420-36430, 36440, 36600, 36640, 37202, 43752, 51701-51703, 62310-62319, 64400-64435, 64445-64450, 64479, 64483, 64490, 64493, 64505-64530, 69990, 76000-76001, 93000-93010, 93040-93042, 93318, 94002, 94200, 94250, 94680-94690, 94770, 95812-95816, 95819, 95822, 95829, 95955, 96360, 96365, 96372, 96374-96376, 99148-99149, 99150, J1644, J2001

Note: These CCI edits are used for Medicare. Other payers may reimburse on codes listed above.

Medicare Edits

	Fac RVU	Non-Fac RVU	FUD	Assist
25246	2.22	4.83	0	N/A

Medicare References: None

25248

25248 Exploration with removal of deep foreign body, forearm or wrist

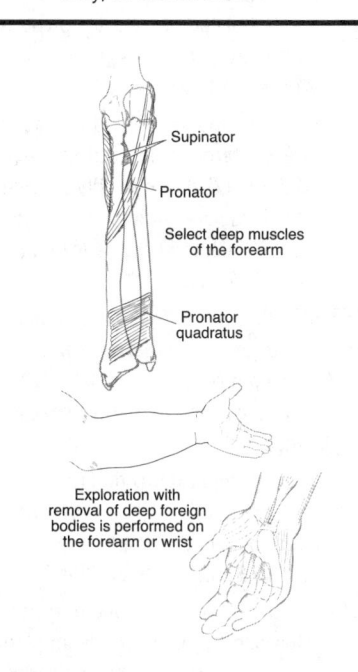

Explanation
The physician removes a deeply implanted foreign body from the forearm or wrist. The physician incises the site and dissects down to reach the area where the foreign object is embedded. Exploration of the site is done. Separately reportable x-rays may be taken to locate the object. All parts of the object are removed. The wound is sutured in layers.

Coding Tips
Local anesthesia is included in this service. However, this procedure may be performed under general anesthesia, depending on the age and/or condition of the patient. For removal of a superficial foreign body, see 20520. For removal, foreign body, wrist joint, requiring arthrotomy, see 25101. For removal of hardware (K-wire, pin, or rod), see 20670 or 20680. For removal of a wrist prosthesis, see 25250 or 25251. For radiology services, see 73060–73080. Surgical trays, A4550, are not separately reimbursed by Medicare; however, other third-party payers may cover them. Check with the specific payer to determine coverage.

ICD-9-CM Procedural
- 81.91 Arthrocentesis
- 83.02 Myotomy
- 83.09 Other incision of soft tissue
- 98.27 Removal of foreign body without incision from upper limb, except hand

Anesthesia
25248 01810

ICD-9-CM Diagnostic
- 728.82 Foreign body granuloma of muscle — (Use additional code to identify foreign body (V90.01-V90.9))
- 729.6 Residual foreign body in soft tissue — (Use additional code to identify foreign body (V90.01-V90.9))
- 881.10 Open wound of forearm, complicated
- 881.12 Open wound of wrist, complicated
- 959.3 Injury, other and unspecified, elbow, forearm, and wrist

Terms To Know

foreign body. Any object or substance found in an organ and tissue that does not belong under normal circumstances.

granuloma. Abnormal, dense collections or cells forming a mass or nodule of chronically inflamed tissue with granulations that is usually associated with an infective process.

open wound. Opening or break of the skin.

soft tissue. Nonepithelial tissues outside of the skeleton that includes subcutaneous adipose tissue, fibrous tissue, fascia, muscles, blood and lymph vessels, and peripheral nervous system tissue.

CCI Version 16.3
01810, 0213T, 0216T, 0228T, 0230T, 20103, 20670, 24300, 25000, 25020, 25115-25116, 25250, 25259, 25295, 36000, 36400-36410, 36420-36430, 36440, 36600, 36640, 37202, 43752, 51701-51703, 62310-62319, 64400-64435, 64445-64450, 64479, 64483, 64490, 64493, 64505-64530, 69990, 93000-93010, 93040-93042, 93318, 94002, 94200, 94250, 94680-94690, 94770, 95812-95816, 95819, 95822, 95829, 95955, 96360, 96365, 96372, 96374-96376, 99148-99149, 99150

Note: These CCI edits are used for Medicare. Other payers may reimburse on codes listed above.

Medicare Edits

	Fac RVU	Non-Fac RVU	FUD	Assist
25248	12.45	12.45	90	N/A

Medicare References: 100-2,15,260; 100-4,12,30; 100-4,12,90.3; 100-4,14,10

25250-25251

25250 Removal of wrist prosthesis; (separate procedure)
25251 complicated, including total wrist

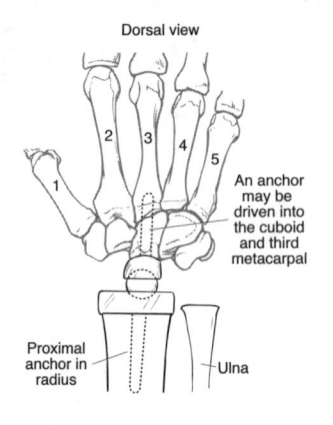

Dorsal view

An anchor may be driven into the cuboid and third metacarpal

Proximal anchor in radius

Ulna

A wrist prosthesis is removed. Report 25251 when removal is complicated, requiring resection of bone from the carpals and/or the radius and ulna

Explanation

In 25250, the physician removes a prosthesis from the wrist. An incision is made overlying the wrist. The physician extends the incision deep to the wrist joint, opening the joint. They physician identifies the artificial joint piece that has failed. Using hand and powered instruments, the physician removes the prosthesis. The joint and incision both are irrigated with antibiotic solution and repaired in multiple layers. If infection is present, the incision is left open to drain temporarily. In 25251, the physician removes all the parts of a wrist joint prosthesis from the wrist. An incision is made overlying the wrist. The physician may use the previous wrist surgery incision. The physician extends the incision down to the wrist joint by dividing and dissecting tissues. Some tissue may require debridement. The joint is entered through an arthrotomy cut. The physician identifies the pieces of artificial joint. Each piece is dissected free from the bone. Any loose pieces are removed. The entire joint is explored. The physician may smooth or debride the ends of the exposed bone. Any nonviable soft tissue and synovium is removed. The joint is irrigated with antibiotic solution. If infection is present, the joint and incision are left open for temporary drainage. Otherwise, the incisions are repaired in multiple layers.

Coding Tips

Note that 25250, a separate procedure by definition, is usually a component of a more complex service and is not identified separately. When performed alone or with other unrelated procedures/services it may be reported. If performed alone, list the code; if performed with other procedures/services, list the code and append modifier 59. According to CPT guidelines, cast application or strapping (including removal) is only reported as a replacement procedure or when the cast application or strapping is an initial service performed without a restorative treatment or procedure. See "Application of Casts and Strapping" in the CPT book in the Surgery Section, under the Musculoskeletal system.

ICD-9-CM Procedural

80.03 Arthrotomy for removal of prosthesis without replacement, wrist
84.57 Removal of (cement) spacer

Anesthesia
01830

ICD-9-CM Diagnostic

731.3 Major osseous defects — (Code first underlying disease: 170.0-170.9, 730.00-730.29, 733.00-733.09, 733.40-733.49, 996.45)
996.40 Unspecified mechanical complication of internal orthopedic device, implant, and graft — (Use additional code to identify prosthetic joint with mechanical complication, V43.60-V43.69)
996.41 Mechanical loosening of prosthetic joint — (Use additional code to identify prosthetic joint with mechanical complication, V43.60-V43.69)
996.42 Dislocation of prosthetic joint — (Use additional code to identify prosthetic joint with mechanical complication, V43.60-V43.69)
996.43 Broken prosthetic joint implant — (Use additional code to identify prosthetic joint with mechanical complication, V43.60-V43.69)
996.44 Peri-prosthetic fracture around prosthetic joint — (Use additional code to identify prosthetic joint with mechanical complication, V43.60-V43.69.
996.45 Peri-prosthetic osteolysis — (Use additional code to identify prosthetic joint with mechanical complication, V43.60-V43.69. Use additional code to identify major osseous defect, if applicable: 731.3)
996.47 Other mechanical complication of prosthetic joint implant — (Use additional code to identify prosthetic joint with mechanical complication, V43.60-V43.69)
996.66 Infection and inflammatory reaction due to internal joint prosthesis — (Use additional code to identify specified infections. Use additional code to identify infected prosthetic joint: V43.60-V43.69)
996.67 Infection and inflammatory reaction due to other internal orthopedic device, implant, and graft — (Use additional code to identify specified infections)
996.77 Other complications due to internal joint prosthesis — (Use additional code to identify complication: 338.18-338.19, 338.28-338.29)
996.78 Other complications due to other internal orthopedic device, implant, and graft — (Use additional code to identify complication: 338.18-338.19, 338.28-338.29)
998.6 Persistent postoperative fistula, not elsewhere classified
998.83 Non-healing surgical wound
V43.63 Wrist joint replacement by other means

CCI Version 16.3

01810, 0213T, 0216T, 0228T, 0230T, 20670, 24300, 25000, 25020, 25040, 25120, 25130, 25150-25151, 25210, 25240, 25259, 25295, 25320, 36000, 36400-36410, 36420-36430, 36440, 36600, 36640, 37202, 43752, 51701-51703, 62310-62319, 64400-64435, 64445-64450, 64479, 64483, 64490, 64493, 64505-64530, 69990, 93000-93010, 93040-93042, 93318, 94002, 94200, 94250, 94680-94690, 94770, 95812-95816, 95819, 95822, 95829, 95955, 96360, 96365, 96372, 96374-96376, 99148-99149, 99150

Also not with 25250: 25085-25100, 25105
Also not with 25251: 25085-25105, 25115-25116, 25145, 25250

Note: These CCI edits are used for Medicare. Other payers may reimburse on codes listed above.

Medicare Edits

	Fac RVU	Non-Fac RVU	FUD	Assist
25250	15.32	15.32	90	80
25251	20.96	20.96	90	80

Medicare References: 100-2,15,260; 100-4,12,30; 100-4,12,90.3; 100-4,14,10

25259

25259 Manipulation, wrist, under anesthesia

Ulnar bursa
Superficialis tendons
Deep profundus flexor tendons

Schematic cross section of the stacked nature of flexor tendons as they enter the wrist

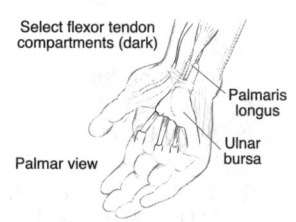

Select flexor tendon compartments (dark)

Palmaris longus
Ulnar bursa
Palmar view

The flexors provide grasping action to the hands. The tendons pass through the wrist and turn muscular in the forearm area. The palmaris longus tendon may be used for grafts

Explanation

Manipulation of the wrist under anesthesia may be necessary to gain the loss of motion following a surgical procedure or due to scar tissue. Following the induction of general anesthesia, the physician evaluates the wrist. The wrist is manipulated by stretching, rotation, and other maneuvers to gain the appropriate range of motion.

Coding Tips

This is a unilateral procedure. If performed bilaterally, some payers require that the service be reported twice with modifier 50 appended to the second code, while others require identification of the service only once with modifier 50 appended. Check with individual payers. Modifier 50 identifies a procedure performed identically on the opposite side of the body (mirror image). For application of external fixation, see 20690 or 20692.

ICD-9-CM Procedural

93.25	Forced extension of limb
93.26	Manual rupture of joint adhesions
93.29	Other forcible correction of musculoskeletal deformity

Anesthesia

25259 01820

ICD-9-CM Diagnostic

357.1	Polyneuropathy in collagen vascular disease — (Code first underlying disease: 446.0, 710.0, 714.0)
359.6	Symptomatic inflammatory myopathy in diseases classified elsewhere — (Code first underlying disease: 135, 140.0-208.9, 277.30-277.39, 446.0, 710.0, 710.1, 710.2, 714.0)
446.0	Polyarteritis nodosa
710.0	Systemic lupus erythematosus — (Use additional code to identify manifestation: 424.91, 581.81, 582.81, 583.81)
710.1	Systemic sclerosis — (Use additional code to identify manifestation: 359.6, 517.2)
710.2	Sicca syndrome
714.0	Rheumatoid arthritis — (Use additional code to identify manifestation: 357.1, 359.6)
715.13	Primary localized osteoarthrosis, forearm
715.93	Osteoarthrosis, unspecified whether generalized or localized, forearm
718.43	Contracture of forearm joint
718.53	Ankylosis of forearm joint
719.23	Villonodular synovitis, forearm
719.53	Stiffness of joint, not elsewhere classified, forearm
726.4	Enthesopathy of wrist and carpus

Terms To Know

adhesion. Abnormal fibrous connection between two structures, soft tissue or bony structures, that may occur as the result of surgery, infection, or trauma.

ankylosis. Abnormal union or fusion of bones in a joint, which is normally moveable.

contracture. Shortening of muscle or connective tissue.

polyarteritis nodosa. Systemic necrotizing vasculitis of small and medium arteries that results in the infarction and scarring within the affected organs.

polyneuropathy. Disease process of severe inflammation of multiple nerves.

synovitis. Inflammation of the synovial membrane that lines a synovial joint, resulting in pain and swelling.

CCI Version 16.3

01810, 0213T, 0216T, 0228T, 0230T, 36000, 36400-36410, 36420-36430, 36440, 36600, 36640, 37202, 43752, 51701-51703, 62310-62319, 64400-64435, 64445-64450, 64479, 64483, 64490, 64493, 64505-64530, 93000-93010, 93040-93042, 93318, 94002, 94200, 94250, 94680-94690, 94770, 95812-95816, 95819, 95822, 95829, 95955, 96360, 96365, 96372, 96374-96376, 99148-99149, 99150

Note: These CCI edits are used for Medicare. Other payers may reimburse on codes listed above.

Medicare Edits

	Fac RVU	Non-Fac RVU	FUD	Assist
25259	11.7	11.7	90	N/A

Medicare References: None

25260-25263

25260 Repair, tendon or muscle, flexor, forearm and/or wrist; primary, single, each tendon or muscle

25263 secondary, single, each tendon or muscle

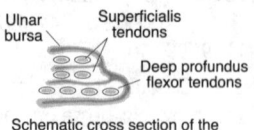

Explanation

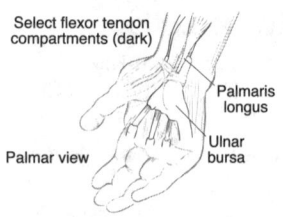

The physician repairs a flexor tendon or muscle of the forearm and/or wrist. The repair is done to restore continuity for normal function by reapproximating the severed ends. Primary tendon repairs can be performed when a clean wound is presented close to the time of injury that can be satisfactorily stabilized for a good end result-such as wounds inflicted with a sharp edge. Secondary tendon repairs are those that must wait because of complicated wounds or those that are performed again after an unsatisfactory first repair. The physician identifies the tendon or muscle by extending the original laceration or making new incisions. The ends of the severed tendon are identified and repaired at the level of separation. The ends are reapproximated using the suture configuration of choice from several different stitching techniques. If the injury occurs in the area of carpal tunnel, at the wrist flexion crease, complete or partial release of the transverse carpal ligament may be necessary. The flexor profundus and sublimis tendons are repaired with attention to proper orientation and location in the carpal tunnel. After the ends are properly matched and sutured, nerves and vessels are repaired as needed. The wound is closed and the limb is immobilized in a posterior splint at approximately 45 degrees of flexion. Involved fingers are held in passive flexion by an elastic band attached at the wrist level and at the fingernail by a wire. Report 25260 for a primary repair, one performed within the first 12-24 hours of injury where tendons are involved. Report 25263 for a secondary repair, one performed 10 or more days out from the injury or a subsequent repair done when the first procedure failed to restore function. Use these codes once for each tendon or muscle repaired.

Coding Tips

These codes should be reported for each tendon repair performed. When multiple tendon repairs are performed, report one tendon as the primary procedure and append modifier 51 to subsequent procedures. For secondary tendon repair with a graft, see 25265. Surgical trays, A4550, are not separately reimbursed by Medicare; however, other third-party payers may cover them. Check with the specific payer to determine coverage.

ICD-9-CM Procedural

- 83.64 Other suture of tendon
- 83.65 Other suture of muscle or fascia
- 83.88 Other plastic operations on tendon
- 83.99 Other operations on muscle, tendon, fascia, and bursa

Anesthesia

01810

ICD-9-CM Diagnostic

- 727.64 Nontraumatic rupture of flexor tendons of hand and wrist
- 727.69 Nontraumatic rupture of other tendon
- 727.9 Unspecified disorder of synovium, tendon, and bursa
- 841.8 Sprain and strain of other specified sites of elbow and forearm
- 842.00 Sprain and strain of unspecified site of wrist
- 842.01 Sprain and strain of carpal (joint) of wrist
- 842.02 Sprain and strain of radiocarpal (joint) (ligament) of wrist
- 842.09 Other wrist sprain and strain
- 881.20 Open wound of forearm, with tendon involvement
- 881.22 Open wound of wrist, with tendon involvement
- 884.2 Multiple and unspecified open wound of upper limb, with tendon involvement
- 905.8 Late effect of tendon injury
- 959.3 Injury, other and unspecified, elbow, forearm, and wrist

Terms To Know

distal. Located farther away from a specified reference point.

proximal. Located closest to a specified reference point, usually the midline.

tendon. Fibrous tissue that connects muscle to bone, consisting primarily of collagen and containing little vasculature.

volar. Palm of the hand (palmar) or sole of the foot (plantar).

CCI Version 16.3

01810, 0213T, 0216T, 0228T, 0230T, 24300, 25000-25001, 25109-25110, 25115, 25259, 25280-25295, 29065-29075, 29105-29125, 35761, 36000, 36400-36410, 36420-36430, 36440, 36600, 36640, 37202, 43752, 51701-51703, 62310-62319, 64400-64435, 64445-64450, 64479, 64483, 64490, 64493, 64505-64530, 64704-64708, 64719-64721, 69990, 93000-93010, 93040-93042, 93318, 94002, 94200, 94250, 94680-94690, 94770, 95812-95816, 95819, 95822, 95829, 95955, 96360, 96365, 96372, 96374-96376, 99148-99149, 99150

Also not with 25260: 12002, 12032-12034, 12037, 13121, 37618

Note: These CCI edits are used for Medicare. Other payers may reimburse on codes listed above.

Medicare Edits

	Fac RVU	Non-Fac RVU	FUD	Assist
25260	19.17	19.17	90	N/A
25263	19.1	19.1	90	80

Medicare References: 100-2,15,260; 100-4,12,30; 100-4,12,90.3; 100-4,14,10

25265

25265 Repair, tendon or muscle, flexor, forearm and/or wrist; secondary, with free graft (includes obtaining graft), each tendon or muscle

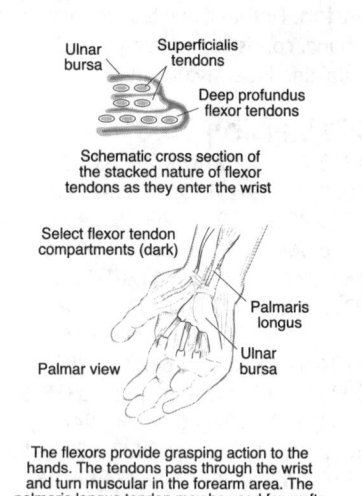

Explanation

The physician performs a secondary repair of a flexor tendon or muscle of the forearm and/or wrist with a free graft. A secondary tendon repair is one performed 10 or more days out from the injury because of complicated wounds that would compromise immediate repair or one performed again after the first procedure failed to restore function. When the flexor tendons in the forearm and wrist area have become tightly contracted, a graft is necessary to bring the ends together. The palmaris longus is the graft of choice. The physician first approaches the involved flexor muscle or tendon through a zigzag incision on the palmar surface of the wrist or forearm, depending on the area of the tendon in need of grafting. The possibly scarred flexor tendon is freed and brought out through the incision, preserving as much healthy sheath as possible. The free graft is obtained by making a transverse incision in the volar wrist, dividing the palmaris longus tendon at its insertion, and while holding tension on the graft at its distal end with a clamp, advancing a tendon stripper into the proximal forearm. The proximal end is mobilized and the graft is withdrawn. Likewise, another incision may be made more proximally in the forearm, the tendon divided, and the segment withdrawn. The transverse skin incision is closed. The tendon graft is threaded through the forearm using a tendon passer. The tendon ends must be attached to the graft under the right tension. The junctures are secured using a monofilament wire and several possible suturing techniques. The wound is closed and dressed. A dorsal splint is applied maintaining wrist flexion to protect repair.

Coding Tips

This code should be reported for each tendon repair performed. When multiple tendon repairs are performed, report one tendon as the primary procedure and append modifier 51 to subsequent procedures. For secondary tendon repair without a graft, see 25263.

ICD-9-CM Procedural

- 83.64 Other suture of tendon
- 83.65 Other suture of muscle or fascia
- 83.81 Tendon graft
- 83.82 Graft of muscle or fascia
- 83.88 Other plastic operations on tendon
- 83.99 Other operations on muscle, tendon, fascia, and bursa

Anesthesia

25265   01810

ICD-9-CM Diagnostic

- 727.64 Nontraumatic rupture of flexor tendons of hand and wrist
- 727.69 Nontraumatic rupture of other tendon
- 727.9 Unspecified disorder of synovium, tendon, and bursa
- 841.8 Sprain and strain of other specified sites of elbow and forearm
- 842.00 Sprain and strain of unspecified site of wrist
- 842.01 Sprain and strain of carpal (joint) of wrist
- 842.02 Sprain and strain of radiocarpal (joint) (ligament) of wrist
- 842.09 Other wrist sprain and strain
- 881.20 Open wound of forearm, with tendon involvement
- 881.22 Open wound of wrist, with tendon involvement
- 884.2 Multiple and unspecified open wound of upper limb, with tendon involvement
- 905.8 Late effect of tendon injury
- 959.3 Injury, other and unspecified, elbow, forearm, and wrist

Terms To Know

distal. Located farther away from a specified reference point.

flexion. Act of bending or being bent.

late effect. Abnormality, dysfunction, or other residual condition produced after the acute phase of an illness, injury, or disease is over. There is no time limit on when late effects can appear.

open wound. Opening or break of the skin.

proximal. Located closest to a specified reference point, usually the midline.

sprain and strain. Injuries to a joint, in which the fibers of supporting ligaments or muscles are overstretched or slightly ruptured, with the ligaments and muscles maintaining continuity.

tendon. Fibrous tissue that connects muscle to bone, consisting primarily of collagen and containing little vasculature.

CCI Version 16.3

01810, 0213T, 0216T, 0228T, 0230T, 20920-20926, 24300, 25000-25001, 25109-25110, 25115, 25259, 25280-25295, 29065-29075, 29105, 35761, 36000, 36400-36410, 36420-36430, 36440, 36600, 36640, 37202, 43752, 51701-51703, 62310-62319, 64400-64435, 64445-64450, 64479, 64483, 64490, 64493, 64505-64530, 64704-64708, 64719-64721, 69990, 93000-93010, 93040-93042, 93318, 94002, 94200, 94250, 94680-94690, 94770, 95812-95816, 95819, 95822, 95829, 95955, 96360, 96365, 96372, 96374-96376, 99148-99149, 99150

Note: These CCI edits are used for Medicare. Other payers may reimburse on codes listed above.

Medicare Edits

	Fac RVU	Non-Fac RVU	FUD	Assist
25265	22.71	22.71	90	80

Medicare References: 100-2,15,260; 100-4,12,30; 100-4,12,90.3; 100-4,14,10

25270-25272

25270 Repair, tendon or muscle, extensor, forearm and/or wrist; primary, single, each tendon or muscle

25272 secondary, single, each tendon or muscle

Extensor digitorum muscles and tendons
Extensor carpi radialis brevis and longus
Extensor carpi ulnaris
Extensor pollicis longus
Select extensor muscles and tendons
Extensor pollicis brevis

The extensor tendons and muscles act to open the hand and extend the fingers

A primary repair of an extensor tendon or muscle of the forearm and/or wrist is performed. Report 25272 for secondary repair of each tendon or muscle

Explanation

The physician repairs an extensor tendon or muscle of the forearm and/or wrist. The repair is done to restore continuity for normal function by reapproximating the severed ends. Primary tendon repairs can be performed when a clean wound is presented close to the time of injury that can be satisfactorily stabilized for a good end result, such as wounds inflicted with a sharp edge. Secondary tendon repairs are those that must wait because of complicated wounds or those that are performed again after an unsatisfactory first repair. The physician identifies the tendon or muscle by extending the original laceration or making new incisions. The ends of the severed tendon are identified and repaired at the level of separation. The ends are reapproximated using the suture configuration of choice from several different stitching techniques. Tendons in the dorsal wrist area are retained by the dorsal carpal ligament (extensor retinaculum) and are encased in fibro-osseous canals. They tend to get stuck in their canals as they heal; therefore, release of the sutured area may be necessary by excising a portion of the overlying carpal ligament. Many extensor tendons in the dorsal forearm are covered by their respective muscles and must be sutured, since sutures placed in muscle tend to pull out of the tissue. The wound is closed and the wrist is immobilized with a volar splint, in moderate or full extension. Report 25270 for a primary repair, one performed within the first 12-24 hours of injury. Report 25272 for a secondary repair, one performed 10 or more days out from the injury or a subsequent repair done when the first procedure failed to restore function. Use these codes once for each tendon or muscle repaired.

Coding Tips

These codes should be reported for each tendon or muscle repair performed. When multiple tendon repairs are performed, report one tendon as the primary procedure and append modifier 51 to subsequent procedures. For secondary repair of the extensor tendon or muscle with a graft, see 25274.

ICD-9-CM Procedural

- 83.64 Other suture of tendon
- 83.65 Other suture of muscle or fascia
- 83.81 Tendon graft
- 83.88 Other plastic operations on tendon
- 83.99 Other operations on muscle, tendon, fascia, and bursa

Anesthesia
01810

ICD-9-CM Diagnostic

- 727.63 Nontraumatic rupture of extensor tendons of hand and wrist
- 727.69 Nontraumatic rupture of other tendon
- 727.9 Unspecified disorder of synovium, tendon, and bursa
- 841.8 Sprain and strain of other specified sites of elbow and forearm
- 842.00 Sprain and strain of unspecified site of wrist
- 842.01 Sprain and strain of carpal (joint) of wrist
- 842.02 Sprain and strain of radiocarpal (joint) (ligament) of wrist
- 842.09 Other wrist sprain and strain
- 881.20 Open wound of forearm, with tendon involvement
- 881.22 Open wound of wrist, with tendon involvement
- 884.2 Multiple and unspecified open wound of upper limb, with tendon involvement
- 905.7 Late effect of sprain and strain without mention of tendon injury
- 905.8 Late effect of tendon injury
- 959.3 Injury, other and unspecified, elbow, forearm, and wrist

Terms To Know

sprain and strain. Injuries to a joint, in which the fibers of supporting ligaments or muscles are overstretched or slightly ruptured, with the ligaments and muscles maintaining continuity.

tendon. Fibrous tissue that connects muscle to bone, consisting primarily of collagen and containing little vasculature.

CCI Version 16.3

01810, 0213T, 0216T, 0228T, 0230T, 24300, 25000, 25109-25110, 25116-25118, 25259, 25275-25295, 29065-29075, 29105, 36000, 36400-36410, 36420-36430, 36440, 36600, 36640, 37202, 43752, 51701-51703, 62310-62319, 64400-64435, 64445-64450, 64479, 64483, 64490, 64493, 64505-64530, 64704-64708, 64719-64721, 69990, 93000-93010, 93040-93042, 93318, 94002, 94200, 94250, 94680-94690, 94770, 95812-95816, 95819, 95822, 95829, 95955, 96360, 96365, 96372, 96374-96376, 99148-99149, 99150

Also not with 25270: 12034, 12037, 37618

Note: These CCI edits are used for Medicare. Other payers may reimburse on codes listed above.

Medicare Edits

	Fac RVU	Non-Fac RVU	FUD	Assist
25270	15.17	15.17	90	80
25272	17.04	17.04	90	80

Medicare References: 100-2,15,260; 100-4,12,30; 100-4,12,90.3; 100-4,14,10

25274

25274 Repair, tendon or muscle, extensor, forearm and/or wrist; secondary, with free graft (includes obtaining graft), each tendon or muscle

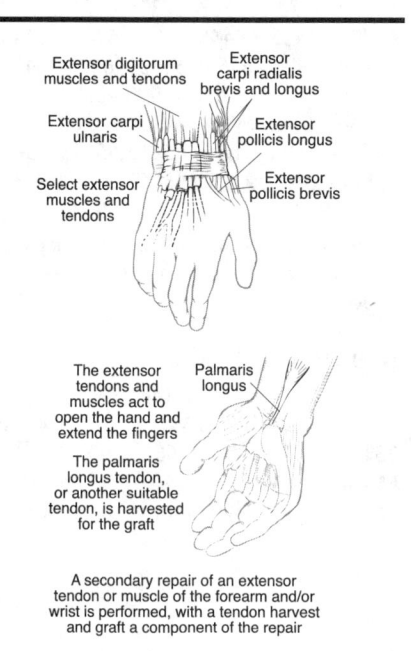

Explanation

The physician performs a secondary repair of an extensor tendon or muscle of the forearm and/or wrist with a free graft. A secondary tendon repair is one performed 10 or more days out from the injury because of complicated wounds that would compromise immediate repair or one performed again after the first procedure failed to restore function. When the extensor tendons in the forearm and wrist area have become tightly contracted or a segment of tendon has been lost, a graft is necessary to bring the ends together. The palmaris longus is the graft of choice. The physician first approaches the involved extensor muscle or tendon through an incision on the dorsal surface of the wrist or forearm, depending on the area of the tendon in need of grafting. The possibly scarred tendon is freed and the ends brought out through the incision for repair. The free graft is obtained by making a transverse incision in the volar wrist, dividing the palmaris longus tendon at its insertion, and while holding tension on the graft at its distal end with a clamp, advancing a tendon stripper into the proximal forearm. The proximal end is mobilized and the graft is withdrawn. Likewise, another incision may be made more proximally in the forearm, the tendon divided, and the segment withdrawn. The transverse skin incision is closed. The tendon graft is threaded through the forearm using a tendon passer. The tendon ends must be attached to the graft under the right tension. The junctures are secured using a monofilament wire and several possible suturing techniques. The wound is closed and the wrist is immobilized with a volar splint, in moderate or full extension.

Coding Tips

This code should be reported for each tendon or muscle repair performed. When multiple tendon repairs are performed, report one tendon as the primary procedure and append modifier 51 to subsequent procedures. Harvesting of graft is included in this code and should not be reported separately. For repair of a tendon or muscle, extensor forearm, primary or secondary without graft, see 25270 and 25272.

ICD-9-CM Procedural

- 83.64 Other suture of tendon
- 83.65 Other suture of muscle or fascia
- 83.81 Tendon graft
- 83.88 Other plastic operations on tendon
- 83.99 Other operations on muscle, tendon, fascia, and bursa

Anesthesia

25274 01810

ICD-9-CM Diagnostic

- 727.63 Nontraumatic rupture of extensor tendons of hand and wrist
- 727.69 Nontraumatic rupture of other tendon
- 727.9 Unspecified disorder of synovium, tendon, and bursa
- 841.8 Sprain and strain of other specified sites of elbow and forearm
- 842.00 Sprain and strain of unspecified site of wrist
- 842.01 Sprain and strain of carpal (joint) of wrist
- 842.02 Sprain and strain of radiocarpal (joint) (ligament) of wrist
- 842.09 Other wrist sprain and strain
- 881.20 Open wound of forearm, with tendon involvement
- 881.22 Open wound of wrist, with tendon involvement
- 884.2 Multiple and unspecified open wound of upper limb, with tendon involvement
- 905.7 Late effect of sprain and strain without mention of tendon injury
- 905.8 Late effect of tendon injury
- 959.3 Injury, other and unspecified, elbow, forearm, and wrist

Terms To Know

distal. Located farther away from a specified reference point.

flexion. Act of bending or being bent.

late effect. Abnormality, dysfunction, or other residual condition produced after the acute phase of an illness, injury, or disease is over. There is no time limit on when late effects can appear.

proximal. Located closest to a specified reference point, usually the midline.

sprain and strain. Injuries to a joint, in which the fibers of supporting ligaments or muscles are overstretched or slightly ruptured, with the ligaments and muscles maintaining continuity.

tendon. Fibrous tissue that connects muscle to bone, consisting primarily of collagen and containing little vasculature.

CCI Version 16.3

01810, 0213T, 0216T, 0228T, 0230T, 20924-20926, 24300, 25000, 25109-25110, 25116, 25259, 25275-25295, 29065-29075, 29105, 36000, 36400-36410, 36420-36430, 36440, 36600, 36640, 37202, 43752, 51701-51703, 62310-62319, 64400-64435, 64445-64450, 64479, 64483, 64490, 64493, 64505-64530, 64704-64708, 64719-64721, 69990, 93000-93010, 93040-93042, 93318, 94002, 94200, 94250, 94680-94690, 94770, 95812-95816, 95819, 95822, 95829, 95955, 96360, 96365, 96372, 96374-96376, 99148-99149, 99150

Note: These CCI edits are used for Medicare. Other payers may reimburse on codes listed above.

Medicare Edits

	Fac RVU	Non-Fac RVU	FUD	Assist
25274	20.4	20.4	90	80

Medicare References: 100-2,15,260; 100-4,12,30; 100-4,12,90.3; 100-4,14,10

25275

25275 Repair, tendon sheath, extensor, forearm and/or wrist, with free graft (includes obtaining graft) (eg, for extensor carpi ulnaris subluxation)

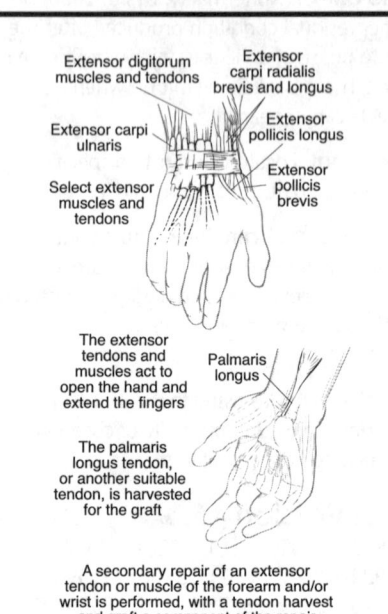

Explanation

The physician repairs an extensor tendon sheath of the forearm and/or wrist with a free graft. This is done for extensor carpi ulnaris (ECU) subluxation. The ECU passes through a groove at the distal end of the ulna and is covered by a ligament. The ECU is the only wrist extensor that lies in its own retaining fibro-osseous sheath tunnel. Disruption of this compartment sheath is what allows the extensor carpi ulnaris to sublux. An incision is made and the underlying tissues are dissected to reach the sheath disruption of the ECU tendon. If the fibro-osseous sheath has ruptured so that the sheath lies under the ECU tendon on its ulnar groove, the sheath is sutured together directly over the tendon. When the fibro-osseous sheath has ruptured so that the sheath lies superficial to the tendon, the sheath is reconstructed with a piece of the extensor retinaculum, the fibrous sheet, or band of fascia overlying the extensor tendons. The subcutaneous tissues and skin are closed and a dressing is applied.

Coding Tips

This is a unilateral procedure. If performed bilaterally, some payers require that the service be reported twice with modifier 50 appended to the second code, while others require identification of the service only once with modifier 50 appended. Check with individual payers. Modifier 50 identifies a procedure performed identically on the opposite side of the body (mirror image).

ICD-9-CM Procedural

83.61	Suture of tendon sheath
83.81	Tendon graft

Anesthesia

25275	01810

ICD-9-CM Diagnostic

727.63	Nontraumatic rupture of extensor tendons of hand and wrist
727.69	Nontraumatic rupture of other tendon
727.9	Unspecified disorder of synovium, tendon, and bursa
841.8	Sprain and strain of other specified sites of elbow and forearm
842.00	Sprain and strain of unspecified site of wrist
842.01	Sprain and strain of carpal (joint) of wrist
842.02	Sprain and strain of radiocarpal (joint) (ligament) of wrist
842.09	Other wrist sprain and strain
881.20	Open wound of forearm, with tendon involvement
881.22	Open wound of wrist, with tendon involvement
884.2	Multiple and unspecified open wound of upper limb, with tendon involvement
905.7	Late effect of sprain and strain without mention of tendon injury
905.8	Late effect of tendon injury
959.3	Injury, other and unspecified, elbow, forearm, and wrist

Terms To Know

dorsum. Back side or back part of the body or individual anatomical structure.

extensor. Any muscle that extends a joint.

rupture. Tearing or breaking open of tissue.

sheath. Covering enclosing an organ or part.

tendon. Fibrous tissue that connects muscle to bone, consisting primarily of collagen and containing little vasculature.

CCI Version 16.3

01810, 0213T, 0216T, 0228T, 0230T, 20924-20926, 25000, 25109-25110, 25280-25295, 29058-29085, 29105-29126, 29260-29280, 36000, 36400-36410, 36420-36430, 36440, 36600, 36640, 37202, 43752, 51701-51703, 62310-62319, 64400-64435, 64445-64450, 64479, 64483, 64490, 64493, 64505-64530, 64704-64708, 64719-64721, 69990, 93000-93010, 93040-93042, 93318, 94002, 94200, 94250, 94680-94690, 94770, 95812-95816, 95819, 95822, 95829, 95955, 96360, 96365, 96372, 96374-96376, 99148-99149, 99150

Note: These CCI edits are used for Medicare. Other payers may reimburse on codes listed above.

Medicare Edits

	Fac RVU	Non-Fac RVU	FUD	Assist
25275	19.66	19.66	90	80

Medicare References: 100-2,15,260; 100-4,12,30; 100-4,12,90.3; 100-4,14,10

25280

25280 Lengthening or shortening of flexor or extensor tendon, forearm and/or wrist, single, each tendon

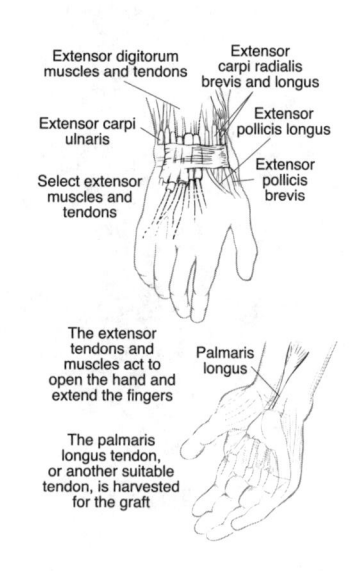

Explanation

The physician lengthens or shortens a flexor or extensor tendon of the forearm and/or wrist. For lengthening, the physician makes an incision in the forearm and down through the tissues to identify the affected tendon. The physician may make a series of small, equal-depth cuts spaced on opposite sides of the tendon to allow it to stretch without tearing through. An elongated Z incision may be cut in the tendon and the ends of the long half of each section are sewn together or an oblique incision is made across the tendon and the ends are slid apart until the pointed tips meet, which are sutured together. Several methods are also used to shorten a tendon that has become too long to function properly. A Z incision may be made in the tendon and the two short sides of the Z brought together and reapproximated. The tendon can be doubled over on itself with a small fold and sutured. A wedge-shaped piece may be excised and the two ends sutured. The soft tissue is closed in layers and a bandage is applied.

Coding Tips

This code should be reported for each tendon lengthening or shortening performed. When multiple tendons are lengthened or shortened, report one tendon as the primary procedure and append modifier 51 to subsequent procedures. According to CPT guidelines, cast application or strapping (including removal) is only reported as a replacement procedure or when the cast application or strapping is an initial service performed without a restorative treatment or procedure. See "Application of Casts and Strapping" in the CPT book in the Surgery Section, under the Musculoskeletal system.

ICD-9-CM Procedural

83.85 Other change in muscle or tendon length

Anesthesia

25280 01810

ICD-9-CM Diagnostic

342.10 Spastic hemiplegia affecting unspecified side
342.11 Spastic hemiplegia affecting dominant side
342.12 Spastic hemiplegia affecting nondominant side
342.80 Other specified hemiplegia affecting unspecified side
342.81 Other specified hemiplegia affecting dominant side
342.82 Other specified hemiplegia affecting nondominant side
343.9 Unspecified infantile cerebral palsy
344.89 Other specified paralytic syndrome
718.33 Recurrent dislocation of forearm joint
718.43 Contracture of forearm joint
727.81 Contracture of tendon (sheath)

Terms To Know

aponeurosis. Flat expansion of white, ribbon-like tendinous tissue that functions as the connection of a muscle to its moving part.

contracture. Shortening of muscle or connective tissue.

dorsiflexion. Position of being bent toward the extensor side of a limb.

extensor. Any muscle that extends a joint.

flexor. Muscle/tendon that bends or flexes a limb or part as opposed to extending it.

soft tissue. Nonepithelial tissues outside of the skeleton that includes subcutaneous adipose tissue, fibrous tissue, fascia, muscles, blood and lymph vessels, and peripheral nervous system tissue.

spastic hemiplegia. Paralytic condition affecting one side of the body marked by spasticity of the impaired muscles and an increase in tendon reflexes.

volar. Palm of the hand (palmar) or sole of the foot (plantar).

CCI Version 16.3

01810, 0213T, 0216T, 0228T, 0230T, 24300, 25000-25001, 25109, 25259, 25295, 29065-29075, 29105-29125, 36000, 36400-36410, 36420-36430, 36440, 36600, 36640, 37202, 43752, 51701-51703, 62310-62319, 64400-64435, 64445-64450, 64479, 64483, 64490, 64493, 64505-64530, 64708, 69990, 93000-93010, 93040-93042, 93318, 94002, 94200, 94250, 94680-94690, 94770, 95812-95816, 95819, 95822, 95829, 95955, 96360, 96365, 96372, 96374-96376, 99148-99149, 99150

Note: These CCI edits are used for Medicare. Other payers may reimburse on codes listed above.

Medicare Edits

	Fac RVU	Non-Fac RVU	FUD	Assist
25280	17.28	17.28	90	80

Medicare References: 100-2,15,260; 100-4,12,30; 100-4,12,90.3; 100-4,14,10

25290

25290 Tenotomy, open, flexor or extensor tendon, forearm and/or wrist, single, each tendon

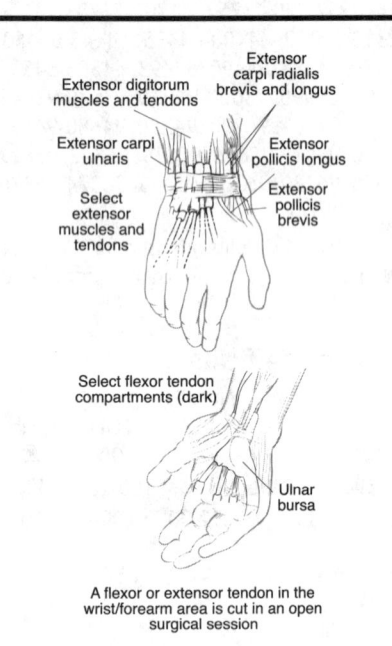

A flexor or extensor tendon in the wrist/forearm area is cut in an open surgical session

Explanation

The physician performs an open tenotomy on a flexor or extensor tendon of the forearm and/or wrist. An incision is made in the wrist or forearm over the site where the tendon to be cut may be accessed. The subcutaneous tissues and fascia are dissected to reach the target tendon. The usual method is to cut into the tendon so as to allow it to expand and heal as a longer tendon, thereby releasing a contracture caused by the tendon. The tissue layers and skin are closed and a dressing is applied.

Coding Tips

This code should be reported for each tendon repaired. When multiple tendons are repaired, report one tendon as the primary procedure and append modifier 51 to subsequent procedures. According to CPT guidelines, cast application or strapping (including removal) is only reported as a replacement procedure or when the cast application or strapping is an initial service performed without a restorative treatment or procedure. See "Application of Casts and Strapping" in the CPT book in the Surgery Section, under the Musculoskeletal system.

ICD-9-CM Procedural

83.13 Other tenotomy

Anesthesia

25290   01810

ICD-9-CM Diagnostic

718.43 Contracture of forearm joint
726.4   Enthesopathy of wrist and carpus
727.00 Unspecified synovitis and tenosynovitis
727.01 Synovitis and tenosynovitis in diseases classified elsewhere — (Code first underlying disease: 015.0-015.9)
727.02 Giant cell tumor of tendon sheath
727.03 Trigger finger (acquired)
727.04 Radial styloid tenosynovitis
727.05 Other tenosynovitis of hand and wrist
727.81 Contracture of tendon (sheath)

Terms To Know

boutonniere deformity. Finger deformity with hyperextension of the distal joint and flexion of the interphalangeal joint.

contracture. Shortening of muscle or connective tissue.

extensor. Any muscle that extends a joint.

flexion. Act of bending or being bent.

flexor. Muscle/tendon that bends or flexes a limb or part as opposed to extending it.

synovitis. Inflammation of the synovial membrane that lines a synovial joint, resulting in pain and swelling.

tendon. Fibrous tissue that connects muscle to bone, consisting primarily of collagen and containing little vasculature.

CCI Version 16.3

01810, 0213T, 0216T, 0228T, 0230T, 24300, 25000-25001, 25109, 25259, 25295, 29065-29075, 29105, 36000, 36400-36410, 36420-36430, 36440, 36600, 36640, 37202, 43752, 51701-51703, 62310-62319, 64400-64435, 64445-64450, 64479, 64483, 64490, 64493, 64505-64530, 69990, 93000-93010, 93040-93042, 93318, 94002, 94200, 94250, 94680-94690, 94770, 95812-95816, 95819, 95822, 95829, 95955, 96360, 96365, 96372, 96374-96376, 99148-99149, 99150

Note: These CCI edits are used for Medicare. Other payers may reimburse on codes listed above.

Medicare Edits

	Fac RVU	Non-Fac RVU	FUD	Assist
25290	14.09	14.09	90	N/A

Medicare References: 100-2,15,260; 100-4,12,30; 100-4,12,90.3; 100-4,14,10

25295

25295 Tenolysis, flexor or extensor tendon, forearm and/or wrist, single, each tendon

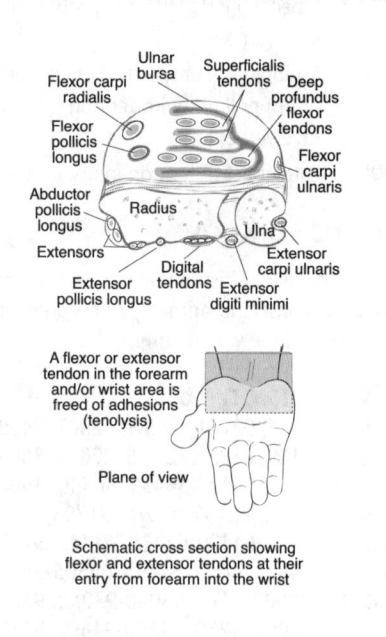

Explanation

Tenolysis of the flexor or extensor tendon is indicated in the case of extrinsic extensor or flexor tendon tightness. In the case of flexor tightness, the physician approaches the involved flexor system through a zigzag incision that is long enough to uncover the entire length of the flexor. The physician excises all limiting adhesions, whether the excess scarring is located proximally in the forearm and/or distally in the wrist. All involved tendons are released of motion-limiting adhesions. The retinacular pulley system is preserved. During the procedure, the patient's active motion is re-evaluated. To achieve this, a local anesthesia is supplemented by an intravenous analgesic-tranquilizer combination drug. After tissue closure, the physician applies a splint over the dressing. These must be applied in a manner that allows continued flexion to maintain tendon gliding through the lysed scars. The above techniques are the same for extrinsic extensors, except there is no critical annular pulley system to preserve, although the sagittal bands must be protected.

Coding Tips

This code should be reported for each tendon involved. When multiple tendons are involved, report one tendon as the primary procedure and append modifier 51 to subsequent procedures. According to CPT guidelines, cast application or strapping (including removal) is only reported as a replacement procedure or when the cast application or strapping is an initial service performed without a restorative treatment or procedure. See "Application of Casts and Strapping" in the CPT book in the Surgery Section, under the Musculoskeletal system.

ICD-9-CM Procedural

83.91 Lysis of adhesions of muscle, tendon, fascia, and bursa

Anesthesia

25295 01810

ICD-9-CM Diagnostic

342.10 Spastic hemiplegia affecting unspecified side
342.11 Spastic hemiplegia affecting dominant side
342.12 Spastic hemiplegia affecting nondominant side
343.9 Unspecified infantile cerebral palsy
344.81 Locked-in state
357.1 Polyneuropathy in collagen vascular disease — (Code first underlying disease: 446.0, 710.0, 714.0)
359.6 Symptomatic inflammatory myopathy in diseases classified elsewhere — (Code first underlying disease: 135, 140.0-208.9, 277.30-277.39, 446.0, 710.0, 710.1, 710.2, 714.0)
446.0 Polyarteritis nodosa
710.0 Systemic lupus erythematosus — (Use additional code to identify manifestation: 424.91, 581.81, 582.81, 583.81)
710.1 Systemic sclerosis — (Use additional code to identify manifestation: 359.6, 517.2)
710.2 Sicca syndrome
714.0 Rheumatoid arthritis — (Use additional code to identify manifestation: 357.1, 359.6)
727.05 Other tenosynovitis of hand and wrist
727.42 Ganglion of tendon sheath
727.81 Contracture of tendon (sheath)
727.82 Calcium deposits in tendon and bursa
727.89 Other disorders of synovium, tendon, and bursa
727.9 Unspecified disorder of synovium, tendon, and bursa
905.8 Late effect of tendon injury

Terms To Know

adhesion. Abnormal fibrous connection between two structures, soft tissue or bony structures, that may occur as the result of surgery, infection, or trauma.

contracture. Shortening of muscle or connective tissue.

flexion. Act of bending or being bent.

polyarteritis nodosa. Systemic necrotizing vasculitis of small and medium arteries that results in the infarction and scarring within the affected organs.

tenosynovitis. Inflammation of a tendon sheath due to infection or disease.

CCI Version 16.3

01810, 0213T, 0216T, 0228T, 0230T, 24300, 25000-25001, 25109, 25118, 25259, 29065-29075, 29105, 35761, 36000, 36400-36410, 36420-36430, 36440, 36600, 36640, 37202, 43752, 51701-51703, 62310-62319, 64400-64435, 64445-64450, 64479, 64483, 64490, 64493, 64505-64530, 69990, 93000-93010, 93040-93042, 93318, 94002, 94200, 94250, 94680-94690, 94770, 95812-95816, 95819, 95822, 95829, 95955, 96360, 96365, 96372, 96374-96376, 99148-99149, 99150

Note: These CCI edits are used for Medicare. Other payers may reimburse on codes listed above.

Medicare Edits

	Fac RVU	Non-Fac RVU	FUD	Assist
25295	16.08	16.08	90	N/A

Medicare References: 100-2,15,260; 100-4,12,30; 100-4,12,90.3; 100-4,14,10

25300-25301

25300 Tenodesis at wrist; flexors of fingers
25301 extensors of fingers

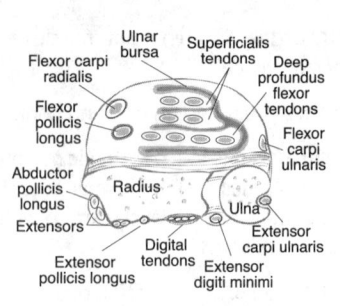

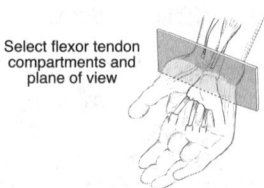

Flexors of the fingers are sutured to bone (tenodesis) in the wrist area. Report 25301 when extensors of the fingers are treated in a similar fashion

Explanation

The physician performs a tenodesis at the wrist. In 25300, the physician exposes the flexor tendons at the wrist level. The terminal phalangeal flexors of the fingers to be tenodesed (usually all four) are identified in the depths of the wound. A window is made in the anterior surface of the distal radius proximal to the wrist. A similar second window is made more proximal. A criss-cross type of suture is passed through all four flexor digitonum profundi tendons side-by-side. The tendon is transected proximal to this suture. The tendons are drawn into the more distal window in the radius, through the medullary canal, out the proximal window, and sutured back to themselves. The tension on the tenodesis is adjusted so that with the wrist in extension, the fingers naturally flex into the palm. With wrist flexion, the fingers can extend through the passive dorsal tenodesis of tension on the extrinsic extensors. All open soft tissues are sutured in layers. The wrist is immobilized in five to 10 degrees of extension and with the metacarpophalangeal joints flexed and the interphalangeal joints extended. Report 25301 if the extensors of the fingers are repaired at the wrist.

Coding Tips

According to CPT guidelines, cast application or strapping (including removal) is only reported as a replacement procedure or when the cast application or strapping is an initial service performed without a restorative treatment or procedure. See "Application of Casts and Strapping" in the CPT book in the Surgery Section, under the Musculoskeletal system.

ICD-9-CM Procedural

- 82.85 Other tenodesis of hand
- 83.88 Other plastic operations on tendon

Anesthesia

01810

ICD-9-CM Diagnostic

- 138 Late effects of acute poliomyelitis — (Note: This category is to be used to indicate conditions classifiable to 045 as the cause of late effects, which are themselves classified elsewhere. The "late effects" include those specified as such, as sequelae, or as due to old or inactive poliomyelitis, without evidence of active disease.)
- 343.8 Other specified infantile cerebral palsy
- 718.73 Developmental dislocation of joint, forearm
- 718.74 Developmental dislocation of joint, hand
- 726.4 Enthesopathy of wrist and carpus
- 727.63 Nontraumatic rupture of extensor tendons of hand and wrist
- 727.64 Nontraumatic rupture of flexor tendons of hand and wrist
- 727.9 Unspecified disorder of synovium, tendon, and bursa
- 833.00 Closed dislocation of wrist, unspecified part
- 833.01 Closed dislocation of distal radioulnar (joint)
- 833.02 Closed dislocation of radiocarpal (joint)
- 833.03 Closed dislocation of midcarpal (joint)
- 833.04 Closed dislocation of carpometacarpal (joint)
- 833.05 Closed dislocation of proximal end of metacarpal (bone)
- 833.09 Closed dislocation of other part of wrist
- 834.00 Closed dislocation of finger, unspecified part
- 834.01 Closed dislocation of metacarpophalangeal (joint)
- 834.02 Closed dislocation of interphalangeal (joint), hand
- 834.10 Open dislocation of finger, unspecified part
- 834.11 Open dislocation of metacarpophalangeal (joint)
- 834.12 Open dislocation interphalangeal (joint), hand
- 881.22 Open wound of wrist, with tendon involvement
- 883.2 Open wound of finger(s), with tendon involvement
- 884.2 Multiple and unspecified open wound of upper limb, with tendon involvement
- 905.8 Late effect of tendon injury

Terms To Know

tendon. Fibrous tissue that connects muscle to bone, consisting primarily of collagen and containing little vasculature.

CCI Version 16.3

01810, 0213T, 0216T, 0228T, 0230T, 24300, 25000, 25109, 25259, 25295, 29075, 36000, 36400-36410, 36420-36430, 36440, 36600, 36640, 37202, 43752, 51701-51703, 62310-62319, 64400-64435, 64445-64450, 64479, 64483, 64490, 64493, 64505-64530, 69990, 93000-93010, 93040-93042, 93318, 94002, 94200, 94250, 94680-94690, 94770, 95812-95816, 95819, 95822, 95829, 95955, 96360, 96365, 96372, 96374-96376, 99148-99149, 99150

Also not with 25300: 25115, 35761
Also not with 25301: 25116-25118
Note: These CCI edits are used for Medicare. Other payers may reimburse on codes listed above.

Medicare Edits

	Fac RVU	Non-Fac RVU	FUD	Assist
25300	20.0	20.0	90	80
25301	18.84	18.84	90	80

Medicare References: 100-2,15,260; 100-4,12,30; 100-4,12,90.3; 100-4,14,10

25310-25312

25310 Tendon transplantation or transfer, flexor or extensor, forearm and/or wrist, single; each tendon

25312 with tendon graft(s) (includes obtaining graft), each tendon

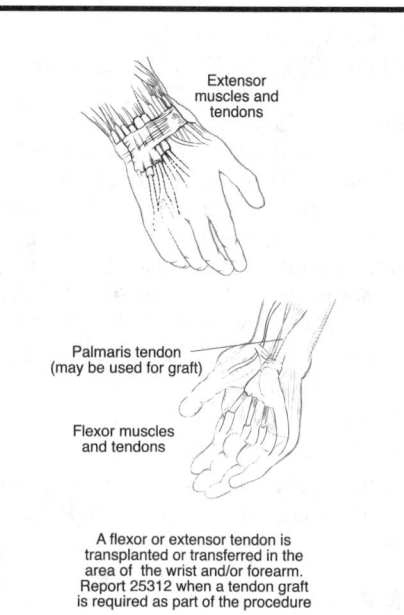

Extensor muscles and tendons

Palmaris tendon (may be used for graft)

Flexor muscles and tendons

A flexor or extensor tendon is transplanted or transferred in the area of the wrist and/or forearm. Report 25312 when a tendon graft is required as part of the procedure

Explanation

The physician performs a flexor or extensor transplantation or transfer in the forearm and wrist. With the patient under anesthesia, the physician exposes the muscle to be transferred by making a longitudinal incision near its insertion. The insertion is released from near its bony attachment for transfer to the involved tendon. The entire tendon may not be released, but rather only the central portion. Through a separate incision, the physician exposes the involved tendon. A tunnel is prepared around or through the arm between the transferred and involved tendons. This tunnel must permit a straight line of pull between the two tendons. The transferred tendon is passed through the tunnel. A small, longitudinal hole is created in the involved tendon. The distal end of the transferred tendon is passed through the involved tendon and sutured to that tendon. After these procedures are complete, all wounds are closed with sutures. Report 25312 if the procedure is performed with tendon grafts, each tendon.

Coding Tips

These codes should be reported for each tendon involved. When multiple tendons are involved, report one tendon as the primary procedure and append modifier 51 to subsequent procedures. According to CPT guidelines, cast application or strapping (including removal) is only reported as a replacement procedure or when the cast application or strapping is an initial service performed without a restorative treatment or procedure. See "Application of Casts and Strapping" in the CPT book in the Surgery Section, under the Musculoskeletal system.

ICD-9-CM Procedural

83.75 Tendon transfer or transplantation
83.81 Tendon graft

Anesthesia

01810

ICD-9-CM Diagnostic

138 Late effects of acute poliomyelitis — (Note: This category is to be used to indicate conditions classifiable to 045 as the cause of late effects, which are themselves classified elsewhere. The "late effects" include those specified as such, as sequelae, or as due to old or inactive poliomyelitis, without evidence of active disease.)
343.8 Other specified infantile cerebral palsy
357.1 Polyneuropathy in collagen vascular disease — (Code first underlying disease: 446.0, 710.0, 714.0)
359.6 Symptomatic inflammatory myopathy in diseases classified elsewhere — (Code first underlying disease: 135, 140.0-208.9, 277.30-277.39, 446.0, 710.0, 710.1, 710.2, 714.0)
446.0 Polyarteritis nodosa
710.0 Systemic lupus erythematosus — (Use additional code to identify manifestation: 424.91, 581.81, 582.81, 583.81)
710.1 Systemic sclerosis — (Use additional code to identify manifestation: 359.6, 517.2)
710.2 Sicca syndrome
714.0 Rheumatoid arthritis — (Use additional code to identify manifestation: 357.1, 359.6)
715.13 Primary localized osteoarthrosis, forearm
715.33 Localized osteoarthrosis not specified whether primary or secondary, forearm
715.93 Osteoarthrosis, unspecified whether generalized or localized, forearm
726.4 Enthesopathy of wrist and carpus
727.63 Nontraumatic rupture of extensor tendons of hand and wrist
727.64 Nontraumatic rupture of flexor tendons of hand and wrist
881.20 Open wound of forearm, with tendon involvement
881.22 Open wound of wrist, with tendon involvement
905.8 Late effect of tendon injury

Terms To Know

osteoarthrosis. Most common form of a noninflammatory degenerative joint disease with degenerating articular cartilage, bone enlargement, and synovial membrane changes.

sicca syndrome. Complex of symptoms of unknown source in middle-aged women in which the following triad exists: keratoconjunctivitis sicca, zerostomia, and connective tissue disease (usually rheumatoid arthritis but sometimes systemic lupus erythematosus).

tendon. Fibrous tissue that connects muscle to bone, consisting primarily of collagen and containing little vasculature.

CCI Version 16.3

01810, 0213T, 0216T, 0228T, 0230T, 24300, 25001, 25109, 25115-25118, 25259, 25295, 29065-29075, 29105, 36000, 36400-36410, 36420-36430, 36440, 36600, 36640, 37202, 43752, 51701-51703, 62310-62319, 64400-64435, 64445-64450, 64479, 64483, 64490, 64493, 64505-64530, 69990, 93000-93010, 93040-93042, 93318, 94002, 94200, 94250, 94680-94690, 94770, 95812-95816, 95819, 95822, 95829, 95955, 96360, 96365, 96372, 96374-96376, 99148-99149, 99150

Also not with 25312: 20924

Note: These CCI edits are used for Medicare. Other payers may reimburse on codes listed above.

Medicare Edits

	Fac RVU	Non-Fac RVU	FUD	Assist
25310	18.83	18.83	90	80
25312	21.86	21.86	90	80

Medicare References: 100-2,15,260; 100-4,12,30; 100-4,12,90.3; 100-4,14,10

25315-25316

25315 Flexor origin slide (eg, for cerebral palsy, Volkmann contracture), forearm and/or wrist;

25316 with tendon(s) transfer

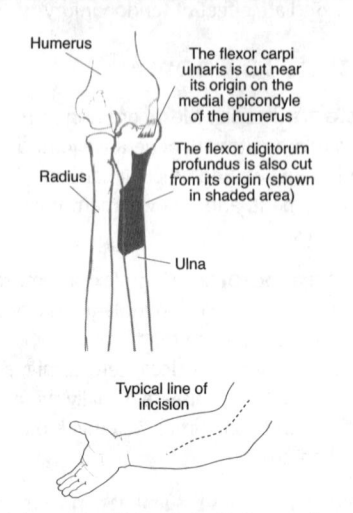

A flexor origin slide is performed in the area of the forearm and/or wrist. Report 25316 when a tendon is transferred. This type of procedure involves releasing flexor muscles near their origins. Severely contracted muscles, as may be found in cerebral palsy, are then relieved

Explanation

The physician performs a flexor origin slide in the forearm or wrist for cerebral palsy. The physician makes a zigzag incision from above the supracondylar region, distally through the middle and lower regions of the forearm. A periosteal elevator is inserted between the brachialis and the common flexor-pronator origin from the medial epicondyle. The elevator is brought out between the numeral and ulnar heads of the flexor carpi ulnaris on the anterior side of the elbow. The origin of the flexors is dissected using a scalpel to detach the muscle subperiosteally. The origins of the pronatorteres flexor carpi radialis, palmaris longus, and the numeral head of the flexor carpi ulnaris are released. The physician dissects the origins of the flexor digitonum superficialis. The ulnar head of the flexor carpi ulnaris is detached subperiosteally. The physician brings together the detached muscles from the proximal and ulnar sides at the interosseous space on the proximal side. Neurolysis of the median and ulnar nerves is performed. The muscles are slid distally the desired amount and are fixed in several places to periosteum and subcutaneous tissue. The ulnar nerve is transposed over the medial epicondyle. The wound is closed in layers. The elbow joint is maintained at 90 degrees, the wrist and fingers in extension, the forearm in supination. Report 25316 if this procedure is performed with a tendon transfer.

Coding Tips

According to CPT guidelines, cast application or strapping (including removal) is only reported as a replacement procedure or when the cast application or strapping is an initial service performed without a restorative treatment or procedure. See "Application of Casts and Strapping" in the CPT book in the Surgery Section, under the Musculoskeletal system. For other tendon transfer, forearm and/or wrist, see 25310 or 25312.

ICD-9-CM Procedural

- 82.85 Other tenodesis of hand
- 83.75 Tendon transfer or transplantation
- 83.88 Other plastic operations on tendon

Anesthesia
01810

ICD-9-CM Diagnostic

- 138 Late effects of acute poliomyelitis — (Note: This category is to be used to indicate conditions classifiable to 045 as the cause of late effects, which are themselves classified elsewhere. The "late effects" include those specified as such, as sequelae, or as due to old or inactive poliomyelitis, without evidence of active disease.)
- 343.0 Diplegic infantile cerebral palsy
- 343.1 Hemiplegic infantile cerebral palsy
- 343.2 Quadriplegic infantile cerebral palsy
- 343.3 Monoplegic infantile cerebral palsy
- 343.4 Infantile hemiplegia
- 343.8 Other specified infantile cerebral palsy
- 343.9 Unspecified infantile cerebral palsy
- 726.4 Enthesopathy of wrist and carpus
- 728.88 Rhabdomyolysis
- 755.26 Congenital longitudinal deficiency, radial, complete or partial (with or without distal deficiencies, incomplete)
- 881.20 Open wound of forearm, with tendon involvement
- 881.22 Open wound of wrist, with tendon involvement
- 905.8 Late effect of tendon injury
- 958.6 Volkmann's ischemic contracture

Terms To Know

cerebral palsy. Brain damage occurring before, during, or shortly after birth that impedes muscle control and tone.

supination. Lying on the back; turning the palm toward the front or upward; raising the medial margin of the foot by an inverting and adducting movement.

Volkmann's contracture. Shortening of the muscles in the fingers or wrist due to injury near the elbow or vascular damage.

CCI Version 16.3

01810, 0213T, 0216T, 0228T, 0230T, 24300, 25001, 25109, 25115, 25259, 25280-25295, 29065-29075, 29105-29126, 36000, 36400-36410, 36420-36430, 36440, 36600, 36640, 37202, 43752, 51701-51703, 62310-62319, 64400-64435, 64445-64450, 64479, 64483, 64490, 64493, 64505-64530, 69990, 93000-93010, 93040-93042, 93318, 94002, 94200, 94250, 94680-94690, 94770, 95812-95816, 95819, 95822, 95829, 95955, 96360, 96365, 96372, 96374-96376, 99148-99149, 99150

Also not with 25315: 64718

Also not with 25316: 25315

Note: These CCI edits are used for Medicare. Other payers may reimburse on codes listed above.

Medicare Edits

	Fac RVU	Non-Fac RVU	FUD	Assist
25315	23.46	23.46	90	80
25316	26.6	26.6	90	80

Medicare References: 100-2,15,260; 100-4,12,30; 100-4,12,90.3; 100-4,14,10

25320

25320 Capsulorrhaphy or reconstruction, wrist, open (eg, capsulodesis, ligament repair, tendon transfer or graft) (includes synovectomy, capsulotomy and open reduction) for carpal instability

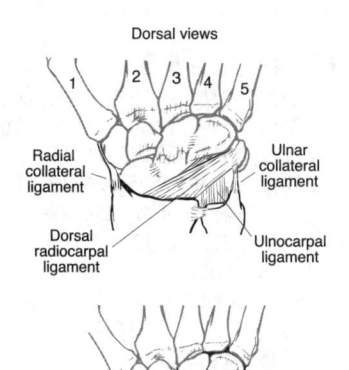

Dorsal views
Radial collateral ligament
Ulnar collateral ligament
Dorsal radiocarpal ligament
Ulnocarpal ligament
Radius — Ulna

Articular spaces of the wrist (containing synovial membranes and fluids)

The wrist capsule is surgically entered and reconstructed (capsulorrhaphy)

Explanation

The physician performs an open capsulorrhaphy or reconstruction of the wrist by any method (capsulodesis, ligament repair, tendon transfer, or graft), including synovectomy, capsulotomy, and open reduction to stem carpal instability. The wrist and finger extensors are retracted laterally and medially. The capsule is longitudinally cut over the involved carpus for exposure. If dislocation was present prior to surgery, this is reduced. The necessary fixation is carried out (i.e., Kirchner wires, screws). Carpal instability may result from dislocation of carpal bones and any number of ligamentous injuries that require reduction and repair, involving the joint capsule. Scapholunate dissociation and instability is one of the most common injuries. Dorsal intercarpal ligament capsulodesis may be performed to reduce the scapholunate gap. A flap of dorsal intercarpal ligament is elevated off the trapezoid and left attached to the triquetrum. The scaphoid inherently tends to sublux in the palmar direction in a flexed posture with dorsal rotational subluxation of the posterior pole. The scaphoid is brought out of its flexed position by applying dorsal pressure to the posterior pole and the scapholunate gap is reduced. The ligamentous flap is rotated down, stretched, and attached to the distal pole of the scaphoid. A flap of wrist capsule may also be created that is left attached to the radius and inserted into the distal pole of the scaphoid to tether it in chronic conditions.

Coding Tips

According to CPT guidelines, cast application or strapping (including removal) is only reported as a replacement procedure or when the cast application or strapping is an initial service performed without a restorative treatment or procedure. See "Application of Casts and Strapping" in the CPT book in the Surgery Section, under the Musculoskeletal system. For reconstruction of distal radial or distal radioulnar joint instability, see 25337.

ICD-9-CM Procedural

- 81.75 Arthroplasty of carpocarpal or carpometacarpal joint without implant
- 81.93 Suture of capsule or ligament of upper extremity
- 83.73 Reattachment of tendon
- 83.75 Tendon transfer or transplantation

Anesthesia
25320 01810

ICD-9-CM Diagnostic

- 170.5 Malignant neoplasm of short bones of upper limb
- 357.1 Polyneuropathy in collagen vascular disease — (Code first underlying disease: 446.0, 710.0, 714.0)
- 359.6 Symptomatic inflammatory myopathy in diseases classified elsewhere — (Code first underlying disease: 135, 140.0-208.9, 277.30-277.39, 446.0, 710.0, 710.1, 710.2, 714.0)
- 446.0 Polyarteritis nodosa
- 710.0 Systemic lupus erythematosus — (Use additional code to identify manifestation: 424.91, 581.81, 582.81, 583.81)
- 710.1 Systemic sclerosis — (Use additional code to identify manifestation: 359.6, 517.2)
- 710.2 Sicca syndrome
- 710.3 Dermatomyositis
- 710.4 Polymyositis
- 710.5 Eosinophilia myalgia syndrome — (Use additional E code to identify drug, if drug-induced)
- 710.8 Other specified diffuse disease of connective tissue
- 710.9 Unspecified diffuse connective tissue disease
- 714.0 Rheumatoid arthritis — (Use additional code to identify manifestation: 357.1, 359.6)
- 714.9 Unspecified inflammatory polyarthropathy
- 715.13 Primary localized osteoarthrosis, forearm
- 715.93 Osteoarthrosis, unspecified whether generalized or localized, forearm
- 718.03 Articular cartilage disorder, forearm
- 718.73 Developmental dislocation of joint, forearm
- 718.83 Other joint derangement, not elsewhere classified, forearm
- 727.63 Nontraumatic rupture of extensor tendons of hand and wrist
- 727.64 Nontraumatic rupture of flexor tendons of hand and wrist
- 727.9 Unspecified disorder of synovium, tendon, and bursa
- 731.1 Osteitis deformans in diseases classified elsewhere — (Code first underlying disease: 170.0-170.9)
- 833.00 Closed dislocation of wrist, unspecified part
- 833.10 Open dislocation of wrist, unspecified part
- 881.12 Open wound of wrist, complicated
- 881.22 Open wound of wrist, with tendon involvement
- 884.1 Multiple and unspecified open wound of upper limb, complicated

CCI Version 16.3

01810, 0213T, 0216T, 0228T, 0230T, 24300, 25000-25001, 25040, 25085-25119, 25259, 25280-25295, 25660, 25670, 29075-29085, 29125-29126, 29260, 36000, 36400-36410, 36420-36430, 36440, 36600, 36640, 37202, 43752, 51701-51703, 62310-62319, 64400-64435, 64445-64450, 64479, 64483, 64490, 64493, 64505-64530, 69990, 93000-93010, 93040-93042, 93318, 94002, 94200, 94250, 94680-94690, 94770, 95812-95816, 95819, 95822, 95829, 95955, 96360, 96365, 96372, 96374-96376, 99148-99149, 99150

Note: These CCI edits are used for Medicare. Other payers may reimburse on codes listed above.

Medicare Edits

	Fac RVU	Non-Fac RVU	FUD	Assist
25320	28.64	28.64	90	80

Medicare References: 100-2,15,260; 100-4,12,30; 100-4,12,90.3; 100-4,14,10

25332

25332 Arthroplasty, wrist, with or without interposition, with or without external or internal fixation

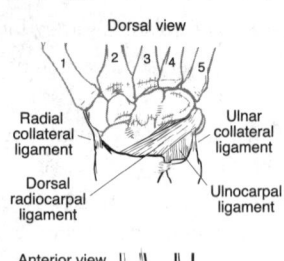

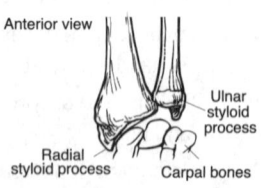

The wrist joint is surgically accessed and manipulated (arthroplasty). The distal radius may be excised, as may the distal ulna. Carpal bones may also be cut as necessary to restore a level of joint function. The radius may be reamed to accept one end of a fixation device; the carpal bones may be prepared to accept the other end. Interposition refers to placing bone or a fixation device between locked carpal bones to restore function

Explanation

The physician performs an arthroplasty of the wrist. The physician makes a straight, dorsal, longitudinal incision centered over the wrist from the middle of the third metacarpal proximally. Skin and subcutaneous tissues are elevated off the fascia and retinaculum. The retinaculum over the fourth dorsal compartment is incised longitudinally and elevated medially and laterally. The extensor pollicis longus is freed, retracted radially, and left in the rerouted position at the end of the procedure. A longitudinal incision is made in the capsule. A capsular periosteal flap is elevated through the dorsal radioulnar ligaments. The distal radius is excised, as is the distal ulna if it is dislocated or severely involved. A cut is made through the hamate, capitate, trapezoid, and distal scapho-trapezoid area. The carpus is removed. The medullary canal of the radius is reamed. A fine awl is used to penetrate the base of the capitate and the shaft of the third metacarpal. The medullary canal of this bone is reamed. If using a double-stemmed component, an additional canal is prepared in the second metacarpal. Appropriate short canals are prepared in the carpal bones. With the wrist in 10 to 20 degree extension, the capsular-periosteal sleeves are repaired over the prosthesis. The extensor retinaculum may be used to reinforce the capsule, or may be repaired anatomically. The skin is closed over a deep and a superficial suction drain.

Coding Tips

According to CPT guidelines, cast application or strapping (including removal) is only reported as a replacement procedure or when the cast application or strapping is an initial service performed without a restorative treatment or procedure. See "Application of Casts and Strapping" in the CPT book in the Surgery Section, under the Musculoskeletal system. Report obtaining fascia for interposition separately, see 20920 and 20922. For prosthetic replacement arthroplasty, see 25441–25446.

ICD-9-CM Procedural

81.74 Arthroplasty of carpocarpal or carpometacarpal joint with implant

Anesthesia

25332 01830

ICD-9-CM Diagnostic

357.1 Polyneuropathy in collagen vascular disease — (Code first underlying disease: 446.0, 710.0, 714.0)
359.6 Symptomatic inflammatory myopathy in diseases classified elsewhere — (Code first underlying disease: 135, 140.0-208.9, 277.30-277.39, 446.0, 710.0, 710.1, 710.2, 714.0)
446.0 Polyarteritis nodosa
710.0 Systemic lupus erythematosus — (Use additional code to identify manifestation: 424.91, 581.81, 582.81, 583.81)
710.1 Systemic sclerosis — (Use additional code to identify manifestation: 359.6, 517.2)
710.2 Sicca syndrome
714.0 Rheumatoid arthritis — (Use additional code to identify manifestation: 357.1, 359.6)
714.9 Unspecified inflammatory polyarthropathy
715.13 Primary localized osteoarthrosis, forearm
715.93 Osteoarthrosis, unspecified whether generalized or localized, forearm
716.93 Unspecified arthropathy, forearm
719.13 Hemarthrosis, forearm
733.81 Malunion of fracture
733.82 Nonunion of fracture
905.2 Late effect of fracture of upper extremities

Terms To Know

arthroplasty. Surgical reconstruction of a joint to improve function and reduce pain; may involve partial or total joint replacement.

hemarthrosis. Occurrence of blood within a joint space.

polyneuropathy. Disease process of severe inflammation of multiple nerves.

CCI Version 16.3

01810, 0213T, 0216T, 0228T, 0230T, 20690, 20692, 20696-20697, 24300, 25000, 25040, 25100-25107, 25110-25145, 25150-25151, 25210-25215, 25240, 25259-25316, 25320, 25441✢, 25446✢, 25449✢, 25492✢, 29075-29085, 29125-29126, 29260, 29844-29845, 36000, 36400-36410, 36420-36430, 36440, 36600, 36640, 37202, 43752, 51701-51703, 62310-62319, 64400-64435, 64445-64450, 64479, 64483, 64490, 64493, 64505-64530, 69990, 93000-93010, 93040-93042, 93318, 94002, 94200, 94250, 94680-94690, 94770, 95812-95816, 95819, 95822, 95829, 95955, 96360, 96365, 96372, 96374-96376, 99148-99149, 99150

Note: These CCI edits are used for Medicare. Other payers may reimburse on codes listed above.

Medicare Edits

	Fac RVU	Non-Fac RVU	FUD	Assist
25332	24.65	24.65	90	80

Medicare References: 100-2,15,260; 100-4,12,30; 100-4,12,90.3; 100-4,14,10

25335

25335 Centralization of wrist on ulna (eg, radial club hand)

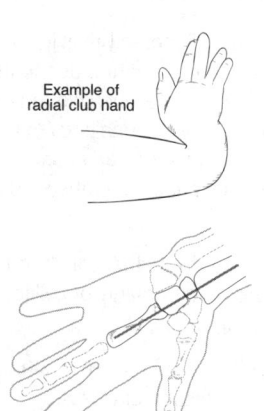

Example of radial club hand

A fixation device stabilizes the hand on the forearm (centralization)

A centralization of the wrist on ulna procedure is performed

Explanation

The physician performs a centralization of the wrist on the ulna for conditions including radial club hand. The physician makes two incisions. A transverse incision is made over the end of the ulna to remove excess skin and fatty tissue and to expose the distal ulna. A Z-plasty incision may be needed on the radial surface of the distal forearm and wrist to give extra length to the tight skin on this side. The physician next incises the capsule, flexes the elbow, and reduces the carpus over the ulna. Insertions of the flexor carpi radialis and brachioradialis are cut. The distal end of the ulna is shaved to flatten its surface and a Kirschner wire is drilled through the capitate and through the base of the third metacarpal. The second wire is removed and the ulnar wire is driven through the hole it created. The distal ulnacarpal capsule is pulled proximally over the ulna and sutured with nonabsorbable suture. The extensor carpi ulnaris is advanced distally over the fifth metacarpal tightly. The flexor carpi ulnaris is sutured with the extensor carpi ulnaris. The two incisions are closed. The wrist is placed in a neutral position and a bulky dressing is applied.

Coding Tips

According to CPT guidelines, cast application or strapping (including removal) is only reported as a replacement procedure or when the cast application or strapping is an initial service performed without a restorative treatment or procedure. See "Application of Casts and Strapping" in the CPT book in the Surgery Section, under the Musculoskeletal system.

ICD-9-CM Procedural

- 78.54 Internal fixation of carpals and metacarpals without fracture reduction
- 80.43 Division of joint capsule, ligament, or cartilage of wrist
- 81.75 Arthroplasty of carpocarpal or carpometacarpal joint without implant

Anesthesia

25335 01830

ICD-9-CM Diagnostic

- 357.1 Polyneuropathy in collagen vascular disease — (Code first underlying disease: 446.0, 710.0, 714.0)
- 359.6 Symptomatic inflammatory myopathy in diseases classified elsewhere — (Code first underlying disease: 135, 140.0-208.9, 277.30-277.39, 446.0, 710.0, 710.1, 710.2, 714.0)
- 446.0 Polyarteritis nodosa
- 710.0 Systemic lupus erythematosus — (Use additional code to identify manifestation: 424.91, 581.81, 582.81, 583.81)
- 710.1 Systemic sclerosis — (Use additional code to identify manifestation: 359.6, 517.2)
- 710.2 Sicca syndrome
- 714.0 Rheumatoid arthritis — (Use additional code to identify manifestation: 357.1, 359.6)
- 736.00 Unspecified deformity of forearm, excluding fingers
- 736.07 Club hand, acquired
- 736.09 Other acquired deformities of forearm, excluding fingers
- 754.89 Other specified nonteratogenic anomalies
- 755.50 Unspecified congenital anomaly of upper limb

Terms To Know

congenital. Present at birth, occurring through heredity or an influence during gestation up to the moment of birth.

deformity. Irregularity or malformation of the body.

distal. Located farther away from a specified reference point.

polyneuropathy. Disease process of severe inflammation of multiple nerves.

CCI Version 16.3

01810, 0213T, 0216T, 0228T, 0230T, 24300, 25000, 25040, 25100-25105, 25115-25118, 25210-25230, 25259, 25290-25295, 25320, 25800-25810, 25820-25825, 29075-29085, 29125-29126, 29260, 29844-29845, 36000, 36400-36410, 36420-36430, 36440, 36600, 36640, 37202, 43752, 51701-51703, 62310-62319, 64400-64435, 64445-64450, 64479, 64483, 64490, 64493, 64505-64530, 69990, 93000-93010, 93040-93042, 93318, 94002, 94200, 94250, 94680-94690, 94770, 95812-95816, 95819, 95822, 95829, 95955, 96360, 96365, 96372, 96374-96376, 99148-99149, 99150

Note: These CCI edits are used for Medicare. Other payers may reimburse on codes listed above.

Medicare Edits

	Fac RVU	Non-Fac RVU	FUD	Assist
25335	24.38	24.38	90	80

Medicare References: 100-2,15,260; 100-4,12,30; 100-4,12,90.3; 100-4,14,10

25337

25337 Reconstruction for stabilization of unstable distal ulna or distal radioulnar joint, secondary by soft tissue stabilization (eg, tendon transfer, tendon graft or weave, or tenodesis) with or without open reduction of distal radioulnar joint

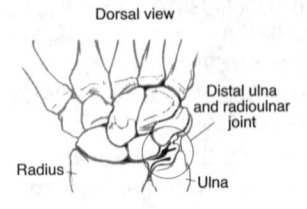

Explanation

Restoring stability to a wrist with an unstable distal ulna or distal radioulnar joint may require just a few procedures or it may dictate many procedures. In all cases, the physician must expose the distal radioulnar joint by making a curvilinear incision on the dorsal wrist starting proximal to the ulna styloid and extending it dorsally, over the ulnar styloid to the carpus. The proximal and ulnar half of the extensor retinaculum is reflected radially. The extensor digiti minimi is retracted, revealing the styloid notch of the radius and the TFC. The capsule is sharply detached from the radius exposing the ulnar head. If a styloid fracture is found, two drill holes are made proximally from the fracture to exit facing the radius. A wire is passed either around or through the styloid using similar drill holes and the two free ends of the wire are passed proximally through the fracture site into the previously drilled holes in the proximal shaft. The wire is twisted, compressing the styloid to the shaft. If the triangular fibrocartilaginous complex is avulsed from the styloid, an intraosseous wiring as described above may be used to restore distal radioulnar stability. If the TFC is not avulsed, an intraosseous wire with a 24-gauge, or larger, should be used. The capsule is sutured closed and the skin is closed in layers. Over the dressing, a long arm cast is applied with the elbow flexed, the forearm in zero degree extension, and the wrist in neutral.

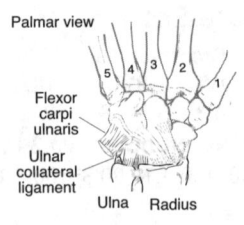

Coding Tips

According to CPT guidelines, cast application or strapping (including removal) is only reported as a replacement procedure or when the cast application or strapping is an initial service performed without a restorative treatment or procedure. See "Application of Casts and Strapping" in the CPT book in the Surgery Section, under the Musculoskeletal system. Report harvesting of fascia lata graft separately, see 20920 and 20922.

ICD-9-CM Procedural

78.43	Other repair or plastic operations on radius and ulna
79.22	Open reduction of fracture of radius and ulna without internal fixation
83.75	Tendon transfer or transplantation
83.81	Tendon graft

Anesthesia

25337   01830

ICD-9-CM Diagnostic

716.13	Traumatic arthropathy, forearm
718.73	Developmental dislocation of joint, forearm
718.83	Other joint derangement, not elsewhere classified, forearm
726.90	Enthesopathy of unspecified site
727.05	Other tenosynovitis of hand and wrist
727.63	Nontraumatic rupture of extensor tendons of hand and wrist
727.64	Nontraumatic rupture of flexor tendons of hand and wrist
728.4	Laxity of ligament
728.5	Hypermobility syndrome
813.43	Closed fracture of distal end of ulna (alone)
813.53	Open fracture of distal end of ulna (alone)
813.92	Open fracture of unspecified part of ulna (alone)
833.01	Closed dislocation of distal radioulnar (joint)
833.09	Closed dislocation of other part of wrist
833.11	Open dislocation of distal radioulnar (joint)
833.19	Open dislocation of other part of wrist
881.20	Open wound of forearm, with tendon involvement
927.10	Crushing injury of forearm — (Use additional code to identify any associated injuries: 800-829, 850.0-854.1, 860.0-869.1)

Terms To Know

open fracture. Exposed break in a bone, always considered compound due to its high risk of infection from the open wound leading to the fracture. Broken bone ends may protrude through the skin and contaminants or foreign bodies are often embedded in the tissues.

tendon. Fibrous tissue that connects muscle to bone, consisting primarily of collagen and containing little vasculature.

tenosynovitis. Inflammation of a tendon sheath due to infection or disease.

CCI Version 16.3

01810, 0213T, 0216T, 0228T, 0230T, 24300, 25000-25001, 25020-25035, 25040, 25065-25066, 25100-25118, 25150, 25248, 25259-25316, 25320, 25676, 26675, 29075-29085, 29125-29126, 29260, 29844-29845, 36000, 36400-36410, 36420-36430, 36440, 36600, 36640, 37202, 43752, 51701-51703, 62310-62319, 64400-64435, 64445-64450, 64479, 64483, 64490, 64493, 64505-64530, 69990, 93000-93010, 93040-93042, 93318, 94002, 94200, 94250, 94680-94690, 94770, 95812-95816, 95819, 95822, 95829, 95955, 96360, 96365, 96372, 96374-96376, 99148-99149, 99150

Note: These CCI edits are used for Medicare. Other payers may reimburse on codes listed above.

Medicare Edits

	Fac RVU	Non-Fac RVU	FUD	Assist
25337	25.96	25.96	90	N/A

Medicare References: 100-2,15,260; 100-4,12,30; 100-4,12,90.3; 100-4,14,10

25350-25355

25350 Osteotomy, radius; distal third
25355   middle or proximal third

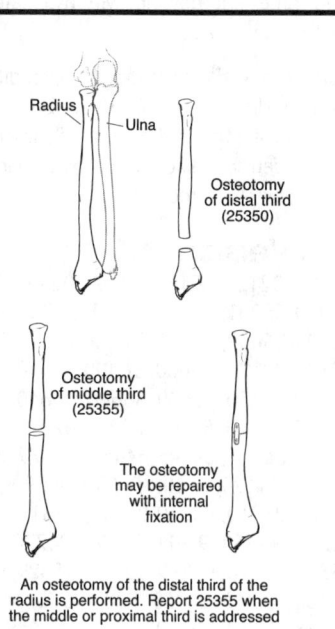

An osteotomy of the distal third of the radius is performed. Report 25355 when the middle or proximal third is addressed

Explanation

The physician performs an osteotomy (bone cut) of the radius. An incision is made in the forearm overlying the distal third area of the radius in 25350 or the middle or proximal third in 25355. The physician performs dissection through the tissue layers and down to the bone. The periosteum is removed from the bone site where the osteotomy will be made. The physician cuts through the radius. The physician realigns the bone to the desired position. Metal plates and screws are typically applied to stabilize the bone. The wound is irrigated with antibiotic solution and repaired in layers. A cast or splint may be applied to further stabilize and support the bone.

Coding Tips

According to CPT guidelines, cast application or strapping (including removal) is only reported as a replacement procedure or when the cast application or strapping is an initial service performed without a restorative treatment or procedure. See "Application of Casts and Strapping" in the CPT book in the Surgery Section, under the Musculoskeletal system. For an osteotomy of the ulna, see 25360. For an osteotomy of the radius and ulna, see 25365.

ICD-9-CM Procedural

- 77.23 Wedge osteotomy of radius and ulna
- 77.33 Other division of radius and ulna

Anesthesia

01830

ICD-9-CM Diagnostic

- 170.4 Malignant neoplasm of scapula and long bones of upper limb
- 198.5 Secondary malignant neoplasm of bone and bone marrow
- 213.4 Benign neoplasm of scapula and long bones of upper limb
- 715.13 Primary localized osteoarthrosis, forearm
- 715.23 Secondary localized osteoarthrosis, forearm
- 718.83 Other joint derangement, not elsewhere classified, forearm
- 731.1 Osteitis deformans in diseases classified elsewhere — (Code first underlying disease: 170.0-170.9)
- 731.3 Major osseous defects — (Code first underlying disease: 170.0-170.9, 730.00-730.29, 733.00-733.09, 733.40-733.49, 996.45)
- 733.12 Pathologic fracture of distal radius and ulna
- 733.49 Aseptic necrosis of other bone site — (Use additional code to identify major osseous defect, if applicable: 731.3)
- 733.81 Malunion of fracture
- 733.82 Nonunion of fracture
- 736.89 Other acquired deformity of other parts of limb
- 755.53 Radioulnar synostosis
- 756.51 Osteogenesis imperfecta
- 813.41 Closed Colles' fracture
- 813.42 Other closed fractures of distal end of radius (alone)
- 813.45 Torus fracture of radius (alone)
- 813.51 Open Colles' fracture
- 813.52 Other open fractures of distal end of radius (alone)
- 905.2 Late effect of fracture of upper extremities

Terms To Know

aseptic necrosis. Death of bone tissue resulting from a disruption in the vascular supply, caused by a noninfectious disease process, such as a fracture or the administration of immunosuppressive drugs.

distal. Located farther away from a specified reference point.

late effect. Abnormality, dysfunction, or other residual condition produced after the acute phase of an illness, injury, or disease is over. There is no time limit on when late effects can appear.

malignant. Any condition tending to progress toward death, specifically an invasive tumor with a loss of cellular differentiation that has the ability to spread or metastasize to other areas in the body.

osteitis deformans. Bone disease characterized by numerous cycles of bone resorption by the body followed by accelerated repair attempts, causing bone deformities and bowing, with associated fractures and pain.

osteogenesis imperfecta. Hereditary collagen disorder that produces brittle, osteoporotic bones that are easily fractured, with hypermobility of points, blue sclerae and a tendency to hemorrhage.

proximal. Located closest to a specified reference point, usually the midline.

CCI Version 16.3

01810, 0213T, 0216T, 0228T, 0230T, 24300, 25100-25107, 25259, 25295, 25600-25609, 36000, 36400-36410, 36420-36430, 36440, 36600, 36640, 37202, 43752, 51701-51703, 62310-62319, 64400-64435, 64445-64450, 64479, 64483, 64490, 64493, 64505-64530, 69990, 93000-93010, 93040-93042, 93318, 94002, 94200, 94250, 94680-94690, 94770, 95812-95816, 95819, 95822, 95829, 95955, 96360, 96365, 96372, 96374-96376, 99148-99149, 99150

Also not with 25350: 25000-25001, 25115-25118, 29075-29085, 29125-29126, 29844, 29855

Also not with 25355: 24665, 25000, 25115-25116, 25526, 29065-29075, 29105

Note: These CCI edits are used for Medicare. Other payers may reimburse on codes listed above.

Medicare Edits

	Fac RVU	Non-Fac RVU	FUD	Assist
25350	20.55	20.55	90	80
25355	23.29	23.29	90	80

Medicare References: 100-2,15,260; 100-4,12,30; 100-4,12,90.3; 100-4,14,10

25360-25365

25360 Osteotomy; ulna
25365 radius AND ulna

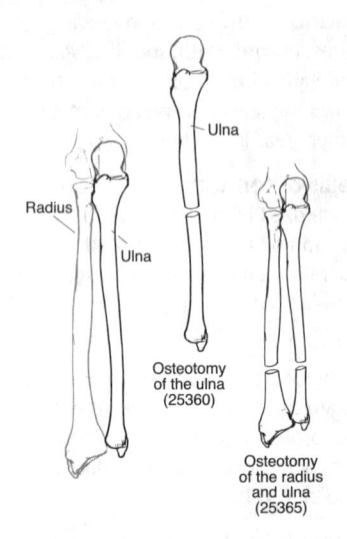

An osteotomy of the ulna is performed. Report 25365 when both the ulna and the radius are addressed.

Explanation

The physician performs an osteotomy of the ulna in 25360 or of both the ulna and radius in 25365. The physician makes a longitudinal incision along the medial border of the forearm to expose the affected part of the ulna. Two separate incisions may be necessary in 25365. An osteotomy is made through the ulna, usually in a wedge shape. This allows the bone to be realigned. The physician applies plates and screws to hold the osteotomy together in the correct position. The incisions are then repaired in multiple layers with sutures, staples, and/or Steri-strips. The arm may be placed in a splint for immobilization.

Coding Tips

According to CPT guidelines, cast application or strapping (including removal) is only reported as a replacement procedure or when the cast application or strapping is an initial service performed without a restorative treatment or procedure. See "Application of Casts and Strapping" in the CPT book in the Surgery Section, under the Musculoskeletal system. For an osteotomy of the distal third of the radius, see 25350. For an osteotomy of the middle or proximal third of the radius, see 25355.

ICD-9-CM Procedural

77.23 Wedge osteotomy of radius and ulna
77.33 Other division of radius and ulna

Anesthesia
01830

ICD-9-CM Diagnostic

170.4 Malignant neoplasm of scapula and long bones of upper limb
198.5 Secondary malignant neoplasm of bone and bone marrow
213.4 Benign neoplasm of scapula and long bones of upper limb
715.13 Primary localized osteoarthrosis, forearm
715.23 Secondary localized osteoarthrosis, forearm
731.1 Osteitis deformans in diseases classified elsewhere — (Code first underlying disease: 170.0-170.9)
731.3 Major osseous defects — (Code first underlying disease: 170.0-170.9, 730.00-730.29, 733.00-733.09, 733.40-733.49, 996.45)
733.49 Aseptic necrosis of other bone site — (Use additional code to identify major osseous defect, if applicable: 731.3)
733.81 Malunion of fracture
733.82 Nonunion of fracture
736.89 Other acquired deformity of other parts of limb
755.53 Radioulnar synostosis
756.51 Osteogenesis imperfecta
905.2 Late effect of fracture of upper extremities

Terms To Know

aseptic necrosis. Death of bone tissue resulting from a disruption in the vascular supply, caused by a noninfectious disease process, such as a fracture or the administration of immunosuppressive drugs.

malignant. Any condition tending to progress toward death, specifically an invasive tumor with a loss of cellular differentiation that has the ability to spread or metastasize to other areas in the body.

malunion. Fracture that has united in a faulty position due to inadequate reduction of the original fracture, insufficient holding of a previously well-reduced fracture, contracture of the soft tissues, or comminuted or osteoporotic bone causing a slow disintegration of the fracture.

nonunion. Failure of two ends of a fracture to mend or completely heal.

osteitis deformans. Bone disease characterized by numerous cycles of bone resorption by the body followed by accelerated repair attempts, causing bone deformities and bowing, with associated fractures and pain.

osteogenesis imperfecta. Hereditary collagen disorder that produces brittle, osteoporotic bones that are easily fractured, with hypermobility of points, blue sclerae and a tendency to hemorrhage.

CCI Version 16.3

01810, 0213T, 0216T, 0228T, 0230T, 24300, 25000-25001, 25100-25107, 25259, 25295, 25600-25609, 25651-25652, 29065-29085, 29105-29126, 36000, 36400-36410, 36420-36430, 36440, 36600, 36640, 37202, 43752, 51701-51703, 62310-62319, 64400-64435, 64445-64450, 64479, 64483, 64490, 64493, 64505-64530, 69990, 93000-93010, 93040-93042, 93318, 94002, 94200, 94250, 94680-94690, 94770, 95812-95816, 95819, 95822, 95829, 95955, 96360, 96365, 96372, 96374-96376, 99148-99149, 99150

Also not with 25360: 24685, 25115-25116, 25545, 64718

Also not with 25365: 25115-25119

Note: These CCI edits are used for Medicare. Other payers may reimburse on codes listed above.

Medicare Edits

	Fac RVU	Non-Fac RVU	FUD	Assist
25360	19.99	19.99	90	80
25365	27.58	27.58	90	80

Medicare References: 100-2,15,260; 100-4,12,30; 100-4,12,90.3; 100-4,14,10

25370-25375

25370 Multiple osteotomies, with realignment on intramedullary rod (Sofield type procedure); radius OR ulna
25375 radius AND ulna

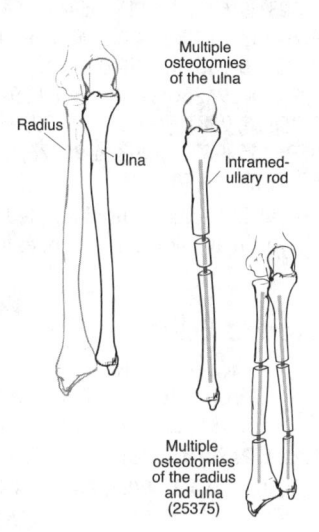

Multiple osteotomies of the ulna are performed with realignment of the shaft on an intramedullary rod. Report 25375 when both radius and ulna are treated.

Explanation

The physician treats the radius or ulna in 25370 or both in 25375. A longitudinal incision is made to expose the entire shaft of the bone. Two separate incisions may be necessary in 25375. The physician makes an osteotomy (bone cut) through the proximal and distal ends of the bone shaft. The bone shaft is then removed from the wound. The physician studies the bone shaft to determine how many times it must be osteotomized so that its segments can be threaded onto a medullary nail. The osteotomies are made and each fragment placed end to end on the medullary nail. Because the cortex of the ulna and radius are very thin, a bone graft is usually added. This may be harvested from the surrounding area or a separate incision may be needed. A separate incision would be made over the iliac crest, bone harvested, and the incision closed. The medullary nail is then inserted into place. The periosteum is sutured into place. The physician repairs the incision in multiple layers with sutures, staples, and/or Steri-strips. The arm is immobilized in a cast.

Coding Tips

According to CPT guidelines, cast application or strapping (including removal) is only reported as a replacement procedure or when the cast application or strapping is an initial service performed without a restorative treatment or procedure. See "Application of Casts and Strapping" in the CPT book in the Surgery Section, under the Musculoskeletal system. For osteotomy, radius, see 25350 or 25355; ulna, see 25360; radius and ulna, see 25365.

ICD-9-CM Procedural

- 77.23 Wedge osteotomy of radius and ulna
- 77.33 Other division of radius and ulna
- 78.43 Other repair or plastic operations on radius and ulna

Anesthesia

01830

ICD-9-CM Diagnostic

- 170.4 Malignant neoplasm of scapula and long bones of upper limb
- 198.5 Secondary malignant neoplasm of bone and bone marrow
- 209.73 Secondary neuroendocrine tumor of bone
- 213.4 Benign neoplasm of scapula and long bones of upper limb
- 715.13 Primary localized osteoarthrosis, forearm
- 716.13 Traumatic arthropathy, forearm
- 716.53 Unspecified polyarthropathy or polyarthritis, forearm
- 716.93 Unspecified arthropathy, forearm
- 731.1 Osteitis deformans in diseases classified elsewhere — (Code first underlying disease: 170.0-170.9)
- 731.3 Major osseous defects — (Code first underlying disease: 170.0-170.9, 730.00-730.29, 733.00-733.09, 733.40-733.49, 996.45)
- 733.81 Malunion of fracture
- 733.82 Nonunion of fracture
- 736.89 Other acquired deformity of other parts of limb
- 755.50 Unspecified congenital anomaly of upper limb
- 755.59 Other congenital anomaly of upper limb, including shoulder girdle
- 756.51 Osteogenesis imperfecta
- 756.53 Osteopoikilosis
- V54.02 Encounter for lengthening/adjustment of growth rod

Terms To Know

benign. Mild or nonmalignant in nature.

malignant. Any condition tending to progress toward death, specifically an invasive tumor with a loss of cellular differentiation that has the ability to spread or metastasize to other areas in the body.

osteogenesis imperfecta. Hereditary collagen disorder that produces brittle, osteoporotic bones that are easily fractured, with hypermobility of points, blue sclerae and a tendency to hemorrhage.

osteopoikilosis. Rare genetic disorder that manifests in multiple areas of sclerotic bone density on the ends of long bones, identified by x-ray and often without symptoms.

secondary. Second in order of occurrence or importance, or appearing during the course of another disease or condition.

CCI Version 16.3

01810, 0213T, 0216T, 0228T, 0230T, 20690, 20692, 24300, 25115-25119, 25259, 25295, 29065-29085, 29105-29126, 36000, 36400-36410, 36420-36430, 36440, 36600, 36640, 37202, 43752, 51701-51703, 62310-62319, 64400-64435, 64445-64450, 64479, 64483, 64490, 64493, 64505-64530, 69990, 93000-93010, 93040-93042, 93318, 94002, 94200, 94250, 94680-94690, 94770, 95812-95816, 95819, 95822, 95829, 95955, 96360, 96365, 96372, 96374-96376, 99148-99149, 99150

Also not with 25370: 25515, 25525-25526, 25545, 25574

Also not with 25375: 25575

Note: These CCI edits are used for Medicare. Other payers may reimburse on codes listed above.

Medicare Edits

	Fac RVU	Non-Fac RVU	FUD	Assist
25370	30.22	30.22	90	80
25375	27.15	27.15	90	80

Medicare References: 100-2,15,260; 100-4,12,30; 100-4,12,90.3; 100-4,14,10

25390

25390 Osteoplasty, radius OR ulna; shortening

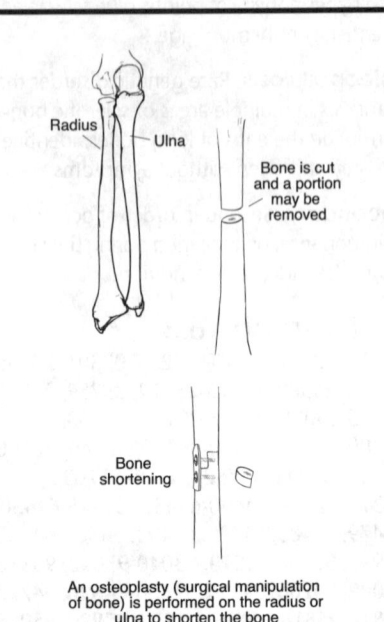

An osteoplasty (surgical manipulation of bone) is performed on the radius or ulna to shorten the bone.

Explanation

The physician shortens the radius or ulna. An incision is made on the anterior aspect of the distal forearm. The radial artery is exposed and carefully retracted. The physician continues dissection to expose the distal shaft of the radius. Based on preoperative x-rays, an osteotomy is made at the distal end of the radius. A more proximal osteotomy is then made, which shortens the radius usually by 2.0 mm to 3.0 mm. The physician removes the bone fragment. A plate is attached to the distal segment with screws. Reduction forceps hold and compress the osteotomy while the plate is attached to the proximal fragment with screws. Separately reportable x-rays are used to check radioulnar length. Drain tubes are inserted. The physician repairs the incision in multiple layers with sutures, staples, and/or Steri-strips. However, the forearm fascia is left open to minimize the chances of compartment syndrome. The forearm is placed in a splint.

Coding Tips

According to CPT guidelines, cast application or strapping (including removal) is only reported as a replacement procedure or when the cast application or strapping is an initial service performed without a restorative treatment or procedure. See "Application of Casts and Strapping" in the CPT book in the Surgery Section, under the Musculoskeletal system. For radius and ulna shortening, see 25392.

ICD-9-CM Procedural

78.23 Limb shortening procedures, radius and ulna

Anesthesia

25390 01830

ICD-9-CM Diagnostic

718.83 Other joint derangement, not elsewhere classified, forearm

732.3 Juvenile osteochondrosis of upper extremity

733.99 Other disorders of bone and cartilage

736.00 Unspecified deformity of forearm, excluding fingers

736.09 Other acquired deformities of forearm, excluding fingers

755.50 Unspecified congenital anomaly of upper limb

755.54 Madelung's deformity

755.59 Other congenital anomaly of upper limb, including shoulder girdle

Terms To Know

anomaly. Irregularity in the structure or position of an organ or tissue.

anterior. Situated in the front area or toward the belly surface of the body; an anatomical reference point used to show the position and relationship of one body structure to another.

congenital. Present at birth, occurring through heredity or an influence during gestation up to the moment of birth.

distal. Located farther away from a specified reference point.

fascia. Fibrous sheet or band of tissue that envelops organs, muscles, and groupings of muscles.

proximal. Located closest to a specified reference point, usually the midline.

CCI Version 16.3

01810, 0213T, 0216T, 0228T, 0230T, 24300, 25115-25119, 25240, 25259, 25295, 25360, 25515, 25525-25526, 25545, 25574, 29065-29085, 29105-29126, 36000, 36400-36410, 36420-36430, 36440, 36600, 36640, 37202, 43752, 51701-51703, 62310-62319, 64400-64435, 64445-64450, 64479, 64483, 64490, 64493, 64505-64530, 69990, 93000-93010, 93040-93042, 93318, 94002, 94200, 94250, 94680-94690, 94770, 95812-95816, 95819, 95822, 95829, 95955, 96360, 96365, 96372, 96374-96376, 99148-99149, 99150

Note: These CCI edits are used for Medicare. Other payers may reimburse on codes listed above.

Medicare Edits

	Fac RVU	Non-Fac RVU	FUD	Assist
25390	23.38	23.38	90	80

Medicare References: 100-2,15,260; 100-4,12,30; 100-4,12,90.3; 100-4,14,10

25391

25391 Osteoplasty, radius OR ulna; lengthening with autograft

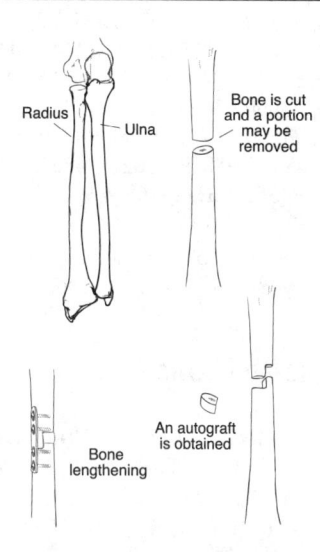

Explanation

The radius or ulna of the forearm is lengthened with an autograft. One bone is often bowed due to the shortened and hypoplastic development of the other, as in congenital pseudoarthrosis. The forearm is incised and the overlying tissue is dissected to reach the bone. A few centimeters of bone may need to be resected to remove the deformity, taking care to preserve the epiphysis is the case of growing children. Surrounding abnormal tissues are also resected. The newly created defect is bridged with a vascularized bone graft from the patient, often taken from the fibula. The autograft is fixed to the bone of the radius and/or ulna with an intramedullary K-wire and may be proximally supported by placing another K-wire. Vascular anastomosis is completed between the artery of the graft and the ulnar or radial artery and the graft vein and the basilic vein. The wound is closed. A skin island that was preserved with the vascularized autograft may also be incorporated in the wound closure. A cast is applied to the forearm.

Coding Tips

According to CPT guidelines, cast application or strapping (including removal) is only reported as a replacement procedure or when the cast application or strapping is an initial service performed without a restorative treatment or procedure. See "Application of Casts and Strapping" in the CPT book in the Surgery Section, under the Musculoskeletal system. For radius and ulna lengthening with autograft, see 25393.

ICD-9-CM Procedural

- 77.79 Excision of other bone for graft, except facial bones
- 78.03 Bone graft of radius and ulna
- 78.13 Application of external fixator device, radius and ulna
- 78.33 Limb lengthening procedures, radius and ulna
- 84.53 Implantation of internal limb lengthening device with kinetic distraction
- 84.54 Implantation of other internal limb lengthening device
- 84.71 Application of external fixator device, monoplanar system
- 84.72 Application of external fixator device, ring system
- 84.73 Application of hybrid external fixator device

Anesthesia

25391 01830

ICD-9-CM Diagnostic

- 718.83 Other joint derangement, not elsewhere classified, forearm
- 733.81 Malunion of fracture
- 733.82 Nonunion of fracture
- 733.99 Other disorders of bone and cartilage
- 736.00 Unspecified deformity of forearm, excluding fingers
- 736.09 Other acquired deformities of forearm, excluding fingers
- 755.20 Congenital unspecified reduction deformity of upper limb
- 755.26 Congenital longitudinal deficiency, radial, complete or partial (with or without distal deficiencies, incomplete)
- 755.27 Congenital longitudinal deficiency, ulnar, complete or partial (with or without distal deficiencies, incomplete)
- 755.50 Unspecified congenital anomaly of upper limb

Terms To Know

anomaly. Irregularity in the structure or position of an organ or tissue.

congenital. Present at birth, occurring through heredity or an influence during gestation up to the moment of birth.

deformity. Irregularity or malformation of the body.

malunion. Fracture that has united in a faulty position due to inadequate reduction of the original fracture, insufficient holding of a previously well-reduced fracture, contracture of the soft tissues, or comminuted or osteoporotic bone causing a slow disintegration of the fracture.

nonunion. Failure of two ends of a fracture to mend or completely heal.

CCI Version 16.3

01810, 0213T, 0216T, 0228T, 0230T, 20900-20902, 24300, 25115-25119, 25259, 25295, 25515, 25525-25526, 25545, 25574, 29065-29085, 29105-29126, 36000, 36400-36410, 36420-36430, 36440, 36600, 36640, 37202, 43752, 51701-51703, 62310-62319, 64400-64435, 64445-64450, 64479, 64483, 64490, 64493, 64505-64530, 69990, 93000-93010, 93040-93042, 93318, 94002, 94200, 94250, 94680-94690, 94770, 95812-95816, 95819, 95822, 95829, 95955, 96360, 96365, 96372, 96374-96376, 99148-99149, 99150

Note: These CCI edits are used for Medicare. Other payers may reimburse on codes listed above.

Medicare Edits

	Fac RVU	Non-Fac RVU	FUD	Assist
25391	30.08	30.08	90	80

Medicare References: 100-2,15,260; 100-4,12,30; 100-4,12,90.3; 100-4,14,10

25392

25392 Osteoplasty, radius AND ulna; shortening (excluding 64876)

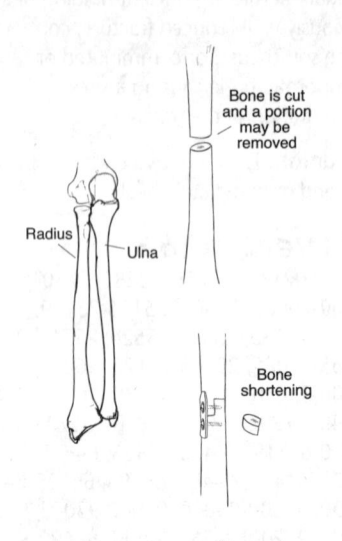

An osteoplasty (surgical manipulation of bone) is performed on both the radius and ulna to shorten the bones

Explanation

The physician shortens the radius and ulna. Incisions are made on the anterior aspect of the distal forearm. The radial artery is exposed and carefully retracted. The physician continues dissection to expose the distal shaft of the radius and ulna. Based on preoperative x-rays, an osteotomy is made at the distal end of the radius. A more proximal osteotomy is then made, which shortens the radius usually by 2.0 mm to 3.0 mm. This procedure is repeated on the ulna. The physician removes the bone fragments. A plate is then attached to the distal segment of the radius and ulna with screws. Reduction forceps hold and compress the osteotomy while the plate is attached to the proximal fragment with screws. Separately reportable x-rays are used to check radioulnar length. Drain tubes are inserted. The physician repairs the incision in multiple layers with sutures, staples, and/or Steri-strips. However, the forearm fascia is left open to minimize the chances of compartment syndrome. The forearm is placed in a splint.

Coding Tips

According to CPT guidelines, cast application or strapping (including removal) is only reported as a replacement procedure or when the cast application or strapping is an initial service performed without a restorative treatment or procedure. See "Application of Casts and Strapping" in the CPT book in the Surgery Section, under the Musculoskeletal system. For radius or ulna shortening, see 25390.

ICD-9-CM Procedural

78.23 Limb shortening procedures, radius and ulna

Anesthesia

25392 01830

ICD-9-CM Diagnostic

718.83 Other joint derangement, not elsewhere classified, forearm
732.3 Juvenile osteochondrosis of upper extremity
733.99 Other disorders of bone and cartilage
736.00 Unspecified deformity of forearm, excluding fingers
736.09 Other acquired deformities of forearm, excluding fingers
755.50 Unspecified congenital anomaly of upper limb
755.59 Other congenital anomaly of upper limb, including shoulder girdle

Terms To Know

anomaly. Irregularity in the structure or position of an organ or tissue.

anterior. Situated in the front area or toward the belly surface of the body; an anatomical reference point used to show the position and relationship of one body structure to another.

congenital. Present at birth, occurring through heredity or an influence during gestation up to the moment of birth.

distal. Located farther away from a specified reference point.

fascia. Fibrous sheet or band of tissue that envelops organs, muscles, and groupings of muscles.

proximal. Located closest to a specified reference point, usually the midline.

CCI Version 16.3

01810, 0213T, 0216T, 0228T, 0230T, 24300, 25115-25119, 25240, 25259, 25295, 25360, 25575, 29065-29085, 29105-29126, 36000, 36400-36410, 36420-36430, 36440, 36600, 36640, 37202, 43752, 51701-51703, 62310-62319, 64400-64435, 64445-64450, 64479, 64483, 64490, 64493, 64505-64530, 69990, 93000-93010, 93040-93042, 93318, 94002, 94200, 94250, 94680-94690, 94770, 95812-95816, 95819, 95822, 95829, 95955, 96360, 96365, 96372, 96374-96376, 99148-99149, 99150

Note: These CCI edits are used for Medicare. Other payers may reimburse on codes listed above.

Medicare Edits

	Fac RVU	Non-Fac RVU	FUD	Assist
25392	30.65	30.65	90	80

Medicare References: 100-2,15,260; 100-4,12,30; 100-4,12,90.3; 100-4,14,10

25393

25393 Osteoplasty, radius AND ulna; lengthening with autograft

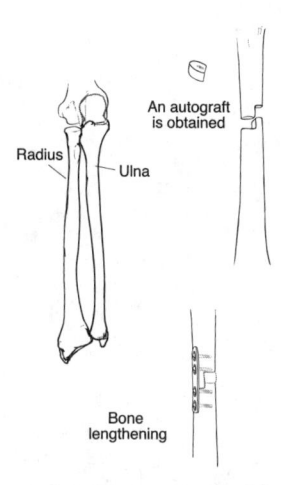

An osteoplasty (surgical manipulation of bone) with autograft is performed on both the radius and ulna to lengthen the bones

Explanation

The radius and the ulna of the forearm are lengthened with an autograft. One bone is often bowed due to the shortened and hypoplastic development of the other, as in congenital pseudoarthrosis. The forearm is incised and the overlying tissue is dissected to reach the bone. A few centimeters of bone may need to be resected to remove the deformity, taking care to preserve the epiphysis is the case of growing children. Surrounding abnormal tissues are also resected. The newly created defect is bridged with a vascularized bone graft from the patient, often taken from the fibula. The autograft is fixed to the bone of the radius and/or ulna with an intramedullary K-wire and may be proximally supported by placing another K-wire. Vascular anastomosis is completed between the artery of the graft and the ulnar or radial artery and the graft vein and the basilic vein. The wound is closed. A skin island that was preserved with the vascularized autograft may also be incorporated in the wound closure. A cast is applied to the forearm.

Coding Tips

According to CPT guidelines, cast application or strapping (including removal) is only reported as a replacement procedure or when the cast application or strapping is an initial service performed without a restorative treatment or procedure. See "Application of Casts and Strapping" in the CPT book in the Surgery Section, under the Musculoskeletal system. For radius or ulna lengthening, see 25391.

ICD-9-CM Procedural

- 77.79 Excision of other bone for graft, except facial bones
- 78.03 Bone graft of radius and ulna
- 78.13 Application of external fixator device, radius and ulna
- 78.33 Limb lengthening procedures, radius and ulna
- 84.53 Implantation of internal limb lengthening device with kinetic distraction
- 84.54 Implantation of other internal limb lengthening device
- 84.71 Application of external fixator device, monoplanar system
- 84.72 Application of external fixator device, ring system
- 84.73 Application of hybrid external fixator device

Anesthesia

25393 01830

ICD-9-CM Diagnostic

- 718.83 Other joint derangement, not elsewhere classified, forearm
- 733.81 Malunion of fracture
- 733.82 Nonunion of fracture
- 733.99 Other disorders of bone and cartilage
- 736.00 Unspecified deformity of forearm, excluding fingers
- 736.09 Other acquired deformities of forearm, excluding fingers
- 755.20 Congenital unspecified reduction deformity of upper limb
- 755.26 Congenital longitudinal deficiency, radial, complete or partial (with or without distal deficiencies, incomplete)
- 755.27 Congenital longitudinal deficiency, ulnar, complete or partial (with or without distal deficiencies, incomplete)
- 755.50 Unspecified congenital anomaly of upper limb

Terms To Know

anomaly. Irregularity in the structure or position of an organ or tissue.

congenital. Present at birth, occurring through heredity or an influence during gestation up to the moment of birth.

deformity. Irregularity or malformation of the body.

distal. Located farther away from a specified reference point.

fracture. Break in bone or cartilage.

malunion. Fracture that has united in a faulty position due to inadequate reduction of the original fracture, insufficient holding of a previously well-reduced fracture, contracture of the soft tissues, or comminuted or osteoporotic bone causing a slow disintegration of the fracture.

nonunion. Failure of two ends of a fracture to mend or completely heal.

CCI Version 16.3

01810, 0213T, 0216T, 0228T, 0230T, 20900-20902, 24300, 25115-25119, 25259, 25295, 25575, 29065-29085, 29105-29126, 36000, 36400-36410, 36420-36430, 36440, 36600, 36640, 37202, 43752, 51701-51703, 62310-62319, 64400-64435, 64445-64450, 64479, 64483, 64490, 64493, 64505-64530, 69990, 93000-93010, 93040-93042, 93318, 94002, 94200, 94250, 94680-94690, 94770, 95812-95816, 95819, 95822, 95829, 95955, 96360, 96365, 96372, 96374-96376, 99148-99149, 99150

Note: These CCI edits are used for Medicare. Other payers may reimburse on codes listed above.

Medicare Edits

	Fac RVU	Non-Fac RVU	FUD	Assist
25393	34.89	34.89	90	80

Medicare References: 100-2,15,260; 100-4,12,30; 100-4,12,90.3; 100-4,14,10

25394

25394 Osteoplasty, carpal bone, shortening

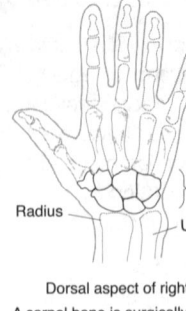

Dorsal aspect of right hand
A carpal bone is surgically shortened

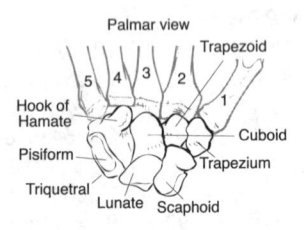

Palmar view

Explanation
The physician shortens a carpal bone. The physician makes the incision over the area of the carpal bone. Dissection is carried down to the level of the carpal bone. The bone is shortened. The amount of bone removed is dependent on the condition treated. The incision is closed with sutures.

Coding Tips
This is a unilateral procedure. If performed bilaterally, some payers require that the service be reported twice with modifier 50 appended to the second code, while others require identification of the service only once with modifier 50 appended. Check with individual payers. Modifier 50 identifies a procedure performed identically on the opposite side of the body (mirror image).

ICD-9-CM Procedural
78.24 Limb shortening procedures, carpals and metacarpals

Anesthesia
25394 01830

ICD-9-CM Diagnostic
718.83 Other joint derangement, not elsewhere classified, forearm
732.3 Juvenile osteochondrosis of upper extremity
733.99 Other disorders of bone and cartilage
736.00 Unspecified deformity of forearm, excluding fingers
736.09 Other acquired deformities of forearm, excluding fingers
755.50 Unspecified congenital anomaly of upper limb
755.59 Other congenital anomaly of upper limb, including shoulder girdle

Terms To Know
anomaly. Irregularity in the structure or position of an organ or tissue.

congenital. Present at birth, occurring through heredity or an influence during gestation up to the moment of birth.

deformity. Irregularity or malformation of the body.

osteochondrosis. Disease manifested by degeneration or necrosis of the growth plate or ossification centers of bones in children, followed by regenerating and reossification.

CCI Version 16.3
01810, 0213T, 0216T, 0228T, 0230T, 11010-11012, 11040-11044, 25115-25119, 25295, 29058-29085, 29105-29126, 29260, 36000, 36400-36410, 36420-36430, 36440, 36600, 36640, 37202, 43752, 51701-51703, 62310-62319, 64400-64435, 64445-64450, 64479, 64483, 64490, 64493, 64505-64530, 69990, 93000-93010, 93040-93042, 93318, 94002, 94200, 94250, 94680-94690, 94770, 95812-95816, 95819, 95822, 95829, 95955, 96360, 96365, 96372, 96374-96376, 99148-99149, 99150

Note: These CCI edits are used for Medicare. Other payers may reimburse on codes listed above.

Medicare Edits

	Fac RVU	Non-Fac RVU	FUD	Assist
25394	22.82	22.82	90	80

Medicare References: None

25400-25405

25400 Repair of nonunion or malunion, radius OR ulna; without graft (eg, compression technique)

25405 with autograft (includes obtaining graft)

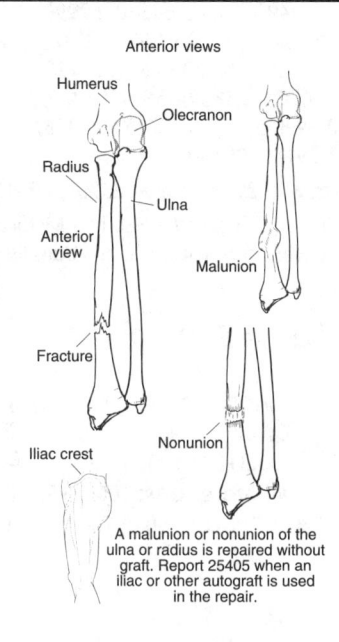

Explanation
The physician exposes a nonunion or malunion of the radius or ulna by making a 10 cm to 15 cm longitudinal incision over the fracture site. With a reciprocating saw, each bone is divided through the nonunion. The fragments are aligned. A compression plate is centered over the fracture and screws are inserted. In 25405, a bone graft is needed to help heal the nonunion due to loss of bone. For example, if the nonunion is old, approximately 0.6 cm to 1.3 cm of bone is resected from the ends of the fragments. Autogenous iliac bone is typically used. Bone from the upper tibia may also be used. This requires an incision over the site of harvest. The physician uses an osteotome to harvest strips of bone. These strips are placed around the ends of the fracture along with the compression plate for internal fixation. The incision is repaired in layers with sutures, staples, and/or Steri-strips. However, the deep fascial layer is not closed because of the potential to develop compartment syndrome. A long arm cast is applied with the elbow at 90 degrees of flexion.

Coding Tips
In 25405, any bone graft harvest is not reported separately. According to CPT guidelines, cast application or strapping (including removal) is only reported as a replacement procedure or when the cast application or strapping is an initial service performed without a restorative treatment or procedure. See "Application of Casts and Strapping" in the CPT book in the Surgery Section, under the Musculoskeletal system. For repair of nonunion or malunion of the radius and ulna, see 25415 and 25420.

ICD-9-CM Procedural
- 77.77 Excision of tibia and fibula for graft
- 77.79 Excision of other bone for graft, except facial bones
- 78.03 Bone graft of radius and ulna
- 78.43 Other repair or plastic operations on radius and ulna

Anesthesia
01830

ICD-9-CM Diagnostic
- 733.81 Malunion of fracture
- 733.82 Nonunion of fracture
- 905.2 Late effect of fracture of upper extremities

Terms To Know
flexion. Act of bending or being bent.

fracture. Break in bone or cartilage.

late effect. Abnormality, dysfunction, or other residual condition produced after the acute phase of an illness, injury, or disease is over. There is no time limit on when late effects can appear.

malunion. Fracture that has united in a faulty position due to inadequate reduction of the original fracture, insufficient holding of a previously well-reduced fracture, contracture of the soft tissues, or comminuted or osteoporotic bone causing a slow disintegration of the fracture.

nonunion. Failure of two ends of a fracture to mend or completely heal.

CCI Version 16.3
01810, 0213T, 0216T, 0228T, 0230T, 20680, 24300, 25040, 25100-25105, 25115-25119, 25259, 25295, 25350-25360, 25515, 25525-25526, 25545, 25574, 29065-29085, 29105-29126, 36000, 36400-36410, 36420-36430, 36440, 36600, 36640, 37202, 43752, 51701-51703, 62310-62319, 64400-64435, 64445-64450, 64479, 64483, 64490, 64493, 64505-64530, 69990, 93000-93010, 93040-93042, 93318, 94002, 94200, 94250, 94680-94690, 94770, 95812-95816, 95819, 95822, 95829, 95955, 96360, 96365, 96372, 96374-96376, 99148-99149, 99150

Also not with 25405: 20900-20902, 25400

Note: These CCI edits are used for Medicare. Other payers may reimburse on codes listed above.

Medicare Edits

	Fac RVU	Non-Fac RVU	FUD	Assist
25400	24.47	24.47	90	80
25405	31.32	31.32	90	80

Medicare References: 100-2,15,260; 100-4,12,30; 100-4,12,90.3; 100-4,14,10

25415-25420

25415 Repair of nonunion or malunion, radius AND ulna; without graft (eg, compression technique)
25420 with autograft (includes obtaining graft)

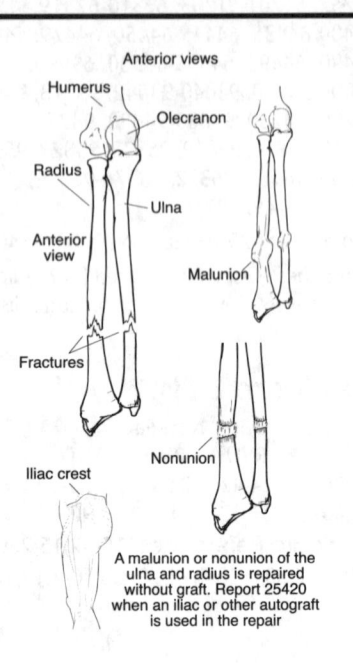

A malunion or nonunion of the ulna and radius is repaired without graft. Report 25420 when an iliac or other autograft is used in the repair

Explanation

The physician exposes the nonunions through two 10 cm to 15 cm longitudinal incisions One incision is made on the lateral aspect and one on the medial aspect of the forearm. With a reciprocating saw, the physician divides each bone through the nonunion. The fragments are aligned. The physician centers a compression plate over the fracture and inserts screws. In 25420, a bone graft is needed to help bone healing of the nonunion due to loss of bone. For example, if the nonunion is old, approximately 0.6 cm to 1.3 cm of bone is resected from the ends of the fragments. Autogenous iliac bone graft is typically used. The physician makes an incision over the iliac crest. Once the bone is exposed, an osteotome is used to harvest strips of bone. These strips are placed around the ends of the fracture. Internal fixation with a compression plate is the same as for 25415. The incision are repaired in layers with sutures, staples, and/or Steri-strips. However, the deep fascial layer is not closed because of the potential to develop compartment syndrome. A long arm cast is applied with the elbow in 90 degrees of flexion.

Coding Tips

Bone graft harvest for 25420 is not reported separately. According to CPT guidelines, cast application or strapping (including removal) is only reported as a replacement procedure or when the cast application or strapping is an initial service performed without a restorative treatment or procedure. See "Application of Casts and Strapping" in the CPT book in the Surgery Section, under the Musculoskeletal system. For repair of nonunion or malunion of the radius or ulna, see 25400 (without graft) or 25405 (with graft).

ICD-9-CM Procedural

77.77 Excision of tibia and fibula for graft
77.79 Excision of other bone for graft, except facial bones
78.03 Bone graft of radius and ulna
78.43 Other repair or plastic operations on radius and ulna

Anesthesia
01830

ICD-9-CM Diagnostic

733.81 Malunion of fracture
733.82 Nonunion of fracture
905.2 Late effect of fracture of upper extremities

Terms To Know

flexion. Act of bending or being bent.

fracture. Break in bone or cartilage.

late effect. Abnormality, dysfunction, or other residual condition produced after the acute phase of an illness, injury, or disease is over. There is no time limit on when late effects can appear.

malunion. Fracture that has united in a faulty position due to inadequate reduction of the original fracture, insufficient holding of a previously well-reduced fracture, contracture of the soft tissues, or comminuted or osteoporotic bone causing a slow disintegration of the fracture.

nonunion. Failure of two ends of a fracture to mend or completely heal.

CCI Version 16.3

01810, 0213T, 0216T, 0228T, 0230T, 20680, 24300, 25040, 25100-25105, 25115-25119, 25259, 25295, 25365, 25575, 29065-29085, 29105-29126, 36000, 36400-36410, 36420-36430, 36440, 36600, 36640, 37202, 43752, 51701-51703, 62310-62319, 64400-64435, 64445-64450, 64479, 64483, 64490, 64493, 64505-64530, 69990, 93000-93010, 93040-93042, 93318, 94002, 94200, 94250, 94680-94690, 94770, 95812-95816, 95819, 95822, 95829, 95955, 96360, 96365, 96372, 96374-96376, 99148-99149, 99150

Also not with 25420: 20900-20902, 25415

Note: These CCI edits are used for Medicare. Other payers may reimburse on codes listed above.

Medicare Edits

	Fac RVU	Non-Fac RVU	FUD	Assist
25415	29.7	29.7	90	80
25420	35.31	35.31	90	80

Medicare References: 100-2,15,260; 100-4,12,30; 100-4,12,90.3; 100-4,14,10

25425-25426

25425 Repair of defect with autograft; radius OR ulna
25426 radius AND ulna

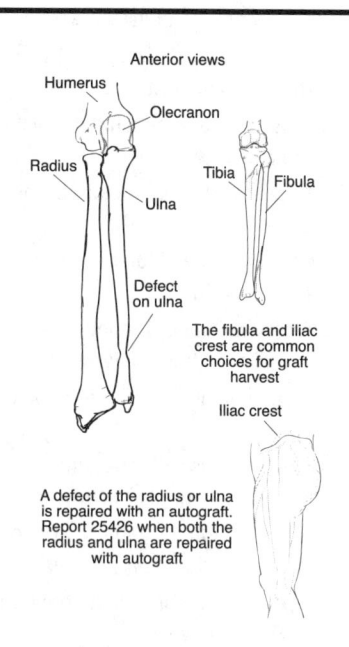

A defect of the radius or ulna is repaired with an autograft. Report 25426 when both the radius and ulna are repaired with autograft.

Explanation

The physician repairs a defect of the radius or ulna in 25425 or of both the radius and ulna in 25426. The physician makes a longitudinal incision along the forearm. An anterior approach is made for the radius, medial for the ulna, or two incisions for both. The defect is exposed through dissection. To harvest the bone graft, the physician makes a separate incision over the iliac crest. Bone from the upper tibia may also be used. The bone is exposed and the physician uses an osteotome to harvest strips of bone. These bone strips are used to fill the defect. A screw or wire wrapped around the defect holds the bone graft in place. The incision is repaired in multiple layers with sutures, staples, and/or Steri-strips. However, the deep fascial layer is not closed because of the potential to develop compartment syndrome. The arm may be placed in a long arm cast with the elbow at 90 degrees of flexion.

Coding Tips

Any bone graft harvest is not reported separately. According to CPT guidelines, cast application or strapping (including removal) is only reported as a replacement procedure or when the cast application or strapping is an initial service performed without a restorative treatment or procedure. See "Application of Casts and Strapping" in the CPT book in the Surgery Section, under the Musculoskeletal system.

ICD-9-CM Procedural

- 77.77 Excision of tibia and fibula for graft
- 77.79 Excision of other bone for graft, except facial bones
- 78.03 Bone graft of radius and ulna
- 78.43 Other repair or plastic operations on radius and ulna

Anesthesia
01830

ICD-9-CM Diagnostic

- 730.13 Chronic osteomyelitis, forearm — (Use additional code to identify organism: 041.1. Use additional code to identify major osseous defect, if applicable: 731.3)
- 730.83 Other infections involving bone in diseases classified elsewhere, forearm — (Use additional code to identify organism: 041.1. Code first underlying disease: 002.0, 015.0-015.9)
- 731.3 Major osseous defects — (Code first underlying disease: 170.0-170.9, 730.00-730.29, 733.00-733.09, 733.40-733.49, 996.45)
- 732.3 Juvenile osteochondrosis of upper extremity
- 733.12 Pathologic fracture of distal radius and ulna
- 733.49 Aseptic necrosis of other bone site — (Use additional code to identify major osseous defect, if applicable: 731.3)
- 733.81 Malunion of fracture
- 733.82 Nonunion of fracture
- 736.00 Unspecified deformity of forearm, excluding fingers
- 736.05 Wrist drop (acquired)
- 736.09 Other acquired deformities of forearm, excluding fingers
- 755.26 Congenital longitudinal deficiency, radial, complete or partial (with or without distal deficiencies, incomplete)
- 755.27 Congenital longitudinal deficiency, ulnar, complete or partial (with or without distal deficiencies, incomplete)
- 905.2 Late effect of fracture of upper extremities
- 996.40 Unspecified mechanical complication of internal orthopedic device, implant, and graft — (Use additional code to identify prosthetic joint with mechanical complication, V43.60-V43.69)
- 996.49 Other mechanical complication of other internal orthopedic device, implant, and graft — (Use additional code to identify prosthetic joint with mechanical complication, V43.60-V43.69)

Terms To Know

aseptic necrosis. Death of bone tissue resulting from a disruption in the vascular supply, caused by a noninfectious disease process, such as a fracture or the administration of immunosuppressive drugs.

osteomyelitis. Inflammation of bone that may remain localized or spread to the marrow, cortex, or periosteum, in response to an infecting organism, usually bacterial and pyogenic.

CCI Version 16.3

01810, 0213T, 0216T, 0228T, 0230T, 20690, 20900-20902, 24300, 25100-25105, 25115-25119, 25259, 25295, 29065-29085, 29105-29126, 36000, 36400-36410, 36420-36430, 36440, 36600, 36640, 37202, 43752, 51701-51703, 62310-62319, 64400-64435, 64445-64450, 64479, 64483, 64490, 64493, 64505-64530, 69990, 93000-93010, 93040-93042, 93318, 94002, 94200, 94250, 94680-94690, 94770, 95812-95816, 95819, 95822, 95829, 95955, 96360, 96365, 96372, 96374-96376, 99148-99149, 99150

Also not with 25425: 25515, 25525-25526, 25545, 25574

Also not with 25426: 25040, 25425, 25575

Note: These CCI edits are used for Medicare. Other payers may reimburse on codes listed above.

Medicare Edits

	Fac RVU	Non-Fac RVU	FUD	Assist
25425	29.87	29.87	90	80
25426	32.86	32.86	90	80

Medicare References: 100-2,15,260; 100-4,12,30; 100-4,12,90.3; 100-4,14,10

25430

25430 Insertion of vascular pedicle into carpal bone (eg, Hori procedure)

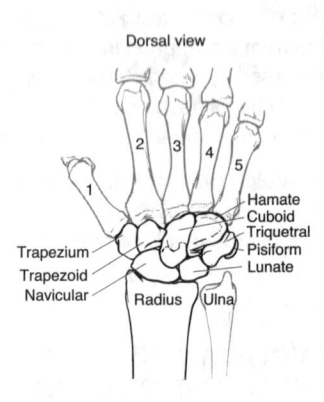

Explanation

The physician makes an incision away from the iliac crest through the external oblique muscle. The internal oblique muscle is incised and isolated from the underlying transversalis muscle. The ascending branch is followed to its junction with the deep circumflex iliac vein, and the dissection proceeds to the isolation of the flap vessels to their origin at the external iliac crest vessels. The physician divides the transversalis muscle, identifies the iliacus muscle, and divides the iliacus at the site of the planned bone cut. The fascia and muscles are released from the lateral surface of the ilium to the level of the planned bone cut. The bone cuts are made with an oscillating saw. The direction and extent depend on the recipient bed defect. Following ligation of the pedicle and transfer, the bone portion of the flap is countered to meet the dimensions of the bone defect. The bone is secured to the plate and the soft tissue inset is completed prior to microvascular anastomosis. Free cancellous bone is packed into the opening osteotomies.

Coding Tips

Any bone graft harvest is not reported separately.

ICD-9-CM Procedural

- 86.73 Attachment of pedicle or flap graft to hand
- 86.74 Attachment of pedicle or flap graft to other sites

Anesthesia

25430 01830

ICD-9-CM Diagnostic

- 170.5 Malignant neoplasm of short bones of upper limb
- 198.5 Secondary malignant neoplasm of bone and bone marrow
- 213.5 Benign neoplasm of short bones of upper limb
- 238.0 Neoplasm of uncertain behavior of bone and articular cartilage
- 239.2 Neoplasms of unspecified nature of bone, soft tissue, and skin
- 730.13 Chronic osteomyelitis, forearm — (Use additional code to identify organism: 041.1. Use additional code to identify major osseous defect, if applicable: 731.3)
- 730.14 Chronic osteomyelitis, hand — (Use additional code to identify organism: 041.1. Use additional code to identify major osseous defect, if applicable: 731.3)
- 730.23 Unspecified osteomyelitis, forearm — (Use additional code to identify organism: 041.1. Use additional code to identify major osseous defect, if applicable: 731.3)
- 730.24 Unspecified osteomyelitis, hand — (Use additional code to identify organism: 041.1. Use additional code to identify major osseous defect, if applicable: 731.3)
- 731.3 Major osseous defects — (Code first underlying disease: 170.0-170.9, 730.00-730.29, 733.00-733.09, 733.40-733.49, 996.45)
- 733.49 Aseptic necrosis of other bone site — (Use additional code to identify major osseous defect, if applicable: 731.3)
- 733.82 Nonunion of fracture
- 733.90 Disorder of bone and cartilage, unspecified
- 733.99 Other disorders of bone and cartilage
- 814.00 Unspecified closed fracture of carpal bone
- 814.01 Closed fracture of navicular (scaphoid) bone of wrist
- 814.02 Closed fracture of lunate (semilunar) bone of wrist
- 814.03 Closed fracture of triquetral (cuneiform) bone of wrist
- 814.04 Closed fracture of pisiform bone of wrist
- 814.05 Closed fracture of trapezium bone (larger multangular) of wrist
- 814.06 Closed fracture of trapezoid bone (smaller multangular) of wrist
- 814.07 Closed fracture of capitate bone (os magnum) of wrist
- 814.08 Closed fracture of hamate (unciform) bone of wrist
- 814.10 Unspecified open fracture of carpal bone
- 814.12 Open fracture of lunate (semilunar) bone of wrist
- 814.13 Open fracture of triquetral (cuneiform) bone of wrist
- 814.14 Open fracture of pisiform bone of wrist
- 814.15 Open fracture of trapezium bone (larger multangular) of wrist
- 814.16 Open fracture of trapezoid bone (smaller multangular) of wrist
- 814.17 Open fracture of capitate bone (os magnum) of wrist
- 814.18 Open fracture of hamate (unciform) bone of wrist
- 814.19 Open fracture of other bone of wrist
- 905.2 Late effect of fracture of upper extremities
- 927.20 Crushing injury of hand(s) — (Use additional code to identify any associated injuries: 800-829, 850.0-854.1, 860.0-869.1)
- 927.21 Crushing injury of wrist — (Use additional code to identify any associated injuries: 800-829, 850.0-854.1, 860.0-869.1)

CCI Version 16.3

01810, 0213T, 0216T, 0228T, 0230T, 29058-29085, 29105-29126, 29260, 36000, 36400-36410, 36420-36430, 36440, 36600, 36640, 37202, 43752, 51701-51703, 62310-62319, 64400-64435, 64445-64450, 64479, 64483, 64490, 64493, 64505-64530, 69990, 93000-93010, 93040-93042, 93318, 94002, 94200, 94250, 94680-94690, 94770, 95812-95816, 95819, 95822, 95829, 95955, 96360, 96365, 96372, 96374-96376, 99148-99149, 99150

Note: These CCI edits are used for Medicare. Other payers may reimburse on codes listed above.

Medicare Edits

	Fac RVU	Non-Fac RVU	FUD	Assist
25430	20.42	20.42	90	N/A

Medicare References: None

25431

25431 Repair of nonunion of carpal bone (excluding carpal scaphoid (navicular)) (includes obtaining graft and necessary fixation), each bone

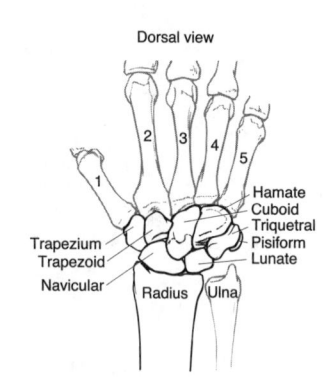

Explanation

Nonunion of the carpal bone refers to fractures that still allow free movement of bone ends more than six months after the injury and the start of treatment. In the case of a complex nonunion, the physician may take a graft from the medial aspect of the ulna and reinsert it into the prepared carpal site. Intravenous anesthesia is administered. An autogenous iliac bone graft is typically used for repair, which is obtained through an incision over the iliac crest. Once the bone is exposed, an osteotome is used to harvest strips of bone. These strips are placed between the carpal bones of the fracture through a 2.0 cm incision made at the base of the involved metacarpus. The physician centers a compression plate over the fracture and inserts screws. Lunate fractures require a short-arm spica cast or splint with thumb immobilization. Fractures of the pisiform can be immobilized with a volar splint. Injuries to the triquetrum are best treated with a sugar tong splint. Treatment of a hamate fracture involves a short-arm cast with the fourth and fifth metacarpophalangeal joints held in flexion.

Coding Tips

This is a unilateral procedure. If performed bilaterally, some payers require that the service be reported twice with modifier 50 appended to the second code, while others require identification of the service only once with modifier 50 appended. Check with individual payers. Modifier 50 identifies a procedure performed identically on the opposite side of the body (mirror image). According to CPT guidelines, cast application or strapping (including removal) is only reported as a replacement procedure or when the cast application or strapping is an initial service performed without a restorative treatment or procedure. See "Application of Casts and Strapping" in the CPT book in the Surgery Section, under the Musculoskeletal system.

ICD-9-CM Procedural

- 77.77 Excision of tibia and fibula for graft
- 78.04 Bone graft of carpals and metacarpals
- 78.79 Osteoclasis of other bone, except facial bones

Anesthesia

25431   01830

ICD-9-CM Diagnostic

- 733.82 Nonunion of fracture
- 905.2 Late effect of fracture of upper extremities

Terms To Know

flexion. Act of bending or being bent.

fracture. Break in bone or cartilage.

late effect. Abnormality, dysfunction, or other residual condition produced after the acute phase of an illness, injury, or disease is over. There is no time limit on when late effects can appear.

nonunion. Failure of two ends of a fracture to mend or completely heal.

CCI Version 16.3

01810, 0213T, 0216T, 0228T, 0230T, 11010-11012, 11040-11044, 20650, 20680, 20900-20902, 20962, 25100-25105, 25118, 25130-25135, 25250, 25320, 25430, 25630-25635, 25645, 25660, 25670, 25680-25695, 29058-29085, 29105-29126, 29260, 36000, 36400-36410, 36420-36430, 36440, 36600, 36640, 37202, 43752, 51701-51703, 62310-62319, 64400-64435, 64445-64450, 64479, 64483, 64490, 64493, 64505-64530, 69990, 93000-93010, 93040-93042, 93318, 94002, 94200, 94250, 94680-94690, 94770, 95812-95816, 95819, 95822, 95829, 95955, 96360, 96365, 96372, 96374-96376, 99148-99149, 99150

Note: These CCI edits are used for Medicare. Other payers may reimburse on codes listed above.

Medicare Edits

	Fac RVU	Non-Fac RVU	FUD	Assist
25431	22.9	22.9	90	80

Medicare References: None

25440

25440 Repair of nonunion, scaphoid carpal (navicular) bone, with or without radial styloidectomy (includes obtaining graft and necessary fixation)

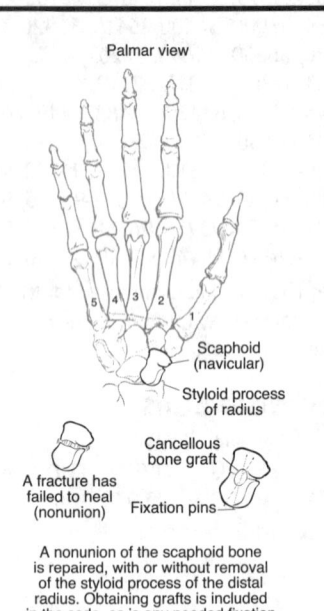

Palmar view

Scaphoid (navicular)
Styloid process of radius
A fracture has failed to heal (nonunion)
Cancellous bone graft
Fixation pins

A nonunion of the scaphoid bone is repaired, with or without removal of the styloid process of the distal radius. Obtaining grafts is included in the code, as is any needed fixation

Explanation

The physician performs this procedure when a scaphoid fracture has not healed and particularly if nonunion is accompanied by displacement of the fracture. The physician makes a 4.0 cm to 5.0 cm longitudinal incision along the radial border of the flexor carpi radialis tendon to expose the fracture site. The capsule is divided longitudinally and the underlying ligaments are retracted. An egg-shaped cavity is created in the fracture fragments. A cancellous bone graft is obtained and the graft is jammed between the fragments as they are distracted. The physician uses internal fixation such as Kirschner wires to affix the bones if instability exists. If a radial styloidectomy is performed, the physician makes an incision on the radial wrist at the base of the thumb. Radial styloid bone is removed. The physician closes the incision with sutures.

Coding Tips

Bone graft harvest for 25440 is not reported separately. According to CPT guidelines, cast application or strapping (including removal) is only reported as a replacement procedure or when the cast application or strapping is an initial service performed without a restorative treatment or procedure. See "Application of Casts and Strapping" in the CPT book in the Surgery Section, under the Musculoskeletal system. For radius and ulna shortening, see 25392.

ICD-9-CM Procedural

- 77.77 Excision of tibia and fibula for graft
- 77.79 Excision of other bone for graft, except facial bones
- 78.04 Bone graft of carpals and metacarpals

Anesthesia

25440 01830

ICD-9-CM Diagnostic

- 733.82 Nonunion of fracture
- 905.2 Late effect of fracture of upper extremities

Terms To Know

fracture. Break in bone or cartilage.

late effect. Abnormality, dysfunction, or other residual condition produced after the acute phase of an illness, injury, or disease is over. There is no time limit on when late effects can appear.

nonunion. Failure of two ends of a fracture to mend or completely heal.

CCI Version 16.3

01810, 0213T, 0216T, 0228T, 0230T, 20650, 20680-20690, 20900-20902, 24300, 25100-25107, 25118, 25130-25135, 25230, 25250, 25259, 25320, 25394, 25430, 25622-25624, 25628, 25670, 25680-25695, 29065-29085, 29105-29126, 29260, 36000, 36400-36410, 36420-36430, 36440, 36600, 36640, 37202, 43752, 51701-51703, 62310-62319, 64400-64435, 64445-64450, 64479, 64483, 64490, 64493, 64505-64530, 69990, 93000-93010, 93040-93042, 93318, 94002, 94200, 94250, 94680-94690, 94770, 95812-95816, 95819, 95822, 95829, 95955, 96360, 96365, 96372, 96374-96376, 99148-99149, 99150

Note: These CCI edits are used for Medicare. Other payers may reimburse on codes listed above.

Medicare Edits

	Fac RVU	Non-Fac RVU	FUD	Assist
25440	22.5	22.5	90	80

Medicare References: 100-2,15,260; 100-4,12,30; 100-4,12,90.3; 100-4,14,10

25441

25441 Arthroplasty with prosthetic replacement; distal radius

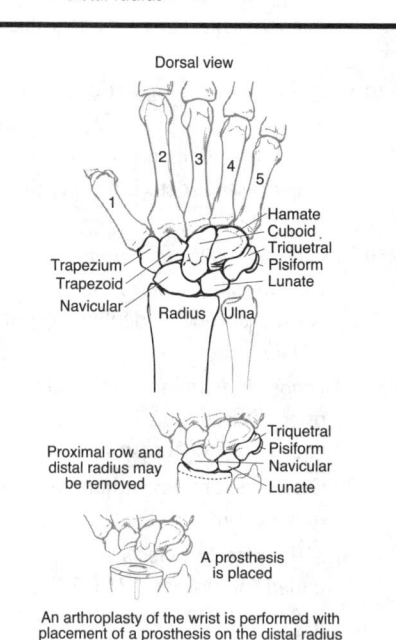

Explanation

The physician performs an arthroplasty on the wrist to relieve function-limiting wrist pain. The physician makes a T-shaped incision overlying the dorsal wrist. The capsule and synovium are incised and elevated. The distal end of the radius and the proximal carpal row are excised to accommodate the implant. The medullary canal of the third metacarpal is exposed and an awl is placed into the canal for reaming. The awl is removed, then the prosthetic awl is impacted into the base of the carpus and third metacarpal shaft. The medullary canal of the radius is reamed and implanted with the prosthesis. Cement is injected into the medullary canal of the third metacarpal after previously inserting a small cancellous bone plug. The distal component is impacted home first. The proximal component is generally not cemented and is impacted only. The capsule is repaired over the prosthesis with strong sutures. A suction drain is placed beneath the capsule. The retinaculum is repaired over all of the extensor tendons. The skin is sutured closed and the wrist is immobilized.

Coding Tips

If significant additional time and effort is documented, append modifier 22 and submit a cover letter and operative report. According to CPT guidelines, cast application or strapping (including removal) is only reported as a replacement procedure or when the cast application or strapping is an initial service performed without a restorative treatment or procedure. See "Application of Casts and Strapping" in the CPT book in the Surgery Section, under the Musculoskeletal system. For removal of an implant, see 25251. For arthroplasty, with prosthetic replacement of the distal ulna, see 25442; scaphoid (navicular), see 25443; lunate, see 25444; trapezium, see 25445; distal radius and partial or entire carpus (total wrist), see 25446.

ICD-9-CM Procedural

81.74 Arthroplasty of carpocarpal or carpometacarpal joint with implant

Anesthesia
25441 01830

ICD-9-CM Diagnostic

- 357.1 Polyneuropathy in collagen vascular disease — (Code first underlying disease: 446.0, 710.0, 714.0)
- 359.6 Symptomatic inflammatory myopathy in diseases classified elsewhere — (Code first underlying disease: 135, 140.0-208.9, 277.30-277.39, 446.0, 710.0, 710.1, 710.2, 714.0)
- 446.0 Polyarteritis nodosa
- 710.0 Systemic lupus erythematosus — (Use additional code to identify manifestation: 424.91, 581.81, 582.81, 583.81)
- 710.1 Systemic sclerosis — (Use additional code to identify manifestation: 359.6, 517.2)
- 710.2 Sicca syndrome
- 711.03 Pyogenic arthritis, forearm — (Use additional code to identify infectious organism: 041.0-041.8)
- 711.93 Unspecified infective arthritis, forearm
- 714.0 Rheumatoid arthritis — (Use additional code to identify manifestation: 357.1, 359.6)
- 715.13 Primary localized osteoarthrosis, forearm
- 715.23 Secondary localized osteoarthrosis, forearm
- 715.33 Localized osteoarthrosis not specified whether primary or secondary, forearm
- 716.13 Traumatic arthropathy, forearm
- 716.23 Allergic arthritis, forearm
- 716.63 Unspecified monoarthritis, forearm
- 716.93 Unspecified arthropathy, forearm
- 730.13 Chronic osteomyelitis, forearm — (Use additional code to identify organism: 041.1. Use additional code to identify major osseous defect, if applicable: 731.3)
- 730.23 Unspecified osteomyelitis, forearm — (Use additional code to identify organism: 041.1. Use additional code to identify major osseous defect, if applicable: 731.3)
- 731.3 Major osseous defects — (Code first underlying disease: 170.0-170.9, 730.00-730.29, 733.00-733.09, 733.40-733.49, 996.45)
- 905.2 Late effect of fracture of upper extremities

Terms To Know

osteomyelitis. Inflammation of bone that may remain localized or spread to the marrow, cortex, or periosteum, in response to an infecting organism, usually bacterial and pyogenic.

polyarteritis nodosa. Systemic necrotizing vasculitis of small and medium arteries that results in the infarction and scarring within the affected organs.

CCI Version 16.3

01810, 0213T, 0216T, 0228T, 0230T, 20650, 24300, 25000, 25040, 25100-25107, 25120, 25130, 25150-25151, 25210-25215, 25259, 25320, 25350, 25365, 25390, 25447-25449❖, 29065-29085, 29105-29126, 29846, 36000, 36400-36410, 36420-36430, 36440, 36600, 36640, 37202, 43752, 51701-51703, 62310-62319, 64400-64435, 64445-64450, 64479, 64483, 64490, 64493, 64505-64530, 64719, 69990, 93000-93010, 93040-93042, 93318, 94002, 94200, 94250, 94680-94690, 94770, 95812-95816, 95819, 95822, 95829, 95955, 96360, 96365, 96372, 96374-96376, 99148-99149, 99150

Note: These CCI edits are used for Medicare. Other payers may reimburse on codes listed above.

Medicare Edits

	Fac RVU	Non-Fac RVU	FUD	Assist
25441	27.07	27.07	90	80

Medicare References: 100-2,15,260; 100-4,12,30; 100-4,12,90.3; 100-4,14,10

25442

25442 Arthroplasty with prosthetic replacement; distal ulna

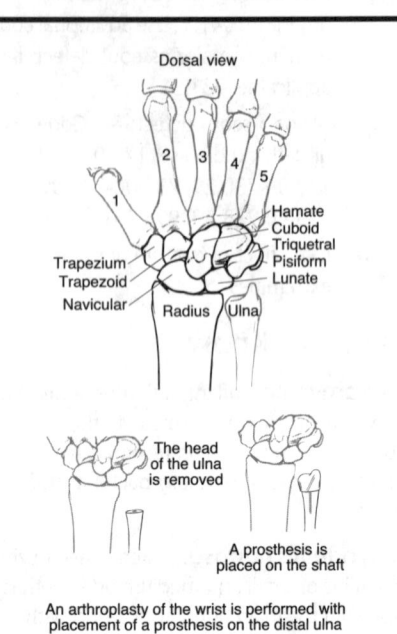

Explanation
The physician performs this arthroplasty to decrease ulnar bone overgrowth following resection of the distal ulna. The physician makes a dorsal ulnar longitudinal incision overlying the ulnar head. The extensor retinaculum is incised. The neck of the ulna is subperiosteally exposed and the ulnar head is resected at the neck. The cut edge of the ulna is smoothed and the medullary canal reamed to accept the stem of the implant. The appropriately sized implant is tested and two drill holes are made 2.0 cm from the resected bone. The physician stabilizes the distal ulna by attaching the base of the sixth dorsal compartment retinaculum to the interosseous membrane with sutures. The distal end of the ulna is pressed volarly and is sutured tightly into the soft tissue on the radial side with the radial itself. The wound is closed with sutures over a drain. A conforming dressing is applied.

Coding Tips
If significant additional time and effort is documented, append modifier 22 and submit a cover letter and operative report. According to CPT guidelines, cast application or strapping (including removal) is only reported as a replacement procedure or when the cast application or strapping is an initial service performed without a restorative treatment or procedure. See "Application of Casts and Strapping" in the CPT book in the Surgery Section, under the Musculoskeletal system. For removal of an implant, see 25251. For arthroplasty, with prosthetic replacement of the distal radius, see 25441; scaphoid (navicular), see 25443; lunate, see 25444; trapezium, see 25445; distal radius and partial or entire carpus (total wrist), see 25446.

ICD-9-CM Procedural
81.74 Arthroplasty of carpocarpal or carpometacarpal joint with implant

Anesthesia
25442   01830

ICD-9-CM Diagnostic
357.1 Polyneuropathy in collagen vascular disease — (Code first underlying disease: 446.0, 710.0, 714.0)
359.6 Symptomatic inflammatory myopathy in diseases classified elsewhere — (Code first underlying disease: 135, 140.0-208.9, 277.30-277.39, 446.0, 710.0, 710.1, 710.2, 714.0)
446.0 Polyarteritis nodosa
710.0 Systemic lupus erythematosus — (Use additional code to identify manifestation: 424.91, 581.81, 582.81, 583.81)
710.1 Systemic sclerosis — (Use additional code to identify manifestation: 359.6, 517.2)
710.2 Sicca syndrome
711.03 Pyogenic arthritis, forearm — (Use additional code to identify infectious organism: 041.0-041.8)
711.04 Pyogenic arthritis, hand — (Use additional code to identify infectious organism: 041.0-041.8)
711.93 Unspecified infective arthritis, forearm
711.94 Unspecified infective arthritis, hand
714.0 Rheumatoid arthritis — (Use additional code to identify manifestation: 357.1, 359.6)
715.13 Primary localized osteoarthrosis, forearm
715.14 Primary localized osteoarthrosis, hand
715.23 Secondary localized osteoarthrosis, forearm
715.24 Secondary localized osteoarthrosis, involving hand
715.33 Localized osteoarthrosis not specified whether primary or secondary, forearm
715.34 Localized osteoarthrosis not specified whether primary or secondary, hand
716.13 Traumatic arthropathy, forearm
716.14 Traumatic arthropathy, hand
719.23 Villonodular synovitis, forearm
719.24 Villonodular synovitis, hand
730.13 Chronic osteomyelitis, forearm — (Use additional code to identify organism: 041.1. Use additional code to identify major osseous defect, if applicable: 731.3)
730.14 Chronic osteomyelitis, hand — (Use additional code to identify organism: 041.1. Use additional code to identify major osseous defect, if applicable: 731.3)
730.33 Periostitis, without mention of osteomyelitis, forearm — (Use additional code to identify organism: 041.1)
730.34 Periostitis, without mention of osteomyelitis, hand — (Use additional code to identify organism: 041.1)
731.0 Osteitis deformans without mention of bone tumor
731.3 Major osseous defects — (Code first underlying disease: 170.0-170.9, 730.00-730.29, 733.00-733.09, 733.40-733.49, 996.45)
733.49 Aseptic necrosis of other bone site — (Use additional code to identify major osseous defect, if applicable: 731.3)
733.82 Nonunion of fracture
756.51 Osteogenesis imperfecta
905.2 Late effect of fracture of upper extremities

CCI Version 16.3
01810, 0213T, 0216T, 0228T, 0230T, 24300, 25040, 25100-25107, 25115, 25118-25120, 25130, 25150-25151, 25210-25215, 25240, 25259, 25295, 25320, 25332❖, 25360-25365, 25390, 25449❖, 29065-29085, 29105-29126, 36000, 36400-36410, 36420-36430, 36440, 36600, 36640, 37202, 43752, 51701-51703, 62310-62319, 64400-64435, 64445-64450, 64479, 64483, 64490, 64493, 64505-64530, 64719, 69990, 93000-93010, 93040-93042, 93318, 94002, 94200, 94250, 94680-94690, 94770, 95812-95816, 95819, 95822, 95829, 95955, 96360, 96365, 96372, 96374-96376, 99148-99149, 99150

Note: These CCI edits are used for Medicare. Other payers may reimburse on codes listed above.

Medicare Edits

	Fac RVU	Non-Fac RVU	FUD	Assist
25442	23.01	23.01	90	80

Medicare References: 100-2,15,260; 100-4,12,30; 100-4,12,90.3; 100-4,14,10

25443

25443 Arthroplasty with prosthetic replacement; scaphoid carpal (navicular)

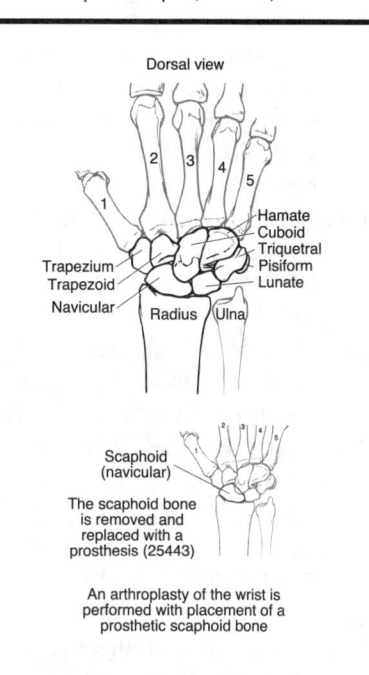

Dorsal view — Hamate, Cuboid, Triquetral, Pisiform, Lunate, Trapezium, Trapezoid, Navicular, Radius, Ulna

Scaphoid (navicular) — The scaphoid bone is removed and replaced with a prosthesis (25443)

An arthroplasty of the wrist is performed with placement of a prosthetic scaphoid bone

Explanation

The physician performs an arthroplasty with prosthetic replacement of the scaphoid. The physician makes a straight, longitudinal, or curvilinear incision over the anatomic snuff-box (superficial to the scaphoid), the "V" between the thumb and index finger. The capsule is incised longitudinally. The scaphoid is removed maintaining ligament stability. If a defect is found in the distal capsule, this is closed with a nonabsorbable suture. A hole is made in the proximal joint surface of the trapezium for insertion of the prosthetic stem. An implant is inserted. The implant is stabilized with sutures through drill holes in the lunate and radial styloid. The implant is also stabilized with a K-wire passed through the implant into an adjacent carpal bone or the radius. The capsule is closed, followed by skin closure. A compression dressing is applied.

Coding Tips

If significant additional time and effort is documented, append modifier 22 and submit a cover letter and operative report. According to CPT guidelines, cast application or strapping (including removal) is only reported as a replacement procedure or when the cast application or strapping is an initial service performed without a restorative treatment or procedure. See "Application of Casts and Strapping" in the CPT book in the Surgery Section, under the Musculoskeletal system. For removal of an implant, see 25251. For arthroplasty, with prosthetic replacement of the distal radius, see 25441; distal ulna, see 25442; lunate, see 25444; trapezium, see 25445; distal radius and partial or entire carpus (total wrist), see 25446.

ICD-9-CM Procedural
81.74 Arthroplasty of carpocarpal or carpometacarpal joint with implant

Anesthesia
25443 01830

ICD-9-CM Diagnostic

357.1 Polyneuropathy in collagen vascular disease — (Code first underlying disease: 446.0, 710.0, 714.0)
359.6 Symptomatic inflammatory myopathy in diseases classified elsewhere — (Code first underlying disease: 135, 140.0-208.9, 277.30-277.39, 446.0, 710.0, 710.1, 710.2, 714.0)
711.03 Pyogenic arthritis, forearm — (Use additional code to identify infectious organism: 041.0-041.8)
711.04 Pyogenic arthritis, hand — (Use additional code to identify infectious organism: 041.0-041.8)
714.0 Rheumatoid arthritis — (Use additional code to identify manifestation: 357.1, 359.6)
715.13 Primary localized osteoarthrosis, forearm
715.14 Primary localized osteoarthrosis, hand
715.23 Secondary localized osteoarthrosis, forearm
715.24 Secondary localized osteoarthrosis, involving hand
715.33 Localized osteoarthrosis not specified whether primary or secondary, forearm
715.34 Localized osteoarthrosis not specified whether primary or secondary, hand
716.13 Traumatic arthropathy, forearm
716.14 Traumatic arthropathy, hand
719.23 Villonodular synovitis, forearm
719.24 Villonodular synovitis, hand
719.64 Other symptoms referable to hand joint
730.13 Chronic osteomyelitis, forearm — (Use additional code to identify organism: 041.1. Use additional code to identify major osseous defect, if applicable: 731.3)
730.14 Chronic osteomyelitis, hand — (Use additional code to identify organism: 041.1. Use additional code to identify major osseous defect, if applicable: 731.3)
730.23 Unspecified osteomyelitis, forearm — (Use additional code to identify organism: 041.1. Use additional code to identify major osseous defect, if applicable: 731.3)
730.24 Unspecified osteomyelitis, hand — (Use additional code to identify organism: 041.1. Use additional code to identify major osseous defect, if applicable: 731.3)
730.33 Periostitis, without mention of osteomyelitis, forearm — (Use additional code to identify organism: 041.1)
730.34 Periostitis, without mention of osteomyelitis, hand — (Use additional code to identify organism: 041.1)
731.0 Osteitis deformans without mention of bone tumor
731.3 Major osseous defects — (Code first underlying disease: 170.0-170.9, 730.00-730.29, 733.00-733.09, 733.40-733.49, 996.45)
733.82 Nonunion of fracture
756.51 Osteogenesis imperfecta
905.2 Late effect of fracture of upper extremities

CCI Version 16.3
01810, 0213T, 0216T, 0228T, 0230T, 20650, 24300, 25040, 25100-25107, 25130, 25210-25215, 25259, 25320, 25332❖, 25394, 25447-25449❖, 29065-29085, 29105-29126, 36000, 36400-36410, 36420-36430, 36440, 36600, 36640, 37202, 43752, 51701-51703, 62310-62319, 64400-64435, 64445-64450, 64479, 64483, 64490, 64493, 64505-64530, 64719-64721, 69990, 93000-93010, 93040-93042, 93318, 94002, 94200, 94250, 94680-94690, 94770, 95812-95816, 95819, 95822, 95829, 95955, 96360, 96365, 96372, 96374-96376, 99148-99149, 99150

Note: These CCI edits are used for Medicare. Other payers may reimburse on codes listed above.

Medicare Edits

	Fac RVU	Non-Fac RVU	FUD	Assist
25443	22.8	22.8	90	80

Medicare References: 100-2,15,260; 100-4,12,30; 100-4,12,90.3; 100-4,14,10

25444

25444 Arthroplasty with prosthetic replacement; lunate

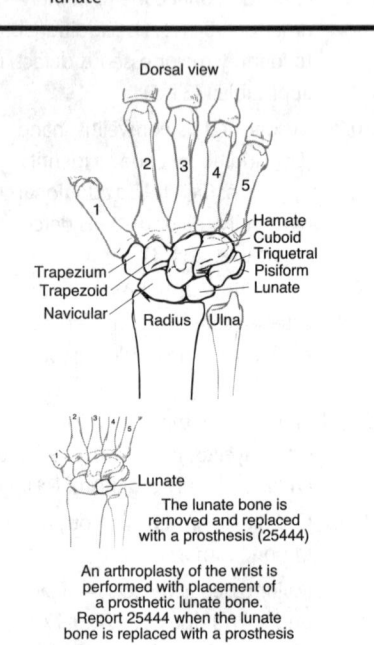

Explanation

The physician performs an arthroplasty with prosthetic replacement of the lunate. The physician makes a straight, longitudinal, or transverse incision over the dorsum of the wrist ulnar to Lister's tubercle of the radius. The fourth dorsal compartment is opened and the radiocarpal joint capsule is transversely cut. The scapholunate and lunate-triquetral interosseous ligaments are cut. The lunate is removed. If a defect in the volar ligamentous capsule is found, it is repaired. A hole is made in the middle of the triquetrum to accept the prosthetic stem. The implant is fixed to the carpus and radius with a K-wire. An absorbable suture may be placed through the scaphoid and prosthesis to increase stability. The distal capsule flap is sutured to the radius with nonabsorbable sutures. The wounds are closed and a bulky compression dressing is applied.

Coding Tips

If significant additional time and effort is documented, append modifier 22 and submit a cover letter and operative report. According to CPT guidelines, cast application or strapping (including removal) is only reported as a replacement procedure or when the cast application or strapping is an initial service performed without a restorative treatment or procedure. See "Application of Casts and Strapping" in the CPT book in the Surgery Section, under the Musculoskeletal system. For removal of an implant, see 25251. For arthroplasty, with prosthetic replacement of the distal radius, see 25441; distal ulna, see 25442; scaphoid (navicular), see 25443; trapezium, see 25445; distal radius and partial or entire carpus (total wrist), see 25446.

ICD-9-CM Procedural

81.74 Arthroplasty of carpocarpal or carpometacarpal joint with implant

Anesthesia
25444 01830

ICD-9-CM Diagnostic

- 357.1 Polyneuropathy in collagen vascular disease — (Code first underlying disease: 446.0, 710.0, 714.0)
- 359.6 Symptomatic inflammatory myopathy in diseases classified elsewhere — (Code first underlying disease: 135, 140.0-208.9, 277.30-277.39, 446.0, 710.0, 710.1, 710.2, 714.0)
- 711.03 Pyogenic arthritis, forearm — (Use additional code to identify infectious organism: 041.0-041.8)
- 711.04 Pyogenic arthritis, hand — (Use additional code to identify infectious organism: 041.0-041.8)
- 714.0 Rheumatoid arthritis — (Use additional code to identify manifestation: 357.1, 359.6)
- 715.13 Primary localized osteoarthrosis, forearm
- 715.14 Primary localized osteoarthrosis, hand
- 715.23 Secondary localized osteoarthrosis, forearm
- 715.24 Secondary localized osteoarthrosis, involving hand
- 715.33 Localized osteoarthrosis not specified whether primary or secondary, forearm
- 715.34 Localized osteoarthrosis not specified whether primary or secondary, hand
- 716.13 Traumatic arthropathy, forearm
- 716.14 Traumatic arthropathy, hand
- 719.23 Villonodular synovitis, forearm
- 719.24 Villonodular synovitis, hand
- 730.13 Chronic osteomyelitis, forearm — (Use additional code to identify organism: 041.1. Use additional code to identify major osseous defect, if applicable: 731.3)
- 730.14 Chronic osteomyelitis, hand — (Use additional code to identify organism: 041.1. Use additional code to identify major osseous defect, if applicable: 731.3)
- 730.23 Unspecified osteomyelitis, forearm — (Use additional code to identify organism: 041.1. Use additional code to identify major osseous defect, if applicable: 731.3)
- 730.24 Unspecified osteomyelitis, hand — (Use additional code to identify organism: 041.1. Use additional code to identify major osseous defect, if applicable: 731.3)
- 730.33 Periostitis, without mention of osteomyelitis, forearm — (Use additional code to identify organism: 041.1)
- 730.34 Periostitis, without mention of osteomyelitis, hand — (Use additional code to identify organism: 041.1)
- 731.0 Osteitis deformans without mention of bone tumor
- 731.3 Major osseous defects — (Code first underlying disease: 170.0-170.9, 730.00-730.29, 733.00-733.09, 733.40-733.49, 996.45)
- 733.49 Aseptic necrosis of other bone site — (Use additional code to identify major osseous defect, if applicable: 731.3)
- 733.82 Nonunion of fracture
- 756.51 Osteogenesis imperfecta
- 905.2 Late effect of fracture of upper extremities

CCI Version 16.3

01810, 0213T, 0216T, 0228T, 0230T, 20650, 24300, 25040, 25100-25107, 25130, 25210-25215, 25259, 25320, 25332❖, 25394, 25449❖, 29065-29085, 29105-29126, 36000, 36400-36410, 36420-36430, 36440, 36600, 36640, 37202, 43752, 51701-51703, 62310-62319, 64400-64435, 64445-64450, 64479, 64483, 64490, 64493, 64505-64530, 64719-64721, 69990, 93000-93010, 93040-93042, 93318, 94002, 94200, 94250, 94680-94690, 94770, 95812-95816, 95819, 95822, 95829, 95955, 96360, 96365, 96372, 96374-96376, 99148-99149, 99150

Note: These CCI edits are used for Medicare. Other payers may reimburse on codes listed above.

Medicare Edits

	Fac RVU	Non-Fac RVU	FUD	Assist
25444	23.14	23.14	90	80

Medicare References: 100-2,15,260; 100-4,12,30; 100-4,12,90.3; 100-4,14,10

25445

25445 Arthroplasty with prosthetic replacement; trapezium

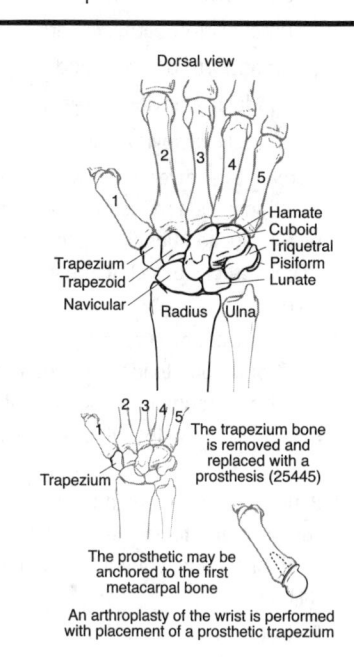

Explanation

The physician performs an arthroplasty with prosthetic replacement of the trapezium. The physician makes a straight, longitudinal cut from the middle of the thumb metacarpal to the radial styloid. The capsule is split longitudinally from the metacarpal to the scaphoid. The capsule and periosteum are elevated off the trapezium. The radial portion of the trapezoid is removed. The base of the first metacarpal is squared off. A triangular hole is made in the base of the metacarpal and the canal is made to accept the implant stem. The size of the implant should be slightly smaller than a tight fit. The capsule is repaired and reinforced by suturing slips of the abductor pollicis and flexor carpi radialis muscles to the capsule. A K-wire is placed through the implant and into the trapezoid or capitate to stabilize the position for six weeks. The skin is closed, leaving the wire protruding through incision, and a bulky dressing is applied to keep the thumb abducted.

Coding Tips

If significant additional time and effort is documented, append modifier 22 and submit a cover letter and operative report. According to CPT guidelines, cast application or strapping (including removal) is only reported as a replacement procedure or when the cast application or strapping is an initial service performed without a restorative treatment or procedure. See "Application of Casts and Strapping" in the CPT book in the Surgery Section, under the Musculoskeletal system. For removal of an implant, see 25251. For arthroplasty, with prosthetic replacement of the distal radius, see 25441; distal ulna, see 25442; scaphoid (navicular), see 25443; lunate, see 25444; distal radius and partial or entire carpus (total wrist), see 25446.

ICD-9-CM Procedural

81.79 Other repair of hand, fingers, and wrist

Anesthesia

25445 01830

ICD-9-CM Diagnostic

357.1 Polyneuropathy in collagen vascular disease — (Code first underlying disease: 446.0, 710.0, 714.0)
359.6 Symptomatic inflammatory myopathy in diseases classified elsewhere — (Code first underlying disease: 135, 140.0-208.9, 277.30-277.39, 446.0, 710.0, 710.1, 710.2, 714.0)
711.03 Pyogenic arthritis, forearm — (Use additional code to identify infectious organism: 041.0-041.8)
711.04 Pyogenic arthritis, hand — (Use additional code to identify infectious organism: 041.0-041.8)
714.0 Rheumatoid arthritis — (Use additional code to identify manifestation: 357.1, 359.6)
715.13 Primary localized osteoarthrosis, forearm
715.14 Primary localized osteoarthrosis, hand
715.23 Secondary localized osteoarthrosis, forearm
715.24 Secondary localized osteoarthrosis, involving hand
715.33 Localized osteoarthrosis not specified whether primary or secondary, forearm
715.34 Localized osteoarthrosis not specified whether primary or secondary, hand
716.13 Traumatic arthropathy, forearm
716.14 Traumatic arthropathy, hand
719.23 Villonodular synovitis, forearm
719.24 Villonodular synovitis, hand
719.63 Other symptoms referable to forearm joint
730.13 Chronic osteomyelitis, forearm — (Use additional code to identify organism: 041.1. Use additional code to identify major osseous defect, if applicable: 731.3)
730.14 Chronic osteomyelitis, hand — (Use additional code to identify organism: 041.1. Use additional code to identify major osseous defect, if applicable: 731.3)
730.33 Periostitis, without mention of osteomyelitis, forearm — (Use additional code to identify organism: 041.1)
730.34 Periostitis, without mention of osteomyelitis, hand — (Use additional code to identify organism: 041.1)
731.0 Osteitis deformans without mention of bone tumor
731.3 Major osseous defects — (Code first underlying disease: 170.0-170.9, 730.00-730.29, 733.00-733.09, 733.40-733.49, 996.45)
733.49 Aseptic necrosis of other bone site — (Use additional code to identify major osseous defect, if applicable: 731.3)
733.82 Nonunion of fracture
756.51 Osteogenesis imperfecta
905.2 Late effect of fracture of upper extremities

CCI Version 16.3

01810, 0213T, 0216T, 0228T, 0230T, 20650, 24300, 25040, 25100-25107, 25130, 25210-25215, 25259, 25320, 25332❖, 25394, 25447-25449❖, 29065-29085, 29105-29126, 36000, 36400-36410, 36420-36430, 36440, 36600, 36640, 37202, 43752, 51701-51703, 62310-62319, 64400-64435, 64445-64450, 64479, 64483, 64490, 64493, 64505-64530, 69990, 93000-93010, 93040-93042, 93318, 94002, 94200, 94250, 94680-94690, 94770, 95812-95816, 95819, 95822, 95829, 95955, 96360, 96365, 96372, 96374-96376, 99148-99149, 99150

Note: These CCI edits are used for Medicare. Other payers may reimburse on codes listed above.

Medicare Edits

	Fac RVU	Non-Fac RVU	FUD	Assist
25445	20.99	20.99	90	N/A

Medicare References: 100-2,15,260; 100-4,12,30; 100-4,12,90.3; 100-4,14,10

25446

25446 Arthroplasty with prosthetic replacement; distal radius and partial or entire carpus (total wrist)

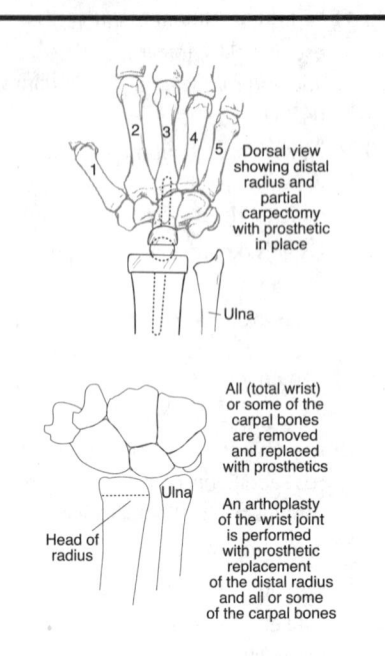

Dorsal view showing distal radius and partial carpectomy with prosthetic in place

Ulna

All (total wrist) or some of the carpal bones are removed and replaced with prosthetics

Ulna

Head of radius

An arthoplasty of the wrist joint is performed with prosthetic replacement of the distal radius and all or some of the carpal bones

Explanation

The physician performs a total wrist arthroplasty. The physician makes a straight, dorsal, longitudinal incision centered over the wrist from the middle of the third metacarpal proximally. The skin and subcutaneous tissues are elevated off the underlying fascia and retinaculum. The retinaculum over the fourth dorsal compartment is incised longitudinally and elevated. The extensor pollicis longus is freed and retracted radically. A longitudinal incision is made in the capsule overlying the distal radius. Ulnarly, a capsular periosteal flap is elevated through the dorsal radioulnar ligaments. Radially, the subperiosteal dissection continues to the radial styloid beneath the first dorsal compartment. The distal radius is excised, as is the distal ulna if it is dislocated or severely involved. A cut, made to match the shape of the prosthesis of choice, is made through the hamate, capitate, trapezoid, and distal scaphotrapezial area. The carpus is removed. The medullary canal of the radius is reamed. A fine awl is used to penetrate the base of the capitate and the shaft of the third metacarpal. The medullary canal of this bone is reamed. If using a double-stemmed component, an additional canal is prepared in the second metacarpal. The component is inserted into the canals. Appropriate short canals are prepared in the carpal bases. The metallic components are inserted. The prosthetic polyethylene ball is placed on the trummion and motion is tested. When desired motion is achieved, cement is mixed and injected into the medullary canals. The capsular-periosteal tissues are repaired over the prosthesis. The extensor retinaculum may be used to reinforce the capsule. The skin is closed over a deep and a superficial suction drain.

Coding Tips

If significant additional time and effort is documented, append modifier 22 and submit a cover letter and operative report. According to CPT guidelines, cast application or strapping (including removal) is only reported as a replacement procedure or when the cast application or strapping is an initial service performed without a restorative treatment or procedure. See "Application of Casts and Strapping" in the CPT book in the Surgery Section, under the Musculoskeletal system. For removal of an implant, see 25251. For arthroplasty, with prosthetic replacement of the distal radius, see 25441; distal ulna, see 25442; scaphoid (navicular), see 25443; lunate, see 25444; trapezium, see 25445.

ICD-9-CM Procedural
81.73 Total wrist replacement

Anesthesia
25446 01832

ICD-9-CM Diagnostic

357.1 Polyneuropathy in collagen vascular disease — (Code first underlying disease: 446.0, 710.0, 714.0)
359.6 Symptomatic inflammatory myopathy in diseases classified elsewhere — (Code first underlying disease: 135, 140.0-208.9, 277.30-277.39, 446.0, 710.0, 710.1, 710.2, 714.0)
446.0 Polyarteritis nodosa
710.0 Systemic lupus erythematosus — (Use additional code to identify manifestation: 424.91, 581.81, 582.81, 583.81)
710.1 Systemic sclerosis — (Use additional code to identify manifestation: 359.6, 517.2)
711.03 Pyogenic arthritis, forearm — (Use additional code to identify infectious organism: 041.0-041.8)
711.04 Pyogenic arthritis, hand — (Use additional code to identify infectious organism: 041.0-041.8)
714.0 Rheumatoid arthritis — (Use additional code to identify manifestation: 357.1, 359.6)
715.13 Primary localized osteoarthrosis, forearm
715.14 Primary localized osteoarthrosis, hand
715.23 Secondary localized osteoarthrosis, forearm
715.24 Secondary localized osteoarthrosis, involving hand
716.13 Traumatic arthropathy, forearm
716.14 Traumatic arthropathy, hand
719.23 Villonodular synovitis, forearm
719.24 Villonodular synovitis, hand
730.13 Chronic osteomyelitis, forearm — (Use additional code to identify organism: 041.1. Use additional code to identify major osseous defect, if applicable: 731.3)
730.14 Chronic osteomyelitis, hand — (Use additional code to identify organism: 041.1. Use additional code to identify major osseous defect, if applicable: 731.3)
730.33 Periostitis, without mention of osteomyelitis, forearm — (Use additional code to identify organism: 041.1)
730.34 Periostitis, without mention of osteomyelitis, hand — (Use additional code to identify organism: 041.1)
731.0 Osteitis deformans without mention of bone tumor
733.82 Nonunion of fracture
756.51 Osteogenesis imperfecta

CCI Version 16.3
01810, 0213T, 0216T, 0228T, 0230T, 20670-20680, 24300, 25040, 25100-25107, 25110, 25115-25118, 25120, 25130, 25150-25151, 25210-25215, 25250, 25259, 25295, 25320, 25350, 25360-25365, 25390, 29065-29085, 29105-29126, 29844, 36000, 36400-36410, 36420-36430, 36440, 36600, 36640, 37202, 43752, 51701-51703, 62310-62319, 64400-64435, 64445-64450, 64479, 64483, 64490, 64493, 64505-64530, 64719, 69990, 93000-93010, 93040-93042, 93318, 94002, 94200, 94250, 94680-94690, 94770, 95812-95816, 95819, 95822, 95829, 95955, 96360, 96365, 96372, 96374-96376, 99148-99149, 99150

Note: These CCI edits are used for Medicare. Other payers may reimburse on codes listed above.

Medicare Edits

	Fac RVU	Non-Fac RVU	FUD	Assist
25446	34.35	34.35	90	80

Medicare References: 100-2,15,260; 100-4,12,30; 100-4,12,90.3; 100-4,14,10

25447

25447 Arthroplasty, interposition, intercarpal or carpometacarpal joints

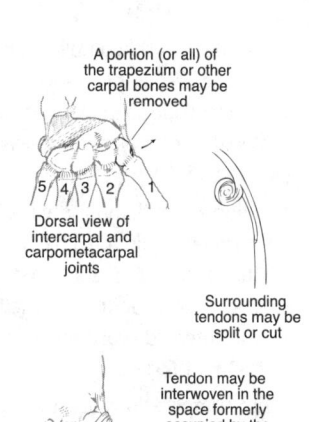

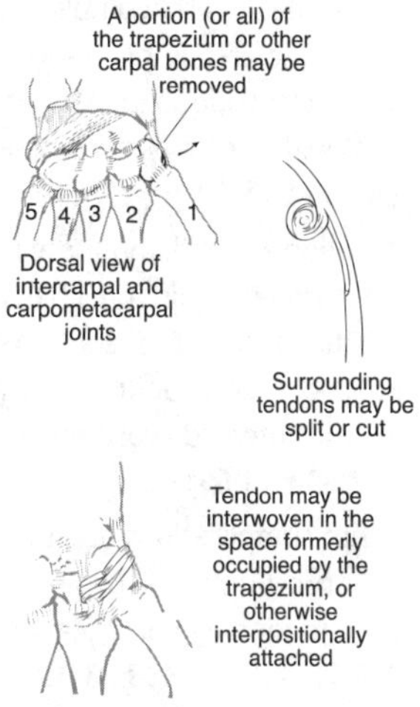

Explanation

The physician performs an interposition arthroplasty of the intercarpal or carpometacarpal joints. The physician makes a zigzag incision over the proximal one third of the first metacarpal and extends it along the first wrist extensor compartment. The metacarpal joint is vertically incised to release the capsule from the base of the metacarpal. The joint is completely dislocated to expose the metacarpal end. The physician resects the metacarpal based perpendicular to its long axis. The base is shaped to allow the insertion of a metacarpal prosthesis. The medullary canal of the metacarpal is reamed to accept the prosthetic stem. The stem is inserted and the base of the prosthesis is seated on the flat surface of the trapezium bone. A Kirschner wire is inserted through the first metacarpal and into the carpus to ensure alignment. The capsule and wounds are sutured closed. This procedure may be referred to as a ligament reconstruction tendon interposition (LRTI) or a Burton LRTI.

Coding Tips

If significant additional time and effort is documented, append modifier 22 and submit a cover letter and operative report. According to CPT guidelines, cast application or strapping (including removal) is only reported as a replacement procedure or when the cast application or strapping is an initial service performed without a restorative treatment or procedure. See "Application of Casts and Strapping" in the CPT book in the Surgery section, under the musculoskeletal system. For wrist arthroplasty, see 25332. Report tendon harvest or transfer from a distant site separately and append modifier 51; see 25310 for the wrist and 26480 for dorsum of the hand.

ICD-9-CM Procedural

81.74 Arthroplasty of carpocarpal or carpometacarpal joint with implant

Anesthesia
25447 01830

ICD-9-CM Diagnostic

357.1 Polyneuropathy in collagen vascular disease — (Code first underlying disease: 446.0, 710.0, 714.0)
359.6 Symptomatic inflammatory myopathy in diseases classified elsewhere — (Code first underlying disease: 135, 140.0-208.9, 277.30-277.39, 446.0, 710.0, 710.1, 710.2, 714.0)
446.0 Polyarteritis nodosa
710.0 Systemic lupus erythematosus — (Use additional code to identify manifestation: 424.91, 581.81, 582.81, 583.81)
710.1 Systemic sclerosis — (Use additional code to identify manifestation: 359.6, 517.2)
710.2 Sicca syndrome
714.0 Rheumatoid arthritis — (Use additional code to identify manifestation: 357.1, 359.6)
715.04 Generalized osteoarthrosis, involving hand
715.14 Primary localized osteoarthrosis, hand
715.94 Osteoarthrosis, unspecified whether generalized or localized, hand
716.14 Traumatic arthropathy, hand
716.94 Unspecified arthropathy, hand
814.00 Unspecified closed fracture of carpal bone
905.2 Late effect of fracture of upper extremities

Terms To Know

myositis. Inflammation of a muscle with voluntary movement.

polyarteritis nodosa. Systemic necrotizing vasculitis of small and medium arteries that results in the infarction and scarring within the affected organs.

polyneuropathy. Disease process of severe inflammation of multiple nerves.

sicca syndrome. Complex of symptoms of unknown source in middle-aged women in which the following triad exists: keratoconjunctivitis sicca, zerostomia, and connective tissue disease (usually rheumatoid arthritis but sometimes systemic lupus erythematosus).

systemic sclerosis. Systemic disease characterized by excess fibrotic collagen build-up, turning the skin thickened and hard. Fibrotic changes also occur in various organs and cause vascular abnormalities and affect more women than men.

CCI Version 16.3

01810, 0213T, 0216T, 0228T, 0230T, 20650, 20690, 20924, 24300, 25040, 25100-25107, 25130, 25210-25215, 25259, 25320, 25394, 26070, 26100, 26130, 26200-26205, 26230, 26615, 26665, 26685, 29065-29085, 29105-29126, 36000, 36400-36410, 36420-36430, 36440, 36600, 36640, 37202, 43752, 51701-51703, 62310-62319, 64400-64435, 64445-64450, 64479, 64483, 64490, 64493, 64505-64530, 69990, 76000-76001, 93000-93010, 93040-93042, 93318, 94002, 94200, 94250, 94680-94690, 94770, 95812-95816, 95819, 95822, 95829, 95955, 96360, 96365, 96372, 96374-96376, 99148-99149, 99150

Note: These CCI edits are used for Medicare. Other payers may reimburse on codes listed above.

Medicare Edits

	Fac RVU	Non-Fac RVU	FUD	Assist
25447	23.98	23.98	90	80

Medicare References: 100-2,15,260; 100-4,12,30; 100-4,12,90.3; 100-4,14,10

25449

25449 Revision of arthroplasty, including removal of implant, wrist joint

Dorsal view

Implants or prosthetics may take several forms

Proximal anchor in radius

Ulna

An arthroplasty of the wrist is revised and an implant (prosthetic) is removed

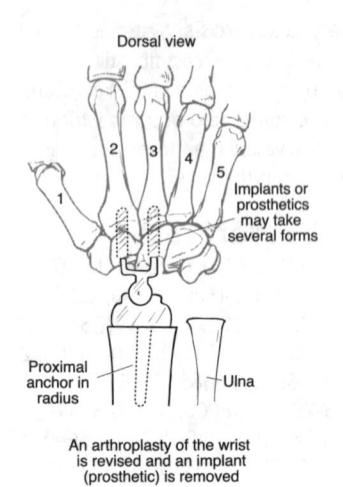

Explanation

The physician revises an arthroplasty, including removal of an implant in the wrist joint. The physician makes an incision over the wrist, reduces the joint if it is not already dislocated, and removes the device from the radius and the one or two metacarpals in which it was implanted. If necessary, a new device is placed into the wrist. The skin is closed in layers and a bulky dressing is applied.

Coding Tips

This code includes implant removal. If significant additional time and effort is documented, append modifier 22 and submit a cover letter and operative report. According to CPT guidelines, cast application or strapping (including removal) is only reported as a replacement procedure or when the cast application or strapping is an initial service performed without a restorative treatment or procedure. See "Application of Casts and Strapping" in the CPT book in the Surgery Section, under the Musculoskeletal system. For wrist arthroplasty, see 25332. For arthroplasty with prosthetic replacement, see 25441–25446.

ICD-9-CM Procedural

- 78.64 Removal of implanted device from carpals and metacarpals
- 81.75 Arthroplasty of carpocarpal or carpometacarpal joint without implant

Anesthesia
25449   01830

ICD-9-CM Diagnostic

- 711.03 Pyogenic arthritis, forearm — (Use additional code to identify infectious organism: 041.0-041.8)
- 711.04 Pyogenic arthritis, hand — (Use additional code to identify infectious organism: 041.0-041.8)
- 711.83 Arthropathy associated with other infectious and parasitic diseases, forearm — (Code first underlying disease: 080-088, 100-104, 130-136)
- 711.84 Arthropathy associated with other infectious and parasitic diseases, hand — (Code first underlying disease: 080-088, 100-104, 130-136)
- 711.93 Unspecified infective arthritis, forearm
- 711.94 Unspecified infective arthritis, hand
- 730.13 Chronic osteomyelitis, forearm — (Use additional code to identify organism: 041.1. Use additional code to identify major osseous defect, if applicable: 731.3)
- 730.14 Chronic osteomyelitis, hand — (Use additional code to identify organism: 041.1. Use additional code to identify major osseous defect, if applicable: 731.3)
- 731.3 Major osseous defects — (Code first underlying disease: 170.0-170.9, 730.00-730.29, 733.00-733.09, 733.40-733.49, 996.45)
- 996.40 Unspecified mechanical complication of internal orthopedic device, implant, and graft — (Use additional code to identify prosthetic joint with mechanical complication, V43.60-V43.69)
- 996.41 Mechanical loosening of prosthetic joint — (Use additional code to identify prosthetic joint with mechanical complication, V43.60-V43.69)
- 996.42 Dislocation of prosthetic joint — (Use additional code to identify prosthetic joint with mechanical complication, V43.60-V43.69)
- 996.43 Broken prosthetic joint implant — (Use additional code to identify prosthetic joint with mechanical complication, V43.60-V43.69)
- 996.44 Peri-prosthetic fracture around prosthetic joint — (Use additional code to identify prosthetic joint with mechanical complication, V43.60-V43.69.
- 996.45 Peri-prosthetic osteolysis — (Use additional code to identify prosthetic joint with mechanical complication, V43.60-V43.69. Use additional code to identify major osseous defect, if applicable: 731.3)
- 996.47 Other mechanical complication of prosthetic joint implant — (Use additional code to identify prosthetic joint with mechanical complication, V43.60-V43.69)
- 996.66 Infection and inflammatory reaction due to internal joint prosthesis — (Use additional code to identify specified infections. Use additional code to identify infected prosthetic joint: V43.60-V43.69)
- 996.77 Other complications due to internal joint prosthesis — (Use additional code to identify complication: 338.18-338.19, 338.28-338.29)
- 998.59 Other postoperative infection — (Use additional code to identify infection)
- 998.6 Persistent postoperative fistula, not elsewhere classified
- V43.63 Wrist joint replacement by other means

CCI Version 16.3

01810, 0213T, 0216T, 0228T, 0230T, 20670-20680, 24300, 25040, 25100-25107, 25111, 25116-25118, 25120, 25130, 25150-25151, 25210-25215, 25250, 25259, 25295, 25320, 25350, 25360-25365, 25390, 25394, 25446❖, 29065-29085, 29105-29126, 36000, 36400-36410, 36420-36430, 36440, 36600, 36640, 37202, 43752, 51701-51703, 62310-62319, 64400-64435, 64445-64450, 64479, 64483, 64490, 64493, 64505-64530, 64719, 69990, 93000-93010, 93040-93042, 93318, 94002, 94200, 94250, 94680-94690, 94770, 95812-95816, 95819, 95822, 95829, 95955, 96360, 96365, 96372, 96374-96376, 99148-99149, 99150

Note: These CCI edits are used for Medicare. Other payers may reimburse on codes listed above.

Medicare Edits

	Fac RVU	Non-Fac RVU	FUD	Assist
25449	30.58	30.58	90	80

Medicare References: 100-2,15,260; 100-4,12,30; 100-4,12,90.3; 100-4,14,10

25450-25455

25450 Epiphyseal arrest by epiphysiodesis or stapling; distal radius OR ulna
25455 distal radius AND ulna

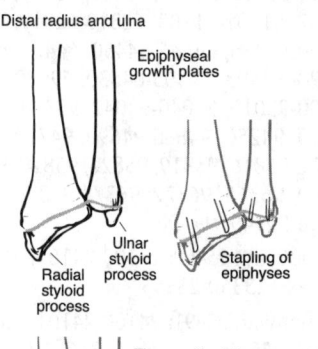

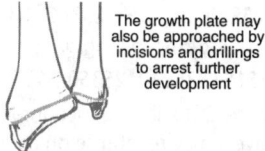

A distal ulnar or radial epiphyseal growth plate is arrested through epiphysiodesis (multiple small incisions and drillings) or by stapling. Report 25455 when both radial and ulnar growth plates are arrested

Explanation

The physician makes an incision overlying the distal forearm and along the medial (ulna) or lateral (radius) aspect in 25450 or both in 25455. The distal epiphyseal plate is located here. Dissection is carried down to expose the epiphyseal plate. The physician may elect to use a curet to scrape out the epiphysis (growth plate). A staple may be placed through the epiphyseal plate instead. Either procedure arrests further growth of that particular bone. The physician then repairs the incision in multiple layers with sutures, staples, and/or Steri-strips. A splint may be placed for immobilization.

Coding Tips

According to CPT guidelines, cast application or strapping (including removal) is only reported as a replacement procedure or when the cast application or strapping is an initial service performed without a restorative treatment or procedure. See "Application of Casts and Strapping" in the CPT book in the Surgery Section, under the Musculoskeletal system.

ICD-9-CM Procedural

78.23 Limb shortening procedures, radius and ulna

Anesthesia

01830

ICD-9-CM Diagnostic

732.3 Juvenile osteochondrosis of upper extremity

Terms To Know

distal. Located farther away from a specified reference point.

epiphysis. End of a long bone.

lateral. To/on the side.

medial. Middle or midline.

osteochondrosis. Disease manifested by degeneration or necrosis of the growth plate or ossification centers of bones in children, followed by regenerating and reossification.

CCI Version 16.3

01810, 0213T, 0216T, 0228T, 0230T, 24300, 25100-25105, 25120, 25150-25151, 25259, 29065-29085, 29105-29126, 36000, 36400-36410, 36420-36430, 36440, 36600, 36640, 37202, 43752, 51701-51703, 62310-62319, 64400-64435, 64445-64450, 64479, 64483, 64490, 64493, 64505-64530, 69990, 93000-93010, 93040-93042, 93318, 94002, 94200, 94250, 94680-94690, 94770, 95812-95816, 95819, 95822, 95829, 95955, 96360, 96365, 96372, 96374-96376, 99148-99149, 99150

Note: These CCI edits are used for Medicare. Other payers may reimburse on codes listed above.

Medicare Edits

	Fac RVU	Non-Fac RVU	FUD	Assist
25450	16.47	16.47	90	N/A
25455	18.14	18.14	90	N/A

Medicare References: 100-2,15,260; 100-4,12,30; 100-4,12,90.3; 100-4,14,10

25490-25492

25490 Prophylactic treatment (nailing, pinning, plating or wiring) with or without methylmethacrylate; radius
25491 ulna
25492 radius AND ulna

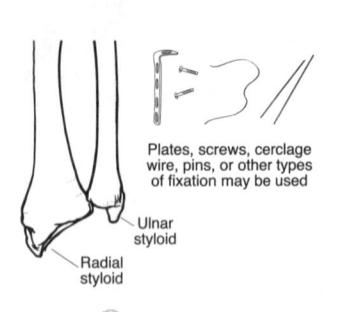

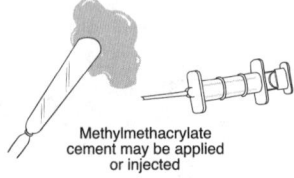

Plates, screws, cerclage wire, pins, or other types of fixation may be used

Ulnar styloid
Radial styloid

Methylmethacrylate cement may be applied or injected

The radius is treated with internal fixation (with or without methylmethacrylate) as a preventive measure. Report 25491 when the treatment is for the ulna. Report 25492 when both radius and ulna are treated

Explanation

The physician applies prophylactic treatment. The physician treats the radius in 25490. A longitudinal incision is made along the forearm. Dissection is carried down to expose the affected part of the radius. In 25491, the ulna is treated. A longitudinal incision is required along the medial aspect of the ulna. In 25492, both the radius and ulna are treated, which may require two separate incisions. Pins or a plate with screws are used to stabilize the bone. If there are defects in the bone, such that the internal fixation does not provide good purchase with the bone, methylmethacrylate (cement) is used to fill in the gaps. Wiring (cerclage) may also be wrapped around the bone to provide additional fixation. The physician may also insert an intramedullary nail through the canal of the radius to provide internal stabilization. This is usually inserted through the distal end of the radius. The incisions are repaired in multiple layers with sutures, staples, and/or Steri-strips.

Coding Tips

According to CPT guidelines, cast application or strapping (including removal) is only reported as a replacement procedure or when the cast application or strapping is an initial service performed without a restorative treatment or procedure. See "Application of Casts and Strapping" in the CPT book in the Surgery Section, under the Musculoskeletal system. For radiology services, see 73090.

ICD-9-CM Procedural

78.53 Internal fixation of radius and ulna without fracture reduction
84.55 Insertion of bone void filler

Anesthesia
01830

ICD-9-CM Diagnostic

170.4 Malignant neoplasm of scapula and long bones of upper limb
198.5 Secondary malignant neoplasm of bone and bone marrow
213.4 Benign neoplasm of scapula and long bones of upper limb
238.0 Neoplasm of uncertain behavior of bone and articular cartilage
239.2 Neoplasms of unspecified nature of bone, soft tissue, and skin
731.3 Major osseous defects — (Code first underlying disease: 170.0-170.9, 730.00-730.29, 733.00-733.09, 733.40-733.49, 996.45)
733.49 Aseptic necrosis of other bone site — (Use additional code to identify major osseous defect, if applicable: 731.3)

Terms To Know

aseptic necrosis. Death of bone tissue resulting from a disruption in the vascular supply, caused by a noninfectious disease process, such as a fracture or the administration of immunosuppressive drugs.

benign. Mild or nonmalignant in nature.

malignant. Any condition tending to progress toward death, specifically an invasive tumor with a loss of cellular differentiation that has the ability to spread or metastasize to other areas in the body.

osteomyelitis. Inflammation of bone that may remain localized or spread to the marrow, cortex, or periosteum, in response to an infecting organism, usually bacterial and pyogenic.

secondary. Second in order of occurrence or importance, or appearing during the course of another disease or condition.

soft tissue. Nonepithelial tissues outside of the skeleton that includes subcutaneous adipose tissue, fibrous tissue, fascia, muscles, blood and lymph vessels, and peripheral nervous system tissue.

CCI Version 16.3

01810, 0213T, 0216T, 0228T, 0230T, 20690, 20692, 20696-20697, 24000, 24006, 24300, 24495, 25020, 25100-25105, 25115-25119, 25259, 25295, 25390, 29065-29085, 29105-29126, 36000, 36400-36410, 36420-36430, 36440, 36600, 36640, 37202, 43752, 51701-51703, 62310-62319, 64400-64435, 64445-64450, 64479, 64483, 64490, 64493, 64505-64530, 69990, 93000-93010, 93040-93042, 93318, 94002, 94200, 94250, 94680-94690, 94770, 95812-95816, 95819, 95822, 95829, 95955, 96360, 96365, 96372, 96374-96376, 99148-99149, 99150

Also not with 25490: 24100-24101, 25151, 25332❖, 25350-25355

Also not with 25491: 24100-24101, 25000, 25150, 25240, 25332❖, 25360

Also not with 25492: 24100-24102, 25000, 25150-25151, 25240, 25350-25365

Note: These CCI edits are used for Medicare. Other payers may reimburse on codes listed above.

Medicare Edits

	Fac RVU	Non-Fac RVU	FUD	Assist
25490	20.54	20.54	90	80
25491	22.52	22.52	90	80
25492	27.26	27.26	90	80

Medicare References: 100-2,15,260; 100-4,12,30; 100-4,12,90.3; 100-4,14,10

25500-25505

25500 Closed treatment of radial shaft fracture; without manipulation
25505 with manipulation

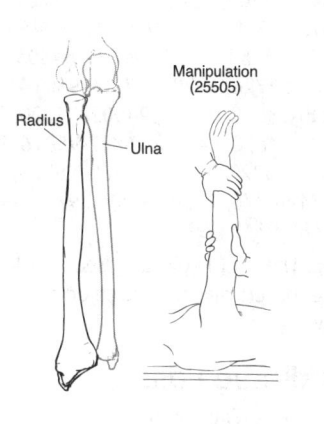

A radial shaft fracture is treated in a closed fashion without manipulation. Report 25505 when manipulation is required to treat the fracture

Explanation

The physician treats a radial shaft fracture without manipulation in 25500 or with manipulation in 25505. No incisions are made. If manipulation is required (25505), anesthesia may be necessary to relax the muscles. With the elbow at 90 degrees of flexion, the physician uses a combination of traction and countertraction while the radius is reduced. The patient may be placed in a long arm cast. The cast is removed after approximately 18 days and a functional brace is applied, allowing wrist and elbow movement, but limited pronation and supination.

Coding Tips

According to CPT guidelines, cast application or strapping (including removal) is only reported as a replacement procedure or when the cast application or strapping is an initial service performed without a restorative treatment or procedure. See "Application of Casts and Strapping" in the CPT book in the Surgery Section, under the Musculoskeletal system. In 25505, local anesthesia is included in the service. However, this procedure may be performed under general anesthesia, depending on the age and/or condition of the patient. For radiology services, see 73090. For closed treatment of a radial shaft fracture, with dislocation of the distal radio-ulnar joint, see 25520. For open treatment of a radial shaft fracture, see 25515. For open treatment of a radial shaft fracture with open treatment of a radio-ulnar dislocation, see 25526. For treatment of a radial and ulnar shaft fracture, see 25560–25575. For an ulnar shaft fracture alone, see 25530–25545.

ICD-9-CM Procedural

- **79.02** Closed reduction of fracture of radius and ulna without internal fixation
- **93.53** Application of other cast

Anesthesia

01820

ICD-9-CM Diagnostic

- **733.19** Pathologic fracture of other specified site
- **813.21** Closed fracture of shaft of radius (alone)

Terms To Know

closed fracture. Break in a bone without a concomitant opening in the skin. A closed fracture is coded when the type of fracture is not specified.

flexion. Act of bending or being bent.

fracture. Break in bone or cartilage.

pathologic fracture. Break in bone due to a disease process that weakens the bone structure, such as osteoporosis, osteomalacia, or neoplasia, and not traumatic injury.

pronation. Lying on the stomach or in a face down position; turning the palm toward the back or downward; lowering of the medial margin of the foot by an everting and abducting movement.

supination. Lying on the back; turning the palm toward the front or upward; raising the medial margin of the foot by an inverting and adducting movement.

CCI Version 16.3

01810, 01820, 0213T, 0216T, 0228T, 0230T, 24300, 25259, 29058-29085, 29105-29126, 29260, 29700-29715, 36000, 36400-36410, 36420-36430, 36440, 36600, 36640, 37202, 43752, 51701-51703, 62310-62319, 64400-64435, 64445-64450, 64479, 64483, 64490, 64493, 64505-64530, 69990, 93000-93010, 93040-93042, 93318, 94002, 94200, 94250, 94680-94690, 94770, 95812-95816, 95819, 95822, 95829, 95955, 96360, 96365, 96372, 96374-96376, 97597-97598, 97602-97606, 99148-99149, 99150

Also not with 25500: 29515

Also not with 25505: 25500, J0670, J2001

Note: These CCI edits are used for Medicare. Other payers may reimburse on codes listed above.

Medicare Edits

	Fac RVU	Non-Fac RVU	FUD	Assist
25500	6.87	7.5	90	N/A
25505	13.15	14.27	90	N/A

Medicare References: 100-2,15,260; 100-4,12,30; 100-4,12,90.3; 100-4,14,10

25515

25515 Open treatment of radial shaft fracture, includes internal fixation, when performed

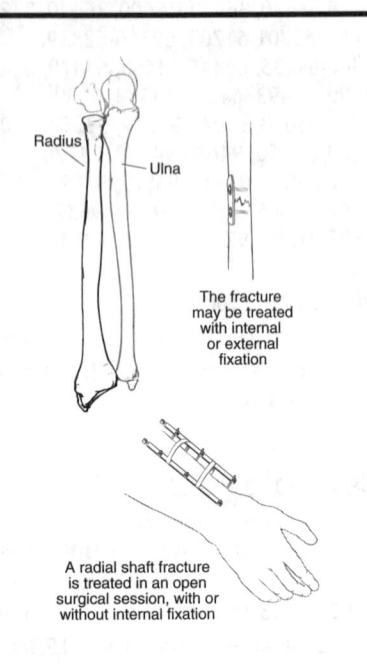

Radius
Ulna
The fracture may be treated with internal or external fixation

A radial shaft fracture is treated in an open surgical session, with or without internal fixation

Explanation
The physician treats a radial shaft fracture. If internal fixation is required, the physician may use plate and screw fixation or a medullary nail. A plate and screw fixation is described. If the fracture is in the lower half of the radius, an anterior forearm incision is made. If the fracture is in the upper half of the radius, a posterior forearm incision is made. Dissection exposes the fractured fragments. The physician uses bone-holding forceps to reduce the fracture. A plate of appropriate length is selected and centered over the fracture. Plates with five or six holes are usually required. The screws are inserted. The incision is repaired in layers. The deep fascia is not closed because of the potential of developing compartment syndrome. Depending on the rigidity of the fixation, a cast or splint may be applied.

Coding Tips
According to CPT guidelines, cast application or strapping (including removal) is only reported as a replacement procedure or when the cast application or strapping is an initial service performed without a restorative treatment or procedure. See "Application of Casts and Strapping" in the CPT book in the Surgery Section, under the Musculoskeletal system. For radiology services, see 73090. For closed treatment of a radial shaft fracture, see 25500–25505. For open treatment of a radial shaft fracture with open treatment of a radio-ulnar dislocation, see 25526. For treatment of a radial and ulnar shaft fracture, see 25560–25575. For an ulnar shaft fracture alone, see 25530–25545.

ICD-9-CM Procedural
- 79.22 Open reduction of fracture of radius and ulna without internal fixation
- 79.32 Open reduction of fracture of radius and ulna with internal fixation

Anesthesia
25515 01830

ICD-9-CM Diagnostic
- 733.19 Pathologic fracture of other specified site
- 733.82 Nonunion of fracture
- 813.21 Closed fracture of shaft of radius (alone)
- 813.31 Open fracture of shaft of radius (alone)

Terms To Know
comminuted fracture. Any type of fracture in which the bone is splintered or crushed, resulting in multiple bone fragments.

fascia. Fibrous sheet or band of tissue that envelops organs, muscles, and groupings of muscles.

nonunion. Failure of two ends of a fracture to mend or completely heal.

open wound. Opening or break of the skin.

pathologic fracture. Break in bone due to a disease process that weakens the bone structure, such as osteoporosis, osteomalacia, or neoplasia, and not traumatic injury.

CCI Version 16.3
01810, 01820, 0213T, 0216T, 0228T, 0230T, 20650, 20902, 24300, 24495, 25020, 25024-25025, 25115-25119, 25259-25260, 25270, 25295, 25500-25505, 29058-29085, 29105-29126, 29260, 29700-29715, 36000, 36400-36410, 36420-36430, 36440, 36600, 36640, 37202, 43752, 51701-51703, 62310-62319, 64400-64435, 64445-64450, 64479, 64483, 64490, 64493, 64505-64530, 64702-64726, 69990, 93000-93010, 93040-93042, 93318, 94002, 94200, 94250, 94680-94690, 94770, 95812-95816, 95819, 95822, 95829, 95955, 96360, 96365, 96372, 96374-96376, 97597-97598, 97602-97606, 99148-99149, 99150

Note: These CCI edits are used for Medicare. Other payers may reimburse on codes listed above.

Medicare Edits

	Fac RVU	Non-Fac RVU	FUD	Assist
25515	19.38	19.38	90	80

Medicare References: 100-2,15,260; 100-4,12,30; 100-4,12,90.3; 100-4,14,10

25520

25520 Closed treatment of radial shaft fracture and closed treatment of dislocation of distal radioulnar joint (Galeazzi fracture/dislocation)

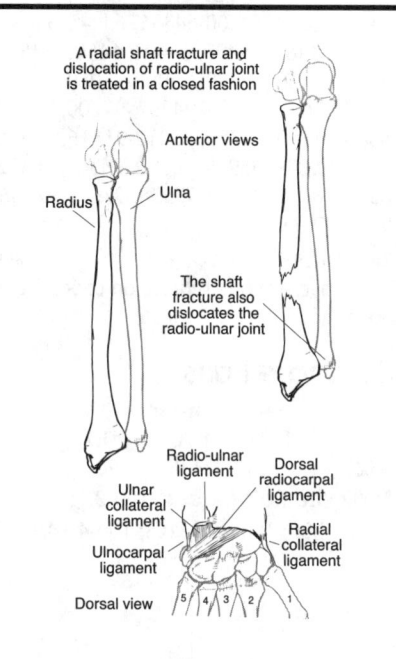

Explanation

The physician treats a radial shaft fracture and a dislocation of the distal radio-ulnar joint. No incisions are made. The physician may reduce the fracture and dislocation by manipulation with traction force. A long arm cast is applied to immobilize the elbow and wrist.

Coding Tips

According to CPT guidelines, cast application or strapping (including removal) is only reported as a replacement procedure or when the cast application or strapping is an initial service performed without a restorative treatment or procedure. See "Application of Casts and Strapping" in the CPT book in the Surgery Section, under the Musculoskeletal system. Local anesthesia is included in this service. However, this procedure may be performed under general anesthesia, depending on the age and/or condition of the patient. For radiology services, see 73090. For closed treatment of a radial shaft fracture, see 25500–25505. For open treatment of a radial shaft fracture, with open treatment of a radio-ulnar dislocation, see 25526. For treatment of a radial and ulnar shaft fracture, see 25560–25575. For an ulnar shaft fracture alone, see 25530–25545.

ICD-9-CM Procedural

- 79.02 Closed reduction of fracture of radius and ulna without internal fixation
- 79.79 Closed reduction of dislocation of other specified site, except temporomandibular

Anesthesia

25520 01820

ICD-9-CM Diagnostic

- 733.19 Pathologic fracture of other specified site
- 813.00 Unspecified fracture of radius and ulna, upper end of forearm, closed
- 813.20 Unspecified closed fracture of shaft of radius or ulna
- 813.21 Closed fracture of shaft of radius (alone)
- 833.01 Closed dislocation of distal radioulnar (joint)

Terms To Know

closed fracture. Break in a bone without a concomitant opening in the skin. A closed fracture is coded when the type of fracture is not specified.

dislocation. Displacement of a bone in relation to its neighboring tissue, especially a joint.

distal. Located farther away from a specified reference point.

fracture. Break in bone or cartilage.

Galeazzi fracture. Break of the radius proximal to the wrist with a distal ulnar dislocation.

CCI Version 16.3

01810, 01820, 0213T, 0216T, 0228T, 0230T, 24300, 25259, 29058-29085, 29105-29126, 29260, 29700-29715, 36000, 36400-36410, 36420-36430, 36440, 36600, 36640, 37202, 43752, 51701-51703, 62310-62319, 64400-64435, 64445-64450, 64479, 64483, 64490, 64493, 64505-64530, 69990, 93000-93010, 93040-93042, 93318, 94002, 94200, 94250, 94680-94690, 94770, 95812-95816, 95819, 95822, 95829, 95955, 96360, 96365, 96372, 96374-96376, 97597-97598, 97602-97606, 99148-99149, 99150

Note: These CCI edits are used for Medicare. Other payers may reimburse on codes listed above.

Medicare Edits

	Fac RVU	Non-Fac RVU	FUD	Assist
25520	15.2	15.98	90	N/A

Medicare References: 100-2,15,260; 100-4,12,30; 100-4,12,90.3; 100-4,14,10

25525

25525 Open treatment of radial shaft fracture, includes internal fixation, when performed, and closed treatment of distal radioulnar joint dislocation (Galeazzi fracture/dislocation), includes percutaneous skeletal fixation, when performed

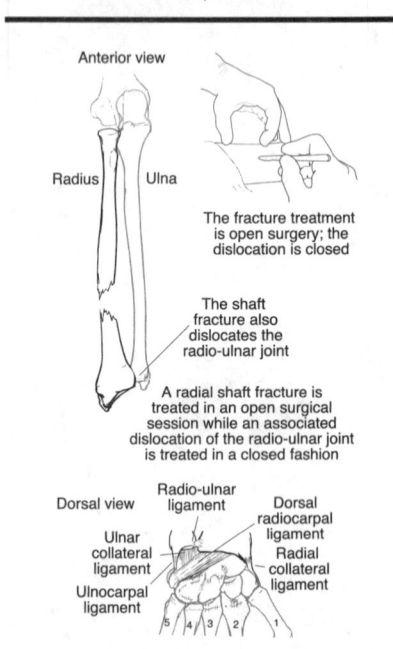

Explanation

The physician makes a 5 to 6 inch longitudinal incision over the anterior aspect of the forearm and centered over the fracture. Dissection exposes the pronator quadratus muscle, which is freed from the radius. The physician reduces the fracture with bone-holding forceps. A plate of appropriate length may be selected and centered over the fracture. The screws are inserted. The pronator quadratus muscle is reattached. The incision is repaired in layers with sutures, staples, and/or Steri-strips. The deep fascia is not closed. The physician places the arm in a cast. The physician may also apply percutaneous skeletal fixation. Kirschner wires are inserted through small stab incisions through the radius and into the ulna to stabilize the radius.

Coding Tips

According to CPT guidelines, cast application or strapping (including removal) is only reported as a replacement procedure or when the cast application or strapping is an initial service performed without a restorative treatment or procedure. See "Application of Casts and Strapping" in the CPT book in the Surgery Section, under the Musculoskeletal system. For radiology services, see 73090. For open treatment of a radial shaft fracture, with open treatment of a radio-ulnar dislocation, see 25526. For closed treatment of a radial shaft fracture, see 25500–25505. For closed treatment of a radial shaft fracture, with closed treatment of a radio-ulnar dislocation, see 25520. For treatment of a radial and ulnar shaft fracture, see 25560–25575. For an ulnar shaft fracture alone, see 25530–25545.

ICD-9-CM Procedural

- 79.22 Open reduction of fracture of radius and ulna without internal fixation
- 79.32 Open reduction of fracture of radius and ulna with internal fixation
- 79.73 Closed reduction of dislocation of wrist
- 84.71 Application of external fixator device, monoplanar system
- 84.72 Application of external fixator device, ring system
- 84.73 Application of hybrid external fixator device

Anesthesia

25525 01830

ICD-9-CM Diagnostic

- 733.19 Pathologic fracture of other specified site
- 813.21 Closed fracture of shaft of radius (alone)
- 813.31 Open fracture of shaft of radius (alone)
- 833.01 Closed dislocation of distal radioulnar (joint)
- 833.11 Open dislocation of distal radioulnar (joint)

Terms To Know

dissection. Separating by cutting tissue or body structures apart.

forceps. Tool used for grasping or compressing tissue.

fracture types. There are three basic degrees of fracture: type I: a small crack in the bone without displacement; type II: a fracture in which the bone is slightly displaced; type III: a fracture in which there are more than three broken pieces of bone that cannot fit together.

Galeazzi fracture. Break of the radius proximal to the wrist with a distal ulnar dislocation.

percutaneous skeletal fixation. Treatment that is neither open nor closed. In this procedure, the injury site is not directly visualized. Instead, fixation devices (pins, screws) are placed to stabilize the dislocation using x-ray guidance.

CCI Version 16.3

01810, 01820, 0213T, 0216T, 0228T, 0230T, 20650, 20902, 24300, 24495, 25115-25119, 25259, 25295, 25520, 29058-29085, 29105-29126, 29260, 29700-29715, 36000, 36400-36410, 36420-36430, 36440, 36600, 36640, 37202, 43752, 51701-51703, 62310-62319, 64400-64435, 64445-64450, 64479, 64483, 64490, 64493, 64505-64530, 64702-64726, 69990, 93000-93010, 93040-93042, 93318, 94002, 94200, 94250, 94680-94690, 94770, 95812-95816, 95819, 95822, 95829, 95955, 96360, 96365, 96372, 96374-96376, 97597-97598, 97602-97606, 99148-99149, 99150

Note: These CCI edits are used for Medicare. Other payers may reimburse on codes listed above.

Medicare Edits

	Fac RVU	Non-Fac RVU	FUD	Assist
25525	23.01	23.01	90	80

Medicare References: 100-2,15,260; 100-4,12,30; 100-4,12,90.3; 100-4,14,10

25526

25526 Open treatment of radial shaft fracture, includes internal fixation, when performed, and open treatment of distal radioulnar joint dislocation (Galeazzi fracture/dislocation), includes internal fixation, when performed, includes repair of triangular fibrocartilage complex

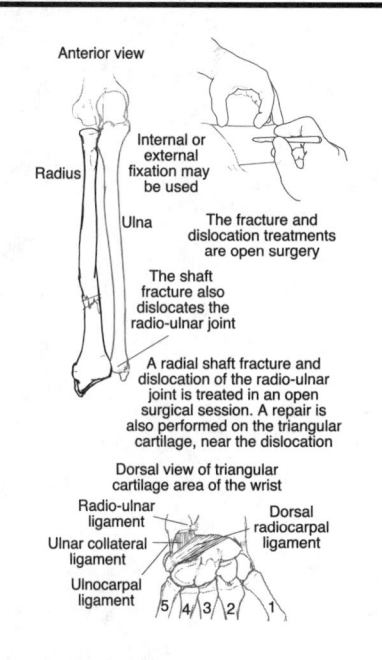

Explanation

The physician treats a radial shaft fracture via an open approach, using internal fixation when required. This procedure includes repair of the triangular fibrocartilage complex. After the affected hand is suspended in finger traps, the physician reduces the fracture and confirms the reduction radiographically. Under separately reportable radiographic guidance, a Kirschner wire is inserted from the tip of the radial styloid obliquely across the fracture site. A second pin is inserted in a slightly more longitudinal direction. Finger traps are removed and the pins are cut off approximately 2 cm above the skin and bent at right angles. If tears are present in the fibrocartilage complex, they are repaired with sutures. Skin incisions may be made to prevent skin tethering. A dressing and splint are applied.

Coding Tips

According to CPT guidelines, cast application or strapping (including removal) is only reported as a replacement procedure or when the cast application or strapping is an initial service performed without a restorative treatment or procedure. See "Application of Casts and Strapping" in the CPT book in the Surgery Section, under the Musculoskeletal system. For radiology services, see 73090. For open treatment of a radial shaft fracture, with closed treatment of a radio-ulnar dislocation, see 25525. For closed treatment of a radial shaft fracture, see 25500–25505. For closed treatment of a radial shaft fracture, with closed treatment of a radio-ulnar dislocation, see 25520. For treatment of a radial and ulnar shaft fracture, see 25560–25575. For an ulnar shaft fracture alone, see 25530–25545.

ICD-9-CM Procedural

79.22 Open reduction of fracture of radius and ulna without internal fixation
79.32 Open reduction of fracture of radius and ulna with internal fixation
79.83 Open reduction of dislocation of wrist

Anesthesia
25526 01830

ICD-9-CM Diagnostic

733.19 Pathologic fracture of other specified site
813.21 Closed fracture of shaft of radius (alone)
813.31 Open fracture of shaft of radius (alone)
833.01 Closed dislocation of distal radioulnar (joint)
833.11 Open dislocation of distal radioulnar (joint)

Terms To Know

fracture types. There are three basic degrees of fracture: type I: a small crack in the bone without displacement; type II: a fracture in which the bone is slightly displaced; type III: a fracture in which there are more than three broken pieces of bone that cannot fit together.

Galeazzi fracture. Break of the radius proximal to the wrist with a distal ulnar dislocation.

open fracture. Exposed break in a bone, always considered compound due to its high risk of infection from the open wound leading to the fracture. Broken bone ends may protrude through the skin and contaminants or foreign bodies are often embedded in the tissues.

CCI Version 16.3

01810, 01820, 0213T, 0216T, 0228T, 0230T, 20650, 20902, 24300, 24495, 25020, 25024-25025, 25100-25107, 25115-25119, 25259, 25295, 25520, 29058-29085, 29105-29126, 29260, 29700-29715, 36000, 36400-36410, 36420-36430, 36440, 36600, 36640, 37202, 43752, 51701-51703, 62310-62319, 64400-64435, 64445-64450, 64479, 64483, 64490, 64493, 64505-64530, 64702-64726, 69990, 93000-93010, 93040-93042, 93318, 94002, 94200, 94250, 94680-94690, 94770, 95812-95816, 95819, 95822, 95829, 95955, 96360, 96365, 96372, 96374-96376, 97597-97598, 97602-97606, 99148-99149, 99150

Note: These CCI edits are used for Medicare. Other payers may reimburse on codes listed above.

Medicare Edits

	Fac RVU	Non-Fac RVU	FUD	Assist
25526	28.34	28.34	90	80

Medicare References: 100-2,15,260; 100-4,12,30; 100-4,12,90.3; 100-4,14,10

25530-25535

25530 Closed treatment of ulnar shaft fracture; without manipulation
25535 with manipulation

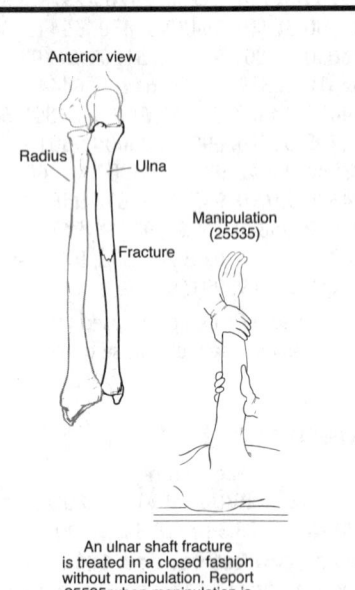

An ulnar shaft fracture is treated in a closed fashion without manipulation. Report 25535 when manipulation is required to treat the fracture

Explanation

The physician treats an ulnar shaft fracture without manipulation in 25530 or with manipulation in 25535. No incisions are made. If manipulation is required, the physician uses a combination of traction and countertraction with manual manipulation of the fracture. The patient is placed in a long arm cast with the elbow at 90 degrees of flexion. A functional splint or brace is applied.

Coding Tips

According to CPT guidelines, cast application or strapping (including removal) is only reported as a replacement procedure or when the cast application or strapping is an initial service performed without a restorative treatment or procedure. See "Application of Casts and Strapping" in the CPT book in the Surgery Section, under the Musculoskeletal system. In 25535, local anesthesia is included in the service. However, this procedure may be performed under general anesthesia, depending on the age and/or condition of the patient. For radiology services, see 73090, and add modifier 26 to identify the professional component only, unless the physician owns the equipment. For open treatment of an ulnar shaft fracture, see 25545. For treatment of radial shaft fractures, see 25500–25526. For treatment of radial and ulnar shaft fractures, see 25560–25575.

ICD-9-CM Procedural

79.02 Closed reduction of fracture of radius and ulna without internal fixation
93.53 Application of other cast

Anesthesia
01820

ICD-9-CM Diagnostic

733.19 Pathologic fracture of other specified site
813.22 Closed fracture of shaft of ulna (alone)

Terms To Know

closed fracture. Break in a bone without a concomitant opening in the skin. A closed fracture is coded when the type of fracture is not specified.

flexion. Act of bending or being bent.

fracture. Break in bone or cartilage.

pathologic fracture. Break in bone due to a disease process that weakens the bone structure, such as osteoporosis, osteomalacia, or neoplasia, and not traumatic injury.

CCI Version 16.3

01810, 01820, 0213T, 0216T, 0228T, 0230T, 24300, 25259, 29058-29085, 29105-29126, 29260, 29700-29715, 36000, 36400-36410, 36420-36430, 36440, 36600, 36640, 37202, 43752, 51701-51703, 62310-62319, 64400-64435, 64445-64450, 64479, 64483, 64490, 64493, 64505-64530, 69990, 93000-93010, 93040-93042, 93318, 94002, 94200, 94250, 94680-94690, 94770, 95812-95816, 95819, 95822, 95829, 95955, 96360, 96365, 96372, 96374-96376, 97597-97598, 97602-97606, 99148-99149, 99150

Also not with 25530: 12002
Also not with 25535: 25530, J0670, J2001
Note: These CCI edits are used for Medicare. Other payers may reimburse on codes listed above.

Medicare Edits

	Fac RVU	Non-Fac RVU	FUD	Assist
25530	6.56	7.27	90	N/A
25535	12.95	13.89	90	N/A

Medicare References: 100-2,15,260; 100-4,12,30; 100-4,12,90.3; 100-4,14,10

25545

25545 Open treatment of ulnar shaft fracture, includes internal fixation, when performed

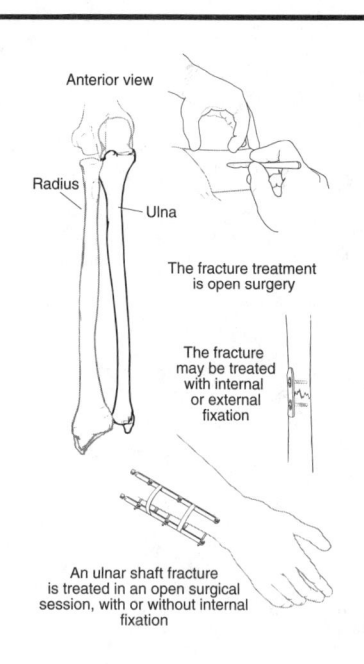

Explanation
The physician makes an incision along the subcutaneous border of the ulna, exposing the shaft fracture. The physician reduces the fracture with bone-holding forceps. If internal fixation is required, a plate of appropriate length is selected and centered over the fracture. The screws are inserted. Only the subcutaneous tissue is closed. The skin incision is repaired with sutures, staples, and/or Steri-strips. Depending on the rigidity of the fixation, a cast or splint may be applied.

Coding Tips
According to CPT guidelines, cast application or strapping (including removal) is only reported as a replacement procedure or when the cast application or strapping is an initial service performed without a restorative treatment or procedure. See "Application of Casts and Strapping" in the CPT book in the Surgery Section, under the Musculoskeletal system. Local anesthesia is included in the service. However, this procedure may be performed under general anesthesia, depending on the age and/or condition of the patient. For radiology services, see 73090. For closed treatment of an ulnar shaft fracture, without manipulation, see 25530; with manipulation, see 25535. For treatment of radial shaft fractures, see 25500–25526. For treatment of radial and ulnar shaft fractures, see 25560–25575.

ICD-9-CM Procedural
- 79.22 Open reduction of fracture of radius and ulna without internal fixation
- 79.32 Open reduction of fracture of radius and ulna with internal fixation

Anesthesia
25545 01830

ICD-9-CM Diagnostic
- 733.19 Pathologic fracture of other specified site
- 733.81 Malunion of fracture
- 733.82 Nonunion of fracture
- 813.22 Closed fracture of shaft of ulna (alone)
- 813.32 Open fracture of shaft of ulna (alone)

Terms To Know

malunion. Fracture that has united in a faulty position due to inadequate reduction of the original fracture, insufficient holding of a previously well-reduced fracture, contracture of the soft tissues, or comminuted or osteoporotic bone causing a slow disintegration of the fracture.

nonunion. Failure of two ends of a fracture to mend or completely heal.

open fracture. Exposed break in a bone, always considered compound due to its high risk of infection from the open wound leading to the fracture. Broken bone ends may protrude through the skin and contaminants or foreign bodies are often embedded in the tissues.

pathologic fracture. Break in bone due to a disease process that weakens the bone structure, such as osteoporosis, osteomalacia, or neoplasia, and not traumatic injury.

CCI Version 16.3
01810, 01820, 0213T, 0216T, 0228T, 0230T, 20520-20525, 20650, 20902, 24300, 24495, 25020, 25024-25025, 25115-25119, 25248, 25259, 25295, 25530-25535, 29058-29085, 29105-29126, 29260, 29700-29715, 36000, 36400-36410, 36420-36430, 36440, 36600, 36640, 37202, 43752, 51701-51703, 62310-62319, 64400-64435, 64445-64450, 64479, 64483, 64490, 64493, 64505-64530, 64702-64726, 69990, 93000-93010, 93040-93042, 93318, 94002, 94200, 94250, 94680-94690, 94770, 95812-95816, 95819, 95822, 95829, 95955, 96360, 96365, 96372, 96374-96376, 97597-97598, 97602-97606, 99148-99149, 99150

Note: These CCI edits are used for Medicare. Other payers may reimburse on codes listed above.

Medicare Edits

	Fac RVU	Non-Fac RVU	FUD	Assist
25545	18.08	18.08	90	80

Medicare References: 100-2,15,260; 100-4,12,30; 100-4,12,90.3; 100-4,14,10

25560-25565

25560 Closed treatment of radial and ulnar shaft fractures; without manipulation
25565 with manipulation

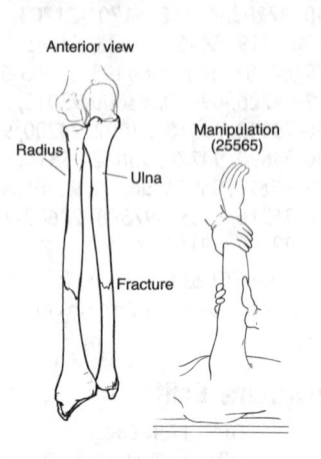

A shaft fracture of both radius and ulna is treated in a closed fashion. Report 25565 when manipulation is required to treat the fracture

Explanation

For undisplaced and stable fractures, the physician immobilizes the elbow and wrist with a long arm cast. Separately reportable x-rays are taken to confirm that displacement does not occur. In 25565, the fractures are displaced and manual reduction is required. Analgesia or a certain degree of sedation may be necessary. The physician uses a combination of traction and manual manipulation to reduce the fractures. A long arm cast immobilizes the elbow and wrist.

Coding Tips

According to CPT guidelines, cast application or strapping (including removal) is only reported as a replacement procedure or when the cast application or strapping is an initial service performed without a restorative treatment or procedure. See "Application of Casts and Strapping" in the CPT book in the Surgery Section, under the Musculoskeletal system. In 25565, local anesthesia is included in the service. However, this procedure may be performed under general anesthesia, depending on the age and/or condition of the patient. For radiology services, see 73090. For open treatment of radial and ulnar shaft fractures, see 25574 and 25575.

ICD-9-CM Procedural

79.02 Closed reduction of fracture of radius and ulna without internal fixation

93.53 Application of other cast

Anesthesia
01820

ICD-9-CM Diagnostic

733.19 Pathologic fracture of other specified site
813.23 Closed fracture of shaft of radius with ulna

Terms To Know

fracture. Break in bone or cartilage.

fracture types. There are three basic degrees of fracture: type I: a small crack in the bone without displacement; type II: a fracture in which the bone is slightly displaced; type III: a fracture in which there are more than three broken pieces of bone that cannot fit together.

CCI Version 16.3

01810, 01820, 0213T, 0216T, 0228T, 0230T, 24300, 25259, 29058-29085, 29105-29126, 29260, 29700-29715, 36000, 36400-36410, 36420-36430, 36440, 36600, 36640, 37202, 43752, 51701-51703, 62310-62319, 64400-64435, 64445-64450, 64479, 64483, 64490, 64493, 64505-64530, 69990, 93000-93010, 93040-93042, 93318, 94002, 94200, 94250, 94680-94690, 94770, 95812-95816, 95819, 95822, 95829, 95955, 96360, 96365, 96372, 96374-96376, 97597-97598, 97602-97606, 99148-99149, 99150

Also not with 25565: 25560, 76000-76001, J0670, J2001

Note: These CCI edits are used for Medicare. Other payers may reimburse on codes listed above.

Medicare Edits

	Fac RVU	Non-Fac RVU	FUD	Assist
25560	6.87	7.62	90	N/A
25565	13.59	14.9	90	N/A

Medicare References: 100-2,15,260; 100-4,12,30; 100-4,12,90.3; 100-4,14,10

25574-25575

25574 Open treatment of radial AND ulnar shaft fractures, with internal fixation, when performed; of radius OR ulna
25575 of radius AND ulna

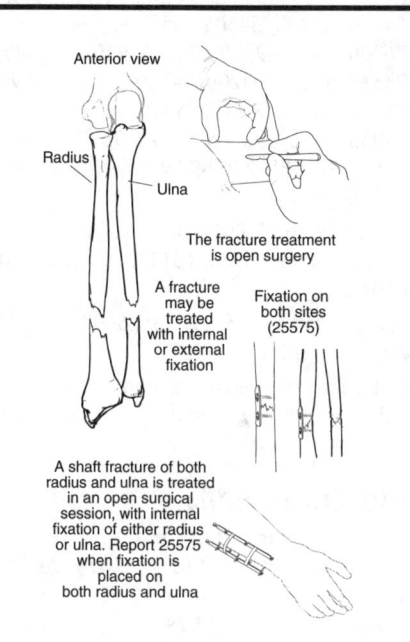

Explanation
When both the radius and ulna are fractured, the physician exposes and reduces both fractures prior to fixation. Separate incisions along the forearm may be needed to expose the fracture. In 25574, only one fracture is stabilized, requiring only one incision. The other fracture is stable and does not require fixation. In 25575, both radial and ulnar fractures require fixation, usually requiring separate incisions. Once the fracture site is exposed and reduced, internal fixation is applied. A plate of appropriate length is selected and centered over the fracture. The physician inserts the screws. The incisions are repaired in layers with sutures, staples, and/or Steri-strips. The deep fascia is not closed, preventing the development of compartment syndrome. Depending upon the rigidity of the fixation, a cast or splint may be applied.

Coding Tips
According to CPT guidelines, cast application or strapping (including removal) is only reported as a replacement procedure or when the cast application or strapping is an initial service performed without a restorative treatment or procedure. See "Application of Casts and Strapping" in the CPT book in the Surgery Section, under the Musculoskeletal system. In 25575, local anesthesia is included in the service. However, this procedure may be performed under general anesthesia, depending on the age and/or condition of the patient. For radiology services, see 73090. For closed treatment of radial and ulnar shaft fractures, see 25560 and 25565.

ICD-9-CM Procedural
79.32 Open reduction of fracture of radius and ulna with internal fixation

Anesthesia
01830

ICD-9-CM Diagnostic
733.19 Pathologic fracture of other specified site
813.23 Closed fracture of shaft of radius with ulna
813.33 Open fracture of shaft of radius with ulna
927.10 Crushing injury of forearm — (Use additional code to identify any associated injuries: 800-829, 850.0-854.1, 860.0-869.1)

Terms To Know
comminuted fracture. Any type of fracture in which the bone is splintered or crushed, resulting in multiple bone fragments.

fascia. Fibrous sheet or band of tissue that envelops organs, muscles, and groupings of muscles.

soft tissue. Nonepithelial tissues outside of the skeleton that includes subcutaneous adipose tissue, fibrous tissue, fascia, muscles, blood and lymph vessels, and peripheral nervous system tissue.

CCI Version 16.3
01810, 01820, 0213T, 0216T, 0228T, 0230T, 20650, 20902, 24300, 24495, 25020, 25024-25025, 25115-25119, 25259, 25295, 25560-25565, 29058-29085, 29105-29126, 29260, 29700-29715, 36000, 36400-36410, 36420-36430, 36440, 36600, 36640, 37202, 43752, 51701-51703, 62310-62319, 64400-64435, 64445-64450, 64479, 64483, 64490, 64493, 64505-64530, 64702-64726, 69990, 93000-93010, 93040-93042, 93318, 94002, 94200, 94250, 94680-94690, 94770, 95812-95816, 95819, 95822, 95829, 95955, 96360, 96365, 96372, 96374-96376, 97597-97598, 97602-97606, 99148-99149, 99150

Also not with 25575: 13121, 25574

Note: These CCI edits are used for Medicare. Other payers may reimburse on codes listed above.

Medicare Edits

	Fac RVU	Non-Fac RVU	FUD	Assist
25574	19.44	19.44	90	80
25575	26.15	26.15	90	80

Medicare References: 100-2,15,260; 100-4,12,30; 100-4,12,90.3; 100-4,14,10

25600-25605

25600 Closed treatment of distal radial fracture (eg, Colles or Smith type) or epiphyseal separation, includes closed treatment of fracture of ulnar styloid, when performed; without manipulation
25605 with manipulation

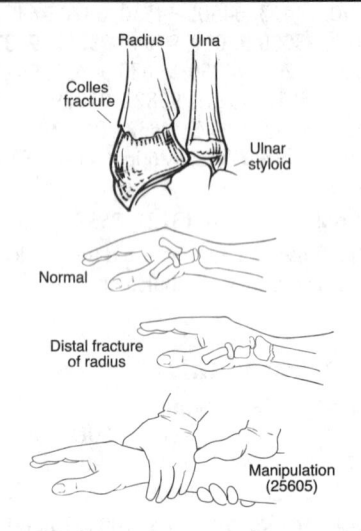

A fracture of the distal radius, or dislocation of the epiphysis, is treated in an open fashion, with or without an associated fracture of the ulnar styloid. Report 25605 when manipulation is required to reduce the fracture or dislocation

Explanation

The physician treats a distal radial fracture. A Colles' fracture is a fracture of the distal radius with dorsal displacement. A Smith fracture is palmar displacement of the distal radius. The ulnar styloid is usually fractured. If good alignment and correct angulation of the distal radial articular surface is present, the physician immobilizes the wrist and forearm in a cast or splint until the fracture or epiphyseal separation is stable. In 25605, manipulation is required to reduce an unstable and/or displaced fracture or epiphyseal separation. For either 25600 or 25605, closed treatment of the ulnar styloid may be performed. Analgesia or sedation may be necessary to achieve reduction. The physician uses a combination of longitudinal distraction of the fracture and manipulation of the distal fragment to achieve reduction. The wrist and forearm are placed in a cast or splint until the fracture or epiphyseal separation is stable.

Coding Tips

According to CPT guidelines, cast application or strapping (including removal) is only reported as a replacement procedure or when the cast application or strapping is an initial service performed without a restorative treatment or procedure. See "Application of Casts and Strapping" in the CPT book in the Surgery Section, under the Musculoskeletal system. In 25605, local anesthesia is included in the service. However, this procedure may be performed under general anesthesia, depending on the age and/or condition of the patient. For radiology services, see 73090. For percutaneous skeletal fixation, see 25606. For open treatment of a distal radial fracture, see 25607–25609. For treatment of radial shaft fractures, see 25500–25515.

ICD-9-CM Procedural

- 79.02 Closed reduction of fracture of radius and ulna without internal fixation
- 79.42 Closed reduction of separated epiphysis of radius and ulna
- 93.53 Application of other cast
- 93.54 Application of splint

Anesthesia
01820

ICD-9-CM Diagnostic

- 732.9 Unspecified osteochondropathy
- 733.12 Pathologic fracture of distal radius and ulna
- 813.40 Unspecified closed fracture of lower end of forearm
- 813.41 Closed Colles' fracture
- 813.42 Other closed fractures of distal end of radius (alone)
- 813.44 Closed fracture of lower end of radius with ulna
- 813.45 Torus fracture of radius (alone)
- 813.47 Torus fracture of radius and ulna

Terms To Know

closed fracture. Break in a bone without a concomitant opening in the skin. A closed fracture is coded when the type of fracture is not specified.

distal. Located farther away from a specified reference point.

dorsal. Pertaining to the back or posterior aspect.

epiphysis. End of a long bone.

osteochondropathy. Any condition in which the bone and cartilage are affected, or in which endochondral ossification occurs.

pathologic fracture. Break in bone due to a disease process that weakens the bone structure, such as osteoporosis, osteomalacia, or neoplasia, and not traumatic injury.

torus fracture. Buckling or bowing of the bone with little or no displacement at the end and no breakage, usually occurring in children due to softer bone tissue.

CCI Version 16.3

01810, 01820, 0213T, 0216T, 0228T, 0230T, 24300, 25259, 25650, 29058-29085, 29260, 29700-29715, 36000, 36400-36410, 36420-36430, 36440, 36600, 36640, 37202, 43752, 51701-51703, 62310-62319, 64400-64435, 64445-64450, 64479, 64483, 64490, 64493, 64505-64530, 69990, 76000-76001, 93000-93010, 93040-93042, 93318, 94002, 94200, 94250, 94680-94690, 94770, 95812-95816, 95819, 95822, 95829, 95955, 96360, 96365, 96372, 96374-96376, 97597-97598, 97602-97606, 99148-99149, 99150

Also not with 25600: 12001-12004, 12032-12034, 13120, 13132, 29105-29130, G0168

Also not with 25605: 12005, 25600, 29105-29126, J0670, J2001

Note: These CCI edits are used for Medicare. Other payers may reimburse on codes listed above.

Medicare Edits

	Fac RVU	Non-Fac RVU	FUD	Assist
25600	7.46	8.2	90	N/A
25605	16.81	17.78	90	N/A

Medicare References: 100-2,15,260; 100-4,12,30; 100-4,12,90.3; 100-4,14,10

25606

25606 Percutaneous skeletal fixation of distal radial fracture or epiphyseal separation

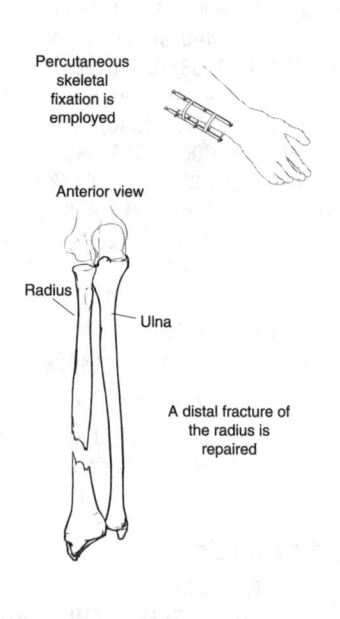

Explanation
The physician treats a fracture of the distal radius. The physician first manipulates the area to reduce the fracture. The physician applies a combination of traction on the wrist and manipulation of the distal radius to reduce the fracture. An assistant maintains the reduction. Using a drill, the physician inserts two Kirschner wires percutaneously (directly through the skin) through the radial styloid, across the fracture, and into the opposite metaphyseal cortex of the ulna. The Kirschner wires are cut off just beneath the skin. The arm is immobilized in a cast. The wires are removed in six weeks. If there is a severely comminuted fracture of the distal radius that is not suitable for percutaneous Kirschner wire stabilization alone, the physician may apply a traction cast or an Ace-Colles external fixator. For application of a traction cast, the fracture or separation is first reduced and a Steinmann pin is inserted transversely through the proximal elbow. A second pin is inserted transversely through the bases of the second and third metacarpals. A plaster cast is applied above and below the elbow and incorporates the two pins. The pins and cast are left in place for approximately eight weeks. With an external fixator, the fracture or separation is first reduced by manipulation and traction. The external fixator is applied to the forearm and wrist to stabilize the fracture or separation.

Coding Tips
Do not report 25606 in conjuction with 25650. For percutaneous treatment of ulnar styloid fracture, see 25651. For open treatment of ulnar styloid fracture, see 25652.

ICD-9-CM Procedural
- 79.12 Closed reduction of fracture of radius and ulna with internal fixation
- 79.42 Closed reduction of separated epiphysis of radius and ulna

Anesthesia
25606 01820

ICD-9-CM Diagnostic
- 732.9 Unspecified osteochondropathy
- 733.12 Pathologic fracture of distal radius and ulna
- 813.41 Closed Colles' fracture
- 813.42 Other closed fractures of distal end of radius (alone)
- 813.44 Closed fracture of lower end of radius with ulna

Terms To Know
fixation. Act or condition of being attached, secured, fastened, or held in position.

manipulation. Skillful treatment by hand to reduce fractures and dislocations, or provide therapy through forceful passive movement of a joint beyond its active limit of motion.

percutaneous skeletal fixation. Treatment that is neither open nor closed. In this procedure, the injury site is not directly visualized. Instead, fixation devices (pins, screws) are placed to stabilize the dislocation using x-ray guidance.

reduction. Correction of a fracture, dislocation, or hernia to the correct place and alignment, manually or by surgery.

traction. Drawing out or holding tension on an area by applying a direct therapeutic pulling force.

CCI Version 16.3
01810, 01820, 0213T, 0216T, 0228T, 0230T, 12001, 13121, 15851, 20650, 24300, 25230, 25259, 25600-25605❖, 25650, 29058-29085, 29105-29126, 29260, 36000, 36400-36410, 36420-36430, 36440, 36600, 36640, 37202, 43752, 51701-51703, 62310-62319, 64400-64435, 64445-64450, 64479, 64483, 64490, 64493, 64505-64530, 64708, 64718, 69990, 76000-76001, 93000-93010, 93040-93042, 93318, 94002, 94200, 94250, 94680-94690, 94770, 95812-95816, 95819, 95822, 95829, 95955, 96360, 96365, 96372, 96374-96376, 97597-97598, 97602-97606, 99148-99149, 99150, G0168, J2001

Note: These CCI edits are used for Medicare. Other payers may reimburse on codes listed above.

Medicare Edits

	Fac RVU	Non-Fac RVU	FUD	Assist
25606	19.3	19.3	90	N/A

Medicare References: None

25607-25609

25607 Open treatment of distal radial extra-articular fracture or epiphyseal separation, with internal fixation

25608 Open treatment of distal radial intra-articular fracture or epiphyseal separation; with internal fixation of 2 fragments

25609 with internal fixation of 3 or more fragments

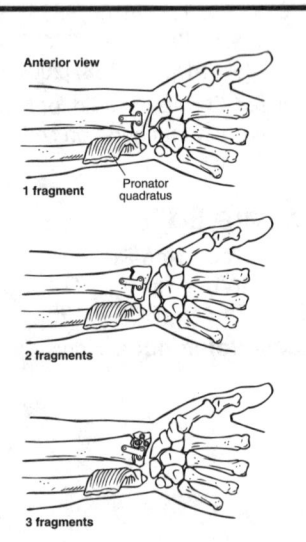

Internal fixation is required to repair a fracture of the bones of the wrist

Report 25608 if internal fixation treats two fragments or 25609 if three or more fragments are treated

Explanation

The physician makes a 7.5 cm longitudinal incision along the anterolateral aspect of the distal forearm. The physician exposes the fracture by dissecting between the planes of muscles and tendons of the lateral wrist area while protecting the median nerve. The pronator quadratus muscle is severed from the radius. The physician reduces the fracture or separation. A small T-plate is fixed to the proximal fragment with one or two screws. Usually no screw is inserted through the distal part of the plate since it acts as a buttress and helps hold the fracture in reduction. Direct visualization and separately reportable x-rays are used to confirm correct reduction and restoration of the joint surface. The pronator quadratus is replaced at its origin on the radius. The incision is repaired in layers using sutures, staples, and/or Steri-strips. The arm is immobilized in a cast. Report 25607 for open treatment of the fracture with internal fixation; 25608 for fracture repair in which two fragments of bone in the joint receive internal fixation; and 25609 for fracture repair in which three or more fragments of bone in the joint receive internal fixation.

Coding Tips

Do not report 25607, 25608, 25609 in conjunction with 25650. For percutaneous treatment of ulnar styloid fracture, see 25651. For open treatment of ulnar styloid fracture, see 25652.

ICD-9-CM Procedural

- **79.32** Open reduction of fracture of radius and ulna with internal fixation
- **79.52** Open reduction of separated epiphysis of radius and ulna

Anesthesia

01830

ICD-9-CM Diagnostic

- **732.9** Unspecified osteochondropathy
- **733.12** Pathologic fracture of distal radius and ulna
- **733.82** Nonunion of fracture
- **813.41** Closed Colles' fracture
- **813.42** Other closed fractures of distal end of radius (alone)
- **813.44** Closed fracture of lower end of radius with ulna
- **813.51** Open Colles' fracture
- **813.52** Other open fractures of distal end of radius (alone)
- **813.54** Open fracture of lower end of radius with ulna

Terms To Know

fixation. Act or condition of being attached, secured, fastened, or held in position.

manipulation. Skillful treatment by hand to reduce fractures and dislocations, or provide therapy through forceful passive movement of a joint beyond its active limit of motion.

reduction. Correction of a fracture, dislocation, or hernia to the correct place and alignment, manually or by surgery.

traction. Drawing out or holding tension on an area by applying a direct therapeutic pulling force.

CCI Version 16.3

01810, 01820, 0213T, 0216T, 0228T, 0230T, 11000, 11040-11042, 13131, 20650, 24300, 25115-25116, 25230, 25259, 25650, 29058-29085, 29105-29126, 29260, 29700-29715, 36000, 36400-36410, 36420-36430, 36440, 36600, 36640, 37202, 43752, 51701-51703, 62310-62319, 64400-64435, 64445-64450, 64479, 64483, 64490, 64493, 64505-64530, 69990, 76000-76001, 93000-93010, 93040-93042, 93318, 94002, 94200, 94250, 94680-94690, 94770, 95812-95816, 95819, 95822, 95829, 95955, 96360, 96365, 96372, 96374-96376, 97597-97598, 97602-97606, 99148-99149, 99150

Also not with 25607: 25600-25606

Also not with 25608: 25600-25607❖

Also not with 25609: 25600-25608, 25830❖

Note: These CCI edits are used for Medicare. Other payers may reimburse on codes listed above.

Medicare Edits

	Fac RVU	Non-Fac RVU	FUD	Assist
25607	21.15	21.15	90	80
25608	23.76	23.76	90	80
25609	30.31	30.31	90	80

Medicare References: None

25622-25624

25622 Closed treatment of carpal scaphoid (navicular) fracture; without manipulation
25624 with manipulation

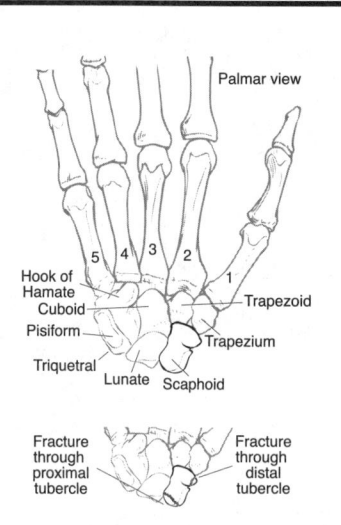

A fracture of the scaphoid (navicular) bone is treated in a closed fashion. Report 25624 when manipulation is required during the treatment

Explanation

The physician treats a scaphoid fracture of the wrist without open surgery or manual manipulation in 25622. Separately reportable x-rays confirm the position and alignment of the bone. In 25624, manipulation of the bone is required. The patient may require anesthesia. The physician manipulates the area by pushing on the wrist bones, particularly the scaphoid. The physician also pulls on the fingers and forearm, moving the fractured area back into position. Separately reportable x-rays confirm alignment. In both 25622 and 25624, a cast is placed on the wrist and forearm with a thumb spica to hold the fracture in position.

Coding Tips

According to CPT guidelines, cast application or strapping (including removal) is only reported as a replacement procedure or when the cast application or strapping is an initial service performed without a restorative treatment or procedure. See "Application of Casts and Strapping" in the CPT book in the Surgery Section, under the Musculoskeletal system. In 25624, local anesthesia is included in the service. However, this procedure may be performed under general anesthesia, depending on the age and/or condition of the patient. For radiology services, see 73100–73115. For open treatment of a navicular fracture, see 25628. For closed treatment of other carpal bone fractures (excluding navicular), see 25630 and 25635.

ICD-9-CM Procedural

79.03 Closed reduction of fracture of carpals and metacarpals without internal fixation
93.53 Application of other cast

Anesthesia
01820

ICD-9-CM Diagnostic

733.19 Pathologic fracture of other specified site
814.01 Closed fracture of navicular (scaphoid) bone of wrist

Terms To Know

closed fracture. Break in a bone without a concomitant opening in the skin. A closed fracture is coded when the type of fracture is not specified.

fracture. Break in bone or cartilage.

pathologic fracture. Break in bone due to a disease process that weakens the bone structure, such as osteoporosis, osteomalacia, or neoplasia, and not traumatic injury.

CCI Version 16.3

01810, 01820, 0213T, 0216T, 0228T, 0230T, 24300, 25259, 29058-29085, 29105-29126, 29260, 29700-29715, 36000, 36400-36410, 36420-36430, 36440, 36600, 36640, 37202, 43752, 51701-51703, 62310-62319, 64400-64435, 64445-64450, 64479, 64483, 64490, 64493, 64505-64530, 69990, 93000-93010, 93040-93042, 93318, 94002, 94200, 94250, 94680-94690, 94770, 95812-95816, 95819, 95822, 95829, 95955, 96360, 96365, 96372, 96374-96376, 97597-97598, 97602-97606, 99148-99149, 99150

Also not with 25624: 25622, J0670, J2001

Note: These CCI edits are used for Medicare. Other payers may reimburse on codes listed above.

Medicare Edits

	Fac RVU	Non-Fac RVU	FUD	Assist
25622	7.7	8.49	90	N/A
25624	11.96	13.1	90	80

Medicare References: 100-2,15,260; 100-4,12,30; 100-4,12,90.3; 100-4,14,10

25628

25628 Open treatment of carpal scaphoid (navicular) fracture, includes internal fixation, when performed

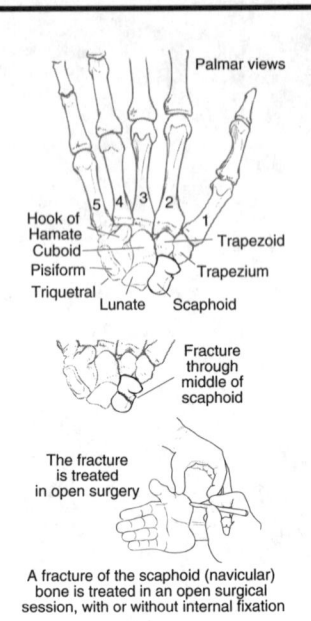

Palmar views

Hook of Hamate, Cuboid, Pisiform, Triquetral, Lunate, Scaphoid, Trapezoid, Trapezium

Fracture through middle of scaphoid

The fracture is treated in open surgery

A fracture of the scaphoid (navicular) bone is treated in an open surgical session, with or without internal fixation

Explanation
The physician treats a fracture of the wrist scaphoid bone. An incision is made over the scaphoid bone. The physician extends the incision down to the bone and the fracture is identified. Soft tissue is debrided as necessary. The physician places the bone fragments in their correct anatomical position. Typically, screws are applied to hold the pieces together. The physician irrigates the wound and closes it in layers. A cast or splint is applied to provide additional support of the area.

Coding Tips
According to CPT guidelines, cast application or strapping (including removal) is only reported as a replacement procedure or when the cast application or strapping is an initial service performed without a restorative treatment or procedure. See "Application of Casts and Strapping" in the CPT book in the Surgery Section, under the Musculoskeletal system. For radiology services, see 73100–73115. For closed treatment of a navicular fracture, without manipulation, see 25622; with manipulation, see 25624. For open treatment of other wrist fractures (excluding navicular), see 25645.

ICD-9-CM Procedural
78.14 Application of external fixator device, carpals and metacarpals
79.23 Open reduction of fracture of carpals and metacarpals without internal fixation
79.33 Open reduction of fracture of carpals and metacarpals with internal fixation

Anesthesia
25628 01830

ICD-9-CM Diagnostic
733.19 Pathologic fracture of other specified site
814.01 Closed fracture of navicular (scaphoid) bone of wrist
814.11 Open fracture of navicular (scaphoid) bone of wrist

Terms To Know

closed fracture. Break in a bone without a concomitant opening in the skin. A closed fracture is coded when the type of fracture is not specified.

fracture. Break in bone or cartilage.

open fracture. Exposed break in a bone, always considered compound due to its high risk of infection from the open wound leading to the fracture. Broken bone ends may protrude through the skin and contaminants or foreign bodies are often embedded in the tissues.

CCI Version 16.3
01810, 01820, 0213T, 0216T, 0228T, 0230T, 20650, 24300, 25085-25105, 25110, 25115-25118, 25259, 25295, 25394, 25622-25624, 29058-29085, 29105-29126, 29260, 29700-29715, 36000, 36400-36410, 36420-36430, 36440, 36600, 36640, 37202, 43752, 51701-51703, 62310-62319, 64400-64435, 64445-64450, 64479, 64483, 64490, 64493, 64505-64530, 69990, 93000-93010, 93040-93042, 93318, 94002, 94200, 94250, 94680-94690, 94770, 95812-95816, 95819, 95822, 95829, 95955, 96360, 96365, 96372, 96374-96376, 97597-97598, 97602-97606, 99148-99149, 99150

Note: These CCI edits are used for Medicare. Other payers may reimburse on codes listed above.

Medicare Edits

	Fac RVU	Non-Fac RVU	FUD	Assist
25628	20.91	20.91	90	80

Medicare References: 100-2,15,260; 100-4,12,30; 100-4,12,90.3; 100-4,14,10

25630-25635

25630 Closed treatment of carpal bone fracture (excluding carpal scaphoid [navicular]); without manipulation, each bone
25635 with manipulation, each bone

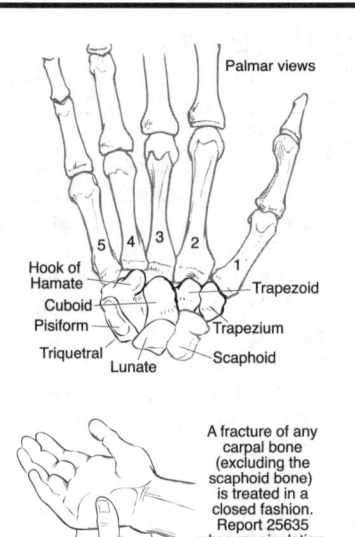

Explanation

The physician performs closed treatment of a fracture of the carpal bone, each bone. Triquetrum fractures are usually nondisplaced and respond well to casting or splinting for six weeks. Capitate fractures are generally treated by conservative casting, immobilizing the wrist and thumb. Hamate fractures are accompanied by fractures at the base of the ulnar metacarpal, and become asymptomatic after a four to six-week period of immobilization. Lunate fractures are similarly treated by immobilization. Report 25630 if no manipulation is performed; report 25635 if manipulation is performed, each bone.

Coding Tips

According to CPT guidelines, cast application or strapping (including removal) is only reported as a replacement procedure or when the cast application or strapping is an initial service performed without a restorative treatment or procedure. See "Application of Casts and Strapping" in the CPT book in the Surgery Section, under the Musculoskeletal system. In 25635, local anesthesia is included in the service. However, this procedure may be performed under general anesthesia, depending on the age and/or condition of the patient. For radiology services, see 73100–73115. For open treatment of a carpal bone fracture (excluding navicular), see 25645. For closed treatment of navicular fracture, see 25622 and 25624.

ICD-9-CM Procedural

- **79.03** Closed reduction of fracture of carpals and metacarpals without internal fixation
- **93.53** Application of other cast
- **93.54** Application of splint

Anesthesia
01820

ICD-9-CM Diagnostic

- **733.19** Pathologic fracture of other specified site
- **814.02** Closed fracture of lunate (semilunar) bone of wrist
- **814.03** Closed fracture of triquetral (cuneiform) bone of wrist
- **814.04** Closed fracture of pisiform bone of wrist
- **814.05** Closed fracture of trapezium bone (larger multangular) of wrist
- **814.06** Closed fracture of trapezoid bone (smaller multangular) of wrist
- **814.07** Closed fracture of capitate bone (os magnum) of wrist
- **814.08** Closed fracture of hamate (unciform) bone of wrist
- **814.09** Closed fracture of other bone of wrist

Terms To Know

closed fracture. Break in a bone without a concomitant opening in the skin. A closed fracture is coded when the type of fracture is not specified.

fracture. Break in bone or cartilage.

fracture types. There are three basic degrees of fracture: type I: a small crack in the bone without displacement; type II: a fracture in which the bone is slightly displaced; type III: a fracture in which there are more than three broken pieces of bone that cannot fit together.

pathologic fracture. Break in bone due to a disease process that weakens the bone structure, such as osteoporosis, osteomalacia, or neoplasia, and not traumatic injury.

CCI Version 16.3

01810, 01820, 0213T, 0216T, 0228T, 0230T, 24300, 25259, 29058-29085, 29260, 29700-29715, 36000, 36400-36410, 36420-36430, 36440, 36600, 36640, 37202, 43752, 51701-51703, 62310-62319, 64400-64435, 64445-64450, 64479, 64483, 64490, 64493, 64505-64530, 69990, 93000-93010, 93040-93042, 93318, 94002, 94200, 94250, 94680-94690, 94770, 95812-95816, 95819, 95822, 95829, 95955, 96360, 96365, 96372, 96374-96376, 97597-97598, 97602-97606, 99148-99149, 99150

Also not with 25630: 12005, 29105-29130

Also not with 25635: 25630, 29105-29126, J0670, J2001

Note: These CCI edits are used for Medicare. Other payers may reimburse on codes listed above.

Medicare Edits

	Fac RVU	Non-Fac RVU	FUD	Assist
25630	7.83	8.59	90	N/A
25635	11.49	12.71	90	80

Medicare References: 100-2,15,260; 100-4,12,30; 100-4,12,90.3; 100-4,14,10

25645

25645 Open treatment of carpal bone fracture (other than carpal scaphoid [navicular]), each bone

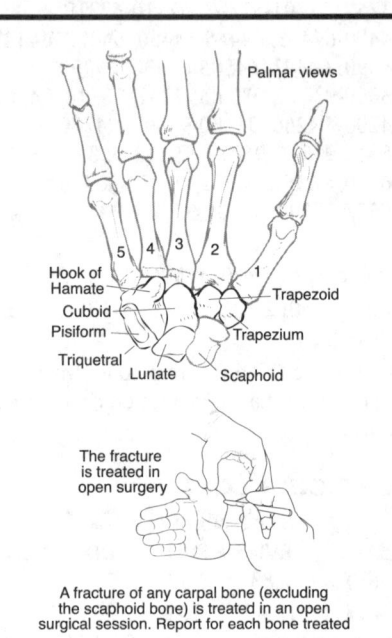

Palmar views

Hook of Hamate, Cuboid, Pisiform, Triquetral, Lunate, Scaphoid, Trapezoid, Trapezium

The fracture is treated in open surgery

A fracture of any carpal bone (excluding the scaphoid bone) is treated in an open surgical session. Report for each bone treated

Explanation

The physician performs open treatment of a fracture of the carpal bone. Only some carpal bones are treated with open procedures. For hook of the hamate fractures, the physician makes an incision over the ulnar aspect of the wrist. The fracture is reduced and fixed with Kirschner wires or the hook is excised. The tissue is closed in layers and a compression dressing is applied. Trapezium fractures are often treated with open surgery and may require secondary surgery to treat symptoms of pain. Capitate fractures - especially if associated with scaphoid fractures - are often treated with reduction and internal fixation via Kirschner wires. In cases in which lunate fractures do not respond well to immobilization, the physician may elect open treatment. An incision is made over the lunate to excise avulsed fragments. The soft tissue is closed in layers and a compression dressing is applied.

Coding Tips

According to CPT guidelines, cast application or strapping (including removal) is only reported as a replacement procedure or when the cast application or strapping is an initial service performed without a restorative treatment or procedure. See "Application of Casts and Strapping" in the CPT book in the Surgery Section, under the Musculoskeletal system. For radiology services, see 73100–73115. For closed treatment of a carpal bone fracture without manipulation, see 25630; with manipulation, see 25635. For open treatment of a navicular fracture, see 25628.

ICD-9-CM Procedural

- 79.23 Open reduction of fracture of carpals and metacarpals without internal fixation
- 79.33 Open reduction of fracture of carpals and metacarpals with internal fixation

Anesthesia

25645   01830

ICD-9-CM Diagnostic

- 733.19 Pathologic fracture of other specified site
- 814.02 Closed fracture of lunate (semilunar) bone of wrist
- 814.03 Closed fracture of triquetral (cuneiform) bone of wrist
- 814.04 Closed fracture of pisiform bone of wrist
- 814.05 Closed fracture of trapezium bone (larger multangular) of wrist
- 814.06 Closed fracture of trapezoid bone (smaller multangular) of wrist
- 814.07 Closed fracture of capitate bone (os magnum) of wrist
- 814.08 Closed fracture of hamate (unciform) bone of wrist
- 814.09 Closed fracture of other bone of wrist
- 814.12 Open fracture of lunate (semilunar) bone of wrist
- 814.13 Open fracture of triquetral (cuneiform) bone of wrist
- 814.14 Open fracture of pisiform bone of wrist
- 814.15 Open fracture of trapezium bone (larger multangular) of wrist
- 814.16 Open fracture of trapezoid bone (smaller multangular) of wrist
- 814.17 Open fracture of capitate bone (os magnum) of wrist
- 814.18 Open fracture of hamate (unciform) bone of wrist
- 814.19 Open fracture of other bone of wrist

Terms To Know

closed fracture. Break in a bone without a concomitant opening in the skin. A closed fracture is coded when the type of fracture is not specified.

open fracture. Exposed break in a bone, always considered compound due to its high risk of infection from the open wound leading to the fracture. Broken bone ends may protrude through the skin and contaminants or foreign bodies are often embedded in the tissues.

CCI Version 16.3

01810, 01820, 0213T, 0216T, 0228T, 0230T, 24300, 25085-25105, 25110, 25115-25118, 25259, 25295, 25394, 25630-25635, 29058-29085, 29105-29126, 29260, 29700-29715, 36000, 36400-36410, 36420-36430, 36440, 36600, 36640, 37202, 43752, 51701-51703, 62310-62319, 64400-64435, 64445-64450, 64479, 64483, 64490, 64493, 64505-64530, 69990, 93000-93010, 93040-93042, 93318, 94002, 94200, 94250, 94680-94690, 94770, 95812-95816, 95819, 95822, 95829, 95955, 96360, 96365, 96372, 96374-96376, 97597-97598, 97602-97606, 99148-99149, 99150

Note: These CCI edits are used for Medicare. Other payers may reimburse on codes listed above.

Medicare Edits

	Fac RVU	Non-Fac RVU	FUD	Assist
25645	16.49	16.49	90	80

Medicare References: 100-2,15,260; 100-4,12,30; 100-4,12,90.3; 100-4,14,10

25650

25650 Closed treatment of ulnar styloid fracture

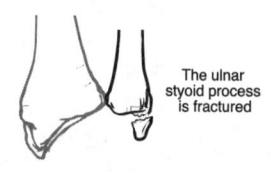

Explanation
The physician treats an ulnar styloid fracture with a cast or splint. No manual manipulation and no incisions are required.

Coding Tips
According to CPT guidelines, cast application or strapping (including removal) is only reported as a replacement procedure or when the cast application or strapping is an initial service performed without a restorative treatment or procedure. See "Application of Casts and Strapping" in the CPT book in the Surgery Section, under the Musculoskeletal system. For radiology services, see 73090 and 73100–73110. Do not report code 25650 with 25600, 25605, 25607-25609.

ICD-9-CM Procedural
- 93.53 Application of other cast
- 93.54 Application of splint

Anesthesia
25650 01820

ICD-9-CM Diagnostic
- 733.12 Pathologic fracture of distal radius and ulna
- 813.43 Closed fracture of distal end of ulna (alone)

Terms To Know

closed fracture. Break in a bone without a concomitant opening in the skin. A closed fracture is coded when the type of fracture is not specified.

pathologic fracture. Break in bone due to a disease process that weakens the bone structure, such as osteoporosis, osteomalacia, or neoplasia, and not traumatic injury.

splint. Brace or support for an anatomical structure after surgery or injury.

strapping. Application of overlapping strips of tape or bandaging to put pressure on the affected area.

CCI Version 16.3
01810, 01820, 0213T, 0216T, 0228T, 0230T, 24300, 25259, 29058-29085, 29105-29126, 29260, 29700-29715, 36000, 36400-36410, 36420-36430, 36440, 36600, 36640, 37202, 43752, 51701-51703, 62310-62319, 64400-64435, 64445-64450, 64479, 64483, 64490, 64493, 64505-64530, 69990, 93000-93010, 93040-93042, 93318, 94002, 94200, 94250, 94680-94690, 94770, 95812-95816, 95819, 95822, 95829, 95955, 96360, 96365, 96372, 96374-96376, 97597-97598, 97602-97606, 99148-99149, 99150

Note: These CCI edits are used for Medicare. Other payers may reimburse on codes listed above.

Medicare Edits

	Fac RVU	Non-Fac RVU	FUD	Assist
25650	8.38	9.01	90	N/A

Medicare References: None

25651

25651 Percutaneous skeletal fixation of ulnar styloid fracture

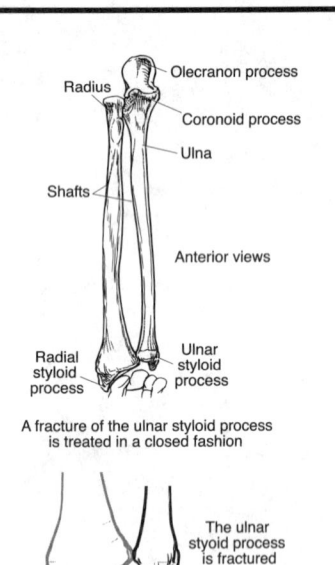

Explanation

The physician performs percutaneous skeletal fixation of an ulnar styloid fracture. Following fixation of the ulnar styloid fragment, the remaining depressed articular fragments are elevated and reduced with traction, direct pressure, or with use of a small incision and application of pointed reduction clamps.

Coding Tips

This is a unilateral procedure. If performed bilaterally, some payers require that the service be reported twice with modifier 50 appended to the second code, while others require identification of the service only once with modifier 50 appended. Check with individual payers. Modifier 50 identifies a procedure performed identically on the opposite side of the body (mirror image). According to CPT guidelines, cast application or strapping (including removal) is only reported as a replacement procedure or when the cast application or strapping is an initial service performed without a restorative treatment or procedure. See "Application of Casts and Strapping" in the CPT book in the Surgery Section, under the Musculoskeletal system.

ICD-9-CM Procedural

- 78.13 Application of external fixator device, radius and ulna
- 79.12 Closed reduction of fracture of radius and ulna with internal fixation

Anesthesia
25651 01820, 01830

ICD-9-CM Diagnostic

- 733.19 Pathologic fracture of other specified site
- 813.43 Closed fracture of distal end of ulna (alone)

Terms To Know

closed fracture. Break in a bone without a concomitant opening in the skin. A closed fracture is coded when the type of fracture is not specified.

distal. Located farther away from a specified reference point.

pathologic fracture. Break in bone due to a disease process that weakens the bone structure, such as osteoporosis, osteomalacia, or neoplasia, and not traumatic injury.

percutaneous skeletal fixation. Treatment that is neither open nor closed. In this procedure, the injury site is not directly visualized. Instead, fixation devices (pins, screws) are placed to stabilize the dislocation using x-ray guidance.

CCI Version 16.3

01810, 01820, 0213T, 0216T, 0228T, 0230T, 12001, 12031, 20650, 20690, 20692, 20696-20697, 25650, 29058-29085, 29105-29126, 29260, 29705-29715, 36000, 36400-36410, 36420-36430, 36440, 36600, 36640, 37202, 43752, 51701-51703, 62310-62319, 64400-64435, 64445-64450, 64479, 64483, 64490, 64493, 64505-64530, 69990, 76000-76001, 93000-93010, 93040-93042, 93318, 94002, 94200, 94250, 94680-94690, 94770, 95812-95816, 95819, 95822, 95829, 95955, 96360, 96365, 96372, 96374-96376, 97597-97598, 97602-97606, 99148-99149, 99150, G0168

Note: These CCI edits are used for Medicare. Other payers may reimburse on codes listed above.

Medicare Edits

	Fac RVU	Non-Fac RVU	FUD	Assist
25651	13.92	13.92	90	80

Medicare References: None

25652

25652 Open treatment of ulnar styloid fracture

A fracture of the ulnar styloid process is treated in an open fashion

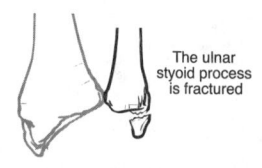

The ulnar styloid process is fractured

Explanation

If closed reduction of the ulnar styloid fracture is not possible, the physician extends an incision down to the bone and identifies the fracture. Soft tissue is debrided as necessary. The physician places the bone fragments in their correct anatomical position. The wound is irrigated and closed in layers. A cast or splint is applied to provide additional support.

Coding Tips

This is a unilateral procedure. If performed bilaterally, some payers require that the service be reported twice with modifier 50 appended to the second code, while others require identification of the service only once with modifier 50 appended. Check with individual payers. Modifier 50 identifies a procedure performed identically on the opposite side of the body (mirror image). According to CPT guidelines, cast application or strapping (including removal) is only reported as a replacement procedure or when the cast application or strapping is an initial service performed without a restorative treatment or procedure. See "Application of Casts and Strapping" in the CPT book in the Surgery Section, under the Musculoskeletal system.

ICD-9-CM Procedural

79.22 Open reduction of fracture of radius and ulna without internal fixation

Anesthesia

25652 01830

ICD-9-CM Diagnostic

733.12 Pathologic fracture of distal radius and ulna
733.81 Malunion of fracture
733.82 Nonunion of fracture
813.43 Closed fracture of distal end of ulna (alone)
813.53 Open fracture of distal end of ulna (alone)

Terms To Know

closed fracture. Break in a bone without a concomitant opening in the skin. A closed fracture is coded when the type of fracture is not specified.

distal. Located farther away from a specified reference point.

malunion. Fracture that has united in a faulty position due to inadequate reduction of the original fracture, insufficient holding of a previously well-reduced fracture, contracture of the soft tissues, or comminuted or osteoporotic bone causing a slow disintegration of the fracture.

nonunion. Failure of two ends of a fracture to mend or completely heal.

open fracture. Exposed break in a bone, always considered compound due to its high risk of infection from the open wound leading to the fracture. Broken bone ends may protrude through the skin and contaminants or foreign bodies are often embedded in the tissues.

pathologic fracture. Break in bone due to a disease process that weakens the bone structure, such as osteoporosis, osteomalacia, or neoplasia, and not traumatic injury.

unilateral. Located on or affecting one side.

CCI Version 16.3

01810, 01820, 0213T, 0216T, 0228T, 0230T, 11000, 11040-11044, 20650, 25105, 25115-25118, 25650-25651, 25830❖, 29058-29085, 29105-29126, 29260, 29700-29715, 36000, 36400-36410, 36420-36430, 36440, 36600, 36640, 37202, 43752, 51701-51703, 62310-62319, 64400-64435, 64445-64450, 64479, 64483, 64490, 64493, 64505-64530, 69990, 76000-76001, 93000-93010, 93040-93042, 93318, 94002, 94200, 94250, 94680-94690, 94770, 95812-95816, 95819, 95822, 95829, 95955, 96360, 96365, 96372, 96374-96376, 97597-97598, 97602-97606, 99148-99149, 99150, G0168

Note: These CCI edits are used for Medicare. Other payers may reimburse on codes listed above.

Medicare Edits

	Fac RVU	Non-Fac RVU	FUD	Assist
25652	18.02	18.02	90	N/A

Medicare References: None

25660

25660 Closed treatment of radiocarpal or intercarpal dislocation, 1 or more bones, with manipulation

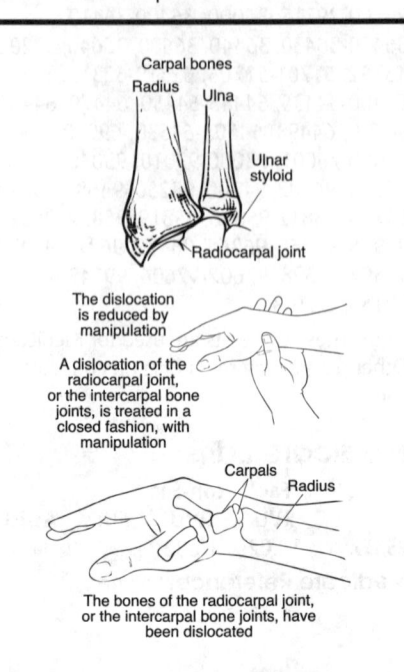

Explanation

The physician repairs the dislocation of radiocarpal or intercarpal bones with manipulation. Sustained traction is held while the physician applies force to reduce the dislocated bone into the proper anatomical position. Immobilization post-reduction depends on the physician's preference.

Coding Tips

Local anesthesia is included in this service. However, this procedure may be performed under general anesthesia, depending on the age and/or condition of the patient. According to CPT guidelines, cast application or strapping (including removal) is only reported as a replacement procedure or when the cast application or strapping is an initial service performed without a restorative treatment or procedure. See "Application of Casts and Strapping" in the CPT book in the Surgery Section, under the Musculoskeletal system. For radiology services, see 73100–73115. For open treatment of a radiocarpal or an intercarpal dislocation, see 25670.

ICD-9-CM Procedural

79.73 Closed reduction of dislocation of wrist

Anesthesia

25660 01820

ICD-9-CM Diagnostic

718.23 Pathological dislocation of forearm joint
718.24 Pathological dislocation of hand joint
718.33 Recurrent dislocation of forearm joint
718.34 Recurrent dislocation of hand joint
718.73 Developmental dislocation of joint, forearm
833.02 Closed dislocation of radiocarpal (joint)
833.03 Closed dislocation of midcarpal (joint)

Terms To Know

closed dislocation. Simple displacement of a body part without an open wound.

developmental dislocation. Displacement of a body part occurring in the developmental phase of childhood.

intercarpal. Between the carpal bones in the wrist.

pathological dislocation. Displacement of a bone or joint caused by a disease process, such as infection, lesions, or muscle weakness, and not traumatic injury.

CCI Version 16.3

01810, 01820, 0213T, 0216T, 0228T, 0230T, 24300, 25259, 29058-29085, 29105-29126, 29260, 29700-29715, 36000, 36400-36410, 36420-36430, 36440, 36600, 36640, 37202, 43752, 51701-51703, 62310-62319, 64400-64435, 64445-64450, 64479, 64483, 64490, 64493, 64505-64530, 69990, 93000-93010, 93040-93042, 93318, 94002, 94200, 94250, 94680-94690, 94770, 95812-95816, 95819, 95822, 95829, 95955, 96360, 96365, 96372, 96374-96376, 97597-97598, 97602-97606, 99148-99149, 99150

Note: These CCI edits are used for Medicare. Other payers may reimburse on codes listed above.

Medicare Edits

	Fac RVU	Non-Fac RVU	FUD	Assist
25660	11.57	11.57	90	80

Medicare References: 100-2,15,260; 100-4,12,30; 100-4,12,90.3; 100-4,14,10

25670

25670 Open treatment of radiocarpal or intercarpal dislocation, 1 or more bones

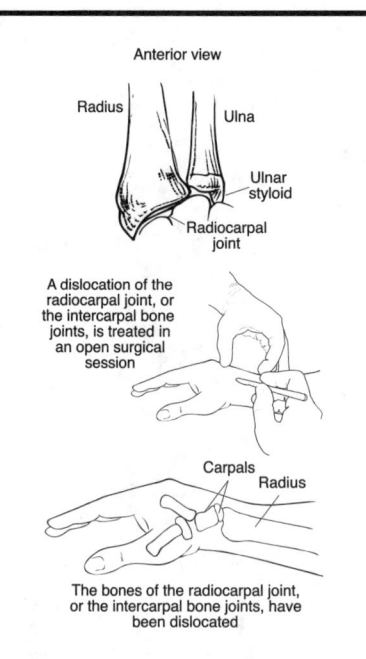

Explanation

The physician performs an open treatment of radiocarpal or intercarpal dislocation, one or more bones. The physician makes a dorsal incision overlying the wrist and the dislocation is reduced. If involved ligaments are torn, they are repaired to stabilize the reduction. The physician may use the overlying capsule to reinforce the stabilization. The soft tissue is closed in layers and a compression dressing is applied.

Coding Tips

According to CPT guidelines, cast application or strapping (including removal) is only reported as a replacement procedure or when the cast application or strapping is an initial service performed without a restorative treatment or procedure. See "Application of Casts and Strapping" in the CPT book in the Surgery Section, under the Musculoskeletal system. For radiology services, see 73100–73115. For closed treatment of a radiocarpal or an intercarpal dislocation, see 25660.

ICD-9-CM Procedural

79.83 Open reduction of dislocation of wrist

Anesthesia

25670 01830

ICD-9-CM Diagnostic

- 718.23 Pathological dislocation of forearm joint
- 718.24 Pathological dislocation of hand joint
- 718.33 Recurrent dislocation of forearm joint
- 718.34 Recurrent dislocation of hand joint
- 718.73 Developmental dislocation of joint, forearm
- 833.02 Closed dislocation of radiocarpal (joint)
- 833.03 Closed dislocation of midcarpal (joint)
- 833.12 Open dislocation of radiocarpal (joint)
- 833.13 Open dislocation of midcarpal (joint)

Terms To Know

developmental dislocation. Displacement of a body part occurring in the developmental phase of childhood.

dorsal. Pertaining to the back or posterior aspect.

pathological dislocation. Displacement of a bone or joint caused by a disease process, such as infection, lesions, or muscle weakness, and not traumatic injury.

soft tissue. Nonepithelial tissues outside of the skeleton that includes subcutaneous adipose tissue, fibrous tissue, fascia, muscles, blood and lymph vessels, and peripheral nervous system tissue.

CCI Version 16.3

01810, 01820, 0213T, 0216T, 0228T, 0230T, 24300, 25085-25105, 25110, 25115-25118, 25259, 25295, 25394, 25660, 29058-29085, 29105-29126, 29260, 29700-29715, 36000, 36400-36410, 36420-36430, 36440, 36600, 36640, 37202, 43752, 51701-51703, 62310-62319, 64400-64435, 64445-64450, 64479, 64483, 64490, 64493, 64505-64530, 69990, 93000-93010, 93040-93042, 93318, 94002, 94200, 94250, 94680-94690, 94770, 95812-95816, 95819, 95822, 95829, 95955, 96360, 96365, 96372, 96374-96376, 97597-97598, 97602-97606, 99148-99149, 99150

Note: These CCI edits are used for Medicare. Other payers may reimburse on codes listed above.

Medicare Edits

	Fac RVU	Non-Fac RVU	FUD	Assist
25670	17.59	17.59	90	80

Medicare References: 100-2,15,260; 100-4,12,30; 100-4,12,90.3; 100-4,14,10

25671

25671 Percutaneous skeletal fixation of distal radioulnar dislocation

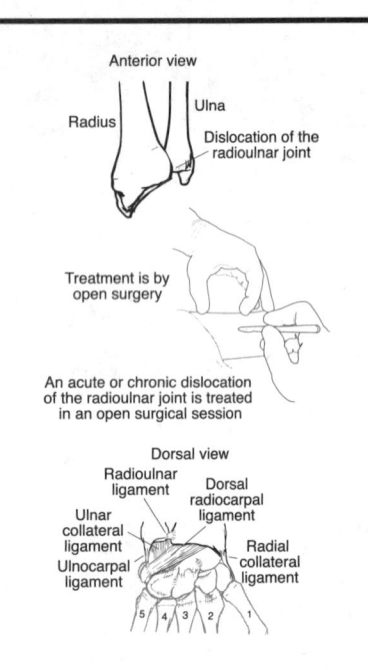

Explanation

Percutaneous pinning with or without bone grafting is commonly performed at 10 days from injury. The physician may use fluoroscopic guidance to perform an initial closed reduction and to insert pins from the radial styloid to the ulnar cortex of the radius for percutaneous fixation.

Coding Tips

This is a unilateral procedure. If performed bilaterally, some payers require that the service be reported twice with modifier 50 appended to the second code, while others require identification of the service only once with modifier 50 appended. Check with individual payers. Modifier 50 identifies a procedure performed identically on the opposite side of the body (mirror image). According to CPT guidelines, cast application or strapping (including removal) is only reported as a replacement procedure or when the cast application or strapping is an initial service performed without a restorative treatment or procedure. See "Application of Casts and Strapping" in the CPT book in the Surgery Section, under the Musculoskeletal system.

ICD-9-CM Procedural

79.73 Closed reduction of dislocation of wrist

Anesthesia

25671 01820, 01830

ICD-9-CM Diagnostic

718.23 Pathological dislocation of forearm joint
718.33 Recurrent dislocation of forearm joint
718.73 Developmental dislocation of joint, forearm
833.01 Closed dislocation of distal radioulnar (joint)

Terms To Know

developmental dislocation. Displacement of a body part occurring in the developmental phase of childhood.

dislocation. Displacement of a bone in relation to its neighboring tissue, especially a joint.

pathological dislocation. Displacement of a bone or joint caused by a disease process, such as infection, lesions, or muscle weakness, and not traumatic injury.

CCI Version 16.3

01810, 01820, 0213T, 0216T, 0228T, 0230T, 12001, 12031, 20650, 20690, 20692, 20696-20697, 25675, 29058-29085, 29105-29126, 29260, 29705-29715, 36000, 36400-36410, 36420-36430, 36440, 36600, 36640, 37202, 43752, 51701-51703, 62310-62319, 64400-64435, 64445-64450, 64479, 64483, 64490, 64493, 64505-64530, 69990, 76000-76001, 93000-93010, 93040-93042, 93318, 94002, 94200, 94250, 94680-94690, 94770, 95812-95816, 95819, 95822, 95829, 95955, 96360, 96365, 96372, 96374-96376, 97597-97598, 97602-97606, 99148-99149, 99150, G0168

Note: These CCI edits are used for Medicare. Other payers may reimburse on codes listed above.

Medicare Edits

	Fac RVU	Non-Fac RVU	FUD	Assist
25671	15.26	15.26	90	N/A

Medicare References: 100-2,15,260; 100-4,12,30; 100-4,12,90.3; 100-4,14,10

25675

25675 Closed treatment of distal radioulnar dislocation with manipulation

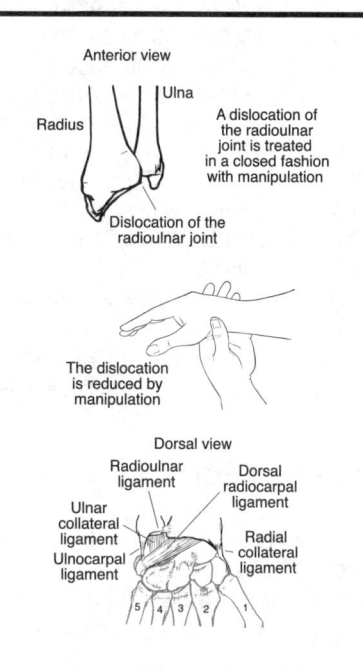

Explanation
The physician performs closed treatment of a distal radioulnar dislocation with manipulation. The physician reduces the dislocation by pronation (if the ulna is involved) and supination (if the ulna is dorsal). The arm is immobilized.

Coding Tips
According to CPT guidelines, cast application or strapping (including removal) is only reported as a replacement procedure or when the cast application or strapping is an initial service performed without a restorative treatment or procedure. See "Application of Casts and Strapping" in the CPT book in the Surgery Section, under the Musculoskeletal system. Local anesthesia is included in this service. However, this procedure may be performed under general anesthesia, depending on the age and/or condition of the patient. For radiology services, see 73090–73092 and 73100–73110. For open treatment of a distal radioulnar dislocation, see 25676.

ICD-9-CM Procedural
79.73 Closed reduction of dislocation of wrist

Anesthesia
25675 01820

ICD-9-CM Diagnostic
718.23 Pathological dislocation of forearm joint
718.33 Recurrent dislocation of forearm joint
718.73 Developmental dislocation of joint, forearm
833.01 Closed dislocation of distal radioulnar (joint)

Terms To Know
developmental dislocation. Displacement of a body part occurring in the developmental phase of childhood.

distal. Located farther away from a specified reference point.

dorsal. Pertaining to the back or posterior aspect.

pathological dislocation. Displacement of a bone or joint caused by a disease process, such as infection, lesions, or muscle weakness, and not traumatic injury.

pronation. Lying on the stomach or in a face down position; turning the palm toward the back or downward; lowering of the medial margin of the foot by an everting and abducting movement.

supination. Lying on the back; turning the palm toward the front or upward; raising the medial margin of the foot by an inverting and adducting movement.

CCI Version 16.3
01810, 01820, 0213T, 0216T, 0228T, 0230T, 24300, 25259, 29058-29085, 29105-29126, 29260, 29700-29715, 36000, 36400-36410, 36420-36430, 36440, 36600, 36640, 37202, 43752, 51701-51703, 62310-62319, 64400-64435, 64445-64450, 64479, 64483, 64490, 64493, 64505-64530, 69990, 93000-93010, 93040-93042, 93318, 94002, 94200, 94250, 94680-94690, 94770, 95812-95816, 95819, 95822, 95829, 95955, 96360, 96365, 96372, 96374-96376, 97597-97598, 97602-97606, 99148-99149, 99150, J0670, J2001

Note: These CCI edits are used for Medicare. Other payers may reimburse on codes listed above.

Medicare Edits

	Fac RVU	Non-Fac RVU	FUD	Assist
25675	11.3	12.29	90	80

Medicare References: 100-2,15,260; 100-4,12,30; 100-4,12,90.3; 100-4,14,10

25676

25676 Open treatment of distal radioulnar dislocation, acute or chronic

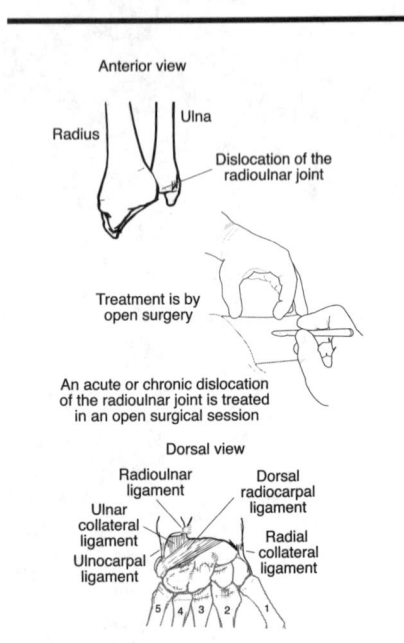

Explanation

The physician performs an open treatment of a distal radioulnar dislocation, acute or chronic. For a locked dislocation or incongruous reduction, the physician opens the joint for reduction and repairs the triangular fibrocartilage (TFC)/ulnar collateral ligament complex (UCLC), stabilizing the repair with Kirschner wires. The physician incises the dorsum of the wrist on the ulnar side. The proximal and ulnar half of the extensor retinaculum is raised radially. The extensor digiti minimi is retracted to reveal the TFC. The capsule is detached from the radius and reflected ulnarly. After the dislocated joint is reduced, the TFC lesion may be repaired or reconstructed using a local or grafted tissue from the retinaculum, extensor carpi ulnaris, or flexor carpi ulnaris. Kirschner wires may be used to stabilize the repair, after which the overlying soft tissue is sutured closed and a bulky dressing is applied.

Coding Tips

According to CPT guidelines, cast application or strapping (including removal) is only reported as a replacement procedure or when the cast application or strapping is an initial service performed without a restorative treatment or procedure. See "Application of Casts and Strapping" in the CPT book in the Surgery Section, under the Musculoskeletal system. For radiology services, see 73090–73092 and 73100–73110. For closed treatment of a distal radioulnar dislocation, see 25675.

ICD-9-CM Procedural

79.83 Open reduction of dislocation of wrist

Anesthesia

25676 01830

ICD-9-CM Diagnostic

718.23 Pathological dislocation of forearm joint
718.33 Recurrent dislocation of forearm joint
718.73 Developmental dislocation of joint, forearm
833.01 Closed dislocation of distal radioulnar (joint)
833.11 Open dislocation of distal radioulnar (joint)

Terms To Know

acute. Sudden, severe. Documentation and reporting of an acute condition is important to establishing medical necessity.

chronic. Persistent, continuing, or recurring.

lesion. Area of damaged tissue that has lost continuity or function, due to disease or trauma. Lesions may be located on internal structures such as the brain, nerves, or kidneys, or visible on the skin.

ligament. Band or sheet of fibrous tissue that connects the articular surfaces of bones or supports visceral organs.

pathological dislocation. Displacement of a bone or joint caused by a disease process, such as infection, lesions, or muscle weakness, and not traumatic injury.

soft tissue. Nonepithelial tissues outside of the skeleton that includes subcutaneous adipose tissue, fibrous tissue, fascia, muscles, blood and lymph vessels, and peripheral nervous system tissue.

CCI Version 16.3

01810, 01820, 0213T, 0216T, 0228T, 0230T, 24300, 25085-25105, 25110, 25115-25119, 25240, 25259, 25295, 25360, 25671-25675, 29058-29085, 29105-29126, 29260, 29700-29715, 36000, 36400-36410, 36420-36430, 36440, 36600, 36640, 37202, 43752, 51701-51703, 62310-62319, 64400-64435, 64445-64450, 64479, 64483, 64490, 64493, 64505-64530, 69990, 93000-93010, 93040-93042, 93318, 94002, 94200, 94250, 94680-94690, 94770, 95812-95816, 95819, 95822, 95829, 95955, 96360, 96365, 96372, 96374-96376, 97597-97598, 97602-97606, 99148-99149, 99150

Note: These CCI edits are used for Medicare. Other payers may reimburse on codes listed above.

Medicare Edits

	Fac RVU	Non-Fac RVU	FUD	Assist
25676	18.32	18.32	90	80

Medicare References: 100-2,15,260; 100-4,12,30; 100-4,12,90.3; 100-4,14,10

25680

25680 Closed treatment of trans-scaphoperilunar type of fracture dislocation, with manipulation

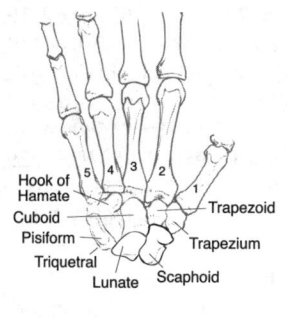

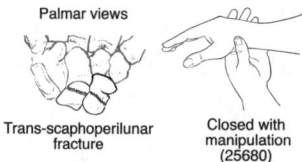

Explanation

The physician performs closed treatment of a trans-scaphoperilunar type of fracture dislocation using manipulation. After being placed in continual traction for five to 10 minutes, the patient's hand is dorsiflexed while maintaining traction. While stabilizing the lunate, volar, gradual palmar flexion reduces the capitate. The wrist is immobilized in a dorsal plaster thumb spica splint at 30 degrees volar flexion. Usually, if the scaphoid is properly reduced (visualized via separately reportable radiographs), the midcarpal joint is adequately reduced as well.

Coding Tips

According to CPT guidelines, cast application or strapping (including removal) is only reported as a replacement procedure or when the cast application or strapping is an initial service performed without a restorative treatment or procedure. See "Application of Casts and Strapping" in the CPT book in the Surgery Section, under the Musculoskeletal system. Local anesthesia is included in this service. However, this procedure may be performed under general anesthesia, depending on the age and/or condition of the patient. For radiology services, see 73100 and 73110. For open treatment of a trans-scaphoperilunar type fracture-dislocation, see 25685.

ICD-9-CM Procedural

79.03 Closed reduction of fracture of carpals and metacarpals without internal fixation
79.73 Closed reduction of dislocation of wrist

Anesthesia

25680 01820

ICD-9-CM Diagnostic

733.19 Pathologic fracture of other specified site
814.01 Closed fracture of navicular (scaphoid) bone of wrist
833.03 Closed dislocation of midcarpal (joint)

Terms To Know

closed fracture. Break in a bone without a concomitant opening in the skin. A closed fracture is coded when the type of fracture is not specified.

dislocation. Displacement of a bone in relation to its neighboring tissue, especially a joint.

dorsiflexion. Position of being bent toward the extensor side of a limb.

flexion. Act of bending or being bent.

fracture. Break in bone or cartilage.

volar. Palm of the hand (palmar) or sole of the foot (plantar).

CCI Version 16.3

01810, 01820, 0213T, 0216T, 0228T, 0230T, 24300, 25259, 29058-29085, 29105-29126, 29260, 29700-29715, 36000, 36400-36410, 36420-36430, 36440, 36600, 36640, 37202, 43752, 51701-51703, 62310-62319, 64400-64435, 64445-64450, 64479, 64483, 64490, 64493, 64505-64530, 69990, 93000-93010, 93040-93042, 93318, 94002, 94200, 94250, 94680-94690, 94770, 95812-95816, 95819, 95822, 95829, 95955, 96360, 96365, 96372, 96374-96376, 97597-97598, 97602-97606, 99148-99149, 99150

Note: These CCI edits are used for Medicare. Other payers may reimburse on codes listed above.

Medicare Edits

	Fac RVU	Non-Fac RVU	FUD	Assist
25680	13.29	13.29	90	80

Medicare References: 100-2,15,260; 100-4,12,30; 100-4,12,90.3; 100-4,14,10

25685

25685 Open treatment of trans-scaphoperilunar type of fracture dislocation

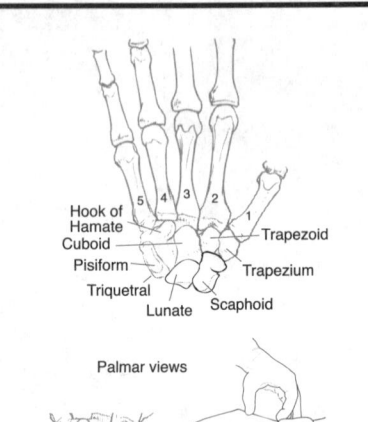

Palmar views

Trans-scaphoperilunar fracture | Open surgery (25685)

A trans-scaphoperilunar type fracture dislocation is treated in a closed fashion with manipulation. Report 25685 when the treatment is open surgery

Explanation

The physician performs open treatment of a trans-scaphoperilunar type of fracture dislocation. The physician makes a longitudinal, volar incision overlying the wrist, radial to the flexor carpi radialis tendon. This muscle is retracted toward the ulnar side and the wrist joint is opened exposing the scaphoid fracture. After the fracture is reduced, Kirschner wires are drilled into the scaphoid to hold the reduction. If fixation of the scaphoid adequately stabilizes the midcarpal joint, no further fixation is required. If separately reportable radiographs visualize even the slightest tendency of volar subluxation or rotary instability of the lunate, the volar incision must be extended and, occasionally, a dorsal incision must be made. In such cases, additional Kirschner wires should be introduced to stabilize the capitate-lunate joint. If this operation is performed within two to three weeks of injury, bone grafting is not used. If open reduction is delayed for more than three weeks post-surgery, bone grafting (reported separately) may be used. Capsular and skin closure is performed.

Coding Tips

According to CPT guidelines, cast application or strapping (including removal) is only reported as a replacement procedure or when the cast application or strapping is an initial service performed without a restorative treatment or procedure. See "Application of Casts and Strapping" in the CPT book in the Surgery Section, under the Musculoskeletal system. For radiology services, see 73100 and 73110. For closed treatment of a trans-scaphoperilunar type fracture-dislocation, see 25680. Surgical trays, A4550, are not separately reimbursed by Medicare; however, other third-party payers may cover them. Check with the specific payer to determine coverage.

ICD-9-CM Procedural

79.83   Open reduction of dislocation of wrist

Anesthesia

25685   01830

ICD-9-CM Diagnostic

733.19 Pathologic fracture of other specified site
814.01 Closed fracture of navicular (scaphoid) bone of wrist
814.11 Open fracture of navicular (scaphoid) bone of wrist
833.03 Closed dislocation of midcarpal (joint)
833.13 Open dislocation of midcarpal (joint)

Terms To Know

closed fracture. Break in a bone without a concomitant opening in the skin. A closed fracture is coded when the type of fracture is not specified.

dislocation. Displacement of a bone in relation to its neighboring tissue, especially a joint.

dorsal. Pertaining to the back or posterior aspect.

fracture. Break in bone or cartilage.

open fracture. Exposed break in a bone, always considered compound due to its high risk of infection from the open wound leading to the fracture. Broken bone ends may protrude through the skin and contaminants or foreign bodies are often embedded in the tissues.

subluxation. Partial or complete dislocation.

volar. Palm of the hand (palmar) or sole of the foot (plantar).

CCI Version 16.3

01810, 01820, 0213T, 0216T, 0228T, 0230T, 24300, 25085-25107, 25110-25119, 25210-25215, 25259, 25295, 25394, 25680, 29058-29085, 29105-29126, 29260, 29700-29715, 36000, 36400-36410, 36420-36430, 36440, 36600, 36640, 37202, 43752, 51701-51703, 62310-62319, 64400-64435, 64445-64450, 64479, 64483, 64490, 64493, 64505-64530, 64702-64726, 69990, 93000-93010, 93040-93042, 93318, 94002, 94200, 94250, 94680-94690, 94770, 95812-95816, 95819, 95822, 95829, 95955, 96360, 96365, 96372, 96374-96376, 97597-97598, 97602-97606, 99148-99149, 99150

Note: These CCI edits are used for Medicare. Other payers may reimburse on codes listed above.

Medicare Edits

	Fac RVU	Non-Fac RVU	FUD	Assist
25685	21.36	21.36	90	80

Medicare References: 100-2,15,260; 100-4,12,30; 100-4,12,90.3; 100-4,14,10

25690

25690 Closed treatment of lunate dislocation, with manipulation

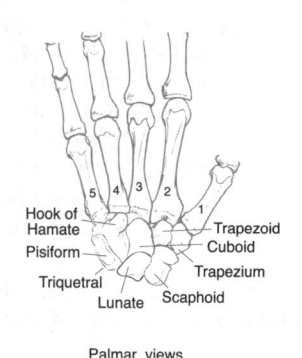

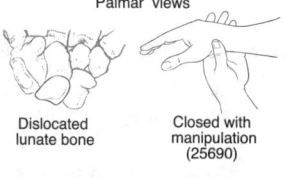

Hook of Hamate, Pisiform, Triquetral, Lunate, Scaphoid, Trapezoid, Cuboid, Trapezium

Palmar views

Dislocated lunate bone

Closed with manipulation (25690)

A dislocated lunate bone is treated in an open fashion with manipulation

Explanation

The physician treats a lunate dislocation with manipulation. During sustained traction, the physician applies force to reduce the dislocated lunate. Immobilization post reduction depends on the physician's preference.

Coding Tips

According to CPT guidelines, cast application or strapping (including removal) is only reported as a replacement procedure or when the cast application or strapping is an initial service performed without a restorative treatment or procedure. See "Application of Casts and Strapping" in the CPT book in the Surgery Section, under the Musculoskeletal system. Local anesthesia is included in this service. However, this procedure may be performed under general anesthesia, depending on the age and/or condition of the patient. For radiology services, see 73100 and 73110. For open treatment of a lunate dislocation, see 25695.

ICD-9-CM Procedural

79.73 Closed reduction of dislocation of wrist

Anesthesia

25690 01820

ICD-9-CM Diagnostic

718.24 Pathological dislocation of hand joint
718.34 Recurrent dislocation of hand joint
718.73 Developmental dislocation of joint, forearm
833.03 Closed dislocation of midcarpal (joint)

Terms To Know

developmental dislocation. Displacement of a body part occurring in the developmental phase of childhood.

dislocation. Displacement of a bone in relation to its neighboring tissue, especially a joint.

pathological dislocation. Displacement of a bone or joint caused by a disease process, such as infection, lesions, or muscle weakness, and not traumatic injury.

CCI Version 16.3

01810, 01820, 0213T, 0216T, 0228T, 0230T, 24300, 25259, 29058-29085, 29105-29126, 29260, 29700-29715, 36000, 36400-36410, 36420-36430, 36440, 36600, 36640, 37202, 43752, 51701-51703, 62310-62319, 64400-64435, 64445-64450, 64479, 64483, 64490, 64493, 64505-64530, 69990, 93000-93010, 93040-93042, 93318, 94002, 94200, 94250, 94680-94690, 94770, 95812-95816, 95819, 95822, 95829, 95955, 96360, 96365, 96372, 96374-96376, 97597-97598, 97602-97606, 99148-99149, 99150

Note: These CCI edits are used for Medicare. Other payers may reimburse on codes listed above.

Medicare Edits

	Fac RVU	Non-Fac RVU	FUD	Assist
25690	13.66	13.66	90	80

Medicare References: 100-2,15,260; 100-4,12,30; 100-4,12,90.3; 100-4,14,10

25695

25695 Open treatment of lunate dislocation

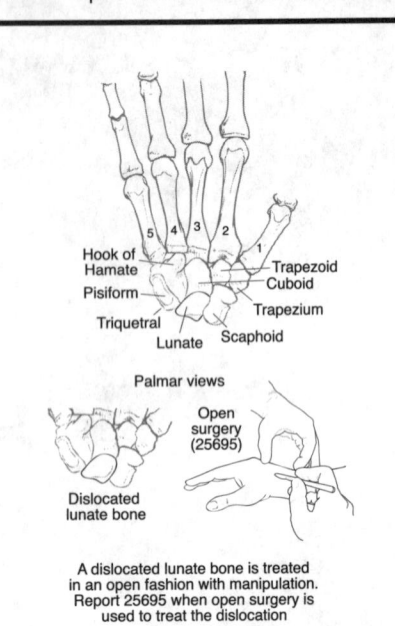

A dislocated lunate bone is treated in an open fashion with manipulation. Report 25695 when open surgery is used to treat the dislocation.

Explanation

The physician performs an open lunate dislocation. The physician makes both dorsal and volar incisions over the wrist. Through the dorsal longitudinal incision, the extensor tendons are retracted. The proximal pole of the scaphoid is retracted to expose the capitate. Through the volar longitudinal incision, the flexor tendons and median nerve are retracted to the radial side exposing a tear in the volar capsule and ligaments. The dislocated lunate is reduced through the volar approach by manually pushing it back between the capitate and radius while an assistant applies axial traction through the hand. The physician repairs the capsular-ligamentous complex tear with nonabsorbable sutures. On the dorsal side, the physician reduces the proximal pole of the capitate into the distal concavity of the lunate. The proximal pole of the scaphoid is reduced. Kirschner wires are drilled into the scaphoid, lunate, and capitate for stabilization. The physician repairs the dorsal ligamentous complex. The skin is closed.

Coding Tips

According to CPT guidelines, cast application or strapping (including removal) is only reported as a replacement procedure or when the cast application or strapping is an initial service performed without a restorative treatment or procedure. See "Application of Casts and Strapping" in the CPT book in the Surgery Section, under the Musculoskeletal system. For radiology services, see 73100 and 73110. For closed treatment of a lunate dislocation, see 25690.

ICD-9-CM Procedural

79.83 Open reduction of dislocation of wrist

Anesthesia

25695 01830

ICD-9-CM Diagnostic

718.24 Pathological dislocation of hand joint
718.34 Recurrent dislocation of hand joint
718.73 Developmental dislocation of joint, forearm
833.03 Closed dislocation of midcarpal (joint)
833.13 Open dislocation of midcarpal (joint)

Terms To Know

developmental dislocation. Displacement of a body part occurring in the developmental phase of childhood.

dislocation. Displacement of a bone in relation to its neighboring tissue, especially a joint.

distal. Located farther away from a specified reference point.

dorsal. Pertaining to the back or posterior aspect.

ligament. Band or sheet of fibrous tissue that connects the articular surfaces of bones or supports visceral organs.

pathological dislocation. Displacement of a bone or joint caused by a disease process, such as infection, lesions, or muscle weakness, and not traumatic injury.

proximal. Located closest to a specified reference point, usually the midline.

volar. Palm of the hand (palmar) or sole of the foot (plantar).

CCI Version 16.3

01810, 01820, 0213T, 0216T, 0228T, 0230T, 24300, 25085-25105, 25110, 25115-25118, 25259, 25295, 25394, 25690, 29058-29085, 29105-29126, 29260, 29700-29715, 36000, 36400-36410, 36420-36430, 36440, 36600, 36640, 37202, 43752, 51701-51703, 62310-62319, 64400-64435, 64445-64450, 64479, 64483, 64490, 64493, 64505-64530, 69990, 93000-93010, 93040-93042, 93318, 94002, 94200, 94250, 94680-94690, 94770, 95812-95816, 95819, 95822, 95829, 95955, 96360, 96365, 96372, 96374-96376, 97597-97598, 97602-97606, 99148-99149, 99150

Note: These CCI edits are used for Medicare. Other payers may reimburse on codes listed above.

Medicare Edits

	Fac RVU	Non-Fac RVU	FUD	Assist
25695	18.41	18.41	90	80

Medicare References: 100-2,15,260; 100-4,12,30; 100-4,12,90.3; 100-4,14,10

25800-25810

25800 Arthrodesis, wrist; complete, without bone graft (includes radiocarpal and/or intercarpal and/or carpometacarpal joints)
25805 with sliding graft
25810 with iliac or other autograft (includes obtaining graft)

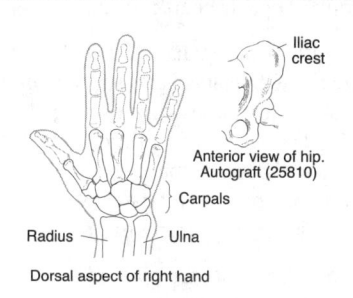

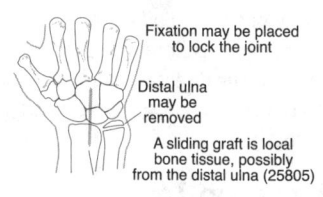

Iliac crest
Anterior view of hip. Autograft (25810)
Carpals
Radius Ulna
Dorsal aspect of right hand

Fixation may be placed to lock the joint
Distal ulna may be removed
A sliding graft is local bone tissue, possibly from the distal ulna (25805)

The total wrist joint is permanently fixed in place (arthrodesis). Report 25805 when a sliding graft is used. Report 25810 when an autograft (from an independent site on the patient) is used to freeze the joint

Explanation

The physician performs fusion of the wrist joint, including the radiocarpal, intercarpal, and/or carpometacarpal joints. The physician exposes the wrist through a dorsal, longitudinal incision. A dorsal tenosynovectomy is performed and the wrist capsule is elevated exposing the radiocarpal joint. The physician excises the distal ulna and performs a synovectomy of the radiocarpal joint. The radial collateral ligament is released from the radial styloid. The cartilage and sclerotic band is removed from the distal radius and proximal carpal row. Using an awl, the physician makes a channel in the medullary canal of the radius, through which a Steinmann pin is used for internal fixation. The pin is drilled through the carpus to exit between the second and third, or between the third and fourth metacarpal, depending on alignment between the carpus and the radius. One or two small staples, or an obliquely-placed Kirschner, may be used to provide additional fixation on the radiocarpal joint. The position of the wrist can be varied only five to 10 degrees by adjusting the direction of the pin as it is driven into the radius. A drain is placed subcutaneously prior to skin closure. A milky compression dressing is applied and the wrist is splinted in the desired position of fusion. Report 25800 if performed without bone graft. Report 25805 if performed with sliding graft. Report 25810 if performed with iliac or other autograft.

Coding Tips

In 25810, any iliac or other autogenous bone graft harvest is not reported separately. According to CPT guidelines, cast application or strapping (including removal) is only reported as a replacement procedure or when the cast application or strapping is an initial service performed without a restorative treatment or procedure. See "Application of Casts and Strapping" in the CPT book in the Surgery Section, under the Musculoskeletal system. For limited wrist arthrodesis, see 25820. For limited wrist arthrodesis with autograft, see 25825.

ICD-9-CM Procedural

81.25 Carporadial fusion
81.26 Metacarpocarpal fusion
81.29 Arthrodesis of other specified joint

Anesthesia

01830

ICD-9-CM Diagnostic

170.5 Malignant neoplasm of short bones of upper limb
171.2 Malignant neoplasm of connective and other soft tissue of upper limb, including shoulder
198.5 Secondary malignant neoplasm of bone and bone marrow
238.0 Neoplasm of uncertain behavior of bone and articular cartilage
710.2 Sicca syndrome
711.03 Pyogenic arthritis, forearm — (Use additional code to identify infectious organism: 041.0-041.8)
711.04 Pyogenic arthritis, hand — (Use additional code to identify infectious organism: 041.0-041.8)
714.0 Rheumatoid arthritis — (Use additional code to identify manifestation: 357.1, 359.6)
714.30 Polyarticular juvenile rheumatoid arthritis, chronic or unspecified
715.13 Primary localized osteoarthrosis, forearm
715.14 Primary localized osteoarthrosis, hand
715.23 Secondary localized osteoarthrosis, forearm
715.24 Secondary localized osteoarthrosis, involving hand
716.04 Kaschin-Beck disease, hand
716.13 Traumatic arthropathy, forearm
716.14 Traumatic arthropathy, hand
718.03 Articular cartilage disorder, forearm
718.04 Articular cartilage disorder, hand
718.33 Recurrent dislocation of forearm joint
718.34 Recurrent dislocation of hand joint
719.23 Villonodular synovitis, forearm
719.24 Villonodular synovitis, hand
733.81 Malunion of fracture

CCI Version 16.3

01810, 0213T, 0216T, 0228T, 0230T, 20650, 20690, 20692, 20696-20697, 20900-20902, 24300, 25110-25120, 25130, 25210-25215, 25259, 25295, 25320, 25660, 25670, 25820-25825, 26843-26844, 36000, 36400-36410, 36420-36430, 36440, 36600, 36640, 37202, 43752, 51701-51703, 62310-62319, 64400-64435, 64445-64450, 64479, 64483, 64490, 64493, 64505-64530, 64702-64726, 69990, 93000-93010, 93040-93042, 93318, 94002, 94200, 94250, 94680-94690, 94770, 95812-95816, 95819, 95822, 95829, 95955, 96360, 96365, 96372, 96374-96376, 99148-99149, 99150

Also not with 25800: 25085-25107, 25151, 29835-29836, 76000-76001

Also not with 25805: 25100-25107, 25151

Also not with 25810: 25085-25107, 26200, 29835-29836

Note: These CCI edits are used for Medicare. Other payers may reimburse on codes listed above.

Medicare Edits

	Fac RVU	Non-Fac RVU	FUD	Assist
25800	21.49	21.49	90	80
25805	24.87	24.87	90	80
25810	25.35	25.35	90	80

Medicare References: 100-2,15,260; 100-4,12,30; 100-4,12,90.3; 100-4,14,10

25820-25825

25820 Arthrodesis, wrist; limited, without bone graft (eg, intercarpal or radiocarpal)
25825 with autograft (includes obtaining graft)

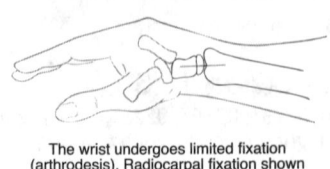

The wrist undergoes limited fixation (arthrodesis). Radiocarpal fixation shown above. Report 25825 when an autograft is used in the procedure

Articular spaces of the wrist. The intercarpal joints only may be fixed as part of a limited procedure

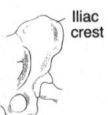

Iliac crest

Anterior view of hip. Autograft (25825)

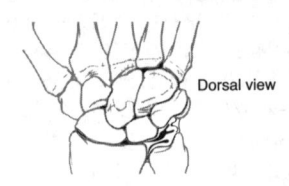

Dorsal view

Explanation

The physician performs intercarpal or radiocarpal fusion. The physician makes a curved dorsal incision from the bases of the second and third metacarpal to the tubercle. The wrist joint capsule is opened via a longitudinal incision centered over the capitate-lunate joint. The dorsal three-quarters of the capitate, lunate, and scaphoid bones are removed. Approximately 25 degrees of wrist dorsiflexion will lock the graft in place. If the graft needs further stabilization, crossed Kirschner wires may be used for fixation. The skin is closed in layers. A long-arm cast is placed for six weeks followed by a short-arm gauntlet for an additional six weeks. Report 25820 if a graft is not used. Report 25825 if a fitted circular or rectangular corticocanulous graft from iliac crest is removed and precisely shaped to fit the recipient. This graft is fit into the proximal row carpal area that has been removed.

Coding Tips

Arthrodesis of the wrist may also be referred to as a "four-corner fusion." In 25825, any bone graft harvest is not reported separately. According to CPT guidelines, cast application or strapping (including removal) is only reported as a replacement procedure or when the cast application or strapping is an initial service performed without a restorative treatment or procedure. See "Application of Casts and Strapping" in the CPT book in the Surgery Section, under the Musculoskeletal system. For arthrodesis, wrist, complete without bone graft, see 25800. For arthrodesis, wrist, complete with sliding graft, see 25805; with iliac or other autograft, see 25810.

ICD-9-CM Procedural

81.25 Carporadial fusion
81.29 Arthrodesis of other specified joint

Anesthesia
01830

ICD-9-CM Diagnostic

357.1 Polyneuropathy in collagen vascular disease — (Code first underlying disease: 446.0, 710.0, 714.0)
359.6 Symptomatic inflammatory myopathy in diseases classified elsewhere — (Code first underlying disease: 135, 140.0-208.9, 277.30-277.39, 446.0, 710.0, 710.1, 710.2, 714.0)
446.0 Polyarteritis nodosa
710.0 Systemic lupus erythematosus — (Use additional code to identify manifestation: 424.91, 581.81, 582.81, 583.81)
710.1 Systemic sclerosis — (Use additional code to identify manifestation: 359.6, 517.2)
710.2 Sicca syndrome
714.0 Rheumatoid arthritis — (Use additional code to identify manifestation: 357.1, 359.6)
714.31 Polyarticular juvenile rheumatoid arthritis, acute
715.04 Generalized osteoarthrosis, involving hand
715.14 Primary localized osteoarthrosis, hand
715.24 Secondary localized osteoarthrosis, involving hand
715.34 Localized osteoarthrosis not specified whether primary or secondary, hand
715.94 Osteoarthrosis, unspecified whether generalized or localized, hand
716.04 Kaschin-Beck disease, hand
716.14 Traumatic arthropathy, hand
718.04 Articular cartilage disorder, hand
718.84 Other joint derangement, not elsewhere classified, hand
731.3 Major osseous defects — (Code first underlying disease: 170.0-170.9, 730.00-730.29, 733.00-733.09, 733.40-733.49, 996.80)
733.49 Aseptic necrosis of other bone site — (Use additional code to identify major osseous defect, if applicable: 731.3)
733.81 Malunion of fracture

Terms To Know

arthrodesis. Surgical fixation or fusion of a joint to reduce pain and improve stability, performed openly or arthroscopically.

malunion. Fracture that has united in a faulty position due to inadequate reduction of the original fracture, insufficient holding of a previously well-reduced fracture, contracture of the soft tissues, or comminuted or osteoporotic bone causing a slow disintegration of the fracture.

sicca syndrome. Complex of symptoms of unknown source in middle-aged women in which the following triad exists: keratoconjunctivitis sicca, zerostomia, and connective tissue disease (usually rheumatoid arthritis but sometimes systemic lupus erythematosus).

CCI Version 16.3

01810, 0213T, 0216T, 0228T, 0230T, 20650, 24300, 25110-25120, 25130, 25210-25215, 25259, 25295, 25320, 25628, 25645, 25660, 25670, 26200, 29835-29836, 36000, 36400-36410, 36420-36430, 36440, 36600, 36640, 37202, 43752, 51701-51703, 62310-62319, 64400-64435, 64445-64450, 64479, 64483, 64490, 64493, 64505-64530, 64719-64721, 69990, 93000-93010, 93040-93042, 93318, 94002, 94200, 94250, 94680-94690, 94770, 95812-95816, 95819, 95822, 95829, 95955, 96360, 96365, 96372, 96374-96376, 99148-99149, 99150

Also not with 25820: 25085-25107, 29125

Also not with 25825: 20900-20902, 25100-25107, 25820

Note: These CCI edits are used for Medicare. Other payers may reimburse on codes listed above.

Medicare Edits

	Fac RVU	Non-Fac RVU	FUD	Assist
25820	17.81	17.81	90	80
25825	21.97	21.97	90	80

Medicare References: 100-2,15,260; 100-4,12,30; 100-4,12,90.3; 100-4,14,10

25830

25830 Arthrodesis, distal radioulnar joint with segmental resection of ulna, with or without bone graft (eg, Sauve-Kapandji procedure)

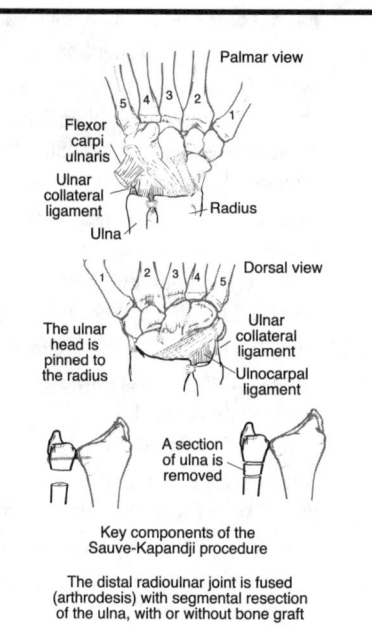

Key components of the Sauve-Kapandji procedure

The distal radioulnar joint is fused (arthrodesis) with segmental resection of the ulna, with or without bone graft

Explanation

The physician performs fusion of the distal radioulnar joint and resection of the ulna, sometimes using a bone graft. The physician makes a dorsal, curvilinear incision over the distal radioulnar joint. The extensor retinaculum is reflected, uncovering the extensor carpi ulnaris and extensor digiti minimi tendons. The capsule is cut and reflected, exposing the ulnar head. A small lamina spreader may be used to view the sigmoid notch of the radius. The periosteum is stripped from the ulna just proximal to the articular surface. The dorsal radioulnar ligaments are stripped sharply. If the distal ulna has been removed, or part of the distal ulna is missing, the remaining portion is decorticated. The radius is prepared by making a notch in the ulnar aspect where the distal ulna can be slotted. The ulna is manually compressed into the notch, holding the forearm in 10-15 degree pronation. The physician drives a Kirschner wire from the ulna into the radius and two compression screws from the outer aspect of the ulna through both cortices of the radius. The extensor retinaculum is reconstructed and the skin is closed.

Coding Tips

According to CPT guidelines, cast application or strapping (including removal) is only reported as a replacement procedure or when the cast application or strapping is an initial service performed without a restorative treatment or procedure. See "Application of Casts and Strapping" in the CPT book in the Surgery Section, under the Musculoskeletal system. For complete wrist arthrodesis, see 25800-25810. For limited wrist arthrodesis, see 25820 and 25825.

ICD-9-CM Procedural

81.29 Arthrodesis of other specified joint

Anesthesia

25830   01830

ICD-9-CM Diagnostic

- 170.5 Malignant neoplasm of short bones of upper limb
- 198.5 Secondary malignant neoplasm of bone and bone marrow
- 238.0 Neoplasm of uncertain behavior of bone and articular cartilage
- 239.2 Neoplasms of unspecified nature of bone, soft tissue, and skin
- 715.33 Localized osteoarthrosis not specified whether primary or secondary, forearm
- 715.93 Osteoarthrosis, unspecified whether generalized or localized, forearm
- 716.13 Traumatic arthropathy, forearm
- 718.33 Recurrent dislocation of forearm joint
- 731.3 Major osseous defects — (Code first underlying disease: 170.0-170.9, 730.00-730.29, 733.00-733.09, 733.40-733.49, 996.45)
- 733.49 Aseptic necrosis of other bone site — (Use additional code to identify major osseous defect, if applicable: 731.3)
- 733.81 Malunion of fracture

Terms To Know

aseptic necrosis. Death of bone tissue resulting from a disruption in the vascular supply, caused by a noninfectious disease process, such as a fracture or the administration of immunosuppressive drugs.

malignant. Any condition tending to progress toward death, specifically an invasive tumor with a loss of cellular differentiation that has the ability to spread or metastasize to other areas in the body.

malunion. Fracture that has united in a faulty position due to inadequate reduction of the original fracture, insufficient holding of a previously well-reduced fracture, contracture of the soft tissues, or comminuted or osteoporotic bone causing a slow disintegration of the fracture.

osteoarthrosis. Most common form of a noninflammatory degenerative joint disease with degenerating articular cartilage, bone enlargement, and synovial membrane changes.

pronation. Lying on the stomach or in a face down position; turning the palm toward the back or downward; lowering of the medial margin of the foot by an everting and abducting movement.

secondary. Second in order of occurrence or importance, or appearing during the course of another disease or condition.

soft tissue. Nonepithelial tissues outside of the skeleton that includes subcutaneous adipose tissue, fibrous tissue, fascia, muscles, blood and lymph vessels, and peripheral nervous system tissue.

CCI Version 16.3

01810, 0213T, 0216T, 0228T, 0230T, 24300, 25100-25105, 25110, 25119, 25240, 25259, 25295, 25320, 25360, 25390, 25500-25505, 25520, 25535, 25560-25565, 25600-25608❖, 25650-25651, 25660, 25675, 25800-25810, 25820-25825, 36000, 36400-36410, 36420-36430, 36440, 36600, 36640, 37202, 43752, 51701-51703, 62310-62319, 64400-64435, 64445-64450, 64479, 64483, 64490, 64493, 64505-64530, 69990, 93000-93010, 93040-93042, 93318, 94002, 94200, 94250, 94680-94690, 94770, 95812-95816, 95819, 95822, 95829, 95955, 96360, 96365, 96372, 96374-96376, 99148-99149, 99150

Note: These CCI edits are used for Medicare. Other payers may reimburse on codes listed above.

Medicare Edits

	Fac RVU	Non-Fac RVU	FUD	Assist
25830	27.69	27.69	90	80

Medicare References: 100-2,15,260; 100-4,12,30; 100-4,12,90.3; 100-4,14,10

25900

25900 Amputation, forearm, through radius and ulna;

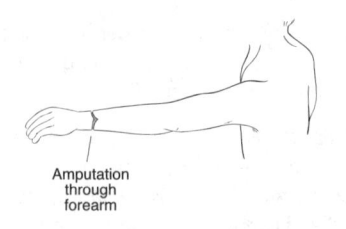

Amputation through forearm

An amputation is performed through the forearem. Report 25900 when the amputation is non-circular

Explanation

In elective below-elbow amputations, the physician cuts the soft tissue flaps distal to the intended level of bone amputation. The physician dissects the superficial veins and cuts them at the level of the amputation. Cutaneous nerves are cut proximal to the level of the amputation. The dorsal and volar antebrachial fascia is cut, and, depending on the level of amputation, either the tendons or muscle bellies are divided after the radial and ulnar vessels are severed. Muscle bellies are incised just distal to the planned level of bony resection. Nerves are cut through a separate incision and brought under the muscle. The anterior and posterior interosseous vessels should be ligated or coagulated with electrocautery. An incision in the periosteum is carried out sharply and circumferentially. The bone is transected at the desired level at this time and the specimen is removed. The bone ends are smoothed with a rasp. Closure is accomplished after hemostasis is obtained following tourniquet release. The skin flaps can be fashioned and subcutaneous tissue and skin are closed in separate layers. A drain is sometimes placed. The stump is dressed and wrapped with an elastic bandage applied more firmly distally than proximally.

Coding Tips

Adjacent tissue transfer is included in this procedure. However, report any free grafts separately. For open, circular (guillotine) amputation, see 25905. For secondary closure or scar revision of a forearm amputation, see 25907. For re-amputation of the forearm, see 25909.

ICD-9-CM Procedural

84.05 Amputation through forearm

Anesthesia

25900 01830

ICD-9-CM Diagnostic

- 170.5 Malignant neoplasm of short bones of upper limb
- 170.9 Malignant neoplasm of bone and articular cartilage, site unspecified
- 198.5 Secondary malignant neoplasm of bone and bone marrow
- 250.70 Diabetes with peripheral circulatory disorders, type II or unspecified type, not stated as uncontrolled — (Use additional code to identify manifestation: 443.81, 785.4)
- 250.71 Diabetes with peripheral circulatory disorders, type I [juvenile type], not stated as uncontrolled — (Use additional code to identify manifestation: 443.81, 785.4)
- 440.24 Atherosclerosis of native arteries of the extremities with gangrene — (Use additional code for any associated ulceration: 707.10-707.9)
- 443.81 Peripheral angiopathy in diseases classified elsewhere — (Code first underlying disease: 249.7, 250.7)
- 446.0 Polyarteritis nodosa
- 682.3 Cellulitis and abscess of upper arm and forearm — (Use additional code to identify organism, such as 041.1, etc.)
- 728.86 Necrotizing fasciitis — (Use additional code to identify infectious organism, 041.00-041.89, 785.4, if applicable)
- 730.13 Chronic osteomyelitis, forearm — (Use additional code to identify organism: 041.1. Use additional code to identify major osseous defect, if applicable: 731.3)
- 731.1 Osteitis deformans in diseases classified elsewhere — (Code first underlying disease: 170.0-170.9)
- 731.3 Major osseous defects — (Code first underlying disease: 170.0-170.9, 730.00-730.29, 733.00-733.09, 733.40-733.49, 996.45)
- 785.4 Gangrene — (Code first any associated underlying condition)
- 887.0 Traumatic amputation of arm and hand (complete) (partial), unilateral, below elbow, without mention of complication
- 887.1 Traumatic amputation of arm and hand (complete) (partial), unilateral, below elbow, complicated
- 887.6 Traumatic amputation of arm and hand (complete) (partial), bilateral (any level), without mention of complication
- 887.7 Traumatic amputation of arm and hand (complete) (partial), bilateral (any level), complicated
- 927.10 Crushing injury of forearm — (Use additional code to identify any associated injuries: 800-829, 850.0-854.1, 860.0-869.1)
- 927.21 Crushing injury of wrist — (Use additional code to identify any associated injuries: 800-829, 850.0-854.1, 860.0-869.1)
- 943.51 Deep necrosis of underlying tissues due to burn (deep third degree) of forearm, with loss of a body part
- 958.3 Posttraumatic wound infection not elsewhere classified

CCI Version 16.3

01810, 0213T, 0216T, 0228T, 0230T, 20103, 24300, 25120, 25150-25151, 25259, 25350-25393, 36000, 36400-36410, 36420-36430, 36440, 36600, 36640, 37202, 37618, 43752, 51701-51703, 62310-62319, 64400-64435, 64445-64450, 64479, 64483, 64490, 64493, 64505-64530, 64704-64708, 64718-64719, 64774-64776, 64782, 64784, 69990, 93000-93010, 93040-93042, 93318, 94002, 94200, 94250, 94680-94690, 94770, 95812-95816, 95819, 95822, 95829, 95955, 96360, 96365, 96372, 96374-96376, 97597-97598, 97602-97606, 99148-99149, 99150

Note: These CCI edits are used for Medicare. Other payers may reimburse on codes listed above.

Medicare Edits

	Fac RVU	Non-Fac RVU	FUD	Assist
25900	21.39	21.39	90	80

Medicare References: None

25905

25905 Amputation, forearm, through radius and ulna; open, circular (guillotine)

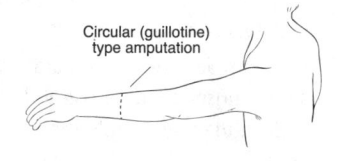

Circular (guillotine) type amputation

An amputation is performed through the forearm. Report 25905 when the amputation is circular (guillotine), straight across, and through the bones of the forearm

Explanation
The physician performs a guillotine amputation. Just distal to the level of intended bone section, the physician incises the skin in a circular manner down to the deep fascia and allows it to retract. The muscles at the edge of the retracted skin are divided. All vessels encountered are ligated and divided. All major nerves are divided at a proximal level so that they retract proximal to the end of the stump. The physician sections the bone at the ends of the retracted muscles. The bone end is covered by the distal muscle bulk, and the skin is stretched over the stump and sutured closed. The stump is covered with a compressive dressing to control post-surgical edema.

Coding Tips
Adjacent tissue transfer is included in this procedure. However, report any free grafts separately. For forearm amputation, see 25900. For secondary closure or scar revision of a forearm amputation, see 25907. For re-amputation of the forearm, see 25909.

ICD-9-CM Procedural
84.05 Amputation through forearm

Anesthesia
25905 01830

ICD-9-CM Diagnostic
170.5 Malignant neoplasm of short bones of upper limb
170.9 Malignant neoplasm of bone and articular cartilage, site unspecified
198.5 Secondary malignant neoplasm of bone and bone marrow
249.70 Secondary diabetes mellitus with peripheral circulatory disorders, not stated as uncontrolled, or unspecified — (Use additional code to identify manifestation: 443.81, 785.4) (Use additional code to identify any associated insulin use: V58.67)
249.71 Secondary diabetes mellitus with peripheral circulatory disorders, uncontrolled — (Use additional code to identify manifestation: 443.81, 785.4) (Use additional code to identify any associated insulin use: V58.67)
250.70 Diabetes with peripheral circulatory disorders, type II or unspecified type, not stated as uncontrolled — (Use additional code to identify manifestation: 443.81, 785.4)
250.71 Diabetes with peripheral circulatory disorders, type I [juvenile type], not stated as uncontrolled — (Use additional code to identify manifestation: 443.81, 785.4)
440.24 Atherosclerosis of native arteries of the extremities with gangrene — (Use additional code for any associated ulceration: 707.10-707.9)
443.81 Peripheral angiopathy in diseases classified elsewhere — (Code first underlying disease: 249.7, 250.7)
446.0 Polyarteritis nodosa
682.3 Cellulitis and abscess of upper arm and forearm — (Use additional code to identify organism, such as 041.1, etc.)
728.86 Necrotizing fasciitis — (Use additional code to identify infectious organism, 041.00-041.89, 785.4, if applicable)
730.13 Chronic osteomyelitis, forearm — (Use additional code to identify organism: 041.1. Use additional code to identify major osseous defect, if applicable: 731.3)
731.1 Osteitis deformans in diseases classified elsewhere — (Code first underlying disease: 170.0-170.9)
731.3 Major osseous defects — (Code first underlying disease: 170.0-170.9, 730.00-730.29, 733.00-733.09, 733.40-733.49, 996.45)
785.4 Gangrene — (Code first any associated underlying condition)
887.0 Traumatic amputation of arm and hand (complete) (partial), unilateral, below elbow, without mention of complication
887.1 Traumatic amputation of arm and hand (complete) (partial), unilateral, below elbow, complicated
887.6 Traumatic amputation of arm and hand (complete) (partial), bilateral (any level), without mention of complication
887.7 Traumatic amputation of arm and hand (complete) (partial), bilateral (any level), complicated
927.10 Crushing injury of forearm — (Use additional code to identify any associated injuries: 800-829, 850.0-854.1, 860.0-869.1)
927.21 Crushing injury of wrist — (Use additional code to identify any associated injuries: 800-829, 850.0-854.1, 860.0-869.1)
943.51 Deep necrosis of underlying tissues due to burn (deep third degree) of forearm, with loss of a body part
958.3 Posttraumatic wound infection not elsewhere classified

Terms To Know
osteomyelitis. Inflammation of bone that may remain localized or spread to the marrow, cortex, or periosteum, in response to an infecting organism, usually bacterial and pyogenic.

CCI Version 16.3
01810, 0213T, 0216T, 0228T, 0230T, 20103, 24300, 25120, 25150-25151, 25259, 25350-25393, 25900, 36000, 36400-36410, 36420-36430, 36440, 36600, 36640, 37202, 37618, 43752, 51701-51703, 62310-62319, 64400-64435, 64445-64450, 64479, 64483, 64490, 64493, 64505-64530, 69990, 93000-93010, 93040-93042, 93318, 94002, 94200, 94250, 94680-94690, 94770, 95812-95816, 95819, 95822, 95829, 95955, 96360, 96365, 96372, 96374-96376, 97597-97598, 97602-97606, 99148-99149, 99150

Note: These CCI edits are used for Medicare. Other payers may reimburse on codes listed above.

Medicare Edits

	Fac RVU	Non-Fac RVU	FUD	Assist
25905	21.08	21.08	90	80

Medicare References: None

25907

25907 Amputation, forearm, through radius and ulna; secondary closure or scar revision

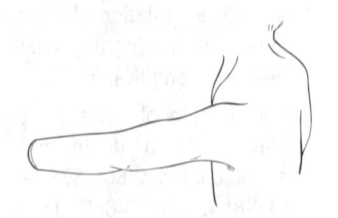

A previous site of an amputation through the forearm is closed secondarily or a scar has formed requiring revision at the site of the previous amputation

Explanation

The physician performs secondary closure or scar revision after the stump has granulated or healed by a scar. In this procedure, no additional bone is sectioned. The physician resects the scar and granulation tissue from the end of the stump. Skin flaps are fashioned as close as possible to the thick scar surrounding the granulating wound. The dense layer of scar tissue is excised from over the end of the bone. Additional muscle may be removed as well. The skin flaps are pulled over the end of the stump and connected with nonabsorbable sutures. A temporary drain or suction tubes may also be used.

Coding Tips

Adjacent tissue transfer is included in this procedure. However, report any free grafts separately. For amputation, forearm, through the radius and ulna, see 25900; open circular (guillotine) method, see 25905. For re-amputation of the forearm, see 25909.

ICD-9-CM Procedural

84.3 Revision of amputation stump

Anesthesia

25907 00400

ICD-9-CM Diagnostic

- 170.5 Malignant neoplasm of short bones of upper limb
- 170.9 Malignant neoplasm of bone and articular cartilage, site unspecified
- 198.5 Secondary malignant neoplasm of bone and bone marrow
- 249.70 Secondary diabetes mellitus with peripheral circulatory disorders, not stated as uncontrolled, or unspecified — (Use additional code to identify manifestation: 443.81, 785.4) (Use additional code to identify any associated insulin use: V58.67)
- 249.71 Secondary diabetes mellitus with peripheral circulatory disorders, uncontrolled — (Use additional code to identify manifestation: 443.81, 785.4) (Use additional code to identify any associated insulin use: V58.67)
- 250.70 Diabetes with peripheral circulatory disorders, type II or unspecified type, not stated as uncontrolled — (Use additional code to identify manifestation: 443.81, 785.4)
- 250.71 Diabetes with peripheral circulatory disorders, type I [juvenile type], not stated as uncontrolled — (Use additional code to identify manifestation: 443.81, 785.4)
- 440.24 Atherosclerosis of native arteries of the extremities with gangrene — (Use additional code for any associated ulceration: 707.10-707.9)
- 443.81 Peripheral angiopathy in diseases classified elsewhere — (Code first underlying disease: 249.7, 250.7)
- 443.9 Unspecified peripheral vascular disease
- 446.0 Polyarteritis nodosa
- 682.3 Cellulitis and abscess of upper arm and forearm — (Use additional code to identify organism, such as 041.1, etc.)
- 707.00 Pressure ulcer, unspecified site — (Use additional code to identify pressure ulcer stage: 707.20-707.25)
- 707.01 Pressure ulcer, elbow — (Use additional code to identify pressure ulcer stage: 707.20-707.25)
- 707.09 Pressure ulcer, other site — (Use additional code to identify pressure ulcer stage: 707.20-707.25)
- 707.8 Chronic ulcer of other specified site
- 709.2 Scar condition and fibrosis of skin
- 728.86 Necrotizing fasciitis — (Use additional code to identify infectious organism, 041.00-041.89, 785.4, if applicable)
- 730.12 Chronic osteomyelitis, upper arm — (Use additional code to identify organism: 041.1. Use additional code to identify major osseous defect, if applicable: 731.3)
- 731.3 Major osseous defects — (Code first underlying disease: 170.0-170.9, 730.00-730.29, 733.00-733.09, 733.40-733.49, 996.45)
- 785.4 Gangrene — (Code first any associated underlying condition)
- 944.58 Deep necrosis of underlying tissues due to burn (deep third degree) of multiple sites of wrist(s) and hand(s), with loss of a body part
- 997.60 Late complications of amputation stump, unspecified — (Use additional code to identify complications)
- 997.61 Neuroma of amputation stump — (Use additional code to identify complications)
- 997.62 Infection (chronic) of amputation stump — (Use additional code to identify complications)
- 997.69 Other late amputation stump complication — (Use additional code to identify complications)
- 998.83 Non-healing surgical wound
- V51.8 Other aftercare involving the use of plastic surgery
- V58.41 Planned postoperative wound closure — (This code should be used in conjunction with other aftercare codes to fully identify the reason for the aftercare encounter)

CCI Version 16.3

01810, 0213T, 0216T, 0228T, 0230T, 24300, 25120, 25150-25151, 25259, 25350-25393, 25900, 36000, 36400-36410, 36420-36430, 36440, 36600, 36640, 37202, 37618, 43752, 51701-51703, 62310-62319, 64400-64435, 64445-64450, 64479, 64483, 64490, 64493, 64505-64530, 69990, 93000-93010, 93040-93042, 93318, 94002, 94200, 94250, 94680-94690, 94770, 95812-95816, 95819, 95822, 95829, 95955, 96360, 96365, 96372, 96374-96376, 97597-97598, 97602-97606, 99148-99149, 99150

Note: These CCI edits are used for Medicare. Other payers may reimburse on codes listed above.

Medicare Edits

	Fac RVU	Non-Fac RVU	FUD	Assist
25907	18.44	18.44	90	80

Medicare References: 100-2,15,260; 100-4,12,30; 100-4,12,90.3; 100-4,14,10

25909

25909 Amputation, forearm, through radius and ulna; re-amputation

The site of a previous amputation through the forearm requires re-amputation

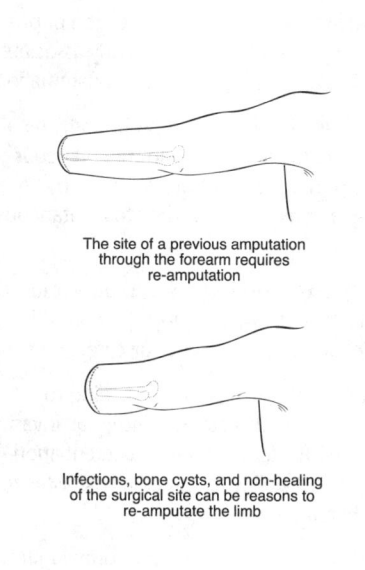

Infections, bone cysts, and non-healing of the surgical site can be reasons to re-amputate the limb

Explanation

The physician performs a reamputation. A reamputation may be necessary at a proximal level to reach healthy tissue. The physician cuts the soft tissue flaps distal to the intended level of bone amputation. The physician dissects the superficial veins and cuts them at the level of the amputation. Cutaneous nerves are cut proximal to the level of the amputation. The dorsal and volar antebrachial fascia is cut, and, depending on the level of amputation, either the tendons or muscle bellies are divided after the radial and ulnar vessels are severed. Muscle bellies are incised just distal to the planned level of bony resection. Nerves are cut through a separate incision and brought under the muscle. The anterior and posterior interosseous vessels should be ligated or coagulated with electrocautery. An incision in the periosteum is carried out sharply and circumferentially. The bone is transected at the desired level at this time and the specimen is removed. The bone ends are smoothed with a rasp. Closure is accomplished after hemostasis is obtained following tourniquet release. The skin flaps can be fashioned and subcutaneous tissue and skin are closed.

Coding Tips

Adjacent tissue transfer is included in this procedure. However, report any free grafts separately. For secondary closure or scar revision of a forearm amputation, see 25907. For amputation, forearm, through the radius and ulna, see 25900; open circular (guillotine) method, see 25905.

ICD-9-CM Procedural

84.05	Amputation through forearm
84.3	Revision of amputation stump

Anesthesia

25909 01830

ICD-9-CM Diagnostic

249.70 Secondary diabetes mellitus with peripheral circulatory disorders, not stated as uncontrolled, or unspecified — (Use additional code to identify manifestation: 443.81, 785.4) (Use additional code to identify any associated insulin use: V58.67)

249.71 Secondary diabetes mellitus with peripheral circulatory disorders, uncontrolled — (Use additional code to identify manifestation: 443.81, 785.4) (Use additional code to identify any associated insulin use: V58.67)

250.70 Diabetes with peripheral circulatory disorders, type II or unspecified type, not stated as uncontrolled — (Use additional code to identify manifestation: 443.81, 785.4)

250.71 Diabetes with peripheral circulatory disorders, type I [juvenile type], not stated as uncontrolled — (Use additional code to identify manifestation: 443.81, 785.4)

785.4 Gangrene — (Code first any associated underlying condition)

997.60 Late complications of amputation stump, unspecified — (Use additional code to identify complications)

997.61 Neuroma of amputation stump — (Use additional code to identify complications)

997.62 Infection (chronic) of amputation stump — (Use additional code to identify complications)

997.69 Other late amputation stump complication — (Use additional code to identify complications)

998.59 Other postoperative infection — (Use additional code to identify infection)

998.6 Persistent postoperative fistula, not elsewhere classified

998.83 Non-healing surgical wound

V49.66 Upper limb amputation, above elbow

V51.8 Other aftercare involving the use of plastic surgery

Terms To Know

fascia. Fibrous sheet or band of tissue that envelops organs, muscles, and groupings of muscles.

fistula. Abnormal tube-like passage between two body cavities or organs or from an organ to the outside surface.

gangrene. Death of tissue, usually resulting from a loss of vascular supply, followed by a bacterial attack or onset of disease.

neuroma. Any type of tumor growing from a nerve or comprised of nerve cells and fibers.

periosteum. Double-layered connective membrane on the outer surface of bone.

CCI Version 16.3

01810, 0213T, 0216T, 0228T, 0230T, 24300, 25120, 25150-25151, 25259, 25350-25393, 25900, 36000, 36400-36410, 36420-36430, 36440, 36600, 36640, 37202, 37618, 43752, 51701-51703, 62310-62319, 64400-64435, 64445-64450, 64479, 64483, 64490, 64493, 64505-64530, 69990, 93000-93010, 93040-93042, 93318, 94002, 94200, 94250, 94680-94690, 94770, 95812-95816, 95819, 95822, 95829, 95955, 96360, 96365, 96372, 96374-96376, 97597-97598, 97602-97606, 99148-99149, 99150

Note: These CCI edits are used for Medicare. Other payers may reimburse on codes listed above.

Medicare Edits

	Fac RVU	Non-Fac RVU	FUD	Assist
25909	20.62	20.62	90	80

Medicare References: None

25915

25915 Krukenberg procedure

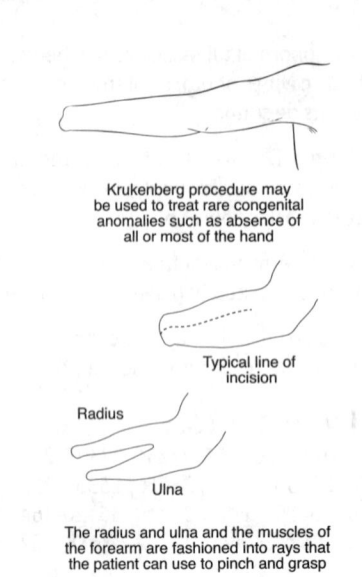

Krukenberg procedure may be used to treat rare congenital anomalies such as absence of all or most of the hand

Typical line of incision
Radius
Ulna

The radius and ulna and the muscles of the forearm are fashioned into rays that the patient can use to pinch and grasp

Explanation
The physician performs the Krukenberg procedure, a forearm amputation. The physician longitudinally splits the stump into radial and ulnar rays by making a dorsal, longitudinal incision toward the ulnar aspect of the forearm. Also, a volar, longitudinal incision is made toward the radial aspect of the forearm. The muscles left or transferred to the radial side of the forearm are the radial wrist extensors and flexors, the flexors of the index and long fingers, the index and long finger extensors, the pronator teres, the palmaris longus, and the brachioradialis. The remaining muscles are left or inserted on the ulnar side of the forearm. On occasion, some muscles need resection to reduce bulk, but the pronator tercs must be preserved. The interosseous membrane is freed along its ulnar border. Skin closure is performed, ensuring the tactile skin is placed over the contact surfaces between the radius and ulna.

Coding Tips
Adjacent tissue transfer is included in this procedure. However, report any free grafts separately. According to CPT guidelines, cast application or strapping (including removal) is only reported as a replacement procedure or when the cast application or strapping is an initial service performed without a restorative treatment or procedure. See "Application of Casts and Strapping" in the CPT book in the Surgery Section, under the Musculoskeletal system.

ICD-9-CM Procedural
82.89 Other plastic operations on hand

Anesthesia
25915 01830

ICD-9-CM Diagnostic
170.5 Malignant neoplasm of short bones of upper limb
198.5 Secondary malignant neoplasm of bone and bone marrow
249.70 Secondary diabetes mellitus with peripheral circulatory disorders, not stated as uncontrolled, or unspecified — (Use additional code to identify manifestation: 443.81, 785.4) (Use additional code to identify any associated insulin use: V58.67)
249.71 Secondary diabetes mellitus with peripheral circulatory disorders, uncontrolled — (Use additional code to identify manifestation: 443.81, 785.4) (Use additional code to identify any associated insulin use: V58.67)
250.70 Diabetes with peripheral circulatory disorders, type II or unspecified type, not stated as uncontrolled — (Use additional code to identify manifestation: 443.81, 785.4)
250.71 Diabetes with peripheral circulatory disorders, type I [juvenile type], not stated as uncontrolled — (Use additional code to identify manifestation: 443.81, 785.4)
440.24 Atherosclerosis of native arteries of the extremities with gangrene — (Use additional code for any associated ulceration: 707.10-707.9)
443.81 Peripheral angiopathy in diseases classified elsewhere — (Code first underlying disease: 249.7, 250.7)
682.3 Cellulitis and abscess of upper arm and forearm — (Use additional code to identify organism, such as 041.1, etc.)
728.86 Necrotizing fasciitis — (Use additional code to identify infectious organism, 041.00-041.89, 785.4, if applicable)
736.00 Unspecified deformity of forearm, excluding fingers
755.50 Unspecified congenital anomaly of upper limb
785.4 Gangrene — (Code first any associated underlying condition)
997.60 Late complications of amputation stump, unspecified — (Use additional code to identify complications)
997.61 Neuroma of amputation stump — (Use additional code to identify complications)

Terms To Know
abscess. Circumscribed collection of pus resulting from bacteria, frequently associated with swelling and other signs of inflammation.

cellulitis. Sudden, severe, suppurative inflammation and edema in subcutaneous tissue or muscle, most often caused by bacterial infection secondary to a cutaneous lesion.

gangrene. Death of tissue, usually resulting from a loss of vascular supply, followed by a bacterial attack or onset of disease.

malignant. Any condition tending to progress toward death, specifically an invasive tumor with a loss of cellular differentiation that has the ability to spread or metastasize to other areas in the body.

neuroma. Any type of tumor growing from a nerve or comprised of nerve cells and fibers.

osteogenesis imperfecta. Hereditary collagen disorder that produces brittle, osteoporotic bones that are easily fractured, with hypermobility of points, blue sclerae and a tendency to hemorrhage.

secondary. Second in order of occurrence or importance, or appearing during the course of another disease or condition.

CCI Version 16.3
01810, 0213T, 0216T, 0228T, 0230T, 24300, 25120, 25150-25151, 25259, 25310-25312, 25350-25393, 36000, 36400-36410, 36420-36430, 36440, 36600, 36640, 37202, 37618, 43752, 51701-51703, 62310-62319, 64400-64435, 64445-64450, 64479, 64483, 64490, 64493, 64505-64530, 69990, 93000-93010, 93040-93042, 93318, 94002, 94200, 94250, 94680-94690, 94770, 95812-95816, 95819, 95822, 95829, 95955, 96360, 96365, 96372, 96374-96376, 97597-97598, 97602-97606, 99148-99149, 99150

Note: These CCI edits are used for Medicare. Other payers may reimburse on codes listed above.

Medicare Edits
	Fac RVU	Non-Fac RVU	FUD	Assist
25915	33.22	33.22	90	80

Medicare References: None

25920-25924

25920 Disarticulation through wrist;
25922 secondary closure or scar revision
25924 re-amputation

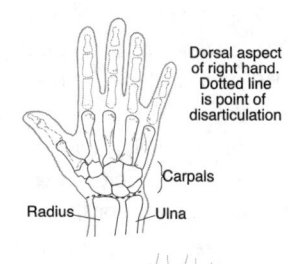

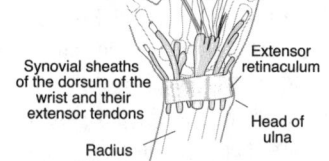

Dorsal aspect of right hand. Dotted line is point of disarticulation
Carpals
Radius — Ulna

Synovial sheaths of the dorsum of the wrist and their extensor tendons
Extensor retinaculum
Head of ulna
Radius

An amputation by disarticulation through the wrist is performed. Report 25922 for secondary closure or scar revision to the site of a previous disarticulation. Report 25924 when a previous disarticulation requires re-amputation of the site

Explanation

The physician disarticulates (amputates) the hand from the forearm through the wrist. The physician makes a long, palmar flap and a short, dorsal flap at a level distal to the radioulnar joint. These flaps are pulled back proximally and all veins are ligated. The physician cuts the superficial branch of the radial nerve and the dorsal sensory branch of the ulnar nerve. The lateral and medial antebrachial cutaneous nerves are cut. The radial and ulnar blood vessels are severed proximate to the wrist. The median nerve is cut while traction is applied. The flexor and extensor tendons are pulled distally and cut. The physician makes a transverse, dorsal incision of the dorsal radiocarpal ligament to view the radiocarpal joint. Circumferential dissection of the radiocarpal capsular and ligamentous attachments are carried out. The amputated specimen is removed. The styloid processes are rounded off and the skin flaps are closed in two layers of subcutaneous tissue and skin. A soft dressing is applied distal to proximal. Report 25920 if an amputation through the wrist is performed. Report 25922 if a secondary closure or scar revision is performed on the stump. Report 25924 if a re-amputation is performed. All use a similar technique.

Coding Tips

Adjacent tissue transfer is included in these procedures. However, report any free grafts separately.

ICD-9-CM Procedural

84.04 Disarticulation of wrist
84.3 Revision of amputation stump

Anesthesia

25920 01830
25922 00400
25924 01830

ICD-9-CM Diagnostic

170.5 Malignant neoplasm of short bones of upper limb
171.2 Malignant neoplasm of connective and other soft tissue of upper limb, including shoulder
195.5 Malignant neoplasm of lower limb
250.70 Diabetes with peripheral circulatory disorders, type II or unspecified type, not stated as uncontrolled — (Use additional code to identify manifestation: 443.81, 785.4)
250.71 Diabetes with peripheral circulatory disorders, type I [juvenile type], not stated as uncontrolled — (Use additional code to identify manifestation: 443.81, 785.4)
440.24 Atherosclerosis of native arteries of the extremities with gangrene — (Use additional code for any associated ulceration: 707.10-707.9)
443.81 Peripheral angiopathy in diseases classified elsewhere — (Code first underlying disease: 249.7, 250.7)
446.0 Polyarteritis nodosa
682.3 Cellulitis and abscess of upper arm and forearm — (Use additional code to identify organism, such as 041.1, etc.)
707.09 Pressure ulcer, other site — (Use additional code to identify pressure ulcer stage: 707.20-707.25)
707.8 Chronic ulcer of other specified site
709.2 Scar condition and fibrosis of skin
728.86 Necrotizing fasciitis — (Use additional code to identify infectious organism, 041.00-041.89, 785.4, if applicable)
785.4 Gangrene — (Code first any associated underlying condition)
817.1 Multiple open fractures of hand bones
887.0 Traumatic amputation of arm and hand (complete) (partial), unilateral, below elbow, without mention of complication
927.21 Crushing injury of wrist — (Use additional code to identify any associated injuries: 800-829, 850.0-854.1, 860.0-869.1)
997.60 Late complications of amputation stump, unspecified — (Use additional code to identify complications)
997.61 Neuroma of amputation stump — (Use additional code to identify complications)
997.62 Infection (chronic) of amputation stump — (Use additional code to identify complications)
997.69 Other late amputation stump complication — (Use additional code to identify complications)
998.59 Other postoperative infection — (Use additional code to identify infection)
998.6 Persistent postoperative fistula, not elsewhere classified
998.83 Non-healing surgical wound
V51.8 Other aftercare involving the use of plastic surgery
V58.41 Planned postoperative wound closure — (This code should be used in conjunction with other aftercare codes to fully identify the reason for the aftercare encounter)

CCI Version 16.3

01810, 0213T, 0216T, 0228T, 0230T, 24300, 25085-25105, 25120, 25150-25151, 25250, 25259, 25320, 36000, 36400-36410, 36420-36430, 36440, 36600, 36640, 37202, 37618, 43752, 51701-51703, 62310-62319, 64400-64435, 64445-64450, 64479, 64483, 64490, 64493, 64505-64530, 69990, 93000-93010, 93040-93042, 93318, 94002, 94200, 94250, 94680-94690, 94770, 95812-95816, 95819, 95822, 95829, 95955, 96360, 96365, 96372, 96374-96376, 97597-97598, 97602-97606, 99148-99149, 99150

Also not with 25920: 20103, 25350-25394
Also not with 25922: 25350-25394, 25920
Also not with 25924: 25350-25393, 25920
Note: These CCI edits are used for Medicare. Other payers may reimburse on codes listed above.

Medicare Edits

	Fac RVU	Non-Fac RVU	FUD	Assist
25920	20.15	20.15	90	80
25922	15.02	15.02	90	80
25924	18.66	18.66	90	80

Medicare References: 100-2,15,260; 100-4,12,30; 100-4,12,90.3; 100-4,14,10

25927-25931

25927 Transmetacarpal amputation;
25929 secondary closure or scar revision
25931 re-amputation

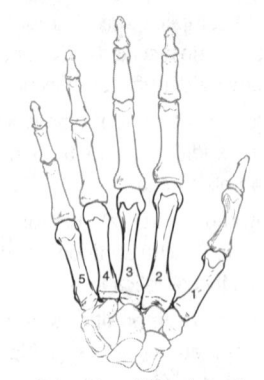

Palmar view of the metacarpal bones of right hand

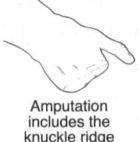

An amputation is performed through the carpal bones. Report 25929 for a secondary closure or a scar revision to the amputation site. Report 25931 when a re-amputation is required.

Amputation includes the knuckle ridge

Explanation

The physician amputates the fingers. The physician makes circumferential incisions around each digit excluding the thumb. These incisions are carried out at the mid-proximophalangeal level. The extensor digitonum communis of each digit (also the extensor indicis proprius of the index and the extensor digiti minimi of the little) are transected at the metacarpal bases. Individually, each metacarpal bone is transected and elevated from its soft tissue bed. The lumbricals and dorsal interossei are sectioned. Identified blood vessels are ligated. Nerves are ligated and transected. The flexor tendons are transected and allowed to retract in the palm. The volar plate, ligaments, and palmar fascia at this level are all cut and amputated digits are removed. The open periosteal tubes are closed. The soft tissue flaps are drawn over the end of the stump and interrupted sutures are used. A soft dressing is applied. Report 25927 if an amputation is performed. Report 25929 if a secondary closure or scar revision is performed. Report 25931 if a re-amputation is performed. All use a similar technique.

Coding Tips

Adjacent tissue transfer is included in these procedures. However, report any free grafts separately.

ICD-9-CM Procedural

84.03	Amputation through hand
84.3	Revision of amputation stump

Anesthesia

25927	01830
25929	00400
25931	01830

ICD-9-CM Diagnostic

170.5	Malignant neoplasm of short bones of upper limb
171.2	Malignant neoplasm of connective and other soft tissue of upper limb, including shoulder
198.5	Secondary malignant neoplasm of bone and bone marrow
249.70	Secondary diabetes mellitus with peripheral circulatory disorders, not stated as uncontrolled, or unspecified — (Use additional code to identify manifestation: 443.81, 785.4) (Use additional code to identify any associated insulin use: V58.67)
249.71	Secondary diabetes mellitus with peripheral circulatory disorders, uncontrolled — (Use additional code to identify manifestation: 443.81, 785.4) (Use additional code to identify any associated insulin use: V58.67)
250.70	Diabetes with peripheral circulatory disorders, type II or unspecified type, not stated as uncontrolled — (Use additional code to identify manifestation: 443.81, 785.4)
250.71	Diabetes with peripheral circulatory disorders, type I [juvenile type], not stated as uncontrolled — (Use additional code to identify manifestation: 443.81, 785.4)
440.24	Atherosclerosis of native arteries of the extremities with gangrene — (Use additional code for any associated ulceration: 707.10-707.9)
443.81	Peripheral angiopathy in diseases classified elsewhere — (Code first underlying disease: 249.7, 250.7)
682.3	Cellulitis and abscess of upper arm and forearm — (Use additional code to identify organism, such as 041.1, etc.)
707.8	Chronic ulcer of other specified site
728.86	Necrotizing fasciitis — (Use additional code to identify infectious organism, 041.00-041.89, 785.4, if applicable)
785.4	Gangrene — (Code first any associated underlying condition)
927.20	Crushing injury of hand(s) — (Use additional code to identify any associated injuries: 800-829, 850.0-854.1, 860.0-869.1)
997.60	Late complications of amputation stump, unspecified — (Use additional code to identify complications)
997.61	Neuroma of amputation stump — (Use additional code to identify complications)
997.62	Infection (chronic) of amputation stump — (Use additional code to identify complications)
997.69	Other late amputation stump complication — (Use additional code to identify complications)
998.59	Other postoperative infection — (Use additional code to identify infection)
998.6	Persistent postoperative fistula, not elsewhere classified
998.83	Non-healing surgical wound
V51.8	Other aftercare involving the use of plastic surgery
V58.41	Planned postoperative wound closure — (This code should be used in conjunction with other aftercare codes to fully identify the reason for the aftercare encounter)

CCI Version 16.3

01810, 0213T, 0216T, 0228T, 0230T, 24300, 25259, 26070-26075, 26100-26105, 26230, 26565, 36000, 36400-36410, 36420-36430, 36440, 36600, 36640, 37202, 37618, 43752, 51701-51703, 62310-62319, 64400-64435, 64445-64450, 64479, 64483, 64490, 64493, 64505-64530, 64704, 64719-64721, 64774-64776, 64782, 64784-64786, 69990, 93000-93010, 93040-93042, 93318, 94002, 94200, 94250, 94680-94690, 94770, 95812-95816, 95819, 95822, 95829, 95955, 96360, 96365, 96372, 96374-96376, 97597-97598, 97602-97606, 99148-99149, 99150

Also not with 25927: 20103, 25250
Also not with 25929: 25250, 25927
Also not with 25931: 25927

Note: These CCI edits are used for Medicare. Other payers may reimburse on codes listed above.

Medicare Edits

	Fac RVU	Non-Fac RVU	FUD	Assist
25927	23.18	23.18	90	80
25929	17.17	17.17	90	80
25931	20.21	20.21	90	N/A

Medicare References: 100-2,15,260; 100-4,12,30; 100-4,12,90.3; 100-4,14,10

26010-26011

26010 Drainage of finger abscess; simple
26011 complicated (eg, felon)

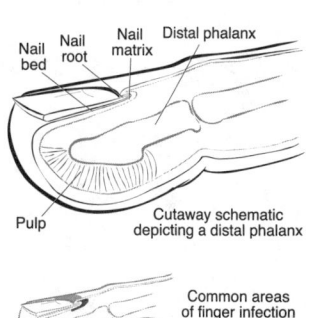

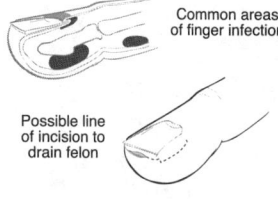

Nail bed, Nail root, Nail matrix, Distal phalanx, Pulp
Cutaway schematic depicting a distal phalanx

Common areas of finger infection

Possible line of incision to drain felon

A felon is an infection of the pulp at the tip of the finger

An abscess of the finger is drained. Report 26011 for complicated drainage

Explanation

The physician drains an abscess located in a finger. In 26010, the physician lances an abscess located in the cutaneous tissue of a finger. In 26011, the abscess just reaches deep subcutaneous tissue and requires debridement and irrigation. The wound may be left open to drain.

Coding Tips

Local anesthesia is included in this service. For drainage of tendon sheath, hand or finger, see 26020. For incision into the bone cortex, and or finger, see 26034. Surgical trays, A4550, are not separately reimbursed by Medicare; however, other third-party payers may cover them. Check with the specific payer to determine coverage.

ICD-9-CM Procedural

86.04 Other incision with drainage of skin and subcutaneous tissue

Anesthesia

00400

ICD-9-CM Diagnostic

681.00 Unspecified cellulitis and abscess of finger — (Use additional code to identify organism: 041.1)
681.01 Felon — (Use additional code to identify organism: 041.1)
681.02 Onychia and paronychia of finger — (Use additional code to identify organism: 041.1)
780.62 Postprocedural fever
883.1 Open wound of finger(s), complicated

Terms To Know

abscess. Circumscribed collection of pus resulting from bacteria, frequently associated with swelling and other signs of inflammation.

carbuncle. Necrotic infection of the skin and subcutaneous tissues, occurring mainly in the neck and back, that produces pus and forms drainage cavities.

cellulitis. Sudden, severe, suppurative inflammation and edema in subcutaneous tissue or muscle, most often caused by bacterial infection secondary to a cutaneous lesion.

felon. Painful abscess on the palmar side of a distal fingertip, usually occurring after inoculation of a disease-causing microorganism, such as Staphylococcus aureus in the closed space of the terminal phalanx.

furuncle. Inflamed, painful cyst or nodule on the skin caused by bacteria, often staphylococcus, entering along the hair follicle.

onychia. Inflammation or infection of the nail matrix leading to a loss of the nail.

open wound. Opening or break of the skin.

paronychia. Infection of nail structures.

subcutaneous tissue. Sheet or wide band of adipose (fat) and areolar connective tissue in two layers attached to the dermis.

CCI Version 16.3

01810, 0213T, 0216T, 0228T, 0230T, 10060, 10140, 10160, 20500, 20526-20553, 25259, 26340, 29086, 36000, 36400-36410, 36420-36430, 36440, 36600, 36640, 37202, 43752, 51701-51703, 62310-62319, 64400-64435, 64445-64450, 64479, 64483, 64490, 64493, 64505-64530, 69990, 93000-93010, 93040-93042, 93318, 94002, 94200, 94250, 94680-94690, 94770, 95812-95816, 95819, 95822, 95829, 95955, 96360, 96365, 96372, 96374-96376, 97597-97598, 97602-97606, 99148-99149, 99150, J0670, J2001

Also not with 26010: 12001, 29130, 76000-76001, G0168

Also not with 26011: 26010

Note: These CCI edits are used for Medicare. Other payers may reimburse on codes listed above.

Medicare Edits

	Fac RVU	Non-Fac RVU	FUD	Assist
26010	3.9	7.33	10	N/A
26011	5.33	11.09	10	N/A

Medicare References: 100-2,15,260; 100-4,12,30; 100-4,12,90.3; 100-4,14,10

26020

26020 Drainage of tendon sheath, digit and/or palm, each

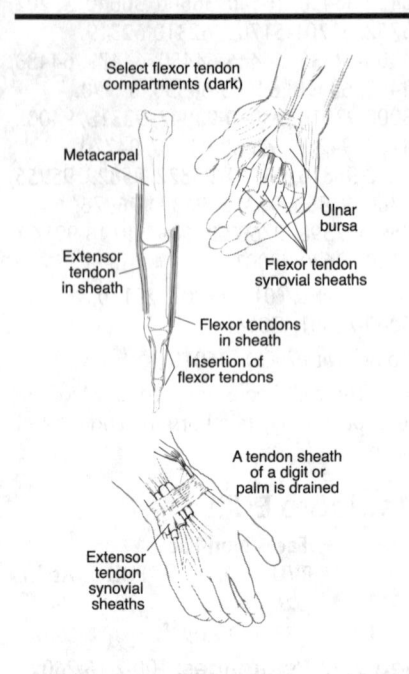

Explanation

The physician drains fluid located in a tendon sheath located in a finger or in the palm. The physician incises the skin above the affected sheath and dissects to the tendon sheath. The sheath is lanced and drained. An irrigation catheter may be placed and the wound is irrigated for up to 48 hours. The operative incision is closed in sutured layers.

Coding Tips

Local anesthesia is included in this service. However, this procedure may be performed under general anesthesia, depending on the age and/or condition of the patient. For drainage of a finger abscess, simple, see 26010; complicated, see 26011. For drainage of a palmar bursa, see 26025 and 26030.

ICD-9-CM Procedural

82.01 Exploration of tendon sheath of hand
83.01 Exploration of tendon sheath

Anesthesia

26020 01810

ICD-9-CM Diagnostic

727.05 Other tenosynovitis of hand and wrist
727.89 Other disorders of synovium, tendon, and bursa
882.1 Open wound of hand except finger(s) alone, complicated
882.2 Open wound of hand except finger(s) alone, with tendon involvement
883.1 Open wound of finger(s), complicated
883.2 Open wound of finger(s), with tendon involvement

Terms To Know

open wound. Opening or break of the skin.

synovia. Clear fluid lubricant of joints, bursae, and tendon sheaths, secreted by the synovial membrane.

tendon. Fibrous tissue that connects muscle to bone, consisting primarily of collagen and containing little vasculature.

tenosynovitis. Inflammation of a tendon sheath due to infection or disease.

CCI Version 16.3

01810, 0213T, 0216T, 0228T, 0230T, 10060, 10140, 10160, 11010-11012❖, 20500, 20526-20553, 25259, 26055, 26115, 26185, 26340, 29086, 29125, 29130, 36000, 36400-36410, 36420-36430, 36440, 36600, 36640, 37202, 43752, 51701-51703, 62310-62319, 64400-64435, 64445-64450, 64479, 64483, 64490, 64493, 64505-64530, 64722, 69990, 93000-93010, 93040-93042, 93318, 94002, 94200, 94250, 94680-94690, 94770, 95812-95816, 95819, 95822, 95829, 95955, 96360, 96365, 96372, 96374-96376, 97597-97598, 97602-97606, 99148-99149, 99150

Note: These CCI edits are used for Medicare. Other payers may reimburse on codes listed above.

Medicare Edits

	Fac RVU	Non-Fac RVU	FUD	Assist
26020	12.47	12.47	90	N/A

Medicare References: 100-2,15,260; 100-4,12,30; 100-4,12,90.3; 100-4,14,10

26025-26030

26025 Drainage of palmar bursa; single, bursa
26030 multiple bursa

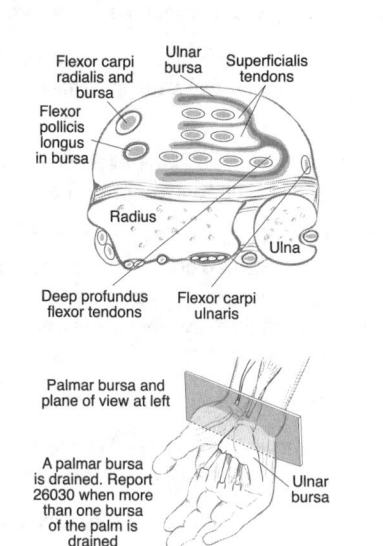

Explanation
The physician drains a palmar bursa or multiple bursas located on the ulnar or radial side of the palm. The physician incises the skin over the bursa and dissects to the bursa. The bursa is lanced and irrigated with a catheter. The catheter is removed and the incision is sutured in layers. Report 26025 for a single bursa, report 26030 for multiple and/or complicated bursas.

Coding Tips
Local anesthesia is included in these services. However, these procedures may be performed under general anesthesia, depending on the age and/or condition of the patient. For drainage of a tendon sheath, palm or digit, see 26020.

ICD-9-CM Procedural
82.03 Bursotomy of hand

Anesthesia
01810

ICD-9-CM Diagnostic
682.4 Cellulitis and abscess of hand, except fingers and thumb — (Use additional code to identify organism, such as 041.1, etc.)
727.05 Other tenosynovitis of hand and wrist
727.3 Other bursitis disorders
727.89 Other disorders of synovium, tendon, and bursa
882.1 Open wound of hand except finger(s) alone, complicated
882.2 Open wound of hand except finger(s) alone, with tendon involvement
958.8 Other early complications of trauma

Terms To Know
abscess. Circumscribed collection of pus resulting from bacteria, frequently associated with swelling and other signs of inflammation.

bursa. Cavity or sac containing fluid that occurs between articulating surfaces and serves to reduce friction from moving parts. An anatomical structure frequently referenced in orthopedic notes as it may become diseased or need removal.

cellulitis. Sudden, severe, suppurative inflammation and edema in subcutaneous tissue or muscle, most often caused by bacterial infection secondary to a cutaneous lesion.

open wound. Opening or break of the skin.

synovia. Clear fluid lubricant of joints, bursae, and tendon sheaths, secreted by the synovial membrane.

tendon. Fibrous tissue that connects muscle to bone, consisting primarily of collagen and containing little vasculature.

tenosynovitis. Inflammation of a tendon sheath due to infection or disease.

CCI Version 16.3
01810, 0213T, 0216T, 0228T, 0230T, 10060, 10140, 10160, 20500, 20526-20553, 25259, 26115, 26185, 26340, 29086, 36000, 36400-36410, 36420-36430, 36440, 36600, 36640, 37202, 43752, 51701-51703, 62310-62319, 64400-64435, 64445-64450, 64479, 64483, 64490, 64493, 64505-64530, 69990, 93000-93010, 93040-93042, 93318, 94002, 94200, 94250, 94680-94690, 94770, 95812-95816, 95819, 95822, 95829, 95955, 96360, 96365, 96372, 96374-96376, 97597-97598, 97602-97606, 99148-99149, 99150

Also not with 26025: 11011-11012❖

Also not with 26030: 11012❖, 26025, 26111

Note: These CCI edits are used for Medicare. Other payers may reimburse on codes listed above.

Medicare Edits

	Fac RVU	Non-Fac RVU	FUD	Assist
26025	12.1	12.1	90	80
26030	14.25	14.25	90	80

Medicare References: 100-2,15,260; 100-4,12,30; 100-4,12,90.3; 100-4,14,10

26034

26034 Incision, bone cortex, hand or finger (eg, osteomyelitis or bone abscess)

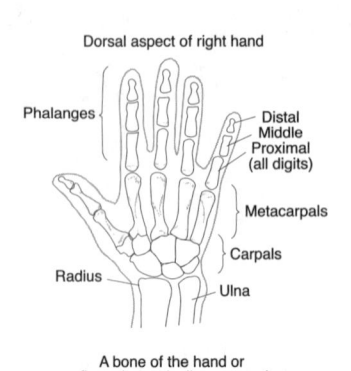

Explanation

The physician incises the bone cortex of infected bone in the hand or finger to treat an abscess or osteomyelitis. The physician makes an incision over the affected area. Dissection is carried down through the soft tissues to expose the bone. The periosteum is split and reflected from the bone overlying the infected area. A curette may be used to scrape away the abscess or infected portion down to healthy bony tissue or drill holes may be made through the cortex into the medullary canal in a window outline around the infected or abscessed bone. The area is drained and debrided of infected bony and soft tissue. The physician irrigates the area with antibiotic solution, the periosteum is closed over the bone, and the soft tissues are sutured closed; or the wound is packed and left open, allowing the area to drain. Secondary closure is performed approximately three weeks later. Dressings are changed daily. A splint may be applied to limit movement.

Coding Tips

Local anesthesia is included in this service. However, this procedure may be performed under general anesthesia, depending on the age and/or condition of the patient.

ICD-9-CM Procedural

- 77.14 Other incision of carpals and metacarpals without division
- 77.19 Other incision of other bone, except facial bones, without division

Anesthesia
26034 01830

ICD-9-CM Diagnostic

- 681.00 Unspecified cellulitis and abscess of finger — (Use additional code to identify organism: 041.1)
- 681.02 Onychia and paronychia of finger — (Use additional code to identify organism: 041.1)
- 682.4 Cellulitis and abscess of hand, except fingers and thumb — (Use additional code to identify organism, such as 041.1, etc.)
- 730.04 Acute osteomyelitis, hand — (Use additional code to identify organism: 041.1. Use additional code to identify major osseous defect, if applicable: 731.3)
- 730.14 Chronic osteomyelitis, hand — (Use additional code to identify organism: 041.1. Use additional code to identify major osseous defect, if applicable: 731.3)
- 730.24 Unspecified osteomyelitis, hand — (Use additional code to identify organism: 041.1. Use additional code to identify major osseous defect, if applicable: 731.3)
- 730.34 Periostitis, without mention of osteomyelitis, hand — (Use additional code to identify organism: 041.1)
- 730.84 Other infections involving diseases classified elsewhere, hand bone — (Use additional code to identify organism: 041.1. Code first underlying disease: 002.0, 015.0-015.9)
- 730.94 Unspecified infection of bone, hand — (Use additional code to identify organism: 041.1)
- 731.3 Major osseous defects — (Code first underlying disease: 170.0-170.9, 730.00-730.29, 733.00-733.09, 733.40-733.49, 996.45)
- 883.1 Open wound of finger(s), complicated

Terms To Know

abscess. Circumscribed collection of pus resulting from bacteria, frequently associated with swelling and other signs of inflammation.

acute. Sudden, severe. Documentation and reporting of an acute condition is important to establishing medical necessity.

cellulitis. Sudden, severe, suppurative inflammation and edema in subcutaneous tissue or muscle, most often caused by bacterial infection secondary to a cutaneous lesion.

chronic. Persistent, continuing, or recurring.

infection. Presence of microorganisms in body tissues that may result in cellular damage.

onychia. Inflammation or infection of the nail matrix leading to a loss of the nail.

osteomyelitis. Inflammation of bone that may remain localized or spread to the marrow, cortex, or periosteum, in response to an infecting organism, usually bacterial and pyogenic.

paronychia. Infection of nail structures.

periosteum. Double-layered connective membrane on the outer surface of bone.

periostitis. Inflammation of the outer layers of bone.

CCI Version 16.3

01810, 0213T, 0216T, 0228T, 0230T, 10060, 10140, 10160, 11012❖, 20000-20005, 20526-20553, 20615, 25259, 26185, 26340, 29086, 36000, 36400-36410, 36420-36430, 36440, 36600, 36640, 37202, 43752, 51701-51703, 62310-62319, 64400-64435, 64445-64450, 64479, 64483, 64490, 64493, 64505-64530, 69990, 93000-93010, 93040-93042, 93318, 94002, 94200, 94250, 94680-94690, 94770, 95812-95816, 95819, 95822, 95829, 95955, 96360, 96365, 96372, 96374-96376, 97597-97598, 97602-97606, 99148-99149, 99150

Note: These CCI edits are used for Medicare. Other payers may reimburse on codes listed above.

Medicare Edits

	Fac RVU	Non-Fac RVU	FUD	Assist
26034	15.49	15.49	90	N/A

Medicare References: 100-2,15,260; 100-4,12,30; 100-4,12,90.3; 100-4,14,10

26035

26035 Decompression fingers and/or hand, injection injury (eg, grease gun)

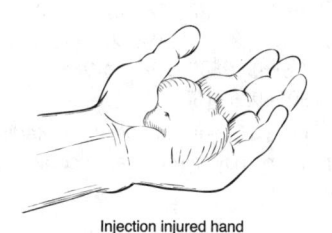

Injection injured hand

Injuries to the hand and fingers of this type include substances injected by pneumatic or hydraulic pressure. The material is injected into the hand, often in significant quantities

A hand or fingers that have been injured by injection are decompressed

Explanation

The physician decompresses fingers and/or a hand damaged due to an injection injury. The physician incises the skin overlying the entry point of the injection injury. The tissue is dissected to the fascial or periosteal layers and injected material is removed. If the injected material has followed the periosteum or fascia proximally, the incision length is increased until all the injected material is removed. The wound is irrigated and closed in sutured layers.

Coding Tips

Local anesthesia is included in this service. However, this procedure may be performed under general anesthesia, depending on the age and/or condition of the patient. For decompressive fasciotomy, hand, see 26037.

ICD-9-CM Procedural

- 77.14 Other incision of carpals and metacarpals without division
- 82.96 Other injection of locally-acting therapeutic substance into soft tissue of hand

Anesthesia

26035 00400, 01830

ICD-9-CM Diagnostic

- 882.1 Open wound of hand except finger(s) alone, complicated
- 882.2 Open wound of hand except finger(s) alone, with tendon involvement
- 883.1 Open wound of finger(s), complicated
- 883.2 Open wound of finger(s), with tendon involvement

Terms To Know

fascia. Fibrous sheet or band of tissue that envelops organs, muscles, and groupings of muscles.

injury. Harm or damage sustained by the body.

open wound. Opening or break of the skin.

proximal. Located closest to a specified reference point, usually the midline.

tendon. Fibrous tissue that connects muscle to bone, consisting primarily of collagen and containing little vasculature.

CCI Version 16.3

01810, 0213T, 0216T, 0228T, 0230T, 20103, 20526-20553, 25259, 26340, 29086, 36000, 36400-36410, 36420-36430, 36440, 36600, 36640, 37202, 43752, 51701-51703, 62310-62319, 64400-64435, 64445-64450, 64479, 64483, 64490, 64493, 64505-64530, 69990, 93000-93010, 93040-93042, 93318, 94002, 94200, 94250, 94680-94690, 94770, 95812-95816, 95819, 95822, 95829, 95955, 96360, 96365, 96372, 96374-96376, 99148-99149, 99150

Note: These CCI edits are used for Medicare. Other payers may reimburse on codes listed above.

Medicare Edits

	Fac RVU	Non-Fac RVU	FUD	Assist
26035	24.57	24.57	90	80

Medicare References: None

26037

26037 Decompressive fasciotomy, hand (excludes 26035)

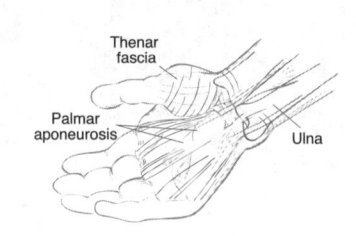

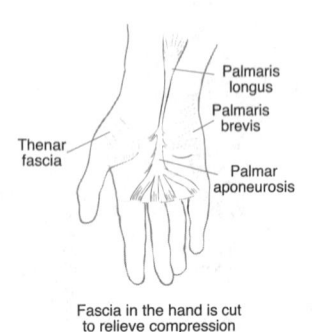

Thenar fascia
Palmar aponeurosis
Ulna
Palmaris longus
Palmaris brevis
Thenar fascia
Palmar aponeurosis

Fascia in the hand is cut to relieve compression

Explanation

The physician decompresses the hand fascia. The physician incises the skin overlying the affected fascia. The fascia is incised and the underlying tissues are irrigated. The operative incision is closed in sutured layers.

Coding Tips

According to CPT guidelines, cast application or strapping (including removal) is only reported as a replacement procedure or when the cast application or strapping is an initial service performed without a restorative treatment or procedure. See "Application of Casts and Strapping" in the CPT book in the Surgery Section, under the Musculoskeletal system. Local anesthesia is included in this service. However, this procedure may be performed under general anesthesia, depending on the age and/or condition of the patient. For injection injury, fingers or hand, see 26035.

ICD-9-CM Procedural

82.12 Fasciotomy of hand

Anesthesia

26037 01810

ICD-9-CM Diagnostic

682.4 Cellulitis and abscess of hand, except fingers and thumb — (Use additional code to identify organism, such as 041.1, etc.)

728.0 Infective myositis
728.86 Necrotizing fasciitis — (Use additional code to identify infectious organism, 041.00-041.89, 785.4, if applicable)
728.88 Rhabdomyolysis
728.89 Other disorder of muscle, ligament, and fascia — (Use additional E code to identify drug, if drug-induced)
729.4 Unspecified fasciitis
729.71 Nontraumatic compartment syndrome of upper extremity — (Code first, if applicable, postprocedural complication: 998.89)
882.1 Open wound of hand except finger(s) alone, complicated
927.20 Crushing injury of hand(s) — (Use additional code to identify any associated injuries: 800-829, 850.0-854.1, 860.0-869.1)
958.8 Other early complications of trauma
958.91 Traumatic compartment syndrome of upper extremity

Terms To Know

abscess. Circumscribed collection of pus resulting from bacteria, frequently associated with swelling and other signs of inflammation.

cellulitis. Sudden, severe, suppurative inflammation and edema in subcutaneous tissue or muscle, most often caused by bacterial infection secondary to a cutaneous lesion.

fascia. Fibrous sheet or band of tissue that envelops organs, muscles, and groupings of muscles.

myositis. Inflammation of a muscle with voluntary movement.

open wound. Opening or break of the skin.

CCI Version 16.3

01810, 0213T, 0216T, 0228T, 0230T, 11012❖, 20526-20553, 25259, 26185, 26340, 29086, 29125, 36000, 36400-36410, 36420-36430, 36440, 36600, 36640, 37202, 43752, 51701-51703, 62310-62319, 64400-64435, 64445-64450, 64479, 64483, 64490, 64493, 64505-64530, 69990, 93000-93010, 93040-93042, 93318, 94002, 94200, 94250, 94680-94690, 94770, 95812-95816, 95819, 95822, 95829, 95955, 96360, 96365, 96372, 96374-96376, 99148-99149, 99150

Note: These CCI edits are used for Medicare. Other payers may reimburse on codes listed above.

Medicare Edits

	Fac RVU	Non-Fac RVU	FUD	Assist
26037	16.59	16.59	90	80

Medicare References: None

26040-26045

26040 Fasciotomy, palmar (eg, Dupuytren's contracture); percutaneous
26045   open, partial

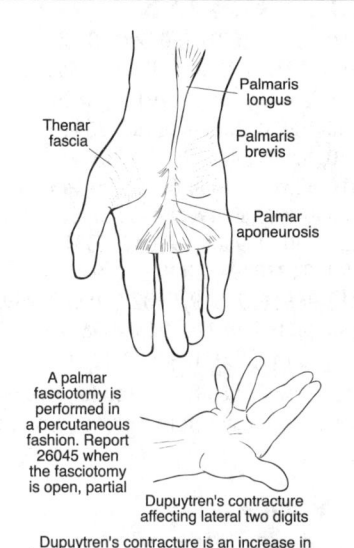

A palmar fasciotomy is performed in a percutaneous fashion. Report 26045 when the fasciotomy is open, partial

Dupuytren's contracture affecting lateral two digits

Dupuytren's contracture is an increase in the fibrous tissues of the palmar aponeurosis, which results in a shortening of the bands that extend from this fascial tissue to the base of the fingers. The result is fixed flexion of digits

Explanation

The physician incises the palmar fascia to release a Dupuytren's contracture. A Dupuytren's contracture is a shortening of the palmar fascia resulting in flexion deformity of a finger. In 26040, the physician makes a stab wound through the subcutaneous to the palmar fascia, which is incised. In 26045, the subcutaneous tissue is incised and retracted to expose the palmar fascia. The palmar fascia is incised to relieve tension and allow the hand to extend correctly. The operative wound is sutured in layers.

Coding Tips

According to CPT guidelines, cast application or strapping (including removal) is only reported as a replacement procedure or when the cast application or strapping is an initial service performed without a restorative treatment or procedure. See "Application of Casts and Strapping" in the CPT book in the Surgery Section, under the Musculoskeletal system. Local anesthesia is included in these services. However, these procedures may be performed under general anesthesia, depending on the age and/or condition of the patient. For fasciectomy, see 26121–26125.

ICD-9-CM Procedural

82.12 Fasciotomy of hand

Anesthesia

01810

ICD-9-CM Diagnostic

728.6 Contracture of palmar fascia

Terms To Know

Dupuytren's contracture. Shortening of the palmar fascia resulting in flexion deformity of a finger.

fascia. Fibrous sheet or band of tissue that envelops organs, muscles, and groupings of muscles.

subcutaneous tissue. Sheet or wide band of adipose (fat) and areolar connective tissue in two layers attached to the dermis.

CCI Version 16.3

01810, 0213T, 0216T, 0228T, 0230T, 20526-20553, 25259, 26055, 26340, 29086, 36000, 36400-36410, 36420-36430, 36440, 36600, 36640, 37202, 43752, 51701-51703, 62310-62319, 64400-64435, 64445-64450, 64479, 64483, 64490, 64493, 64505-64530, 69990, 93000-93010, 93040-93042, 93318, 94002, 94200, 94250, 94680-94690, 94770, 95812-95816, 95819, 95822, 95829, 95955, 96360, 96365, 96372, 96374-96376, 99148-99149, 99150

Also not with 26040: 11010-11012❖

Also not with 26045: 11012❖, 26040, 26185, 64718

Note: These CCI edits are used for Medicare. Other payers may reimburse on codes listed above.

Medicare Edits

	Fac RVU	Non-Fac RVU	FUD	Assist
26040	8.9	8.9	90	N/A
26045	13.49	13.49	90	N/A

Medicare References: 100-2,15,260; 100-4,12,30; 100-4,12,90.3; 100-4,14,10

26055

26055 Tendon sheath incision (eg, for trigger finger)

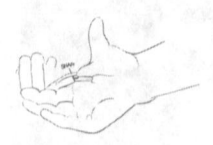

A snapping sound may be heard when the trigger finger is forced into extension

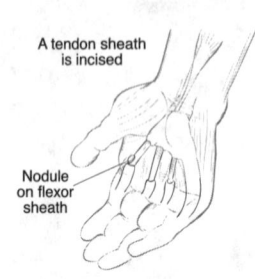

A tendon sheath is incised

Nodule on flexor sheath

Trigger finger may be caused by a nodule on the flexor tendon that has difficulty entering the narrow sheath. A popping sound is often heard upon flexion or extension of the finger

Explanation

The physician makes an incision in a tendon sheath to release tension in the tendon. (For example, this procedure would be performed to relieve trigger finger.) The physician incises the skin overlying the tendon and dissects to the tendon sheath. The sheath is incised lengthwise allowing the tendon to move. The operative incision is closed in sutured layers.

Coding Tips

Local anesthesia is included in this service. However, this procedure may be performed under general anesthesia, depending on the age and/or condition of the patient. For percutaneous tenotomy, digits, see 26060. Surgical trays, A4550, are not separately reimbursed by Medicare; however, other third-party payers may cover them. Check with the specific payer to determine coverage.

ICD-9-CM Procedural

82.01   Exploration of tendon sheath of hand

Anesthesia

26055   01810

ICD-9-CM Diagnostic

357.1   Polyneuropathy in collagen vascular disease — (Code first underlying disease: 446.0, 710.0, 714.0)

359.6   Symptomatic inflammatory myopathy in diseases classified elsewhere — (Code first underlying disease: 135, 140.0-208.9, 277.30-277.39, 446.0, 710.0, 710.1, 710.2, 714.0)

446.0   Polyarteritis nodosa

710.0   Systemic lupus erythematosus — (Use additional code to identify manifestation: 424.91, 581.81, 582.81, 583.81)

710.1   Systemic sclerosis — (Use additional code to identify manifestation: 359.6, 517.2)

710.2   Sicca syndrome

711.04 Pyogenic arthritis, hand — (Use additional code to identify infectious organism: 041.0-041.8)

711.84 Arthropathy associated with other infectious and parasitic diseases, hand — (Code first underlying disease: 080-088, 100-104, 130-136)

711.94 Unspecified infective arthritis, hand

714.0   Rheumatoid arthritis — (Use additional code to identify manifestation: 357.1, 359.6)

716.04 Kaschin-Beck disease, hand

716.14 Traumatic arthropathy, hand

716.54 Unspecified polyarthropathy or polyarthritis, hand

716.64 Unspecified monoarthritis, hand

716.84 Other specified arthropathy, hand

716.94 Unspecified arthropathy, hand

718.44 Contracture of hand joint

718.94 Unspecified derangement of hand joint

727.00 Unspecified synovitis and tenosynovitis

727.01 Synovitis and tenosynovitis in diseases classified elsewhere — (Code first underlying disease: 015.0-015.9)

727.03 Trigger finger (acquired)

727.04 Radial styloid tenosynovitis

727.05 Other tenosynovitis of hand and wrist

727.89 Other disorders of synovium, tendon, and bursa

736.20 Unspecified deformity of finger

736.29 Other acquired deformity of finger

756.89 Other specified congenital anomaly of muscle, tendon, fascia, and connective tissue

905.8   Late effect of tendon injury

Terms To Know

contracture. Shortening of muscle or connective tissue.

late effect. Abnormality, dysfunction, or other residual condition produced after the acute phase of an illness, injury, or disease is over. There is no time limit on when late effects can appear.

CCI Version 16.3

01810, 0213T, 0216T, 0228T, 0230T, 11010-11012❖, 12042, 20526-20553, 25259, 26185, 26340, 29086, 29125, 36000, 36400-36410, 36420-36430, 36440, 36600, 36640, 37202, 43752, 51701-51703, 62310-62319, 64400-64435, 64445-64450, 64479, 64483, 64490, 64493, 64505-64530, 93000-93010, 93040-93042, 93318, 94002, 94200, 94250, 94680-94690, 94770, 95812-95816, 95819, 95822, 95829, 95955, 96360, 96365, 96372, 96374-96376, 99148-99149, 99150, J0670, J2001

Note: These CCI edits are used for Medicare. Other payers may reimburse on codes listed above.

Medicare Edits

	Fac RVU	Non-Fac RVU	FUD	Assist
26055	8.76	16.14	90	N/A

Medicare References: 100-2,15,260; 100-4,12,30; 100-4,12,90.3; 100-4,14,10

26060

26060 Tenotomy, percutaneous, single, each digit

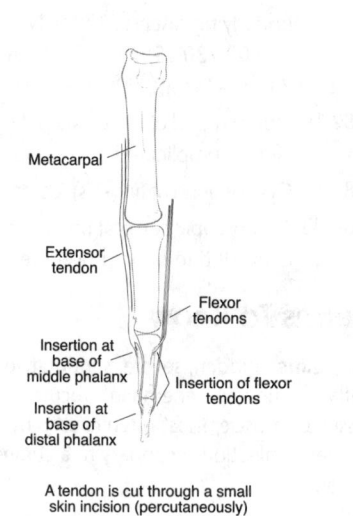

Metacarpal
Extensor tendon
Flexor tendons
Insertion at base of middle phalanx
Insertion of flexor tendons
Insertion at base of distal phalanx

A tendon is cut through a small skin incision (percutaneously)

Explanation

The physician incises a tendon at the subcutaneous level. The physician incises the overlying skin. The tendon is severed through the subcutaneous tissue. The operative incision is closed in sutured layers. A splint may be applied for immobilization. Report each digit separately.

Coding Tips

This procedure is for tenotomy for each digit. When multiple digits are involved, report one digit as the primary procedure and append modifier 51 to subsequent procedures. Some payers may require the use of HCPCS Level II modifiers FA-F9 to identify the specific finger involved. According to CPT guidelines, cast application or strapping (including removal) is only reported as a replacement procedure or when the cast application or strapping is an initial service performed without a restorative treatment or procedure. See "Application of Casts and Strapping" in the CPT book in the Surgery Section, under the Musculoskeletal system. Local anesthesia is included in this service. However, this procedure may be performed under general anesthesia, depending on the age and/or condition of the patient. For incision of a tendon sheath, see 26055. Surgical trays, A4550, are not separately reimbursed by Medicare; however, other third-party payers may cover them. Check with the specific payer to determine coverage.

ICD-9-CM Procedural

82.11 Tenotomy of hand

Anesthesia

26060 01810

ICD-9-CM Diagnostic

727.00 Unspecified synovitis and tenosynovitis
727.01 Synovitis and tenosynovitis in diseases classified elsewhere — (Code first underlying disease: 015.0-015.9)
727.02 Giant cell tumor of tendon sheath
727.03 Trigger finger (acquired)
727.04 Radial styloid tenosynovitis
727.05 Other tenosynovitis of hand and wrist
727.09 Other synovitis and tenosynovitis
727.81 Contracture of tendon (sheath)
727.82 Calcium deposits in tendon and bursa
727.89 Other disorders of synovium, tendon, and bursa

Terms To Know

bursa. Cavity or sac containing fluid that occurs between articulating surfaces and serves to reduce friction from moving parts. An anatomical structure frequently referenced in orthopedic notes as it may become diseased or need removal.

contracture. Shortening of muscle or connective tissue.

subcutaneous tissue. Sheet or wide band of adipose (fat) and areolar connective tissue in two layers attached to the dermis.

synovia. Clear fluid lubricant of joints, bursae, and tendon sheaths, secreted by the synovial membrane.

synovitis. Inflammation of the synovial membrane that lines a synovial joint, resulting in pain and swelling.

tendon. Fibrous tissue that connects muscle to bone, consisting primarily of collagen and containing little vasculature.

CCI Version 16.3

01810, 0213T, 0216T, 0228T, 0230T, 11010-11012❖, 20526-20553, 25259, 26340, 29086, 29125, 36000, 36400-36410, 36420-36430, 36440, 36600, 36640, 37202, 43752, 51701-51703, 62310-62319, 64400-64435, 64445-64450, 64479, 64483, 64490, 64493, 64505-64530, 69990, 93000-93010, 93040-93042, 93318, 94002, 94200, 94250, 94680-94690, 94770, 95812-95816, 95819, 95822, 95829, 95955, 96360, 96365, 96372, 96374-96376, 99148-99149, 99150

Note: These CCI edits are used for Medicare. Other payers may reimburse on codes listed above.

Medicare Edits

	Fac RVU	Non-Fac RVU	FUD	Assist
26060	7.67	7.67	90	80

Medicare References: 100-2,15,260; 100-4,12,30; 100-4,12,90.3; 100-4,14,10

26070-26080

26070 Arthrotomy, with exploration, drainage, or removal of loose or foreign body; carpometacarpal joint
26075 metacarpophalangeal joint, each
26080 interphalangeal joint, each

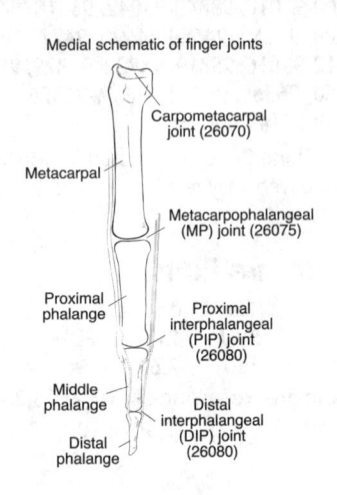

A joint of the finger is incised and explored; drainage is performed if necessary as is removal of loose or foreign bodies. Report 26070 for the carpometacarpal joint. Report 26075 for each metacarpophalangeal joint. Report 26080 for each interphalangeal joint

Explanation

The physician performs an arthrotomy of a carpometacarpal joint in 26070, a metacarpophalangeal joint in 26075, or an interphalangeal joint in 26080 that includes exploration, drainage, or removal of any loose or foreign body. An incision is made over the joint to be exposed. The soft tissues are dissected away and the joint capsule is exposed and incised. The joint space is explored, any necrotic tissue is removed, and infection or abnormal fluid is drained. If a foreign body is present (e.g., bullet, nail, gravel), it is exposed and removed. The wound is irrigated with antibiotic solution. The physician may leave the wound packed open with daily dressing changes to allow for drainage and secondary healing by granulation. If the incision is repaired, drain tubes may be inserted and the incision closed in layers with sutures, staples, and/or Steri-strips. Report 26075 and 26080 once for each specified joint.

Coding Tips

For 26080, some payers may require the use of HCPCS Level II modifiers FA-F9 to identify the specific finger involved. According to CPT guidelines, cast application or strapping (including removal) is only reported as a replacement procedure or when the cast application or strapping is an initial service performed without a restorative treatment or procedure. See "Application of Casts and Strapping" in the CPT book in the Surgery Section, under the Musculoskeletal system. Local anesthesia is included in these services. However, these procedures may be performed under general anesthesia, depending on the age and/or condition of the patient.

ICD-9-CM Procedural

80.14 Other arthrotomy of hand and finger

Anesthesia
01830

ICD-9-CM Diagnostic

- 682.4 Cellulitis and abscess of hand, except fingers and thumb — (Use additional code to identify organism, such as 041.1, etc.)
- 709.4 Foreign body granuloma of skin and subcutaneous tissue — (Use additional code to identify foreign body (V90.01-V90.9))
- 711.04 Pyogenic arthritis, hand — (Use additional code to identify infectious organism: 041.0-041.8)
- 716.14 Traumatic arthropathy, hand
- 728.0 Infective myositis
- 728.82 Foreign body granuloma of muscle — (Use additional code to identify foreign body (V90.01-V90.9))
- 728.89 Other disorder of muscle, ligament, and fascia — (Use additional E code to identify drug, if drug-induced)
- 729.4 Unspecified fasciitis
- 729.6 Residual foreign body in soft tissue — (Use additional code to identify foreign body (V90.01-V90.9))
- 730.04 Acute osteomyelitis, hand — (Use additional code to identify organism: 041.1. Use additional code to identify major osseous defect, if applicable: 731.3)
- 730.14 Chronic osteomyelitis, hand — (Use additional code to identify organism: 041.1. Use additional code to identify major osseous defect, if applicable: 731.3)
- 730.24 Unspecified osteomyelitis, hand — (Use additional code to identify organism: 041.1. Use additional code to identify major osseous defect, if applicable: 731.3)
- 730.34 Periostitis, without mention of osteomyelitis, hand — (Use additional code to identify organism: 041.1)
- 730.84 Other infections involving diseases classified elsewhere, hand bone — (Use additional code to identify organism: 041.1. Code first underlying disease: 002.0, 015.0-015.9)
- 731.3 Major osseous defects — (Code first underlying disease: 170.0-170.9, 730.00-730.29, 733.00-733.09, 733.40-733.49, 996.45)
- 882.1 Open wound of hand except finger(s) alone, complicated
- 883.1 Open wound of finger(s), complicated
- V64.43 Arthroscopic surgical procedure converted to open procedure

Terms To Know

cellulitis. Sudden, severe, suppurative inflammation and edema in subcutaneous tissue or muscle, most often caused by bacterial infection secondary to a cutaneous lesion.

periostitis. Inflammation of the outer layers of bone.

CCI Version 16.3

01810, 0213T, 0216T, 0228T, 0230T, 10060, 10140, 10160, 11010-11012❖, 20103, 20500, 20526-20553, 25259, 26185, 26340, 29086, 36000, 36400-36410, 36420-36430, 36440, 36600, 36640, 37202, 43752, 51701-51703, 62310-62319, 64400-64435, 64445-64450, 64479, 64483, 64490, 64493, 64505-64530, 69990, 93000-93010, 93040-93042, 93318, 94002, 94200, 94250, 94680-94690, 94770, 95812-95816, 95819, 95822, 95829, 95955, 96360, 96365, 96372, 96374-96376, 99148-99149, 99150

Also not with 26070: 26100❖, 29125

Also not with 26075: 26105❖, 29900-29901

Note: These CCI edits are used for Medicare. Other payers may reimburse on codes listed above.

Medicare Edits

	Fac RVU	Non-Fac RVU	FUD	Assist
26070	8.79	8.79	90	N/A
26075	9.23	9.23	90	N/A
26080	11.13	11.13	90	N/A

Medicare References: 100-2,15,260; 100-4,12,30; 100-4,12,90.3; 100-4,14,10

26100-26110

26100	Arthrotomy with biopsy; carpometacarpal joint, each
26105	metacarpophalangeal joint, each
26110	interphalangeal joint, each

A finger joint is incised and a biopsy is collected. Report 26100 for a carpometacarpal joint. Report 26105 for a metacarpophalangeal joint. And report 26110 for an interphalangeal joint.

Explanation

The physician performs an arthrotomy of a carpometacarpal joint in 26100, a metacarpophalangeal joint in 26105, or an interphalangeal joint in 26110 with biopsy. An incision is made over the joint to be exposed. The soft tissues are dissected away and the joint capsule is exposed and incised. The joint space is explored and a biopsy sample, such as from the synovial membrane, or fluid is removed. The wound is irrigated and may be left open with daily dressing changes to allow for secondary healing. If the incision is repaired, drain tubes may be inserted and the incision closed in layers with sutures, staples, and/or Steri-strips. Report codes 26100-26110 once for each specified joint.

Coding Tips

For 26110, some payers may require the use of HCPCS Level II modifiers FA-F9 to identify the specific finger involved. According to CPT guidelines, cast application or strapping (including removal) is only reported as a replacement procedure or when the cast application or strapping is an initial service performed without a restorative treatment or procedure. See "Application of Casts and Strapping" in the CPT book in the Surgery Section, under the Musculoskeletal system. Local anesthesia is included in these services. However, these procedures may be performed under general anesthesia, depending on the age and/or condition of the patient.

ICD-9-CM Procedural

80.34 Biopsy of joint structure of hand and finger

Anesthesia

01830

ICD-9-CM Diagnostic

357.1 Polyneuropathy in collagen vascular disease — (Code first underlying disease: 446.0, 710.0, 714.0)
359.6 Symptomatic inflammatory myopathy in diseases classified elsewhere — (Code first underlying disease: 135, 140.0-208.9, 277.30-277.39, 446.0, 710.0, 710.1, 710.2, 714.0)
446.0 Polyarteritis nodosa
710.0 Systemic lupus erythematosus — (Use additional code to identify manifestation: 424.91, 581.81, 582.81, 583.81)
710.1 Systemic sclerosis — (Use additional code to identify manifestation: 359.6, 517.2)
710.2 Sicca syndrome
711.04 Pyogenic arthritis, hand — (Use additional code to identify infectious organism: 041.0-041.8)
711.44 Arthropathy, associated with other bacterial diseases, hand — (Code first underlying disease, such as diseases classifiable to 010-040 (except 036.82), 090-099 (except 098.50))
711.54 Arthropathy associated with other viral diseases, hand — (Code first underlying disease: 045-049, 050-079, 480, 487)
711.64 Arthropathy associated with mycoses, hand — (Code first underlying disease: 110.0-118)
713.8 Arthropathy associated with other conditions classifiable elsewhere — (Code first underlying disease as conditions classifiable elsewhere except as in: 711.1-711.8, 712, 713.0-713.7)
714.0 Rheumatoid arthritis — (Use additional code to identify manifestation: 357.1, 359.6)
714.30 Polyarticular juvenile rheumatoid arthritis, chronic or unspecified
714.9 Unspecified inflammatory polyarthropathy
716.04 Kaschin-Beck disease, hand
716.64 Unspecified monoarthritis, hand
719.24 Villonodular synovitis, hand
726.4 Enthesopathy of wrist and carpus
727.00 Unspecified synovitis and tenosynovitis
727.01 Synovitis and tenosynovitis in diseases classified elsewhere — (Code first underlying disease: 015.0-015.9)
727.05 Other tenosynovitis of hand and wrist
V64.43 Arthroscopic surgical procedure converted to open procedure

Terms To Know

arthrotomy. Surgical incision into a joint that may include exploration, drainage, or removal of a foreign body. Coding depends upon site and intent.

sicca syndrome. Complex of symptoms of unknown source in middle-aged women in which the following triad exists: keratoconjunctivitis sicca, zerostomia, and connective tissue disease (usually rheumatoid arthritis but sometimes systemic lupus erythematosus).

tenosynovitis. Inflammation of a tendon sheath due to infection or disease.

villonodular synovitis. Inflammation of the synovial membrane due to excessive synovial tissue formation, especially in the knee.

CCI Version 16.3

01810, 0213T, 0216T, 0228T, 0230T, 10060, 10140, 10160, 11010-11012❖, 20526-20553, 25259, 26185, 26340, 29086, 36000, 36400-36410, 36420-36430, 36440, 36600, 36640, 37202, 43752, 51701-51703, 62310-62319, 64400-64435, 64445-64450, 64479, 64483, 64490, 64493, 64505-64530, 69990, 93000-93010, 93040-93042, 93318, 94002, 94200, 94250, 94680-94690, 94770, 95812-95816, 95819, 95822, 95829, 95955, 96360, 96365, 96372, 96374-96376, 99148-99149, 99150

Also not with 26105: 29900-29901

Also not with 26110: 26080❖

Note: These CCI edits are used for Medicare. Other payers may reimburse on codes listed above.

Medicare Edits

	Fac RVU	Non-Fac RVU	FUD	Assist
26100	9.47	9.47	90	80
26105	9.61	9.61	90	80
26110	9.2	9.2	90	N/A

Medicare References: 100-2,15,260; 100-4,12,30; 100-4,12,90.3; 100-4,14,10

26115-26116 (26111, 26113)

26115 Excision, tumor or vascular malformation, soft tissue of hand or finger, subcutaneous; less than 1.5 cm
26111 1.5 cm or greater
26116 Excision, tumor, soft tissue, or vascular malformation, of hand or finger, subfascial (eg, intramuscular); less than 1.5 cm
26113 1.5 cm or greater

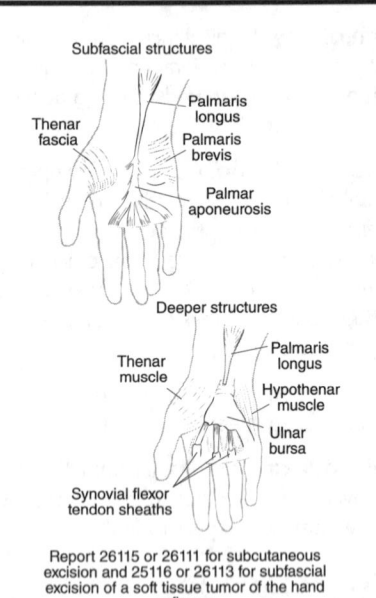

Explanation
The physician removes a tumor or vascular malformation from the soft tissue of the hand or finger that is located in the subcutaneous tissue in 26111 and 26115 and in the deep soft tissue below the fascial plane, or within the muscle, in 26113 or 26116. With the proper anesthesia administered, the physician makes an incision in the skin overlying the mass and dissects down to the tumor or malformation. The extent of the tumor is identified and a dissection is undertaken all the way around the tumor. The blood vessels are ligated and the defective tissue of the vascular malformation is excised. A portion of neighboring soft tissue may also be removed to ensure adequate removal of all tumor tissue. A drain may be inserted, and the incision is repaired with layers of sutures, staples, or Steri-strips. Report 26115 for excision of subcutaneous tumors less than 1.5 cm and 26111 for excision of subcutaneous tumors 1.5 cm or greater. Report 26116 for excision of subfascial or intramuscular tumors less than 1.5 cm and 26113 for excision of subfascial or intramuscular tumors 1.5 cm or greater.

Coding Tips
Codes 26111 and 26113 are resequenced codes and will not display in numeric order. According to CPT guidelines, cast application or strapping (including removal) is only reported as a replacement procedure or when the cast application or strapping is an initial service performed without a restorative treatment or procedure. See "Application of Casts and Strapping" in the CPT book in the Surgery Section, under the Musculoskeletal system. When medically necessary, report moderate (conscious) sedation provided by the performing physician with 99143–99145. When provided by another physician, report 99148–99150.

ICD-9-CM Procedural
- 82.21 Excision of lesion of tendon sheath of hand
- 82.22 Excision of lesion of muscle of hand
- 82.29 Excision of other lesion of soft tissue of hand
- 83.49 Other excision of soft tissue
- 86.3 Other local excision or destruction of lesion or tissue of skin and subcutaneous tissue
- 86.4 Radical excision of skin lesion

Anesthesia
- **26111** 00400, 01810, 01840, 01850
- **26113** 01810, 01840, 01850
- **26115** 00400, 01810, 01840, 01850
- **26116** 01810

ICD-9-CM Diagnostic
- 171.2 Malignant neoplasm of connective and other soft tissue of upper limb, including shoulder
- 172.6 Malignant melanoma of skin of upper limb, including shoulder
- 173.6 Other malignant neoplasm of skin of upper limb, including shoulder
- 195.4 Malignant neoplasm of upper limb
- 198.89 Secondary malignant neoplasm of other specified sites
- 209.33 Merkel cell carcinoma of the upper limb
- 209.75 Secondary Merkel cell carcinoma
- 214.1 Lipoma of other skin and subcutaneous tissue
- 215.2 Other benign neoplasm of connective and other soft tissue of upper limb, including shoulder
- 228.01 Hemangioma of skin and subcutaneous tissue
- 238.1 Neoplasm of uncertain behavior of connective and other soft tissue
- 239.2 Neoplasms of unspecified nature of bone, soft tissue, and skin
- 686.1 Pyogenic granuloma of skin and subcutaneous tissue — (Use additional code to identify any infectious organism: 041.0-041.8)
- 727.02 Giant cell tumor of tendon sheath
- 728.79 Other fibromatoses of muscle, ligament, and fascia
- 747.63 Congenital upper limb vessel anomaly
- 747.69 Congenital anomaly of other specified site of peripheral vascular system
- 782.2 Localized superficial swelling, mass, or lump

CCI Version 16.3
01810, 0228T, 0230T, 10060, 10140, 10160, 11010-11012❖, 11040-11044, 12001-12007, 12020-12021, 12041-12047, 13131-13132, 20526-20553, 25259, 26340, 29086, 36000, 36400-36410, 36420-36430, 36440, 36600, 36640, 37202, 37618, 43752, 51701-51703, 62310-62319, 64400-64435, 64445-64450, 64479, 64483, 64505-64530, 64702-64704, 93000-93010, 93040-93042, 93318, 94002, 94200, 94250, 94680-94690, 94770, 95812-95816, 95819, 95822, 95829, 95955, 96360, 96365, 96372, 96374-96376, 99148-99149, 99150

Also not with 26111: 0213T, 0216T, 26010-26025, 26055-26110, 26115, 26160-26185, 26520-26525, 64490, 64493, 69990

Also not with 26113: 0213T, 0216T, 13121, 26010-26030, 26055, 26070-26080, 26110-26111, 26115-26116, 26140-26185, 26455-26460, 26520-26525❖, 26535-26536❖, 64490, 64493, 69990

Also not with 26115: 26010-26011, 26055-26110, 26160, 26185, 26520-26525, 69990, J0670, J2001

Also not with 26116: 13121, 26010-26030, 26055, 26070-26080, 26110-26111, 26115, 26140-26185, 26455-26460, 26520-26525, 26535-26536❖

Note: These CCI edits are used for Medicare. Other payers may reimburse on codes listed above.

Medicare Edits

	Fac RVU	Non-Fac RVU	FUD	Assist
26111	12.5	12.5	90	80
26113	16.38	16.38	90	80
26115	9.95	16.1	90	N/A
26116	15.23	15.23	90	N/A

Medicare References: 100-2,15,260; 100-4,12,30; 100-4,12,90.3; 100-4,14,10

26117-26118

26117 Radical resection of tumor (eg, malignant neoplasm), soft tissue of hand or finger; less than 3 cm

26118 3 cm or greater

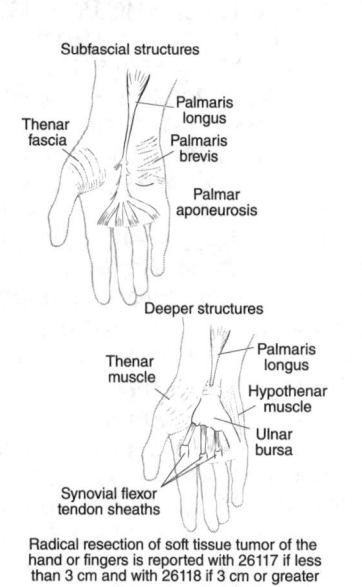

Radical resection of soft tissue tumor of the hand or fingers is reported with 26117 if less than 3 cm and with 26118 if 3 cm or greater

Explanation

The physician removes a malignant soft tissue tumor from the hand or finger, not involving bone. An incision is made over the tumor and dissection exposes it. The tumor and any adjacent tissue that may be affected by the spread of the neoplasm are excised. Large resections may be needed. The type and stage of the lesion determines the extent of the tumor margin resection area. Muscle or fascia may need to be repaired and drains may be placed. The surgical wound is repaired by intermediate or complex closure, adjacent tissue transfer, or graft. Report 26117 for excision of tumors less than 3 cm, and 26118 for excision of tumors 3 cm or greater.

Coding Tips

For radical resection of a tumor of the soft tissue of the forearm or wrist area, see 25077–25078.

ICD-9-CM Procedural

- 82.21 Excision of lesion of tendon sheath of hand
- 82.22 Excision of lesion of muscle of hand
- 82.29 Excision of other lesion of soft tissue of hand
- 83.49 Other excision of soft tissue
- 86.3 Other local excision or destruction of lesion or tissue of skin and subcutaneous tissue
- 86.4 Radical excision of skin lesion

Anesthesia

01810

ICD-9-CM Diagnostic

- 171.2 Malignant neoplasm of connective and other soft tissue of upper limb, including shoulder
- 172.6 Malignant melanoma of skin of upper limb, including shoulder
- 173.6 Other malignant neoplasm of skin of upper limb, including shoulder
- 195.4 Malignant neoplasm of upper limb
- 198.89 Secondary malignant neoplasm of other specified sites
- 209.33 Merkel cell carcinoma of the upper limb
- 209.75 Secondary Merkel cell carcinoma
- 214.1 Lipoma of other skin and subcutaneous tissue
- 215.2 Other benign neoplasm of connective and other soft tissue of upper limb, including shoulder
- 228.01 Hemangioma of skin and subcutaneous tissue
- 238.1 Neoplasm of uncertain behavior of connective and other soft tissue
- 239.2 Neoplasms of unspecified nature of bone, soft tissue, and skin
- 686.1 Pyogenic granuloma of skin and subcutaneous tissue — (Use additional code to identify any infectious organism: 041.0-041.8)
- 727.02 Giant cell tumor of tendon sheath
- 728.79 Other fibromatoses of muscle, ligament, and fascia
- 747.63 Congenital upper limb vessel anomaly
- 747.69 Congenital anomaly of other specified site of peripheral vascular system
- 782.2 Localized superficial swelling, mass, or lump

Terms To Know

radical resection. Removal of an entire tumor (e.g., malignant neoplasm) along with a large area of surrounding tissue, including adjacent lymph nodes that may have been infiltrated.

soft tissue. Nonepithelial tissues outside of the skeleton that includes subcutaneous adipose tissue, fibrous tissue, fascia, muscles, blood and lymph vessels, and peripheral nervous system tissue.

CCI Version 16.3

01810, 0228T, 0230T, 10060, 10140, 10160, 11010-11012❖, 11040-11044, 12001-12007, 12020-12021, 12041-12047, 13131-13132, 20526-20553, 25259, 26010-26030, 26160-26185, 26340, 29086, 36000, 36400-36410, 36420-36430, 36440, 36600, 36640, 37202, 43752, 51701-51703, 62310-62319, 64400-64435, 64445-64450, 64479, 64483, 64505-64530, 69990, 93000-93010, 93040-93042, 93318, 94002, 94200, 94250, 94680-94690, 94770, 95812-95816, 95819, 95822, 95829, 95955, 96360, 96365, 96372, 96374-96376, 99148-99149, 99150

Also not with 26117: 26055-26116

Also not with 26118: 0213T, 0216T, 26055-26117, 26260, 26262, 64490, 64493

Note: These CCI edits are used for Medicare. Other payers may reimburse on codes listed above.

Medicare Edits

	Fac RVU	Non-Fac RVU	FUD	Assist
26117	21.27	21.27	90	N/A
26118	32.02	32.02	90	80

Medicare References: 100-2,15,260; 100-4,12,30; 100-4,12,90.3; 100-4,14,10

26121-26125

26121 Fasciectomy, palm only, with or without Z-plasty, other local tissue rearrangement, or skin grafting (includes obtaining graft)

26123 Fasciectomy, partial palmar with release of single digit including proximal interphalangeal joint, with or without Z-plasty, other local tissue rearrangement, or skin grafting (includes obtaining graft);

26125 each additional digit (List separately in addition to code for primary procedure)

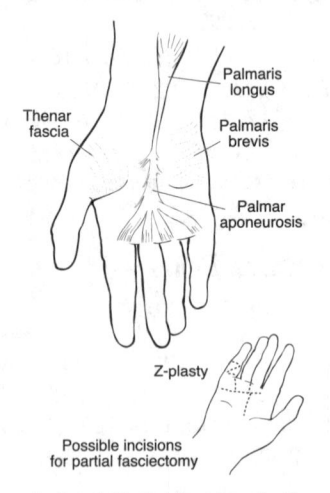

A palmar fasciectomy is performed, with or without Z-plasty, other local tissue rearrangement, or skin grafting. Report 26123 for a partial palmar fasciectomy with release of a single digit, including proximal interphalangeal joint. And report 26125 for each additional digit

Explanation

The physician removes the palmar fascia. The physician incises the overlying skin and subcutaneous tissue. The palmar fascia is exposed and resected. Tendon sheaths are freed. The operative incision is closed in sutured layers if possible. Z-plasties are performed or skin grafts are obtained to close the wound if necessary. In 26121, the entire palmar fascia is removed. In 26123, part of the palmar fascia is removed and flexor tendons at proximal interphalangeal joints are released. Use 26125 to report additional digits.

Coding Tips

Use 26125 in conjunction with 26123. As an "add-on" code, 26125 is not subject to multiple procedure rules. No reimbursement reduction or modifier 51 is applied. Add-on codes describe additional intra-service work associated with the primary procedure. They are performed by the same physician on the same date of service as the primary service/procedure, and must never be reported as a stand-alone code. For palmar fasciotomy, see 26040 or 26045.

ICD-9-CM Procedural

82.35	Other fasciectomy of hand
86.61	Full-thickness skin graft to hand
86.84	Relaxation of scar or web contracture of skin

Anesthesia

26121	01810
26123	01810
26125	N/A

ICD-9-CM Diagnostic

239.2	Neoplasms of unspecified nature of bone, soft tissue, and skin
682.4	Cellulitis and abscess of hand, except fingers and thumb — (Use additional code to identify organism, such as 041.1, etc.)
718.44	Contracture of hand joint
727.03	Trigger finger (acquired)
727.81	Contracture of tendon (sheath)
728.0	Infective myositis
728.6	Contracture of palmar fascia
729.4	Unspecified fasciitis
736.29	Other acquired deformity of finger
882.1	Open wound of hand except finger(s) alone, complicated

Terms To Know

abscess. Circumscribed collection of pus resulting from bacteria, frequently associated with swelling and other signs of inflammation.

cellulitis. Sudden, severe, suppurative inflammation and edema in subcutaneous tissue or muscle, most often caused by bacterial infection secondary to a cutaneous lesion.

contracture. Shortening of muscle or connective tissue.

deformity. Irregularity or malformation of the body.

fascia. Fibrous sheet or band of tissue that envelops organs, muscles, and groupings of muscles.

open wound. Opening or break of the skin.

CCI Version 16.3

25259, 26340

Also not with 26121: 01810, 0213T, 0216T, 0228T, 0230T, 14000-14001, 14020-14061, 14301, 14350, 15002, 15004, 15050-15100, 15110, 15115, 15120, 15130, 15135, 15150, 15155, 15170, 15175, 15200, 15220, 15240, 15260, 15300, 15335, 15340, 15360, 15365, 15400, 15570-15576, 15600-15620, 15630-15650, 15734-15740, 15750, 15756-15776, 20526-20553, 26040, 26055, 26123❖, 26145, 26185, 26440, 29086, 36000, 36400-36410, 36420-36430, 36440, 36600, 36640, 37202, 43752, 51701-51703, 62310-62319, 64400-64435, 64445-64450, 64479, 64483, 64490, 64493, 64505-64530, 64704, 64721, 69990, 93000-93010, 93040-93042, 93318, 94002, 94200, 94250, 94680-94690, 94770, 95812-95816, 95819, 95822, 95829, 95955, 96360, 96365, 96372, 96374-96376, 99148-99149, 99150

Also not with 26123: 01810, 0213T, 0216T, 0228T, 0230T, 10060, 10140, 10160, 11000, 11040-11042, 14000-14001, 14020-14061, 14301, 14350, 15002, 15004, 15050-15100, 15110, 15115, 15120, 15130, 15135, 15150, 15155, 15170, 15175, 15200, 15220, 15240, 15260, 15300, 15335, 15340, 15360, 15365, 15400, 15570-15576, 15600-15620, 15630-15650, 15734-15740, 15750, 15756-15776, 20526-20553, 26055, 26145-26160, 26185, 26440-26442, 26520-26525, 26546, 26706, 26785, 29085-29086, 29125, 36000, 36400-36410, 36420-36430, 36440, 36600, 36640, 37202, 43752, 51701-51703, 62310-62319, 64400-64435, 64445-64450, 64479, 64483, 64490, 64493, 64505-64530, 64702-64704, 64718, 69990, 93000-93010, 93040-93042, 93318, 94002, 94200, 94250, 94680-94690, 94770, 95812-95816, 95819, 95822, 95829, 95955, 96360, 96365, 96372, 96374-96376, 99148-99149, 99150

Also not with 26125: 20526, 29086

Note: These CCI edits are used for Medicare. Other payers may reimburse on codes listed above.

Medicare Edits

	Fac RVU	Non-Fac RVU	FUD	Assist
26121	17.34	17.34	90	N/A
26123	24.08	24.08	90	N/A
26125	8.19	8.19	N/A	N/A

Medicare References: 100-2,15,260; 100-4,12,30; 100-4,12,90.3; 100-4,14,10

26130

26130 Synovectomy, carpometacarpal joint

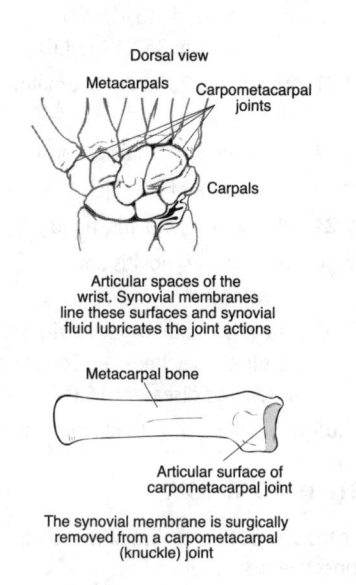

Dorsal view
Metacarpals
Carpometacarpal joints
Carpals

Articular spaces of the wrist. Synovial membranes line these surfaces and synovial fluid lubricates the joint actions

Metacarpal bone

Articular surface of carpometacarpal joint

The synovial membrane is surgically removed from a carpometacarpal (knuckle) joint

Explanation
The physician removes the synovial membrane from the carpometacarpal joint. The physician incises the skin overlying the affected joint. The joint capsule is exposed by dissecting down through the soft tissues and freeing and reflecting the muscles. The joint capsule is incised to expose the synovium, the inner membrane of the articular capsule that lines the joint cavity. The inflamed or enlarged synovium is dissected away from the capsule and the bones and removed. A drain tube may be placed and the incision is repaired in layers with sutures, staples, and/or Steri-strips. A splint may be applied to limit movement.

Coding Tips
This code should be reported for each joint involved. When multiple joints are involved, report one joint synovectomy as the primary procedure and append modifier 51 to subsequent procedures. Local anesthesia is included in this service. However, this procedure may be performed under general anesthesia, depending on the age and/or condition of the patient. For synovectomy, metacarpophalangeal joint, see 26135.

ICD-9-CM Procedural
80.79 Synovectomy of other specified site

Anesthesia
26130 01810

ICD-9-CM Diagnostic
275.40 Unspecified disorder of calcium metabolism — (Use additional code to identify any associated mental retardation)
275.42 Hypercalcemia — (Use additional code to identify any associated mental retardation)
275.49 Other disorders of calcium metabolism — (Use additional code to identify any associated mental retardation)
357.1 Polyneuropathy in collagen vascular disease — (Code first underlying disease: 446.0, 710.0, 714.0)
359.6 Symptomatic inflammatory myopathy in diseases classified elsewhere — (Code first underlying disease: 135, 140.0-208.9, 277.30-277.39, 446.0, 710.0, 710.1, 710.2, 714.0)
446.0 Polyarteritis nodosa
710.0 Systemic lupus erythematosus — (Use additional code to identify manifestation: 424.91, 581.81, 582.81, 583.81)
710.1 Systemic sclerosis — (Use additional code to identify manifestation: 359.6, 517.2)
710.2 Sicca syndrome
711.04 Pyogenic arthritis, hand — (Use additional code to identify infectious organism: 041.0-041.8)
711.44 Arthropathy, associated with other bacterial diseases, hand — (Code first underlying disease, such as diseases classifiable to 010-040 (except 036.82), 090-099 (except 098.50))
711.54 Arthropathy associated with other viral diseases, hand — (Code first underlying disease: 045-049, 050-079, 480, 487)
711.94 Unspecified infective arthritis, hand
712.84 Other specified crystal arthropathies, hand
713.8 Arthropathy associated with other conditions classifiable elsewhere — (Code first underlying disease as conditions classifiable elsewhere except as in: 711.1-711.8, 712, 713.0-713.7)
714.0 Rheumatoid arthritis — (Use additional code to identify manifestation: 357.1, 359.6)
714.30 Polyarticular juvenile rheumatoid arthritis, chronic or unspecified
714.31 Polyarticular juvenile rheumatoid arthritis, acute
714.32 Pauciarticular juvenile rheumatoid arthritis
714.33 Monoarticular juvenile rheumatoid arthritis
714.9 Unspecified inflammatory polyarthropathy
716.04 Kaschin-Beck disease, hand
716.14 Traumatic arthropathy, hand
716.64 Unspecified monoarthritis, hand
719.24 Villonodular synovitis, hand
726.4 Enthesopathy of wrist and carpus
727.00 Unspecified synovitis and tenosynovitis
727.50 Unspecified rupture of synovium

Terms To Know
hypercalcemia. Abnormally high levels of calcium in the blood, resulting in symptoms of muscle weakness, fatigue, nausea, depression, and constipation.

systemic sclerosis. Systemic disease characterized by excess fibrotic collagen build-up, turning the skin thickened and hard. Fibrotic changes also occur in various organs and cause vascular abnormalities and affect more women than men.

tenosynovitis. Inflammation of a tendon sheath due to infection or disease.

villonodular synovitis. Inflammation of the synovial membrane due to excessive synovial tissue formation, especially in the knee.

CCI Version 16.3
01810, 0213T, 0216T, 0228T, 0230T, 10060, 10140, 10160, 11012❖, 20526-20553, 25259, 26100, 26185, 26340, 29086, 36000, 36400-36410, 36420-36430, 36440, 36600, 36640, 37202, 43752, 51701-51703, 62310-62319, 64400-64435, 64445-64450, 64479, 64483, 64490, 64493, 64505-64530, 69990, 93000-93010, 93040-93042, 93318, 94002, 94200, 94250, 94680-94690, 94770, 95812-95816, 95819, 95822, 95829, 95955, 96360, 96365, 96372, 96374-96376, 99148-99149, 99150

Note: These CCI edits are used for Medicare. Other payers may reimburse on codes listed above.

Medicare Edits

	Fac RVU	Non-Fac RVU	FUD	Assist
26130	13.27	13.27	90	N/A

Medicare References: 100-2,15,260; 100-4,12,30; 100-4,12,90.3; 100-4,14,10

26135

26135 Synovectomy, metacarpophalangeal joint including intrinsic release and extensor hood reconstruction, each digit

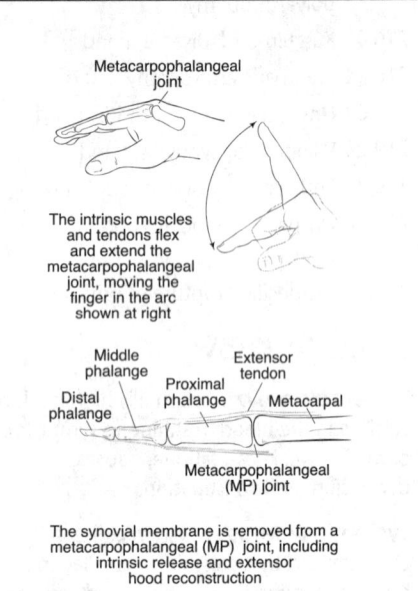

Explanation
The physician removes the synovial membrane from the metacarpophalangeal joint, releases intrinsic musculature, and reconstructs the extensor hood. The physician incises the skin overlying the affected joint and dissects down through the soft tissues to the joint capsule. The joint capsule is incised and the synovium, the inner membrane of the articular capsule that lines the joint cavity, is removed. Intrinsic muscle contractions are released by exposing the extensor aponeurosis and incising the fibers at their insertion down into the tendon with a parallel incision, while preserving the transverse fibers. The adequacy of the dissection is tested and adjusted before the remaining flap part of the extensor hood is resected. The incision is closed with running sutures and a plaster splint is applied to hold the metacarpophalangeal joints in extension but allow full movement of the interphalangeal joints. Report each finger separately.

Coding Tips
This code should be reported for each joint involved. When multiple joints are involved, report one joint synovectomy as the primary procedure and append modifier 51 to subsequent procedures. Local anesthesia is included in this service. However, this procedure may be performed under general anesthesia, depending on the age and/or condition of the patient. For synovectomy of the carpometacarpal joint, see 26130.

ICD-9-CM Procedural
80.74 Synovectomy of hand and finger

Anesthesia
26135 01810

ICD-9-CM Diagnostic
- 275.40 Unspecified disorder of calcium metabolism — (Use additional code to identify any associated mental retardation)
- 275.42 Hypercalcemia — (Use additional code to identify any associated mental retardation)
- 275.49 Other disorders of calcium metabolism — (Use additional code to identify any associated mental retardation)
- 275.5 Hungry bone syndrome
- 357.1 Polyneuropathy in collagen vascular disease — (Code first underlying disease: 446.0, 710.0, 714.0)
- 359.6 Symptomatic inflammatory myopathy in diseases classified elsewhere — (Code first underlying disease: 135, 140.0-208.9, 277.30-277.39, 446.0, 710.0, 710.1, 710.2, 714.0)
- 446.0 Polyarteritis nodosa
- 710.0 Systemic lupus erythematosus — (Use additional code to identify manifestation: 424.91, 581.81, 582.81, 583.81)
- 710.1 Systemic sclerosis — (Use additional code to identify manifestation: 359.6, 517.2)
- 710.2 Sicca syndrome
- 711.04 Pyogenic arthritis, hand — (Use additional code to identify infectious organism: 041.0-041.8)
- 711.44 Arthropathy, associated with other bacterial diseases, hand — (Code first underlying disease, such as diseases classifiable to 010-040 (except 036.82), 090-099 (except 098.50))
- 711.54 Arthropathy associated with other viral diseases, hand — (Code first underlying disease: 045-049, 050-079, 480, 487)
- 711.64 Arthropathy associated with mycoses, hand — (Code first underlying disease: 110.0-118)
- 711.94 Unspecified infective arthritis, hand
- 712.84 Other specified crystal arthropathies, hand
- 713.8 Arthropathy associated with other conditions classifiable elsewhere — (Code first underlying disease as conditions classifiable elsewhere except as in: 711.1-711.8, 712, 713.0-713.7)
- 714.0 Rheumatoid arthritis — (Use additional code to identify manifestation: 357.1, 359.6)
- 714.31 Polyarticular juvenile rheumatoid arthritis, acute
- 716.14 Traumatic arthropathy, hand
- 718.44 Contracture of hand joint
- 719.24 Villonodular synovitis, hand
- 727.00 Unspecified synovitis and tenosynovitis
- 727.01 Synovitis and tenosynovitis in diseases classified elsewhere — (Code first underlying disease: 015.0-015.9)
- 727.05 Other tenosynovitis of hand and wrist

Terms To Know
contracture. Shortening of muscle or connective tissue.

hypercalcemia. Abnormally high levels of calcium in the blood, resulting in symptoms of muscle weakness, fatigue, nausea, depression, and constipation.

polyarteritis nodosa. Systemic necrotizing vasculitis of small and medium arteries that results in the infarction and scarring within the affected organs.

tenosynovitis. Inflammation of a tendon sheath due to infection or disease.

villonodular synovitis. Inflammation of the synovial membrane due to excessive synovial tissue formation, especially in the knee.

CCI Version 16.3
01810, 0213T, 0216T, 0228T, 0230T, 10060, 10140, 10160, 11012✣, 20526-20553, 25259, 26075, 26105, 26185, 26340, 26520, 29086, 29125, 29900-29901, 36000, 36400-36410, 36420-36430, 36440, 36600, 36640, 37202, 43752, 51701-51703, 62310-62319, 64400-64435, 64445-64450, 64479, 64483, 64490, 64493, 64505-64530, 69990, 93000-93010, 93040-93042, 93318, 94002, 94200, 94250, 94680-94690, 94770, 95812-95816, 95819, 95822, 95829, 95955, 96360, 96365, 96372, 96374-96376, 99148-99149, 99150

Note: These CCI edits are used for Medicare. Other payers may reimburse on codes listed above.

Medicare Edits

	Fac RVU	Non-Fac RVU	FUD	Assist
26135	15.97	15.97	90	80

Medicare References: 100-2,15,260; 100-4,12,30; 100-4,12,90.3; 100-4,14,10

26140

26140 Synovectomy, proximal interphalangeal joint, including extensor reconstruction, each interphalangeal joint

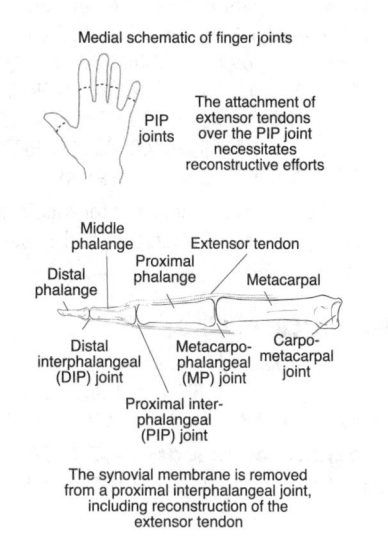

Medial schematic of finger joints

The attachment of extensor tendons over the PIP joint necessitates reconstructive efforts

PIP joints

Middle phalange
Distal phalange
Proximal phalange
Extensor tendon
Metacarpal

Distal interphalangeal (DIP) joint
Metacarpophalangeal (MP) joint
Carpometacarpal joint
Proximal interphalangeal (PIP) joint

The synovial membrane is removed from a proximal interphalangeal joint, including reconstruction of the extensor tendon

Explanation

The physician removes the synovial membrane from the proximal interphalangeal joint and reconstructs the extensor tendon. The physician makes a midlateral incision overlying the proximal interphalangeal joint, severs the attachment of the transverse retinacular ligament, and elevates the extensor hood. The collateral ligament and central tendon are identified and the joint is entered. The synovium, the inner membrane of the articular capsule that lines the joint cavity, is removed. The transverse retinacular ligament is relocated and the extensor tendons over the dorsum of the finger are repaired as needed and reattached to the joint. The incision is sutured in layers. Report each finger separately.

Coding Tips

This code should be reported for each joint involved. When multiple joints are involved, report one joint synovectomy as the primary procedure and append modifier 51 to subsequent procedures. Some payers may require the use of HCPCS Level II modifiers FA-F9 to identify the specific finger involved. Local anesthesia is included in this service. However, this procedure may be performed under general anesthesia, depending on the age and/or condition of the patient.

ICD-9-CM Procedural

80.74 Synovectomy of hand and finger

Anesthesia

26140 01810

ICD-9-CM Diagnostic

275.40 Unspecified disorder of calcium metabolism — (Use additional code to identify any associated mental retardation)
275.42 Hypercalcemia — (Use additional code to identify any associated mental retardation)
275.49 Other disorders of calcium metabolism — (Use additional code to identify any associated mental retardation)
277.30 Amyloidosis, unspecified — (Use additional code to identify any associated mental retardation)
277.31 Familial Mediterranean fever — (Use additional code to identify any associated mental retardation)
277.39 Other amyloidosis — (Use additional code to identify any associated mental retardation)
357.1 Polyneuropathy in collagen vascular disease — (Code first underlying disease: 446.0, 710.0, 714.0)
359.6 Symptomatic inflammatory myopathy in diseases classified elsewhere — (Code first underlying disease: 135, 140.0-208.9, 277.30-277.39, 446.0, 710.0, 710.1, 710.2, 714.0)
446.0 Polyarteritis nodosa
710.0 Systemic lupus erythematosus — (Use additional code to identify manifestation: 424.91, 581.81, 582.81, 583.81)
710.1 Systemic sclerosis — (Use additional code to identify manifestation: 359.6, 517.2)
710.2 Sicca syndrome
711.04 Pyogenic arthritis, hand — (Use additional code to identify infectious organism: 041.0-041.8)
711.44 Arthropathy, associated with other bacterial diseases, hand — (Code first underlying disease, such as diseases classifiable to 010-040 (except 036.82), 090-099 (except 098.50))
711.54 Arthropathy associated with other viral diseases, hand — (Code first underlying disease: 045-049, 050-079, 480, 487)
711.64 Arthropathy associated with mycoses, hand — (Code first underlying disease: 110.0-118)
711.94 Unspecified infective arthritis, hand

712.84 Other specified crystal arthropathies, hand
713.8 Arthropathy associated with other conditions classifiable elsewhere — (Code first underlying disease as conditions classifiable elsewhere except as in: 711.1-711.8, 712, 713.0-713.7)
714.0 Rheumatoid arthritis — (Use additional code to identify manifestation: 357.1, 359.6)
714.1 Felty's syndrome
718.44 Contracture of hand joint
727.00 Unspecified synovitis and tenosynovitis
727.01 Synovitis and tenosynovitis in diseases classified elsewhere — (Code first underlying disease: 015.0-015.9)
727.05 Other tenosynovitis of hand and wrist
736.21 Boutonniere deformity

Terms To Know

amyloidosis. Condition in which insoluble, fibril-like proteins (amyloid) build up in one or more organs and tissues within the body.

Felty's syndrome. Splenomegaly, leukopenia, arthritis, hypersplenism, anemia and other symptoms.

hypercalcemia. Abnormally high levels of calcium in the blood, resulting in symptoms of muscle weakness, fatigue, nausea, depression, and constipation.

CCI Version 16.3

01810, 0213T, 0216T, 0228T, 0230T, 10060, 10140, 10160, 20526-20553, 25259, 26080, 26185, 26340, 26525, 29086-29105, 36000, 36400-36410, 36420-36430, 36440, 36600, 36640, 37202, 43752, 51701-51703, 62310-62319, 64400-64435, 64445-64450, 64479, 64483, 64490, 64493, 64505-64530, 69990, 93000-93010, 93040-93042, 93318, 94002, 94200, 94250, 94680-94690, 94770, 95812-95816, 95819, 95822, 95829, 95955, 96360, 96365, 96372, 96374-96376, 99148-99149, 99150

Note: These CCI edits are used for Medicare. Other payers may reimburse on codes listed above.

Medicare Edits

	Fac RVU	Non-Fac RVU	FUD	Assist
26140	14.61	14.61	90	N/A

Medicare References: 100-2,15,260; 100-4,12,30; 100-4,12,90.3; 100-4,14,10

26145

26145 Synovectomy, tendon sheath, radical (tenosynovectomy), flexor tendon, palm and/or finger, each tendon

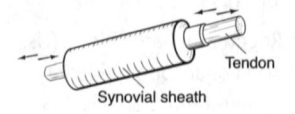

Schematic of flexor tendon in its synovial sheath

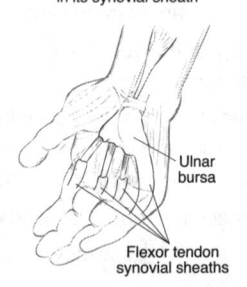

A synovial sheath from a flexor tendon of the palm or a finger is removed in a radical surgical procedure

Explanation
The physician removes the synovial membrane from a flexor tendon sheath (tenosynovectomy) at the palm or finger. The physician incises the skin of the affected finger on the palmar side in a zigzag fashion and exposes the flexor tendon sheath. Taking care not to damage neurovascular bundles, the sheath is excised, except for a small area in the middle of the phalanx sections. The synovium is removed as much as possible and the incision is closed with interrupted sutures. A compression dressing and supportive wrist splint are applied.

Coding Tips
This code should be reported for each tendon involved. When multiple tendons are involved, report one tendon sheath synovectomy as the primary procedure and append modifier 51 to subsequent procedures. Local anesthesia is included in this service. However, this procedure may be performed under general anesthesia, depending on the age and/or condition of the patient. For tendon sheath synovectomies at the wrist, see 25115 and 25116.

ICD-9-CM Procedural
80.74 Synovectomy of hand and finger

Anesthesia
26145 01810

ICD-9-CM Diagnostic
- 171.2 Malignant neoplasm of connective and other soft tissue of upper limb, including shoulder
- 238.1 Neoplasm of uncertain behavior of connective and other soft tissue
- 239.2 Neoplasms of unspecified nature of bone, soft tissue, and skin
- 357.1 Polyneuropathy in collagen vascular disease — (Code first underlying disease: 446.0, 710.0, 714.0)
- 359.6 Symptomatic inflammatory myopathy in diseases classified elsewhere — (Code first underlying disease: 135, 140.0-208.9, 277.30-277.39, 446.0, 710.0, 710.1, 710.2, 714.0)
- 446.0 Polyarteritis nodosa
- 710.0 Systemic lupus erythematosus — (Use additional code to identify manifestation: 424.91, 581.81, 582.81, 583.81)
- 710.1 Systemic sclerosis — (Use additional code to identify manifestation: 359.6, 517.2)
- 710.2 Sicca syndrome
- 714.0 Rheumatoid arthritis — (Use additional code to identify manifestation: 357.1, 359.6)
- 714.1 Felty's syndrome

Terms To Know
Felty's syndrome. Splenomegaly, leukopenia, arthritis, hypersplenism, anemia and other symptoms.

malignant. Any condition tending to progress toward death, specifically an invasive tumor with a loss of cellular differentiation that has the ability to spread or metastasize to other areas in the body.

soft tissue. Nonepithelial tissues outside of the skeleton that includes subcutaneous adipose tissue, fibrous tissue, fascia, muscles, blood and lymph vessels, and peripheral nervous system tissue.

tendon. Fibrous tissue that connects muscle to bone, consisting primarily of collagen and containing little vasculature.

CCI Version 16.3
01810, 0213T, 0216T, 0228T, 0230T, 10060, 10140, 10160, 11420-11426, 20526-20553, 25000, 25259, 26055, 26185, 26340, 26440-26442, 29085-29086, 36000, 36400-36410, 36420-36430, 36440, 36600, 36640, 37202, 43752, 51701-51703, 62310-62319, 64400-64435, 64445-64450, 64479, 64483, 64490, 64493, 64505-64530, 64704, 64718, 69990, 93000-93010, 93040-93042, 93318, 94002, 94200, 94250, 94680-94690, 94770, 95812-95816, 95819, 95822, 95829, 95955, 96360, 96365, 96372, 96374-96376, 99148-99149, 99150

Note: These CCI edits are used for Medicare. Other payers may reimburse on codes listed above.

Medicare Edits

	Fac RVU	Non-Fac RVU	FUD	Assist
26145	14.83	14.83	90	N/A

Medicare References: 100-2,15,260; 100-4,12,30; 100-4,12,90.3; 100-4,14,10

26160

26160 Excision of lesion of tendon sheath or joint capsule (eg, cyst, mucous cyst, or ganglion), hand or finger

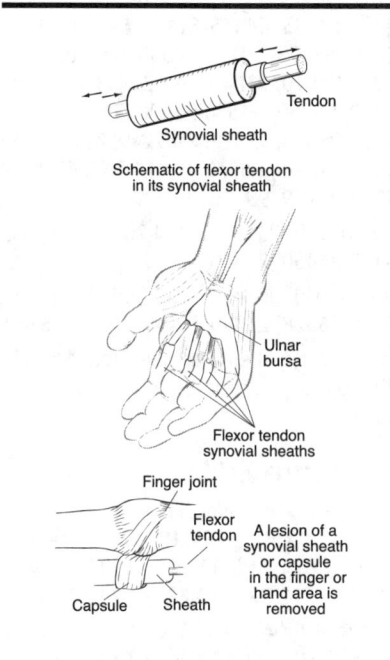

Explanation

The physician excises a lesion of the tendon sheath or joint capsule in the hand or finger, such as a cyst or ganglion. The physician incises the overlying skin and dissects to locate the affected area. The lesion, cyst, or ganglion is identified and excised from the tendon sheath or joint capsule. The incision is sutured in layers.

Coding Tips

Local anesthesia is included in this service. However, this procedure may be performed under general anesthesia, depending on the age and/or condition of the patient. For excision of a wrist ganglion, see 25111 or 25112. For a tendon sheath incision, without excision of a lesion (e.g., for trigger finger), see 26055.

ICD-9-CM Procedural

82.21 Excision of lesion of tendon sheath of hand

Anesthesia

26160 01810

ICD-9-CM Diagnostic

215.2 Other benign neoplasm of connective and other soft tissue of upper limb, including shoulder
229.8 Benign neoplasm of other specified sites
238.8 Neoplasm of uncertain behavior of other specified sites
239.2 Neoplasms of unspecified nature of bone, soft tissue, and skin
727.00 Unspecified synovitis and tenosynovitis
727.02 Giant cell tumor of tendon sheath
727.04 Radial styloid tenosynovitis
727.41 Ganglion of joint
727.42 Ganglion of tendon sheath
727.9 Unspecified disorder of synovium, tendon, and bursa
782.2 Localized superficial swelling, mass, or lump

Terms To Know

benign. Mild or nonmalignant in nature.

bursa. Cavity or sac containing fluid that occurs between articulating surfaces and serves to reduce friction from moving parts. An anatomical structure frequently referenced in orthopedic notes as it may become diseased or need removal.

cyst. Elevated encapsulated mass containing fluid, semisolid, or solid material with a membranous lining.

ganglion. Fluid-filled, benign cyst appearing on a tendon sheath or aponeurosis, frequently found in the hand, wrist, or foot and connecting to an underlying joint.

lesion. Area of damaged tissue that has lost continuity or function, due to disease or trauma. Lesions may be located on internal structures such as the brain, nerves, or kidneys, or visible on the skin.

soft tissue. Nonepithelial tissues outside of the skeleton that includes subcutaneous adipose tissue, fibrous tissue, fascia, muscles, blood and lymph vessels, and peripheral nervous system tissue.

synovia. Clear fluid lubricant of joints, bursae, and tendon sheaths, secreted by the synovial membrane.

synovitis. Inflammation of the synovial membrane that lines a synovial joint, resulting in pain and swelling.

tendon. Fibrous tissue that connects muscle to bone, consisting primarily of collagen and containing little vasculature.

CCI Version 16.3

01810, 0213T, 0216T, 0228T, 0230T, 10060, 10140, 10160, 11010❖, 11420-11426, 12001-12007, 12020-12021, 12041-12047, 13131-13132, 20526-20553, 25259, 26020, 26055, 26070-26110, 26130-26145, 26170-26185, 26340, 26440-26442, 29086, 36000, 36400-36410, 36420-36430, 36440, 36600, 36640, 37202, 43752, 51701-51703, 62310-62319, 64400-64435, 64445-64450, 64479, 64483, 64490, 64493, 64505-64530, 69990, 93000-93010, 93040-93042, 93318, 94002, 94200, 94250, 94680-94690, 94770, 95812-95816, 95819, 95822, 95829, 95955, 96360, 96365, 96372, 96374-96376, 99148-99149, 99150, J0670, J2001

Note: These CCI edits are used for Medicare. Other payers may reimburse on codes listed above.

Medicare Edits

	Fac RVU	Non-Fac RVU	FUD	Assist
26160	9.49	16.38	90	N/A

Medicare References: 100-2,15,260; 100-4,12,30; 100-4,12,90.3; 100-4,14,10

26170-26180

26170 Excision of tendon, palm, flexor or extensor, single, each tendon

26180 Excision of tendon, finger, flexor or extensor, each tendon

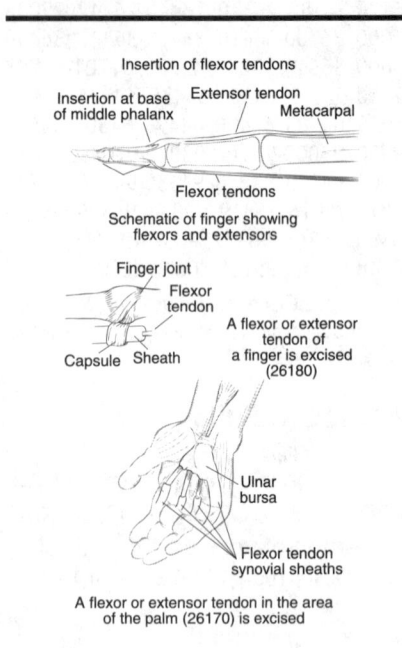

Explanation

The physician excises a flexor or extensor tendon in the hand or finger. Included in these codes are flexor tendons extending from the palm of the hand to the fingertips, essential to grasping motion, and extensor tendons stretching from the wrist along the back of the hand to the fingertips, essential to opening the hand. The physician incises the overlying skin and dissects to the flexor or extensor tendon. The tendon is freed and resected. The incision is sutured in layers. Report 26170 for each flexor or extensor tendon of the hand and 26180 for each flexor or extensor tendon of the finger.

Coding Tips

Code 26170 should not be reported in conjunction with 26390, 26415. For 26180, some payers may require the use of HCPCS Level II modifiers FA–F9 to identify the specific finger involved.

ICD-9-CM Procedural

82.33 Other tenonectomy of hand

Anesthesia

01810

ICD-9-CM Diagnostic

357.1 Polyneuropathy in collagen vascular disease — (Code first underlying disease: 446.0, 710.0, 714.0)

359.6 Symptomatic inflammatory myopathy in diseases classified elsewhere — (Code first underlying disease: 135, 140.0-208.9, 277.30-277.39, 446.0, 710.0, 710.1, 710.2, 714.0)

446.0 Polyarteritis nodosa

682.4 Cellulitis and abscess of hand, except fingers and thumb — (Use additional code to identify organism, such as 041.1, etc.)

710.0 Systemic lupus erythematosus — (Use additional code to identify manifestation: 424.91, 581.81, 582.81, 583.81)

710.1 Systemic sclerosis — (Use additional code to identify manifestation: 359.6, 517.2)

710.2 Sicca syndrome

714.0 Rheumatoid arthritis — (Use additional code to identify manifestation: 357.1, 359.6)

716.14 Traumatic arthropathy, hand

727.81 Contracture of tendon (sheath)

727.89 Other disorders of synovium, tendon, and bursa

728.6 Contracture of palmar fascia

882.2 Open wound of hand except finger(s) alone, with tendon involvement

905.8 Late effect of tendon injury

Terms To Know

cellulitis. Sudden, severe, suppurative inflammation and edema in subcutaneous tissue or muscle, most often caused by bacterial infection secondary to a cutaneous lesion.

contracture. Shortening of muscle or connective tissue.

late effect. Abnormality, dysfunction, or other residual condition produced after the acute phase of an illness, injury, or disease is over. There is no time limit on when late effects can appear.

systemic sclerosis. Systemic disease characterized by excess fibrotic collagen build-up, turning the skin thickened and hard. Fibrotic changes also occur in various organs and cause vascular abnormalities and affect more women than men.

tendon. Fibrous tissue that connects muscle to bone, consisting primarily of collagen and containing little vasculature.

CCI Version 16.3

01810, 0213T, 0216T, 0228T, 0230T, 20526-20553, 25259, 26115, 26185, 26340, 26500-26502, 29086, 36000, 36400-36410, 36420-36430, 36440, 36600, 36640, 37202, 43752, 51701-51703, 62310-62319, 64400-64435, 64445-64450, 64479, 64483, 64490, 64493, 64505-64530, 69990, 93000-93010, 93040-93042, 93318, 94002, 94200, 94250, 94680-94690, 94770, 95812-95816, 95819, 95822, 95829, 95955, 96360, 96365, 96372, 96374-96376, 99148-99149, 99150

Also not with 26170: 26410-26412, 26440-26450, 26460

Also not with 26180: 26055-26060, 26170, 26418-26428, 26440-26449, 26455-26460

Note: These CCI edits are used for Medicare. Other payers may reimburse on codes listed above.

Medicare Edits

	Fac RVU	Non-Fac RVU	FUD	Assist
26170	11.71	11.71	90	80
26180	12.72	12.72	90	80

Medicare References: 100-2,15,260; 100-4,12,30; 100-4,12,90.3; 100-4,14,10

26185

26185 Sesamoidectomy, thumb or finger (separate procedure)

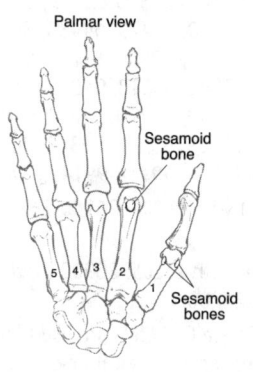

Palmar view

A sesamoid bone is removed from the thumb or finger

Sesamoid bones are round or ovular bony nodes that may normally appear in certain tendons. They often serve to protect the tendons from wear and also change the course of the tendon as it approaches insertion. This offers a greater degree of leverage

Explanation

This procedure is rarely performed, but may be necessary in cases of sesamoid fracture or when performing a metacarpal-sesamoid synostosis. The physician makes a midlateral incision over the metacarpophalangeal joint of the thumb on the radial side. The radial side of the extensor apparatus is opened, and the radial carpal ligament is dissected. The opponens pollicis muscle is separated from its attachment to the metacarpal neck. The metacarpophalangeal joint is opened through incision. In the case of a fracture, the fractured bone is exposed and removed. In a synostosis, the lateral sesamoid bone is exposed, its cartilage is removed along with the cortex of the first metacarpal neck. Drill holes are placed in the metacarpal neck and a wire suture is passed around the sesamoid bone. The capsule and overlying tissue are sutured closed.

Coding Tips

This procedure is rarely performed, but may be necessary in cases of a sesamoid fracture or when performing a metacarpal-sesamoid synostosis. This separate procedure by definition is usually a component of a more complex service and is not identified separately. When performed alone or with other unrelated procedures/services, it may be reported. If performed alone, list the code; if performed with other procedures/services, list the code and append modifier 59. Some payers may require the use of HCPCS Level II modifiers FA–F9 to identify the specific finger involved.

ICD-9-CM Procedural

77.99 Total ostectomy of other bone, except facial bones

Anesthesia

26185 01830

ICD-9-CM Diagnostic

170.5 Malignant neoplasm of short bones of upper limb
213.5 Benign neoplasm of short bones of upper limb
357.1 Polyneuropathy in collagen vascular disease — (Code first underlying disease: 446.0, 710.0, 714.0)
359.6 Symptomatic inflammatory myopathy in diseases classified elsewhere — (Code first underlying disease: 135, 140.0-208.9, 277.30-277.39, 446.0, 710.0, 710.1, 710.2, 714.0)
446.0 Polyarteritis nodosa
710.0 Systemic lupus erythematosus — (Use additional code to identify manifestation: 424.91, 581.81, 582.81, 583.81)
710.1 Systemic sclerosis — (Use additional code to identify manifestation: 359.6, 517.2)
710.2 Sicca syndrome
714.0 Rheumatoid arthritis — (Use additional code to identify manifestation: 357.1, 359.6)
715.09 Generalized osteoarthrosis, involving multiple sites
715.14 Primary localized osteoarthrosis, hand
726.4 Enthesopathy of wrist and carpus
726.90 Enthesopathy of unspecified site
732.9 Unspecified osteochondropathy
733.99 Other disorders of bone and cartilage

Terms To Know

polyneuropathy. Disease process of severe inflammation of multiple nerves.

systemic sclerosis. Systemic disease characterized by excess fibrotic collagen build-up, turning the skin thickened and hard. Fibrotic changes also occur in various organs and cause vascular abnormalities and affect more women than men.

CCI Version 16.3

01810, 0213T, 0216T, 0228T, 0230T, 11900-11901, 12001-12007, 12011-12057, 13100-13101, 13120-13121, 13131-13132, 13150-13152, 15851-15860, 20500-20501, 20526-20553, 25259, 26340, 26910❖, 26952❖, 29075-29131, 29280, 29705, 29730-29740, 35761, 36000, 36400-36410, 36420-36430, 36440, 36600, 36640, 37202, 37618, 43752, 51701-51703, 62310-62319, 64400-64435, 64445-64450, 64479, 64483, 64490, 64493, 64505-64560, 64565, 64573-64580, 64585-64595, 64702-64708, 64719-64726, 69990, 76000-76001, 76080, 77002, 87070, 87076-87077, 87102, 93000-93010, 93040-93042, 93318, 94002, 94200, 94250, 94680-94690, 94770, 95812-95816, 95819, 95822, 95829, 95860, 95900, 95955, 96360, 96365, 96372, 96374-96376, 99148-99149, 99150, G0168

Note: These CCI edits are used for Medicare. Other payers may reimburse on codes listed above.

Medicare Edits

	Fac RVU	Non-Fac RVU	FUD	Assist
26185	15.7	15.7	90	80

Medicare References: 100-2,15,260; 100-4,12,30; 100-4,12,90.3; 100-4,14,10

26200-26205

26200 Excision or curettage of bone cyst or benign tumor of metacarpal;
26205 with autograft (includes obtaining graft)

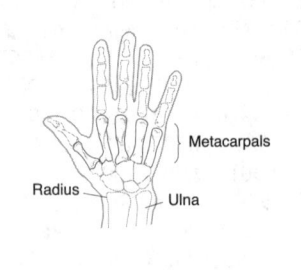

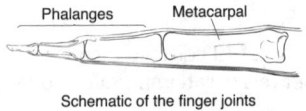

A benign tumor or cyst of a metacarpal bone is excised or removed using curett. Report 26205 when an autograft (from the patient) is used in the repair

Explanation
A bone cyst or benign tumor of the metacarpal bones is removed. The physician makes an incision in the hand overlying the cyst or tumor. The skin and underlying soft tissues are reflected to expose the periosteum, which is separated from the bone. Curettes or osteotomes are used to scrape or cut the lesion from the bone. Once the benign tumor or cyst is removed and healthy bone tissue is present, the periosteum is repositioned and the incision is repaired in layers. If the bone defect created requires a graft for repair, the physician may obtain the necessary size bone graft from a separate donor site on the patient and pack it into the site where the tumor or bone cyst was removed. Report 26205 if an autograft is obtained.

Coding Tips
Any bone graft harvest is not reported separately for 26205. According to CPT guidelines, cast application or strapping (including removal) is only reported as a replacement procedure or when the cast application or strapping is an initial service performed without a restorative treatment or procedure. See "Application of Casts and Strapping" in the CPT book in the Surgery Section, under the Musculoskeletal system. For excision or curettage of a bone cyst or a benign tumor of the finger, see 26210 or 26215.

ICD-9-CM Procedural
77.64 Local excision of lesion or tissue of carpals and metacarpals

Anesthesia
01830

ICD-9-CM Diagnostic
- 213.5 Benign neoplasm of short bones of upper limb
- 238.0 Neoplasm of uncertain behavior of bone and articular cartilage
- 239.2 Neoplasms of unspecified nature of bone, soft tissue, and skin
- 726.91 Exostosis of unspecified site
- 733.21 Solitary bone cyst
- 733.22 Aneurysmal bone cyst
- 733.29 Other cyst of bone

Terms To Know

aneurysmal bone cyst. Solitary bone lesion that bulges into the periosteum, marked by a calcified rim.

benign. Mild or nonmalignant in nature.

cyst. Elevated encapsulated mass containing fluid, semisolid, or solid material with a membranous lining.

distal. Located farther away from a specified reference point.

exostosis. Abnormal formation of a benign bony growth.

neoplasm. New abnormal growth, tumor.

soft tissue. Nonepithelial tissues outside of the skeleton that includes subcutaneous adipose tissue, fibrous tissue, fascia, muscles, blood and lymph vessels, and peripheral nervous system tissue.

tumor. Pathological swelling or enlargement; a neoplastic growth of uncontrolled, abnormal multiplication of cells.

CCI Version 16.3
01810, 0213T, 0216T, 0228T, 0230T, 10060, 10140, 10160, 20000-20005, 20526-20553, 20615, 25259, 26111-26116, 26230, 26340, 29086, 36000, 36400-36410, 36420-36430, 36440, 36600, 36640, 37202, 43752, 51701-51703, 62310-62319, 64400-64435, 64445-64450, 64479, 64483, 64490, 64493, 64505-64530, 69990, 93000-93010, 93040-93042, 93318, 94002, 94200, 94250, 94680-94690, 94770, 95812-95816, 95819, 95822, 95829, 95955, 96360, 96365, 96372, 96374-96376, 99148-99149, 99150

Also not with 26200: 26145-26160, 26185, 75716

Also not with 26205: 20900-20902, 26160, 26185-26200

Note: These CCI edits are used for Medicare. Other payers may reimburse on codes listed above.

Medicare Edits

	Fac RVU	Non-Fac RVU	FUD	Assist
26200	13.04	13.04	90	80
26205	17.5	17.5	90	N/A

Medicare References: 100-2,15,260; 100-4,12,30; 100-4,12,90.3; 100-4,14,10

26210-26215

26210 Excision or curettage of bone cyst or benign tumor of proximal, middle, or distal phalanx of finger;
26215 with autograft (includes obtaining graft)

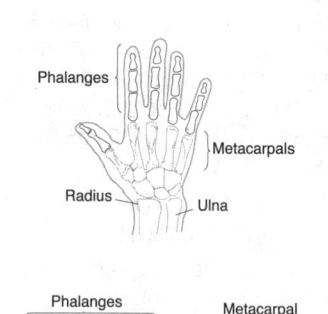

A benign tumor or cyst of a phalangeal bone is excised or removed using currett. Report 26215 when an autograft (from the patient) is used in the repair

Explanation
A bone cyst or benign tumor of the proximal, middle, or distal phalanx of the finger is removed. The physician makes an incision in the finger overlying the cyst or tumor. The skin and underlying soft tissues are reflected to expose the periosteum, which is separated from the bone. Curettes or osteotomes are used to scrape or cut the lesion from the bone. Once the benign tumor or cyst is removed and healthy bone tissue is present, the periosteum is repositioned and the incision is repaired in layers. If the bone defect created requires a graft for repair, the physician may obtain the necessary size bone graft from a separate donor site on the patient and pack it into the site where the tumor or bone cyst was removed. Report 26215 if an autograph is obtained.

Coding Tips
Any bone graft harvest is not reported separately for 26215. Some payers may require the use of HCPCS Level II modifiers FA-F9 to identify the specific finger involved. According to CPT guidelines, cast application or strapping (including removal) is only reported as a replacement procedure or when the cast application or strapping is an initial service performed without a restorative treatment or procedure. See "Application of Casts and Strapping" in the CPT book in the Surgery Section, under the Musculoskeletal system. For excision or curettage of a bone cyst or a benign tumor of the metacarpal, see 26200 or 26205.

ICD-9-CM Procedural
77.64   Local excision of lesion or tissue of carpals and metacarpals

Anesthesia
01830

ICD-9-CM Diagnostic
213.5   Benign neoplasm of short bones of upper limb
238.0   Neoplasm of uncertain behavior of bone and articular cartilage
239.2   Neoplasms of unspecified nature of bone, soft tissue, and skin
726.91 Exostosis of unspecified site
733.21 Solitary bone cyst
733.22 Aneurysmal bone cyst
733.29 Other cyst of bone

Terms To Know
aneurysmal bone cyst. Solitary bone lesion that bulges into the periosteum, marked by a calcified rim.

benign. Mild or nonmalignant in nature.

cyst. Elevated encapsulated mass containing fluid, semisolid, or solid material with a membranous lining.

distal. Located farther away from a specified reference point.

exostosis. Abnormal formation of a benign bony growth.

lesion. Area of damaged tissue that has lost continuity or function, due to disease or trauma. Lesions may be located on internal structures such as the brain, nerves, or kidneys, or visible on the skin.

proximal. Located closest to a specified reference point, usually the midline.

soft tissue. Nonepithelial tissues outside of the skeleton that includes subcutaneous adipose tissue, fibrous tissue, fascia, muscles, blood and lymph vessels, and peripheral nervous system tissue.

tumor. Pathological swelling or enlargement; a neoplastic growth of uncontrolled, abnormal multiplication of cells.

CCI Version 16.3
01810, 0213T, 0216T, 0228T, 0230T, 10060, 10140, 10160, 20526-20553, 20615, 25259, 26111-26116, 26160, 26185, 26235-26236, 26340, 29086, 36000, 36400-36410, 36420-36430, 36440, 36600, 36640, 37202, 43752, 51701-51703, 62310-62319, 64400-64435, 64445-64450, 64479, 64483, 64490, 64493, 64505-64530, 69990, 93000-93010, 93040-93042, 93318, 94002, 94200, 94250, 94680-94690, 94770, 95812-95816, 95819, 95822, 95829, 95955, 96360, 96365, 96372, 96374-96376, 99148-99149, 99150

Also not with 26210: 20000-20005
Also not with 26215: 20900-20902, 26210
Note: These CCI edits are used for Medicare. Other payers may reimburse on codes listed above.

Medicare Edits

	Fac RVU	Non-Fac RVU	FUD	Assist
26210	12.74	12.74	90	N/A
26215	16.26	16.26	90	N/A

Medicare References: 100-2,15,260; 100-4,12,30; 100-4,12,90.3; 100-4,14,10

26230-26236

26230 Partial excision (craterization, saucerization, or diaphysectomy) bone (eg, osteomyelitis); metacarpal
26235 proximal or middle phalanx of finger
26236 distal phalanx of finger

Schematic of the finger joints

A partial excision of a finger bone is performed. Report 26230 when a metacarpal bone is partially excised. Report 26235 when a proximal phalangeal bone is addressed. Report 26236 when the distal phalanx is treated.

Explanation
The physician performs a partial excision of a metacarpal bone in 26230, the proximal or middle phalanx of a finger in 26235, or the distal phalanx of a finger in 26236 to remove infected bone. An incision is made over the infected part of the hand or finger and the underlying soft tissues are divided to expose the bone. The periosteum is reflected and the infected portion of bone is removed and irrigated. The excavation of bone may excise a crater-like piece, leave a small saucer-like shelf depression in the bone, or may remove a portion of the shaft (diaphysis) of a long bone. If a significant portion of bone is removed, the physician may use bone graft material to fill the cavity left in the bone. The periosteum is closed over the bone, the soft tissues are sutured closed, and a soft dressing is applied.

Coding Tips
For 26235 and 26236, some payers may require the use of HCPCS Level II modifiers FA-F9 to identify the specific finger involved. According to CPT guidelines, cast application or strapping (including removal) is only reported as a replacement procedure or when the cast application or strapping is an initial service performed without a restorative treatment or procedure. See "Application of Casts and Strapping" in the CPT book in the Surgery Section, under the Musculoskeletal system.

ICD-9-CM Procedural
77.89 Other partial ostectomy of other bone, except facial bones

Anesthesia
01830

ICD-9-CM Diagnostic
730.14 Chronic osteomyelitis, hand — (Use additional code to identify organism: 041.1. Use additional code to identify major osseous defect, if applicable: 731.3)
730.18 Chronic osteomyelitis, other specified sites — (Use additional code to identify organism: 041.1. Use additional code to identify major osseous defect, if applicable: 731.3)
730.24 Unspecified osteomyelitis, hand — (Use additional code to identify organism: 041.1. Use additional code to identify major osseous defect, if applicable: 731.3)
730.84 Other infections involving diseases classified elsewhere, hand bone — (Use additional code to identify organism: 041.1. Code first underlying disease: 002.0, 015.0-015.9)
731.3 Major osseous defects — (Code first underlying disease: 170.0-170.9, 730.00-730.29, 733.00-733.09, 733.40-733.49, 996.45)
733.49 Aseptic necrosis of other bone site — (Use additional code to identify major osseous defect, if applicable: 731.3)

Terms To Know
aseptic necrosis. Death of bone tissue resulting from a disruption in the vascular supply, caused by a noninfectious disease process, such as a fracture or the administration of immunosuppressive drugs.

chronic. Persistent, continuing, or recurring.

distal. Located farther away from a specified reference point.

infection. Presence of microorganisms in body tissues that may result in cellular damage.

osteomyelitis. Inflammation of bone that may remain localized or spread to the marrow, cortex, or periosteum, in response to an infecting organism, usually bacterial and pyogenic.

proximal. Located closest to a specified reference point, usually the midline.

CCI Version 16.3
01810, 0213T, 0216T, 0228T, 0230T, 10060, 10140, 10160, 20526-20553, 25259, 26111-26116, 26160, 26185, 26340, 29086, 36000, 36400-36410, 36420-36430, 36440, 36600, 36640, 37202, 43752, 51701-51703, 62310-62319, 64400-64435, 64445-64450, 64479, 64483, 64490, 64493, 64505-64530, 69990, 93000-93010, 93040-93042, 93318, 94002, 94200, 94250, 94680-94690, 94770, 95812-95816, 95819, 95822, 95829, 95955, 96360, 96365, 96372, 96374-96376, 99148-99149, 99150

Also not with 26230: 20670, 29125

Also not with 26235: 26034

Note: These CCI edits are used for Medicare. Other payers may reimburse on codes listed above.

Medicare Edits

	Fac RVU	Non-Fac RVU	FUD	Assist
26230	14.48	14.48	90	80
26235	14.32	14.32	90	80
26236	12.75	12.75	90	N/A

Medicare References: 100-2,15,260; 100-4,12,30; 100-4,12,90.3; 100-4,14,10

26250-26262

26250 Radical resection of tumor, metacarpal
26260 Radical resection of tumor, proximal or middle phalanx of finger
26262 Radical resection of tumor, distal phalanx of finger

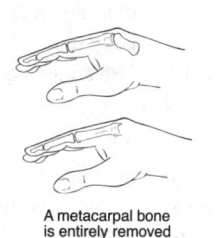

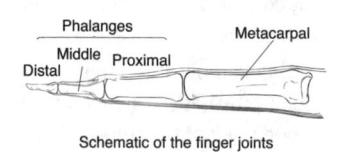

A radical excision of a metacarpal bone is performed. Report 26255 when an autograft (from the patient) is used in the repair of the surgical defect

Explanation
The physician performs a radical resection of a tumor. The physician incises the overlying skin and dissects to determine the extent of invasion. The bone and surrounding tissues are resected. If a graft is needed for reconstruction, it is obtained from the distal radius or iliac crest. Skin is approximated over the surgical defect and sutured in layers. In 26250, a tumor of the metacarpal bone is excised. In 26260, a tumor of the proximal or middle phalanx of a finger is excised. In 26262, a tumor of the distal phalanx of a finger is excised.

Coding Tips
According to CPT guidelines, cast application or strapping (including removal) is only reported as a replacement procedure or when the cast application or strapping is an initial service performed without a restorative treatment or procedure. See "Application of Casts and Strapping" in the CPT book in the Surgery Section, under the Musculoskeletal system.

ICD-9-CM Procedural
77.64 Local excision of lesion or tissue of carpals and metacarpals

Anesthesia
01830

ICD-9-CM Diagnostic
170.5 Malignant neoplasm of short bones of upper limb
195.4 Malignant neoplasm of upper limb
198.5 Secondary malignant neoplasm of bone and bone marrow
198.89 Secondary malignant neoplasm of other specified sites
209.73 Secondary neuroendocrine tumor of bone
238.0 Neoplasm of uncertain behavior of bone and articular cartilage
238.1 Neoplasm of uncertain behavior of connective and other soft tissue
239.2 Neoplasms of unspecified nature of bone, soft tissue, and skin

Terms To Know
distal. Located farther away from a specified reference point.

lesion. Area of damaged tissue that has lost continuity or function, due to disease or trauma.

malignant. Any condition tending to progress toward death, specifically an invasive tumor with a loss of cellular differentiation that has the ability to spread or metastasize to other areas in the body.

radical resection. Removal of an entire tumor (e.g., malignant neoplasm) along with a large area of surrounding tissue, including adjacent lymph nodes that may have been infiltrated.

secondary. Second in order of occurrence or importance, or appearing during the course of another disease or condition.

tumor. Pathological swelling or enlargement; a neoplastic growth of uncontrolled, abnormal multiplication of cells.

CCI Version 16.3
01810, 0213T, 0216T, 0228T, 0230T, 10060, 10140, 10160, 11010-11012❖, 11040-11044, 12001-12007, 12020-12021, 12041-12047, 13131-13132, 20220-20225, 20526-20553, 25259, 26010-26030, 26034, 26340, 26546❖, 29086, 36000, 36400-36410, 36420-36430, 36440, 36600, 36640, 37202, 43752, 51701-51703, 62310-62319, 64400-64435, 64445-64450, 64479, 64483, 64490, 64493, 64505-64530, 69990, 93000-93010, 93040-93042, 93318, 94002, 94200, 94250, 94680-94690, 94770, 95812-95816, 95819, 95822, 95829, 95955, 96360, 96365, 96372, 96374-96376, 99148-99149, 99150

Also not with 26250: 20240-20245, 26070-26075, 26100-26105, 26111-26118, 26130-26135, 26160-26205, 26230, 26565

Also not with 26260: 20240-20245, 20690, 26075-26080, 26105-26117, 26135-26140, 26160-26185, 26210-26215, 26235-26236, 26567

Also not with 26262: 20240, 26075-26080, 26105-26117, 26135-26140, 26160-26185, 26210-26215, 26235-26236, 26567

Note: These CCI edits are used for Medicare. Other payers may reimburse on codes listed above.

Medicare Edits

	Fac RVU	Non-Fac RVU	FUD	Assist
26250	28.87	28.87	90	80
26260	22.64	22.64	90	80
26262	17.4	17.4	90	80

Medicare References: 100-2,15,260; 100-4,12,30; 100-4,12,90.3; 100-4,14,10

26320

26320 Removal of implant from finger or hand

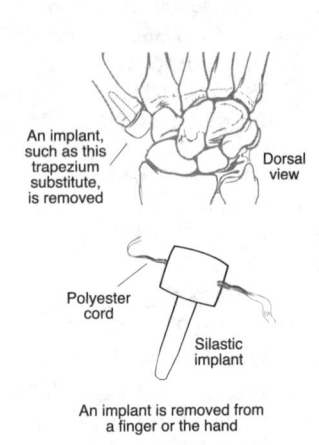

An implant, such as this trapezium substitute, is removed. Dorsal view.

An implant is removed from a finger or the hand (Polyester cord, Silastic implant).

Explanation

The physician removes a previously placed implant from a finger or hand. The physician incises the overlying skin and dissects to the implant. The implant is removed and the operative incision is closed in sutured layers.

Coding Tips

According to CPT guidelines, cast application or strapping (including removal) is only reported as a replacement procedure or when the cast application or strapping is an initial service performed without a restorative treatment or procedure. See "Application of Casts and Strapping" in the CPT book in the Surgery Section, under the Musculoskeletal system. Local anesthesia is included in this service. However, this procedure may be performed under general anesthesia, depending on the age and/or condition of the patient. For removal of a foreign body in the muscle or tendon sheath, see 20520 or 20525.

ICD-9-CM Procedural

- 78.64 Removal of implanted device from carpals and metacarpals
- 80.04 Arthrotomy for removal of prosthesis without replacement, hand and finger
- 84.57 Removal of (cement) spacer

Anesthesia

26320   01830

ICD-9-CM Diagnostic

- 359.6 Symptomatic inflammatory myopathy in diseases classified elsewhere — (Code first underlying disease: 135, 140.0-208.9, 277.30-277.39, 446.0, 710.0, 710.1, 710.2, 714.0)
- 446.0 Polyarteritis nodosa
- 710.0 Systemic lupus erythematosus — (Use additional code to identify manifestation: 424.91, 581.81, 582.81, 583.81)
- 710.1 Systemic sclerosis — (Use additional code to identify manifestation: 359.6, 517.2)
- 710.2 Sicca syndrome
- 714.0 Rheumatoid arthritis — (Use additional code to identify manifestation: 357.1, 359.6)
- 731.3 Major osseous defects — (Code first underlying disease: 170.0-170.9, 730.00-730.29, 733.00-733.09, 733.40-733.49, 996.45)
- 905.2 Late effect of fracture of upper extremities
- 996.40 Unspecified mechanical complication of internal orthopedic device, implant, and graft — (Use additional code to identify prosthetic joint with mechanical complication, V43.60-V43.69)
- 996.41 Mechanical loosening of prosthetic joint — (Use additional code to identify prosthetic joint with mechanical complication, V43.60-V43.69)
- 996.42 Dislocation of prosthetic joint — (Use additional code to identify prosthetic joint with mechanical complication, V43.60-V43.69)
- 996.43 Broken prosthetic joint implant — (Use additional code to identify prosthetic joint with mechanical complication, V43.60-V43.69)
- 996.44 Peri-prosthetic fracture around prosthetic joint — (Use additional code to identify prosthetic joint with mechanical complication, V43.60-V43.69.
- 996.45 Peri-prosthetic osteolysis — (Use additional code to identify prosthetic joint with mechanical complication, V43.60-V43.69. Use additional code to identify major osseous defect, if applicable: 731.3)
- 996.47 Other mechanical complication of prosthetic joint implant — (Use additional code to identify prosthetic joint with mechanical complication, V43.60-V43.69)
- 996.49 Other mechanical complication of other internal orthopedic device, implant, and graft — (Use additional code to identify prosthetic joint with mechanical complication, V43.60-V43.69)
- 996.66 Infection and inflammatory reaction due to internal joint prosthesis — (Use additional code to identify specified infections. Use additional code to identify infected prosthetic joint: V43.60-V43.69)
- 996.67 Infection and inflammatory reaction due to other internal orthopedic device, implant, and graft — (Use additional code to identify specified infections)
- 996.77 Other complications due to internal joint prosthesis — (Use additional code to identify complication: 338.18-338.19, 338.28-338.29)
- 996.78 Other complications due to other internal orthopedic device, implant, and graft — (Use additional code to identify complication: 338.18-338.19, 338.28-338.29)
- 998.51 Infected postoperative seroma — (Use additional code to identify organism)
- 998.59 Other postoperative infection — (Use additional code to identify infection)
- V43.69 Other joint replacement by other means

CCI Version 16.3

01810, 0213T, 0216T, 0228T, 0230T, 11010❖, 20526-20553, 20670, 25259, 26340-26410❖, 29086, 36000, 36400-36410, 36420-36430, 36440, 36600, 36640, 37202, 43752, 51701-51703, 62310-62319, 64400-64435, 64445-64450, 64479, 64483, 64490, 64493, 64505-64530, 69990, 93000-93010, 93040-93042, 93318, 94002, 94200, 94250, 94680-94690, 94770, 95812-95816, 95819, 95822, 95829, 95955, 96360, 96365, 96372, 96374-96376, 99148-99149, 99150

Note: These CCI edits are used for Medicare. Other payers may reimburse on codes listed above.

Medicare Edits

	Fac RVU	Non-Fac RVU	FUD	Assist
26320	9.99	9.99	90	N/A

Medicare References: 100-2,15,260; 100-4,12,30; 100-4,12,90.3; 100-4,14,10

26340

26340 Manipulation, finger joint, under anesthesia, each joint

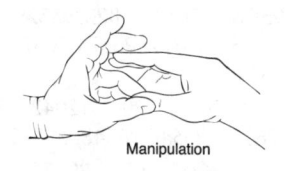

Manipulation

A finger joint is manipulated while under anesthesia

Explanation

Manipulation of the finger joint under anesthesia may be necessary to gain the loss of motion following a surgical procedure or due to scar tissue. Following the induction of general anesthesia, the physician evaluates the finger. The finger is manipulated by stretching, rotation, and other maneuvers to gain the appropriate range of motion.

Coding Tips

Some payers may require the use of HCPCS Level II modifiers FA–F9 to identify the specific finger involved. For application of external fixation, see 20690 and 20692.

ICD-9-CM Procedural

93.25	Forced extension of limb
93.26	Manual rupture of joint adhesions
93.29	Other forcible correction of musculoskeletal deformity

Anesthesia

26340 01820

ICD-9-CM Diagnostic

357.1	Polyneuropathy in collagen vascular disease — (Code first underlying disease: 446.0, 710.0, 714.0)
359.6	Symptomatic inflammatory myopathy in diseases classified elsewhere — (Code first underlying disease: 135, 140.0-208.9, 277.30-277.39, 446.0, 710.0, 710.1, 710.2, 714.0)
446.0	Polyarteritis nodosa
710.0	Systemic lupus erythematosus — (Use additional code to identify manifestation: 424.91, 581.81, 582.81, 583.81)
710.1	Systemic sclerosis — (Use additional code to identify manifestation: 359.6, 517.2)
710.2	Sicca syndrome
714.0	Rheumatoid arthritis — (Use additional code to identify manifestation: 357.1, 359.6)
715.14	Primary localized osteoarthrosis, hand
715.94	Osteoarthrosis, unspecified whether generalized or localized, hand
718.44	Contracture of hand joint
718.54	Ankylosis of hand joint
719.24	Villonodular synovitis, hand
719.54	Stiffness of joint, not elsewhere classified, hand
726.8	Other peripheral enthesopathies

Terms To Know

adhesion. Abnormal fibrous connection between two structures, soft tissue or bony structures, that may occur as the result of surgery, infection, or trauma.

ankylosis. Abnormal union or fusion of bones in a joint, which is normally moveable.

contracture. Shortening of muscle or connective tissue.

myopathy. Any disease process within muscle tissue.

osteoarthrosis. Most common form of a noninflammatory degenerative joint disease with degenerating articular cartilage, bone enlargement, and synovial membrane changes.

polyarteritis nodosa. Systemic necrotizing vasculitis of small and medium arteries that results in the infarction and scarring within the affected organs.

polyneuropathy. Disease process of severe inflammation of multiple nerves.

sicca syndrome. Complex of symptoms of unknown source in middle-aged women in which the following triad exists: keratoconjunctivitis sicca, zerostomia, and connective tissue disease (usually rheumatoid arthritis but sometimes systemic lupus erythematosus).

synovitis. Inflammation of the synovial membrane that lines a synovial joint, resulting in pain and swelling.

systemic sclerosis. Systemic disease characterized by excess fibrotic collagen build-up, turning the skin thickened and hard. Fibrotic changes also occur in various organs and cause vascular abnormalities and affect more women than men.

villonodular synovitis. Inflammation of the synovial membrane due to excessive synovial tissue formation, especially in the knee.

CCI Version 16.3

01810, 0213T, 0216T, 0228T, 0230T, 36000, 36400-36410, 36420-36430, 36440, 36600, 36640, 37202, 43752, 51701-51703, 62310-62319, 64400-64435, 64445-64450, 64479, 64483, 64490, 64493, 64505-64530, 93000-93010, 93040-93042, 93318, 94002, 94200, 94250, 94680-94690, 94770, 95812-95816, 95819, 95822, 95829, 95955, 96360, 96365, 96372, 96374-96376, 99148-99149, 99150

Note: These CCI edits are used for Medicare. Other payers may reimburse on codes listed above.

Medicare Edits

	Fac RVU	Non-Fac RVU	FUD	Assist
26340	9.4	9.4	90	N/A

Medicare References: None

26350-26352

26350 Repair or advancement, flexor tendon, not in zone 2 digital flexor tendon sheath (eg, no man's land); primary or secondary without free graft, each tendon

26352 secondary with free graft (includes obtaining graft), each tendon

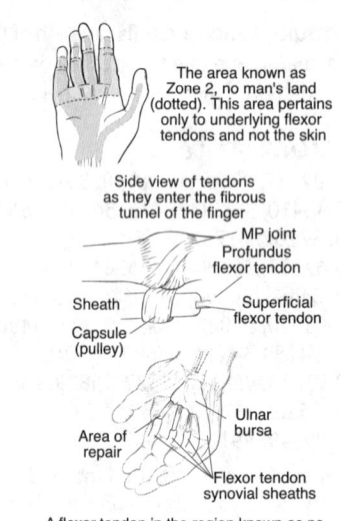

The area known as Zone 2, no man's land (dotted). This area pertains only to underlying flexor tendons and not the skin

Side view of tendons as they enter the fibrous tunnel of the finger

MP joint
Profundus flexor tendon
Sheath
Superficial flexor tendon
Capsule (pulley)
Area of repair
Ulnar bursa
Flexor tendon synovial sheaths

A flexor tendon in the region known as no man's land (but not in the tendon sheath) is repaired or advanced, either as primary or secondary (first or subsequent) procedure. Report 26352 when secondary with use of a free graft in the repair or advancement

Explanation

The physician repairs or advances a single tendon NOT located in "no man's land." "No man's land" is located between the A1 pulley and the insertion of the superficialis tendon. The physician incises the skin overlying the proximal or distal phalanx and dissects to the tendon. The tendon is repaired with sutures or advanced to improve joint function. Primary repair is done immediately after injury. Secondary repair is done sometime after the incident of injury. If a graft is needed for secondary repair, it is obtained from the palmaris longus tendon or from the foot. The operative incision is closed in sutured layers. Report 26350 for each primary or secondary tendon repair without autograft. Report 26352 for each secondary tendon repair with autograft.

Coding Tips

These codes are used once for each tendon repair performed. When multiple tendons are repaired, report one tendon as the primary procedure and append modifier 51 to subsequent procedures. In 26352, any tendon graft harvest is not reported separately. According to CPT guidelines, cast application or strapping (including removal) is only reported as a replacement procedure or when the cast application or strapping is an initial service performed without a restorative treatment or procedure. See "Application of Casts and Strapping" in the CPT book in the Surgery Section, under the Musculoskeletal system. These codes report tendon repair that is not in "no man's land." For repair of tendons in "no man's land," see 26356–26358.

ICD-9-CM Procedural

- 82.42 Delayed suture of flexor tendon of hand
- 82.44 Other suture of flexor tendon of hand
- 82.51 Advancement of tendon of hand
- 83.71 Advancement of tendon
- 83.88 Other plastic operations on tendon

Anesthesia
01810

ICD-9-CM Diagnostic

- 357.1 Polyneuropathy in collagen vascular disease — (Code first underlying disease: 446.0, 710.0, 714.0)
- 359.6 Symptomatic inflammatory myopathy in diseases classified elsewhere — (Code first underlying disease: 135, 140.0-208.9, 277.30-277.39, 446.0, 710.0, 710.1, 710.2, 714.0)
- 446.0 Polyarteritis nodosa
- 710.0 Systemic lupus erythematosus — (Use additional code to identify manifestation: 424.91, 581.81, 582.81, 583.81)
- 710.1 Systemic sclerosis — (Use additional code to identify manifestation: 359.6, 517.2)
- 710.2 Sicca syndrome
- 714.0 Rheumatoid arthritis — (Use additional code to identify manifestation: 357.1, 359.6)
- 727.64 Nontraumatic rupture of flexor tendons of hand and wrist
- 881.22 Open wound of wrist, with tendon involvement
- 882.2 Open wound of hand except finger(s) alone, with tendon involvement
- 883.2 Open wound of finger(s), with tendon involvement
- 884.2 Multiple and unspecified open wound of upper limb, with tendon involvement
- 886.1 Traumatic amputation of other finger(s) (complete) (partial), complicated
- 959.4 Injury, other and unspecified, hand, except finger
- 998.2 Accidental puncture or laceration during procedure

CCI Version 16.3

01810, 0213T, 0216T, 0228T, 0230T, 20526-20553, 25000, 25259, 26055, 26145-26185, 26440-26442, 26450-26455, 26478-26479, 29075, 29086, 29130-29131, 29280, 36000, 36400-36410, 36420-36430, 36440, 36600, 36640, 37202, 43752, 51701-51703, 62310-62319, 64400-64435, 64445-64450, 64479, 64483, 64490, 64493, 64505-64530, 64702-64704, 69990, 93000-93010, 93040-93042, 93318, 94002, 94200, 94250, 94680-94690, 94770, 95812-95816, 95819, 95822, 95829, 95955, 96360, 96365, 96372, 96374-96376, 99148-99149, 99150

Also not with 26350: 12041-12042, 12045, 12047, 26340, 26546-26548, 29125

Also not with 26352: 20924-20926, 26340-26350, 26546❖

Note: These CCI edits are used for Medicare. Other payers may reimburse on codes listed above.

Medicare Edits

	Fac RVU	Non-Fac RVU	FUD	Assist
26350	20.51	20.51	90	N/A
26352	23.42	23.42	90	80

Medicare References: 100-2,15,260; 100-4,12,30; 100-4,12,90.3; 100-4,14,10

26356-26358

26356 Repair or advancement, flexor tendon, in zone 2 digital flexor tendon sheath (eg, no man's land); primary, without free graft, each tendon

26357 secondary, without free graft, each tendon

26358 secondary, with free graft (includes obtaining graft), each tendon

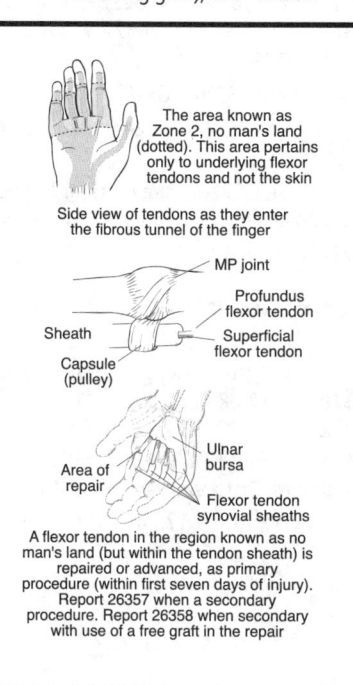

The area known as Zone 2, no man's land (dotted). This area pertains only to underlying flexor tendons and not the skin

Side view of tendons as they enter the fibrous tunnel of the finger

- MP joint
- Profundus flexor tendon
- Sheath
- Superficial flexor tendon
- Capsule (pulley)
- Area of repair
- Ulnar bursa
- Flexor tendon synovial sheaths

A flexor tendon in the region known as no man's land (but within the tendon sheath) is repaired or advanced, as primary procedure (within first seven days of injury). Report 26357 when a secondary procedure. Report 26358 when secondary with use of a free graft in the repair

Explanation

The physician repairs or advances a single flexor tendon located in "no man's land." "No man's land" is located between the A1 pulley and the insertion of the superficialis tendon. The physician incises the skin overlying the medial phalanx and dissects to the tendon. The tendon is repaired with sutures or advanced and sutured to improve joint function. Primary repair is done immediately after injury. Secondary repair is done sometime after the incident of injury or following a previous surgical repair. If a graft is needed for secondary repair, it is obtained from the palmaris longus tendon or from the foot. The incision is sutured in layers. Report 26356 for each primary flexor tendon repair or advancement without a free graft. Report 26357 for each secondary flexor tendon repair or advancement without a free graft and 26358 for each secondary tendon repair with a free graft (includes harvesting the graft).

Coding Tips

These codes are used once for each tendon repair performed. When multiple tendons are repaired, report one tendon as the primary procedure and append modifier 51 to subsequent procedures. In 26358, any tendon graft harvest is not reported separately. According to CPT guidelines, cast application or strapping (including removal) is only reported as a replacement procedure or when the cast application or strapping is an initial service performed without a restorative treatment or procedure. See "Application of Casts and Strapping" in the CPT book in the Surgery Section, under the Musculoskeletal system. For tendon repair not in "no man's land," see 26350-26352.

ICD-9-CM Procedural

- 82.42 Delayed suture of flexor tendon of hand
- 82.44 Other suture of flexor tendon of hand
- 82.51 Advancement of tendon of hand
- 83.71 Advancement of tendon
- 83.88 Other plastic operations on tendon

Anesthesia
01810

ICD-9-CM Diagnostic

- 357.1 Polyneuropathy in collagen vascular disease — (Code first underlying disease: 446.0, 710.0, 714.0)
- 359.6 Symptomatic inflammatory myopathy in diseases classified elsewhere — (Code first underlying disease: 135, 140.0-208.9, 277.30-277.39, 446.0, 710.0, 710.1, 710.2, 714.0)
- 446.0 Polyarteritis nodosa
- 710.0 Systemic lupus erythematosus — (Use additional code to identify manifestation: 424.91, 581.81, 582.81, 583.81)
- 710.1 Systemic sclerosis — (Use additional code to identify manifestation: 359.6, 517.2)
- 710.2 Sicca syndrome
- 714.0 Rheumatoid arthritis — (Use additional code to identify manifestation: 357.1, 359.6)
- 727.64 Nontraumatic rupture of flexor tendons of hand and wrist
- 881.22 Open wound of wrist, with tendon involvement
- 882.2 Open wound of hand except finger(s) alone, with tendon involvement
- 883.2 Open wound of finger(s), with tendon involvement
- 884.2 Multiple and unspecified open wound of upper limb, with tendon involvement
- 886.1 Traumatic amputation of other finger(s) (complete) (partial), complicated
- 959.4 Injury, other and unspecified, hand, except finger
- 998.2 Accidental puncture or laceration during procedure

CCI Version 16.3

01810, 0213T, 0216T, 0228T, 0230T, 20526-20553, 25000, 25259, 26055, 26145-26185, 26340, 26440-26442, 26450-26455, 26478-26479, 29075, 29086, 29130-29131, 29280, 36000, 36400-36410, 36420-36430, 36440, 36600, 36640, 37202, 43752, 51701-51703, 62310-62319, 64400-64435, 64445-64450, 64479, 64483, 64490, 64493, 64505-64530, 64702-64704, 69990, 93000-93010, 93040-93042, 93318, 94002, 94200, 94250, 94680-94690, 94770, 95812-95816, 95819, 95822, 95829, 95955, 96360, 96365, 96372, 96374-96376, 99148-99149, 99150

Also not with 26356: 12001, 26500, 26546-26548, 76000-76001, G0168

Also not with 26357: 26546❖

Also not with 26358: 20924-20926, 26357

Note: These CCI edits are used for Medicare. Other payers may reimburse on codes listed above.

Medicare Edits

	Fac RVU	Non-Fac RVU	FUD	Assist
26356	31.29	31.29	90	N/A
26357	25.02	25.02	90	80
26358	26.72	26.72	90	80

Medicare References: 100-2,15,260; 100-4,12,30; 100-4,12,90.3; 100-4,14,10

26370-26373

26370 Repair or advancement of profundus tendon, with intact superficialis tendon; primary, each tendon
26372 secondary with free graft (includes obtaining graft), each tendon
26373 secondary without free graft, each tendon

A profundus (deep) flexor tendon is repaired or advanced for the first time, while the superficial tendon remains intact. Report 26372 for a secondary repair that requires a free graft. And report 26373 for a secondary repair without a free graft

Explanation

The physician repairs or advances the profundus flexor tendon; the superficialis tendon is intact. The physician incises the skin overlying the damaged tendon. The tendon is repaired with sutures or advanced to improve joint function. Primary repair is done immediately after injury. Secondary repair is done sometime after the incident of injury or following a previous surgical repair. If a graft is needed for secondary repair, it is obtained from the palmaris longus tendon or from the foot. The incision is sutured in layers. Report 26370 for each primary tendon repair without graft. Report 26372 for each secondary tendon repair with free graft. Report 26373 for each secondary tendon repair without free graft.

Coding Tips

These codes are used once for each tendon repair performed. When multiple tendons are repaired, report one tendon as the primary procedure and append modifier 51 to subsequent procedures. In 26372, any tendon graft harvest is not reported separately. According to CPT guidelines, cast application or strapping (including removal) is only reported as a replacement procedure or when the cast application or strapping is an initial service performed without a restorative treatment or procedure. See "Application of Casts and Strapping" in the CPT book in the Surgery section, under the musculoskeletal system.

ICD-9-CM Procedural

- **82.42** Delayed suture of flexor tendon of hand
- **82.44** Other suture of flexor tendon of hand
- **82.51** Advancement of tendon of hand
- **83.71** Advancement of tendon
- **83.88** Other plastic operations on tendon

Anesthesia
01810

ICD-9-CM Diagnostic

- **357.1** Polyneuropathy in collagen vascular disease — (Code first underlying disease: 446.0, 710.0, 714.0)
- **359.6** Symptomatic inflammatory myopathy in diseases classified elsewhere — (Code first underlying disease: 135, 140.0-208.9, 277.30-277.39, 446.0, 710.0, 710.1, 710.2, 714.0)
- **446.0** Polyarteritis nodosa
- **710.0** Systemic lupus erythematosus — (Use additional code to identify manifestation: 424.91, 581.81, 582.81, 583.81)
- **710.1** Systemic sclerosis — (Use additional code to identify manifestation: 359.6, 517.2)
- **710.2** Sicca syndrome
- **714.0** Rheumatoid arthritis — (Use additional code to identify manifestation: 357.1, 359.6)
- **727.64** Nontraumatic rupture of flexor tendons of hand and wrist
- **881.22** Open wound of wrist, with tendon involvement
- **882.2** Open wound of hand except finger(s) alone, with tendon involvement
- **883.2** Open wound of finger(s), with tendon involvement
- **884.2** Multiple and unspecified open wound of upper limb, with tendon involvement
- **886.1** Traumatic amputation of other finger(s) (complete) (partial), complicated
- **959.4** Injury, other and unspecified, hand, except finger
- **998.2** Accidental puncture or laceration during procedure

CCI Version 16.3

01810, 0213T, 0216T, 0228T, 0230T, 20526-20553, 25259, 26170-26185, 26340, 29075, 29086, 29130-29131, 29280, 36000, 36400-36410, 36420-36430, 36440, 36600, 36640, 37202, 43752, 51701-51703, 62310-62319, 64400-64435, 64445-64450, 64479, 64483, 64490, 64493, 64505-64530, 69990, 93000-93010, 93040-93042, 93318, 94002, 94200, 94250, 94680-94690, 94770, 95812-95816, 95819, 95822, 95829, 95955, 96360, 96365, 96372, 96374-96376, 99148-99149, 99150

Also not with 26370: 26548

Also not with 26372: 20924-20926, 26373, 29125

Note: These CCI edits are used for Medicare. Other payers may reimburse on codes listed above.

Medicare Edits

	Fac RVU	Non-Fac RVU	FUD	Assist
26370	22.08	22.08	90	80
26372	25.59	25.59	90	80
26373	24.44	24.44	90	80

Medicare References: 100-2,15,260; 100-4,12,30; 100-4,12,90.3; 100-4,14,10

26390-26392

26390 Excision flexor tendon, with implantation of synthetic rod for delayed tendon graft, hand or finger, each rod

26392 Removal of synthetic rod and insertion of flexor tendon graft, hand or finger (includes obtaining graft), each rod

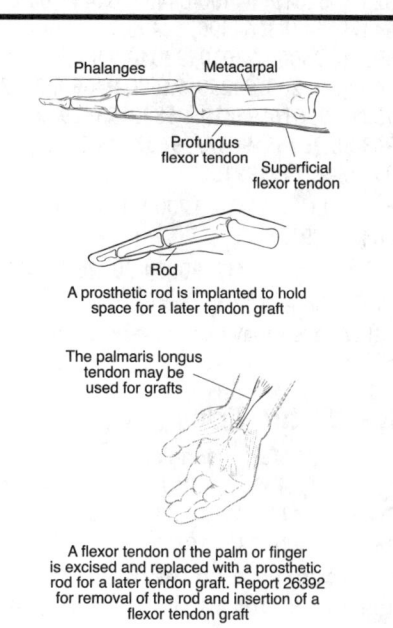

Explanation

The physician excises a flexor tendon in a finger or hand and implants a synthetic rod for a delayed tendon graft. The physician incises the overlying skin and dissects to the tendon. The tendon is freed, the proximal and distal ends are severed, and the tendon is removed. The physician implants a prosthesis so the surrounding tissue will form a natural tube for a tendon graft to be performed at a later operative session. The operative incision is closed in sutured layers. In the later operative session, the physician incises the overlying skin and dissects to the tube or rod. The tube or rod is removed. A graft is obtained from the palmaris longus tendon or from the foot and inserted in the new position. The proximal and distal ends are sutured into place and the operative incision is closed in sutured layers.

Coding Tips

These codes are used once for each tendon repair performed. When multiple tendons are repaired, report one tendon as the primary procedure and append modifier 51 to subsequent procedures. In 26392, harvesting of a tendon graft is not reported separately. According to CPT guidelines, cast application or strapping (including removal) is only reported as a replacement procedure or when the cast application or strapping is an initial service performed without a restorative treatment or procedure. See "Application of Casts and Strapping" in the CPT book in the Surgery section, under the musculoskeletal system.

ICD-9-CM Procedural

- 78.64 Removal of implanted device from carpals and metacarpals
- 82.33 Other tenonectomy of hand
- 82.79 Plastic operation on hand with other graft or implant
- 83.81 Tendon graft

Anesthesia
01810

ICD-9-CM Diagnostic

- 727.64 Nontraumatic rupture of flexor tendons of hand and wrist
- 727.69 Nontraumatic rupture of other tendon
- 881.22 Open wound of wrist, with tendon involvement
- 882.2 Open wound of hand except finger(s) alone, with tendon involvement
- 883.2 Open wound of finger(s), with tendon involvement
- 884.2 Multiple and unspecified open wound of upper limb, with tendon involvement
- 906.1 Late effect of open wound of extremities without mention of tendon injury
- 998.2 Accidental puncture or laceration during procedure
- V51.8 Other aftercare involving the use of plastic surgery
- V54.01 Encounter for removal of internal fixation device
- V54.02 Encounter for lengthening/adjustment of growth rod
- V54.09 Other aftercare involving internal fixation device

CCI Version 16.3

01810, 0213T, 0216T, 0228T, 0230T, 20526-20553, 25259, 29075, 29086, 29130-29131, 29280, 36000, 36400-36410, 36420-36430, 36440, 36600, 36640, 37202, 43752, 51701-51703, 62310-62319, 64400-64435, 64445-64450, 64479, 64483, 64490, 64493, 64505-64530, 69990, 93000-93010, 93040-93042, 93318, 94002, 94200, 94250, 94680-94690, 94770, 95812-95816, 95819, 95822, 95829, 95955, 96360, 96365, 96372, 96374-96376, 99148-99149, 99150

Also not with 26390: 25000, 26055, 26113❖, 26116❖, 26145-26185, 26340-26358, 26440-26442, 26450-26455, 26478-26479, 64702-64704

Also not with 26392: 20924, 26185, 26340

Note: These CCI edits are used for Medicare. Other payers may reimburse on codes listed above.

Medicare Edits

	Fac RVU	Non-Fac RVU	FUD	Assist
26390	24.05	24.05	90	80
26392	28.04	28.04	90	80

Medicare References: 100-2,15,260; 100-4,12,30; 100-4,12,90.3; 100-4,14,10

26410-26412

26410 Repair, extensor tendon, hand, primary or secondary; without free graft, each tendon
26412 with free graft (includes obtaining graft), each tendon

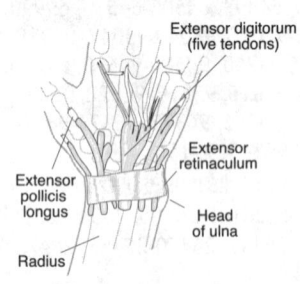

The six synovial sheaths of the dorsum of the wrist branch into nine extensor tendons

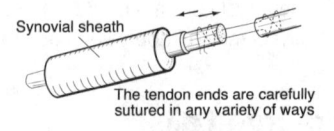

The tendon ends are carefully sutured in any variety of ways

Primary surgery of the tendons is usually considered to occur in the first seven days following injury

An extensor tendon of the hand is repaired, either primary or secondary. Report 26412 when a free graft is required to complete the repair

Explanation

The physician repairs or advances a single extensor tendon located in the hand. The physician incises the skin overlying the tendon. The tendon is repaired with sutures or advanced to improve joint function. Primary repair is done immediately after injury. Secondary repair is done sometime after the incident of injury. If a graft is needed for secondary repair, it is obtained from the palmaris longus tendon or from the foot. The operative incision is closed in sutured layers. Report 26410 for each primary or secondary tendon repair without free graft. Report 26412 for each secondary tendon repair with free graft.

Coding Tips

These codes are used once for each tendon repair performed. When multiple tendons are repaired, report one tendon as the primary procedure and append modifier 51 to subsequent procedures. In 26410, harvesting of a tendon graft is not reported separately. According to CPT guidelines, cast application or strapping (including removal) is only reported as a replacement procedure or when the cast application or strapping is an initial service performed without a restorative treatment or procedure. See "Application of Casts and Strapping" in the CPT book in the Surgery section, under the musculoskeletal system.

ICD-9-CM Procedural

- 82.43 Delayed suture of other tendon of hand
- 82.45 Other suture of other tendon of hand
- 83.81 Tendon graft
- 83.88 Other plastic operations on tendon

Anesthesia
01810

ICD-9-CM Diagnostic

- 727.63 Nontraumatic rupture of extensor tendons of hand and wrist
- 881.22 Open wound of wrist, with tendon involvement
- 882.2 Open wound of hand except finger(s) alone, with tendon involvement
- 884.2 Multiple and unspecified open wound of upper limb, with tendon involvement
- 927.20 Crushing injury of hand(s) — (Use additional code to identify any associated injuries: 800-829, 850.0-854.1, 860.0-869.1)
- 959.4 Injury, other and unspecified, hand, except finger
- 998.2 Accidental puncture or laceration during procedure

Terms To Know

injury. Harm or damage sustained by the body.

laceration. Tearing injury; a torn, ragged-edged wound.

tendon. Fibrous tissue that connects muscle to bone, consisting primarily of collagen and containing little vasculature.

CCI Version 16.3

01810, 0213T, 0216T, 0228T, 0230T, 20526-20553, 25000, 25118, 25259, 26055, 26130-26135, 26160, 26185, 26340, 26445-26449, 26460, 26476-26477, 29075, 29086, 29130-29131, 29280, 36000, 36400-36410, 36420-36430, 36440, 36600, 36640, 37202, 43752, 51701-51703, 62310-62319, 64400-64435, 64445-64450, 64479, 64483, 64490, 64493, 64505-64530, 69990, 93000-93010, 93040-93042, 93318, 94002, 94200, 94250, 94680-94690, 94770, 95812-95816, 95819, 95822, 95829, 95955, 96360, 96365, 96372, 96374-96376, 99148-99149, 99150

Also not with 26410: 12002, 13131-13132, 26437, 29125

Also not with 26412: 20924-20926, 26410

Note: These CCI edits are used for Medicare. Other payers may reimburse on codes listed above.

Medicare Edits

	Fac RVU	Non-Fac RVU	FUD	Assist
26410	16.28	16.28	90	N/A
26412	19.73	19.73	90	80

Medicare References: 100-2,15,260; 100-4,12,30; 100-4,12,90.3; 100-4,14,10

26415-26416

26415 Excision of extensor tendon, with implantation of synthetic rod for delayed tendon graft, hand or finger, each rod

26416 Removal of synthetic rod and insertion of extensor tendon graft (includes obtaining graft), hand or finger, each rod

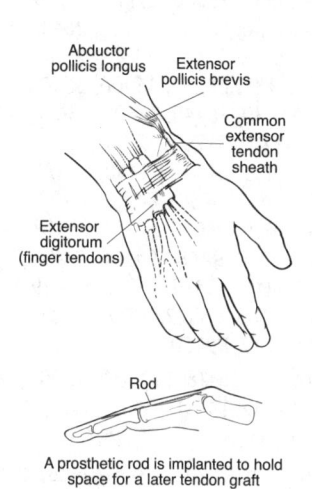

A prosthetic rod is implanted to hold space for a later tendon graft

An extensor tendon of the hand or finger is removed and a prosthetic rod implanted. Report code 26416 for the later removal of the rod and subsequent insertion of a tendon graft

Explanation

The physician excises an extensor tendon in a finger or hand and implants a synthetic rod for a delayed tendon graft. The physician incises the overlying skin and dissects to the tendon. The tendon is freed, the proximal and distal ends are severed, and the tendon is removed. The physician implants a prosthetic rod so the surrounding tissue will form a natural tube for a tendon graft to be performed at a later operative session. The operative incision is closed in sutured layers. In a later operative session (26416), the physician incises the overlying skin and dissects to the tube or rod. The tube or rod is removed. A graft is obtained from the palmaris longus tendon or from the foot and inserted in the new position. The proximal and distal ends are sutured into place and the operative incision is closed in sutured layers.

Coding Tips

These codes are used once for each tendon repair performed. When multiple tendons are repaired, report one tendon as the primary procedure and append modifier 51 to subsequent procedures. In 26416, harvesting of a tendon graft is not reported separately. According to CPT guidelines, cast application or strapping (including removal) is only reported as a replacement procedure or when the cast application or strapping is an initial service performed without a restorative treatment or procedure. See "Application of Casts and Strapping" in the CPT book in the Surgery section, under the musculoskeletal system.

ICD-9-CM Procedural

- **78.64** Removal of implanted device from carpals and metacarpals
- **82.33** Other tenonectomy of hand
- **82.79** Plastic operation on hand with other graft or implant

Anesthesia
01810

ICD-9-CM Diagnostic

- **727.63** Nontraumatic rupture of extensor tendons of hand and wrist
- **881.22** Open wound of wrist, with tendon involvement
- **882.2** Open wound of hand except finger(s) alone, with tendon involvement
- **883.2** Open wound of finger(s), with tendon involvement
- **884.2** Multiple and unspecified open wound of upper limb, with tendon involvement
- **887.1** Traumatic amputation of arm and hand (complete) (partial), unilateral, below elbow, complicated
- **998.2** Accidental puncture or laceration during procedure
- **V51.8** Other aftercare involving the use of plastic surgery
- **V54.01** Encounter for removal of internal fixation device
- **V54.02** Encounter for lengthening/adjustment of growth rod
- **V54.09** Other aftercare involving internal fixation device

Terms To Know

distal. Located farther away from a specified reference point.

extensor. Any muscle that extends a joint.

laceration. Tearing injury; a torn, ragged-edged wound.

open wound. Opening or break of the skin.

proximal. Located closest to a specified reference point, usually the midline.

rupture. Tearing or breaking open of tissue.

tendon. Fibrous tissue that connects muscle to bone, consisting primarily of collagen and containing little vasculature.

CCI Version 16.3

01810, 0213T, 0216T, 0228T, 0230T, 20526-20553, 25259, 26340, 29075, 29086, 29130-29131, 29280, 36000, 36400-36410, 36420-36430, 36440, 36600, 36640, 37202, 43752, 51701-51703, 62310-62319, 64400-64435, 64445-64450, 64479, 64483, 64490, 64493, 64505-64530, 69990, 93000-93010, 93040-93042, 93318, 94002, 94200, 94250, 94680-94690, 94770, 95812-95816, 95819, 95822, 95829, 95955, 96360, 96365, 96372, 96374-96376, 99148-99149, 99150

Also not with 26415: 25000, 26055, 26113❖, 26116❖, 26145-26185, 26410-26412, 26418-26437, 26445-26449, 26460, 26476-26477, 64702-64704

Also not with 26416: 20924, 26170-26185

Note: These CCI edits are used for Medicare. Other payers may reimburse on codes listed above.

Medicare Edits

	Fac RVU	Non-Fac RVU	FUD	Assist
26415	20.13	20.13	90	80
26416	24.17	24.17	90	N/A

Medicare References: 100-2,15,260; 100-4,12,30; 100-4,12,90.3; 100-4,14,10

26418-26420

26418 Repair, extensor tendon, finger, primary or secondary; without free graft, each tendon

26420 with free graft (includes obtaining graft) each tendon

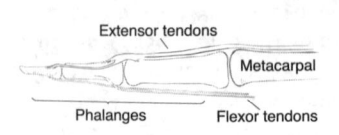

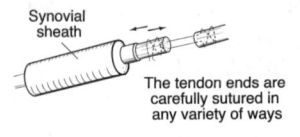

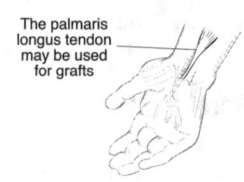

Explanation

The physician repairs or advances a single extensor tendon located in the finger. The physician incises the skin overlying the tendon. The tendon is repaired with sutures or advanced to improve joint function. Primary repair is done immediately after injury. Secondary repair is done sometime after the incident of injury. If a graft is needed for secondary repair, it is obtained from the palmaris longus tendon or from the foot. The operative incision is closed in sutured layers. Report 26418 for each primary or secondary tendon repair without free graft. Report 26420 for each secondary tendon repair with free graft.

Coding Tips

These codes are used once for each tendon repair performed. When multiple tendons are repaired, report one tendon as the primary procedure and append modifier 51 to subsequent procedures. In 26420, harvesting of a tendon graft is not reported separately. Some payers may require the use of HCPCS Level II modifiers FA-F9 to identify the specific finger involved. According to CPT guidelines, cast application or strapping (including removal) is only reported as a replacement procedure or when the cast application or strapping is an initial service performed without a restorative treatment or procedure.

See "Application of Casts and Strapping" in the CPT book in the Surgery section, under the musculoskeletal system.

ICD-9-CM Procedural

- 82.43 Delayed suture of other tendon of hand
- 82.45 Other suture of other tendon of hand
- 82.51 Advancement of tendon of hand

Anesthesia

01810

ICD-9-CM Diagnostic

- 357.1 Polyneuropathy in collagen vascular disease — (Code first underlying disease: 446.0, 710.0, 714.0)
- 359.6 Symptomatic inflammatory myopathy in diseases classified elsewhere — (Code first underlying disease: 135, 140.0-208.9, 277.30-277.39, 446.0, 710.0, 710.1, 710.2, 714.0)
- 446.0 Polyarteritis nodosa
- 710.0 Systemic lupus erythematosus — (Use additional code to identify manifestation: 424.91, 581.81, 582.81, 583.81)
- 710.1 Systemic sclerosis — (Use additional code to identify manifestation: 359.6, 517.2)
- 710.2 Sicca syndrome
- 714.0 Rheumatoid arthritis — (Use additional code to identify manifestation: 357.1, 359.6)
- 727.63 Nontraumatic rupture of extensor tendons of hand and wrist
- 727.9 Unspecified disorder of synovium, tendon, and bursa
- 883.2 Open wound of finger(s), with tendon involvement

Terms To Know

myopathy. Any disease process within muscle tissue.

polyneuropathy. Disease process of severe inflammation of multiple nerves.

sicca syndrome. Complex of symptoms of unknown source in middle-aged women in which the following triad exists: keratoconjunctivitis sicca, zerostomia, and connective tissue disease (usually rheumatoid arthritis but sometimes systemic lupus erythematosus).

systemic sclerosis. Systemic disease characterized by excess fibrotic collagen build-up, turning the skin thickened and hard. Fibrotic changes also occur in various organs and cause vascular abnormalities and affect more women than men.

CCI Version 16.3

01810, 0213T, 0216T, 0228T, 0230T, 20526-20553, 25000, 25118, 25259, 26055, 26135-26160, 26185, 26340, 26445-26449, 26460, 26476-26477, 29075, 29086, 29130-29131, 29280, 36000, 36400-36410, 36420-36430, 36440, 36600, 36640, 37202, 43752, 51701-51703, 62310-62319, 64400-64435, 64445-64450, 64479, 64483, 64490, 64493, 64505-64530, 69990, 93000-93010, 93040-93042, 93318, 94002, 94200, 94250, 94680-94690, 94770, 95812-95816, 95819, 95822, 95829, 95955, 96360, 96365, 96372, 96374-96376, 99148-99149, 99150

Also not with 26418: 11010❖, 12001-12004, 12042, 12047, 13131-13132, 26426-26428❖, 29125, G0168

Also not with 26420: 20924-20926, 26418

Note: These CCI edits are used for Medicare. Other payers may reimburse on codes listed above.

Medicare Edits

	Fac RVU	Non-Fac RVU	FUD	Assist
26418	16.52	16.52	90	N/A
26420	20.48	20.48	90	80

Medicare References: 100-2,15,260; 100-4,12,30; 100-4,12,90.3; 100-4,14,10

26426-26428

26426 Repair of extensor tendon, central slip, secondary (eg, boutonniere deformity); using local tissue(s), including lateral band(s), each finger

26428 with free graft (includes obtaining graft), each finger

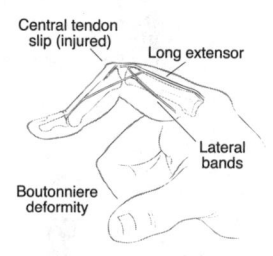

Central tendon slip (injured) — Long extensor — Lateral bands — Boutonniere deformity

Disruption of the central tendon slip causes the finger to drop. Tension from the lateral bands causes the finger tip to be fully extended

An extensor tendon central slip is repaired in a secondary procedure (more than 72 hours following injury) using local tissue graft. Report 26428 when a free graft is used in the repair

Explanation

The physician repairs a Boutonniere, or buttonhole, deformity of the central slip extensor tendon with a soft tissue procedure that reconstructs the central slip using the lateral band in 26426 or a free tendon graft in 26428. In this deformity, the tendons are imbalanced due to synovitis in the proximal interphalangeal (PIP) joint that causes a stretching of the central slip and subluxation of the lateral bands, which become tight from the swollen joint pressure and act as flexors to the PIP joint. This causes hyperextension deformities in the distal interphalangeal and metacarpophalangeal joints. The physician makes a dorsal, longitudinal incision over the proximal interphalangeal joint to the distal IP joint. The displaced lateral bands are mobilized and a tenotomy is done on the two lateral tendons next to the distal IP joint. The functionality of the central tendon must be restored. The lateral bands are aligned with the central tendon and used as local tissue to reconstruct the central slip. Report 26428 if a separate free tendon graft must be harvested to repair the central slip. A synovectomy is done. Tendon balance must be assured before the proximal IP joint is fixed in extension. The finger is later placed in a dynamic extension splint after removal of the fixation wire.

Coding Tips

These codes are used once for each tendon repair performed. When multiple tendons are repaired, report one tendon as the primary procedure and append modifier 51 to subsequent procedures. In 26428, harvesting of a tendon graft is not reported separately. Some payers may require the use of HCPCS Level II modifiers FA–F9 to identify the specific finger involved. According to CPT guidelines, cast application or strapping (including removal) is only reported as a replacement procedure or when the cast application or strapping is an initial service performed without a restorative treatment or procedure. See "Application of Casts and Strapping" in the CPT book in the Surgery section, under the musculoskeletal system.

ICD-9-CM Procedural

83.88 Other plastic operations on tendon

Anesthesia

01810

ICD-9-CM Diagnostic

357.1 Polyneuropathy in collagen vascular disease — (Code first underlying disease: 446.0, 710.0, 714.0)

359.6 Symptomatic inflammatory myopathy in diseases classified elsewhere — (Code first underlying disease: 135, 140.0-208.9, 277.30-277.39, 446.0, 710.0, 710.1, 710.2, 714.0)

446.0 Polyarteritis nodosa

710.0 Systemic lupus erythematosus — (Use additional code to identify manifestation: 424.91, 581.81, 582.81, 583.81)

710.1 Systemic sclerosis — (Use additional code to identify manifestation: 359.6, 517.2)

710.2 Sicca syndrome

714.0 Rheumatoid arthritis — (Use additional code to identify manifestation: 357.1, 359.6)

714.1 Felty's syndrome

736.21 Boutonniere deformity

883.2 Open wound of finger(s), with tendon involvement

905.2 Late effect of fracture of upper extremities

Terms To Know

boutonniere deformity. Finger deformity with hyperextension of the distal joint and flexion of the interphalangeal joint.

Felty's syndrome. Splenomegaly, leukopenia, arthritis, hypersplenism, anemia and other symptoms.

myopathy. Any disease process within muscle tissue.

polyneuropathy. Disease process of severe inflammation of multiple nerves.

sicca syndrome. Complex of symptoms of unknown source in middle-aged women in which the following triad exists: keratoconjunctivitis sicca, zerostomia, and connective tissue disease (usually rheumatoid arthritis but sometimes systemic lupus erythematosus).

systemic sclerosis. Systemic disease characterized by excess fibrotic collagen build-up, turning the skin thickened and hard. Fibrotic changes also occur in various organs and cause vascular abnormalities and affect more women than men.

CCI Version 16.3

01810, 0213T, 0216T, 0228T, 0230T, 20526-20553, 25000, 25259, 26055, 26185, 26340, 29075, 29086, 29130-29131, 29280, 36000, 36400-36410, 36420-36430, 36440, 36600, 36640, 37202, 43752, 51701-51703, 62310-62319, 64400-64435, 64445-64450, 64479, 64483, 64490, 64493, 64505-64530, 69990, 93000-93010, 93040-93042, 93318, 94002, 94200, 94250, 94680-94690, 94770, 95812-95816, 95819, 95822, 95829, 95955, 96360, 96365, 96372, 96374-96376, 99148-99149, 99150

Also not with 26426: 13131-13132, 29125, 76000-76001

Also not with 26428: 20924-20926, 26426

Note: These CCI edits are used for Medicare. Other payers may reimburse on codes listed above.

Medicare Edits

	Fac RVU	Non-Fac RVU	FUD	Assist
26426	15.61	15.61	90	N/A
26428	21.72	21.72	90	80

Medicare References: 100-2,15,260; 100-4,12,30; 100-4,12,90.3; 100-4,14,10

26432

26432 Closed treatment of distal extensor tendon insertion, with or without percutaneous pinning (eg, mallet finger)

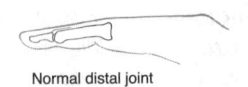

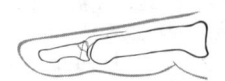

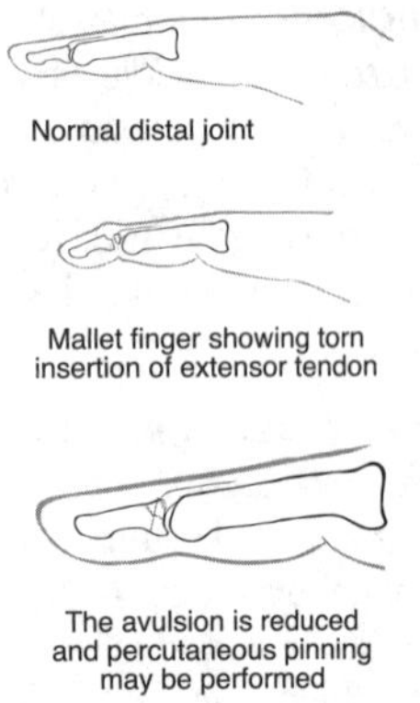

Normal distal joint

Mallet finger showing torn insertion of extensor tendon

The avulsion is reduced and percutaneous pinning may be performed

A torn or avulsed distal extensor tendon insertion is treated in a closed fashion, with or without percutaneous (through the skin) pin fixation

Explanation
The physician repairs the distal insertion extensor tendon without incising the skin. The physician uses a splint to hold the finger in an extended position. If extensive damage occurred during injury, pins may be used to stabilize the joint.

Coding Tips
This code is used once for each tendon repair performed. When multiple tendons are repaired, report one tendon as the primary procedure and append modifier 51 to subsequent procedures. According to CPT guidelines, cast application or strapping (including removal) is only reported as a replacement procedure or when the cast application or strapping is an initial service performed without a restorative treatment or procedure. See "Application of Casts and Strapping" in the CPT book in the Surgery section, under the musculoskeletal system.

ICD-9-CM Procedural
82.84 Repair of mallet finger
83.88 Other plastic operations on tendon

Anesthesia
26432 01810

ICD-9-CM Diagnostic
736.1 Mallet finger

Terms To Know
extensor. Any muscle that extends a joint.

mallet finger. Congenital or acquired flexion deformity of the terminal interphalangeal joint that causes bowing of the fingertip and an inability to extend the fingertip.

tendon. Fibrous tissue that connects muscle to bone, consisting primarily of collagen and containing little vasculature.

CCI Version 16.3
01810, 0213T, 0216T, 0228T, 0230T, 11010❖, 20526-20553, 20690, 20692, 20696-20697, 25000, 25259, 26055, 26180-26185, 26340, 29075, 29086, 29130-29131, 29280, 36000, 36400-36410, 36420-36430, 36440, 36600, 36640, 37202, 43752, 51701-51703, 62310-62319, 64400-64435, 64445-64450, 64479, 64483, 64490, 64493, 64505-64530, 69990, 76000-76001, 93000-93010, 93040-93042, 93318, 94002, 94200, 94250, 94680-94690, 94770, 95812-95816, 95819, 95822, 95829, 95955, 96360, 96365, 96372, 96374-96376, 99148-99149, 99150

Note: These CCI edits are used for Medicare. Other payers may reimburse on codes listed above.

Medicare Edits
	Fac RVU	Non-Fac RVU	FUD	Assist
26432	14.29	14.29	90	N/A

Medicare References: 100-2,15,260; 100-4,12,30; 100-4,12,90.3; 100-4,14,10

26433-26434

26433 Repair of extensor tendon, distal insertion, primary or secondary; without graft (eg, mallet finger)

26434 with free graft (includes obtaining graft)

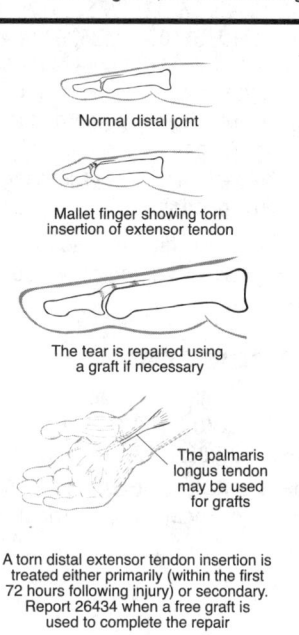

Normal distal joint

Mallet finger showing torn insertion of extensor tendon

The tear is repaired using a graft if necessary

The palmaris longus tendon may be used for grafts

A torn distal extensor tendon insertion is treated either primarily (within the first 72 hours following injury) or secondary. Report 26434 when a free graft is used to complete the repair

Explanation
The physician repairs the distal insertion of an extensor tendon (mallet finger), using a graft if necessary. The physician incises the overlying skin and dissects to the damaged tendon. The tendon is repaired with sutures to improve joint function. If a graft is needed for repair, it is obtained from the palmaris longus tendon or from the foot. The incision is sutured in layers. Primary repair is done immediately after injury. Secondary repair is done sometime after the incident of injury or following a previous surgical repair. Report 26433 for primary or secondary repair without a graft and 26434 for primary or secondary repair requiring a graft.

Coding Tips
These codes are used once for each tendon repair performed. When multiple tendons are repaired, report one tendon as the primary procedure and append modifier 51 to subsequent procedures. In 26434, harvesting of a tendon graft is not reported separately. According to CPT guidelines, cast application or strapping (including removal) is only reported as a replacement procedure or when the cast application or strapping is an initial service performed without a restorative treatment or procedure. See "Application of Casts and Strapping" in the CPT book in the Surgery section, under the musculoskeletal system. For tenovaginotomy for trigger finger, see 26055.

ICD-9-CM Procedural
82.84 Repair of mallet finger
83.88 Other plastic operations on tendon

Anesthesia
01810

ICD-9-CM Diagnostic
736.1 Mallet finger

Terms To Know
mallet finger. Congenital or acquired flexion deformity of the terminal interphalangeal joint that causes bowing of the fingertip and an inability to extend the fingertip.

tendon. Fibrous tissue that connects muscle to bone, consisting primarily of collagen and containing little vasculature.

CCI Version 16.3
01810, 0213T, 0216T, 0228T, 0230T, 20526-20553, 25000, 25259, 26055, 26180-26185, 26340, 29075, 29086, 29130-29131, 29280, 36000, 36400-36410, 36420-36430, 36440, 36600, 36640, 37202, 43752, 51701-51703, 62310-62319, 64400-64435, 64445-64450, 64479, 64483, 64490, 64493, 64505-64530, 69990, 93000-93010, 93040-93042, 93318, 94002, 94200, 94250, 94680-94690, 94770, 95812-95816, 95819, 95822, 95829, 95955, 96360, 96365, 96372, 96374-96376, 99148-99149, 99150

Also not with 26433: 13132, 26432, 26746, 26785, 29125

Also not with 26434: 20924-20926, 26432-26433

Note: These CCI edits are used for Medicare. Other payers may reimburse on codes listed above.

Medicare Edits

	Fac RVU	Non-Fac RVU	FUD	Assist
26433	15.29	15.29	90	N/A
26434	18.5	18.5	90	80

Medicare References: 100-2,15,260; 100-4,12,30; 100-4,12,90.3; 100-4,14,10

26437

26437 Realignment of extensor tendon, hand, each tendon

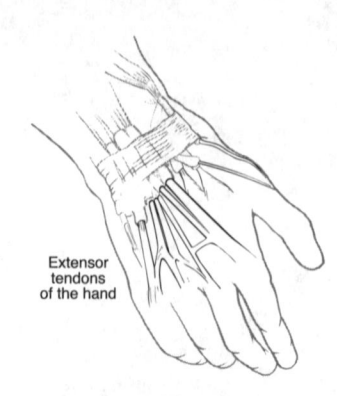

Extensor tendons of the hand

The extensor tendons act to open the hand and spread the fingers

An extensor tendon of the hand is realigned

Explanation
The physician realigns an extensor tendon in the hand. The physician incises the overlying skin and dissects to the damaged tendon. The tendon is realigned to correct finger position. The operative incision is closed in sutured layers. Report each tendon separately.

Coding Tips
This code is used once for each tendon repair performed. When multiple tendons are repaired, report one tendon as the primary procedure and append modifier 51 to subsequent procedures. According to CPT guidelines, cast application or strapping (including removal) is only reported as a replacement procedure or when the cast application or strapping is an initial service performed without a restorative treatment or procedure. See "Application of Casts and Strapping" in the CPT book in the Surgery section, under the musculoskeletal system.

ICD-9-CM Procedural
83.88 Other plastic operations on tendon

Anesthesia
26437 01810

ICD-9-CM Diagnostic
357.1 Polyneuropathy in collagen vascular disease — (Code first underlying disease: 446.0, 710.0, 714.0)
359.6 Symptomatic inflammatory myopathy in diseases classified elsewhere — (Code first underlying disease: 135, 140.0-208.9, 277.30-277.39, 446.0, 710.0, 710.1, 710.2, 714.0)
446.0 Polyarteritis nodosa
710.0 Systemic lupus erythematosus — (Use additional code to identify manifestation: 424.91, 581.81, 582.81, 583.81)
710.1 Systemic sclerosis — (Use additional code to identify manifestation: 359.6, 517.2)
710.2 Sicca syndrome
714.0 Rheumatoid arthritis — (Use additional code to identify manifestation: 357.1, 359.6)
882.2 Open wound of hand except finger(s) alone, with tendon involvement

Terms To Know
extensor. Any muscle that extends a joint.

myopathy. Any disease process within muscle tissue.

open wound. Opening or break of the skin.

polyneuropathy. Disease process of severe inflammation of multiple nerves.

systemic sclerosis. Systemic disease characterized by excess fibrotic collagen build-up, turning the skin thickened and hard. Fibrotic changes also occur in various organs and cause vascular abnormalities and affect more women than men.

tendon. Fibrous tissue that connects muscle to bone, consisting primarily of collagen and containing little vasculature.

CCI Version 16.3
01810, 0213T, 0216T, 0228T, 0230T, 20526-20553, 25000, 25259, 26055, 26170❖, 26185, 26340, 26520, 26546❖, 29075, 29086, 29125, 29130-29131, 29280, 36000, 36400-36410, 36420-36430, 36440, 36600, 36640, 37202, 43752, 51701-51703, 62310-62319, 64400-64435, 64445-64450, 64479, 64483, 64490, 64493, 64505-64530, 69990, 93000-93010, 93040-93042, 93318, 94002, 94200, 94250, 94680-94690, 94770, 95812-95816, 95819, 95822, 95829, 95955, 96360, 96365, 96372, 96374-96376, 99148-99149, 99150

Note: These CCI edits are used for Medicare. Other payers may reimburse on codes listed above.

Medicare Edits

	Fac RVU	Non-Fac RVU	FUD	Assist
26437	17.88	17.88	90	N/A

Medicare References: 100-2,15,260; 100-4,12,30; 100-4,12,90.3; 100-4,14,10

26440-26442

26440 Tenolysis, flexor tendon; palm OR finger, each tendon
26442 palm AND finger, each tendon

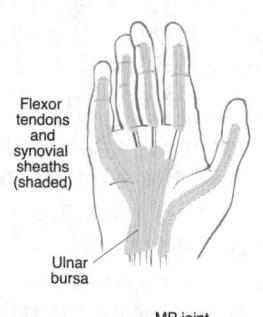

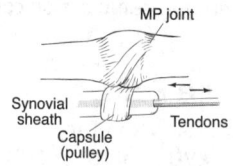

Flexor tendons and synovial sheaths (shaded)
Ulnar bursa
MP joint
Synovial sheath
Capsule (pulley)
Tendons

Adhesions or scar tissue affecting the action of the flexor tendons are removed

A flexor tendon in the palm or finger area is lysed of scar tissue or adhesions. Report 26442 when the lysis extends to both the palm and a finger

Explanation

The physician removes scar tissue to release a flexor tendon in a finger or palm. The physician incises the overlying tissue and dissects to the affected tendon. The scar tissue is debrided and removed, freeing the tendon. The operative incision is closed in sutured layers. In 26440, repair is limited to the palm or finger. In 26442, repair extends to the hand and finger. Report each tendon separately.

Coding Tips

These codes are used once for each tendon repair performed. When multiple tendons are repaired, report one tendon as the primary procedure and append modifier 51 to subsequent procedures. According to CPT guidelines, cast application or strapping (including removal) is only reported as a replacement procedure or when the cast application or strapping is an initial service performed without a restorative treatment or procedure. See "Application of Casts and Strapping" in the CPT book in the Surgery section, under the musculoskeletal system.

ICD-9-CM Procedural

82.91 Lysis of adhesions of hand
83.91 Lysis of adhesions of muscle, tendon, fascia, and bursa

Anesthesia

01810

ICD-9-CM Diagnostic

357.1 Polyneuropathy in collagen vascular disease — (Code first underlying disease: 446.0, 710.0, 714.0)
359.6 Symptomatic inflammatory myopathy in diseases classified elsewhere — (Code first underlying disease: 135, 140.0-208.9, 277.30-277.39, 446.0, 710.0, 710.1, 710.2, 714.0)
446.0 Polyarteritis nodosa
710.0 Systemic lupus erythematosus — (Use additional code to identify manifestation: 424.91, 581.81, 582.81, 583.81)
710.1 Systemic sclerosis — (Use additional code to identify manifestation: 359.6, 517.2)
710.2 Sicca syndrome
714.0 Rheumatoid arthritis — (Use additional code to identify manifestation: 357.1, 359.6)
727.00 Unspecified synovitis and tenosynovitis
727.05 Other tenosynovitis of hand and wrist
727.81 Contracture of tendon (sheath)
727.89 Other disorders of synovium, tendon, and bursa
736.29 Other acquired deformity of finger
883.2 Open wound of finger(s), with tendon involvement
905.8 Late effect of tendon injury

Terms To Know

adhesion. Abnormal fibrous connection between two structures, soft tissue or bony structures, that may occur as the result of surgery, infection, or trauma.

contracture. Shortening of muscle or connective tissue.

synovitis. Inflammation of the synovial membrane that lines a synovial joint, resulting in pain and swelling.

systemic sclerosis. Systemic disease characterized by excess fibrotic collagen build-up, turning the skin thickened and hard. Fibrotic changes also occur in various organs and cause vascular abnormalities and affect more women than men.

tendon. Fibrous tissue that connects muscle to bone, consisting primarily of collagen and containing little vasculature.

tenosynovitis. Inflammation of a tendon sheath due to infection or disease.

CCI Version 16.3

01810, 0213T, 0216T, 0228T, 0230T, 20526-20553, 25259, 26055, 26185, 26340, 26450-26455, 26546❖, 29075, 29086, 29125, 29130-29131, 29280, 36000, 36400-36410, 36420-36430, 36440, 36600, 36640, 37202, 43752, 51701-51703, 62310-62319, 64400-64435, 64445-64450, 64479, 64483, 64490, 64493, 64505-64530, 69990, 93000-93010, 93040-93042, 93318, 94002, 94200, 94250, 94680-94690, 94770, 95812-95816, 95819, 95822, 95829, 95955, 96360, 96365, 96372, 96374-96376, 99148-99149, 99150

Also not with 26440: 12032, 64708
Also not with 26442: 26440

Note: These CCI edits are used for Medicare. Other payers may reimburse on codes listed above.

Medicare Edits

	Fac RVU	Non-Fac RVU	FUD	Assist
26440	17.9	17.9	90	N/A
26442	27.68	27.68	90	N/A

Medicare References: 100-2,15,260; 100-4,12,30; 100-4,12,90.3; 100-4,14,10

26445-26449

26445 Tenolysis, extensor tendon, hand OR finger, each tendon

26449 Tenolysis, complex, extensor tendon, finger, including forearm, each tendon

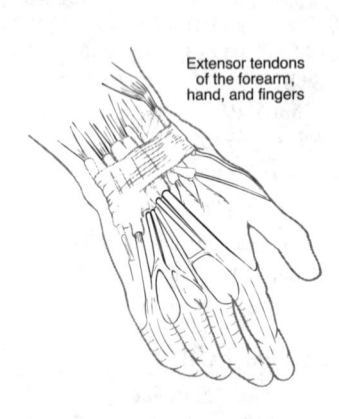

Extensor tendons of the forearm, hand, and fingers

Scar tissue or adhesions of an extensor tendon of the hand or finger are surgically removed (lysed). Report 26449 when the procedure is complex and the lysis extends to the tendons of the forearm

Explanation

The physician removes scar tissue to release an extensor tendon in a finger or the dorsum of hand. The physician incises the overlying tissue and dissects to the affected tendon. The scar tissue is debrided and removed, freeing the tendon. The operative incision is closed in sutured layers. In 26445, repair is limited to the hand or finger. In 26449, repair extends to the finger, including the forearm. Report each tendon separately.

Coding Tips

These codes are used once for each tendon repair performed. When multiple tendons are repaired, report one tendon as the primary procedure and append modifier 51 to subsequent procedures. For 26449, some payers may require the use of HCPCS Level II modifiers FA-F9 to identify the specific finger involved. According to CPT guidelines, cast application or strapping (including removal) is only reported as a replacement procedure or when the cast application or strapping is an initial service performed without a restorative treatment or procedure. See "Application of Casts and Strapping" in the CPT book in the Surgery section, under the musculoskeletal system.

ICD-9-CM Procedural

82.91 Lysis of adhesions of hand

83.91 Lysis of adhesions of muscle, tendon, fascia, and bursa

Anesthesia

01810

ICD-9-CM Diagnostic

357.1 Polyneuropathy in collagen vascular disease — (Code first underlying disease: 446.0, 710.0, 714.0)

359.6 Symptomatic inflammatory myopathy in diseases classified elsewhere — (Code first underlying disease: 135, 140.0-208.9, 277.30-277.39, 446.0, 710.0, 710.1, 710.2, 714.0)

446.0 Polyarteritis nodosa

710.0 Systemic lupus erythematosus — (Use additional code to identify manifestation: 424.91, 581.81, 582.81, 583.81)

710.1 Systemic sclerosis — (Use additional code to identify manifestation: 359.6, 517.2)

710.2 Sicca syndrome

714.0 Rheumatoid arthritis — (Use additional code to identify manifestation: 357.1, 359.6)

727.00 Unspecified synovitis and tenosynovitis

727.04 Radial styloid tenosynovitis

727.05 Other tenosynovitis of hand and wrist

727.89 Other disorders of synovium, tendon, and bursa

736.29 Other acquired deformity of finger

882.2 Open wound of hand except finger(s) alone, with tendon involvement

883.2 Open wound of finger(s), with tendon involvement

905.8 Late effect of tendon injury

Terms To Know

late effect. Abnormality, dysfunction, or other residual condition produced after the acute phase of an illness, injury, or disease is over. There is no time limit on when late effects can appear.

systemic sclerosis. Systemic disease characterized by excess fibrotic collagen build-up, turning the skin thickened and hard. Fibrotic changes also occur in various organs and cause vascular abnormalities and affect more women than men.

CCI Version 16.3

01810, 0213T, 0216T, 0228T, 0230T, 20526-20553, 25259, 26185, 26340, 26460, 26546✣, 29075, 29086, 29130-29131, 29280, 36000, 36400-36410, 36420-36430, 36440, 36600, 36640, 37202, 43752, 51701-51703, 62310-62319, 64400-64435, 64445-64450, 64479, 64483, 64490, 64493, 64505-64530, 69990, 93000-93010, 93040-93042, 93318, 94002, 94200, 94250, 94680-94690, 94770, 95812-95816, 95819, 95822, 95829, 95955, 96360, 96365, 96372, 96374-96376, 99148-99149, 99150

Also not with 26445: 12032, 25000

Also not with 26449: 26445

Note: These CCI edits are used for Medicare. Other payers may reimburse on codes listed above.

Medicare Edits

	Fac RVU	Non-Fac RVU	FUD	Assist
26445	16.65	16.65	90	N/A
26449	21.29	21.29	90	80

Medicare References: 100-2,15,260; 100-4,12,30; 100-4,12,90.3; 100-4,14,10

26450-26460

26450 Tenotomy, flexor, palm, open, each tendon
26455 Tenotomy, flexor, finger, open, each tendon
26460 Tenotomy, extensor, hand or finger, open, each tendon

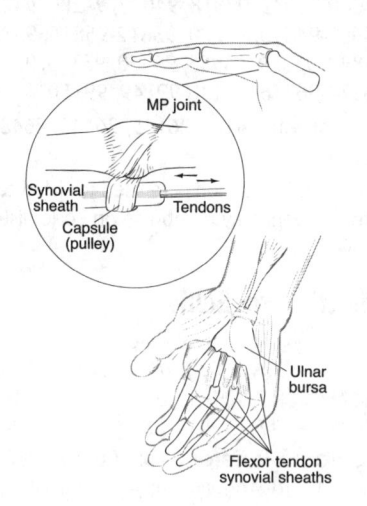

A flexor tendon in the area of the palm is cut (tenotomy) in an open surgical session. Report 26455 when the tenotomy is in a finger. Report 26460 when the tendon is cut in an open surgical session

Explanation

The physician incises a flexor tendon. The physician incises the overlying skin and dissects to the flexor tendon. The tendon is incised. The operative incision is closed in sutured layers. In 26450, the tendon is located in the palm. In 26455, the tendon is located in a finger. In 26460, the physician incises an extensor tendon in a hand or finger. The physician incises the overlying skin and dissects to the extensor tendon. The tendon is incised. The operative incision is closed in sutured layers. Report each tendon separately.

Coding Tips

These codes are used once for each tendon repair performed. When multiple tendons are repaired, report one tendon as the primary procedure and append modifier 51 to subsequent procedures. For 26455, some payers may require the use of HCPCS Level II modifiers FA–F9 to identify the specific finger involved. According to CPT guidelines, cast application or strapping (including removal) is only reported as a replacement procedure or when the cast application or strapping is an initial service performed without a restorative treatment or procedure. See "Application of Casts and Strapping" in the CPT book in the Surgery Section, under the Musculoskeletal system.

ICD-9-CM Procedural
82.11 Tenotomy of hand

Anesthesia
01810

ICD-9-CM Diagnostic
- 718.44 Contracture of hand joint
- 727.00 Unspecified synovitis and tenosynovitis
- 727.05 Other tenosynovitis of hand and wrist
- 727.81 Contracture of tendon (sheath)
- 728.6 Contracture of palmar fascia
- 736.29 Other acquired deformity of finger
- 755.50 Unspecified congenital anomaly of upper limb
- 883.2 Open wound of finger(s), with tendon involvement
- 905.8 Late effect of tendon injury

Terms To Know

contracture. Shortening of muscle or connective tissue.

extensor. Any muscle that extends a joint.

fascia. Fibrous sheet or band of tissue that envelops organs, muscles, and groupings of muscles.

flexor. Muscle/tendon that bends or flexes a limb or part as opposed to extending it.

late effect. Abnormality, dysfunction, or other residual condition produced after the acute phase of an illness, injury, or disease is over. There is no time limit on when late effects can appear.

synovitis. Inflammation of the synovial membrane that lines a synovial joint, resulting in pain and swelling.

tendon. Fibrous tissue that connects muscle to bone, consisting primarily of collagen and containing little vasculature.

tenosynovitis. Inflammation of a tendon sheath due to infection or disease.

CCI Version 16.3

01810, 0213T, 0216T, 0228T, 0230T, 11010❖, 20526-20553, 25259, 26185, 26340, 26546❖, 29075, 29086, 29130-29131, 29280, 36000, 36400-36410, 36420-36430, 36440, 36600, 36640, 37202, 43752, 51701-51703, 62310-62319, 64400-64435, 64445-64450, 64479, 64483, 64490, 64493, 64505-64530, 69990, 93000-93010, 93040-93042, 93318, 94002, 94200, 94250, 94680-94690, 94770, 95812-95816, 95819, 95822, 95829, 95955, 96360, 96365, 96372, 96374-96376, 99148-99149, 99150

Also not with 26455: 26055

Note: These CCI edits are used for Medicare. Other payers may reimburse on codes listed above.

Medicare Edits

	Fac RVU	Non-Fac RVU	FUD	Assist
26450	11.6	11.6	90	80
26455	11.56	11.56	90	80
26460	11.24	11.24	90	N/A

Medicare References: 100-2,15,260; 100-4,12,30; 100-4,12,90.3; 100-4,14,10

26471-26474

26471 Tenodesis; of proximal interphalangeal joint, each joint
26474 of distal joint, each joint

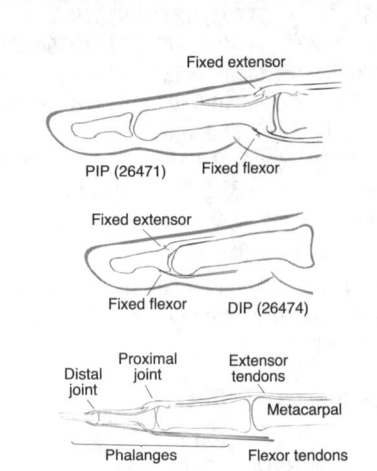

A finger tendon (or tendons) is sutured to bone (tenodesis) near the tip of the finger. Report 26471 when fixation occurs at the proximal phalangeal joint (PIP). And report 26474 when the fixation occurs at the distal phalangeal joint (DIP)

Explanation

The physician sutures the tendon to the proximal or distal interphalangeal joint for stabilization. The physician incises the overlying skin and dissects to the joint. The tendon is incised and sutured over the joint space, providing joint stabilization. The operative incision is closed in sutured layers. In 26471, the proximal joint is stabilized. In 26474, the distal joint is stabilized. Report each tendon separately.

Coding Tips

These codes are used once for each tendon repair performed. When multiple tendons are repaired, report one tendon as the primary procedure and append modifier 51 to subsequent procedures. Some payers may require the use of HCPCS Level II modifiers FA–F9 to identify the specific finger involved. According to CPT guidelines, cast application or strapping (including removal) is only reported as a replacement procedure or when the cast application or strapping is an initial service performed without a restorative treatment or procedure. See "Application of Casts and Strapping" in the CPT book in the Surgery Section, under the Musculoskeletal system.

ICD-9-CM Procedural

82.85 Other tenodesis of hand

Anesthesia
01810

ICD-9-CM Diagnostic

714.1 Felty's syndrome
715.14 Primary localized osteoarthrosis, hand
718.44 Contracture of hand joint
718.84 Other joint derangement, not elsewhere classified, hand
727.64 Nontraumatic rupture of flexor tendons of hand and wrist
816.11 Open fracture of middle or proximal phalanx or phalanges of hand
816.12 Open fracture of distal phalanx or phalanges of hand
833.15 Open dislocation of proximal end of metacarpal (bone)
834.11 Open dislocation of metacarpophalangeal (joint)
883.2 Open wound of finger(s), with tendon involvement
886.1 Traumatic amputation of other finger(s) (complete) (partial), complicated
927.3 Crushing injury of finger(s) — (Use additional code to identify any associated injuries: 800-829, 850.0-854.1, 860.0-869.1)

Terms To Know

contracture. Shortening of muscle or connective tissue.

distal. Located farther away from a specified reference point.

Felty's syndrome. Splenomegaly, leukopenia, arthritis, hypersplenism, anemia and other symptoms.

fracture. Break in bone or cartilage.

primary localized osteoarthrosis. Degenerative joint disease confined to a specific area.

proximal. Located closest to a specified reference point, usually the midline.

rupture. Tearing or breaking open of tissue.

tendon. Fibrous tissue that connects muscle to bone, consisting primarily of collagen and containing little vasculature.

traumatic amputation. Removal of a part or limb from accidental injury.

CCI Version 16.3

01810, 0213T, 0216T, 0228T, 0230T, 20526-20553, 25259, 26180-26185, 26340, 26546❖, 29075, 29086, 29130-29131, 29280, 36000, 36400-36410, 36420-36430, 36440, 36600, 36640, 37202, 43752, 51701-51703, 62310-62319, 64400-64435, 64445-64450, 64479, 64483, 64490, 64493, 64505-64530, 69990, 93000-93010, 93040-93042, 93318, 94002, 94200, 94250, 94680-94690, 94770, 95812-95816, 95819, 95822, 95829, 95955, 96360, 96365, 96372, 96374-96376, 99148-99149, 99150

Also not with 26474: 26145, 26440, 26485, 29125

Note: These CCI edits are used for Medicare. Other payers may reimburse on codes listed above.

Medicare Edits

	Fac RVU	Non-Fac RVU	FUD	Assist
26471	17.67	17.67	90	80
26474	17.23	17.23	90	80

Medicare References: 100-2,15,260; 100-4,12,30; 100-4,12,90.3; 100-4,14,10

26476

26476 Lengthening of tendon, extensor, hand or finger, each tendon

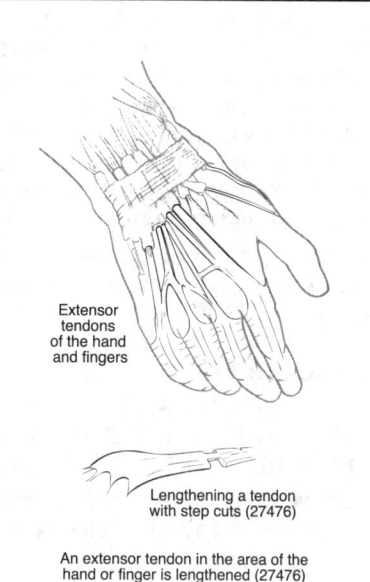

Extensor tendons of the hand and fingers

Lengthening a tendon with step cuts (27476)

An extensor tendon in the area of the hand or finger is lengthened (27476)

Explanation

The physician lengthens an extensor tendon in a hand or a finger. The physician incises the overlying skin and dissects to the tendon. The physician performs step cuts to lengthen the tendon. The operative incision is closed in sutured layers. Report each tendon separately.

Coding Tips

This code is used once for each tendon lengthening performed. When multiple tendons are lengthened, report one tendon as the primary procedure and append modifier 51 to subsequent procedures. According to CPT guidelines, cast application or strapping (including removal) is only reported as a replacement procedure or when the cast application or strapping is an initial service performed without a restorative treatment or procedure. See "Application of Casts and Strapping" in the CPT book in the Surgery Section, under the Musculoskeletal system. For lengthening of a flexor tendon, hand or finger, see 26478.

ICD-9-CM Procedural

82.55 Other change in muscle or tendon length of hand

Anesthesia

26476 01810

ICD-9-CM Diagnostic

715.14 Primary localized osteoarthrosis, hand
718.44 Contracture of hand joint
755.50 Unspecified congenital anomaly of upper limb
816.00 Closed fracture of unspecified phalanx or phalanges of hand
816.01 Closed fracture of middle or proximal phalanx or phalanges of hand
816.10 Open fracture of phalanx or phalanges of hand, unspecified
816.11 Open fracture of middle or proximal phalanx or phalanges of hand
834.01 Closed dislocation of metacarpophalangeal (joint)
883.2 Open wound of finger(s), with tendon involvement
886.1 Traumatic amputation of other finger(s) (complete) (partial), complicated
905.2 Late effect of fracture of upper extremities
906.4 Late effect of crushing
927.3 Crushing injury of finger(s) — (Use additional code to identify any associated injuries: 800-829, 850.0-854.1, 860.0-869.1)

Terms To Know

congenital. Present at birth, occurring through heredity or an influence during gestation up to the moment of birth.

contracture. Shortening of muscle or connective tissue.

extensor. Any muscle that extends a joint.

fracture. Break in bone or cartilage.

late effect. Abnormality, dysfunction, or other residual condition produced after the acute phase of an illness, injury, or disease is over. There is no time limit on when late effects can appear.

primary localized osteoarthrosis. Degenerative joint disease confined to a specific area.

tendon. Fibrous tissue that connects muscle to bone, consisting primarily of collagen and containing little vasculature.

CCI Version 16.3

01810, 0213T, 0216T, 0228T, 0230T, 20526-20553, 25259, 26170-26185, 26340, 29075, 29086, 29130-29131, 29280, 36000, 36400-36410, 36420-36430, 36440, 36600, 36640, 37202, 43752, 51701-51703, 62310-62319, 64400-64435, 64445-64450, 64479, 64483, 64490, 64493, 64505-64530, 69990, 93000-93010, 93040-93042, 93318, 94002, 94200, 94250, 94680-94690, 94770, 95812-95816, 95819, 95822, 95829, 95955, 96360, 96365, 96372, 96374-96376, 99148-99149, 99150

Note: These CCI edits are used for Medicare. Other payers may reimburse on codes listed above.

Medicare Edits

	Fac RVU	Non-Fac RVU	FUD	Assist
26476	16.87	16.87	90	N/A

Medicare References: 100-2,15,260; 100-4,12,30; 100-4,12,90.3; 100-4,14,10

26477

26477 Shortening of tendon, extensor, hand or finger, each tendon

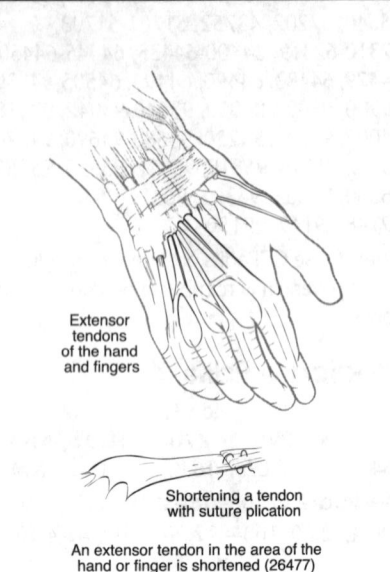

Extensor tendons of the hand and fingers

Shortening a tendon with suture plication

An extensor tendon in the area of the hand or finger is shortened (26477)

Explanation

The physician shortens an extensor tendon in a hand or a finger. The physician incises the overlying skin and dissects to the tendon. The physician removes a section of the tendon and sutures the ends back together, shortening the tendon. The operative incision is closed in sutured layers. Report each tendon separately.

Coding Tips

This code is used once for each tendon that is shortened. When multiple tendons are shortened, report one tendon as the primary procedure and append modifier 51 to subsequent procedures. According to CPT guidelines, cast application or strapping (including removal) is only reported as a replacement procedure or when the cast application or strapping is an initial service performed without a restorative treatment or procedure. See "Application of Casts and Strapping" in the CPT book in the Surgery Section, under the Musculoskeletal system. For shortening of a flexor tendon, hand or finger, see 26479.

ICD-9-CM Procedural

82.55 Other change in muscle or tendon length of hand

Anesthesia

26477 01810

ICD-9-CM Diagnostic

715.14 Primary localized osteoarthrosis, hand
755.50 Unspecified congenital anomaly of upper limb
816.00 Closed fracture of unspecified phalanx or phalanges of hand
816.01 Closed fracture of middle or proximal phalanx or phalanges of hand
816.10 Open fracture of phalanx or phalanges of hand, unspecified
816.11 Open fracture of middle or proximal phalanx or phalanges of hand
833.15 Open dislocation of proximal end of metacarpal (bone)
834.01 Closed dislocation of metacarpophalangeal (joint)
834.11 Open dislocation of metacarpophalangeal (joint)
842.12 Sprain and strain of metacarpophalangeal (joint) of hand
883.2 Open wound of finger(s), with tendon involvement
886.1 Traumatic amputation of other finger(s) (complete) (partial), complicated
905.2 Late effect of fracture of upper extremities
906.4 Late effect of crushing
927.3 Crushing injury of finger(s) — (Use additional code to identify any associated injuries: 800-829, 850.0-854.1, 860.0-869.1)

Terms To Know

anomaly. Irregularity in the structure or position of an organ or tissue.

congenital. Present at birth, occurring through heredity or an influence during gestation up to the moment of birth.

dislocation. Displacement of a bone in relation to its neighboring tissue, especially a joint.

extensor. Any muscle that extends a joint.

fracture. Break in bone or cartilage.

late effect. Abnormality, dysfunction, or other residual condition produced after the acute phase of an illness, injury, or disease is over. There is no time limit on when late effects can appear.

primary localized osteoarthrosis. Degenerative joint disease confined to a specific area.

tendon. Fibrous tissue that connects muscle to bone, consisting primarily of collagen and containing little vasculature.

CCI Version 16.3

01810, 0213T, 0216T, 0228T, 0230T, 20526-20553, 25259, 26170-26185, 26340, 26476❖, 29075, 29086, 29130-29131, 29280, 36000, 36400-36410, 36420-36430, 36440, 36600, 36640, 37202, 43752, 51701-51703, 62310-62319, 64400-64435, 64445-64450, 64479, 64483, 64490, 64493, 64505-64530, 69990, 93000-93010, 93040-93042, 93318, 94002, 94200, 94250, 94680-94690, 94770, 95812-95816, 95819, 95822, 95829, 95955, 96360, 96365, 96372, 96374-96376, 99148-99149, 99150

Note: These CCI edits are used for Medicare. Other payers may reimburse on codes listed above.

Medicare Edits

	Fac RVU	Non-Fac RVU	FUD	Assist
26477	16.74	16.74	90	N/A

Medicare References: 100-2,15,260; 100-4,12,30; 100-4,12,90.3; 100-4,14,10

26478

26478 Lengthening of tendon, flexor, hand or finger, each tendon

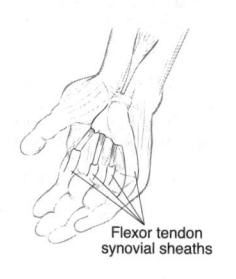

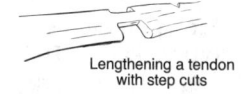

A flexor tendon in the area of the hand or finger is lengthened (26478)

Explanation

The physician lengthens a flexor tendon in a hand or a finger. The physician incises the overlying skin and dissects to the tendon. The physician performs step cuts to lengthen the tendon. The operative incision is closed in sutured layers. Report each tendon separately.

Coding Tips

This code is used once for each tendon lengthening performed. When multiple tendons are lengthened, report one tendon as the primary procedure and append modifier 51 to subsequent procedures. According to CPT guidelines, cast application or strapping (including removal) is only reported as a replacement procedure or when the cast application or strapping is an initial service performed without a restorative treatment or procedure. See "Application of Casts and Strapping" in the CPT book in the Surgery Section, under the Musculoskeletal system. For lengthening of an extensor tendon, hand or finger, see 26476.

ICD-9-CM Procedural

82.55 Other change in muscle or tendon length of hand

Anesthesia

26478 01810

ICD-9-CM Diagnostic

718.44 Contracture of hand joint
727.64 Nontraumatic rupture of flexor tendons of hand and wrist
728.6 Contracture of palmar fascia
755.50 Unspecified congenital anomaly of upper limb
816.11 Open fracture of middle or proximal phalanx or phalanges of hand
833.15 Open dislocation of proximal end of metacarpal (bone)
834.11 Open dislocation of metacarpophalangeal (joint)
842.12 Sprain and strain of metacarpophalangeal (joint) of hand
882.2 Open wound of hand except finger(s) alone, with tendon involvement
883.2 Open wound of finger(s), with tendon involvement
886.1 Traumatic amputation of other finger(s) (complete) (partial), complicated
905.2 Late effect of fracture of upper extremities
906.4 Late effect of crushing

Terms To Know

anomaly. Irregularity in the structure or position of an organ or tissue.

congenital. Present at birth, occurring through heredity or an influence during gestation up to the moment of birth.

contracture. Shortening of muscle or connective tissue.

dislocation. Displacement of a bone in relation to its neighboring tissue, especially a joint.

fascia. Fibrous sheet or band of tissue that envelops organs, muscles, and groupings of muscles.

flexor. Muscle/tendon that bends or flexes a limb or part as opposed to extending it.

tendon. Fibrous tissue that connects muscle to bone, consisting primarily of collagen and containing little vasculature.

CCI Version 16.3

01810, 0213T, 0216T, 0228T, 0230T, 20526-20553, 25259, 26055, 26170-26185, 26340, 29075, 29086, 29130-29131, 29280, 36000, 36400-36410, 36420-36430, 36440, 36600, 36640, 37202, 43752, 51701-51703, 62310-62319, 64400-64435, 64445-64450, 64479, 64483, 64490, 64493, 64505-64530, 69990, 93000-93010, 93040-93042, 93318, 94002, 94200, 94250, 94680-94690, 94770, 95812-95816, 95819, 95822, 95829, 95955, 96360, 96365, 96372, 96374-96376, 99148-99149, 99150

Note: These CCI edits are used for Medicare. Other payers may reimburse on codes listed above.

Medicare Edits

	Fac RVU	Non-Fac RVU	FUD	Assist
26478	17.97	17.97	90	80

Medicare References: 100-2,15,260; 100-4,12,30; 100-4,12,90.3; 100-4,14,10

26479

26479 Shortening of tendon, flexor, hand or finger, each tendon

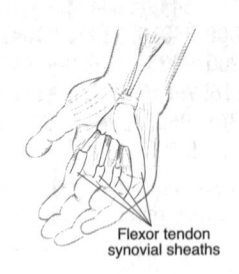

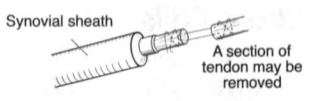

Explanation

The physician shortens a flexor tendon in the hand or finger. The physician incises the overlying skin and dissects to the tendon. The physician removes a section of the tendon and sutures the ends back together, shortening the tendon. The incision is sutured in layers. Report each tendon separately.

Coding Tips

This code is used once for each tendon that is shortened. When multiple tendons are shortened, report one tendon as the primary procedure and append modifier 51 to subsequent procedures. According to CPT guidelines, cast application or strapping (including removal) is only reported as a replacement procedure or when the cast application or strapping is an initial service performed without a restorative treatment or procedure. See "Application of Casts and Strapping" in the CPT book in the Surgery Section, under the Musculoskeletal system. For shortening of an extensor tendon, hand or finger, see 26477.

ICD-9-CM Procedural

82.55 Other change in muscle or tendon length of hand

Anesthesia

26479   01810

ICD-9-CM Diagnostic

727.64 Nontraumatic rupture of flexor tendons of hand and wrist
728.6 Contracture of palmar fascia
755.50 Unspecified congenital anomaly of upper limb
816.11 Open fracture of middle or proximal phalanx or phalanges of hand
833.15 Open dislocation of proximal end of metacarpal (bone)
834.11 Open dislocation of metacarpophalangeal (joint)
842.12 Sprain and strain of metacarpophalangeal (joint) of hand
882.2 Open wound of hand except finger(s) alone, with tendon involvement
883.2 Open wound of finger(s), with tendon involvement
886.1 Traumatic amputation of other finger(s) (complete) (partial), complicated
905.2 Late effect of fracture of upper extremities
906.4 Late effect of crushing

Terms To Know

anomaly. Irregularity in the structure or position of an organ or tissue.

congenital. Present at birth, occurring through heredity or an influence during gestation up to the moment of birth.

contracture. Shortening of muscle or connective tissue.

fascia. Fibrous sheet or band of tissue that envelops organs, muscles, and groupings of muscles.

flexor. Muscle/tendon that bends or flexes a limb or part as opposed to extending it.

late effect. Abnormality, dysfunction, or other residual condition produced after the acute phase of an illness, injury, or disease is over. There is no time limit on when late effects can appear.

rupture. Tearing or breaking open of tissue.

tendon. Fibrous tissue that connects muscle to bone, consisting primarily of collagen and containing little vasculature.

CCI Version 16.3

01810, 0213T, 0216T, 0228T, 0230T, 20526-20553, 25259, 26170-26185, 26340, 26478❖, 29075, 29086, 29130-29131, 29280, 36000, 36400-36410, 36420-36430, 36440, 36600, 36640, 37202, 43752, 51701-51703, 62310-62319, 64400-64435, 64445-64450, 64479, 64483, 64490, 64493, 64505-64530, 69990, 93000-93010, 93040-93042, 93318, 94002, 94200, 94250, 94680-94690, 94770, 95812-95816, 95819, 95822, 95829, 95955, 96360, 96365, 96372, 96374-96376, 99148-99149, 99150

Note: These CCI edits are used for Medicare. Other payers may reimburse on codes listed above.

Medicare Edits

	Fac RVU	Non-Fac RVU	FUD	Assist
26479	17.92	17.92	90	80

Medicare References: 100-2,15,260; 100-4,12,30; 100-4,12,90.3; 100-4,14,10

26480-26483

26480 Transfer or transplant of tendon, carpometacarpal area or dorsum of hand; without free graft, each tendon
26483 with free tendon graft (includes obtaining graft), each tendon

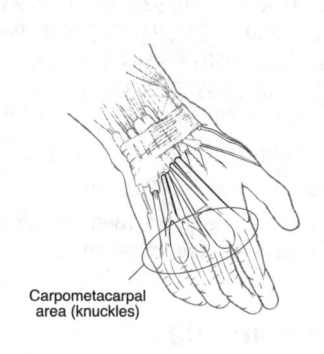

Carpometacarpal area (knuckles)

Extensor tendons of the hand and fingers

Performing a free graft repair (26483)

An extensor tendon in the carpometacarpal area of the hand, or the dorsum (back) of the hand, is transferred or transplanted. Report 26483 when a free tendon graft is required for the repair

Explanation

The physician transfers or transplants a tendon from the carpometacarpal area or dorsum of the hand. A free tendon graft may be used if necessary. The physician incises the overlying skin and dissects to the tendon to be moved. The tendon is freed, transferred, and sutured into place. If a free tendon graft is used, report 26483. The graft is obtained from the palmaris longus tendon or from the foot. The operative incision is closed in sutured layers.

Coding Tips

These codes are used once for each tendon transfer or transplant performed. When multiple tendons are transferred or transplanted, report one tendon as the primary procedure and append modifier 51 to subsequent procedures. According to CPT guidelines, cast application or strapping (including removal) is only reported as a replacement procedure or when the cast application or strapping is an initial service performed without a restorative treatment or procedure. See "Application of Casts and Strapping" in the CPT book in the Surgery Section, under the Musculoskeletal system. For tendon transfer or transplant, palmar, see 26485 and 26489.

ICD-9-CM Procedural

82.56 Other hand tendon transfer or transplantation

Anesthesia

01810

ICD-9-CM Diagnostic

138 Late effects of acute poliomyelitis — (Note: This category is to be used to indicate conditions classifiable to 045 as the cause of late effects, which are themselves classified elsewhere. The "late effects" include those specified as such, as sequelae, or as due to old or inactive poliomyelitis, without evidence of active disease.)
343.0 Diplegic infantile cerebral palsy
714.4 Chronic postrheumatic arthropathy
716.14 Traumatic arthropathy, hand
718.54 Ankylosis of hand joint
718.84 Other joint derangement, not elsewhere classified, hand
719.14 Hemarthrosis, hand
727.63 Nontraumatic rupture of extensor tendons of hand and wrist
755.50 Unspecified congenital anomaly of upper limb
842.12 Sprain and strain of metacarpophalangeal (joint) of hand
882.2 Open wound of hand except finger(s) alone, with tendon involvement
883.2 Open wound of finger(s), with tendon involvement
886.1 Traumatic amputation of other finger(s) (complete) (partial), complicated
905.2 Late effect of fracture of upper extremities
906.4 Late effect of crushing

Terms To Know

ankylosis. Abnormal union or fusion of bones in a joint, which is normally moveable.

diplegic infantile cerebral palsy. Bilateral paralysis and delayed or abnormal motor development caused by trauma at birth or intrauterine pathology.

hemarthrosis. Occurrence of blood within a joint space.

CCI Version 16.3

01810, 0213T, 0216T, 0228T, 0230T, 20526-20553, 25259, 26170❖, 26185, 26340, 29065-29126, 29260, 36000, 36400-36410, 36420-36430, 36440, 36600, 36640, 37202, 43752, 51701-51703, 62310-62319, 64400-64435, 64445-64450, 64479, 64483, 64490, 64493, 64505-64530, 69990, 93000-93010, 93040-93042, 93318, 94002, 94200, 94250, 94680-94690, 94770, 95812-95816, 95819, 95822, 95829, 95955, 96360, 96365, 96372, 96374-96376, 99148-99149, 99150

Also not with 26480: 26445
Also not with 26483: 20924, 26480
Note: These CCI edits are used for Medicare. Other payers may reimburse on codes listed above.

Medicare Edits

	Fac RVU	Non-Fac RVU	FUD	Assist
26480	21.67	21.67	90	80
26483	24.36	24.36	90	80

Medicare References: 100-2,15,260; 100-4,12,30; 100-4,12,90.3; 100-4,14,10

26485-26489

26485 Transfer or transplant of tendon, palmar; without free tendon graft, each tendon
26489 with free tendon graft (includes obtaining graft), each tendon

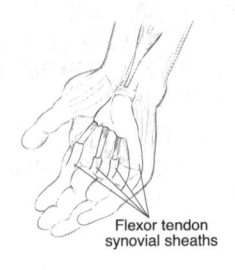

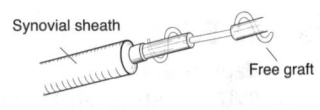

Flexor tendon synovial sheaths

Synovial sheath
Free graft

Performing a free graft repair to a flexor tendon (26489)

A flexor tendon in the palm area of the hand is transferred or transplanted. Report 26489 when a free graft is required for the repair

Explanation
The physician transfers or transplants the palmar tendon; a free tendon graft may be used if necessary. The physician incises the overlying skin and dissects to the tendon to be moved. The tendon is freed, transferred and sutured into place. For transfer or transplant of a palmar tendon without a free graft, report 26485 for each tendon; if a free tendon graft is used, report 26489. The graft is obtained from the palmaris longus tendon or from the foot. The operative incision is closed in sutured layers.

Coding Tips
These codes are used once for each tendon transfer or transplant performed. When multiple tendons are transferred or transplanted, report one tendon as the primary procedure and append modifier 51 to subsequent procedures. According to CPT guidelines, cast application or strapping (including removal) is only reported as a replacement procedure or when the cast application or strapping is an initial service performed without a restorative treatment or procedure. See "Application of Casts and Strapping" in the CPT book in the Surgery Section, under the Musculoskeletal system. For tendon transfer or transplant of the carpometacarpal area or dorsum of hand, see 26480 and 26483.

ICD-9-CM Procedural
82.56 Other hand tendon transfer or transplantation
82.79 Plastic operation on hand with other graft or implant

Anesthesia
01810

ICD-9-CM Diagnostic
138 Late effects of acute poliomyelitis — (Note: This category is to be used to indicate conditions classifiable to 045 as the cause of late effects, which are themselves classified elsewhere. The "late effects" include those specified as such, as sequelae, or as due to old or inactive poliomyelitis, without evidence of active disease.)
343.0 Diplegic infantile cerebral palsy
714.4 Chronic postrheumatic arthropathy
716.14 Traumatic arthropathy, hand
718.54 Ankylosis of hand joint
718.84 Other joint derangement, not elsewhere classified, hand
719.14 Hemarthrosis, hand
727.63 Nontraumatic rupture of extensor tendons of hand and wrist
755.50 Unspecified congenital anomaly of upper limb
842.12 Sprain and strain of metacarpophalangeal (joint) of hand
882.2 Open wound of hand except finger(s) alone, with tendon involvement
883.2 Open wound of finger(s), with tendon involvement
886.1 Traumatic amputation of other finger(s) (complete) (partial), complicated
905.2 Late effect of fracture of upper extremities
906.4 Late effect of crushing

Terms To Know
ankylosis. Abnormal union or fusion of bones in a joint, which is normally moveable.

diplegic infantile cerebral palsy. Bilateral paralysis and delayed or abnormal motor development caused by trauma at birth or intrauterine pathology.

tendon. Fibrous tissue that connects muscle to bone, consisting primarily of collagen and containing little vasculature.

CCI Version 16.3
01810, 0213T, 0216T, 0228T, 0230T, 20526-20553, 25259, 26170❖, 26185, 26340, 29075, 29086, 29130-29131, 29280, 36000, 36400-36410, 36420-36430, 36440, 36600, 36640, 37202, 43752, 51701-51703, 62310-62319, 64400-64435, 64445-64450, 64479, 64483, 64490, 64493, 64505-64530, 69990, 93000-93010, 93040-93042, 93318, 94002, 94200, 94250, 94680-94690, 94770, 95812-95816, 95819, 95822, 95829, 95955, 96360, 96365, 96372, 96374-96376, 99148-99149, 99150
Also not with 26485: 26440, 29125
Also not with 26489: 20924, 26485
Note: These CCI edits are used for Medicare. Other payers may reimburse on codes listed above.

Medicare Edits

	Fac RVU	Non-Fac RVU	FUD	Assist
26485	23.34	23.34	90	80
26489	26.2	26.2	90	80

Medicare References: 100-2,15,260; 100-4,12,30; 100-4,12,90.3; 100-4,14,10

26490-26494

26490 Opponensplasty; superficialis tendon transfer type, each tendon
26492 tendon transfer with graft (includes obtaining graft), each tendon
26494 hypothenar muscle transfer

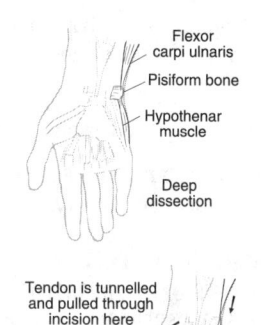

A single superficialis tendon type transfer opponensplasty is performed. Report 26492 when a tendon graft is necessary for the procedure. Report 26494 when the hypothenar muscle is transferred.

Explanation

The physician transfers the superficialis tendon to restore palmar abduction to the thumb. The physician incises the overlying skin and dissects to the superficialis tendon. The tendon is freed and transferred to restore function. If a graft is used, the graft is obtained from the palmaris longus or the abductor digiti minimi. The graft is approximated and sutured into place. The operative incision is closed in sutured layers. Report 26490 if no graft is used. Report 26492 if a graft is used. Report each tendon separately. In 26494, the hypothenar muscle is transferred. The muscle tendon is resected from its distal attachment, transferred to the site, and sutured into place.

Coding Tips

These codes are used once for each tendon repair performed. When multiple tendons are repaired, report one tendon as the primary procedure and append modifier 51 to subsequent procedures. In 26492, harvesting of a tendon graft is not reported separately. According to CPT guidelines, cast application or strapping (including removal) is only reported as a replacement procedure or when the cast application or strapping is an initial service performed without a restorative treatment or procedure. See "Application of Casts and Strapping" in the CPT book in the Surgery Section, under the Musculoskeletal system.

ICD-9-CM Procedural

82.56 Other hand tendon transfer or transplantation

Anesthesia
01810

ICD-9-CM Diagnostic

138 Late effects of acute poliomyelitis — (Note: This category is to be used to indicate conditions classifiable to 045 as the cause of late effects, which are themselves classified elsewhere. The "late effects" include those specified as such, as sequelae, or as due to old or inactive poliomyelitis, without evidence of active disease.)
718.44 Contracture of hand joint
718.84 Other joint derangement, not elsewhere classified, hand
727.63 Nontraumatic rupture of extensor tendons of hand and wrist
728.6 Contracture of palmar fascia
736.29 Other acquired deformity of finger
755.21 Congenital transverse deficiency of upper limb
755.50 Unspecified congenital anomaly of upper limb
816.00 Closed fracture of unspecified phalanx or phalanges of hand
816.01 Closed fracture of middle or proximal phalanx or phalanges of hand
816.03 Closed fracture of multiple sites of phalanx or phalanges of hand
816.10 Open fracture of phalanx or phalanges of hand, unspecified
816.11 Open fracture of middle or proximal phalanx or phalanges of hand
816.12 Open fracture of distal phalanx or phalanges of hand
816.13 Open fractures of multiple sites of phalanx or phalanges of hand
842.01 Sprain and strain of carpal (joint) of wrist
883.2 Open wound of finger(s), with tendon involvement
886.1 Traumatic amputation of other finger(s) (complete) (partial), complicated
905.2 Late effect of fracture of upper extremities
905.9 Late effect of traumatic amputation
906.4 Late effect of crushing
927.3 Crushing injury of finger(s) — (Use additional code to identify any associated injuries: 800-829, 850.0-854.1, 860.0-869.1)

Terms To Know

acute. Sudden, severe. Documentation and reporting of an acute condition is important to establishing medical necessity.

contracture. Shortening of muscle or connective tissue.

fascia. Fibrous sheet or band of tissue that envelops organs, muscles, and groupings of muscles.

tendon. Fibrous tissue that connects muscle to bone, consisting primarily of collagen and containing little vasculature.

CCI Version 16.3

01810, 0213T, 0216T, 0228T, 0230T, 20526-20553, 25259, 26170-26185, 26340, 29075, 29086, 29130-29131, 29280, 36000, 36400-36410, 36420-36430, 36440, 36600, 36640, 37202, 43752, 51701-51703, 62310-62319, 64400-64435, 64445-64450, 64479, 64483, 64490, 64493, 64505-64530, 69990, 93000-93010, 93040-93042, 93318, 94002, 94200, 94250, 94680-94690, 94770, 95812-95816, 95819, 95822, 95829, 95955, 96360, 96365, 96372, 96374-96376, 99148-99149, 99150

Also not with 26492: 20924-20926

Note: These CCI edits are used for Medicare. Other payers may reimburse on codes listed above.

Medicare Edits

	Fac RVU	Non-Fac RVU	FUD	Assist
26490	22.89	22.89	90	80
26492	25.37	25.37	90	80
26494	22.97	22.97	90	80

Medicare References: 100-2,15,260; 100-4,12,30; 100-4,12,90.3; 100-4,14,10

26496

26496 Opponensplasty; other methods

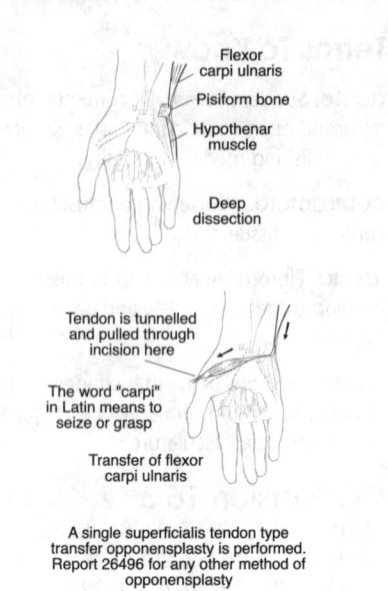

Flexor carpi ulnaris
Pisiform bone
Hypothenar muscle
Deep dissection

Tendon is tunnelled and pulled through incision here
The word "carpi" in Latin means to seize or grasp
Transfer of flexor carpi ulnaris

A single superficialis tendon type transfer opponensplasty is performed. Report 26496 for any other method of opponensplasty

Explanation

The physician performs this procedure when opposition of the thumb is lost because of median nerve paralysis. Methods described using this code include (1) attaching the extensor pollicis brevis to the extensor carpi ulnaris around the ulnar border of the wrist; (2) attaching the extensor carpi radialis longus to the extensor pollicis longus around the ulnar border of the wrist; (3) attaching the extensor indicis proprius tendon, with a small portion of the extensor hood, to the flexor pollicis longus tendon just distal to the metacarpophalangeal (MP) joint; (4) attachment of the extensor digiti minimi around the ulnar border of the wrist to the thumb MP joint; (5) attachment of the extensor indicis proprius with a small portion of the extensor hood around the ulnar border of the wrist to the thumb MP joint; (6) transfer of the adductor pollicis to the tendon of the superficial head of the flexor pollicis brevis; (7) attachment of the flexor pollicis longus around the ulnar aspect of the flexor carpi ulnaris into the abductor pollicis brevis of the interphalangeal joint.

Coding Tips

According to CPT guidelines, cast application or strapping (including removal) is only reported as a replacement procedure or when the cast application or strapping is an initial service performed without a restorative treatment or procedure. See "Application of Casts and Strapping" in the CPT book in the Surgery Section, under the Musculoskeletal system. For thumb fusion in opposition, see 26820.

ICD-9-CM Procedural

82.56 Other hand tendon transfer or transplantation

Anesthesia

26496 01810

ICD-9-CM Diagnostic

138	Late effects of acute poliomyelitis — (Note: This category is to be used to indicate conditions classifiable to 045 as the cause of late effects, which are themselves classified elsewhere. The "late effects" include those specified as such, as sequelae, or as due to old or inactive poliomyelitis, without evidence of active disease.)
718.44	Contracture of hand joint
718.84	Other joint derangement, not elsewhere classified, hand
727.63	Nontraumatic rupture of extensor tendons of hand and wrist
728.6	Contracture of palmar fascia
736.29	Other acquired deformity of finger
755.21	Congenital transverse deficiency of upper limb
755.50	Unspecified congenital anomaly of upper limb
816.00	Closed fracture of unspecified phalanx or phalanges of hand
816.01	Closed fracture of middle or proximal phalanx or phalanges of hand
816.03	Closed fracture of multiple sites of phalanx or phalanges of hand
816.10	Open fracture of phalanx or phalanges of hand, unspecified
816.11	Open fracture of middle or proximal phalanx or phalanges of hand
816.12	Open fracture of distal phalanx or phalanges of hand
816.13	Open fractures of multiple sites of phalanx or phalanges of hand
842.01	Sprain and strain of carpal (joint) of wrist
883.2	Open wound of finger(s), with tendon involvement
886.1	Traumatic amputation of other finger(s) (complete) (partial), complicated
905.2	Late effect of fracture of upper extremities
905.9	Late effect of traumatic amputation
906.4	Late effect of crushing
927.3	Crushing injury of finger(s) — (Use additional code to identify any associated injuries: 800-829, 850.0-854.1, 860.0-869.1)

Terms To Know

contracture. Shortening of muscle or connective tissue.

fascia. Fibrous sheet or band of tissue that envelops organs, muscles, and groupings of muscles.

rupture. Tearing or breaking open of tissue.

traumatic amputation. Removal of a part or limb from accidental injury.

CCI Version 16.3

01810, 0213T, 0216T, 0228T, 0230T, 20526-20553, 25259, 26170-26185, 26340, 29075, 29086, 29130-29131, 29280, 36000, 36400-36410, 36420-36430, 36440, 36600, 36640, 37202, 43752, 51701-51703, 62310-62319, 64400-64435, 64445-64450, 64479, 64483, 64490, 64493, 64505-64530, 69990, 93000-93010, 93040-93042, 93318, 94002, 94200, 94250, 94680-94690, 94770, 95812-95816, 95819, 95822, 95829, 95955, 96360, 96365, 96372, 96374-96376, 99148-99149, 99150

Note: These CCI edits are used for Medicare. Other payers may reimburse on codes listed above.

Medicare Edits

	Fac RVU	Non-Fac RVU	FUD	Assist
26496	24.69	24.69	90	80

Medicare References: 100-2,15,260; 100-4,12,30; 100-4,12,90.3; 100-4,14,10

26497-26498

26497 Transfer of tendon to restore intrinsic function; ring and small finger
26498 all 4 fingers

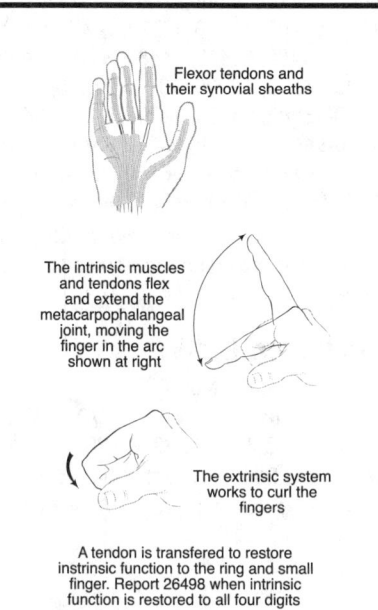

Flexor tendons and their synovial sheaths

The intrinsic muscles and tendons flex and extend the metacarpophalangeal joint, moving the finger in the arc shown at right

The extrinsic system works to curl the fingers

A tendon is transferred to restore instrinsic function to the ring and small finger. Report 26498 when intrinsic function is restored to all four digits

Explanation

The physician transfers a tendon to restore intrinsic function to the fingers. The physician incises the overlying skin and dissects to the affected tendon. The tendon is freed, transferred, and sutured into place to restore function of the flexor digitorum profundus. The operative incision is closed in sutured layers. In 26497, intrinsic function is restored to the ring and small finger. In 26498, intrinsic function is restored to all four fingers.

Coding Tips

According to CPT guidelines, cast application or strapping (including removal) is only reported as a replacement procedure or when the cast application or strapping is an initial service performed without a restorative treatment or procedure. See "Application of Casts and Strapping" in the CPT book in the Surgery Section, under the Musculoskeletal system.

ICD-9-CM Procedural

82.56 Other hand tendon transfer or transplantation

Anesthesia

01810

ICD-9-CM Diagnostic

138 Late effects of acute poliomyelitis — (Note: This category is to be used to indicate conditions classifiable to 045 as the cause of late effects, which are themselves classified elsewhere. The "late effects" include those specified as such, as sequelae, or as due to old or inactive poliomyelitis, without evidence of active disease.)

343.0 Diplegic infantile cerebral palsy
718.44 Contracture of hand joint
718.84 Other joint derangement, not elsewhere classified, hand
727.63 Nontraumatic rupture of extensor tendons of hand and wrist
736.29 Other acquired deformity of finger
755.21 Congenital transverse deficiency of upper limb
816.00 Closed fracture of unspecified phalanx or phalanges of hand
816.01 Closed fracture of middle or proximal phalanx or phalanges of hand
816.03 Closed fracture of multiple sites of phalanx or phalanges of hand
816.10 Open fracture of phalanx or phalanges of hand, unspecified
816.11 Open fracture of middle or proximal phalanx or phalanges of hand
816.12 Open fracture of distal phalanx or phalanges of hand
816.13 Open fractures of multiple sites of phalanx or phalanges of hand
883.2 Open wound of finger(s), with tendon involvement
886.1 Traumatic amputation of other finger(s) (complete) (partial), complicated
905.2 Late effect of fracture of upper extremities
905.9 Late effect of traumatic amputation
906.4 Late effect of crushing
927.3 Crushing injury of finger(s) — (Use additional code to identify any associated injuries: 800-829, 850.0-854.1, 860.0-869.1)

Terms To Know

acute. Sudden, severe. Documentation and reporting of an acute condition is important to establishing medical necessity.

congenital. Present at birth, occurring through heredity or an influence during gestation up to the moment of birth.

contracture. Shortening of muscle or connective tissue.

diplegic infantile cerebral palsy. Bilateral paralysis and delayed or abnormal motor development caused by trauma at birth or intrauterine pathology.

late effect. Abnormality, dysfunction, or other residual condition produced after the acute phase of an illness, injury, or disease is over. There is no time limit on when late effects can appear.

open wound. Opening or break of the skin.

CCI Version 16.3

01810, 0213T, 0216T, 0228T, 0230T, 20526-20553, 25259, 26180-26185, 26340, 26500-26502, 29075, 29086, 29130-29131, 29280, 36000, 36400-36410, 36420-36430, 36440, 36600, 36640, 37202, 43752, 51701-51703, 62310-62319, 64400-64435, 64445-64450, 64479, 64483, 64490, 64493, 64505-64530, 69990, 93000-93010, 93040-93042, 93318, 94002, 94200, 94250, 94680-94690, 94770, 95812-95816, 95819, 95822, 95829, 95955, 96360, 96365, 96372, 96374-96376, 99148-99149, 99150

Note: These CCI edits are used for Medicare. Other payers may reimburse on codes listed above.

Medicare Edits

	Fac RVU	Non-Fac RVU	FUD	Assist
26497	24.92	24.92	90	80
26498	33.13	33.13	90	80

Medicare References: 100-2,15,260; 100-4,12,30; 100-4,12,90.3; 100-4,14,10

26499

26499 Correction claw finger, other methods

Claw finger, or claw hand, is a disorder where the fingers are locked in flexion

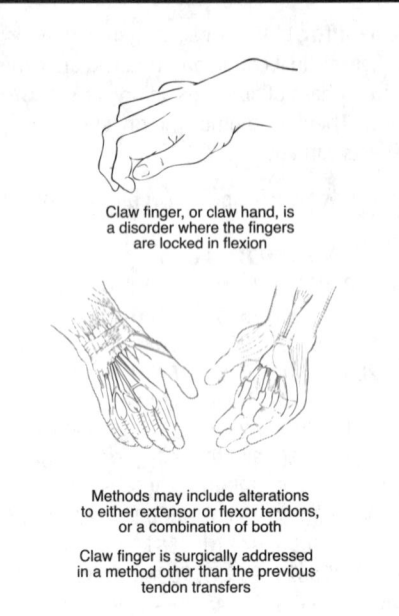

Methods may include alterations to either extensor or flexor tendons, or a combination of both

Claw finger is surgically addressed in a method other than the previous tendon transfers

Explanation

The physician corrects a claw finger. The superficialis technique involves splitting the flexor digitorum superficialis of the long finger into four slips. One slip is passed through the lumbrical canal of each finger to be inserted into the radial lateral band of the dorsal apparatus. This slip is sutured with the wrist in 30 degrees palmar flexion, the MP joints in 80 to 90 degree flexion, and the interphalangeal joints in full extension. In the dorsal approach, the tendon slips of the extensor carpi radialis brevis are passed superficial to the dorsal carpal ligament, through the intermetacarpal spaces, through the lumbrical canal volar to the deep transverse metacarpal ligament. The tendon is attached to the radial lateral bands of the long ring and little fingers and the ulnar lateral band of the index finger. A modification of the latter procedure involves detaching the extensor carpi radialis longus at its insertion and passing it deep to the brachioradialis to the volar sides of the forearm proximate to the wrist. The grafts of the plantaris or palmaris tendons are used. The lateral bands are identified through dorsoradial incisions over the proximal phalanx (except the index finger, which has the ulnar lateral band exposed). The tendon slips are directed through the carpal tunnel volar to the deep transverse metacarpal ligament and into the lateral bands. The tendons are sutured with the wrist dorsiflexed 45 degrees, the MP joints are flexed 70 degrees, and the interphalangeal joints are fixed at zero degrees. Incisions are closed.

Coding Tips

Some payers may require the use of HCPCS Level II modifiers FA–F9 to identify the specific finger involved. According to CPT guidelines, cast application or strapping (including removal) is only reported as a replacement procedure or when the cast application or strapping is an initial service performed without a restorative treatment or procedure. See "Application of Casts and Strapping" in the CPT book in the Surgery Section, under the Musculoskeletal system.

ICD-9-CM Procedural

80.44 Division of joint capsule, ligament, or cartilage of hand and finger
81.28 Interphalangeal fusion
82.55 Other change in muscle or tendon length of hand

Anesthesia
26499 01810

ICD-9-CM Diagnostic
736.06 Claw hand (acquired)

Terms To Know

claw hand deformity. Abnormal positioning of the hand and fingers usually associated with ulnar nerve palsy, in which the metacarpal phalangeal joints are hyperextended with concomitant flexion of the proximal and distal interphalangeal joints.

dorsal. Pertaining to the back or posterior aspect.

dorsiflexion. Position of being bent toward the extensor side of a limb.

fascia. Fibrous sheet or band of tissue that envelops organs, muscles, and groupings of muscles.

flexion. Act of bending or being bent.

flexor. Muscle/tendon that bends or flexes a limb or part as opposed to extending it.

proximal. Located closest to a specified reference point, usually the midline.

tendon. Fibrous tissue that connects muscle to bone, consisting primarily of collagen and containing little vasculature.

volar. Palm of the hand (palmar) or sole of the foot (plantar).

CCI Version 16.3

01810, 0213T, 0216T, 0228T, 0230T, 20526-20553, 25259, 26180❖, 26340, 26500-26502, 29075, 29086, 29130-29131, 29280, 36000, 36400-36410, 36420-36430, 36440, 36600, 36640, 37202, 43752, 51701-51703, 62310-62319, 64400-64435, 64445-64450, 64479, 64483, 64490, 64493, 64505-64530, 69990, 93000-93010, 93040-93042, 93318, 94002, 94200, 94250, 94680-94690, 94770, 95812-95816, 95819, 95822, 95829, 95955, 96360, 96365, 96372, 96374-96376, 99148-99149, 99150

Note: These CCI edits are used for Medicare. Other payers may reimburse on codes listed above.

Medicare Edits

	Fac RVU	Non-Fac RVU	FUD	Assist
26499	23.87	23.87	90	80

Medicare References: 100-2,15,260; 100-4,12,30; 100-4,12,90.3; 100-4,14,10

26500-26502

26500 Reconstruction of tendon pulley, each tendon; with local tissues (separate procedure)
26502 with tendon or fascial graft (includes obtaining graft) (separate procedure)

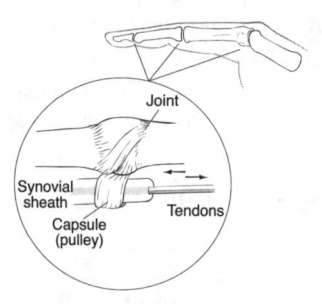

The main tendon pulleys occur at the metacarpophalangeal joint and the interphalangeal joints. However, as many as seven pulleys are described in certain texts

A tendon pulley is reconstructed using local tissues. Report 26502 when a tendon or fascial graft is used in the repair. Report 26504 when a tendon prosthesis is used in the repair

Explanation
The physician reconstructs a tendon pulley. The physician incises the overlying skin and dissects to the damaged pulley located in the A1 position or the distal interphalangeal joint position. In 26500, the tendon pulley is reconstructed using neighboring tissue. In 26502, the physician obtains a fascial graft for reconstruction.

Coding Tips
These separate procedures by definition are usually a component of a more complex service and are not identified separately. When performed alone or with other unrelated procedures/services, they may be reported. If performed alone, list the code; if performed with other procedures/services, list the code and append modifier 59. These codes are used once for each tendon repair performed. When multiple tendons are repaired, report one tendon as the primary procedure and append modifier 51 to subsequent procedures. In 26502, harvesting of a tendon graft is not reported separately. According to CPT guidelines, cast application or strapping (including removal) is only reported as a replacement procedure or when the cast application or strapping is an initial service performed without a restorative treatment or procedure. See "Application of Casts and Strapping" in the CPT book in the Surgery section, under the musculoskeletal system.

ICD-9-CM Procedural
- 82.71 Tendon pulley reconstruction on hand
- 82.79 Plastic operation on hand with other graft or implant
- 83.83 Tendon pulley reconstruction on muscle, tendon, and fascia

Anesthesia
01810

ICD-9-CM Diagnostic
- 138 Late effects of acute poliomyelitis — (Note: This category is to be used to indicate conditions classifiable to 045 as the cause of late effects, which are themselves classified elsewhere. The "late effects" include those specified as such, as sequelae, or as due to old or inactive poliomyelitis, without evidence of active disease.)
- 344.89 Other specified paralytic syndrome
- 715.14 Primary localized osteoarthrosis, hand
- 718.44 Contracture of hand joint
- 718.84 Other joint derangement, not elsewhere classified, hand
- 727.64 Nontraumatic rupture of flexor tendons of hand and wrist
- 727.89 Other disorders of synovium, tendon, and bursa
- 816.00 Closed fracture of unspecified phalanx or phalanges of hand
- 816.01 Closed fracture of middle or proximal phalanx or phalanges of hand
- 816.02 Closed fracture of distal phalanx or phalanges of hand
- 816.03 Closed fracture of multiple sites of phalanx or phalanges of hand
- 816.10 Open fracture of phalanx or phalanges of hand, unspecified
- 816.11 Open fracture of middle or proximal phalanx or phalanges of hand
- 816.12 Open fracture of distal phalanx or phalanges of hand
- 816.13 Open fractures of multiple sites of phalanx or phalanges of hand
- 842.13 Sprain and strain of interphalangeal (joint) of hand
- 883.2 Open wound of finger(s), with tendon involvement
- 886.1 Traumatic amputation of other finger(s) (complete) (partial), complicated
- 905.2 Late effect of fracture of upper extremities
- 905.8 Late effect of tendon injury
- 905.9 Late effect of traumatic amputation
- 927.3 Crushing injury of finger(s) — (Use additional code to identify any associated injuries: 800-829, 850.0-854.1, 860.0-869.1)

Terms To Know
contracture. Shortening of muscle or connective tissue.

late effect. Abnormality, dysfunction, or other residual condition produced after the acute phase of an illness, injury, or disease is over. There is no time limit on when late effects can appear.

tendon. Fibrous tissue that connects muscle to bone, consisting primarily of collagen and containing little vasculature.

CCI Version 16.3
01810, 0213T, 0216T, 0228T, 0230T, 20526-20553, 25259, 26185, 26340, 29075, 29086, 29130-29131, 29280, 36000, 36400-36410, 36420-36430, 36440, 36600, 36640, 37202, 43752, 51701-51703, 62310-62319, 64400-64435, 64445-64450, 64479, 64483, 64490, 64493, 64505-64530, 69990, 93000-93010, 93040-93042, 93318, 94002, 94200, 94250, 94680-94690, 94770, 95812-95816, 95819, 95822, 95829, 95955, 96360, 96365, 96372, 96374-96376, 99148-99149, 99150

Also not with 26500: 64718

Also not with 26502: 20920-20926

Note: These CCI edits are used for Medicare. Other payers may reimburse on codes listed above.

Medicare Edits

	Fac RVU	Non-Fac RVU	FUD	Assist
26500	18.07	18.07	90	80
26502	20.57	20.57	90	80

Medicare References: 100-2,15,260; 100-4,12,30; 100-4,12,90.3; 100-4,14,10

26508

26508 Release of thenar muscle(s) (eg, thumb contracture)

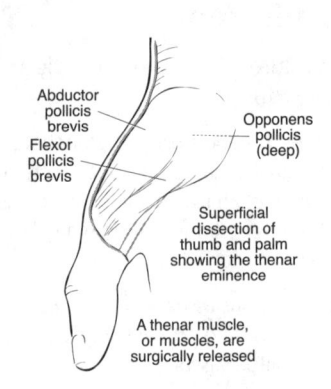

Abductor pollicis brevis
Flexor pollicis brevis
Opponens pollicis (deep)
Superficial dissection of thumb and palm showing the thenar eminence
A thenar muscle, or muscles, are surgically released

The thenar muscles are the abductor pollicis brevis, the opponens pollicis, and the flexor pollicis brevis

Explanation
The physician incises the thenar muscle to release, for example, thumb contracture. The physician incises the overlying skin and dissects to the thenar muscle. The scarred muscle tissue is incised to release contracture. The incision is sutured in layers.

Coding Tips
According to CPT guidelines, cast application or strapping (including removal) is only reported as a replacement procedure or when the cast application or strapping is an initial service performed without a restorative treatment or procedure. See "Application of Casts and Strapping" in the CPT book in the Surgery Section, under the Musculoskeletal system.

ICD-9-CM Procedural
82.19 Other division of soft tissue of hand

Anesthesia
26508 01810

ICD-9-CM Diagnostic
344.89 Other specified paralytic syndrome
357.1 Polyneuropathy in collagen vascular disease — (Code first underlying disease: 446.0, 710.0, 714.0)
359.6 Symptomatic inflammatory myopathy in diseases classified elsewhere — (Code first underlying disease: 135, 140.0-208.9, 277.30-277.39, 446.0, 710.0, 710.1, 710.2, 714.0)
446.0 Polyarteritis nodosa
710.0 Systemic lupus erythematosus — (Use additional code to identify manifestation: 424.91, 581.81, 582.81, 583.81)
710.1 Systemic sclerosis — (Use additional code to identify manifestation: 359.6, 517.2)
710.2 Sicca syndrome
714.0 Rheumatoid arthritis — (Use additional code to identify manifestation: 357.1, 359.6)
715.14 Primary localized osteoarthrosis, hand
718.44 Contracture of hand joint
728.2 Muscular wasting and disuse atrophy, not elsewhere classified
728.88 Rhabdomyolysis
728.89 Other disorder of muscle, ligament, and fascia — (Use additional E code to identify drug, if drug-induced)
736.29 Other acquired deformity of finger
905.8 Late effect of tendon injury
906.4 Late effect of crushing
906.6 Late effect of burn of wrist and hand
909.3 Late effect of complications of surgical and medical care
958.6 Volkmann's ischemic contracture

Terms To Know

atrophy. Reduction in size or activity in an anatomic structure, due to wasting away from disease or other factors.

late effect. Abnormality, dysfunction, or other residual condition produced after the acute phase of an illness, injury, or disease is over. There is no time limit on when late effects can appear.

osteoarthrosis. Most common form of a noninflammatory degenerative joint disease with degenerating articular cartilage, bone enlargement, and synovial membrane changes.

Volkmann's contracture. Shortening of the muscles in the fingers or wrist due to injury near the elbow or vascular damage.

CCI Version 16.3
01810, 0213T, 0216T, 0228T, 0230T, 14040, 20526-20553, 25259, 26185, 26340, 26478, 29075, 29086, 29130-29131, 29280, 36000, 36400-36410, 36420-36430, 36440, 36600, 36640, 37202, 43752, 51701-51703, 62310-62319, 64400-64435, 64445-64450, 64479, 64483, 64490, 64493, 64505-64530, 69990, 93000-93010, 93040-93042, 93318, 94002, 94200, 94250, 94680-94690, 94770, 95812-95816, 95819, 95822, 95829, 95955, 96360, 96365, 96372, 96374-96376, 99148-99149, 99150

Note: These CCI edits are used for Medicare. Other payers may reimburse on codes listed above.

Medicare Edits

	Fac RVU	Non-Fac RVU	FUD	Assist
26508	18.14	18.14	90	80

Medicare References: 100-2,15,260; 100-4,12,30; 100-4,12,90.3; 100-4,14,10

26510

26510 Cross intrinsic transfer, each tendon

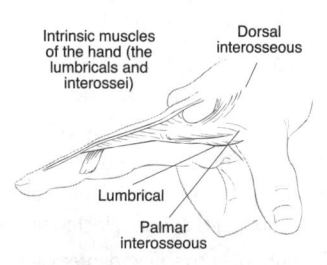

A cross intrinsic transfer is performed. Intrinsic muscles of a finger are incised and their insertions relocated to improve finger function

Explanation

The physician performs a cross intrinsic transfer to restore anatomic position and intrinsic function to the fingers. The physician incises the overlying skin and dissects to the affected tendons. The ulnar tendon is resected and transferred to the radial side of the joint, where it is sutured into place. The incision is sutured in layers.

Coding Tips

According to CPT guidelines, cast application or strapping (including removal) is only reported as a replacement procedure or when the cast application or strapping is an initial service performed without a restorative treatment or procedure. See "Application of Casts and Strapping" in the CPT book in the Surgery section, under the musculoskeletal system.

ICD-9-CM Procedural

83.75 Tendon transfer or transplantation

Anesthesia

26510 01810

ICD-9-CM Diagnostic

- 344.89 Other specified paralytic syndrome
- 357.1 Polyneuropathy in collagen vascular disease — (Code first underlying disease: 446.0, 710.0, 714.0)
- 359.6 Symptomatic inflammatory myopathy in diseases classified elsewhere — (Code first underlying disease: 135, 140.0-208.9, 277.30-277.39, 446.0, 710.0, 710.1, 710.2, 714.0)
- 446.0 Polyarteritis nodosa
- 710.0 Systemic lupus erythematosus — (Use additional code to identify manifestation: 424.91, 581.81, 582.81, 583.81)
- 710.1 Systemic sclerosis — (Use additional code to identify manifestation: 359.6, 517.2)
- 710.2 Sicca syndrome
- 714.0 Rheumatoid arthritis — (Use additional code to identify manifestation: 357.1, 359.6)
- 715.14 Primary localized osteoarthrosis, hand
- 718.44 Contracture of hand joint
- 727.63 Nontraumatic rupture of extensor tendons of hand and wrist
- 727.64 Nontraumatic rupture of flexor tendons of hand and wrist
- 728.2 Muscular wasting and disuse atrophy, not elsewhere classified
- 728.88 Rhabdomyolysis
- 728.89 Other disorder of muscle, ligament, and fascia — (Use additional E code to identify drug, if drug-induced)
- 842.12 Sprain and strain of metacarpophalangeal (joint) of hand
- 883.2 Open wound of finger(s), with tendon involvement
- 886.1 Traumatic amputation of other finger(s) (complete) (partial), complicated
- 905.8 Late effect of tendon injury
- 905.9 Late effect of traumatic amputation
- 906.4 Late effect of crushing
- 906.6 Late effect of burn of wrist and hand
- 927.3 Crushing injury of finger(s) — (Use additional code to identify any associated injuries: 800-829, 850.0-854.1, 860.0-869.1)
- 958.6 Volkmann's ischemic contracture

Terms To Know

contracture. Shortening of muscle or connective tissue.

dissection. Separating by cutting tissue or body structures apart.

dorsal. Pertaining to the back or posterior aspect.

CCI Version 16.3

01810, 0213T, 0216T, 0228T, 0230T, 20526-20553, 25259, 26170-26185, 26340, 26480, 29075, 29086, 29125, 29130-29131, 29280, 36000, 36400-36410, 36420-36430, 36440, 36600, 36640, 37202, 43752, 51701-51703, 62310-62319, 64400-64435, 64445-64450, 64479, 64483, 64490, 64493, 64505-64530, 69990, 93000-93010, 93040-93042, 93318, 94002, 94200, 94250, 94680-94690, 94770, 95812-95816, 95819, 95822, 95829, 95955, 96360, 96365, 96372, 96374-96376, 99148-99149, 99150

Note: These CCI edits are used for Medicare. Other payers may reimburse on codes listed above.

Medicare Edits

	Fac RVU	Non-Fac RVU	FUD	Assist
26510	17.14	17.14	90	80

Medicare References: 100-2,15,260; 100-4,12,30; 100-4,12,90.3; 100-4,14,10

26516-26518

26516 Capsulodesis, metacarpophalangeal joint; single digit
26517 2 digits
26518 3 or 4 digits

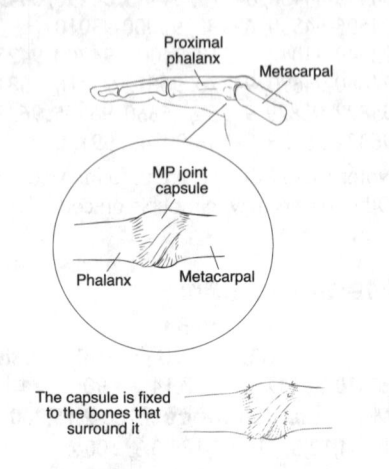

A metacarpophalangeal (MP) joint capsule is sutured to surrounding bone (capsulodesis). Report 26517 when two digits are addressed. Report 26518 when three or four digits are addressed

Explanation

The physician performs a capsulodesis to stabilize the metacarpophalangeal joint. The physician incises the overlying skin and dissects to the MP joint. The capsule of the joint is sutured to the proximal and distal bones to stabilize the joint. The operative incision is closed in sutured layers. In 26516, one digit is repaired. In 26517, two digits are repaired. In 26518, three or four digits are repaired.

Coding Tips

According to CPT guidelines, cast application or strapping (including removal) is only reported as a replacement procedure or when the cast application or strapping is an initial service performed without a restorative treatment or procedure. See "Application of Casts and Strapping" in the CPT book in the Surgery Section, under the Musculoskeletal system.

ICD-9-CM Procedural

81.29 Arthrodesis of other specified joint

Anesthesia
01810

ICD-9-CM Diagnostic

- **343.0** Diplegic infantile cerebral palsy
- **343.1** Hemiplegic infantile cerebral palsy
- **343.2** Quadriplegic infantile cerebral palsy
- **343.3** Monoplegic infantile cerebral palsy
- **343.4** Infantile hemiplegia
- **343.8** Other specified infantile cerebral palsy
- **343.9** Unspecified infantile cerebral palsy
- **344.81** Locked-in state
- **344.89** Other specified paralytic syndrome
- **357.1** Polyneuropathy in collagen vascular disease — (Code first underlying disease: 446.0, 710.0, 714.0)
- **359.6** Symptomatic inflammatory myopathy in diseases classified elsewhere — (Code first underlying disease: 135, 140.0-208.9, 277.30-277.39, 446.0, 710.0, 710.1, 710.2, 714.0)
- **446.0** Polyarteritis nodosa
- **710.0** Systemic lupus erythematosus — (Use additional code to identify manifestation: 424.91, 581.81, 582.81, 583.81)
- **710.1** Systemic sclerosis — (Use additional code to identify manifestation: 359.6, 517.2)
- **710.2** Sicca syndrome
- **714.0** Rheumatoid arthritis — (Use additional code to identify manifestation: 357.1, 359.6)
- **715.14** Primary localized osteoarthrosis, hand
- **718.44** Contracture of hand joint
- **718.74** Developmental dislocation of joint, hand
- **718.84** Other joint derangement, not elsewhere classified, hand
- **719.94** Unspecified disorder of hand joint
- **728.2** Muscular wasting and disuse atrophy, not elsewhere classified
- **728.88** Rhabdomyolysis
- **728.89** Other disorder of muscle, ligament, and fascia — (Use additional E code to identify drug, if drug-induced)
- **736.06** Claw hand (acquired)
- **834.11** Open dislocation of metacarpophalangeal (joint)
- **882.1** Open wound of hand except finger(s) alone, complicated
- **882.2** Open wound of hand except finger(s) alone, with tendon involvement
- **883.1** Open wound of finger(s), complicated
- **883.2** Open wound of finger(s), with tendon involvement
- **886.1** Traumatic amputation of other finger(s) (complete) (partial), complicated
- **906.1** Late effect of open wound of extremities without mention of tendon injury
- **906.4** Late effect of crushing
- **906.6** Late effect of burn of wrist and hand
- **927.20** Crushing injury of hand(s) — (Use additional code to identify any associated injuries: 800-829, 850.0-854.1, 860.0-869.1)
- **927.3** Crushing injury of finger(s) — (Use additional code to identify any associated injuries: 800-829, 850.0-854.1, 860.0-869.1)
- **944.04** Burn of unspecified degree of two or more digits of hand, including thumb
- **944.08** Burn of unspecified degree of multiple sites of wrist(s) and hand(s)
- **944.42** Deep necrosis of underlying tissues due to burn (deep third degree) of thumb (nail), without mention of loss of a body part
- **955.4** Injury to musculocutaneous nerve
- **958.6** Volkmann's ischemic contracture

CCI Version 16.3

01810, 0213T, 0216T, 0228T, 0230T, 20526-20553, 25259, 26185, 26340, 26500-26502, 29075, 29086, 29130-29131, 29280, 36000, 36400-36410, 36420-36430, 36440, 36600, 36640, 37202, 43752, 51701-51703, 62310-62319, 64400-64435, 64445-64450, 64479, 64483, 64490, 64493, 64505-64530, 69990, 93000-93010, 93040-93042, 93318, 94002, 94200, 94250, 94680-94690, 94770, 95812-95816, 95819, 95822, 95829, 95955, 96360, 96365, 96372, 96374-96376, 99148-99149, 99150

Note: These CCI edits are used for Medicare. Other payers may reimburse on codes listed above.

Medicare Edits

	Fac RVU	Non-Fac RVU	FUD	Assist
26516	20.17	20.17	90	80
26517	23.78	23.78	90	80
26518	24.2	24.2	90	80

Medicare References: 100-2,15,260; 100-4,12,30; 100-4,12,90.3; 100-4,14,10

26520-26525

26520 Capsulectomy or capsulotomy; metacarpophalangeal joint, each joint
26525 interphalangeal joint, each joint

Explanation

The physician removes or incises the joint capsule to release contracture and restore function. The physician incises the overlying skin and dissects to the metacarpophalangeal joint. The capsule of the joint is incised or resected and removed. The operative incision is closed in sutured layers. In 26520, the capsulectomy or capsulotomy is performed on the metacarpophalangeal joint. In 26525, the capsulectomy or capsulotomy is performed on the interphalangeal joint. Report each joint separately.

Coding Tips

These codes are used once for each joint. When capsulectomy or capsulotomy is performed on multiple joints, report one capsulectomy/capsulotomy as the primary procedure and append modifier 51 to subsequent procedures. For 26525, some payers may require the use of HCPCS Level II modifiers FA–F9 to identify the specific finger involved. According to CPT guidelines, cast application or strapping (including removal) is only reported as a replacement procedure or when the cast application or strapping is an initial service performed without a restorative treatment or procedure. See "Application of Casts and Strapping" in the CPT book in the Surgery Section, under the Musculoskeletal system. For carpometacarpal joint arthroplasty, see 25447.

ICD-9-CM Procedural

- 80.44 Division of joint capsule, ligament, or cartilage of hand and finger
- 80.94 Other excision of joint of hand and finger

Anesthesia

- **26520** 01810
- **26525** 01830

ICD-9-CM Diagnostic

- 357.1 Polyneuropathy in collagen vascular disease — (Code first underlying disease: 446.0, 710.0, 714.0)
- 359.6 Symptomatic inflammatory myopathy in diseases classified elsewhere — (Code first underlying disease: 135, 140.0-208.9, 277.30-277.39, 446.0, 710.0, 710.1, 710.2, 714.0)
- 446.0 Polyarteritis nodosa
- 710.0 Systemic lupus erythematosus — (Use additional code to identify manifestation: 424.91, 581.81, 582.81, 583.81)
- 710.1 Systemic sclerosis — (Use additional code to identify manifestation: 359.6, 517.2)
- 710.2 Sicca syndrome
- 714.0 Rheumatoid arthritis — (Use additional code to identify manifestation: 357.1, 359.6)
- 714.4 Chronic postrheumatic arthropathy
- 715.14 Primary localized osteoarthrosis, hand
- 716.14 Traumatic arthropathy, hand
- 718.44 Contracture of hand joint
- 719.54 Stiffness of joint, not elsewhere classified, hand
- 728.89 Other disorder of muscle, ligament, and fascia — (Use additional E code to identify drug, if drug-induced)
- 736.20 Unspecified deformity of finger
- 736.29 Other acquired deformity of finger
- 756.89 Other specified congenital anomaly of muscle, tendon, fascia, and connective tissue
- 906.4 Late effect of crushing
- 959.5 Injury, other and unspecified, finger
- 996.92 Complications of reattached hand
- 996.93 Complications of reattached finger(s)
- 998.59 Other postoperative infection — (Use additional code to identify infection)

Terms To Know

contracture. Shortening of muscle or connective tissue.

CCI Version 16.3

01810, 0213T, 0216T, 0228T, 0230T, 11900, 20526-20553, 25259, 26185, 26340, 26440-26442, 26502, 29075, 29086, 29130-29131, 29280, 36000, 36400-36410, 36420-36430, 36440, 36600, 36640, 37202, 43752, 51701-51703, 62310-62319, 64400-64435, 64445-64450, 64479, 64483, 64490, 64493, 64505-64530, 69990, 93000-93010, 93040-93042, 93318, 94002, 94200, 94250, 94680-94690, 94770, 95812-95816, 95819, 95822, 95829, 95955, 96360, 96365, 96372, 96374-96376, 99148-99149, 99150

Also not with 26520: 26055, 26075, 26145-26160, 26593, 29900-29902

Also not with 26525: 26080, 26160, 76000-76001

Note: These CCI edits are used for Medicare. Other payers may reimburse on codes listed above.

Medicare Edits

	Fac RVU	Non-Fac RVU	FUD	Assist
26520	18.8	18.8	90	N/A
26525	18.81	18.81	90	N/A

Medicare References: 100-2,15,260; 100-4,12,30; 100-4,12,90.3; 100-4,14,10

26530-26531

26530 Arthroplasty, metacarpophalangeal joint; each joint
26531 with prosthetic implant, each joint

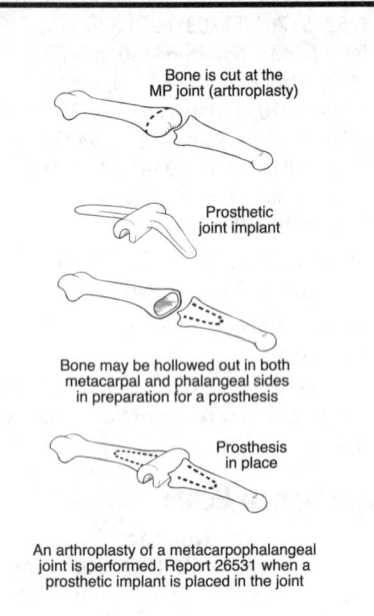

An arthroplasty of a metacarpophalangeal joint is performed. Report 26531 when a prosthetic implant is placed in the joint

Explanation

The physician performs an arthroplasty on the metacarpophalangeal joint. The physician incises the overlying skin and dissects to the MP joint. In 26530, the joint is reconstructed using neighboring tissue. In 26531, a prosthetic joint is used to replace the diseased joint. Report each joint separately.

Coding Tips

These codes are used once for each arthroplasty performed. When arthroplasty is performed on multiple joints, report one procedure as the primary procedure and append modifier 51 to subsequent procedures. According to CPT guidelines, cast application or strapping (including removal) is only reported as a replacement procedure or when the cast application or strapping is an initial service performed without a restorative treatment or procedure. See "Application of Casts and Strapping" in the CPT book in the Surgery Section, under the Musculoskeletal system.

ICD-9-CM Procedural

- 81.71 Arthroplasty of metacarpophalangeal and interphalangeal joint with implant
- 81.72 Arthroplasty of metacarpophalangeal and interphalangeal joint without implant

Anesthesia

01830

ICD-9-CM Diagnostic

- 357.1 Polyneuropathy in collagen vascular disease — (Code first underlying disease: 446.0, 710.0, 714.0)
- 359.6 Symptomatic inflammatory myopathy in diseases classified elsewhere — (Code first underlying disease: 135, 140.0-208.9, 277.30-277.39, 446.0, 710.0, 710.1, 710.2, 714.0)
- 446.0 Polyarteritis nodosa
- 710.0 Systemic lupus erythematosus — (Use additional code to identify manifestation: 424.91, 581.81, 582.81, 583.81)
- 710.1 Systemic sclerosis — (Use additional code to identify manifestation: 359.6, 517.2)
- 710.2 Sicca syndrome
- 714.0 Rheumatoid arthritis — (Use additional code to identify manifestation: 357.1, 359.6)
- 714.4 Chronic postrheumatic arthropathy
- 715.14 Primary localized osteoarthrosis, hand
- 715.94 Osteoarthrosis, unspecified whether generalized or localized, hand
- 716.14 Traumatic arthropathy, hand
- 718.04 Articular cartilage disorder, hand
- 718.74 Developmental dislocation of joint, hand
- 730.14 Chronic osteomyelitis, hand — (Use additional code to identify organism: 041.1. Use additional code to identify major osseous defect, if applicable: 731.3)
- 731.3 Major osseous defects — (Code first underlying disease: 170.0-170.9, 730.00-730.29, 733.00-733.09, 733.40-733.49, 996.45)
- 733.82 Nonunion of fracture
- 815.02 Closed fracture of base of other metacarpal bone(s)
- 815.12 Open fracture of base of other metacarpal bone(s)
- 834.01 Closed dislocation of metacarpophalangeal (joint)
- 834.11 Open dislocation of metacarpophalangeal (joint)
- 882.1 Open wound of hand except finger(s) alone, complicated
- 882.2 Open wound of hand except finger(s) alone, with tendon involvement
- 905.2 Late effect of fracture of upper extremities
- 927.20 Crushing injury of hand(s) — (Use additional code to identify any associated injuries: 800-829, 850.0-854.1, 860.0-869.1)
- 927.3 Crushing injury of finger(s) — (Use additional code to identify any associated injuries: 800-829, 850.0-854.1, 860.0-869.1)

Terms To Know

nonunion. Failure of two ends of a fracture to mend or completely heal.

primary localized osteoarthrosis. Degenerative joint disease confined to a specific area.

CCI Version 16.3

01810, 0213T, 0216T, 0228T, 0230T, 20526-20553, 25259, 26075, 26105, 26135, 26185, 26210-26215, 26235-26236, 26340, 26437, 26520, 26593, 26715, 26746, 29075, 29130-29131, 29280, 29900-29902, 36000, 36400-36410, 36420-36430, 36440, 36600, 36640, 37202, 43752, 51701-51703, 62310-62319, 64400-64435, 64445-64450, 64479, 64483, 64490, 64493, 64505-64530, 69990, 93000-93010, 93040-93042, 93318, 94002, 94200, 94250, 94680-94690, 94770, 95812-95816, 95819, 95822, 95829, 95955, 96360, 96365, 96372, 96374-96376, 99148-99149, 99150

Also not with 26530: 26055, 26410, 26418, 26480, 29086

Also not with 26531: 26410-26412, 26418-26420, 26449, 26852❖, 29086-29125

Note: These CCI edits are used for Medicare. Other payers may reimburse on codes listed above.

Medicare Edits

	Fac RVU	Non-Fac RVU	FUD	Assist
26530	15.52	15.52	90	80
26531	18.06	18.06	90	80

Medicare References: 100-2,15,260; 100-4,12,30; 100-4,12,90.3; 100-4,14,10

26535-26536

26535 Arthroplasty, interphalangeal joint; each joint
26536 with prosthetic implant, each joint

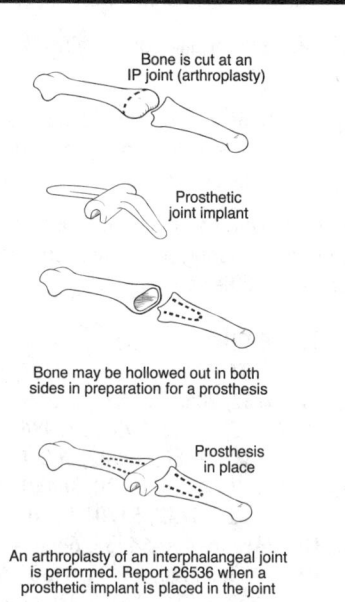

An arthroplasty of an interphalangeal joint is performed. Report 26536 when a prosthetic implant is placed in the joint.

Explanation

The physician performs an arthroplasty on the interphalangeal joint. The physician incises the overlying skin and dissects to the IP joint. In 26535, the joint is reconstructed using neighboring tissue. In 26536, a prosthetic joint is used to replace the diseased joint. Report each joint separately.

Coding Tips

These codes are used once for each arthroplasty performed. When arthroplasty is performed on multiple joints, report one procedure as the primary procedure and append modifier 51 to subsequent procedures. Some payers may require the use of HCPCS Level II modifiers FA–F9 to identify the specific finger involved. According to CPT guidelines, cast application or strapping (including removal) is only reported as a replacement procedure or when the cast application or strapping is an initial service performed without a restorative treatment or procedure. See "Application of Casts and Strapping" in the CPT book in the Surgery Section, under the Musculoskeletal system.

ICD-9-CM Procedural

81.71 Arthroplasty of metacarpophalangeal and interphalangeal joint with implant
81.72 Arthroplasty of metacarpophalangeal and interphalangeal joint without implant

Anesthesia
01830

ICD-9-CM Diagnostic

357.1 Polyneuropathy in collagen vascular disease — (Code first underlying disease: 446.0, 710.0, 714.0)
359.6 Symptomatic inflammatory myopathy in diseases classified elsewhere — (Code first underlying disease: 135, 140.0-208.9, 277.30-277.39, 446.0, 710.0, 710.1, 710.2, 714.0)
446.0 Polyarteritis nodosa
710.0 Systemic lupus erythematosus — (Use additional code to identify manifestation: 424.91, 581.81, 582.81, 583.81)
710.1 Systemic sclerosis — (Use additional code to identify manifestation: 359.6, 517.2)
710.2 Sicca syndrome
714.0 Rheumatoid arthritis — (Use additional code to identify manifestation: 357.1, 359.6)
714.4 Chronic postrheumatic arthropathy
715.14 Primary localized osteoarthrosis, hand
715.94 Osteoarthrosis, unspecified whether generalized or localized, hand
716.14 Traumatic arthropathy, hand
718.44 Contracture of hand joint
718.74 Developmental dislocation of joint, hand
730.14 Chronic osteomyelitis, hand — (Use additional code to identify organism: 041.1. Use additional code to identify major osseous defect, if applicable: 731.3)
731.3 Major osseous defects — (Code first underlying disease: 170.0-170.9, 730.00-730.29, 733.00-733.09, 733.40-733.49, 996.45)
736.29 Other acquired deformity of finger
816.11 Open fracture of middle or proximal phalanx or phalanges of hand
816.12 Open fracture of distal phalanx or phalanges of hand
816.13 Open fractures of multiple sites of phalanx or phalanges of hand
817.1 Multiple open fractures of hand bones
834.02 Closed dislocation of interphalangeal (joint), hand
834.12 Open dislocation interphalangeal (joint), hand
883.1 Open wound of finger(s), complicated
883.2 Open wound of finger(s), with tendon involvement
905.2 Late effect of fracture of upper extremities
905.9 Late effect of traumatic amputation
906.4 Late effect of crushing
927.3 Crushing injury of finger(s) — (Use additional code to identify any associated injuries: 800-829, 850.0-854.1, 860.0-869.1)

Terms To Know

contracture. Shortening of muscle or connective tissue.

osteomyelitis. Inflammation of bone that may remain localized or spread to the marrow, cortex, or periosteum, in response to an infecting organism, usually bacterial and pyogenic.

CCI Version 16.3

01810, 0213T, 0216T, 0228T, 0230T, 20526-20553, 25259, 26080, 26110, 26140, 26185, 26210-26215, 26235-26236, 26340, 26437, 26545, 26548, 26593, 26735, 26746, 26765, 26785, 29075, 29086, 29130-29131, 29280, 36000, 36400-36410, 36420-36430, 36440, 36600, 36640, 37202, 43752, 51701-51703, 62310-62319, 64400-64435, 64445-64450, 64479, 64483, 64490, 64493, 64505-64530, 69990, 93000-93010, 93040-93042, 93318, 94002, 94200, 94250, 94680-94690, 94770, 95812-95816, 95819, 95822, 95829, 95955, 96360, 96365, 96372, 96374-96376, 99148-99149, 99150

Also not with 26535: 26160, 26410, 26418, 26525, 29125

Also not with 26536: 26055, 26410-26412, 26418-26420, 26520-26525

Note: These CCI edits are used for Medicare. Other payers may reimburse on codes listed above.

Medicare Edits

	Fac RVU	Non-Fac RVU	FUD	Assist
26535	11.79	11.79	90	N/A
26536	19.92	19.92	90	80

Medicare References: 100-2,15,260; 100-4,12,30; 100-4,12,90.3; 100-4,14,10

26540

26540 Repair of collateral ligament, metacarpophalangeal or interphalangeal joint

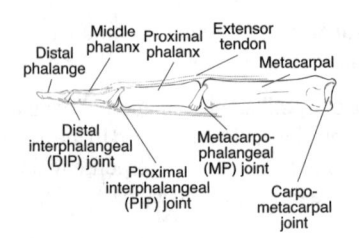

Collateral ligaments occur on both sides of the joint capsule. The structure is similar for the interphalangeal joints and the metacarpophalangeal joint

Explanation
The physician performs a primary repair on a collateral ligament of a metacarpophalangeal joint, possibly using a graft or advancement. The physician incises the overlying the skin and dissects to the MP joint. In 26540, the ligament is repaired with sutures.

Coding Tips
If significant additional time and effort is documented, append modifier 22 and submit a cover letter and operative report. Code 26540 should be reported for each collateral ligament in the metacarpophalangeal or interphalangeal joint repaired. When repair is performed on multiple joints, report one procedure as the primary procedure and append modifier 51 to subsequent procedures. According to CPT guidelines, cast application or strapping (including removal) is only reported as a replacement procedure or when the cast application or strapping is an initial service performed without a restorative treatment or procedure. See "Application of Casts and Strapping" in the CPT book in the Surgery Section, under the Musculoskeletal system. For reconstruction of the collateral ligament in the metacarpophalangeal joint with a tendon or facial graft, see 26541–26542. For reconstruction of the collateral joint of the interphalangeal joint, see 26545.

ICD-9-CM Procedural
81.93 Suture of capsule or ligament of upper extremity

Anesthesia
26540 01810

ICD-9-CM Diagnostic
- 716.14 Traumatic arthropathy, hand
- 718.34 Recurrent dislocation of hand joint
- 718.74 Developmental dislocation of joint, hand
- 718.84 Other joint derangement, not elsewhere classified, hand
- 728.89 Other disorder of muscle, ligament, and fascia — (Use additional E code to identify drug, if drug-induced)
- 816.01 Closed fracture of middle or proximal phalanx or phalanges of hand
- 816.02 Closed fracture of distal phalanx or phalanges of hand
- 816.03 Closed fracture of multiple sites of phalanx or phalanges of hand
- 816.11 Open fracture of middle or proximal phalanx or phalanges of hand
- 816.12 Open fracture of distal phalanx or phalanges of hand
- 816.13 Open fractures of multiple sites of phalanx or phalanges of hand
- 834.01 Closed dislocation of metacarpophalangeal (joint)
- 834.02 Closed dislocation of interphalangeal (joint), hand
- 834.11 Open dislocation of metacarpophalangeal (joint)
- 834.12 Open dislocation interphalangeal (joint), hand
- 842.12 Sprain and strain of metacarpophalangeal (joint) of hand
- 842.13 Sprain and strain of interphalangeal (joint) of hand
- 882.1 Open wound of hand except finger(s) alone, complicated
- 882.2 Open wound of hand except finger(s) alone, with tendon involvement
- 883.1 Open wound of finger(s), complicated
- 883.2 Open wound of finger(s), with tendon involvement
- 927.3 Crushing injury of finger(s) — (Use additional code to identify any associated injuries: 800-829, 850.0-854.1, 860.0-869.1)

Terms To Know

fascia. Fibrous sheet or band of tissue that envelops organs, muscles, and groupings of muscles.

fracture. Break in bone or cartilage.

injury. Harm or damage sustained by the body.

ligament. Band or sheet of fibrous tissue that connects the articular surfaces of bones or supports visceral organs.

tendon. Fibrous tissue that connects muscle to bone, consisting primarily of collagen and containing little vasculature.

CCI Version 16.3
01810, 0213T, 0216T, 0228T, 0230T, 12042, 13131-13132, 20526-20553, 25259, 26185, 26340, 26502, 26746, 29075, 29086, 29125, 29130-29131, 29280, 29902, 36000, 36400-36410, 36420-36430, 36440, 36600, 36640, 37202, 43752, 51701-51703, 62310-62319, 64400-64435, 64445-64450, 64479, 64483, 64490, 64493, 64505-64530, 69990, 93000-93010, 93040-93042, 93318, 94002, 94200, 94250, 94680-94690, 94770, 95812-95816, 95819, 95822, 95829, 95955, 96360, 96365, 96372, 96374-96376, 99148-99149, 99150

Note: These CCI edits are used for Medicare. Other payers may reimburse on codes listed above.

Medicare Edits

	Fac RVU	Non-Fac RVU	FUD	Assist
26540	18.97	18.97	90	80

Medicare References: 100-2,15,260; 100-4,12,30; 100-4,12,90.3; 100-4,14,10

26541-26542

26541 Reconstruction, collateral ligament, metacarpophalangeal joint, single; with tendon or fascial graft (includes obtaining graft)

26542 with local tissue (eg, adductor advancement)

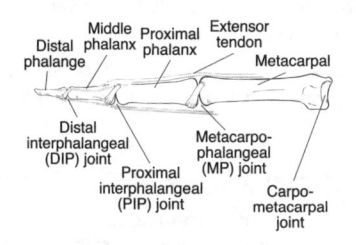

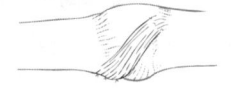

Explanation

The physician performs a primary repair on a collateral ligament of a metacarpophalangeal joint, possibly using a graft or advancement. The physician incises the overlying skin and dissects to the M-P joint. In 26541, a palmaris longus tendon or fascial graft is obtained. The graft is sutured into place. In 26542, an adductor tendon is advanced and sutured into place to stabilize the joint. The operative incision is closed in sutured layers.

Coding Tips

If significant additional time and effort is documented, append modifier 22 and submit a cover letter and operative report. Code 26541 or 26542 should be reported for each collateral ligament in the metacarpophalangeal joint repaired. When repair is performed on multiple joints, report one procedure as the primary procedure and append modifier 51 to subsequent procedures. According to CPT guidelines, cast application or strapping (including removal) is only reported as a replacement procedure or when the cast application or strapping is an initial service performed without a restorative treatment or procedure. See "Application of Casts and Strapping" in the CPT book in the Surgery section, under the musculoskeletal system. For repair of the collateral ligament, metacarpophalangeal joint, see 26540.

ICD-9-CM Procedural

- 81.93 Suture of capsule or ligament of upper extremity
- 82.72 Plastic operation on hand with graft of muscle or fascia
- 83.41 Excision of tendon for graft
- 83.81 Tendon graft

Anesthesia
01810

ICD-9-CM Diagnostic

- 716.14 Traumatic arthropathy, hand
- 718.34 Recurrent dislocation of hand joint
- 718.74 Developmental dislocation of joint, hand
- 718.84 Other joint derangement, not elsewhere classified, hand
- 728.89 Other disorder of muscle, ligament, and fascia — (Use additional E code to identify drug, if drug-induced)
- 816.01 Closed fracture of middle or proximal phalanx or phalanges of hand
- 816.02 Closed fracture of distal phalanx or phalanges of hand
- 816.03 Closed fracture of multiple sites of phalanx or phalanges of hand
- 816.11 Open fracture of middle or proximal phalanx or phalanges of hand
- 816.12 Open fracture of distal phalanx or phalanges of hand
- 816.13 Open fractures of multiple sites of phalanx or phalanges of hand
- 834.01 Closed dislocation of metacarpophalangeal (joint)
- 834.02 Closed dislocation of interphalangeal (joint), hand
- 834.11 Open dislocation of metacarpophalangeal (joint)
- 834.12 Open dislocation interphalangeal (joint), hand
- 842.12 Sprain and strain of metacarpophalangeal (joint) of hand
- 842.13 Sprain and strain of interphalangeal (joint) of hand
- 882.1 Open wound of hand except finger(s) alone, complicated
- 882.2 Open wound of hand except finger(s) alone, with tendon involvement
- 883.1 Open wound of finger(s), complicated
- 883.2 Open wound of finger(s), with tendon involvement
- 927.3 Crushing injury of finger(s) — (Use additional code to identify any associated injuries: 800-829, 850.0-854.1, 860.0-869.1)

Terms To Know

dislocation. Displacement of a bone in relation to its neighboring tissue, especially a joint.

CCI Version 16.3

01810, 0213T, 0216T, 0228T, 0230T, 20526-20553, 25259, 26185, 26340, 26502, 29075, 29086, 29130-29131, 29280, 29902, 36000, 36400-36410, 36420-36430, 36440, 36600, 36640, 37202, 43752, 51701-51703, 62310-62319, 64400-64435, 64445-64450, 64479, 64483, 64490, 64493, 64505-64530, 69990, 93000-93010, 93040-93042, 93318, 94002, 94200, 94250, 94680-94690, 94770, 95812-95816, 95819, 95822, 95829, 95955, 96360, 96365, 96372, 96374-96376, 99148-99149, 99150

Also not with 26541: 20920-20926, 26440, 26540, 76000-76001

Also not with 26542: 26480, 26531, 26593, 29125

Note: These CCI edits are used for Medicare. Other payers may reimburse on codes listed above.

Medicare Edits

	Fac RVU	Non-Fac RVU	FUD	Assist
26541	23.03	23.03	90	80
26542	19.64	19.64	90	80

Medicare References: 100-2,15,260; 100-4,12,30; 100-4,12,90.3; 100-4,14,10

26545

26545 Reconstruction, collateral ligament, interphalangeal joint, single, including graft, each joint

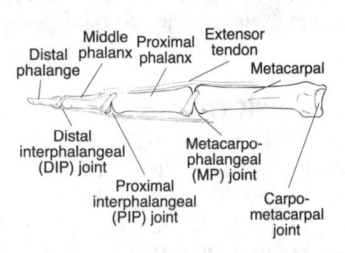

Collateral ligaments occur on both sides of the joint capsule. The structure is similar for the interphalangeal joints and the metacarpophalangeal joint

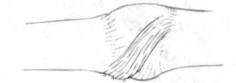

An MP collateral ligament is reconstructed using a tendon or fascial graft. Report 26545 when the reconstruction is on an interphalangeal joint, including graft

Explanation

The physician uses a graft to repair a collateral ligament of an interphalangeal joint. The physician incises the overlying the skin and dissects to the I-P joint. A palmaris longus tendon or fascial graft is obtained and sutured into place. to stabilize the joint. The incision is sutured in layers. Report each joint separately.

Coding Tips

If significant additional time and effort are documented, append modifier 22 and submit a cover letter and operative report. Code 26545 should be reported for each collateral ligament in the interphalangeal joint repaired. When repair is performed on multiple joints, report one procedure as the primary procedure and append modifier 51 to subsequent procedures. According to CPT guidelines, cast application or strapping (including removal) is only reported as a replacement procedure or when the cast application or strapping is an initial service performed without a restorative treatment or procedure. See "Application of Casts and Strapping" in the CPT book in the Surgery section, under the musculoskeletal system. For reconstruction of the collateral ligament of the metacarpophalangeal joint, 26541–26542.

ICD-9-CM Procedural

81.93 Suture of capsule or ligament of upper extremity

82.72 Plastic operation on hand with graft of muscle or fascia
83.41 Excision of tendon for graft
83.81 Tendon graft

Anesthesia
26545 01810

ICD-9-CM Diagnostic

716.14 Traumatic arthropathy, hand
718.34 Recurrent dislocation of hand joint
718.74 Developmental dislocation of joint, hand
718.84 Other joint derangement, not elsewhere classified, hand
728.89 Other disorder of muscle, ligament, and fascia — (Use additional E code to identify drug, if drug-induced)
816.01 Closed fracture of middle or proximal phalanx or phalanges of hand
816.02 Closed fracture of distal phalanx or phalanges of hand
816.03 Closed fracture of multiple sites of phalanx or phalanges of hand
816.11 Open fracture of middle or proximal phalanx or phalanges of hand
816.12 Open fracture of distal phalanx or phalanges of hand
816.13 Open fractures of multiple sites of phalanx or phalanges of hand
834.01 Closed dislocation of metacarpophalangeal (joint)
834.02 Closed dislocation of interphalangeal (joint), hand
834.11 Open dislocation of metacarpophalangeal (joint)
834.12 Open dislocation interphalangeal (joint), hand
842.12 Sprain and strain of metacarpophalangeal (joint) of hand
842.13 Sprain and strain of interphalangeal (joint) of hand
882.1 Open wound of hand except finger(s) alone, complicated
882.2 Open wound of hand except finger(s) alone, with tendon involvement
883.1 Open wound of finger(s), complicated
883.2 Open wound of finger(s), with tendon involvement
927.3 Crushing injury of finger(s) — (Use additional code to identify any associated injuries: 800-829, 850.0-854.1, 860.0-869.1)

CCI Version 16.3

01810, 0213T, 0216T, 0228T, 0230T, 20526-20553, 25259, 26185, 26340, 29075, 29086, 29130-29131, 29280, 36000, 36400-36410, 36420-36430, 36440, 36600, 36640, 37202, 43752, 51701-51703, 62310-62319, 64400-64435, 64445-64450, 64479, 64483, 64490, 64493, 64505-64530, 69990, 93000-93010, 93040-93042, 93318, 94002, 94200, 94250, 94680-94690, 94770, 95812-95816, 95819, 95822, 95829, 95955, 96360, 96365, 96372, 96374-96376, 99148-99149, 99150

Note: These CCI edits are used for Medicare. Other payers may reimburse on codes listed above.

Medicare Edits

	Fac RVU	Non-Fac RVU	FUD	Assist
26545	20.05	20.05	90	80

Medicare References: 100-2,15,260; 100-4,12,30; 100-4,12,90.3; 100-4,14,10

26546

26546 Repair non-union, metacarpal or phalanx (includes obtaining bone graft with or without external or internal fixation)

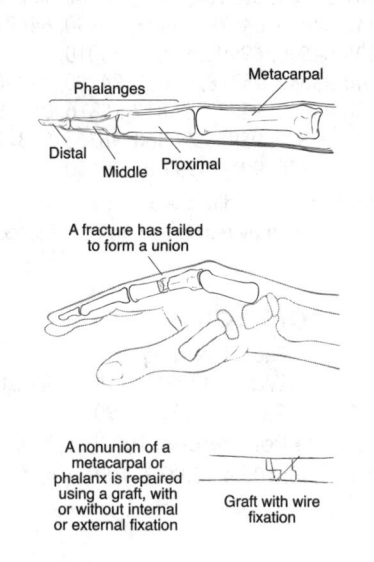

Explanation

The physician performs this procedure to promote healing of a fractured phalanx or metacarpal that fails to heal. The physician makes an incision overlying the dorsal aspect of the fracture of the digit. The extensor mechanism is retracted and the fracture is exposed. Surgical resection of the nonunion itself may be performed. If this resection takes place, fibrous tissue must be removed until there are freshened fracture ends. If a resultant gap produces unacceptable shortening, fixation such as Kirschner wires or pins or AO plates is applied. The physician closes the incision with sutures.

Coding Tips

Any bone graft harvest is not reported separately. According to CPT guidelines, cast application or strapping (including removal) is only reported as a replacement procedure or when the cast application or strapping is an initial service performed without a restorative treatment or procedure. See "Application of Casts and Strapping" in the CPT book in the Surgery Section, under the Musculoskeletal system.

ICD-9-CM Procedural

77.77	Excision of tibia and fibula for graft
77.78	Excision of tarsals and metatarsals for graft
77.99	Total ostectomy of other bone, except facial bones
78.09	Bone graft of other bone, except facial bones
78.44	Other repair or plastic operations on carpals and metacarpals
78.49	Other repair or plastic operations on other bone, except facial bones

Anesthesia

26546 01830

ICD-9-CM Diagnostic

733.82	Nonunion of fracture
905.2	Late effect of fracture of upper extremities

Terms To Know

dorsal. Pertaining to the back or posterior aspect.

extensor. Any muscle that extends a joint.

fibrous tissue. Connective tissues.

fracture. Break in bone or cartilage.

late effect. Abnormality, dysfunction, or other residual condition produced after the acute phase of an illness, injury, or disease is over. There is no time limit on when late effects can appear.

nonunion. Failure of two ends of a fracture to mend or completely heal.

CCI Version 16.3

01810, 0213T, 0216T, 0228T, 0230T, 11900-11901, 12001-12007, 12020-12047, 13120-13121, 13131-13132, 15852, 20500-20501, 20526-20553, 20680-20690, 20692, 20696-20697, 20900-20902, 25259, 26010-26030, 26034❖, 26055, 26070, 26121, 26130-26160, 26185-26205, 26210-26215, 26230-26236, 26340, 26358❖, 26392❖, 26516-26518, 26530, 26535, 29065-29131, 29260-29280, 35761, 36000, 36400-36410, 36420-36430, 36440, 36600, 36640, 37202, 37618, 43752, 51701-51703, 62310-62319, 64400-64435, 64445-64450, 64479, 64483, 64490, 64493, 64505-64560, 64565, 64573-64580, 64585-64595, 64702-64708, 64718-64726, 69990, 76000-76001, 76080, 77002, 87070, 87076-87077, 87102, 93000-93010, 93040-93042, 93318, 94002, 94200, 94250, 94680-94690, 94770, 95812-95816, 95819, 95822, 95829, 95860, 95900, 95955, 96360, 96365, 96372, 96374-96376, 99148-99149, 99150, G0168

Note: These CCI edits are used for Medicare. Other payers may reimburse on codes listed above.

Medicare Edits

	Fac RVU	Non-Fac RVU	FUD	Assist
26546	28.41	28.41	90	80

Medicare References: 100-2,15,260; 100-4,12,30; 100-4,12,90.3; 100-4,14,10

26548

26548 Repair and reconstruction, finger, volar plate, interphalangeal joint

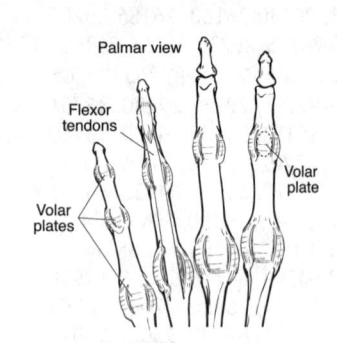

Palmar view
Flexor tendons
Volar plates
Volar plate

The volar plates are the bases of the fibrous sheaths that house the flexor tendons as they pass under the finger joints

An interphalangeal volar plate is repaired and reconstructed

Explanation

The physician repairs a volar plate of an interphalangeal joint. The physician incises the overlying skin and dissects to the IP joint. The plate of the joint is sutured to the proximal and distal bones to stabilize the joint. The operative incision is closed in sutured layers.

Coding Tips

Some payers may require the use of HCPCS Level II modifiers FA–F9 to identify the specific finger involved. According to CPT guidelines, cast application or strapping (including removal) is only reported as a replacement procedure or when the cast application or strapping is an initial service performed without a restorative treatment or procedure. See "Application of Casts and Strapping" in the CPT book in the Surgery Section, under the Musculoskeletal system.

ICD-9-CM Procedural

81.96 Other repair of joint

Anesthesia

26548 01810

ICD-9-CM Diagnostic

716.14 Traumatic arthropathy, hand
718.04 Articular cartilage disorder, hand
718.24 Pathological dislocation of hand joint
718.34 Recurrent dislocation of hand joint
718.74 Developmental dislocation of joint, hand
718.84 Other joint derangement, not elsewhere classified, hand
816.01 Closed fracture of middle or proximal phalanx or phalanges of hand
816.02 Closed fracture of distal phalanx or phalanges of hand
816.03 Closed fracture of multiple sites of phalanx or phalanges of hand
816.11 Open fracture of middle or proximal phalanx or phalanges of hand
816.12 Open fracture of distal phalanx or phalanges of hand
816.13 Open fractures of multiple sites of phalanx or phalanges of hand
834.02 Closed dislocation of interphalangeal (joint), hand
834.12 Open dislocation interphalangeal (joint), hand
842.13 Sprain and strain of interphalangeal (joint) of hand
883.2   Open wound of finger(s), with tendon involvement
905.9   Late effect of traumatic amputation
927.3   Crushing injury of finger(s) — (Use additional code to identify any associated injuries: 800-829, 850.0-854.1, 860.0-869.1)

Terms To Know

dislocation. Displacement of a bone in relation to its neighboring tissue, especially a joint.

distal. Located farther away from a specified reference point.

fracture. Break in bone or cartilage.

injury. Harm or damage sustained by the body.

late effect. Abnormality, dysfunction, or other residual condition produced after the acute phase of an illness, injury, or disease is over. There is no time limit on when late effects can appear.

proximal. Located closest to a specified reference point, usually the midline.

volar. Palm of the hand (palmar) or sole of the foot (plantar).

CCI Version 16.3

01810, 0213T, 0216T, 0228T, 0230T, 20526-20553, 25259, 26185, 26340, 26442, 26746, 29075, 29086, 29125, 29130-29131, 29280, 36000, 36400-36410, 36420-36430, 36440, 36600, 36640, 37202, 43752, 51701-51703, 62310-62319, 64400-64435, 64445-64450, 64479, 64483, 64490, 64493, 64505-64530, 69990, 93000-93010, 93040-93042, 93318, 94002, 94200, 94250, 94680-94690, 94770, 95812-95816, 95819, 95822, 95829, 95955, 96360, 96365, 96372, 96374-96376, 99148-99149, 99150

Note: These CCI edits are used for Medicare. Other payers may reimburse on codes listed above.

Medicare Edits

	Fac RVU	Non-Fac RVU	FUD	Assist
26548	22.03	22.03	90	80

Medicare References: 100-2,15,260; 100-4,12,30; 100-4,12,90.3; 100-4,14,10

26550

26550 Pollicization of a digit

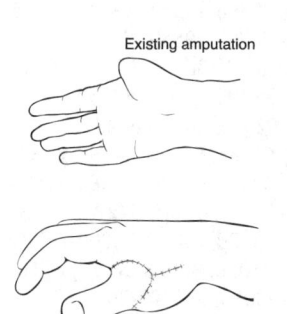

Existing amputation

Pollicized thumb

An amputated or absent thumb is reconstructed using a great toe, a forefinger, or other digit

Explanation

The physician replaces all or part of a thumb with the index finger. The extent of an index finger used is determined by the size of the defect. The physician harvests the index finger with its tendons, blood vessels, and nerves intact and transfers the digit to the thenar eminence. If the thenar eminence must be created, the physician will transfer the index metacarpal along with the digit. If the index metacarpal is not needed, it is removed to provide space for function. The tendons are sutured to the new digit to provide abduction function. The skin is reapproximated and closed in sutured layers.

Coding Tips

According to CPT guidelines, cast application or strapping (including removal) is only reported as a replacement procedure or when the cast application or strapping is an initial service performed without a restorative treatment or procedure. See "Application of Casts and Strapping" in the CPT book in the Surgery Section, under the Musculoskeletal system.

ICD-9-CM Procedural

82.61 Pollicization operation carrying over nerves and blood supply

Anesthesia

26550 01810

ICD-9-CM Diagnostic

755.29 Congenital longitudinal deficiency, phalanges, complete or partial
906.4 Late effect of crushing
906.6 Late effect of burn of wrist and hand
V10.81 Personal history of malignant neoplasm of bone
V49.61 Upper limb amputation, thumb
V49.62 Upper limb amputation, other finger(s)
V51.8 Other aftercare involving the use of plastic surgery

Terms To Know

abduction. Pulling away from a central reference line, such as moving away from the midline of the body.

late effect. Abnormality, dysfunction, or other residual condition produced after the acute phase of an illness, injury, or disease is over. There is no time limit on when late effects can appear.

malignant. Any condition tending to progress toward death, specifically an invasive tumor with a loss of cellular differentiation that has the ability to spread or metastasize to other areas in the body.

tendon. Fibrous tissue that connects muscle to bone, consisting primarily of collagen and containing little vasculature.

CCI Version 16.3

01810, 0213T, 0216T, 0228T, 0230T, 20526-20553, 25259, 26185, 26340, 29075, 29086, 29130-29131, 29280, 36000, 36400-36410, 36420-36430, 36440, 36600, 36640, 37202, 43752, 51701-51703, 62310-62319, 64400-64435, 64445-64450, 64479, 64483, 64490, 64493, 64505-64530, 69990, 93000-93010, 93040-93042, 93318, 94002, 94200, 94250, 94680-94690, 94770, 95812-95816, 95819, 95822, 95829, 95955, 96360, 96365, 96372, 96374-96376, 99148-99149, 99150

Note: These CCI edits are used for Medicare. Other payers may reimburse on codes listed above.

Medicare Edits

	Fac RVU	Non-Fac RVU	FUD	Assist
26550	45.66	45.66	90	80

Medicare References: 100-2,15,260; 100-4,12,30; 100-4,12,90.3; 100-4,14,10

26551

26551 Transfer, toe-to-hand with microvascular anastomosis; great toe wrap-around with bone graft

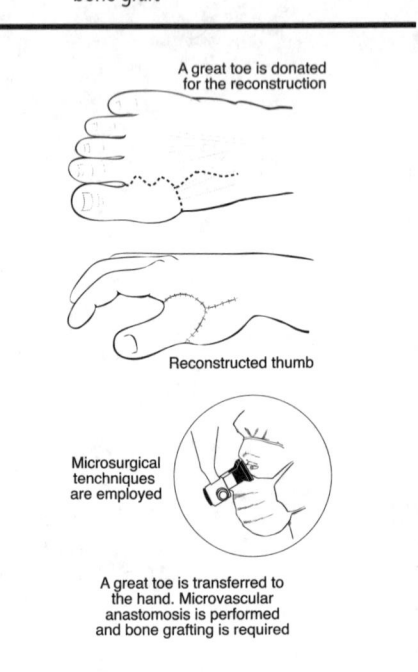

Explanation

The physician performs this procedure to provide functional thumb reconstruction in cases of traumatic thumb amputation or congenital absence. Two surgical teams are employed, one at the hand and the other at the foot. One physician makes a linear incision over the dorsal aspect of the foot, stopping at the base of the toe. A circular incision is made around the toe. The first dorsal metatarsal artery (FDMA) and deep peroneal nerve (DPN) are identified and exposed. The portion of the dorsalis pedis artery that passes to the plantar side of the foot is ligated. The flexor hallucis longus (FHL) is identified along with the plantar digital nerves and arteries. The physician dissects into the web space between the great and second toes where the first plantar metatarsal artery (FPMA) is divided, as are vessels to the second toe. The DPN is split and the fibers to the great toe are divided as well as the digital nerves. The FHL is divided through a separate incision in the midfoot and is pulled into the distal wound. The tourniquet is released and adequate circulation is confirmed. The great toe is perfused for 20 minutes prior to completion of the dissection and transfer to the hand. The second surgical team begins preparing the hand soon after toe dissection begins. The physicians on this team make a palmar thumb skin flap. The dorsal incision extends into the wrist area where the cephalic vein, superficial radial nerve, dorsal dominant branch of the radial artery, and extensor tendons are identified. A transverse incision is made over the volar wrist to allow identification of the flexor pollicis longus (FPL). The thumb metacarpal or phalanx is cut squarely at a right angle to two vertically placed interosseous compression wires and longitudinally placed K-wire, which helps hold the digit in extension. Tendon repairs are performed. The vascular repairs are completed using standard microvascular techniques. The superficial radial nerve and DPN are joined dorsally and the digital nerve repairs are completed volarly. The skin is closed with drains. If a skin graft is necessary, it is placed dorsally over the area of the veins. The donor site is closed by removal of the metatarsal condyles and suturing of the volar plate and sesamoids to the distal metatarsal.

Coding Tips

Do not report 69990 in addition to 26551. The use of the operating microscope is considered a part of the procedure. Head gear and magnifying loupes are also included. For toe-to-hand transfer with other than the great toe, single, see 26553; double, see 26554.

ICD-9-CM Procedural

82.69 Other reconstruction of thumb
84.11 Amputation of toe

Anesthesia

26551 01840

ICD-9-CM Diagnostic

755.29 Congenital longitudinal deficiency, phalanges, complete or partial
906.4 Late effect of crushing
906.6 Late effect of burn of wrist and hand
V10.81 Personal history of malignant neoplasm of bone
V49.61 Upper limb amputation, thumb
V51.8 Other aftercare involving the use of plastic surgery

Terms To Know

congenital. Present at birth, occurring through heredity or an influence during gestation up to the moment of birth.

extensor. Any muscle that extends a joint.

malignant. Any condition tending to progress toward death, specifically an invasive tumor with a loss of cellular differentiation that has the ability to spread or metastasize to other areas in the body.

tendon. Fibrous tissue that connects muscle to bone, consisting primarily of collagen and containing little vasculature.

CCI Version 16.3

01810, 0213T, 0216T, 0228T, 0230T, 11900-11901, 12001-12007, 12020-12047, 13120-13121, 13131-13132, 15757, 15851-15860, 20500-20501, 20526-20553, 25259, 26010-26030, 26034, 26055-26080, 26185, 26340, 26910-26952❖, 29065-29131, 29280, 29345-29358, 29405-29425, 29450, 29505-29515, 29550-29581, 35761, 36000, 36400-36410, 36420-36430, 36440, 36600, 36640, 37202, 37618, 43752, 51701-51703, 62310-62319, 64400-64435, 64445-64450, 64479, 64483, 64490, 64493, 64505-64560, 64565, 64573-64580, 64585-64590, 64702-64708, 64719-64726, 69990, 75710, 75716, 75820, 75822, 76000-76001, 76080, 77002, 87070, 87076-87077, 87102, 93000-93010, 93040-93042, 93318, 94002, 94200, 94250, 94680-94690, 94770, 95812-95816, 95819, 95822, 95829, 95860, 95900, 95955, 96360, 96365, 96372, 96374-96376, 99148-99149, 99150, G0168

Note: These CCI edits are used for Medicare. Other payers may reimburse on codes listed above.

Medicare Edits

	Fac RVU	Non-Fac RVU	FUD	Assist
26551	88.89	88.89	90	80

Medicare References: None

26553-26554

26553 Transfer, toe-to-hand with microvascular anastomosis; other than great toe, single
26554 other than great toe, double

Explanation

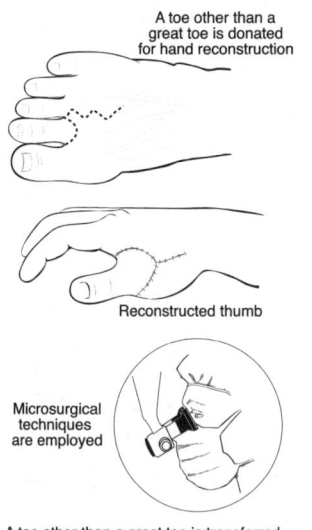

The physician sometimes uses these procedures in cases of traumatic thumb amputation or congenital absence. Two surgical teams are used to complete the transfer. The first team makes a linear incision over the dorsal aspect of the foot, lateral to the dorsalis pedis artery (DPA), traveling from proximal to distal, aiming toward the second toe. Depending on the joint used, the physician may save skin for a graft. The physician harvests two veins in the foot, the dorsalis pedis and metatarsal arteries, the deep peroneal nerve branch, and the extensor tendon to the second toe, and performs an osteotomy at the joint needed. Digital nerves are harvested from the plantar surface. The second team prepares for the toe by making an incision over the wrist where the cephalic vein, superficial radial nerve, dorsal dominant branch of the radial artery, and the flexor pollicis longus (FPL) are identified. The thumb metacarpal or phalanx is cut squarely at a right angle to its long axis after appropriate measurement. If the toe is being transferred to a different finger position, the vein, superficial nerve, digital artery, and extensor tendon are all dissected. To attach the toe to the needed position, the physician affixes the bones by crossed Kirschner wires. The flexor muscles are attached to those of the toe. The digital nerves are repaired and the palmar wounds are closed. The extensor tendons are attached, followed by the approximation of the dorsal sensory nerves, followed by vascular anastomoses. Incisions are closed using sutures. Report 26554 if more than one toe must be transferred because of finger/thumb deficit.

Coding Tips

Do not report 69990 in addition to 26553 or 26554. The use of the operating microscope is considered a part of the procedure. Head gear and magnifying loupes are also included. According to CPT guidelines, cast application or strapping (including removal) is only reported as a replacement procedure or when the cast application or strapping is an initial service performed without a restorative treatment or procedure. See "Application of Casts and Strapping" in the CPT book in the Surgery Section, under the Musculoskeletal system. For toe-to-hand transfer with the great toe, see 26551.

ICD-9-CM Procedural

82.81 Transfer of finger, except thumb
82.89 Other plastic operations on hand

Anesthesia
01840

ICD-9-CM Diagnostic

755.29 Congenital longitudinal deficiency, phalanges, complete or partial
906.1 Late effect of open wound of extremities without mention of tendon injury
906.4 Late effect of crushing
906.6 Late effect of burn of wrist and hand
V10.81 Personal history of malignant neoplasm of bone
V49.62 Upper limb amputation, other finger(s)
V51.8 Other aftercare involving the use of plastic surgery

Terms To Know

congenital. Present at birth, occurring through heredity or an influence during gestation up to the moment of birth.

extensor. Any muscle that extends a joint.

flexor. Muscle/tendon that bends or flexes a limb or part as opposed to extending it.

late effect. Abnormality, dysfunction, or other residual condition produced after the acute phase of an illness, injury, or disease is over. There is no time limit on when late effects can appear.

CCI Version 16.3

01810, 0213T, 0216T, 0228T, 0230T, 11900-11901, 12001-12007, 12020-12047, 13120-13121, 13131-13132, 15852, 20500-20501, 20526-20553, 25259, 26010-26030, 26034, 26055-26080, 26185, 26340, 26910-26952, 29065-29131, 29280, 29345-29358, 29405-29425, 29450, 29505-29515, 35761, 36000, 36400-36410, 36420-36430, 36440, 36600, 36640, 37202, 37618, 43752, 51701-51703, 62310-62319, 64400-64435, 64445-64450, 64479, 64483, 64490, 64493, 64505-64560, 64573-64580, 64585-64595, 64702-64708, 64719-64726, 69990, 75710, 75716, 75820, 75822, 76000-76001, 76080, 77002, 87070, 87076-87077, 87102, 93000-93010, 93040-93042, 93318, 94002, 94200, 94250, 94680-94690, 94770, 95812-95816, 95819, 95822, 95829, 95860, 95900, 95955, 96360, 96365, 96372, 96374-96376, 99148-99149, 99150, G0168

Also not with 26553: 29580-29581
Also not with 26554: 29550-29581, 64565

Note: These CCI edits are used for Medicare. Other payers may reimburse on codes listed above.

Medicare Edits

	Fac RVU	Non-Fac RVU	FUD	Assist
26553	86.86	86.86	90	80
26554	95.28	95.28	90	80

Medicare References: None

26555

26555 Transfer, finger to another position without microvascular anastomosis

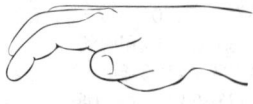

A congenitally malaligned digit

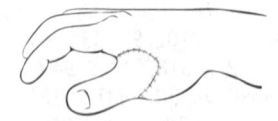

The digit is transferred to another position

A finger is transferred to another position without microvascular anastomosis

Explanation

The physician removes a digit, including the metacarpal bone, and transfers it to another location to improve hand function following trauma or disease. The physician incises the skin overlying the damaged bone. The bone, tendons, nerves, and muscles are removed. The remaining fingers are reapproximated and sutured to provide correct positioning. The skin is reapproximated and closed in sutured layers.

Coding Tips

According to CPT guidelines, cast application or strapping (including removal) is only reported as a replacement procedure or when the cast application or strapping is an initial service performed without a restorative treatment or procedure. See "Application of Casts and Strapping" in the CPT book in the Surgery Section, under the Musculoskeletal system.

ICD-9-CM Procedural

- 82.81 Transfer of finger, except thumb
- 82.89 Other plastic operations on hand

Anesthesia

26555 01830

ICD-9-CM Diagnostic

- 755.29 Congenital longitudinal deficiency, phalanges, complete or partial
- 906.1 Late effect of open wound of extremities without mention of tendon injury
- 906.4 Late effect of crushing
- 906.6 Late effect of burn of wrist and hand
- V10.81 Personal history of malignant neoplasm of bone
- V49.62 Upper limb amputation, other finger(s)
- V51.8 Other aftercare involving the use of plastic surgery

Terms To Know

late effect. Abnormality, dysfunction, or other residual condition produced after the acute phase of an illness, injury, or disease is over. There is no time limit on when late effects can appear.

malignant. Any condition tending to progress toward death, specifically an invasive tumor with a loss of cellular differentiation that has the ability to spread or metastasize to other areas in the body.

tendon. Fibrous tissue that connects muscle to bone, consisting primarily of collagen and containing little vasculature.

CCI Version 16.3

01810, 0213T, 0216T, 0228T, 0230T, 11900, 12020-12021, 13131-13132, 15852, 20526-20553, 25259, 26055-26060, 26075-26080, 26185, 26340, 26910-26952, 29075, 29086, 29130-29131, 29280, 36000, 36400-36410, 36420-36430, 36440, 36600, 36640, 37202, 43752, 51701-51703, 62310-62319, 64400-64435, 64445-64450, 64479, 64483, 64490, 64493, 64505-64530, 64702-64708, 64719-64722, 69990, 75710, 75716, 75820, 75822, 76000-76001, 76080, 77002, 87070, 87076-87077, 87102, 93000-93010, 93040-93042, 93318, 94002, 94200, 94250, 94680-94690, 94770, 95812-95816, 95819, 95822, 95829, 95860, 95900, 95955, 96360, 96365, 96372, 96374-96376, 99148-99149, 99150

Note: These CCI edits are used for Medicare. Other payers may reimburse on codes listed above.

Medicare Edits

	Fac RVU	Non-Fac RVU	FUD	Assist
26555	39.76	39.76	90	80

Medicare References: 100-2,15,260; 100-4,12,30; 100-4,12,90.3; 100-4,14,10

26556

26556 Transfer, free toe joint, with microvascular anastomosis

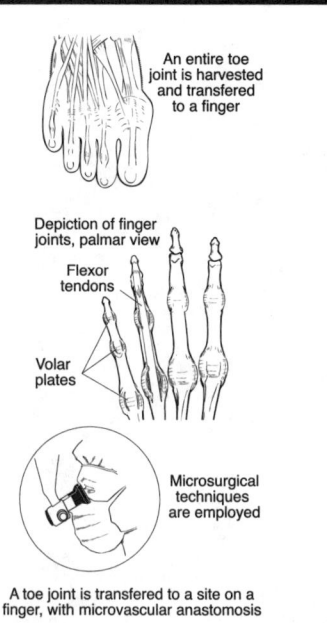

Explanation

The physician performs this procedure if finger joint function is absent, disturbed, or destroyed because of congenital malformation, trauma, or disease. The graft may be an autograft or allograft. Techniques include (1) toe proximal interphalangeal joint (PIPJ) transfer for finger metacarpophalangeal joint (MPJ) and PIPJ reconstruction; (2) metatarsophalangeal (MTPJ) transfer for MPJ or trapeziometacarpal (TMJ) reconstruction; (3) PIPJ or digital interphalangeal joint (DIPJ) "finger bank" transfer. If performing the toe PIPJ transfer for finger PIPJ reconstruction, the physician will engage two teams to prepare the donor and recipient sites simultaneously. One physician makes a longitudinal dorsal incision overlying the toe. The dorsalis pedis and first dorsal metatarsal arteries are dissected, as are dorsal veins. The tibial-side digital artery is divided distally at the level of the DIPJ. The fibular side artery is ligated. The extensor mechanism is cut proximally and distally and the joint is isolated by distal disarticulation through the DIPJ and proximal osteotomy through the first phalanx. The second team prepares the hand by excising the involved PIPJ and dissecting a suitable artery. The toe joint is transferred and stabilized with an intraosseous wire and longitudinal Kirschner wire. The extensor mechanism from the toe is attached to that of the finger. The artery from the toe is attached to that of the finger. At least two veins from the foot are sutured to veins of the hand. The foot wound is closed. The hand wound is also sutured closed. If performing the toe MTPJ transfer for MPJ reconstruction, the physician makes a curved incision to expose the finger joint. The ulnar side of the extensor hood is incised and retracted, and the joint is resected. The radial artery and the cephalic vein are identified through a separate incision. A small branch of the superficial radial nerve is dissected at the wrist level to be sutured to the nerve of the transplanted joint. The donor site is prepared by dissection of the great saphenous vein and first dorsal metatarsal artery. The terminal branch of the deep peroneal nerve is dissected. The toe graft is turned 180 degrees around its longitudinal axis, from dorsal to volar, and attached to the finger. The physician uses a Kirschner wire and anastomoses the vessels. The extensor mechanism is sutured and the skin is closed. The donor site is filled with the finger joint or by bone graft.

Coding Tips

Do not report 69990 in addition to 26556. The use of the operating microscope is considered a part of the procedure. Head gear and magnifying loupes are also included. To report great-toe-to-hand transfer, see 20973.

ICD-9-CM Procedural

- 80.98 Other excision of joint of foot and toe
- 81.72 Arthroplasty of metacarpophalangeal and interphalangeal joint without implant

Anesthesia

26556 01840

ICD-9-CM Diagnostic

- 755.29 Congenital longitudinal deficiency, phalanges, complete or partial
- 755.50 Unspecified congenital anomaly of upper limb
- 755.8 Other specified congenital anomalies of unspecified limb
- 906.4 Late effect of crushing
- 906.6 Late effect of burn of wrist and hand
- V10.81 Personal history of malignant neoplasm of bone
- V49.61 Upper limb amputation, thumb
- V49.62 Upper limb amputation, other finger(s)
- V51.8 Other aftercare involving the use of plastic surgery

CCI Version 16.3

01810, 0213T, 0216T, 0228T, 0230T, 11900-11901, 12001-12007, 12020-12021, 12041-12047, 13131-13132, 15852, 20500-20501, 20526-20553, 25259, 26010-26030, 26034, 26055-26080, 26185, 26340, 26910-26952, 29065-29131, 29280, 29345-29358, 29405-29425, 29450, 29505-29515, 29580-29581, 35761, 36000, 36400-36410, 36420-36430, 36440, 36600, 36640, 37202, 37618, 43752, 51701-51703, 62310-62319, 64400-64435, 64445-64450, 64479, 64483, 64490, 64493, 64505-64560, 64565, 64573-64580, 64585-64595, 64702-64708, 64719-64726, 69990, 75710, 75716, 75820, 75822, 76000-76001, 76080, 77002, 87070, 87076-87077, 87102, 93000-93010, 93040-93042, 93318, 94002, 94200, 94250, 94680-94690, 94770, 95812-95816, 95819, 95822, 95829, 95860, 95900, 95955, 96360, 96365, 96372, 96374-96376, 99148-99149, 99150, G0168

Note: These CCI edits are used for Medicare. Other payers may reimburse on codes listed above.

Medicare Edits

	Fac RVU	Non-Fac RVU	FUD	Assist
26556	83.18	83.18	90	80

Medicare References: None

26560-26562

26560 Repair of syndactyly (web finger) each web space; with skin flaps
26561 with skin flaps and grafts
26562 complex (eg, involving bone, nails)

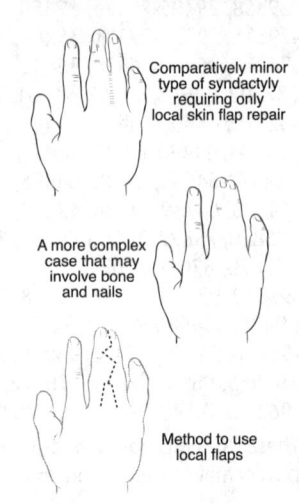

The common congenital abnormality of a webbed finger (syndactyly) is repaired using skin flaps. Report 26561 when skin flaps and grafts are required for the repair. Report 26562 for complex cases involving bone and nails.

Explanation

The physician repairs a syndactyly using skin flaps and grafts. The physician incises the skin of the web for digital release and the underlying tissues are freed. In 26560, the repair is accomplished with skin flaps from the incision area. In 26561, the physician obtains grafts to provide skin coverage. In 26562, the syndactyly is complex and involves the phalangeal bones and fingernails. When possible, the bones are separated. Bone grafts are obtained when necessary for reconstruction. When reconstruction is complete, the skin is reapproximated and closed in sutured layers.

Coding Tips

These codes may be reported multiple times if syndactyly involves more than one web space. Report the specific procedure performed for each web space. When web spaces are repaired, report one web space as the primary procedure and append modifier 51 to subsequent procedures. According to CPT guidelines, cast application or strapping (including removal) is only reported as a replacement procedure or when the cast application or strapping is an initial service performed without a restorative treatment or procedure. See "Application of Casts and Strapping" in the CPT book in the Surgery Section, under the Musculoskeletal system.

ICD-9-CM Procedural

86.85 Correction of syndactyly

Anesthesia

26560 00400
26561 00400
26562 01830

ICD-9-CM Diagnostic

755.10 Syndactyly of multiple and unspecified sites
755.11 Syndactyly of fingers without fusion of bone
755.12 Syndactyly of fingers with fusion of bone

Terms To Know

congenital. Present at birth, occurring through heredity or an influence during gestation up to the moment of birth.

syndactyly. Fusion or webbing of two or more digits.

CCI Version 16.3

01810, 0213T, 0216T, 0228T, 0230T, 20526-20553, 25259, 26185, 26340, 29075, 29086, 29130-29131, 29280, 36000, 36400-36410, 36420-36430, 36440, 36600, 36640, 37202, 43752, 51701-51703, 62310-62319, 64400-64435, 64445-64450, 64479, 64483, 64490, 64493, 64505-64530, 93000-93010, 93040-93042, 93318, 94002, 94200, 94250, 94680-94690, 94770, 95812-95816, 95819, 95822, 95829, 95955, 96360, 96365, 96372, 96374-96376, 99148-99149, 99150

Also not with 26560: 11012❖, 69990

Also not with 26561: 26560

Also not with 26562: 20690, 26561❖, 69990

Note: These CCI edits are used for Medicare. Other payers may reimburse on codes listed above.

Medicare Edits

	Fac RVU	Non-Fac RVU	FUD	Assist
26560	16.79	16.79	90	80
26561	27.37	27.37	90	80
26562	36.55	36.55	90	80

Medicare References: 100-2,15,260; 100-4,12,30; 100-4,12,90.3; 100-4,14,10

26565-26567

26565 Osteotomy; metacarpal, each
26567 phalanx of finger, each

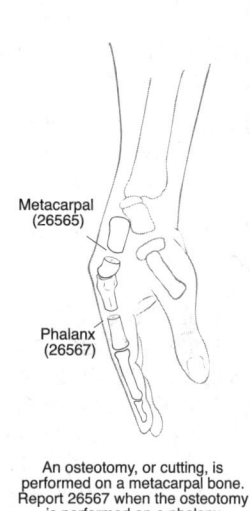

An osteotomy, or cutting, is performed on a metacarpal bone. Report 26567 when the osteotomy is performed on a phalanx

Explanation

The physician performs an osteotomy to correct the metacarpal or phalanx. The physician incises the skin and dissects to the bone. The bone is incised and removed. The operative incision is closed in sutured layers. In 26565, a metacarpal is corrected. In 26567, a phalanx of the finger is corrected.

Coding Tips

These codes are used once for each metacarpal bone (26565) or phalanx of finger (26567) where osteotomy is performed. When multiple osteotomies are performed, report one osteotomy as the primary procedure and append modifier 51 to subsequent procedures. For 26567, some payers may require the use of HCPCS Level II modifiers FA–F9 to identify the specific finger involved. According to CPT guidelines, cast application or strapping (including removal) is only reported as a replacement procedure or when the cast application or strapping is an initial service performed without a restorative treatment or procedure. See "Application of Casts and Strapping" in the CPT book in the Surgery Section, under the Musculoskeletal system.

ICD-9-CM Procedural

- 77.24 Wedge osteotomy of carpals and metacarpals
- 77.34 Other division of carpals and metacarpals
- 77.39 Other division of other bone, except facial bones

Anesthesia
01830

ICD-9-CM Diagnostic

- 357.1 Polyneuropathy in collagen vascular disease — (Code first underlying disease: 446.0, 710.0, 714.0)
- 359.6 Symptomatic inflammatory myopathy in diseases classified elsewhere — (Code first underlying disease: 135, 140.0-208.9, 277.30-277.39, 446.0, 710.0, 710.1, 710.2, 714.0)
- 446.0 Polyarteritis nodosa
- 710.0 Systemic lupus erythematosus — (Use additional code to identify manifestation: 424.91, 581.81, 582.81, 583.81)
- 710.1 Systemic sclerosis — (Use additional code to identify manifestation: 359.6, 517.2)
- 710.2 Sicca syndrome
- 714.0 Rheumatoid arthritis — (Use additional code to identify manifestation: 357.1, 359.6)
- 714.4 Chronic postrheumatic arthropathy
- 715.14 Primary localized osteoarthrosis, hand
- 716.14 Traumatic arthropathy, hand
- 736.00 Unspecified deformity of forearm, excluding fingers
- 736.07 Club hand, acquired
- 736.09 Other acquired deformities of forearm, excluding fingers
- 736.20 Unspecified deformity of finger
- 736.29 Other acquired deformity of finger
- 738.9 Acquired musculoskeletal deformity of unspecified site
- 754.89 Other specified nonteratogenic anomalies
- 755.28 Congenital longitudinal deficiency, carpals or metacarpals, complete or partial (with or without incomplete phalangeal deficiency)
- 756.9 Other and unspecified congenital anomaly of musculoskeletal system
- 905.2 Late effect of fracture of upper extremities
- 909.3 Late effect of complications of surgical and medical care
- 998.59 Other postoperative infection — (Use additional code to identify infection)

Terms To Know

anomaly. Irregularity in the structure or position of an organ or tissue.

dissection. Separating by cutting tissue or body structures apart.

osteotomy. Surgical cutting of a bone.

CCI Version 16.3

01810, 0213T, 0216T, 0228T, 0230T, 11012❖, 20526-20553, 25259, 26185, 26340, 29075, 29086, 29280, 36000, 36400-36410, 36420-36430, 36440, 36600, 36640, 37202, 43752, 51701-51703, 62310-62319, 64400-64435, 64445-64450, 64479, 64483, 64490, 64493, 64505-64530, 69990, 93000-93010, 93040-93042, 93318, 94002, 94200, 94250, 94680-94690, 94770, 95812-95816, 95819, 95822, 95829, 95955, 96360, 96365, 96372, 96374-96376, 99148-99149, 99150

Also not with 26567: 29130-29131

Note: These CCI edits are used for Medicare. Other payers may reimburse on codes listed above.

Medicare Edits

	Fac RVU	Non-Fac RVU	FUD	Assist
26565	19.57	19.57	90	80
26567	19.58	19.58	90	80

Medicare References: 100-2,15,260; 100-4,12,30; 100-4,12,90.3; 100-4,14,10

26568

26568 Osteoplasty, lengthening, metacarpal or phalanx

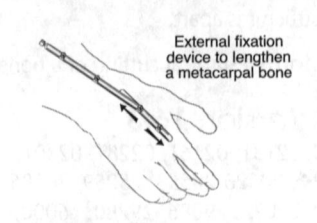

External fixation device to lengthen a metacarpal bone

A metacarpal or phalangeal bone is surgically manipulated (osteoplasty) in order to lengthen the bone

The bone is generally cut to allow the lengthening

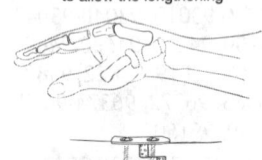

Any variety of approaches may be used, including packing the space with cancellous bone grafts and fixing the site with plates and screws

Explanation

The physician performs an osteoplasty to lengthen a metacarpal or phalanx. The physician incises the skin and dissects to the defective bone. The periosteum is incised and pulled away from the bone. The bone is cut and the proximal and distal ends are distanced. The periosteum is laid over the bone and the operative incision is closed in sutured layers. The hand is splinted in anatomic position until bone callous is formed.

Coding Tips

According to CPT guidelines, cast application or strapping (including removal) is only reported as a replacement procedure or when the cast application or strapping is an initial service performed without a restorative treatment or procedure. See "Application of Casts and Strapping" in the CPT book in the Surgery Section, under the Musculoskeletal system.

ICD-9-CM Procedural

78.14	Application of external fixator device, carpals and metacarpals
78.19	Application of external fixator device, other
78.34	Limb lengthening procedures, carpals and metacarpals
78.39	Other limb lengthening procedures
84.53	Implantation of internal limb lengthening device with kinetic distraction
84.54	Implantation of other internal limb lengthening device
84.71	Application of external fixator device, monoplanar system
84.72	Application of external fixator device, ring system
84.73	Application of hybrid external fixator device

Anesthesia

26568 01830

ICD-9-CM Diagnostic

714.4	Chronic postrheumatic arthropathy
715.14	Primary localized osteoarthrosis, hand
716.14	Traumatic arthropathy, hand
733.81	Malunion of fracture
736.06	Claw hand (acquired)
736.20	Unspecified deformity of finger
736.29	Other acquired deformity of finger
738.9	Acquired musculoskeletal deformity of unspecified site
755.28	Congenital longitudinal deficiency, carpals or metacarpals, complete or partial (with or without incomplete phalangeal deficiency)
756.9	Other and unspecified congenital anomaly of musculoskeletal system
905.2	Late effect of fracture of upper extremities

Terms To Know

claw hand deformity. Abnormal positioning of the hand and fingers usually associated with ulnar nerve palsy, in which the metacarpal phalangeal joints are hyperextended with concomitant flexion of the proximal and distal interphalangeal joints.

congenital. Present at birth, occurring through heredity or an influence during gestation up to the moment of birth.

distal. Located farther away from a specified reference point.

late effect. Abnormality, dysfunction, or other residual condition produced after the acute phase of an illness, injury, or disease is over. There is no time limit on when late effects can appear.

malunion. Fracture that has united in a faulty position due to inadequate reduction of the original fracture, insufficient holding of a previously well-reduced fracture, contracture of the soft tissues, or comminuted or osteoporotic bone causing a slow disintegration of the fracture.

periosteum. Double-layered connective membrane on the outer surface of bone.

primary localized osteoarthrosis. Degenerative joint disease confined to a specific area.

proximal. Located closest to a specified reference point, usually the midline.

CCI Version 16.3

01810, 0213T, 0216T, 0228T, 0230T, 20526-20553, 25259, 26185, 26340, 29075, 29086, 29280, 36000, 36400-36410, 36420-36430, 36440, 36600, 36640, 37202, 43752, 51701-51703, 62310-62319, 64400-64435, 64445-64450, 64479, 64483, 64490, 64493, 64505-64530, 69990, 93000-93010, 93040-93042, 93318, 94002, 94200, 94250, 94680-94690, 94770, 95812-95816, 95819, 95822, 95829, 95955, 96360, 96365, 96372, 96374-96376, 99148-99149, 99150

Note: These CCI edits are used for Medicare. Other payers may reimburse on codes listed above.

Medicare Edits

	Fac RVU	Non-Fac RVU	FUD	Assist
26568	25.86	25.86	90	80

Medicare References: 100-2,15,260; 100-4,12,30; 100-4,12,90.3; 100-4,14,10

26580

26580 Repair cleft hand

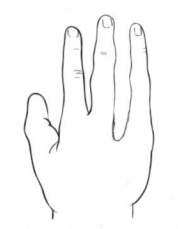

Cleft hand with missing digit

Any variety of techniques may be employed depending on the nature and extent of the cleft

A cleft hand abnormality is repaired

Explanation

The physician repairs a cleft hand. A cleft hand is a malformation where the division between the fingers extends into the metacarpus. The middle digits may be absent and remaining digits are abnormally large. The physician incises the overlying skin and dissects to the deformity. The tissues are brought together with sutures and the tendons are approximated to produce tensor and extensor function. Following correction of the metacarpus, the skin is reapproximated, reduced, and closed in sutured layers.

Coding Tips

According to CPT guidelines, cast application or strapping (including removal) is only reported as a replacement procedure or when the cast application or strapping is an initial service performed without a restorative treatment or procedure. See "Application of Casts and Strapping" in the CPT book in the Surgery Section, under the Musculoskeletal system.

ICD-9-CM Procedural

82.82   Repair of cleft hand

Anesthesia

26580   01830

ICD-9-CM Diagnostic

755.58   Congenital cleft hand

Terms To Know

congenital. Present at birth, occurring through heredity or an influence during gestation up to the moment of birth.

extensor. Any muscle that extends a joint.

tendon. Fibrous tissue that connects muscle to bone, consisting primarily of collagen and containing little vasculature.

CCI Version 16.3

01810, 0213T, 0216T, 0228T, 0230T, 20526-20553, 20690, 25259, 26185, 26340, 26502, 29075, 29086, 29280, 36000, 36400-36410, 36420-36430, 36440, 36600, 36640, 37202, 43752, 51701-51703, 62310-62319, 64400-64435, 64445-64450, 64479, 64483, 64490, 64493, 64505-64530, 69990, 93000-93010, 93040-93042, 93318, 94002, 94200, 94250, 94680-94690, 94770, 95812-95816, 95819, 95822, 95829, 95955, 96360, 96365, 96372, 96374-96376, 99148-99149, 99150

Note: These CCI edits are used for Medicare. Other payers may reimburse on codes listed above.

Medicare Edits

	Fac RVU	Non-Fac RVU	FUD	Assist
26580	39.52	39.52	90	80

Medicare References: 100-2,15,260; 100-4,12,30; 100-4,12,90.3; 100-4,14,10

26587

26587 Reconstruction of polydactylous digit, soft tissue and bone

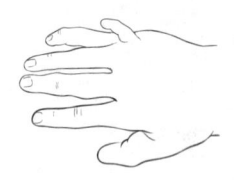

Supernumerary digit

A supernumerary (extra) digit is reconstructed, including soft tissue and bone

Explanation
The physician reconstructs the hand by removing a polydactylous (extra) digit where the digit contains both soft tissue and bone. Excision of a digit containing soft tissue only is reported using 11200. The physician incises the skin at the base of the supernumerary digit. The bone is cut and the digit is resected. The skin is reapproximated, reduced, and sutured in layers.

Coding Tips
According to CPT guidelines, cast application or strapping (including removal) is only reported as a replacement procedure or when the cast application or strapping is an initial service performed without a restorative treatment or procedure. See "Application of Casts and Strapping" in the CPT book in the Surgery Section, under the Musculoskeletal system. For excision of polydactylous digit, soft tissue only, see 11200.

ICD-9-CM Procedural
82.89 Other plastic operations on hand

Anesthesia
26587 01830

ICD-9-CM Diagnostic
755.01 Polydactyly of fingers

Terms To Know

polydactyly. Congenital condition in which there are six or more digits on the hand or foot.

soft tissue. Nonepithelial tissues outside of the skeleton that includes subcutaneous adipose tissue, fibrous tissue, fascia, muscles, blood and lymph vessels, and peripheral nervous system tissue.

CCI Version 16.3
01810, 0213T, 0216T, 0228T, 0230T, 20526-20553, 20690, 25259, 26185, 26340, 26500-26502, 29075, 29086, 29130-29131, 29280, 36000, 36400-36410, 36420-36430, 36440, 36600, 36640, 37202, 43752, 51701-51703, 62310-62319, 64400-64435, 64445-64450, 64479, 64483, 64490, 64493, 64505-64530, 69990, 93000-93010, 93040-93042, 93318, 94002, 94200, 94250, 94680-94690, 94770, 95812-95816, 95819, 95822, 95829, 95955, 96360, 96365, 96372, 96374-96376, 99148-99149, 99150

Note: These CCI edits are used for Medicare. Other payers may reimburse on codes listed above.

Medicare Edits

	Fac RVU	Non-Fac RVU	FUD	Assist
26587	30.12	30.12	90	80

Medicare References: 100-2,15,260; 100-4,12,30; 100-4,12,90.3; 100-4,14,10

26590

26590 Repair macrodactylia, each digit

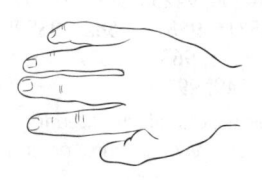

Macrodactylia (abnormally large fingers)

Abnormally large fingers (macrodactylia) are surgically repaired

Explanation
The physician corrects macrodactylia, which is an abnormal largeness of the fingers. The physician incises and retracts the skin to expose the underlying tissue. Reduction is accomplished by removing excess connective tissue and bone if necessary. The tissues are reanastomosed and secured with sutures. The incisions are sutured in layers.

Coding Tips
Some payers may require the use of HCPCS Level II modifiers FA–F9 to identify the specific finger involved. According to CPT guidelines, cast application or strapping (including removal) is only reported as a replacement procedure or when the cast application or strapping is an initial service performed without a restorative treatment or procedure. See "Application of Casts and Strapping" in the CPT book in the Surgery Section, under the Musculoskeletal system.

ICD-9-CM Procedural
82.83   Repair of macrodactyly

Anesthesia
26590   01830

ICD-9-CM Diagnostic
755.57   Macrodactylia (fingers)

Terms To Know

connective tissue. Body tissue made from fibroblasts, collagen, and elastic fibrils that connects, supports, and holds together other tissues and cells and includes cartilage, collagenous, fibrous, elastic, and osseous tissue.

macrodactylia. Abnormal largeness of the fingers.

CCI Version 16.3
01810, 0213T, 0216T, 0228T, 0230T, 20526-20553, 25259, 26185, 26340, 29075, 29086, 29130-29131, 29280, 36000, 36400-36410, 36420-36430, 36440, 36600, 36640, 37202, 43752, 51701-51703, 62310-62319, 64400-64435, 64445-64450, 64479, 64483, 64490, 64493, 64505-64530, 69990, 93000-93010, 93040-93042, 93318, 94002, 94200, 94250, 94680-94690, 94770, 95812-95816, 95819, 95822, 95829, 95955, 96360, 96365, 96372, 96374-96376, 99148-99149, 99150

Note: These CCI edits are used for Medicare. Other payers may reimburse on codes listed above.

Medicare Edits

	Fac RVU	Non-Fac RVU	FUD	Assist
26590	36.76	36.76	90	80

Medicare References: 100-2,15,260; 100-4,12,30; 100-4,12,90.3; 100-4,14,10

26591

26591 Repair, intrinsic muscles of hand, each muscle

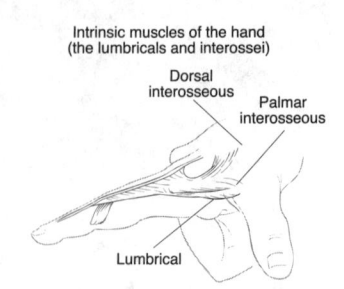

Intrinsic muscles of the hand (the lumbricals and interossei)
Dorsal interosseous
Palmar interosseous
Lumbrical

The lumbricals serve to flex the digits at the metacarpophalangeal joint and extend the interphalangeal joints

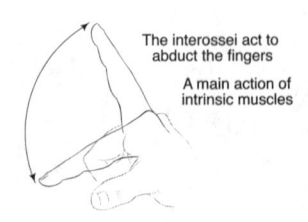

The interossei act to abduct the fingers
A main action of intrinsic muscles

An intrinsic muscle is repaired

Explanation

The physician repairs the intrinsic muscles of the hand to restore intrinsic function. The physician incises the overlying skin and dissects to the damaged muscle. The integrity of the tendons and muscles are tested. Defects are corrected to restore function. The operative incision is closed in sutured layers. When reporting this procedure, indicate which intrinsic muscle was repaired (interossei or lumbricales). Report each muscle separately.

Coding Tips

When multiple muscles are repaired, report one muscle repair as the primary procedure and append modifier 51 to subsequent procedures. According to CPT guidelines, cast application or strapping (including removal) is only reported as a replacement procedure or when the cast application or strapping is an initial service performed without a restorative treatment or procedure. See "Application of Casts and Strapping" in the CPT book in the Surgery Section, under the Musculoskeletal system.

ICD-9-CM Procedural

82.46 Suture of muscle or fascia of hand
82.72 Plastic operation on hand with graft of muscle or fascia
82.89 Other plastic operations on hand

Anesthesia

26591 01810

ICD-9-CM Diagnostic

727.64 Nontraumatic rupture of flexor tendons of hand and wrist
728.2 Muscular wasting and disuse atrophy, not elsewhere classified
728.83 Rupture of muscle, nontraumatic
842.12 Sprain and strain of metacarpophalangeal (joint) of hand
882.1 Open wound of hand except finger(s) alone, complicated
882.2 Open wound of hand except finger(s) alone, with tendon involvement
927.20 Crushing injury of hand(s) — (Use additional code to identify any associated injuries: 800-829, 850.0-854.1, 860.0-869.1)

Terms To Know

atrophy. Reduction in size or activity in an anatomic structure, due to wasting away from disease or other factors.

flexor. Muscle/tendon that bends or flexes a limb or part as opposed to extending it.

injury. Harm or damage sustained by the body.

open wound. Opening or break of the skin.

rupture. Tearing or breaking open of tissue.

sprain and strain. Injuries to a joint, in which the fibers of supporting ligaments or muscles are overstretched or slightly ruptured, with the ligaments and muscles maintaining continuity.

tendon. Fibrous tissue that connects muscle to bone, consisting primarily of collagen and containing little vasculature.

CCI Version 16.3

01810, 0213T, 0216T, 0228T, 0230T, 11010-11012❖, 20526-20553, 25259, 26185, 26340, 26498, 29075, 29086, 29280, 36000, 36400-36410, 36420-36430, 36440, 36600, 36640, 37202, 43752, 51701-51703, 62310-62319, 64400-64435, 64445-64450, 64479, 64483, 64490, 64493, 64505-64530, 69990, 93000-93010, 93040-93042, 93318, 94002, 94200, 94250, 94680-94690, 94770, 95812-95816, 95819, 95822, 95829, 95955, 96360, 96365, 96372, 96374-96376, 99148-99149, 99150

Note: These CCI edits are used for Medicare. Other payers may reimburse on codes listed above.

Medicare Edits

	Fac RVU	Non-Fac RVU	FUD	Assist
26591	12.57	12.57	90	80

Medicare References: 100-2,15,260; 100-4,12,30; 100-4,12,90.3; 100-4,14,10

26593

26593 Release, intrinsic muscles of hand, each muscle

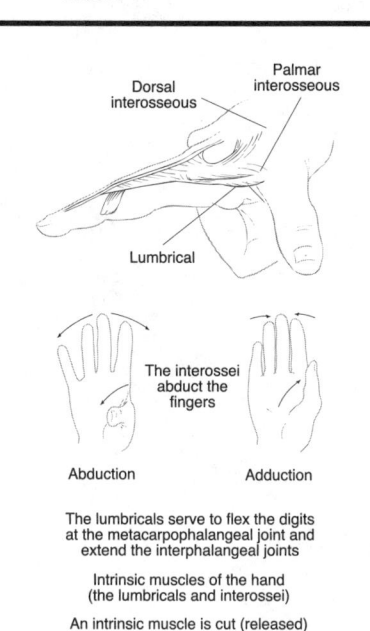

Dorsal interosseous
Palmar interosseous
Lumbrical

The interossei abduct the fingers
Abduction *Adduction*

The lumbricals serve to flex the digits at the metacarpophalangeal joint and extend the interphalangeal joints

Intrinsic muscles of the hand (the lumbricals and interossei)

An intrinsic muscle is cut (released)

Explanation
The physician releases the intrinsic muscles of the hand to restore intrinsic function. The physician incises the overlying skin and dissects to the contracted muscle. The intrinsic muscle is incised to release contracture. The incision is sutured in layers. When reporting this procedure, indicate which intrinsic muscle was released (interossei or lumbricals). If microsurgery is used, report using modifier -20 or 09920. Report each muscle separately.

Coding Tips
When multiple muscles are repaired, report one muscle repair as the primary procedure and append modifier 51 to subsequent procedures. According to CPT guidelines, cast application or strapping (including removal) is only reported as a replacement procedure or when the cast application or strapping is an initial service performed without a restorative treatment or procedure. See "Application of Casts and Strapping" in the CPT book in the Surgery Section, under the Musculoskeletal system.

ICD-9-CM Procedural
82.19 Other division of soft tissue of hand

Anesthesia
26593 01810

ICD-9-CM Diagnostic
343.0 Diplegic infantile cerebral palsy
343.3 Monoplegic infantile cerebral palsy
344.89 Other specified paralytic syndrome
714.4 Chronic postrheumatic arthropathy
728.6 Contracture of palmar fascia
728.88 Rhabdomyolysis
728.89 Other disorder of muscle, ligament, and fascia — (Use additional E code to identify drug, if drug-induced)
736.06 Claw hand (acquired)
756.89 Other specified congenital anomaly of muscle, tendon, fascia, and connective tissue
905.2 Late effect of fracture of upper extremities
905.7 Late effect of sprain and strain without mention of tendon injury
905.8 Late effect of tendon injury
905.9 Late effect of traumatic amputation
906.1 Late effect of open wound of extremities without mention of tendon injury
906.6 Late effect of burn of wrist and hand
907.4 Late effect of injury to peripheral nerve of shoulder girdle and upper limb
927.20 Crushing injury of hand(s) — (Use additional code to identify any associated injuries: 800-829, 850.0-854.1, 860.0-869.1)
958.6 Volkmann's ischemic contracture

Terms To Know

claw hand deformity. Abnormal positioning of the hand and fingers usually associated with ulnar nerve palsy, in which the metacarpal phalangeal joints are hyperextended with concomitant flexion of the proximal and distal interphalangeal joints.

fascia. Fibrous sheet or band of tissue that envelops organs, muscles, and groupings of muscles.

late effect. Abnormality, dysfunction, or other residual condition produced after the acute phase of an illness, injury, or disease is over. There is no time limit on when late effects can appear.

muscle tissue. Network of specialized cells for performing contraction to produce voluntary or involuntary movement of body parts, and skeletal, cardiac, or visceral muscles.

Volkmann's contracture. Shortening of the muscles in the fingers or wrist due to injury near the elbow or vascular damage.

CCI Version 16.3
01810, 0213T, 0216T, 0228T, 0230T, 11011-11012❖, 20526-20553, 25259, 26185, 26340, 29075, 29086, 29280, 36000, 36400-36410, 36420-36430, 36440, 36600, 36640, 37202, 43752, 51701-51703, 62310-62319, 64400-64435, 64445-64450, 64479, 64483, 64490, 64493, 64505-64530, 69990, 93000-93010, 93040-93042, 93318, 94002, 94200, 94250, 94680-94690, 94770, 95812-95816, 95819, 95822, 95829, 95955, 96360, 96365, 96372, 96374-96376, 99148-99149, 99150

Note: These CCI edits are used for Medicare. Other payers may reimburse on codes listed above.

Medicare Edits

	Fac RVU	Non-Fac RVU	FUD	Assist
26593	17.18	17.18	90	N/A

Medicare References: 100-2,15,260; 100-4,12,30; 100-4,12,90.3; 100-4,14,10

26596

26596 Excision of constricting ring of finger, with multiple Z-plasties

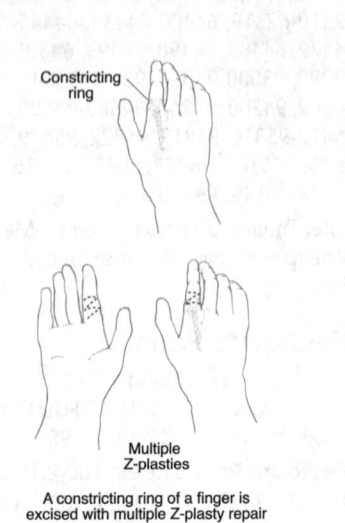

Constricting ring

Multiple Z-plasties

A constricting ring of a finger is excised with multiple Z-plasty repair

Explanation

The physician excises a constricting ring of finger using multiple Z-plasties. The physician cuts the restricted skin in Z-shaped incisions. The Z-flaps are reapproximated, increasing skin surface area without using grafts. The flaps are sutured closed.

Coding Tips

According to CPT guidelines, cast application or strapping (including removal) is only reported as a replacement procedure or when the cast application or strapping is an initial service performed without a restorative treatment or procedure. See "Application of Casts and Strapping" in the CPT book in the Surgery Section, under the Musculoskeletal System. For release of scar contracture or graft repairs, see 11041–11042, 14040–14041, 15120, or 15240.

ICD-9-CM Procedural

86.84 Relaxation of scar or web contracture of skin

Anesthesia

26596 00400

ICD-9-CM Diagnostic

709.2 Scar condition and fibrosis of skin
718.44 Contracture of hand joint
727.81 Contracture of tendon (sheath)
728.6 Contracture of palmar fascia
905.8 Late effect of tendon injury
905.9 Late effect of traumatic amputation
906.1 Late effect of open wound of extremities without mention of tendon injury
906.4 Late effect of crushing
906.6 Late effect of burn of wrist and hand

Terms To Know

contracture. Shortening of muscle or connective tissue.

fascia. Fibrous sheet or band of tissue that envelops organs, muscles, and groupings of muscles.

fibrosis. Formation of fibrous tissue as part of the restorative process.

late effect. Abnormality, dysfunction, or other residual condition produced after the acute phase of an illness, injury, or disease is over. There is no time limit on when late effects can appear.

tendon. Fibrous tissue that connects muscle to bone, consisting primarily of collagen and containing little vasculature.

traumatic amputation. Removal of a part or limb from accidental injury.

CCI Version 16.3

01810, 0213T, 0216T, 0228T, 0230T, 20526-20553, 25259, 26185, 26340, 29075, 29086, 29130-29131, 29280, 36000, 36400-36410, 36420-36430, 36440, 36600, 36640, 37202, 43752, 51701-51703, 62310-62319, 64400-64435, 64445-64450, 64479, 64483, 64490, 64493, 64505-64530, 69990, 93000-93010, 93040-93042, 93318, 94002, 94200, 94250, 94680-94690, 94770, 95812-95816, 95819, 95822, 95829, 95955, 96360, 96365, 96372, 96374-96376, 99148-99149, 99150

Note: These CCI edits are used for Medicare. Other payers may reimburse on codes listed above.

Medicare Edits

	Fac RVU	Non-Fac RVU	FUD	Assist
26596	21.59	21.59	90	80

Medicare References: 100-2,15,260; 100-4,12,30; 100-4,12,90.3; 100-4,14,10

26600-26607

26600 Closed treatment of metacarpal fracture, single; without manipulation, each bone
26605 with manipulation, each bone
26607 Closed treatment of metacarpal fracture, with manipulation, with external fixation, each bone

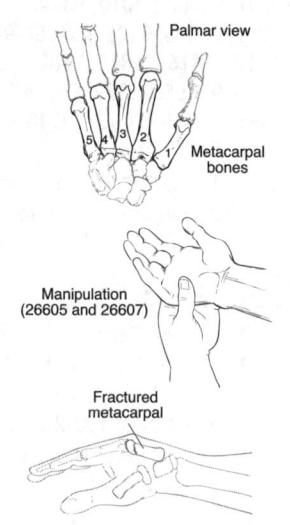

A metacarpal bone fracture is treated without manipulation. Report 26605 when manipulation is required to reduce the fracture. Report 26607 when internal or external fixation is required, with manipulation

Explanation

The physician uses an x-ray to determine the location and severity of the fracture. In 26600, the fracture does not require realignment. In 26605, the proximal and distal ends of the fracture are not in correct anatomical position and the physician reduces the fracture to correct alignment. In 26607, the physician reduces the fracture to correct alignment of the proximal and distal ends of the bone. Internal or external fixation is used to stabilize the fracture. If internal fixation is necessary, the physician percutaneously places a stabilizing wire. The bones are splinted in anatomic position.

Coding Tips

When multiple fractures are treated, report one fracture treatment as the primary procedure and append modifier 51 to subsequent procedures. According to CPT guidelines, cast application or strapping (including removal) is only reported as a replacement procedure or when the cast application or strapping is an initial service performed without a restorative treatment or procedure. See "Application of Casts and Strapping" in the CPT book in the Surgery Section, under the Musculoskeletal system. For radiology services, see 73100 and 73110. For radiology services, add modifier 26 to identify the professional component only unless the physician owns the equipment. For percutaneous skeletal fixation of a metacarpal fracture, see 26608. For open treatment of a metacarpal fracture, see 26615.

ICD-9-CM Procedural

79.03 Closed reduction of fracture of carpals and metacarpals without internal fixation
79.13 Closed reduction of fracture of carpals and metacarpals with internal fixation
79.14 Closed reduction of fracture of phalanges of hand with internal fixation
93.54 Application of splint

Anesthesia
01820

ICD-9-CM Diagnostic

733.19 Pathologic fracture of other specified site
815.00 Closed fracture of metacarpal bone(s), site unspecified
815.02 Closed fracture of base of other metacarpal bone(s)
815.03 Closed fracture of shaft of metacarpal bone(s)
815.04 Closed fracture of neck of metacarpal bone(s)
815.09 Closed fracture of multiple sites of metacarpus
817.0 Multiple closed fractures of hand bones

Terms To Know

closed fracture. Break in a bone without a concomitant opening in the skin. A closed fracture is coded when the type of fracture is not specified.

distal. Located farther away from a specified reference point.

fracture. Break in bone or cartilage.

proximal. Located closest to a specified reference point, usually the midline.

CCI Version 16.3

01810, 01820, 0213T, 0216T, 0228T, 0230T, 20526-20553, 25259, 26340, 26546❖, 29065-29131, 29700-29715, 36000, 36400-36410, 36420-36430, 36440, 36600, 36640, 37202, 43752, 51701-51703, 62310-62319, 64400-64435, 64445-64450, 64479, 64483, 64490, 64493, 64505-64530, 69990, 93000-93010, 93040-93042, 93318, 94002, 94200, 94250, 94680-94690, 94770, 95812-95816, 95819, 95822, 95829, 95955, 96360, 96365, 96372, 96374-96376, 97597-97598, 97602-97606, 99148-99149, 99150

Also not with 26600: 29260-29280

Also not with 26605: 26600, 29280, J0670, J2001

Also not with 26607: 20650, 20690, 20692, 20696-20697, 29280

Note: These CCI edits are used for Medicare. Other payers may reimburse on codes listed above.

Medicare Edits

	Fac RVU	Non-Fac RVU	FUD	Assist
26600	7.56	8.09	90	N/A
26605	8.25	9.04	90	N/A
26607	12.92	12.92	90	80

Medicare References: 100-2,15,260; 100-4,12,30; 100-4,12,90.3; 100-4,14,10

26608

26608 Percutaneous skeletal fixation of metacarpal fracture, each bone

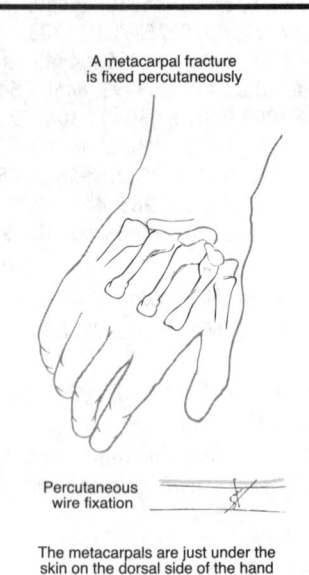

A metacarpal fracture is fixed percutaneously

Percutaneous wire fixation

The metacarpals are just under the skin on the dorsal side of the hand and fractures may be easily fixed subcutaneously

Explanation

The physician fixates a metacarpal fracture using a percutaneously placed wire. The physician uses an x-ray to determine the location and severity of the fracture. The physician reduces the fracture to correct alignment of the proximal and distal ends of the bone. The physician drills a wire through the metacarpophalangeal joint, through the fracture, and into the proximal bone. The drill entry point is dressed and the hand is splinted.

Coding Tips

When multiple fractures are treated, report one fracture treatment as the primary procedure and append modifier 51 to subsequent procedures. According to CPT guidelines, cast application or strapping (including removal) is only reported as a replacement procedure or when the cast application or strapping is an initial service performed without a restorative treatment or procedure. See "Application of Casts and Strapping" in the CPT book in the Surgery Section, under the Musculoskeletal system. For radiology services, see 73100 and 73110. For closed treatment of a metacarpal fracture without manipulation, see 26600; with manipulation, see 26605. For closed treatment with manipulation and internal or external fixation, see 26607. For open treatment of a metacarpal fracture, see 26615.

ICD-9-CM Procedural

78.54 Internal fixation of carpals and metacarpals without fracture reduction

Anesthesia

26608 01820

ICD-9-CM Diagnostic

733.19 Pathologic fracture of other specified site
815.00 Closed fracture of metacarpal bone(s), site unspecified
815.02 Closed fracture of base of other metacarpal bone(s)
815.03 Closed fracture of shaft of metacarpal bone(s)
815.04 Closed fracture of neck of metacarpal bone(s)
815.09 Closed fracture of multiple sites of metacarpus
817.0 Multiple closed fractures of hand bones

Terms To Know

closed fracture. Break in a bone without a concomitant opening in the skin. A closed fracture is coded when the type of fracture is not specified.

distal. Located farther away from a specified reference point.

fracture. Break in bone or cartilage.

proximal. Located closest to a specified reference point, usually the midline.

CCI Version 16.3

01810, 01820, 0213T, 0216T, 0228T, 0230T, 12042, 20526-20553, 20650, 25259, 26340, 26546❖, 26600-26607, 29065-29131, 29280, 29700-29715, 36000, 36400-36410, 36420-36430, 36440, 36600, 36640, 37202, 43752, 51701-51703, 62310-62319, 64400-64435, 64445-64450, 64479, 64483, 64490, 64493, 64505-64530, 69990, 76000-76001, 93000-93010, 93040-93042, 93318, 94002, 94200, 94250, 94680-94690, 94770, 95812-95816, 95819, 95822, 95829, 95955, 96360, 96365, 96372, 96374-96376, 97597-97598, 97602-97606, 99148-99149, 99150, J0670, J2001

Note: These CCI edits are used for Medicare. Other payers may reimburse on codes listed above.

Medicare Edits

	Fac RVU	Non-Fac RVU	FUD	Assist
26608	13.75	13.75	90	80

Medicare References: 100-2,15,260; 100-4,12,30; 100-4,12,90.3; 100-4,14,10

26615

26615 Open treatment of metacarpal fracture, single, includes internal fixation, when performed, each bone

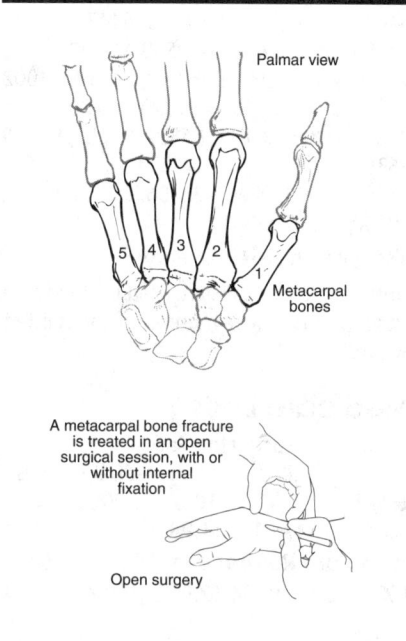

Explanation

The physician performs open correction of a metacarpal fracture. Internal fixation may be used. The physician uses an x-ray to determine the location and severity of the fracture. The physician incises the overlying skin to expose the fracture. A wire or plate may be placed for internal fixation. The incision is sutured in layers and the hand is splinted.

Coding Tips

When multiple fractures are treated, report one fracture treatment as the primary procedure and append modifier 51 to subsequent procedures. According to CPT guidelines, cast application or strapping (including removal) is only reported as a replacement procedure or when the cast application or strapping is an initial service performed without a restorative treatment or procedure. See "Application of Casts and Strapping" in the CPT book in the Surgery Section, under the Musculoskeletal system. For radiology services, see 73100 and 73110. For closed treatment of a metacarpal fracture without manipulation, see 26600; with manipulation, see 26605. For closed treatment with manipulation and internal or external fixation, see 26607. For percutaneous skeletal fixation of a metacarpal fracture, see 26608.

ICD-9-CM Procedural

79.23 Open reduction of fracture of carpals and metacarpals without internal fixation
79.33 Open reduction of fracture of carpals and metacarpals with internal fixation

Anesthesia

26615 01830

ICD-9-CM Diagnostic

733.19 Pathologic fracture of other specified site
733.81 Malunion of fracture
733.82 Nonunion of fracture
815.00 Closed fracture of metacarpal bone(s), site unspecified
815.02 Closed fracture of base of other metacarpal bone(s)
815.03 Closed fracture of shaft of metacarpal bone(s)
815.04 Closed fracture of neck of metacarpal bone(s)
815.09 Closed fracture of multiple sites of metacarpus
815.10 Open fracture of metacarpal bone(s), site unspecified
815.12 Open fracture of base of other metacarpal bone(s)
815.13 Open fracture of shaft of metacarpal bone(s)
815.14 Open fracture of neck of metacarpal bone(s)
815.19 Open fracture of multiple sites of metacarpus
817.0 Multiple closed fractures of hand bones
817.1 Multiple open fractures of hand bones

Terms To Know

closed fracture. Break in a bone without a concomitant opening in the skin. A closed fracture is coded when the type of fracture is not specified.

fracture. Break in bone or cartilage.

open fracture. Exposed break in a bone, always considered compound due to its high risk of infection from the open wound leading to the fracture. Broken bone ends may protrude through the skin and contaminants or foreign bodies are often embedded in the tissues.

CCI Version 16.3

01810, 01820, 0213T, 0216T, 0228T, 0230T, 12004, 12045, 12047, 20526-20553, 20650, 25259, 26055, 26185, 26340, 26546❖, 26600-26608, 29065-29131, 29280, 29700-29715, 36000, 36400-36410, 36420-36430, 36440, 36600, 36640, 37202, 43752, 51701-51703, 62310-62319, 64400-64435, 64445-64450, 64479, 64483, 64490, 64493, 64505-64530, 69990, 76000-76001, 93000-93010, 93040-93042, 93318, 94002, 94200, 94250, 94680-94690, 94770, 95812-95816, 95819, 95822, 95829, 95955, 96360, 96365, 96372, 96374-96376, 97597-97598, 97602-97606, 99148-99149, 99150

Note: These CCI edits are used for Medicare. Other payers may reimburse on codes listed above.

Medicare Edits

	Fac RVU	Non-Fac RVU	FUD	Assist
26615	16.39	16.39	90	N/A

Medicare References: 100-2,15,260; 100-4,12,30; 100-4,12,90.3; 100-4,14,10

26641-26645

26641 Closed treatment of carpometacarpal dislocation, thumb, with manipulation
26645 Closed treatment of carpometacarpal fracture dislocation, thumb (Bennett fracture), with manipulation

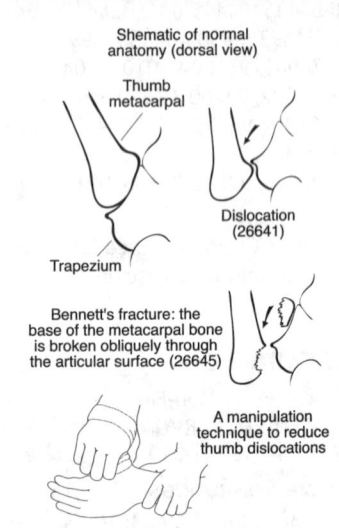

Shematic of normal anatomy (dorsal view)
Thumb metacarpal
Dislocation (26641)
Trapezium

Bennett's fracture: the base of the metacarpal bone is broken obliquely through the articular surface (26645)

A manipulation technique to reduce thumb dislocations

A dislocation of the carpometacarpal joint of the thumb is reduced in a closed fashion with manipulation. Report 26645 when the dislocation is classified as a Bennett's fracture, closed treatment with manipulation

Explanation
The physician manipulates a carpometacarpal dislocation or fracture dislocation of the thumb to restore anatomical position. The physician determines the dislocated position of the bone. The bone is relocated to correct anatomical position using external manipulation, and the hand is splinted. Report 26641 for dislocation without fracture, report 26645 for dislocation including fracture (Bennett fracture).

Coding Tips
When multiple fractures or dislocations are treated, report one fracture or dislocation treatment as the primary procedure and append modifier 51 to subsequent procedures. According to CPT guidelines, cast application or strapping (including removal) is only reported as a replacement procedure or when the cast application or strapping is an initial service performed without a restorative treatment or procedure. See "Application of Casts and Strapping" in the CPT book in the Surgery Section, under the Musculoskeletal system. Local anesthesia is included in these services. However, these procedures may be performed under general anesthesia, depending on the age and/or condition of the patient. For radiology services, see 73100, 73110, and 73120–73140. For percutaneous skeletal fixation of a carpometacarpal fracture dislocation, thumb (Bennett fracture), see 26650. For open treatment of a carpometacarpal fracture dislocation, thumb (Bennett fracture), see 26665.

ICD-9-CM Procedural
79.03 Closed reduction of fracture of carpals and metacarpals without internal fixation
79.13 Closed reduction of fracture of carpals and metacarpals with internal fixation
79.74 Closed reduction of dislocation of hand and finger

Anesthesia
01820

ICD-9-CM Diagnostic
718.24 Pathological dislocation of hand joint
718.30 Recurrent dislocation of joint, site unspecified
718.34 Recurrent dislocation of hand joint
718.74 Developmental dislocation of joint, hand
733.19 Pathologic fracture of other specified site
815.01 Closed fracture of base of thumb (first) metacarpal bone(s)
833.04 Closed dislocation of carpometacarpal (joint)

Terms To Know
closed fracture. Break in a bone without a concomitant opening in the skin. A closed fracture is coded when the type of fracture is not specified.

developmental dislocation. Displacement of a body part occurring in the developmental phase of childhood.

dislocation. Displacement of a bone in relation to its neighboring tissue, especially a joint.

fracture. Break in bone or cartilage.

pathological dislocation. Displacement of a bone or joint caused by a disease process, such as infection, lesions, or muscle weakness, and not traumatic injury.

CCI Version 16.3
01810, 01820, 0213T, 0216T, 0228T, 0230T, 20526-20553, 25259, 26340, 29065-29131, 29280, 29700-29715, 36000, 36400-36410, 36420-36430, 36440, 36600, 36640, 37202, 43752, 51701-51703, 62310-62319, 64400-64435, 64445-64450, 64479, 64483, 64490, 64493, 64505-64530, 69990, 93000-93010, 93040-93042, 93318, 94002, 94200, 94250, 94680-94690, 94770, 95812-95816, 95819, 95822, 95829, 95955, 96360, 96365, 96372, 96374-96376, 97597-97598, 97602-97606, 99148-99149, 99150, J0670, J2001

Also not with 26645: 26546❖

Note: These CCI edits are used for Medicare. Other payers may reimburse on codes listed above.

Medicare Edits

	Fac RVU	Non-Fac RVU	FUD	Assist
26641	9.37	10.2	90	80
26645	11.01	11.95	90	80

Medicare References: 100-2,15,260; 100-4,12,30; 100-4,12,90.3; 100-4,14,10

26650

26650 Percutaneous skeletal fixation of carpometacarpal fracture dislocation, thumb (Bennett fracture), with manipulation

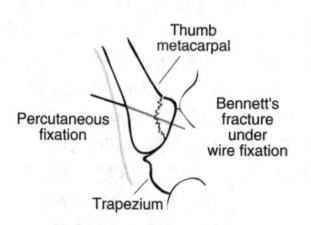

One manipulation technique involves wrapping the thumb in a bandage. The other end is wrapped around the physician's wrist for stability while reducing the fracture/dislocation

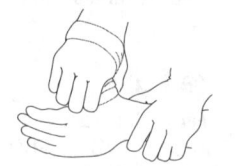

A Bennett's fracture/dislocation of the carpometacarpal joint of the thumb is reduced in a closed fashion with manipulation and percutaneous (through the skin) skeletal fixation

Explanation

The physician manipulates a carpometacarpal fracture dislocation of the thumb to restore anatomical position and secures the bone with a wire. The physician determines the dislocated position of the bone. The bone is relocated to correct anatomical position using external manipulation. The physician drills a wire through the metacarpophalangeal joint, through the fracture, and into the proximal bone. The drill entry point is dressed and the hand is splinted.

Coding Tips

When multiple fractures or dislocations are treated, report one fracture or dislocation treatment as the primary procedure and append modifier 51 to subsequent procedures. According to CPT guidelines, cast application or strapping (including removal) is only reported as a replacement procedure or when the cast application or strapping is an initial service performed without a restorative treatment or procedure. See "Application of Casts and Strapping" in the CPT book in the Surgery Section, under the Musculoskeletal system. For radiology services, see 73100, 73110, and 73120–73140. For closed treatment of a carpometacarpal dislocation, thumb, see 26641. For closed treatment of a Bennett fracture, thumb, see 26645. For open treatment of a carpometacarpal fracture dislocation, thumb (Bennett fracture), see 26665.

ICD-9-CM Procedural

78.14 Application of external fixator device, carpals and metacarpals

79.03 Closed reduction of fracture of carpals and metacarpals without internal fixation

Anesthesia

26650 01820

ICD-9-CM Diagnostic

733.19 Pathologic fracture of other specified site

815.01 Closed fracture of base of thumb (first) metacarpal bone(s)

815.11 Open fracture of base of thumb (first) metacarpal bone(s)

Terms To Know

closed fracture. Break in a bone without a concomitant opening in the skin. A closed fracture is coded when the type of fracture is not specified.

fracture. Break in bone or cartilage.

open fracture. Exposed break in a bone, always considered compound due to its high risk of infection from the open wound leading to the fracture. Broken bone ends may protrude through the skin and contaminants or foreign bodies are often embedded in the tissues.

CCI Version 16.3

01810, 01820, 0213T, 0216T, 0228T, 0230T, 20526-20553, 20650, 25259, 26340, 26546✦, 26641-26645, 29065-29131, 29280, 29700-29715, 36000, 36400-36410, 36420-36430, 36440, 36600, 36640, 37202, 43752, 51701-51703, 62310-62319, 64400-64435, 64445-64450, 64479, 64483, 64490, 64493, 64505-64530, 69990, 93000-93010, 93040-93042, 93318, 94002, 94200, 94250, 94680-94690, 94770, 95812-95816, 95819, 95822, 95829, 95955, 96360, 96365, 96372, 96374-96376, 97597-97598, 97602-97606, 99148-99149, 99150, J0670, J2001

Note: These CCI edits are used for Medicare. Other payers may reimburse on codes listed above.

Medicare Edits

	Fac RVU	Non-Fac RVU	FUD	Assist
26650	13.77	13.77	90	N/A

Medicare References: 100-2,15,260; 100-4,12,30; 100-4,12,90.3; 100-4,14,10

26665

26665 Open treatment of carpometacarpal fracture dislocation, thumb (Bennett fracture), includes internal fixation, when performed

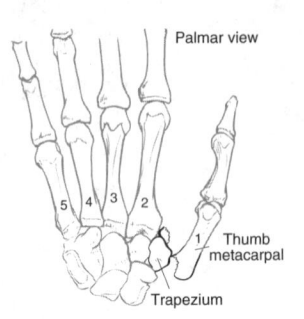

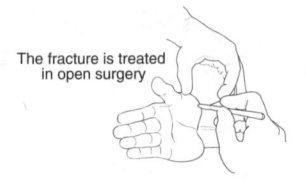

Bennett's fracture (Palmar view, showing bones 5, 4, 3, 2, 1, Thumb metacarpal, Trapezium)

A fracture/dislocation of the thumb metacarpal (Bennett's fracture) is treated in an open surgical session with or without internal fixation

Explanation
The physician performs open reduction of a carpometacarpal fracture dislocation of the thumb. The physician uses an x-ray to determine the position and severity of the defect. The physician incises the overlying skin to expose the fracture and the bones are reapproximated. A wire or plate may be placed for internal fixation. The incision is sutured in layers and the hand is splinted.

Coding Tips
When multiple fractures or dislocations are treated, report one fracture or dislocation treatment as the primary procedure and append modifier 51 to subsequent procedures. According to CPT guidelines, cast application or strapping (including removal) is only reported as a replacement procedure or when the cast application or strapping is an initial service performed without a restorative treatment or procedure. See "Application of Casts and Strapping" in the CPT book in the Surgery Section, under the Musculoskeletal system. For radiology services, see 73100, 73110, and 73120–73140. For closed treatment of a carpometacarpal dislocation, thumb, see 26641. For closed treatment of a Bennett fracture, thumb, see 26645. For percutaneous skeletal fixation of a carpometacarpal fracture dislocation, thumb (Bennett fracture), see 26650.

ICD-9-CM Procedural
79.23 Open reduction of fracture of carpals and metacarpals without internal fixation
79.33 Open reduction of fracture of carpals and metacarpals with internal fixation
79.84 Open reduction of dislocation of hand and finger

Anesthesia
26665 01830

ICD-9-CM Diagnostic
733.19 Pathologic fracture of other specified site
733.81 Malunion of fracture
733.82 Nonunion of fracture
815.01 Closed fracture of base of thumb (first) metacarpal bone(s)
815.11 Open fracture of base of thumb (first) metacarpal bone(s)

Terms To Know
closed fracture. Break in a bone without a concomitant opening in the skin. A closed fracture is coded when the type of fracture is not specified.

fracture. Break in bone or cartilage.

open fracture. Exposed break in a bone, always considered compound due to its high risk of infection from the open wound leading to the fracture. Broken bone ends may protrude through the skin and contaminants or foreign bodies are often embedded in the tissues.

CCI Version 16.3
01810, 01820, 0213T, 0216T, 0228T, 0230T, 20526-20553, 20650, 25000, 25100-25105, 25115-25119, 25259, 25295, 25320, 26185, 26340, 26546❖, 26641-26650, 26727, 29065-29131, 29280, 29700-29715, 36000, 36400-36410, 36420-36430, 36440, 36600, 36640, 37202, 43752, 51701-51703, 62310-62319, 64400-64435, 64445-64450, 64479, 64483, 64490, 64493, 64505-64530, 64702-64704, 69990, 76000-76001, 93000-93010, 93040-93042, 93318, 94002, 94200, 94250, 94680-94690, 94770, 95812-95816, 95819, 95822, 95829, 95955, 96360, 96365, 96372, 96374-96376, 97597-97598, 97602-97606, 99148-99149, 99150

Note: These CCI edits are used for Medicare. Other payers may reimburse on codes listed above.

Medicare Edits

	Fac RVU	Non-Fac RVU	FUD	Assist
26665	18.02	18.02	90	N/A

Medicare References: 100-2,15,260; 100-4,12,30; 100-4,12,90.3; 100-4,14,10

26670-26675

26670 Closed treatment of carpometacarpal dislocation, other than thumb, with manipulation, each joint; without anesthesia

26675 requiring anesthesia

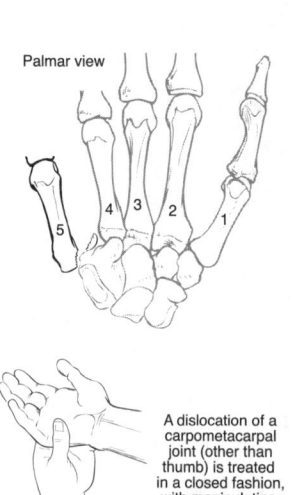

Explanation

The physician treats a carpometacarpal (other than the thumb) dislocation using manipulation; anesthesia may be used if necessary. The physician determines the dislocated position of the bone. The physician uses external manipulation to relocate the bone. In 26670, dislocation is minor and no anesthesia is needed. In 26675, dislocation is major and anesthesia is required.

Coding Tips

When multiple dislocations are treated, report one dislocation treatment as the primary procedure and append modifier 51 to subsequent procedures. According to CPT guidelines, cast application or strapping (including removal) is only reported as a replacement procedure or when the cast application or strapping is an initial service performed without a restorative treatment or procedure. See "Application of Casts and Strapping" in the CPT book in the Surgery Section, under the Musculoskeletal system. For radiology services, see 73100, 73110, and 73120–73140. For open treatment of a carpometacarpal dislocation, other than thumb (Bennett fracture), see 26685; complex, multiple or delayed reduction, see 26686. For percutaneous skeletal fixation, see 26676.

ICD-9-CM Procedural

79.74 Closed reduction of dislocation of hand and finger

Anesthesia
26670 N/A
26675 01820

ICD-9-CM Diagnostic

718.24 Pathological dislocation of hand joint
718.30 Recurrent dislocation of joint, site unspecified
718.34 Recurrent dislocation of hand joint
718.74 Developmental dislocation of joint, hand
833.04 Closed dislocation of carpometacarpal (joint)

Terms To Know

developmental dislocation. Displacement of a body part occurring in the developmental phase of childhood.

pathological dislocation. Displacement of a bone or joint caused by a disease process, such as infection, lesions, or muscle weakness, and not traumatic injury.

CCI Version 16.3

01810, 01820, 0213T, 0216T, 0228T, 0230T, 20526-20553, 25259, 26340, 29065-29131, 29280, 29700-29715, 36000, 36400-36410, 36420-36430, 36440, 36600, 36640, 37202, 43752, 51701-51703, 62310-62319, 64400-64435, 64445-64450, 64479, 64483, 64490, 64493, 64505-64530, 69990, 93000-93010, 93040-93042, 93318, 94002, 94200, 94250, 94680-94690, 94770, 95812-95816, 95819, 95822, 95829, 95955, 96360, 96365, 96372, 96374-96376, 97597-97598, 97602-97606, 99148-99149, 99150, J0670, J2001

Also not with 26670: 26546❖

Also not with 26675: 26670

Note: These CCI edits are used for Medicare. Other payers may reimburse on codes listed above.

Medicare Edits

	Fac RVU	Non-Fac RVU	FUD	Assist
26670	8.46	9.32	90	80
26675	11.75	12.73	90	80

Medicare References: 100-2,15,260; 100-4,12,30; 100-4,12,90.3; 100-4,14,10

26676

26676 Percutaneous skeletal fixation of carpometacarpal dislocation, other than thumb, with manipulation, each joint

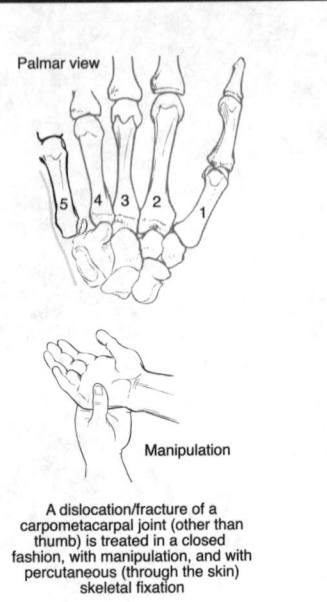

Palmar view

Manipulation

A dislocation/fracture of a carpometacarpal joint (other than thumb) is treated in a closed fashion, with manipulation, and with percutaneous (through the skin) skeletal fixation

Explanation

The physician manipulates a carpometacarpal dislocation (other than the thumb) to restore anatomical position and secures the bone with a wire. The physician determines the dislocated position of the bone. The bone is relocated to correct anatomical position using external manipulation. The physician drills a wire through the metacarpophalangeal joint, through the fracture, and into the proximal bone. The drill entry point is dressed and the hand is splinted.

Coding Tips

When multiple dislocations are treated, report one dislocation treatment as the primary procedure and append modifier 51 to subsequent procedures. According to CPT guidelines, cast application or strapping (including removal) is only reported as a replacement procedure or when the cast application or strapping is an initial service performed without a restorative treatment or procedure. See "Application of Casts and Strapping" in the CPT book in the Surgery Section, under the Musculoskeletal system. For radiology services, see 73100, 73110, and 73120–73140. For open treatment of a carpometacarpal dislocation, other than thumb (Bennett fracture), see 26685; complex, multiple or delayed reduction, see 26686. For closed treatment of a carpometacarpal dislocation, other than thumb (Bennett fracture), without anesthesia, see 26670; with anesthesia, see 26675.

ICD-9-CM Procedural

78.54 Internal fixation of carpals and metacarpals without fracture reduction
79.74 Closed reduction of dislocation of hand and finger

Anesthesia

26676 01820

ICD-9-CM Diagnostic

718.24 Pathological dislocation of hand joint
718.34 Recurrent dislocation of hand joint
718.74 Developmental dislocation of joint, hand
833.04 Closed dislocation of carpometacarpal (joint)
833.14 Open dislocation of carpometacarpal (joint)

Terms To Know

developmental dislocation. Displacement of a body part occurring in the developmental phase of childhood.

pathological dislocation. Displacement of a bone or joint caused by a disease process, such as infection, lesions, or muscle weakness, and not traumatic injury.

proximal. Located closest to a specified reference point, usually the midline.

CCI Version 16.3

01810, 01820, 0213T, 0216T, 0228T, 0230T, 20526-20553, 20650, 25259, 26340, 26670-26675, 29065-29131, 29280, 29700-29715, 36000, 36400-36410, 36420-36430, 36440, 36600, 36640, 37202, 43752, 51701-51703, 62310-62319, 64400-64435, 64445-64450, 64479, 64483, 64490, 64493, 64505-64530, 69990, 93000-93010, 93040-93042, 93318, 94002, 94200, 94250, 94680-94690, 94770, 95812-95816, 95819, 95822, 95829, 95955, 96360, 96365, 96372, 96374-96376, 97597-97598, 97602-97606, 99148-99149, 99150, J0670, J2001

Note: These CCI edits are used for Medicare. Other payers may reimburse on codes listed above.

Medicare Edits

	Fac RVU	Non-Fac RVU	FUD	Assist
26676	14.41	14.41	90	N/A

Medicare References: 100-2,15,260; 100-4,12,30; 100-4,12,90.3; 100-4,14,10

26685-26686

26685 Open treatment of carpometacarpal dislocation, other than thumb; includes internal fixation, when performed, each joint

26686   complex, multiple, or delayed reduction

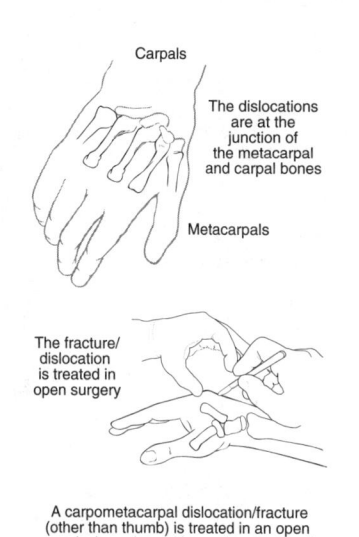

A carpometacarpal dislocation/fracture (other than thumb) is treated in an open surgical session, with or without internal fixation. Report 26686 for complex, multiple, or delayed reduction

Explanation

The physician performs open reduction of a carpometacarpal dislocation on a joint other than the thumb. The physician uses a separately reportable x-ray to determine the position and severity of the defect. The physician incises the overlying skin to expose the dislocation. A wire or plates may be placed for internal fixation. The incision is sutured in layers and the hand is splinted. Report 26685 for each joint that is repaired simply. Report 26686 for complex or multiple dislocations, or when delayed treatment of the dislocation is performed.

Coding Tips

When multiple dislocations are treated, report one dislocation treatment as the primary procedure and append modifier 51 to subsequent procedures. According to CPT guidelines, cast application or strapping (including removal) is only reported as a replacement procedure or when the cast application or strapping is an initial service performed without a restorative treatment or procedure. See "Application of Casts and Strapping" in the CPT book in the Surgery Section, under the Musculoskeletal system. For radiology services, see 73100, 73110, and 73120–73140. For closed treatment of a carpometacarpal dislocation, other than thumb (Bennett fracture), without anesthesia, see 26670; with anesthesia, see 26675. For percutaneous skeletal fixation of a carpometacarpal dislocation, other than thumb (Bennett fracture), see 26676.

ICD-9-CM Procedural

78.54 Internal fixation of carpals and metacarpals without fracture reduction

79.84 Open reduction of dislocation of hand and finger

Anesthesia

01830

ICD-9-CM Diagnostic

718.24 Pathological dislocation of hand joint

718.34 Recurrent dislocation of hand joint

718.74 Developmental dislocation of joint, hand

833.04 Closed dislocation of carpometacarpal (joint)

833.14 Open dislocation of carpometacarpal (joint)

Terms To Know

developmental dislocation. Displacement of a body part occurring in the developmental phase of childhood.

pathological dislocation. Displacement of a bone or joint caused by a disease process, such as infection, lesions, or muscle weakness, and not traumatic injury.

CCI Version 16.3

01810, 01820, 0213T, 0216T, 0228T, 0230T, 20526-20553, 20650, 25000, 25100-25105, 25115-25119, 25259, 25295, 25320, 26185, 26340, 26670-26676, 26727, 29065-29131, 29280, 29700-29715, 36000, 36400-36410, 36420-36430, 36440, 36600, 36640, 37202, 43752, 51701-51703, 62310-62319, 64400-64435, 64445-64450, 64479, 64483, 64490, 64493, 64505-64530, 64702-64704, 69990, 93000-93010, 93040-93042, 93318, 94002, 94200, 94250, 94680-94690, 94770, 95812-95816, 95819, 95822, 95829, 95955, 96360, 96365, 96372, 96374-96376, 97597-97598, 97602-97606, 99148-99149, 99150

Also not with 26686: 26685

Note: These CCI edits are used for Medicare. Other payers may reimburse on codes listed above.

Medicare Edits

	Fac RVU	Non-Fac RVU	FUD	Assist
26685	16.57	16.57	90	N/A
26686	18.05	18.05	90	80

Medicare References: 100-2,15,260; 100-4,12,30; 100-4,12,90.3; 100-4,14,10

26700-26705

26700 Closed treatment of metacarpophalangeal dislocation, single, with manipulation; without anesthesia
26705 requiring anesthesia

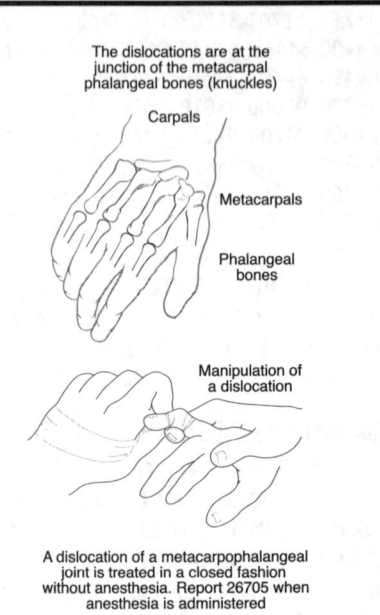

The dislocations are at the junction of the metacarpal phalangeal bones (knuckles)

Manipulation of a dislocation

A dislocation of a metacarpophalangeal joint is treated in a closed fashion without anesthesia. Report 26705 when anesthesia is administered

Explanation

The physician treats a metacarpophalangeal dislocation using manipulation; anesthesia may be used if necessary. The physician determines the dislocated position of the bone. The physician uses external manipulation to relocate the bone. In 26700, dislocation is minor and no anesthesia is needed. In 26705, dislocation is major and anesthesia is required.

Coding Tips

When multiple dislocations are treated, report one dislocation treatment as the primary procedure and append modifier 51 to subsequent procedures. According to CPT guidelines, cast application or strapping (including removal) is only reported as a replacement procedure or when the cast application or strapping is an initial service performed without a restorative treatment or procedure. See "Application of Casts and Strapping" in the CPT book in the Surgery Section, under the Musculoskeletal system. For radiology services, see 73120–73140. For percutaneous skeletal fixation of a metacarpophalangeal dislocation, see 26706. For open treatment of a metacarpophalangeal dislocation, see 26715.

ICD-9-CM Procedural

79.74 Closed reduction of dislocation of hand and finger

Anesthesia

26700 N/A
26705 01820

ICD-9-CM Diagnostic

718.24 Pathological dislocation of hand joint
718.34 Recurrent dislocation of hand joint
718.74 Developmental dislocation of joint, hand
834.01 Closed dislocation of metacarpophalangeal (joint)

Terms To Know

developmental dislocation. Displacement of a body part occurring in the developmental phase of childhood.

pathological dislocation. Displacement of a bone or joint caused by a disease process, such as infection, lesions, or muscle weakness, and not traumatic injury.

CCI Version 16.3

01810, 01820, 0213T, 0216T, 0228T, 0230T, 20526-20553, 25259, 26340, 26546❖, 29065-29131, 29280, 29700-29715, 36000, 36400-36410, 36420-36430, 36440, 36600, 36640, 37202, 43752, 51701-51703, 62310-62319, 64400-64435, 64445-64450, 64479, 64483, 64490, 64493, 64505-64530, 69990, 93000-93010, 93040-93042, 93318, 94002, 94200, 94250, 94680-94690, 94770, 95812-95816, 95819, 95822, 95829, 95955, 96360, 96365, 96372, 96374-96376, 97597-97598, 97602-97606, 99148-99149, 99150, J2001

Also not with 26705: 26700, J0670

Note: These CCI edits are used for Medicare. Other payers may reimburse on codes listed above.

Medicare Edits

	Fac RVU	Non-Fac RVU	FUD	Assist
26700	8.35	8.91	90	N/A
26705	10.75	11.71	90	80

Medicare References: 100-2,15,260; 100-4,12,30; 100-4,12,90.3; 100-4,14,10

26706

26706 Percutaneous skeletal fixation of metacarpophalangeal dislocation, single, with manipulation

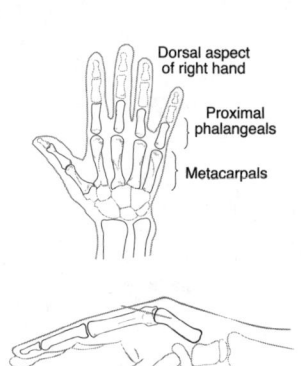

Dorsal aspect of right hand
Proximal phalangeals
Metacarpals

The joint is fixed percutaneously

A metacarpophalangeal dislocation is treated using manipulation and fixed percutaneously (through the skin)

Explanation

The physician manipulates a metacarpophalangeal dislocation to restore anatomical position and secures the bone with a wire. The physician determines the dislocated position of the bone. The bone is relocated to correct anatomical position using external manipulation. The physician drills a wire into the metacarpophalangeal joint, through the fracture, and into the proximal bone. The drill entry point is dressed and the hand is splinted.

Coding Tips

When multiple dislocations are treated, report one dislocation treatment as the primary procedure and append modifier 51 to subsequent procedures. According to CPT guidelines, cast application or strapping (including removal) is only reported as a replacement procedure or when the cast application or strapping is an initial service performed without a restorative treatment or procedure. See "Application of Casts and Strapping" in the CPT book in the Surgery Section, under the Musculoskeletal system. For radiology services, see 73120–73140. For closed treatment of a metacarpophalangeal dislocation, without anesthesia, see 26700; with anesthesia, see 26705. For open treatment of a metacarpophalangeal dislocation, see 26715.

ICD-9-CM Procedural

78.54 Internal fixation of carpals and metacarpals without fracture reduction
79.74 Closed reduction of dislocation of hand and finger

Anesthesia
26706 01820

ICD-9-CM Diagnostic

718.24 Pathological dislocation of hand joint
718.34 Recurrent dislocation of hand joint
718.74 Developmental dislocation of joint, hand
834.01 Closed dislocation of metacarpophalangeal (joint)

Terms To Know

developmental dislocation. Displacement of a body part occurring in the developmental phase of childhood.

pathological dislocation. Displacement of a bone or joint caused by a disease process, such as infection, lesions, or muscle weakness, and not traumatic injury.

proximal. Located closest to a specified reference point, usually the midline.

CCI Version 16.3

01810, 01820, 0213T, 0216T, 0228T, 0230T, 20526-20553, 20650, 25259, 26340, 26546❖, 26700-26705, 29065-29131, 29280, 29700-29715, 36000, 36400-36410, 36420-36430, 36440, 36600, 36640, 37202, 43752, 51701-51703, 62310-62319, 64400-64435, 64445-64450, 64479, 64483, 64490, 64493, 64505-64530, 69990, 93000-93010, 93040-93042, 93318, 94002, 94200, 94250, 94680-94690, 94770, 95812-95816, 95819, 95822, 95829, 95955, 96360, 96365, 96372, 96374-96376, 97597-97598, 97602-97606, 99148-99149, 99150

Note: These CCI edits are used for Medicare. Other payers may reimburse on codes listed above.

Medicare Edits

	Fac RVU	Non-Fac RVU	FUD	Assist
26706	12.6	12.6	90	N/A

Medicare References: 100-2,15,260; 100-4,12,30; 100-4,12,90.3; 100-4,14,10

26715

26715 Open treatment of metacarpophalangeal dislocation, single, includes internal fixation, when performed

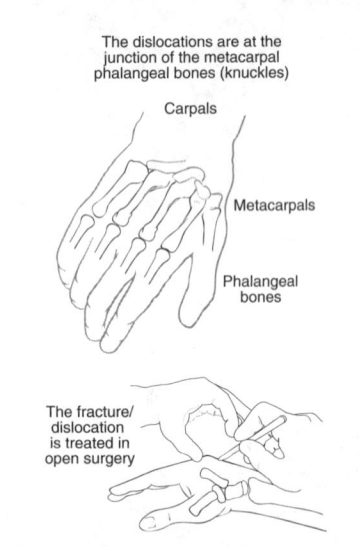

The dislocations are at the junction of the metacarpal phalangeal bones (knuckles)

The fracture/dislocation is treated in open surgery

A dislocation of a metacarpophalangeal joint is treated in an open surgical session, with or without internal fixation

Explanation
The physician performs open reduction of a metacarpophalangeal fracture dislocation. The physician uses an x-ray to determine the position and severity of the defect. An incision is made on the overlying skin to expose the fracture and the bones are reapproximated. A wire or plate may be placed for internal fixation. The incision is sutured in layers and the hand is splinted.

Coding Tips
When multiple dislocations are treated, report one dislocation treatment as the primary procedure and append modifier 51 to subsequent procedures. According to CPT guidelines, cast application or strapping (including removal) is only reported as a replacement procedure or when the cast application or strapping is an initial service performed without a restorative treatment or procedure. See "Application of Casts and Strapping" in the CPT book in the Surgery Section, under the Musculoskeletal system. For radiology services, see 73120–73140. For closed treatment of a metacarpophalangeal dislocation, without anesthesia, see 26700; with anesthesia, see 26705. For percutaneous skeletal fixation of a metacarpophalangeal dislocation, see 26706.

ICD-9-CM Procedural
79.84 Open reduction of dislocation of hand and finger

Anesthesia
26715 01830

ICD-9-CM Diagnostic
718.24 Pathological dislocation of hand joint
718.74 Developmental dislocation of joint, hand
834.01 Closed dislocation of metacarpophalangeal (joint)
834.11 Open dislocation of metacarpophalangeal (joint)

Terms To Know
developmental dislocation. Displacement of a body part occurring in the developmental phase of childhood.

pathological dislocation. Displacement of a bone or joint caused by a disease process, such as infection, lesions, or muscle weakness, and not traumatic injury.

CCI Version 16.3
01810, 01820, 0213T, 0216T, 0228T, 0230T, 20526-20553, 20650, 25259, 26185, 26340, 26546❖, 26700-26706, 29065-29131, 29280, 29700-29715, 36000, 36400-36410, 36420-36430, 36440, 36600, 36640, 37202, 43752, 51701-51703, 62310-62319, 64400-64435, 64445-64450, 64479, 64483, 64490, 64493, 64505-64530, 69990, 93000-93010, 93040-93042, 93318, 94002, 94200, 94250, 94680-94690, 94770, 95812-95816, 95819, 95822, 95829, 95955, 96360, 96365, 96372, 96374-96376, 97597-97598, 97602-97606, 99148-99149, 99150

Note: These CCI edits are used for Medicare. Other payers may reimburse on codes listed above.

Medicare Edits

	Fac RVU	Non-Fac RVU	FUD	Assist
26715	16.32	16.32	90	80

Medicare References: 100-2,15,260; 100-4,12,30; 100-4,12,90.3; 100-4,14,10

26720-26725

26720 Closed treatment of phalangeal shaft fracture, proximal or middle phalanx, finger or thumb; without manipulation, each

26725 with manipulation, with or without skin or skeletal traction, each

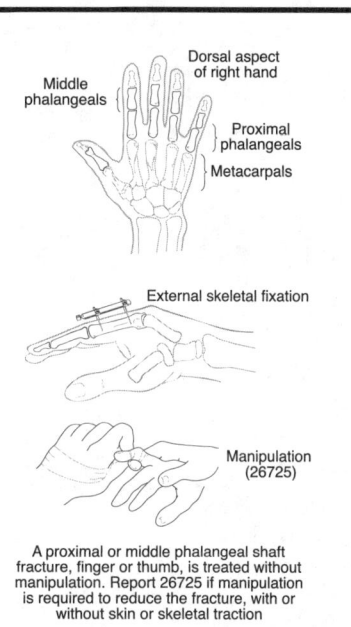

A proximal or middle phalangeal shaft fracture, finger or thumb, is treated without manipulation. Report 26725 if manipulation is required to reduce the fracture, with or without skin or skeletal traction

Explanation

The physician treats a phalangeal shaft fracture of the proximal or middle phalanx, finger or thumb, with or without manipulation. In 26720, no manipulation is necessary. In 26725, the physician manipulates the bones to restore anatomical position. The hand is splinted for stabilization.

Coding Tips

When multiple fractures are treated, report one fracture treatment as the primary procedure and append modifier 51 to subsequent procedures. According to CPT guidelines, cast application or strapping (including removal) is only reported as a replacement procedure or when the cast application or strapping is an initial service performed without a restorative treatment or procedure. Some payers may require the use of HCPCS Level II modifiers FA–F9 to identify the specific finger involved. See "Application of Casts and Strapping" in the CPT book in the Surgery Section, under the Musculoskeletal system. Local anesthesia is included in these services. For radiology services, see 73140. For percutaneous skeletal fixation of an unstable phalangeal shaft fracture, see 26727. For open treatment, see 26735.

ICD-9-CM Procedural

- 79.04 Closed reduction of fracture of phalanges of hand without internal fixation
- 93.54 Application of splint

Anesthesia
01820

ICD-9-CM Diagnostic

- 733.19 Pathologic fracture of other specified site
- 816.01 Closed fracture of middle or proximal phalanx or phalanges of hand
- 816.03 Closed fracture of multiple sites of phalanx or phalanges of hand
- 817.0 Multiple closed fractures of hand bones
- 927.3 Crushing injury of finger(s) — (Use additional code to identify any associated injuries: 800-829, 850.0-854.1, 860.0-869.1)

Terms To Know

closed fracture. Break in a bone without a concomitant opening in the skin. A closed fracture is coded when the type of fracture is not specified.

fracture. Break in bone or cartilage.

phalanx. Bones of the digits (fingers or toes).

proximal. Located closest to a specified reference point, usually the midline.

CCI Version 16.3

01810, 01820, 0213T, 0216T, 0228T, 0230T, 20526-20553, 25259, 26340, 26546❖, 29065-29131, 29280, 29700-29715, 36000, 36400-36410, 36420-36430, 36440, 36600, 36640, 37202, 43752, 51701-51703, 62310-62319, 64400-64435, 64445-64450, 64479, 64483, 64490, 64493, 64505-64530, 69990, 93000-93010, 93040-93042, 93318, 94002, 94200, 94250, 94680-94690, 94770, 95812-95816, 95819, 95822, 95829, 95955, 96360, 96365, 96372, 96374-96376, 97597-97598, 97602-97606, 99148-99149, 99150

Also not with 26725: 20650, 26720, 76000-76001, J0670, J2001

Note: These CCI edits are used for Medicare. Other payers may reimburse on codes listed above.

Medicare Edits

	Fac RVU	Non-Fac RVU	FUD	Assist
26720	5.07	5.48	90	N/A
26725	8.64	9.58	90	N/A

Medicare References: None

26727

26727 Percutaneous skeletal fixation of unstable phalangeal shaft fracture, proximal or middle phalanx, finger or thumb, with manipulation, each

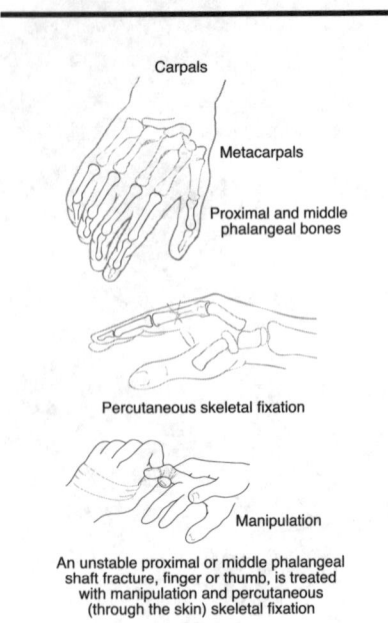

Explanation

The physician treats a phalangeal shaft fracture of the proximal or middle phalanx, finger or thumb, with manipulation and secures it with a wire. The physician drills a wire into the tip of the finger bone, through the fracture, and into the proximal bone. The drill entry point is dressed and the hand is splinted.

Coding Tips

When multiple fractures are treated, report one fracture treatment as the primary procedure and append modifier 51 to subsequent procedures. Some payers may require the use of HCPCS Level II modifiers FA-F9 to identify the specific finger involved. According to CPT guidelines, cast application or strapping (including removal) is only reported as a replacement procedure or when the cast application or strapping is an initial service performed without a restorative treatment or procedure. See "Application of Casts and Strapping" in the CPT book in the Surgery Section, under the Musculoskeletal system. For radiology services, see 73140. For closed treatment of a phalangeal shaft fracture, without manipulation, see 26720; with manipulation, see 26725. For open treatment, see 26735.

ICD-9-CM Procedural

79.14 Closed reduction of fracture of phalanges of hand with internal fixation

Anesthesia

26727 01820

ICD-9-CM Diagnostic

733.19 Pathologic fracture of other specified site
816.01 Closed fracture of middle or proximal phalanx or phalanges of hand
816.03 Closed fracture of multiple sites of phalanx or phalanges of hand
817.0 Multiple closed fractures of hand bones
927.3 Crushing injury of finger(s) — (Use additional code to identify any associated injuries: 800-829, 850.0-854.1, 860.0-869.1)

Terms To Know

closed fracture. Break in a bone without a concomitant opening in the skin. A closed fracture is coded when the type of fracture is not specified.

fracture. Break in bone or cartilage.

phalanx. Bones of the digits (fingers or toes).

proximal. Located closest to a specified reference point, usually the midline.

CCI Version 16.3

01810, 01820, 0213T, 0216T, 0228T, 0230T, 12002, 12005, 20526-20553, 20650, 20690, 20692, 20696-20697, 25259, 26340, 26546❖, 26720-26725, 29065-29131, 29280, 29700-29715, 36000, 36400-36410, 36420-36430, 36440, 36600, 36640, 37202, 43752, 51701-51703, 62310-62319, 64400-64435, 64445-64450, 64479, 64483, 64490, 64493, 64505-64530, 69990, 76000-76001, 93000-93010, 93040-93042, 93318, 94002, 94200, 94250, 94680-94690, 94770, 95812-95816, 95819, 95822, 95829, 95955, 96360, 96365, 96372, 96374-96376, 97597-97598, 97602-97606, 99148-99149, 99150, J0670, J2001

Note: These CCI edits are used for Medicare. Other payers may reimburse on codes listed above.

Medicare Edits

	Fac RVU	Non-Fac RVU	FUD	Assist
26727	13.53	13.53	90	N/A

Medicare References: 100-2,15,260; 100-4,12,30; 100-4,12,90.3; 100-4,14,10

26735

26735 Open treatment of phalangeal shaft fracture, proximal or middle phalanx, finger or thumb, includes internal fixation, when performed, each

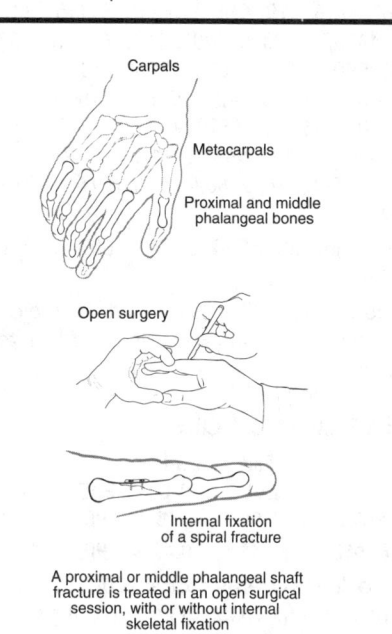

Explanation

The physician performs open correction of a phalangeal shaft fracture. The physician uses an x-ray to determine the position and severity of the defect. The physician incises the overlying skin to expose the fracture and the bones are reapproximated. A wire or plate may be placed for internal fixation. The incision is sutured in layers and the hand is splinted.

Coding Tips

When multiple fractures are treated, report one fracture treatment as the primary procedure and append modifier 51 to subsequent procedures. Some payers may require the use of HCPCS Level II modifiers FA–F9 to identify the specific finger involved. According to CPT guidelines, cast application or strapping (including removal) is only reported as a replacement procedure or when the cast application or strapping is an initial service performed without a restorative treatment or procedure. See "Application of Casts and Strapping" in the CPT book in the Surgery Section, under the Musculoskeletal system. For radiology services, see 73140. For closed treatment of a phalangeal shaft fracture, without manipulation, see 26720; with manipulation, see 26725. For percutaneous skeletal fixation of an unstable phalangeal shaft fracture, see 26727.

ICD-9-CM Procedural

- 79.24 Open reduction of fracture of phalanges of hand without internal fixation
- 79.34 Open reduction of fracture of phalanges of hand with internal fixation
- 79.80 Open reduction of dislocation of unspecified site

Anesthesia

26735   01830

ICD-9-CM Diagnostic

- 733.19 Pathologic fracture of other specified site
- 733.81 Malunion of fracture
- 816.01 Closed fracture of middle or proximal phalanx or phalanges of hand
- 816.03 Closed fracture of multiple sites of phalanx or phalanges of hand
- 816.11 Open fracture of middle or proximal phalanx or phalanges of hand
- 816.13 Open fractures of multiple sites of phalanx or phalanges of hand
- 817.0 Multiple closed fractures of hand bones
- 817.1 Multiple open fractures of hand bones
- 927.3 Crushing injury of finger(s) — (Use additional code to identify any associated injuries: 800-829, 850.0-854.1, 860.0-869.1)

Terms To Know

closed fracture. Break in a bone without a concomitant opening in the skin. A closed fracture is coded when the type of fracture is not specified.

fracture. Break in bone or cartilage.

open fracture. Exposed break in a bone, always considered compound due to its high risk of infection from the open wound leading to the fracture. Broken bone ends may protrude through the skin and contaminants or foreign bodies are often embedded in the tissues.

proximal. Located closest to a specified reference point, usually the midline.

CCI Version 16.3

01810, 01820, 0213T, 0216T, 0228T, 0230T, 12001-12007, 12020-12021, 12041-12047, 13131-13132, 20526-20553, 20650, 25259, 26055, 26080, 26110, 26140-26145, 26185, 26340, 26440-26449, 26525, 26540, 26545-26548, 26720-26727, 29065-29131, 29280, 29700-29715, 36000, 36400-36410, 36420-36430, 36440, 36600, 36640, 37202, 43752, 51701-51703, 62310-62319, 64400-64435, 64445-64450, 64479, 64483, 64490, 64493, 64505-64530, 64702-64704, 69990, 76000-76001, 93000-93010, 93040-93042, 93318, 94002, 94200, 94250, 94680-94690, 94770, 95812-95816, 95819, 95822, 95829, 95955, 96360, 96365, 96372, 96374-96376, 97597-97598, 97602-97606, 99148-99149, 99150, G0168

Note: These CCI edits are used for Medicare. Other payers may reimburse on codes listed above.

Medicare Edits

	Fac RVU	Non-Fac RVU	FUD	Assist
26735	17.02	17.02	90	N/A

Medicare References: 100-2,15,260; 100-4,12,30; 100-4,12,90.3; 100-4,14,10

26740-26742

26740 Closed treatment of articular fracture, involving metacarpophalangeal or interphalangeal joint; without manipulation, each

26742 with manipulation, each

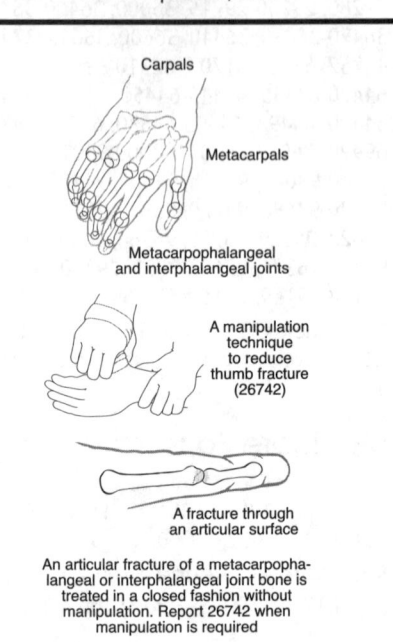

Carpals

Metacarpals

Metacarpophalangeal and interphalangeal joints

A manipulation technique to reduce thumb fracture (26742)

A fracture through an articular surface

An articular fracture of a metacarpophalangeal or interphalangeal joint bone is treated in a closed fashion without manipulation. Report 26742 when manipulation is required.

Explanation

The physician treats an articular fracture involving a metacarpophalangeal or interphalangeal joint with or without manipulation. In 26740, no manipulation is necessary. In 26742, the physician manipulates the bones to restore anatomical position. The hand is splinted for stabilization.

Coding Tips

When multiple fractures are treated, report one fracture treatment as the primary procedure and append modifier 51 to subsequent procedures. According to CPT guidelines, cast application or strapping (including removal) is only reported as a replacement procedure or when the cast application or strapping is an initial service performed without a restorative treatment or procedure. See "Application of Casts and Strapping" in the CPT book in the Surgery Section, under the Musculoskeletal system. Local anesthesia is included in these services. However, 26742 may be performed under general anesthesia, depending on the age and/or condition of the patient. For radiology services, see 73120–73140. For open treatment of an articular fracture, involving the metacarpophalangeal or interphalangeal joint, see 26746.

ICD-9-CM Procedural

79.04 Closed reduction of fracture of phalanges of hand without internal fixation

93.54 Application of splint

Anesthesia

01820

ICD-9-CM Diagnostic

733.19 Pathologic fracture of other specified site

815.01 Closed fracture of base of thumb (first) metacarpal bone(s)

815.02 Closed fracture of base of other metacarpal bone(s)

815.04 Closed fracture of neck of metacarpal bone(s)

815.09 Closed fracture of multiple sites of metacarpus

816.01 Closed fracture of middle or proximal phalanx or phalanges of hand

816.03 Closed fracture of multiple sites of phalanx or phalanges of hand

817.0 Multiple closed fractures of hand bones

927.20 Crushing injury of hand(s) — (Use additional code to identify any associated injuries: 800-829, 850.0-854.1, 860.0-869.1)

927.3 Crushing injury of finger(s) — (Use additional code to identify any associated injuries: 800-829, 850.0-854.1, 860.0-869.1)

Terms To Know

closed fracture. Break in a bone without a concomitant opening in the skin. A closed fracture is coded when the type of fracture is not specified.

fracture. Break in bone or cartilage.

proximal. Located closest to a specified reference point, usually the midline.

CCI Version 16.3

01810, 01820, 0213T, 0216T, 0228T, 0230T, 20526-20553, 25259, 26340, 26546❖, 29065-29131, 29280, 29700-29715, 36000, 36400-36410, 36420-36430, 36440, 36600, 36640, 37202, 43752, 51701-51703, 62310-62319, 64400-64435, 64445-64450, 64479, 64483, 64490, 64493, 64505-64530, 69990, 93000-93010, 93040-93042, 93318, 94002, 94200, 94250, 94680-94690, 94770, 95812-95816, 95819, 95822, 95829, 95955, 96360, 96365, 96372, 96374-96376, 97597-97598, 97602-97606, 99148-99149, 99150

Also not with 26742: 26740, 76000-76001, J0670, J2001

Note: These CCI edits are used for Medicare. Other payers may reimburse on codes listed above.

Medicare Edits

	Fac RVU	Non-Fac RVU	FUD	Assist
26740	5.99	6.38	90	N/A
26742	9.48	10.42	90	N/A

Medicare References: 100-2,15,260; 100-4,12,30; 100-4,12,90.3; 100-4,14,10

26746

26746 Open treatment of articular fracture, involving metacarpophalangeal or interphalangeal joint, includes internal fixation, when performed, each

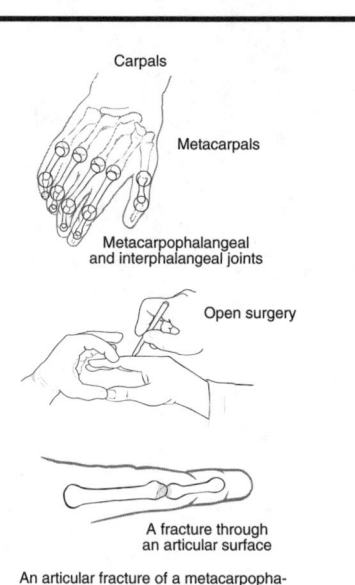

An articular fracture of a metacarpophalangeal or interphalangeal joint bone is treated in an open surgical session, with or without internal fixation

Explanation
The physician performs open reduction of an articular fracture involving a metacarpophalangeal or interphalangeal joint. The physician uses an x-ray to determine the position and severity of the defect. An incision is made on the overlying skin to expose the fracture and the bones are reapproximated. A wire or plate may be placed for internal fixation. The incision is sutured in layers and the hand is splinted.

Coding Tips
When multiple fractures are treated, report one fracture treatment as the primary procedure and append modifier 51 to subsequent procedures. According to CPT guidelines, cast application or strapping (including removal) is only reported as a replacement procedure or when the cast application or strapping is an initial service performed without a restorative treatment or procedure. See "Application of Casts and Strapping" in the CPT book in the Surgery Section, under the Musculoskeletal system. For radiology services, see 73120–73140. For closed treatment of an articular fracture, involving the metacarpophalangeal or interphalangeal joint, without manipulation, see 26740; with manipulation, see 26742.

ICD-9-CM Procedural
- 79.24 Open reduction of fracture of phalanges of hand without internal fixation
- 79.34 Open reduction of fracture of phalanges of hand with internal fixation

Anesthesia
26746 01830

ICD-9-CM Diagnostic
- 733.19 Pathologic fracture of other specified site
- 815.04 Closed fracture of neck of metacarpal bone(s)
- 815.09 Closed fracture of multiple sites of metacarpus
- 815.11 Open fracture of base of thumb (first) metacarpal bone(s)
- 815.14 Open fracture of neck of metacarpal bone(s)
- 815.19 Open fracture of multiple sites of metacarpus
- 816.01 Closed fracture of middle or proximal phalanx or phalanges of hand
- 816.03 Closed fracture of multiple sites of phalanx or phalanges of hand
- 817.0 Multiple closed fractures of hand bones
- 817.1 Multiple open fractures of hand bones

Terms To Know

closed fracture. Break in a bone without a concomitant opening in the skin. A closed fracture is coded when the type of fracture is not specified.

fracture. Break in bone or cartilage.

open fracture. Exposed break in a bone, always considered compound due to its high risk of infection from the open wound leading to the fracture. Broken bone ends may protrude through the skin and contaminants or foreign bodies are often embedded in the tissues.

proximal. Located closest to a specified reference point, usually the midline.

CCI Version 16.3
01810, 01820, 0213T, 0216T, 0228T, 0230T, 13131, 20526-20553, 20650, 25259, 26055, 26075-26080, 26105-26110, 26140-26145, 26185, 26340, 26440-26449, 26520-26525, 26542-26546❖, 26725, 26740-26742, 26750-26756, 26770-26776, 29065-29131, 29280, 29700-29715, 36000, 36400-36410, 36420-36430, 36440, 36600, 36640, 37202, 43752, 51701-51703, 62310-62319, 64400-64435, 64445-64450, 64479, 64483, 64490, 64493, 64505-64530, 64702-64704, 69990, 76000-76001, 93000-93010, 93040-93042, 93318, 94002, 94200, 94250, 94680-94690, 94770, 95812-95816, 95819, 95822, 95829, 95955, 96360, 96365, 96372, 96374-96376, 97597-97598, 97602-97606, 99148-99149, 99150

Note: These CCI edits are used for Medicare. Other payers may reimburse on codes listed above.

Medicare Edits

	Fac RVU	Non-Fac RVU	FUD	Assist
26746	21.13	21.13	90	N/A

Medicare References: 100-2,15,260; 100-4,12,30; 100-4,12,90.3; 100-4,14,10

26750-26755

26750 Closed treatment of distal phalangeal fracture, finger or thumb; without manipulation, each
26755 with manipulation, each

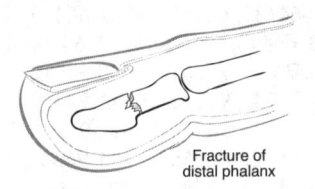

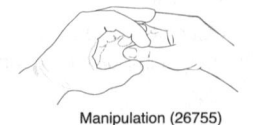

Fracture of distal phalanx

Manipulation (26755)

A fracture of the distal phalanx, whether finger or thumb, is treated in a closed fashion, with or without manipulation. Report 26755 when manipulation is required during the treatment

Explanation

The physician treats a distal phalangeal fracture of the finger or thumb, with or without manipulation. In 26750, no manipulation is necessary. In 26755, the physician manipulates the bones to restore anatomical position. The hand is splinted for stabilization.

Coding Tips

When multiple fractures are treated, report one fracture treatment as the primary procedure and append modifier 51 to subsequent procedures. Some payers may require the use of HCPCS Level II modifiers FA–F9 to identify the specific finger involved. According to CPT guidelines, cast application or strapping (including removal) is only reported as a replacement procedure or when the cast application or strapping is an initial service performed without a restorative treatment or procedure. See "Application of Casts and Strapping" in the CPT book in the Surgery Section, under the Musculoskeletal system. Local anesthesia is included in these services. For radiology services, see 73140. For percutaneous skeletal fixation of a distal phalangeal fracture, see 26756. For open treatment of a distal phalangeal fracture, see 26765.

ICD-9-CM Procedural

79.04 Closed reduction of fracture of phalanges of hand without internal fixation
93.54 Application of splint

Anesthesia
01820

ICD-9-CM Diagnostic

733.19 Pathologic fracture of other specified site
816.02 Closed fracture of distal phalanx or phalanges of hand
816.03 Closed fracture of multiple sites of phalanx or phalanges of hand
817.0 Multiple closed fractures of hand bones

Terms To Know

closed fracture. Break in a bone without a concomitant opening in the skin. A closed fracture is coded when the type of fracture is not specified.

distal. Located farther away from a specified reference point.

fracture. Break in bone or cartilage.

phalanx. Bones of the digits (fingers or toes).

CCI Version 16.3

01810, 01820, 0213T, 0216T, 0228T, 0230T, 20526-20553, 25259, 26340, 26546❖, 29065-29131, 29280, 29700-29715, 36000, 36400-36410, 36420-36430, 36440, 36600, 36640, 37202, 43752, 51701-51703, 62310-62319, 64400-64435, 64445-64450, 64479, 64483, 64490, 64493, 64505-64530, 69990, 93000-93010, 93040-93042, 93318, 94002, 94200, 94250, 94680-94690, 94770, 95812-95816, 95819, 95822, 95829, 95955, 96360, 96365, 96372, 96374-96376, 97597-97598, 97602-97606, 99148-99149, 99150

Also not with 26750: 12041, 13131
Also not with 26755: 26750, J0670, J2001

Note: These CCI edits are used for Medicare. Other payers may reimburse on codes listed above.

Medicare Edits

	Fac RVU	Non-Fac RVU	FUD	Assist
26750	5.04	5.1	90	N/A
26755	7.7	8.81	90	N/A

Medicare References: None

26756

26756 Percutaneous skeletal fixation of distal phalangeal fracture, finger or thumb, each

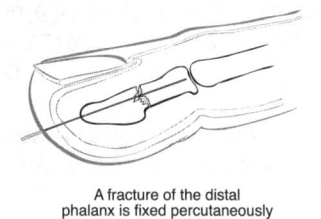

A fracture of the distal phalanx is fixed percutaneously

Explanation

The physician treats a distal phalangeal fracture of the finger or thumb with manipulation and secures it with a wire. The physician drills a wire into the tip of the finger bone, through the fracture, and into the proximal bone. The drill entry point is dressed and the hand is splinted.

Coding Tips

When multiple fractures are treated, report one fracture treatment as the primary procedure and append modifier 51 to subsequent procedures. Some payers may require the use of HCPCS Level II modifiers FA–F9 to identify the specific finger involved. According to CPT guidelines, cast application or strapping (including removal) is only reported as a replacement procedure or when the cast application or strapping is an initial service performed without a restorative treatment or procedure. See "Application of Casts and Strapping" in the CPT book in the Surgery Section, under the Musculoskeletal system. For radiology services, see 73140. For closed treatment of a distal phalangeal fracture, without manipulation, see 26750; with manipulation, see 26755. For open treatment of a distal phalangeal fracture, see 26765.

ICD-9-CM Procedural

78.59 Internal fixation of other bone, except facial bones, without fracture reduction

Anesthesia

26756 01820

ICD-9-CM Diagnostic

733.19 Pathologic fracture of other specified site
816.02 Closed fracture of distal phalanx or phalanges of hand
816.03 Closed fracture of multiple sites of phalanx or phalanges of hand
816.12 Open fracture of distal phalanx or phalanges of hand
816.13 Open fractures of multiple sites of phalanx or phalanges of hand
817.0 Multiple closed fractures of hand bones

Terms To Know

closed fracture. Break in a bone without a concomitant opening in the skin. A closed fracture is coded when the type of fracture is not specified.

distal. Located farther away from a specified reference point.

fracture. Break in bone or cartilage.

manipulation. Skillful treatment by hand to reduce fractures and dislocations, or provide therapy through forceful passive movement of a joint beyond its active limit of motion.

open fracture. Exposed break in a bone, always considered compound due to its high risk of infection from the open wound leading to the fracture. Broken bone ends may protrude through the skin and contaminants or foreign bodies are often embedded in the tissues.

phalanx. Bones of the digits (fingers or toes).

proximal. Located closest to a specified reference point, usually the midline.

CCI Version 16.3

01810, 01820, 0213T, 0216T, 0228T, 0230T, 13132, 20526-20553, 20650, 20690, 20692, 20696-20697, 25259, 26340, 26546❖, 26750-26755, 29065-29131, 29280, 29700-29715, 36000, 36400-36410, 36420-36430, 36440, 36600, 36640, 37202, 43752, 51701-51703, 62310-62319, 64400-64435, 64445-64450, 64479, 64483, 64490, 64493, 64505-64530, 69990, 93000-93010, 93040-93042, 93318, 94002, 94200, 94250, 94680-94690, 94770, 95812-95816, 95819, 95822, 95829, 95955, 96360, 96365, 96372, 96374-96376, 97597-97598, 97602-97606, 99148-99149, 99150, J0670, J2001

Note: These CCI edits are used for Medicare. Other payers may reimburse on codes listed above.

Medicare Edits

	Fac RVU	Non-Fac RVU	FUD	Assist
26756	11.99	11.99	90	80

Medicare References: 100-2,15,260; 100-4,12,30; 100-4,12,90.3; 100-4,14,10

26765

26765 Open treatment of distal phalangeal fracture, finger or thumb, includes internal fixation, when performed, each

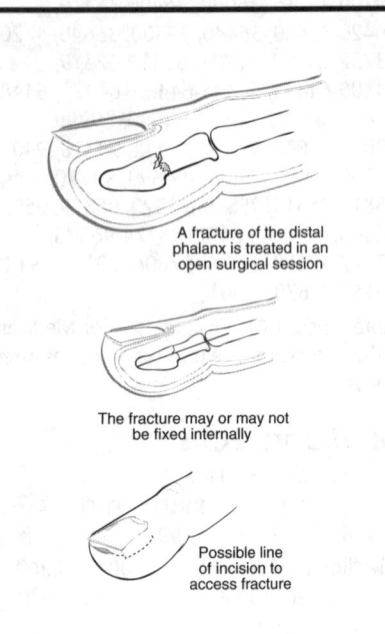

A fracture of the distal phalanx is treated in an open surgical session

The fracture may or may not be fixed internally

Possible line of incision to access fracture

Explanation
The physician performs open reduction of a distal phalangeal fracture of the finger or thumb. The physician uses an x-ray to determine the position and severity of the defect. An incision is made on the overlying skin to expose the fracture and the bones are reapproximated. A wire or plate may be placed for internal fixation. The incision is sutured in layers and the hand is splinted.

Coding Tips
When multiple fractures are treated, report one fracture treatment as the primary procedure and append modifier 51 to subsequent procedures. Some payers may require the use of HCPCS Level II modifiers FA–F9 to identify the specific finger involved. According to CPT guidelines, cast application or strapping (including removal) is only reported as a replacement procedure or when the cast application or strapping is an initial service performed without a restorative treatment or procedure. See "Application of Casts and Strapping" in the CPT book in the Surgery Section, under the Musculoskeletal system. For radiology services, see 73140. For closed treatment of a distal phalangeal fracture, without manipulation, see 26750; with manipulation, see 26755. For percutaneous skeletal fixation of a distal phalangeal fracture, see 26756.

ICD-9-CM Procedural
- 79.24 Open reduction of fracture of phalanges of hand without internal fixation
- 79.34 Open reduction of fracture of phalanges of hand with internal fixation

Anesthesia
26765 01830

ICD-9-CM Diagnostic
- 733.19 Pathologic fracture of other specified site
- 816.02 Closed fracture of distal phalanx or phalanges of hand
- 816.03 Closed fracture of multiple sites of phalanx or phalanges of hand
- 816.12 Open fracture of distal phalanx or phalanges of hand
- 816.13 Open fractures of multiple sites of phalanx or phalanges of hand
- 817.0 Multiple closed fractures of hand bones
- 817.1 Multiple open fractures of hand bones

Terms To Know
closed fracture. Break in a bone without a concomitant opening in the skin. A closed fracture is coded when the type of fracture is not specified.

distal. Located farther away from a specified reference point.

fracture. Break in bone or cartilage.

open fracture. Exposed break in a bone, always considered compound due to its high risk of infection from the open wound leading to the fracture. Broken bone ends may protrude through the skin and contaminants or foreign bodies are often embedded in the tissues.

CCI Version 16.3
01810, 01820, 0213T, 0216T, 0228T, 0230T, 12001-12007, 12020-12021, 12041-12047, 13131-13132, 20526-20553, 20650, 25259, 26185, 26340, 26546✤, 26746-26756, 29065-29131, 29280, 29700-29715, 36000, 36400-36410, 36420-36430, 36440, 36600, 36640, 37202, 43752, 51701-51703, 62310-62319, 64400-64435, 64445-64450, 64479, 64483, 64490, 64493, 64505-64530, 69990, 93000-93010, 93040-93042, 93318, 94002, 94200, 94250, 94680-94690, 94770, 95812-95816, 95819, 95822, 95829, 95955, 96360, 96365, 96372, 96374-96376, 97597-97598, 97602-97606, 99148-99149, 99150, G0168

Note: These CCI edits are used for Medicare. Other payers may reimburse on codes listed above.

Medicare Edits

	Fac RVU	Non-Fac RVU	FUD	Assist
26765	14.14	14.14	90	N/A

Medicare References: 100-2,15,260; 100-4,12,30; 100-4,12,90.3; 100-4,14,10

26770-26775

26770 Closed treatment of interphalangeal joint dislocation, single, with manipulation; without anesthesia
26775 requiring anesthesia

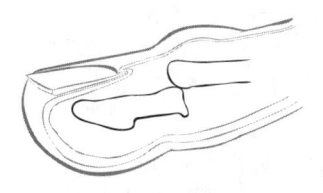

A dislocation of an interphalangeal joint is treated in a closed fashion with manipulation. Report 26775 when anesthesia is required

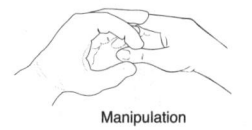

Manipulation

Explanation

The physician treats an interphalangeal joint dislocation using manipulation; anesthesia may be used if necessary. The physician determines the dislocated position of the bone and uses external manipulation to relocate the bone. In 26770, dislocation is minor and no anesthesia is needed. In 26775, dislocation is major and anesthesia is required.

Coding Tips

When multiple dislocations are treated, report one dislocation treatment as the primary procedure and append modifier 51 to subsequent procedures. Some payers may require the use of HCPCS Level II modifiers FA–F9 to identify the specific finger involved. According to CPT guidelines, cast application or strapping (including removal) is only reported as a replacement procedure or when the cast application or strapping is an initial service performed without a restorative treatment or procedure. See "Application of Casts and Strapping" in the CPT book in the Surgery Section, under the Musculoskeletal system. For radiology services, see 73140. For percutaneous skeletal fixation of an interphalangeal joint dislocation, see 26776. For open treatment of an interphalangeal joint dislocation, see 26785.

ICD-9-CM Procedural

79.70 Closed reduction of dislocation of unspecified site

Anesthesia

26770 N/A
26775 01820

ICD-9-CM Diagnostic

718.24 Pathological dislocation of hand joint
718.34 Recurrent dislocation of hand joint
718.74 Developmental dislocation of joint, hand
834.02 Closed dislocation of interphalangeal (joint), hand

Terms To Know

developmental dislocation. Displacement of a body part occurring in the developmental phase of childhood.

manipulation. Skillful treatment by hand to reduce fractures and dislocations, or provide therapy through forceful passive movement of a joint beyond its active limit of motion.

pathological dislocation. Displacement of a bone or joint caused by a disease process, such as infection, lesions, or muscle weakness, and not traumatic injury.

CCI Version 16.3

01810, 01820, 0213T, 0216T, 0228T, 0230T, 20526-20553, 25259, 26340, 26546❖, 29065-29131, 29280, 29700-29715, 36000, 36400-36410, 36420-36430, 36440, 36600, 36640, 37202, 43752, 51701-51703, 62310-62319, 64400-64435, 64445-64450, 64479, 64483, 64490, 64493, 64505-64530, 69990, 93000-93010, 93040-93042, 93318, 94002, 94200, 94250, 94680-94690, 94770, 95812-95816, 95819, 95822, 95829, 95955, 96360, 96365, 96372, 96374-96376, 97597-97598, 97602-97606, 99148-99149, 99150, J2001

Also not with 26775: 26770, J0670

Note: These CCI edits are used for Medicare. Other payers may reimburse on codes listed above.

Medicare Edits

	Fac RVU	Non-Fac RVU	FUD	Assist
26770	7.01	7.59	90	N/A
26775	9.73	10.77	90	N/A

Medicare References: None

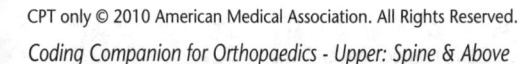

26776

26776 Percutaneous skeletal fixation of interphalangeal joint dislocation, single, with manipulation

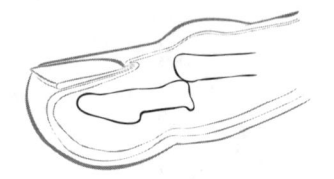

A dislocation of an interphalangeal joint is treated in a closed fashion with manipulation and percutaneous (through the skin) skeletal fixation

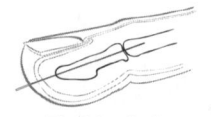

The dislocation is fixed percutaneously

Explanation
The physician manipulates an interphalangeal joint dislocation to restore anatomical position and secures the bone with a wire. The physician determines the dislocated position of the bone. The bone is relocated to correct anatomical position using external manipulation. The physician drills a wire through the interphalangeal joint for stabilization and the hand is splinted.

Coding Tips
When multiple fractures are treated, report one fracture treatment as the primary procedure and append modifier 51 to subsequent procedures. Some payers may require the use of HCPCS Level II modifiers FA–F9 to identify the specific finger involved. According to CPT guidelines, cast application or strapping (including removal) is only reported as a replacement procedure or when the cast application or strapping is an initial service performed without a restorative treatment or procedure. See "Application of Casts and Strapping" in the CPT book in the Surgery Section, under the Musculoskeletal system. For radiology services, see 73140. For closed treatment of an interphalangeal joint dislocation, without anesthesia, see 26770; with anesthesia, see 26775. For open treatment of an interphalangeal joint dislocation, see 26785.

ICD-9-CM Procedural
- 78.59 Internal fixation of other bone, except facial bones, without fracture reduction
- 79.74 Closed reduction of dislocation of hand and finger

Anesthesia
26776 01820

ICD-9-CM Diagnostic
- 718.24 Pathological dislocation of hand joint
- 718.34 Recurrent dislocation of hand joint
- 718.74 Developmental dislocation of joint, hand
- 834.02 Closed dislocation of interphalangeal (joint), hand

Terms To Know

developmental dislocation. Displacement of a body part occurring in the developmental phase of childhood.

manipulation. Skillful treatment by hand to reduce fractures and dislocations, or provide therapy through forceful passive movement of a joint beyond its active limit of motion.

pathological dislocation. Displacement of a bone or joint caused by a disease process, such as infection, lesions, or muscle weakness, and not traumatic injury.

CCI Version 16.3
01810, 01820, 0213T, 0216T, 0228T, 0230T, 20526-20553, 20650, 20690, 25259, 26340, 26546❖, 26770-26775, 29065-29131, 29280, 29700-29715, 36000, 36400-36410, 36420-36430, 36440, 36600, 36640, 37202, 43752, 51701-51703, 62310-62319, 64400-64435, 64445-64450, 64479, 64483, 64490, 64493, 64505-64530, 69990, 93000-93010, 93040-93042, 93318, 94002, 94200, 94250, 94680-94690, 94770, 95812-95816, 95819, 95822, 95829, 95955, 96360, 96365, 96372, 96374-96376, 97597-97598, 97602-97606, 99148-99149, 99150, J0670, J2001

Note: These CCI edits are used for Medicare. Other payers may reimburse on codes listed above.

Medicare Edits

	Fac RVU	Non-Fac RVU	FUD	Assist
26776	12.72	12.72	90	N/A

Medicare References: 100-2,15,260; 100-4,12,30; 100-4,12,90.3; 100-4,14,10

26785

26785 Open treatment of interphalangeal joint dislocation, includes internal fixation, when performed, single

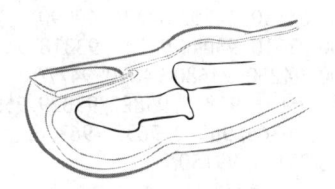

A dislocation of an interphalangeal joint is treated in an open surgical session, with or without internal fixation

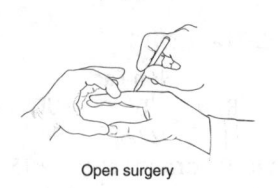

Open surgery

Explanation
The physician performs open correction of an interphalangeal joint dislocation. The physician uses an x-ray to determine the position and severity of the defect. An incision is made on the overlying skin to expose the dislocated joint and the bones are reapproximated. A wire may be placed for internal fixation. The incision is sutured in layers and the hand is splinted.

Coding Tips
When multiple fractures are treated, report one fracture treatment as the primary procedure and append modifier 51 to subsequent procedures. Some payers may require the use of HCPCS Level II modifiers FA–F9 to identify the specific finger involved. According to CPT guidelines, cast application or strapping (including removal) is only reported as a replacement procedure or when the cast application or strapping is an initial service performed without a restorative treatment or procedure. See "Application of Casts and Strapping" in the CPT book in the Surgery Section, under the Musculoskeletal system. For radiology services, see 73140. For closed treatment of an interphalangeal joint dislocation, without anesthesia, see 26770; with anesthesia, see 26775. For percutaneous skeletal fixation of an interphalangeal joint dislocation, see 26776.

ICD-9-CM Procedural
79.80 Open reduction of dislocation of unspecified site

Anesthesia
26785 01830

ICD-9-CM Diagnostic
718.24 Pathological dislocation of hand joint
718.34 Recurrent dislocation of hand joint
718.74 Developmental dislocation of joint, hand
834.02 Closed dislocation of interphalangeal (joint), hand
834.12 Open dislocation interphalangeal (joint), hand

Terms To Know

developmental dislocation. Displacement of a body part occurring in the developmental phase of childhood.

pathological dislocation. Displacement of a bone or joint caused by a disease process, such as infection, lesions, or muscle weakness, and not traumatic injury.

CCI Version 16.3
01810, 01820, 0213T, 0216T, 0228T, 0230T, 12042, 20526-20553, 20650, 25259, 26185, 26340, 26546❖, 26770-26776, 29065-29131, 29280, 29700-29715, 36000, 36400-36410, 36420-36430, 36440, 36600, 36640, 37202, 43752, 51701-51703, 62310-62319, 64400-64435, 64445-64450, 64479, 64483, 64490, 64493, 64505-64530, 69990, 93000-93010, 93040-93042, 93318, 94002, 94200, 94250, 94680-94690, 94770, 95812-95816, 95819, 95822, 95829, 95955, 96360, 96365, 96372, 96374-96376, 97597-97598, 97602-97606, 99148-99149, 99150

Note: These CCI edits are used for Medicare. Other payers may reimburse on codes listed above.

Medicare Edits

	Fac RVU	Non-Fac RVU	FUD	Assist
26785	15.42	15.42	90	N/A

Medicare References: 100-2,15,260; 100-4,12,30; 100-4,12,90.3; 100-4,14,10

26820

26820 Fusion in opposition, thumb, with autogenous graft (includes obtaining graft)

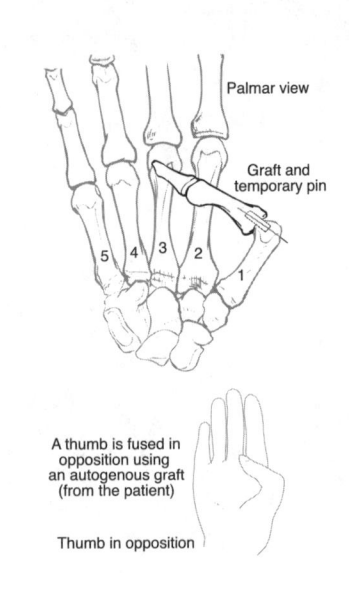

Palmar view

Graft and temporary pin

A thumb is fused in opposition using an autogenous graft (from the patient)

Thumb in opposition

Explanation
The physician fuses the thumb in opposition. The physician incises the overlying skin and dissects to the metacarpophalangeal joint. A bone graft is obtained from the distal radius or iliac crest and placed to secure the joint. A wire is placed through the joint until fusion is complete. The operative incision is closed in sutured layers and the thumb is splinted for stabilization.

Coding Tips
Any bone graft harvest is not reported separately. According to CPT guidelines, cast application or strapping (including removal) is only reported as a replacement procedure or when the cast application or strapping is an initial service performed without a restorative treatment or procedure. See "Application of Casts and Strapping" in the CPT book in the Surgery Section, under the Musculoskeletal system.

ICD-9-CM Procedural
81.29 Arthrodesis of other specified joint

Anesthesia
26820 01830

ICD-9-CM Diagnostic
357.1 Polyneuropathy in collagen vascular disease — (Code first underlying disease: 446.0, 710.0, 714.0)
359.6 Symptomatic inflammatory myopathy in diseases classified elsewhere — (Code first underlying disease: 135, 140.0-208.9, 277.30-277.39, 446.0, 710.0, 710.1, 710.2, 714.0)
446.0 Polyarteritis nodosa
710.0 Systemic lupus erythematosus — (Use additional code to identify manifestation: 424.91, 581.81, 582.81, 583.81)
710.1 Systemic sclerosis — (Use additional code to identify manifestation: 359.6, 517.2)
710.2 Sicca syndrome
714.0 Rheumatoid arthritis — (Use additional code to identify manifestation: 357.1, 359.6)
715.34 Localized osteoarthrosis not specified whether primary or secondary, hand
716.14 Traumatic arthropathy, hand
718.24 Pathological dislocation of hand joint
718.34 Recurrent dislocation of hand joint
726.4 Enthesopathy of wrist and carpus
733.81 Malunion of fracture
905.2 Late effect of fracture of upper extremities
905.6 Late effect of dislocation
906.4 Late effect of crushing

Terms To Know
autogenous transplant. Tissue, such as bone, that is harvested from the patient and used for transplantation back into the same patient.

fusion. Union of adjacent tissues, especially bone.

late effect. Abnormality, dysfunction, or other residual condition produced after the acute phase of an illness, injury, or disease is over. There is no time limit on when late effects can appear.

pathological dislocation. Displacement of a bone or joint caused by a disease process, such as infection, lesions, or muscle weakness, and not traumatic injury.

polyneuropathy. Disease process of severe inflammation of multiple nerves.

systemic sclerosis. Systemic disease characterized by excess fibrotic collagen build-up, turning the skin thickened and hard. Fibrotic changes also occur in various organs and cause vascular abnormalities and affect more women than men.

CCI Version 16.3
01810, 0213T, 0216T, 0228T, 0230T, 20526-20553, 20690, 20692, 20696-20697, 20900-20902, 25259, 26111-26116, 26160, 26185, 26340, 26440-26449, 26546❖, 29086, 36000, 36400-36410, 36420-36430, 36440, 36600, 36640, 37202, 43752, 51701-51703, 62310-62319, 64400-64435, 64445-64450, 64479, 64483, 64490, 64493, 64505-64530, 64702-64726, 69990, 93000-93010, 93040-93042, 93318, 94002, 94200, 94250, 94680-94690, 94770, 95812-95816, 95819, 95822, 95829, 95955, 96360, 96365, 96372, 96374-96376, 99148-99149, 99150

Note: These CCI edits are used for Medicare. Other payers may reimburse on codes listed above.

Medicare Edits

	Fac RVU	Non-Fac RVU	FUD	Assist
26820	22.68	22.68	90	80

Medicare References: 100-2,15,260; 100-4,12,30; 100-4,12,90.3; 100-4,14,10

26841-26842

26841 Arthrodesis, carpometacarpal joint, thumb, with or without internal fixation;

26842 with autograft (includes obtaining graft)

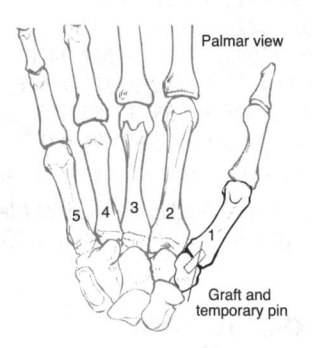

A thumb is fused (arthrodesis) at the carpometacarpal joint, with or without internal fixation. Report 26842 when an autograft (from the patient) is used

Explanation

The physician fuses the carpometacarpal joint of a finger or the thumb. Internal or external fixation may be used. The physician incises the overlying skin and dissects to the carpometacarpal joint. The joint is fixated with a wire, screws, or plates. The incision is sutured in layers and the hand is splinted. If a graft is obtained, the physician harvests bone from the distal radius or iliac crest. The graft is interposed between the two bones to prevent movement and a wire is placed through the joint until fusion is complete. In 26841, the thumb is treated; report 26842 if an autograft is obtained and used. The incision is sutured in layers and the hand is splinted.

Coding Tips

Any bone graft harvest is not reported separately for 26842. According to CPT guidelines, cast application or strapping (including removal) is only reported as a replacement procedure or when the cast application or strapping is an initial service performed without a restorative treatment or procedure. See "Application of Casts and Strapping" in the CPT book in the Surgery Section, under the Musculoskeletal system. For arthrodesis of the carpometacarpal joint, other than thumb, with or without internal fixation, see 26843; with autograft, see 26844.

ICD-9-CM Procedural

81.29 Arthrodesis of other specified joint

Anesthesia

01830

ICD-9-CM Diagnostic

357.1 Polyneuropathy in collagen vascular disease — (Code first underlying disease: 446.0, 710.0, 714.0)

359.6 Symptomatic inflammatory myopathy in diseases classified elsewhere — (Code first underlying disease: 135, 140.0-208.9, 277.30-277.39, 446.0, 710.0, 710.1, 710.2, 714.0)

446.0 Polyarteritis nodosa

710.0 Systemic lupus erythematosus — (Use additional code to identify manifestation: 424.91, 581.81, 582.81, 583.81)

710.1 Systemic sclerosis — (Use additional code to identify manifestation: 359.6, 517.2)

710.2 Sicca syndrome

714.0 Rheumatoid arthritis — (Use additional code to identify manifestation: 357.1, 359.6)

715.34 Localized osteoarthrosis not specified whether primary or secondary, hand

716.14 Traumatic arthropathy, hand

718.24 Pathological dislocation of hand joint

718.34 Recurrent dislocation of hand joint

726.4 Enthesopathy of wrist and carpus

727.00 Unspecified synovitis and tenosynovitis

733.81 Malunion of fracture

755.56 Accessory carpal bones

905.2 Late effect of fracture of upper extremities

905.6 Late effect of dislocation

906.4 Late effect of crushing

Terms To Know

arthrodesis. Surgical fixation or fusion of a joint to reduce pain and improve stability, performed openly or arthroscopically.

autograft. Any tissue harvested from one anatomical site of a person and grafted to another anatomical site of the same person. Most commonly, blood vessels, skin, tendons, fascia, and bone are used as autografts.

fixation. Act or condition of being attached, secured, fastened, or held in position.

CCI Version 16.3

01810, 0213T, 0216T, 0228T, 0230T, 20526-20553, 20690, 20692, 20696-20697, 25259, 26070, 26100, 26111-26116, 26130, 26160, 26185, 26230, 26340, 26440-26449, 26546❖, 26641-26650, 26665-26676, 26685-26686, 29086, 29900-29902, 36000, 36400-36410, 36420-36430, 36440, 36600, 36640, 37202, 43752, 51701-51703, 62310-62319, 64400-64435, 64445-64450, 64479, 64483, 64490, 64493, 64505-64530, 64702-64726, 69990, 93000-93010, 93040-93042, 93318, 94002, 94200, 94250, 94680-94690, 94770, 95812-95816, 95819, 95822, 95829, 95955, 96360, 96365, 96372, 96374-96376, 99148-99149, 99150

Also not with 26841: 11012❖

Also not with 26842: 20900-20902, 26055, 26841

Note: These CCI edits are used for Medicare. Other payers may reimburse on codes listed above.

Medicare Edits

	Fac RVU	Non-Fac RVU	FUD	Assist
26841	21.01	21.01	90	80
26842	22.78	22.78	90	80

Medicare References: 100-2,15,260; 100-4,12,30; 100-4,12,90.3; 100-4,14,10

26843-26844

26843 Arthrodesis, carpometacarpal joint, digit, other than thumb, each;
26844 with autograft (includes obtaining graft)

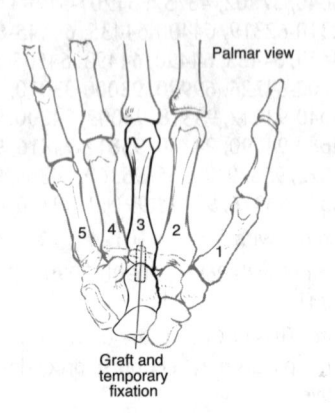

Palmar view

A digit other than a thumb is fused (arthrodesis) at the carpometacarpal joint, with or without internal fixation. Report 26844 when an autograft (from the patient) is used

Explanation
The physician fuses the carpometacarpal joint of a finger or the thumb. Internal or external fixation may be used. The physician incises the overlying skin and dissects to the carpometacarpal joint. The joint is fixated with a wire, screws, or plates. The incision is sutured in layers and the hand is splinted. If a graft is obtained, the physician harvests bone from the distal radius or iliac crest. The graft is interposed between the two bones to prevent movement and a wire is placed through the joint until fusion is complete. In 26843, a finger joint is treated; report 26844 if an autograft is obtained and used. The incision is sutured in layers and the hand is splinted.

Coding Tips
Any bone graft harvest is not reported separately for 26844. According to CPT guidelines, cast application or strapping (including removal) is only reported as a replacement procedure or when the cast application or strapping is an initial service performed without a restorative treatment or procedure. See "Application of Casts and Strapping" in the CPT book in the Surgery Section, under the Musculoskeletal system. For arthrodesis of the carpometacarpal joint, thumb, with or without internal fixation, see 26841; with autograft, see 26842.

ICD-9-CM Procedural
81.29 Arthrodesis of other specified joint

Anesthesia
01830

ICD-9-CM Diagnostic
357.1 Polyneuropathy in collagen vascular disease — (Code first underlying disease: 446.0, 710.0, 714.0)
359.6 Symptomatic inflammatory myopathy in diseases classified elsewhere — (Code first underlying disease: 135, 140.0-208.9, 277.30-277.39, 446.0, 710.0, 710.1, 710.2, 714.0)
446.0 Polyarteritis nodosa
710.0 Systemic lupus erythematosus — (Use additional code to identify manifestation: 424.91, 581.81, 582.81, 583.81)
710.1 Systemic sclerosis — (Use additional code to identify manifestation: 359.6, 517.2)
710.2 Sicca syndrome
714.0 Rheumatoid arthritis — (Use additional code to identify manifestation: 357.1, 359.6)
715.34 Localized osteoarthrosis not specified whether primary or secondary, hand
716.14 Traumatic arthropathy, hand
718.24 Pathological dislocation of hand joint
718.34 Recurrent dislocation of hand joint
726.4 Enthesopathy of wrist and carpus
727.00 Unspecified synovitis and tenosynovitis
733.81 Malunion of fracture
755.56 Accessory carpal bones
905.2 Late effect of fracture of upper extremities
905.6 Late effect of dislocation
906.4 Late effect of crushing

Terms To Know
arthrodesis. Surgical fixation or fusion of a joint to reduce pain and improve stability, performed openly or arthroscopically.

autograft. Any tissue harvested from one anatomical site of a person and grafted to another anatomical site of the same person. Most commonly, blood vessels, skin, tendons, fascia, and bone are used as autografts.

harvest. Removal of cells or tissue from their native site to be used as a graft or transplant to another part of the donor's body or placed into another person.

CCI Version 16.3
01810, 0213T, 0216T, 0228T, 0230T, 20526-20553, 20690, 20692, 20696-20697, 25259, 26070, 26100, 26111-26116, 26130, 26160, 26185, 26230, 26340, 26440-26449, 26546❖, 26641-26650, 26665-26676, 26685-26686, 29086, 29900-29902, 36000, 36400-36410, 36420-36430, 36440, 36600, 36640, 37202, 43752, 51701-51703, 62310-62319, 64400-64435, 64445-64450, 64479, 64483, 64490, 64493, 64505-64530, 64702-64726, 69990, 93000-93010, 93040-93042, 93318, 94002, 94200, 94250, 94680-94690, 94770, 95812-95816, 95819, 95822, 95829, 95955, 96360, 96365, 96372, 96374-96376, 99148-99149, 99150

Also not with 26844: 20900-20902, 26843

Note: These CCI edits are used for Medicare. Other payers may reimburse on codes listed above.

Medicare Edits

	Fac RVU	Non-Fac RVU	FUD	Assist
26843	21.2	21.2	90	80
26844	23.61	23.61	90	80

Medicare References: 100-2,15,260; 100-4,12,30; 100-4,12,90.3; 100-4,14,10

26850-26852

26850 Arthrodesis, metacarpophalangeal joint, with or without internal fixation;
26852 with autograft (includes obtaining graft)

Palmar view

The joint is accessed and the articular surfaces prepared. The joint may fuse over time with splints or casts, without use of internal fixation or grafts

A metacarpophalangeal joint is fused (arthrodesis), with or without internal fixation. Report 26852 when an autograft (from the patient) is used

Explanation

The physician fuses a metacarpophalangeal joint. Internal or external fixation may be used. The physician incises the overlying skin and dissects to the metacarpophalangeal joint. The physician may use a wire to stabilize the joint until fusion is complete. Report 26852 if an autograft is obtained and used. Bone is harvested from the distal radius or iliac crest and interposed between the two bones to prevent movement. The incision is sutured in layers and the hand is splinted.

Coding Tips

Any bone graft harvest is not reported separately for 26852. According to CPT guidelines, cast application or strapping (including removal) is only reported as a replacement procedure or when the cast application or strapping is an initial service performed without a restorative treatment or procedure. See "Application of Casts and Strapping" in the CPT book in the Surgery Section, under the Musculoskeletal system.

ICD-9-CM Procedural

81.27 Metacarpophalangeal fusion

Anesthesia

01830

ICD-9-CM Diagnostic

357.1 Polyneuropathy in collagen vascular disease — (Code first underlying disease: 446.0, 710.0, 714.0)
359.6 Symptomatic inflammatory myopathy in diseases classified elsewhere — (Code first underlying disease: 135, 140.0-208.9, 277.30-277.39, 446.0, 710.0, 710.1, 710.2, 714.0)
446.0 Polyarteritis nodosa
710.0 Systemic lupus erythematosus — (Use additional code to identify manifestation: 424.91, 581.81, 582.81, 583.81)
710.1 Systemic sclerosis — (Use additional code to identify manifestation: 359.6, 517.2)
710.2 Sicca syndrome
714.0 Rheumatoid arthritis — (Use additional code to identify manifestation: 357.1, 359.6)
715.34 Localized osteoarthrosis not specified whether primary or secondary, hand
716.14 Traumatic arthropathy, hand
718.24 Pathological dislocation of hand joint
718.34 Recurrent dislocation of hand joint
726.91 Exostosis of unspecified site
727.00 Unspecified synovitis and tenosynovitis
733.81 Malunion of fracture
905.2 Late effect of fracture of upper extremities
905.6 Late effect of dislocation
906.4 Late effect of crushing

Terms To Know

dissection. Separating by cutting tissue or body structures apart.

exostosis. Abnormal formation of a benign bony growth.

incision. Act of cutting into tissue or an organ.

polyneuropathy. Disease process of severe inflammation of multiple nerves.

systemic sclerosis. Systemic disease characterized by excess fibrotic collagen build-up, turning the skin thickened and hard. Fibrotic changes also occur in various organs and cause vascular abnormalities and affect more women than men.

CCI Version 16.3

01810, 0213T, 0216T, 0228T, 0230T, 20526-20553, 20690, 20692, 20696-20697, 25259, 26075, 26105, 26111-26116, 26135, 26185, 26235-26236, 26340, 26440-26449, 26520, 26546❖, 26700-26706, 26715, 26740-26742, 26746, 29086, 29900-29902, 36000, 36400-36410, 36420-36430, 36440, 36600, 36640, 37202, 43752, 51701-51703, 62310-62319, 64400-64435, 64445-64450, 64479, 64483, 64490, 64493, 64505-64530, 69990, 93000-93010, 93040-93042, 93318, 94002, 94200, 94250, 94680-94690, 94770, 95812-95816, 95819, 95822, 95829, 95955, 96360, 96365, 96372, 96374-96376, 99148-99149, 99150

Also not with 26850: 11012❖, 26160, 26531❖, 29125, 64702-64726

Also not with 26852: 20900-20902, 26145-26160, 26850, 64702-64704, 64712-64718, 64721-64726

Note: These CCI edits are used for Medicare. Other payers may reimburse on codes listed above.

Medicare Edits

	Fac RVU	Non-Fac RVU	FUD	Assist
26850	19.96	19.96	90	80
26852	22.9	22.9	90	80

Medicare References: 100-2,15,260; 100-4,12,30; 100-4,12,90.3; 100-4,14,10

26860-26863

26860 Arthrodesis, interphalangeal joint, with or without internal fixation;
26861 each additional interphalangeal joint (List separately in addition to code for primary procedure)
26862 with autograft (includes obtaining graft)
26863 with autograft (includes obtaining graft), each additional joint (List separately in addition to code for primary procedure)

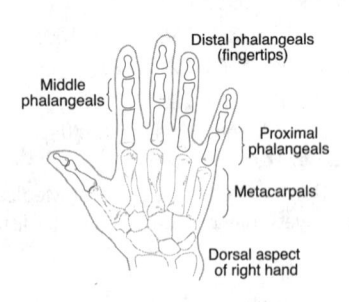

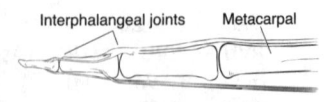

An interphalangeal joint is fused (arthodesis), with or without internal fixation. Report 26861 for each additional digit treated. Report 26862 when an autograft is used in the treatment. Report 26863 when an autograft is used for each additional digit treated

Explanation

The physician fuses an interphalangeal joint. Internal or external fixation may be used. The physician incises the overlying skin and dissects to the interphalangeal joint. The physician may use a wire to stabilize the joint until fusion is complete. Report 26861 for each additional interphalangeal joint. Report 26862 if an autograft is obtained and used. A graft is harvested from the distal radius or iliac crest and interposed between the bones to prevent movement. Report 26863 for autografts on each additional interphalangeal joints. The incision is sutured in layers and the hand is splinted.

Coding Tips

Use 26861 in conjunction with 26860. Use 26863 in conjunction with 26862. As "add-on" codes, 26861 and 26863 are not subject to multiple procedure rules. No reimbursement reduction or modifier 51 is applied. Add-on codes describe additional intra-service work associated with the primary procedure. They are performed by the same physician on the same date of service as the primary service/procedure, and must never be reported as a stand-alone code. Any bone graft harvest is not reported separately. According to CPT guidelines, cast application or strapping (including removal) is only reported as a replacement procedure or when the cast application or strapping is an initial service performed without a restorative treatment or procedure. See "Application of Casts and Strapping" in the CPT book in the Surgery Section, under the Musculoskeletal system.

ICD-9-CM Procedural

81.28   Interphalangeal fusion

Anesthesia

26860   01830
26861   N/A
26862   01830
26863   N/A

ICD-9-CM Diagnostic

357.1   Polyneuropathy in collagen vascular disease — (Code first underlying disease: 446.0, 710.0, 714.0)
359.6   Symptomatic inflammatory myopathy in diseases classified elsewhere — (Code first underlying disease: 135, 140.0-208.9, 277.30-277.39, 446.0, 710.0, 710.1, 710.2, 714.0)
446.0   Polyarteritis nodosa
710.0   Systemic lupus erythematosus — (Use additional code to identify manifestation: 424.91, 581.81, 582.81, 583.81)
710.1   Systemic sclerosis — (Use additional code to identify manifestation: 359.6, 517.2)
710.2   Sicca syndrome
714.0   Rheumatoid arthritis — (Use additional code to identify manifestation: 357.1, 359.6)
715.14   Primary localized osteoarthrosis, hand
715.34   Localized osteoarthrosis not specified whether primary or secondary, hand
716.14   Traumatic arthropathy, hand
718.24   Pathological dislocation of hand joint
718.34   Recurrent dislocation of hand joint
718.94   Unspecified derangement of hand joint
733.81   Malunion of fracture
736.1   Mallet finger
736.20   Unspecified deformity of finger
736.29   Other acquired deformity of finger
905.2   Late effect of fracture of upper extremities
905.6   Late effect of dislocation
906.4   Late effect of crushing
927.3   Crushing injury of finger(s) — (Use additional code to identify any associated injuries: 800-829, 850.0-854.1, 860.0-869.1)
959.5   Injury, other and unspecified, finger

CCI Version 16.3

20690, 25259, 26340, 29086
Also not with 26860: 01810, 0213T, 0216T, 0228T, 0230T, 11011-11012❖, 11420-11426, 12004, 13132, 20526-20553, 20692, 20696-20697, 26080, 26110-26116, 26140-26160, 26185, 26235-26236, 26440-26449, 26525, 26546❖, 26740-26742, 26746, 26770-26776, 26785, 29130, 36000, 36400-36410, 36420-36430, 36440, 36600, 36640, 37202, 43752, 51701-51703, 62310-62319, 64400-64435, 64445-64450, 64479, 64483, 64490, 64493, 64505-64530, 64702-64726, 69990, 76000-76001, 93000-93010, 93040-93042, 93318, 94002, 94200, 94250, 94680-94690, 94770, 95812-95816, 95819, 95822, 95829, 95955, 96360, 96365, 96372, 96374-96376, 99148-99149, 99150

Also not with 26861: 20526
Also not with 26862: 01810, 0213T, 0216T, 0228T, 0230T, 11420-11426, 20526-20553, 20650, 20692, 20696-20697, 20900-20902, 26080, 26110-26116, 26140-26160, 26185, 26235-26236, 26440-26449, 26525, 26546❖, 26740-26742, 26746, 26770-26776, 26785, 26860, 29125, 36000, 36400-36410, 36420-36430, 36440, 36600, 36640, 37202, 43752, 51701-51703, 62310-62319, 64400-64435, 64445-64450, 64479, 64483, 64490, 64493, 64505-64530, 64702-64726, 69990, 93000-93010, 93040-93042, 93318, 94002, 94200, 94250, 94680-94690, 94770, 95812-95816, 95819, 95822, 95829, 95955, 96360, 96365, 96372, 96374-96376, 99148-99149, 99150

Also not with 26863: 20526
Note: These CCI edits are used for Medicare. Other payers may reimburse on codes listed above.

Medicare Edits

	Fac RVU	Non-Fac RVU	FUD	Assist
26860	16.15	16.15	90	N/A
26861	3.09	3.09	N/A	N/A
26862	20.87	20.87	90	80
26863	6.9	6.9	N/A	80

Medicare References: 100-2,15,260; 100-4,12,30; 100-4,12,90.3; 100-4,14,10

26910

26910 Amputation, metacarpal, with finger or thumb (ray amputation), single, with or without interosseous transfer

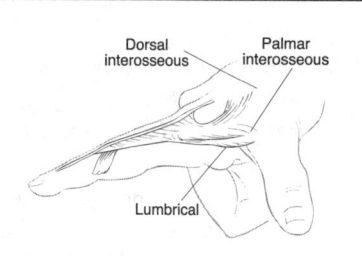

The interossei muscles may be rearranged to preserve intrinsic function of the remaining digits

The amputation occurs at the metacarpal level, usually proximal; a finger or thumb will also be removed

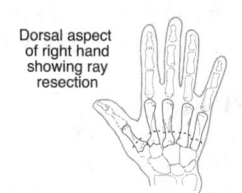

Dorsal aspect of right hand showing ray resection

Explanation
The physician amputates a metacarpal bone including a finger or the thumb. An interosseous transfer may be performed. The physician incises the overlying skin and dissects to the defective metacarpal bone. The bone is freed of all muscular and vascular attachments and removed. Tissues that are no longer necessary for anatomical function are removed. Interossei muscles may be transferred to adjacent metacarpals to retain intrinsic muscle function. Soft tissue structures are returned to anatomic position; the skin is reapproximated, reduced and sutured in layers.

Coding Tips
For repair of soft tissue defects that require a split or full-thickness graft or other pedicle flaps, see 15050–15758. For amputation of the hand through metacarpal bones, see 25927. For repositioning by policization of a digit, see 26550. For repositioning by transfer of a digit, see 26555.

ICD-9-CM Procedural
84.01	Amputation and disarticulation of finger
84.03	Amputation through hand
84.91	Amputation, not otherwise specified

Anesthesia
26910 01830

ICD-9-CM Diagnostic
170.5	Malignant neoplasm of short bones of upper limb
198.5	Secondary malignant neoplasm of bone and bone marrow
238.0	Neoplasm of uncertain behavior of bone and articular cartilage
239.2	Neoplasms of unspecified nature of bone, soft tissue, and skin
250.70	Diabetes with peripheral circulatory disorders, type II or unspecified type, not stated as uncontrolled — (Use additional code to identify manifestation: 443.81, 785.4)
250.71	Diabetes with peripheral circulatory disorders, type I [juvenile type], not stated as uncontrolled — (Use additional code to identify manifestation: 443.81, 785.4)
250.72	Diabetes with peripheral circulatory disorders, type II or unspecified type, uncontrolled — (Use additional code to identify manifestation: 443.81, 785.4)
250.73	Diabetes with peripheral circulatory disorders, type I [juvenile type], uncontrolled — (Use additional code to identify manifestation: 443.81, 785.4)
443.81	Peripheral angiopathy in diseases classified elsewhere — (Code first underlying disease: 249.7, 250.7)
443.9	Unspecified peripheral vascular disease
730.14	Chronic osteomyelitis, hand — (Use additional code to identify organism: 041.1. Use additional code to identify major osseous defect, if applicable: 731.3)
731.3	Major osseous defects — (Code first underlying disease: 170.0-170.9, 730.00-730.29, 733.00-733.09, 733.40-733.49, 996.45)
755.01	Polydactyly of fingers
785.4	Gangrene — (Code first any associated underlying condition)
882.1	Open wound of hand except finger(s) alone, complicated
883.1	Open wound of finger(s), complicated
885.0	Traumatic amputation of thumb (complete) (partial), without mention of complication
886.0	Traumatic amputation of other finger(s) (complete) (partial), without mention of complication
906.4	Late effect of crushing
906.6	Late effect of burn of wrist and hand
927.20	Crushing injury of hand(s) — (Use additional code to identify any associated injuries: 800-829, 850.0-854.1, 860.0-869.1)
927.3	Crushing injury of finger(s) — (Use additional code to identify any associated injuries: 800-829, 850.0-854.1, 860.0-869.1)
944.41	Deep necrosis of underlying tissues due to burn (deep third degree) of single digit [finger (nail)] other than thumb, without mention of loss of a body part
944.42	Deep necrosis of underlying tissues due to burn (deep third degree) of thumb (nail), without mention of loss of a body part
991.1	Frostbite of hand
998.59	Other postoperative infection — (Use additional code to identify infection)

CCI Version 16.3
01810, 0213T, 0216T, 0228T, 0230T, 11040-11044, 11730, 11740-11765, 13131, 20103, 20526-20553, 25259, 26340, 26546❖, 29086, 29125, 36000, 36400-36410, 36420-36430, 36440, 36600, 36640, 37202, 43752, 51701-51703, 62310-62319, 64400-64435, 64445-64450, 64479, 64483, 64490, 64493, 64505-64530, 69990, 93000-93010, 93040-93042, 93318, 94002, 94200, 94250, 94680-94690, 94770, 95812-95816, 95819, 95822, 95829, 95955, 96360, 96365, 96372, 96374-96376, 97597-97598, 97602-97606, 99148-99149, 99150

Note: These CCI edits are used for Medicare. Other payers may reimburse on codes listed above.

Medicare Edits

	Fac RVU	Non-Fac RVU	FUD	Assist
26910	20.65	20.65	90	N/A

Medicare References: 100-2,15,260; 100-4,12,30; 100-4,12,90.3; 100-4,14,10

26951-26952

26951 Amputation, finger or thumb, primary or secondary, any joint or phalanx, single, including neurectomies; with direct closure

26952 with local advancement flaps (V-Y, hood)

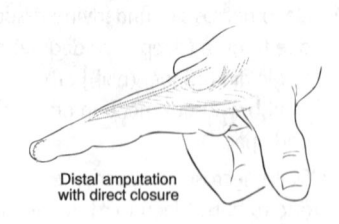

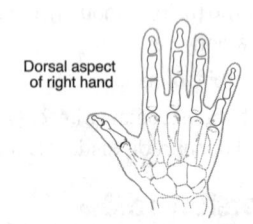

Distal amputation with direct closure

Dorsal aspect of right hand

The amputation may occur at any joint or phalanx and be performed as a primary (immediately following injury) or secondary procedure. Removal of nerves is included. Report 26951 when a direct closure is possible. Report 26952 when local advancement flaps are used

Explanation

The physician amputates a finger or thumb, primary or secondary to injury. Neurectomies are performed. The overlying skin is incised and the tissues are dissected to the bone. The bone is removed, using a saw if necessary. The vessels and nerves are ligated using microsurgical techniques. Primary amputation is removal of the digit following an acute injury or infection. Secondary amputation is removal of the digit after conservative methods to preserve the digit have failed. In 26951, the skin is approximated, reduced, and closed in sutured layers. In 26952, local advancement flaps are necessary for closure.

Coding Tips

For repair of soft tissue defects that require a split or full-thickness graft or other pedicle flaps, see 15050–15758. For amputation of the hand through metacarpal bones, see 25927.

ICD-9-CM Procedural

- 84.01 Amputation and disarticulation of finger
- 84.02 Amputation and disarticulation of thumb
- 84.91 Amputation, not otherwise specified

Anesthesia
01830

ICD-9-CM Diagnostic

- 170.5 Malignant neoplasm of short bones of upper limb
- 198.5 Secondary malignant neoplasm of bone and bone marrow
- 238.0 Neoplasm of uncertain behavior of bone and articular cartilage
- 250.70 Diabetes with peripheral circulatory disorders, type II or unspecified type, not stated as uncontrolled — (Use additional code to identify manifestation: 443.81, 785.4)
- 250.71 Diabetes with peripheral circulatory disorders, type I [juvenile type], not stated as uncontrolled — (Use additional code to identify manifestation: 443.81, 785.4)
- 730.14 Chronic osteomyelitis, hand — (Use additional code to identify organism: 041.1. Use additional code to identify major osseous defect, if applicable: 731.3)
- 730.24 Unspecified osteomyelitis, hand — (Use additional code to identify organism: 041.1. Use additional code to identify major osseous defect, if applicable: 731.3)
- 731.3 Major osseous defects — (Code first underlying disease: 170.0-170.9, 730.00-730.29, 733.00-733.09, 733.40-733.49, 996.45)
- 733.49 Aseptic necrosis of other bone site — (Use additional code to identify major osseous defect, if applicable: 731.3)
- 736.20 Unspecified deformity of finger
- 755.01 Polydactyly of fingers
- 785.4 Gangrene — (Code first any associated underlying condition)
- 883.1 Open wound of finger(s), complicated
- 883.2 Open wound of finger(s), with tendon involvement
- 885.0 Traumatic amputation of thumb (complete) (partial), without mention of complication
- 886.0 Traumatic amputation of other finger(s) (complete) (partial), without mention of complication
- 906.1 Late effect of open wound of extremities without mention of tendon injury
- 906.4 Late effect of crushing
- 906.6 Late effect of burn of wrist and hand
- 927.3 Crushing injury of finger(s) — (Use additional code to identify any associated injuries: 800-829, 850.0-854.1, 860.0-869.1)
- 944.41 Deep necrosis of underlying tissues due to burn (deep third degree) of single digit [finger (nail)] other than thumb, without mention of loss of a body part
- 944.42 Deep necrosis of underlying tissues due to burn (deep third degree) of thumb (nail), without mention of loss of a body part
- 944.43 Deep necrosis of underlying tissues due to burn (deep third degree) of two or more digits of hand, not including thumb, without mention of loss of a body part
- 991.1 Frostbite of hand
- 998.59 Other postoperative infection — (Use additional code to identify infection)

CCI Version 16.3

01810, 0213T, 0216T, 0228T, 0230T, 11040-11044, 11420-11426, 11730, 11740-11765, 12001-12007, 12020-12021, 12041-12047, 13131-13132, 20103, 20526-20553, 25259, 26080, 26320-26340, 26546❖, 29086, 29125, 36000, 36400-36410, 36420-36430, 36440, 36600, 36640, 37202, 43752, 51701-51703, 62310-62319, 64400-64435, 64445-64450, 64479, 64483, 64490, 64493, 64505-64530, 64774-64776, 64782, 64786, 69990, 93000-93010, 93040-93042, 93318, 94002, 94200, 94250, 94680-94690, 94770, 95812-95816, 95819, 95822, 95829, 95955, 96360, 96365, 96372, 96374-96376, 97597-97598, 97602-97606, 99148-99149, 99150, G0168

Also not with 26951: 11011-11012❖, 26185, 26540, 29130

Also not with 26952: 11012❖, 26230

Note: These CCI edits are used for Medicare. Other payers may reimburse on codes listed above.

Medicare Edits

	Fac RVU	Non-Fac RVU	FUD	Assist
26951	18.44	18.44	90	N/A
26952	18.68	18.68	90	N/A

Medicare References: 100-2,15,260; 100-4,12,30; 100-4,12,90.3; 100-4,14,10

29000

29000 Application of halo type body cast (see 20661-20663 for insertion)

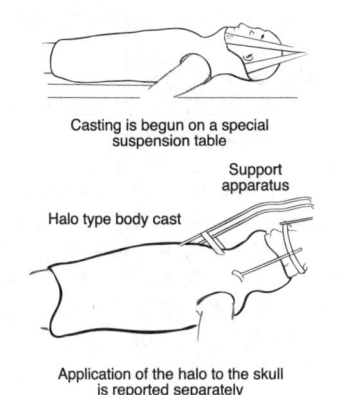

Casting is begun on a special suspension table

Halo type body cast

Support apparatus

Application of the halo to the skull is reported separately

Explanation

The physician constructs this body cast to provide a foundation for a halo in which the cervical spine must be stabilized. This involves use of a torso body cast to which the halo is attached. Casting material is applied tightly, beginning at the pelvis and extending up the torso to the upper chest. Extenders from the halo, which are already inserted around the head, can be attached to the body cast. This holds the halo very securely. An alternative is to use a prefabricated torso/chest brace that is placed on the upper torso. The previously applied halo is attached.

Coding Tips

Application of a halo device is reported separately; see 20661 and 20664. According to CPT guidelines, cast application or strapping (including removal) is only reported as a replacement procedure or when the cast application or strapping is an initial service performed without a restorative treatment or procedure. See "Application of Casts and Strapping" in the CPT book in the Surgery Section, under the Musculoskeletal system.

ICD-9-CM Procedural

- 93.51 Application of plaster jacket
- 93.52 Application of neck support
- 97.13 Replacement of other cast

Anesthesia
29000 01130

ICD-9-CM Diagnostic

- 805.01 Closed fracture of first cervical vertebra without mention of spinal cord injury
- 805.02 Closed fracture of second cervical vertebra without mention of spinal cord injury
- 805.03 Closed fracture of third cervical vertebra without mention of spinal cord injury
- 805.04 Closed fracture of fourth cervical vertebra without mention of spinal cord injury
- 805.05 Closed fracture of fifth cervical vertebra without mention of spinal cord injury
- 805.06 Closed fracture of sixth cervical vertebra without mention of spinal cord injury
- 805.07 Closed fracture of seventh cervical vertebra without mention of spinal cord injury
- 805.08 Closed fracture of multiple cervical vertebrae without mention of spinal cord injury
- 805.11 Open fracture of first cervical vertebra without mention of spinal cord injury
- 805.12 Open fracture of second cervical vertebra without mention of spinal cord injury
- 805.13 Open fracture of third cervical vertebra without mention of spinal cord injury
- 805.14 Open fracture of fourth cervical vertebra without mention of spinal cord injury
- 805.15 Open fracture of fifth cervical vertebra without mention of spinal cord injury
- 805.16 Open fracture of sixth cervical vertebra without mention of spinal cord injury
- 805.17 Open fracture of seventh cervical vertebra without mention of spinal cord injury
- 805.18 Open fracture of multiple cervical vertebrae without mention of spinal cord injury
- 806.00 Closed fracture of C1-C4 level with unspecified spinal cord injury
- 806.01 Closed fracture of C1-C4 level with complete lesion of cord
- 806.02 Closed fracture of C1-C4 level with anterior cord syndrome
- 806.03 Closed fracture of C1-C4 level with central cord syndrome
- 806.04 Closed fracture of C1-C4 level with other specified spinal cord injury
- 806.05 Closed fracture of C5-C7 level with unspecified spinal cord injury
- 806.06 Closed fracture of C5-C7 level with complete lesion of cord
- 806.07 Closed fracture of C5-C7 level with anterior cord syndrome
- 806.08 Closed fracture of C5-C7 level with central cord syndrome
- 806.09 Closed fracture of C5-C7 level with other specified spinal cord injury
- 806.10 Open fracture of C1-C4 level with unspecified spinal cord injury
- 806.11 Open fracture of C1-C4 level with complete lesion of cord
- 806.12 Open fracture of C1-C4 level with anterior cord syndrome
- 806.13 Open fracture of C1-C4 level with central cord syndrome
- 806.14 Open fracture of C1-C4 level with other specified spinal cord injury
- 806.15 Open fracture of C5-C7 level with unspecified spinal cord injury
- 806.16 Open fracture of C5-C7 level with complete lesion of cord
- 806.17 Open fracture of C5-C7 level with anterior cord syndrome
- 806.18 Open fracture of C5-C7 level with central cord syndrome
- 806.19 Open fracture of C5-C7 level with other specified spinal cord injury

CCI Version 16.3

0213T, 0216T, 0228T, 0230T, 22505, 36000, 36400-36410, 36420-36430, 36440, 36600, 36640, 37202, 43752, 51701-51703, 62310-62319, 64400-64435, 64445-64450, 64479, 64483, 64490, 64493, 64505-64530, 69990, 93000-93010, 93040-93042, 93318, 94002, 94200, 94250, 94680-94690, 94770, 95812-95816, 95819, 95822, 95829, 95955, 96360, 96365, 96372, 96374-96376, 99148-99149, 99150

Note: These CCI edits are used for Medicare. Other payers may reimburse on codes listed above.

Medicare Edits

	Fac RVU	Non-Fac RVU	FUD	Assist
29000	4.9	8.39	0	80

Medicare References: 100-2,15,100; 100-4,4,240; 100-4,5,100.7; 100-4,12,30

29010-29015

29010 Application of Risser jacket, localizer, body; only
29015 including head

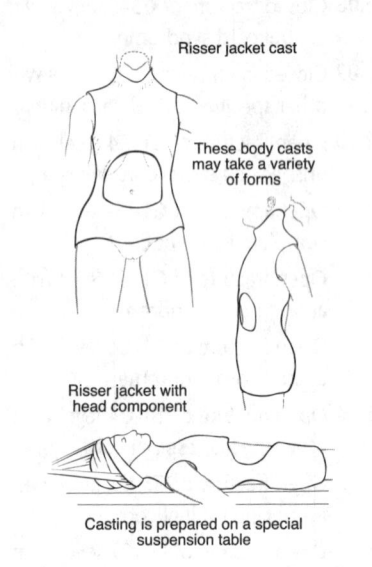

Explanation

The physician applies a Risser jacket, a method of correction for a scoliotic curve. The physician places the patient face up on a canvas strap tied to a rectangular frame. A stockinette is stretched over the patient from the head to the knees. A metallic half-circle carrying a moveable jack with a metal plate to be directed toward the apex of the angulation of the ribs is suspended beneath the frame. The rib angulation area is protected by a heavy piece of felt covered with a contoured square piece of plaster that rests on the plate. The jack is turned so that it presses the plate in a direction on the rib angulation that corrects the scoliotic curvature. A second jack may be applied to correct a double primary curve or a secondary lumbar curve. The cast is applied in sections while traction is applied to the head with a hatter and the pelvis with a pelvic belt attached to the plaster girdle. The casting begins with a well-molded neck and shoulder section and finishes with incorporating the entire trunk. Separately reportable spinal instrumentation largely eliminates the use of the Risser jacket. Report 29015 if this jacket includes the head.

Coding Tips

According to CPT guidelines, cast application or strapping (including removal) is only reported as a replacement procedure or when the cast application or strapping is an initial service performed without a restorative treatment or procedure. See "Application of Casts and Strapping" in the CPT book in the Surgery Section, under the Musculoskeletal system.

ICD-9-CM Procedural

93.51 Application of plaster jacket
93.52 Application of neck support
97.13 Replacement of other cast

Anesthesia

01130

ICD-9-CM Diagnostic

268.1 Rickets, late effect — (Use additional code to identify the nature of late effect)
737.0 Adolescent postural kyphosis
737.10 Kyphosis (acquired) (postural)
737.11 Kyphosis due to radiation
737.12 Kyphosis, postlaminectomy
737.19 Other kyphosis (acquired)
737.20 Lordosis (acquired) (postural)
737.21 Lordosis, postlaminectomy
737.22 Other postsurgical lordosis
737.29 Other lordosis (acquired)
737.30 Scoliosis (and kyphoscoliosis), idiopathic
737.34 Thoracogenic scoliosis
737.39 Other kyphoscoliosis and scoliosis
738.5 Other acquired deformity of back or spine
756.19 Other congenital anomaly of spine
V54.17 Aftercare for healing traumatic fracture of vertebrae
V54.19 Aftercare for healing traumatic fracture of other bone
V54.27 Aftercare for healing pathologic fracture of vertebrae
V54.29 Aftercare for healing pathologic fracture of other bone

Terms To Know

anomaly. Irregularity in the structure or position of an organ or tissue.

congenital. Present at birth, occurring through heredity or an influence during gestation up to the moment of birth.

kyphosis. Abnormal posterior convex curvature of the spine, usually in the thoracic region, resembling a hunchback.

lordosis. Congenital condition in which there is an exaggerated inward curvature of the lower back.

Rickets. Softening or weakening of the bones due to a lack of vitamin D, calcium, and phosphate.

scoliosis. Congenital condition of lateral curvature of the spine, often associated with other spinal column defects, congenital heart disease, or genitourinary abnormalities. It may also be associated with spinal muscular atrophy, cerebral palsy, or muscular dystrophy.

CCI Version 16.3

0213T, 0216T, 0228T, 0230T, 22505, 36000, 36400-36410, 36420-36430, 36440, 36600, 36640, 37202, 43752, 51701-51703, 62310-62319, 64400-64435, 64445-64450, 64479, 64483, 64490, 64493, 64505-64530, 69990, 93000-93010, 93040-93042, 93318, 94002, 94200, 94250, 94680-94690, 94770, 95812-95816, 95819, 95822, 95829, 95955, 96360, 96365, 96372, 96374-96376, 99148-99149, 99150

Note: These CCI edits are used for Medicare. Other payers may reimburse on codes listed above.

Medicare Edits

	Fac RVU	Non-Fac RVU	FUD	Assist
29010	4.76	8.11	0	80
29015	4.67	6.83	0	80

Medicare References: 100-4,4,240; 100-4,5,100.7; 100-4,12,30

29020-29025

29020 Application of turnbuckle jacket, body; only
29025 including head

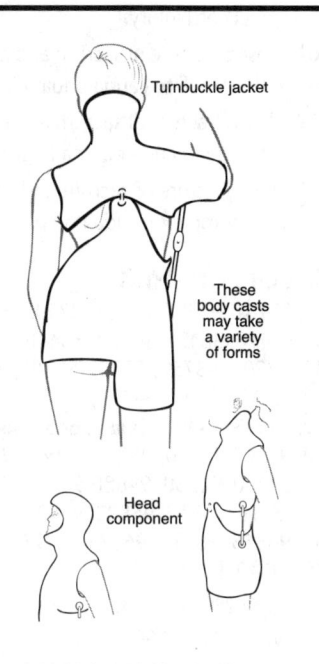

Explanation

The physician applies a turnbuckle jacket to treat scoliotic curves. The physician places the patient face up on a horizontal canvas strap attached to a rectangular frame. Traction is applied by pulling distally on the pelvis on the convex side of the scoliotic curve and the head is pulled toward the concave side. All bony prominences are padded well and two or three layers of felt are placed under the proposed location of the anterior hinge. A body cast is applied extending from the neck to above the knee on the convex side of the curve. Metal hinges are placed in the front and back of the cast toward the convex side of the curve. The cast is allowed to dry for three to five days, cut at the level of the hinges on the concave side forward and back to the hinges. Turnbuckle lugs are inserted into these cuts. A turnbuckle is attached to these edges. From the opposite side of the cast, the physician removes a large elliptical window between the hinges. The turnbuckle is turned each morning. When x-rays (reported separately) indicate the hinges are on the convex side of the curve, no further correction may be obtained by traction. The sides of the cast are reinforced with plaster and wood strips. The turnbuckle and lugs are removed. A large window is cut in the cast over the area of fusion. Report 29020 for application of the jacket. Report 29025 if the head is included in the jacket.

Coding Tips

According to CPT guidelines, cast application or strapping (including removal) is only reported as a replacement procedure or when the cast application or strapping is an initial service performed without a restorative treatment or procedure. See "Application of Casts and Strapping" in the CPT book in the Surgery Section, under the Musculoskeletal system.

ICD-9-CM Procedural

- 93.51 Application of plaster jacket
- 93.52 Application of neck support
- 97.13 Replacement of other cast

Anesthesia
01130

ICD-9-CM Diagnostic

- 268.1 Rickets, late effect — (Use additional code to identify the nature of late effect)
- 737.0 Adolescent postural kyphosis
- 737.10 Kyphosis (acquired) (postural)
- 737.11 Kyphosis due to radiation
- 737.12 Kyphosis, postlaminectomy
- 737.19 Other kyphosis (acquired)
- 737.20 Lordosis (acquired) (postural)
- 737.21 Lordosis, postlaminectomy
- 737.22 Other postsurgical lordosis
- 737.29 Other lordosis (acquired)
- 737.30 Scoliosis (and kyphoscoliosis), idiopathic
- 737.32 Progressive infantile idiopathic scoliosis
- 737.34 Thoracogenic scoliosis
- 737.39 Other kyphoscoliosis and scoliosis
- 738.5 Other acquired deformity of back or spine
- 756.19 Other congenital anomaly of spine
- V54.17 Aftercare for healing traumatic fracture of vertebrae
- V54.19 Aftercare for healing traumatic fracture of other bone
- V54.27 Aftercare for healing pathologic fracture of vertebrae
- V54.29 Aftercare for healing pathologic fracture of other bone

Terms To Know

anomaly. Irregularity in the structure or position of an organ or tissue.

congenital. Present at birth, occurring through heredity or an influence during gestation up to the moment of birth.

kyphosis. Abnormal posterior convex curvature of the spine, usually in the thoracic region, resembling a hunchback.

lordosis. Congenital condition in which there is an exaggerated inward curvature of the lower back.

Rickets. Softening or weakening of the bones due to a lack of vitamin D, calcium, and phosphate.

scoliosis. Congenital condition of lateral curvature of the spine, often associated with other spinal column defects, congenital heart disease, or genitourinary abnormalities. It may also be associated with spinal muscular atrophy, cerebral palsy, or muscular dystrophy.

CCI Version 16.3

0213T, 0216T, 0228T, 0230T, 22505, 36000, 36400-36410, 36420-36430, 36440, 36600, 36640, 37202, 43752, 51701-51703, 62310-62319, 64400-64435, 64445-64450, 64479, 64483, 64490, 64493, 64505-64530, 69990, 93000-93010, 93040-93042, 93318, 94002, 94200, 94250, 94680-94690, 94770, 95812-95816, 95819, 95822, 95829, 95955, 96360, 96365, 96372, 96374-96376, 99148-99149, 99150

Note: These CCI edits are used for Medicare. Other payers may reimburse on codes listed above.

Medicare Edits

	Fac RVU	Non-Fac RVU	FUD	Assist
29020	3.78	6.11	0	80
29025	4.94	7.2	0	80

Medicare References: 100-4,4,240; 100-4,5,100.7; 100-4,12,30

29035-29046

29035 Application of body cast, shoulder to hips;
29040 including head, Minerva type
29044 including 1 thigh
29046 including both thighs

Shoulder to hip body cast

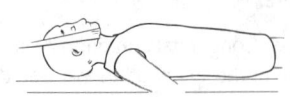

Casting is prepared on a special suspension table

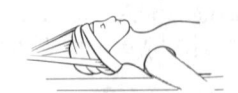

Body cast with head component under preparation (29040)

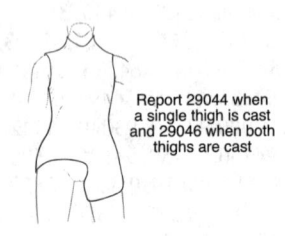

Report 29044 when a single thigh is cast and 29046 when both thighs are cast

Explanation

The physician applies a body cast, shoulder to hips. The physician applies two layers of stockinette to the patient's torso (armpits to hips), adding cotton and felt padding over bony prominences. Fiberglass or plaster cast is applied over the stockinette to create a rigid cast. Report 29035 for application of the cast. Report 29040 if the cast includes the head, Minerva type. Report 29044 if the cast includes one thigh. Report 29046 if the cast includes both thighs.

Coding Tips

According to CPT guidelines, cast application or strapping (including removal) is only reported as a replacement procedure or when the cast application or strapping is an initial service performed without a restorative treatment or procedure. See "Application of Casts and Strapping" in the CPT book in the Surgery Section, under the Musculoskeletal system.

ICD-9-CM Procedural

93.52 Application of neck support
93.53 Application of other cast
97.13 Replacement of other cast

Anesthesia

01130

ICD-9-CM Diagnostic

805.01 Closed fracture of first cervical vertebra without mention of spinal cord injury
805.02 Closed fracture of second cervical vertebra without mention of spinal cord injury
805.03 Closed fracture of third cervical vertebra without mention of spinal cord injury
805.04 Closed fracture of fourth cervical vertebra without mention of spinal cord injury
805.05 Closed fracture of fifth cervical vertebra without mention of spinal cord injury
805.06 Closed fracture of sixth cervical vertebra without mention of spinal cord injury
805.07 Closed fracture of seventh cervical vertebra without mention of spinal cord injury
805.2 Closed fracture of dorsal (thoracic) vertebra without mention of spinal cord injury
805.3 Open fracture of dorsal (thoracic) vertebra without mention of spinal cord injury
805.4 Closed fracture of lumbar vertebra without mention of spinal cord injury
805.5 Open fracture of lumbar vertebra without mention of spinal cord injury
805.6 Closed fracture of sacrum and coccyx without mention of spinal cord injury
805.7 Open fracture of sacrum and coccyx without mention of spinal cord injury
806.01 Closed fracture of C1-C4 level with complete lesion of cord
806.02 Closed fracture of C1-C4 level with anterior cord syndrome
806.03 Closed fracture of C1-C4 level with central cord syndrome
806.06 Closed fracture of C5-C7 level with complete lesion of cord
806.07 Closed fracture of C5-C7 level with anterior cord syndrome
806.08 Closed fracture of C5-C7 level with central cord syndrome
806.21 Closed fracture of T1-T6 level with complete lesion of cord
806.22 Closed fracture of T1-T6 level with anterior cord syndrome
806.23 Closed fracture of T1-T6 level with central cord syndrome
806.26 Closed fracture of T7-T12 level with complete lesion of cord
806.27 Closed fracture of T7-T12 level with anterior cord syndrome
806.28 Closed fracture of T7-T12 level with central cord syndrome
806.4 Closed fracture of lumbar spine with spinal cord injury
806.61 Closed fracture of sacrum and coccyx with complete cauda equina lesion
806.62 Closed fracture of sacrum and coccyx with other cauda equina injury
806.71 Open fracture of sacrum and coccyx with complete cauda equina lesion

CCI Version 16.3

0213T, 0216T, 0228T, 0230T, 22505, 36000, 36400-36410, 36420-36430, 36440, 36600, 36640, 37202, 43752, 51701-51703, 62310-62319, 64400-64435, 64445-64450, 64479, 64483, 64490, 64493, 64505-64530, 69990, 93000-93010, 93040-93042, 93318, 94002, 94200, 94250, 94680-94690, 94770, 95812-95816, 95819, 95822, 95829, 95955, 96360, 96365, 96372, 96374-96376, 99148-99149, 99150

Also not with 29040: 29035
Also not with 29044: 29035
Also not with 29046: 29035, 29044

Note: These CCI edits are used for Medicare. Other payers may reimburse on codes listed above.

Medicare Edits

	Fac RVU	Non-Fac RVU	FUD	Assist
29035	4.14	7.09	0	80
29040	4.53	6.79	0	80
29044	4.83	7.82	0	80
29046	5.14	7.72	0	80

Medicare References: 100-4,4,240; 100-4,5,100.7; 100-4,12,30

29049-29085

29049 Application, cast; figure-of-eight
29055 shoulder spica
29058 plaster Velpeau
29065 shoulder to hand (long arm)
29075 elbow to finger (short arm)
29085 hand and lower forearm (gauntlet)

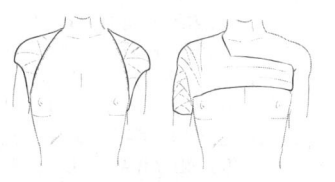

A figure-of-eight plaster cast

A shoulder spica plaster cast

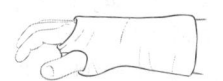

A hand and lower forearm plaster cast

Plaster casts are applied as specified. Report 29049 for a plaster figure-of-eight cast. Report 29055 for a shoulder spica plaster cast. Report 29058 for a plaster Velpeau cast. Report 29065 for a shoulder to hand plaster cast. Report 29075 for an elbow to finger plaster cast. Report 29085 for a hand and lower forearm plaster cast

Explanation

The physician applies a figure-of-eight cast to maintain shoulder retraction while a clavicle fracture heals. A cast method is seldom used; shoulder retraction is maintained with a figure-of-eight shoulder strap. Report 29049 for the cast itself. Report 29055 if the cast includes a shoulder spica. Report 29058 if the cast includes a plaster Velpeau. Report 29065 if the cast is constructed from shoulder to hand. Report 29075 if the cast is constructed from the elbow to finger. Report 29085 if the cast is constructed over the hand and lower forearm.

Coding Tips

According to CPT guidelines, cast application or strapping (including removal) is only reported as a replacement procedure or when the cast application or strapping is an initial service performed without a restorative treatment or procedure. See "Application of Casts and Strapping" in the CPT book in the Surgery Section, under the Musculoskeletal system.

ICD-9-CM Procedural

93.53 Application of other cast
97.11 Replacement of cast on upper limb

Anesthesia

29049 01680
29055 01682
29058 01680
29065 01680
29075 01860
29085 01860

ICD-9-CM Diagnostic

The application of this code is too broad to adequately present ICD-9-CM diagnostic code links here. Refer to your ICD-9-CM book.

CCI Version 16.3

0213T, 0216T, 0228T, 0230T, 36000, 36400-36410, 36420-36430, 36440, 36600, 36640, 37202, 43752, 51701-51703, 62310-62319, 64400-64435, 64445-64450, 64479, 64483, 64490, 64493, 64505-64530, 69990, 93000-93010, 93040-93042, 93318, 94002, 94200, 94250, 94680-94690, 94770, 95812-95816, 95819, 95822, 95829, 95955, 96360, 96365, 96372, 96374-96376, 99148-99149, 99150

Also not with 29049: 22505

Also not with 29065: 29075-29085, 29105-29126, 29705, 76000-76001

Also not with 29075: 12001, 28190-28193, 29085, 29125-29131, 29260, 29700-29705, 76000-76001, G0168

Note: These CCI edits are used for Medicare. Other payers may reimburse on codes listed above.

Medicare Edits

	Fac RVU	Non-Fac RVU	FUD	Assist
29049	1.92	2.66	0	80
29055	3.98	6.12	0	80
29058	2.34	2.93	0	80
29065	1.97	2.7	0	N/A
29075	1.79	2.52	0	N/A
29085	1.92	2.66	0	N/A

Medicare References: 100-2,15,100; 100-4,4,240; 100-4,5,100.7; 100-4,12,30

29086

29086 Application, cast; finger (eg, contracture)

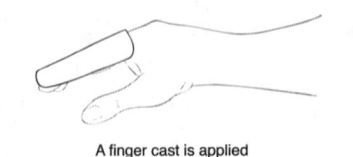

A finger cast is applied

Explanation

The hand is placed in the functioning position, with the thumb opposed. The physician extends a synthetic stockinette from the proximal interphalangeal (PIP) joints of the hand to the wrist joint and cuts a hole for the thumb. The physician covers the gap at the thumb MCP joint by splitting the thumb tube to extend it proximal to the MCP joint. Synthetic cast padding is wrapped to cover the cast area two to three layers thick, with extra layers at the proximal wrist to protect the wrist joint during flexion and extension. The physician uses 1-inch or 2-inch casting tape to wrap the hand and thumb in a thumb spica. The wrapping starts with one full around the metacarpals and then wrapping the tape around the thumb and hand in a figure-eight pattern, alternating the direction of the wrap around the thumb. The free ends of the stockinette are tucked under the second layer of wrap.

Coding Tips

According to CPT guidelines, cast application or strapping (including removal) is only reported as a replacement procedure or when the cast application or strapping is an initial service performed without a restorative treatment or procedure. See "Application of Casts and Strapping" in the CPT book in the Surgery Section, under the Musculoskeletal system.

ICD-9-CM Procedural

93.53 Application of other cast

Anesthesia

29086 01860

ICD-9-CM Diagnostic

718.74	Developmental dislocation of joint, hand
727.03	Trigger finger (acquired)
727.05	Other tenosynovitis of hand and wrist
728.6	Contracture of palmar fascia
736.1	Mallet finger
736.20	Unspecified deformity of finger
736.21	Boutonniere deformity
736.22	Swan-neck deformity
736.29	Other acquired deformity of finger
816.00	Closed fracture of unspecified phalanx or phalanges of hand
816.01	Closed fracture of middle or proximal phalanx or phalanges of hand
816.02	Closed fracture of distal phalanx or phalanges of hand
816.03	Closed fracture of multiple sites of phalanx or phalanges of hand
834.00	Closed dislocation of finger, unspecified part
834.01	Closed dislocation of metacarpophalangeal (joint)
834.02	Closed dislocation of interphalangeal (joint), hand
842.12	Sprain and strain of metacarpophalangeal (joint) of hand
842.13	Sprain and strain of interphalangeal (joint) of hand
883.0	Open wound of finger(s), without mention of complication
883.1	Open wound of finger(s), complicated
883.2	Open wound of finger(s), with tendon involvement
927.3	Crushing injury of finger(s) — (Use additional code to identify any associated injuries: 800-829, 850.0-854.1, 860.0-869.1)
959.5	Injury, other and unspecified, finger
V54.19	Aftercare for healing traumatic fracture of other bone
V54.29	Aftercare for healing pathologic fracture of other bone

Terms To Know

boutonniere deformity. Finger deformity with hyperextension of the distal joint and flexion of the interphalangeal joint.

closed fracture. Break in a bone without a concomitant opening in the skin. A closed fracture is coded when the type of fracture is not specified.

contracture. Shortening of muscle or connective tissue.

dislocation. Displacement of a bone in relation to its neighboring tissue, especially a joint.

flexion. Act of bending or being bent.

proximal. Located closest to a specified reference point, usually the midline.

CCI Version 16.3

0213T, 0216T, 0228T, 0230T, 36000, 36400-36410, 36420-36430, 36440, 36600, 36640, 37202, 43752, 51701-51703, 62310-62319, 64400-64435, 64445-64450, 64479, 64483, 64490, 64493, 64505-64530, 93000-93010, 93040-93042, 93318, 94002, 94200, 94250, 94680-94690, 94770, 95812-95816, 95819, 95822, 95829, 95955, 96360, 96365, 96372, 96374-96376, 99148-99149, 99150

Note: These CCI edits are used for Medicare. Other payers may reimburse on codes listed above.

Medicare Edits

	Fac RVU	Non-Fac RVU	FUD	Assist
29086	1.44	2.12	0	N/A

Medicare References: 100-2,15,100; 100-4,4,240; 100-4,5,100.7; 100-4,12,30

29105-29126

29105 Application of long arm splint (shoulder to hand)
29125 Application of short arm splint (forearm to hand); static
29126 dynamic

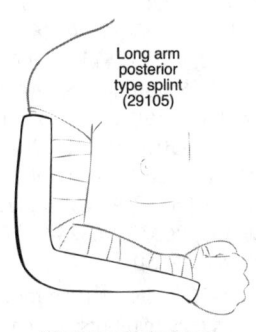

Long arm posterior type splint (29105)

A final wrapping is placed over the splint to hold position

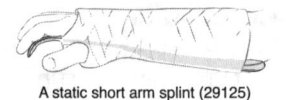

A static short arm splint (29125)

A long arm splint is applied. Report 29125 when a static short arm splint is applied. Report 29126 when a dynamic short arm splint is applied

Explanation

A long arm splint is applied from the shoulder to hand (29105) or a short arm splint from forearm to hand (29125, 29126). Cotton padding is wrapped around the area to be splinted. Plaster strips or fiberglass splint material is applied along the back of the midarm, forearm, and palm side of the hand to maintain the extremity in the desired position. An Ace wrap is applied to hold the splint material in position. Report 29105 for a long arm splint. Report 29125 for a short arm static splint, keeping the wrist totally immobilized. Report 29126 for a short arm dynamic splint, allowing some movement.

Coding Tips

According to CPT guidelines, cast application or strapping (including removal) is only reported as a replacement procedure or when the cast application or strapping is an initial service performed without a restorative treatment or procedure. See "Application of Casts and Strapping" in the CPT book in the Surgery Section, under the Musculoskeletal system.

ICD-9-CM Procedural

93.54 Application of splint
97.14 Replacement of other device for musculoskeletal immobilization

Anesthesia

29105 01680
29125 01860
29126 01860

ICD-9-CM Diagnostic

354.0 Carpal tunnel syndrome
357.1 Polyneuropathy in collagen vascular disease — (Code first underlying disease: 446.0, 710.0, 714.0)
359.6 Symptomatic inflammatory myopathy in diseases classified elsewhere — (Code first underlying disease: 135, 140.0-208.9, 277.30-277.39, 446.0, 710.0, 710.1, 710.2, 714.0)
715.14 Primary localized osteoarthrosis, hand
727.05 Other tenosynovitis of hand and wrist
813.21 Closed fracture of shaft of radius (alone)
813.22 Closed fracture of shaft of ulna (alone)
813.23 Closed fracture of shaft of radius with ulna
813.40 Unspecified closed fracture of lower end of forearm
813.41 Closed Colles' fracture
813.42 Other closed fractures of distal end of radius (alone)
813.43 Closed fracture of distal end of ulna (alone)
813.44 Closed fracture of lower end of radius with ulna
813.45 Torus fracture of radius (alone)
813.47 Torus fracture of radius and ulna
814.01 Closed fracture of navicular (scaphoid) bone of wrist
814.02 Closed fracture of lunate (semilunar) bone of wrist
814.03 Closed fracture of triquetral (cuneiform) bone of wrist
814.04 Closed fracture of pisiform bone of wrist
814.05 Closed fracture of trapezium bone (larger multangular) of wrist
814.06 Closed fracture of trapezoid bone (smaller multangular) of wrist
814.07 Closed fracture of capitate bone (os magnum) of wrist
814.08 Closed fracture of hamate (unciform) bone of wrist
815.01 Closed fracture of base of thumb (first) metacarpal bone(s)
815.02 Closed fracture of base of other metacarpal bone(s)
815.03 Closed fracture of shaft of metacarpal bone(s)
815.04 Closed fracture of neck of metacarpal bone(s)
815.09 Closed fracture of multiple sites of metacarpus
817.0 Multiple closed fractures of hand bones
842.11 Sprain and strain of carpometacarpal (joint) of hand
842.12 Sprain and strain of metacarpophalangeal (joint) of hand
842.13 Sprain and strain of interphalangeal (joint) of hand
923.10 Contusion of forearm
923.20 Contusion of hand(s)
923.21 Contusion of wrist

CCI Version 16.3

0213T, 0216T, 0228T, 0230T, 36000, 36400-36410, 36420-36430, 36440, 36600, 36640, 37202, 43752, 51701-51703, 62310-62319, 64400-64435, 64445-64450, 64479, 64483, 64490, 64493, 64505-64530, 69990, 93000-93010, 93040-93042, 93318, 94002, 94200, 94250, 94680-94690, 94770, 95812-95816, 95819, 95822, 95829, 95955, 96360, 96365, 96372, 96374-96376, 99148-99149, 99150

Also not with 29105: 12001-12002, 12035, 29075, 29125, 29705, G0168

Also not with 29125: 12001-12002, 12032, 12042-12044, 13121, 13132, 29130, 29260, G0168

Note: These CCI edits are used for Medicare. Other payers may reimburse on codes listed above.

Medicare Edits

	Fac RVU	Non-Fac RVU	FUD	Assist
29105	1.71	2.45	0	N/A
29125	1.25	1.95	0	N/A
29126	1.53	2.23	0	N/A

Medicare References: 100-2,15,100; 100-4,4,240; 100-4,5,100.7; 100-4,12,30

29130-29131

29130 Application of finger splint; static
29131 dynamic

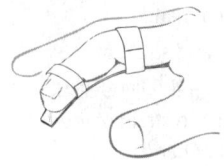

Static finger splint

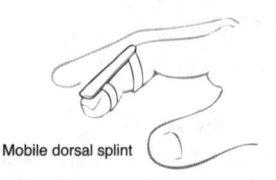

Mobile dorsal splint

A finger splint is applied. Report 29130 for a static type splint. Report 29131 for a dynamic finger splint

Explanation

The physician applies a finger splint. This type of splint is applied to immobilize the digits. A twin layer of cotton padding is applied by the physician to the digit, covering the last two joints of that digit. Plaster casting or fiberglass splint material is applied to the finger from just beyond the knuckle to the tip of the finger. Usually the finger is immobilized in a straight position. Report 29130 if the splint applied is static for full immobilization. Report 29131 if the splint applied is dynamic for some movement.

Coding Tips

Some payers may require the use of HCPCS Level II modifiers FA–F9 to identify the specific finger involved. According to CPT guidelines, cast application or strapping (including removal) is only reported as a replacement procedure or when the cast application or strapping is an initial service performed without a restorative treatment or procedure. See "Application of Casts and Strapping" in the CPT book in the Surgery Section, under the Musculoskeletal system.

ICD-9-CM Procedural

93.54 Application of splint
97.14 Replacement of other device for musculoskeletal immobilization

Anesthesia

01860

ICD-9-CM Diagnostic

718.74 Developmental dislocation of joint, hand
727.03 Trigger finger (acquired)
727.05 Other tenosynovitis of hand and wrist
728.6 Contracture of palmar fascia
736.1 Mallet finger
736.20 Unspecified deformity of finger
736.21 Boutonniere deformity
736.22 Swan-neck deformity
736.29 Other acquired deformity of finger
816.00 Closed fracture of unspecified phalanx or phalanges of hand
816.01 Closed fracture of middle or proximal phalanx or phalanges of hand
816.02 Closed fracture of distal phalanx or phalanges of hand
816.03 Closed fracture of multiple sites of phalanx or phalanges of hand
834.00 Closed dislocation of finger, unspecified part
834.01 Closed dislocation of metacarpophalangeal (joint)
834.02 Closed dislocation of interphalangeal (joint), hand
842.12 Sprain and strain of metacarpophalangeal (joint) of hand
842.13 Sprain and strain of interphalangeal (joint) of hand
883.0 Open wound of finger(s), without mention of complication
883.1 Open wound of finger(s), complicated
883.2 Open wound of finger(s), with tendon involvement
927.3 Crushing injury of finger(s) — (Use additional code to identify any associated injuries: 800-829, 850.0-854.1, 860.0-869.1)
959.5 Injury, other and unspecified, finger
V54.19 Aftercare for healing traumatic fracture of other bone
V54.29 Aftercare for healing pathologic fracture of other bone

Terms To Know

boutonniere deformity. Finger deformity with hyperextension of the distal joint and flexion of the interphalangeal joint.

closed fracture. Break in a bone without a concomitant opening in the skin. A closed fracture is coded when the type of fracture is not specified.

dislocation. Displacement of a bone in relation to its neighboring tissue, especially a joint.

open wound. Opening or break of the skin.

sprain and strain. Injuries to a joint, in which the fibers of supporting ligaments or muscles are overstretched or slightly ruptured, with the ligaments and muscles maintaining continuity.

CCI Version 16.3

0213T, 0216T, 0228T, 0230T, 36000, 36400-36410, 36420-36430, 36440, 36600, 36640, 37202, 43752, 51701-51703, 62310-62319, 64400-64435, 64445-64450, 64479, 64483, 64490, 64493, 64505-64530, 69990, 93000-93010, 93040-93042, 93318, 94002, 94200, 94250, 94680-94690, 94770, 95812-95816, 95819, 95822, 95829, 95955, 96360, 96365, 96372, 96374-96376, 99148-99149, 99150

Note: These CCI edits are used for Medicare. Other payers may reimburse on codes listed above.

Medicare Edits

	Fac RVU	Non-Fac RVU	FUD	Assist
29130	0.83	1.15	0	N/A
29131	0.97	1.46	0	N/A

Medicare References: 100-2,15,100; 100-4,4,240; 100-4,5,100.7; 100-4,12,30

29240-29280

29240 Strapping; shoulder (eg, Velpeau)
29260 elbow or wrist
29280 hand or finger

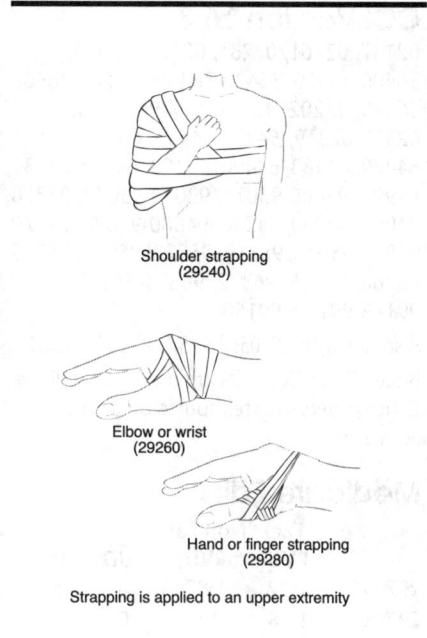

Shoulder strapping (29240)

Elbow or wrist (29260)

Hand or finger strapping (29280)

Strapping is applied to an upper extremity

Explanation

The physician or a medical professional under the physician's direction performs strapping with tape on a patient of any age. This technique was once more frequently used to compress the thorax offering some support and to limit deep inhalation following fracture. This support does not promote healing, but provides palliative relief. A thoracic elastic or canvas binder is more commonly used. Report 29240 if the strapping is applied to the shoulder; report 29260 if strapping is applied to the elbow or wrist; and report 29280 if strapping is applied to the hand or finger.

Coding Tips

According to CPT guidelines, cast application or strapping (including removal) is only reported as a replacement procedure or when the cast application or strapping is an initial service performed without a restorative treatment or procedure. See "Application of Casts and Strapping" in the CPT book in the Surgery Section, under the Musculoskeletal system.

ICD-9-CM Procedural

93.59 Other immobilization, pressure, and attention to wound
97.14 Replacement of other device for musculoskeletal immobilization

Anesthesia

29240 01620
29260 01820
29280 01820

ICD-9-CM Diagnostic

354.0 Carpal tunnel syndrome
718.72 Developmental dislocation of joint, upper arm
718.73 Developmental dislocation of joint, forearm
718.74 Developmental dislocation of joint, hand
727.05 Other tenosynovitis of hand and wrist
810.03 Closed fracture of acromial end of clavicle
811.01 Closed fracture of acromial process of scapula
811.03 Closed fracture of glenoid cavity and neck of scapula
812.01 Closed fracture of surgical neck of humerus
812.02 Closed fracture of anatomical neck of humerus
812.03 Closed fracture of greater tuberosity of humerus
814.01 Closed fracture of navicular (scaphoid) bone of wrist
815.00 Closed fracture of metacarpal bone(s), site unspecified
815.01 Closed fracture of base of thumb (first) metacarpal bone(s)
815.02 Closed fracture of base of other metacarpal bone(s)
815.03 Closed fracture of shaft of metacarpal bone(s)
815.04 Closed fracture of neck of metacarpal bone(s)
815.09 Closed fracture of multiple sites of metacarpus
816.00 Closed fracture of unspecified phalanx or phalanges of hand
816.01 Closed fracture of middle or proximal phalanx or phalanges of hand
816.02 Closed fracture of distal phalanx or phalanges of hand
816.03 Closed fracture of multiple sites of phalanx or phalanges of hand
817.0 Multiple closed fractures of hand bones
833.05 Closed dislocation of proximal end of metacarpal (bone)
834.00 Closed dislocation of finger, unspecified part
834.01 Closed dislocation of metacarpophalangeal (joint)
834.02 Closed dislocation of interphalangeal (joint), hand
834.11 Open dislocation of metacarpophalangeal (joint)
842.10 Sprain and strain of unspecified site of hand
842.11 Sprain and strain of carpometacarpal (joint) of hand
842.12 Sprain and strain of metacarpophalangeal (joint) of hand
842.13 Sprain and strain of interphalangeal (joint) of hand
842.19 Other hand sprain and strain
927.20 Crushing injury of hand(s) — (Use additional code to identify any associated injuries: 800-829, 850.0-854.1, 860.0-869.1)
927.3 Crushing injury of finger(s) — (Use additional code to identify any associated injuries: 800-829, 850.0-854.1, 860.0-869.1)
959.4 Injury, other and unspecified, hand, except finger
959.5 Injury, other and unspecified, finger

CCI Version 16.3

0213T, 0216T, 0228T, 0230T, 36000, 36400-36410, 36420-36430, 36440, 36600, 36640, 37202, 43752, 51701-51703, 62310-62319, 64400-64435, 64445-64450, 64479, 64483, 64490, 64493, 64505-64530, 69990, 93000-93010, 93040-93042, 93318, 94002, 94200, 94250, 94680-94690, 94770, 95812-95816, 95819, 95822, 95829, 95955, 96360, 96365, 96372, 96374-96376, 99148-99149, 99150

Note: These CCI edits are used for Medicare. Other payers may reimburse on codes listed above.

Medicare Edits

	Fac RVU	Non-Fac RVU	FUD	Assist
29240	1.25	1.63	0	N/A
29260	1.07	1.46	0	N/A
29280	1.03	1.43	0	N/A

Medicare References: 100-2,15,100; 100-4,5,100.7; 100-4,12,30

29700-29715

- **29700** Removal or bivalving; gauntlet, boot or body cast
- **29705** full arm or full leg cast
- **29710** shoulder or hip spica, Minerva, or Risser jacket, etc.
- **29715** turnbuckle jacket

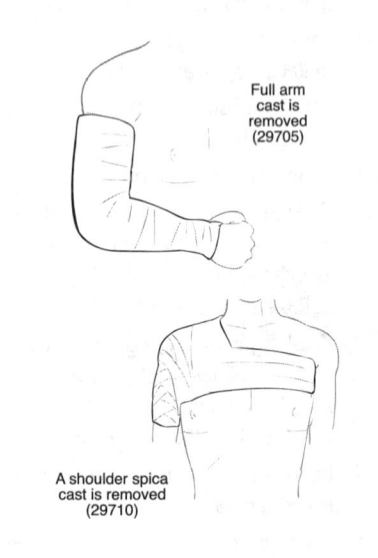

Full arm cast is removed (29705)

A shoulder spica cast is removed (29710)

Explanation

The physician removes or bivalves a cast. These codes are used to remove a cast or to simply cut it in half for the purpose of either using one half the cast as a splint or for intermittent immobilization. A manual cast saw is used to make two cuts in the cast. One cut is extended along the medial edge of the cast. The second cut is extended along the lateral edge of the cast. These cuts are started proximally and are extended distally. Once the cuts are made, the cast may be removed. The front and back portion of the cast may be applied and secured using an Ace bandage intermittently for immobilization. Only one half may be Ace wrapped for splinting purposes. Report 29700 if the cast is a gauntlet, boot, or body cast. Report 29705 if a full arm or full leg cast is removed. Report 29710 if a shoulder cast or hip spica, Minerva, or Risser jacket is removed. Report 29715 if a turnbuckle jacket is removed.

Coding Tips

According to CPT guidelines, cast application or strapping (including removal) is only reported as a replacement procedure or when the cast application or strapping is an initial service performed without a restorative treatment or procedure. See "Application of Casts and Strapping" in the CPT book in the Surgery Section, under the Musculoskeletal system.

ICD-9-CM Procedural
- **97.88** Removal of external immobilization device

Anesthesia
- **29700** 01130
- **29705** 01420
- **29710** 01680
- **29715** 01130

ICD-9-CM Diagnostic
- **V54.10** Aftercare for healing traumatic fracture of arm, unspecified
- **V54.11** Aftercare for healing traumatic fracture of upper arm
- **V54.12** Aftercare for healing traumatic fracture of lower arm
- **V54.19** Aftercare for healing traumatic fracture of other bone
- **V54.20** Aftercare for healing pathologic fracture of arm, unspecified
- **V54.21** Aftercare for healing pathologic fracture of upper arm
- **V54.22** Aftercare for healing pathologic fracture of lower arm
- **V54.29** Aftercare for healing pathologic fracture of other bone
- **V54.89** Other orthopedic aftercare
- **V67.4** Treatment of healed fracture follow-up examination

Terms To Know

distal. Located farther away from a specified reference point.

fracture. Break in bone or cartilage.

lateral. To/on the side.

medial. Middle or midline.

Minerva jacket. Spinal cast or brace that includes a sternal plate, dorsal plate, bonnet, and mandible piece attached to the superstructure of the sternal plate for cervical or high thoracic stability.

proximal. Located closest to a specified reference point, usually the midline.

Risser jacket. Extended body cast with hinges and buckles that covers the neck, extends down to one knee, and sometimes includes an arm to the elbow. This is applied in cases of scoliosis.

turnbuckle jacket. Spinal cast of plaster and hinges applied from the chin and base of the skull down past one thigh, sometimes including one arm, used in the correction of spinal curvature.

CCI Version 16.3

0213T, 0216T, 0228T, 0230T, 36000, 36400-36410, 36420-36430, 36440, 36600, 36640, 37202, 43752, 51701-51703, 62310-62319, 64400-64435, 64445-64450, 64479, 64483, 64490, 64493, 64505-64530, 69990, 93000-93010, 93040-93042, 93318, 94002, 94200, 94250, 94680-94690, 94770, 95812-95816, 95819, 95822, 95829, 95955, 96360, 96365, 96372, 96374-96376, 99148-99149, 99150

Also not with 29705: 15852, 29580-29581

Note: These CCI edits are used for Medicare. Other payers may reimburse on codes listed above.

Medicare Edits

	Fac RVU	Non-Fac RVU	FUD	Assist
29700	1.02	1.87	0	N/A
29705	1.38	1.9	0	N/A
29710	2.46	3.48	0	80
29715	1.6	2.44	0	80

Medicare References: None

29720

29720 Repair of spica, body cast or jacket

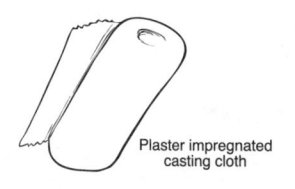

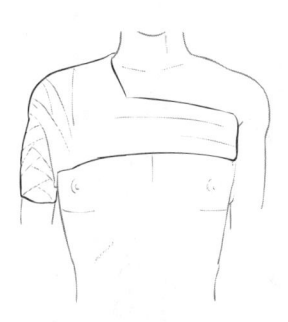

Plaster impregnated casting cloth

Explanation

The physician repairs a spica, body cast, or jacket due to normal wear and tear, revision of the cast or jacket, or the cutting of a window to check the status of a wound, incision, or other area. Additional casting material is applied in the normal manner.

Coding Tips

According to CPT guidelines, cast application or strapping (including removal) is only reported as a replacement procedure or when the cast application or strapping is an initial service performed without a restorative treatment or procedure. See "Application of Casts and Strapping" in the CPT book in the Surgery Section, under the Musculoskeletal system.

ICD-9-CM Procedural

93.59 Other immobilization, pressure, and attention to wound

Anesthesia

29720 01130

ICD-9-CM Diagnostic

V54.19 Aftercare for healing traumatic fracture of other bone
V54.29 Aftercare for healing pathologic fracture of other bone
V54.89 Other orthopedic aftercare
V67.4 Treatment of healed fracture follow-up examination

Terms To Know

fracture. Break in bone or cartilage.

fracture types. There are three basic degrees of fracture: type I: a small crack in the bone without displacement; type II: a fracture in which the bone is slightly displaced; type III: a fracture in which there are more than three broken pieces of bone that cannot fit together.

CCI Version 16.3

0213T, 0216T, 0228T, 0230T, 36000, 36400-36410, 36420-36430, 36440, 36600, 36640, 37202, 43752, 51701-51703, 62310-62319, 64400-64435, 64445-64450, 64479, 64483, 64490, 64493, 64505-64530, 69990, 93000-93010, 93040-93042, 93318, 94002, 94200, 94250, 94680-94690, 94770, 95812-95816, 95819, 95822, 95829, 95955, 96360, 96365, 96372, 96374-96376, 99148-99149, 99150

Note: These CCI edits are used for Medicare. Other payers may reimburse on codes listed above.

Medicare Edits

	Fac RVU	Non-Fac RVU	FUD	Assist
29720	1.28	2.32	0	N/A

Medicare References: None

29730

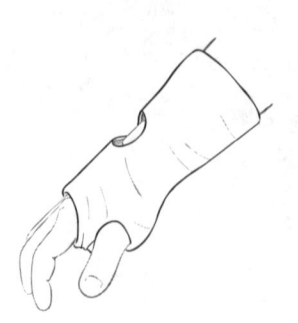

29730 Windowing of cast

A window is cut into a cast, usually to access the site of an open fracture

Explanation
The physician chooses this procedure to check the status of a wound that is underneath the cast or to visualize an area under the cast where infection may exist. A cast saw is used to cut an appropriately-sized section in the cast. This is removed to create a window. Once the status is determined, the physician may reinsert the section and hold it in place with casting material.

Coding Tips
According to CPT guidelines, cast application or strapping (including removal) is only reported as a replacement procedure or when the cast application or strapping is an initial service performed without a restorative treatment or procedure. See "Application of Casts and Strapping" in the CPT book in the Surgery Section, under the Musculoskeletal system.

ICD-9-CM Procedural
- 93.59 Other immobilization, pressure, and attention to wound

Anesthesia
29730 01130, 01420, 01490, 01680, 01682, 01820, 01860

ICD-9-CM Diagnostic
- V54.10 Aftercare for healing traumatic fracture of arm, unspecified
- V54.11 Aftercare for healing traumatic fracture of upper arm
- V54.12 Aftercare for healing traumatic fracture of lower arm
- V54.19 Aftercare for healing traumatic fracture of other bone
- V54.20 Aftercare for healing pathologic fracture of arm, unspecified
- V54.21 Aftercare for healing pathologic fracture of upper arm
- V54.22 Aftercare for healing pathologic fracture of lower arm
- V54.29 Aftercare for healing pathologic fracture of other bone
- V54.89 Other orthopedic aftercare

Terms To Know
fracture. Break in bone or cartilage.

fracture types. There are three basic degrees of fracture: type I: a small crack in the bone without displacement; type II: a fracture in which the bone is slightly displaced; type III: a fracture in which there are more than three broken pieces of bone that cannot fit together.

infection. Presence of microorganisms in body tissues that may result in cellular damage.

open fracture. Exposed break in a bone, always considered compound due to its high risk of infection from the open wound leading to the fracture. Broken bone ends may protrude through the skin and contaminants or foreign bodies are often embedded in the tissues.

CCI Version 16.3
0213T, 0216T, 0228T, 0230T, 36000, 36400-36410, 36420-36430, 36440, 36600, 36640, 37202, 43752, 51701-51703, 62310-62319, 64400-64435, 64445-64450, 64479, 64483, 64490, 64493, 64505-64530, 69990, 93000-93010, 93040-93042, 93318, 94002, 94200, 94250, 94680-94690, 94770, 95812-95816, 95819, 95822, 95829, 95955, 96360, 96365, 96372, 96374-96376, 99148-99149, 99150

Note: These CCI edits are used for Medicare. Other payers may reimburse on codes listed above.

Medicare Edits

	Fac RVU	Non-Fac RVU	FUD	Assist
29730	1.32	1.84	0	N/A

Medicare References: None

29740

29740 Wedging of cast (except clubfoot casts)

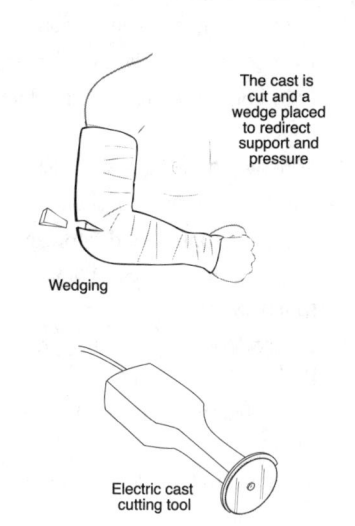

Wedging

The cast is cut and a wedge placed to redirect support and pressure

Electric cast cutting tool

A cast is wedged

Explanation

The physician wedges a cast. X-rays (reported separately) of a casted, fractured extremity may show slight malalignment. Wedging of the cast may correct this malalignment without having to remove the cast. The bony deformities identified by the physician and the necessary direction and amount of correction is decided. The necessary cut is made in the cast using a cast saw. A wedge of plastic or wood is wedged into the cast cut to redirect the pressure of the cast on the fracture site to correct the bony deformity.

Coding Tips

According to CPT guidelines, cast application or strapping (including removal) is only reported as a replacement procedure or when the cast application or strapping is an initial service performed without a restorative treatment or procedure. See "Application of Casts and Strapping" in the CPT book in the Surgery Section, under the Musculoskeletal system.

ICD-9-CM Procedural

93.59 Other immobilization, pressure, and attention to wound

Anesthesia

29740 01130, 01420, 01490, 01680, 01682, 01860

ICD-9-CM Diagnostic

V54.10 Aftercare for healing traumatic fracture of arm, unspecified
V54.11 Aftercare for healing traumatic fracture of upper arm
V54.12 Aftercare for healing traumatic fracture of lower arm
V54.19 Aftercare for healing traumatic fracture of other bone
V54.20 Aftercare for healing pathologic fracture of arm, unspecified
V54.21 Aftercare for healing pathologic fracture of upper arm
V54.22 Aftercare for healing pathologic fracture of lower arm
V54.29 Aftercare for healing pathologic fracture of other bone
V54.89 Other orthopedic aftercare

Terms To Know

deformity. Irregularity or malformation of the body.

fracture. Break in bone or cartilage.

fracture types. There are three basic degrees of fracture: type I: a small crack in the bone without displacement; type II: a fracture in which the bone is slightly displaced; type III: a fracture in which there are more than three broken pieces of bone that cannot fit together.

CCI Version 16.3

0213T, 0216T, 0228T, 0230T, 29405, 36000, 36400-36410, 36420-36430, 36440, 36600, 36640, 37202, 43752, 51701-51703, 62310-62319, 64400-64435, 64445-64450, 64479, 64483, 64490, 64493, 64505-64530, 69990, 93000-93010, 93040-93042, 93318, 94002, 94200, 94250, 94680-94690, 94770, 95812-95816, 95819, 95822, 95829, 95955, 96360, 96365, 96372, 96374-96376, 99148-99149, 99150

Note: These CCI edits are used for Medicare. Other payers may reimburse on codes listed above.

Medicare Edits

	Fac RVU	Non-Fac RVU	FUD	Assist
29740	1.89	2.59	0	N/A

Medicare References: None

29805

29805 Arthroscopy, shoulder, diagnostic, with or without synovial biopsy (separate procedure)

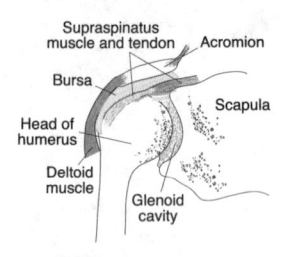

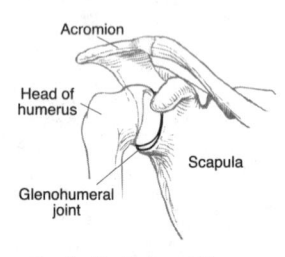

Explanation

A general anesthetic is commonly administered for shoulder arthroscopic procedures. Two to four small poke hole incisions are made above the joint and sterile fluid is introduced into the joint space to provide a better view. A band is placed to restrict blood flow. A small incision is made on one side of the joint and the arthroscope is inserted. The inside of the joint may be viewed through the eyepiece or the image can be reproduced on a screen. A cannula is introduced to take a synovial biopsy. Once the biopsy is completed, the physician irrigates the joint until it is clear of blood and loose particles. A long acting local anesthetic may be injected into the joint to help with post-operative pain. The joint is irrigated and suture or Steri-strip closes the incisions. The area is covered with a sterile dressing and a sling or shoulder immobilizer is applied.

Coding Tips

This separate procedure by definition is usually a component of a more complex service and is not identified separately. When performed alone or with other unrelated procedures/services, it may be reported. If performed alone, list the code; if performed with other procedures/services, list the code and append modifier 59. This is a unilateral procedure. If performed bilaterally, some payers require that the service be reported twice with modifier 50 appended to the second code, while others require identification of the service only once with modifier 50 appended. Check with individual payers. Modifier 50 identifies a procedure performed identically on the opposite side of the body (mirror image). When 29805 is performed with another separately identifiable procedure, the highest dollar value code is listed as the primary procedure and subsequent procedures are appended with modifier 51. When arthroscopy is performed in conjunction with arthrotomy, add modifier 51. Surgical arthroscopy always includes diagnostic arthroscopy. For an open procedure, see 23065–23066 and 23100–23101.

ICD-9-CM Procedural

- 80.21 Arthroscopy of shoulder
- 80.31 Biopsy of joint structure of shoulder

Anesthesia

29805 01622

ICD-9-CM Diagnostic

- 170.4 Malignant neoplasm of scapula and long bones of upper limb
- 195.4 Malignant neoplasm of upper limb
- 213.4 Benign neoplasm of scapula and long bones of upper limb
- 215.2 Other benign neoplasm of connective and other soft tissue of upper limb, including shoulder
- 710.0 Systemic lupus erythematosus — (Use additional code to identify manifestation: 424.91, 581.81, 582.81, 583.81)
- 710.1 Systemic sclerosis — (Use additional code to identify manifestation: 359.6, 517.2)
- 710.2 Sicca syndrome
- 711.01 Pyogenic arthritis, shoulder region — (Use additional code to identify infectious organism: 041.0-041.8)
- 714.0 Rheumatoid arthritis — (Use additional code to identify manifestation: 357.1, 359.6)
- 715.11 Primary localized osteoarthrosis, shoulder region
- 715.21 Secondary localized osteoarthrosis, shoulder region
- 715.91 Osteoarthrosis, unspecified whether generalized or localized, shoulder region
- 716.11 Traumatic arthropathy, shoulder region
- 718.01 Articular cartilage disorder, shoulder region
- 718.21 Pathological dislocation of shoulder joint
- 718.31 Recurrent dislocation of shoulder joint
- 718.41 Contracture of shoulder joint
- 718.71 Developmental dislocation of joint, shoulder region
- 719.11 Hemarthrosis, shoulder region
- 719.21 Villonodular synovitis, shoulder region
- 719.31 Palindromic rheumatism, shoulder region
- 726.0 Adhesive capsulitis of shoulder
- 726.11 Calcifying tendinitis of shoulder
- 727.61 Complete rupture of rotator cuff
- 840.0 Acromioclavicular (joint) (ligament) sprain and strain
- 840.1 Coracoclavicular (ligament) sprain and strain
- 840.2 Coracohumeral (ligament) sprain and strain
- 840.3 Infraspinatus (muscle) (tendon) sprain and strain
- 840.4 Rotator cuff (capsule) sprain and strain
- 840.5 Subscapularis (muscle) sprain and strain
- 840.6 Supraspinatus (muscle) (tendon) sprain and strain

CCI Version 16.3

0213T, 0216T, 0228T, 0230T, 11012❖, 23700, 36000, 36400-36410, 36420-36430, 36440, 36600, 36640, 37202, 43752, 51701-51703, 62310-62319, 64400-64435, 64445-64450, 64479, 64483, 64490, 64493, 64505-64530, 69990, 76000-76001, 93000-93010, 93040-93042, 93318, 94002, 94200, 94250, 94680-94690, 94770, 95812-95816, 95819, 95822, 95829, 95955, 96360, 96365, 96372, 96374-96376, 99148-99149, 99150

Note: These CCI edits are used for Medicare. Other payers may reimburse on codes listed above.

Medicare Edits

	Fac RVU	Non-Fac RVU	FUD	Assist
29805	13.71	13.71	90	N/A

Medicare References: 100-2,15,260; 100-3,100.2; 100-4,12,30; 100-4,12,90.3; 100-4,14,10

29806

29806 Arthroscopy, shoulder, surgical; capsulorrhaphy

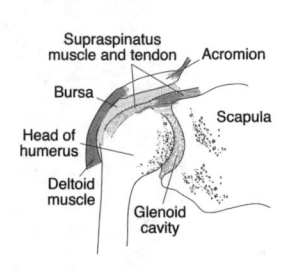

Suprapinatus muscle and tendon; Acromion; Bursa; Head of humerus; Deltoid muscle; Scapula; Glenoid cavity

Anterior views of right shoulder

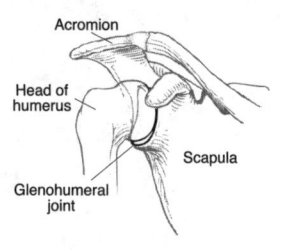

Acromion; Head of humerus; Scapula; Glenohumeral joint

The shoulder is accessed by scope (arthroscopy) for surgical purposes. A capsulorrhapy is performed

Explanation

The patient is positioned side-lying with arm suspended using a weight and a pulley system. An anesthetic is administered. Two to four small poke hole incisions are made around the shoulder joint to allow access to all areas of the shoulder joint. A solution is pumped through one of these incisions and into the joint to expand the joint for better visualization and to cleanse the joint. The arthroscope is inserted through a hole allowing the physician to perform a diagnostic arthroscopic exam by visualizing the shoulder joint. The corticoid process is identified and the tendon of the biceps (short head) is at times incised distal to corticoid for exposure. The anterior capsule is visualized through a small transverse incision of the subscapularis tendon which is tagged for identification and removed from its attachment on the capsule. The quality and laxity of the capsule are assessed and the joint is explored for damage to the labrum or glenoid. The joint is irrigated to remove any loose bodies. If there is no other abnormal laxity, the capsule is advance superiorly and attached to the labrum with sutures. An appropriate amount of slack is taken up to provide stability within the joint. Once the capsule is reattached, the subscapularis tendon is reapproximated but not tightened and repaired. A long acting local anesthetic may be injected into the joint to help with post-operative pain. The joint is irrigated and suture or Steri-strip closes the incisions. The area is covered with a dressing and a sling or shoulder immobilizer is applied.

Coding Tips

This is a unilateral procedure. If performed bilaterally, some payers require that the service be reported twice with modifier 50 appended to the second code, while others require identification of the service only once with modifier 50 appended. Check with individual payers. Modifier 50 identifies a procedure performed identically on the opposite side of the body (mirror image). When 29806 is performed with another separately identifiable procedure, the highest dollar value code is listed as the primary procedure and subsequent procedures are appended with modifier 51. Local anesthesia is included in this service. When arthroscopy is performed in conjunction with arthrotomy, add modifier 51. Surgical arthroscopy always includes diagnostic arthroscopy. For an open procedure, see 23450–23466. For open thermal capsulorrhaphy, use unlisted procedure code 23929. For arthroscopic thermal capsulorrhaphy, use unlisted procedure code 29999, or some non-Medicare payers may requre S2300. Check with non-Medicare payers to determine their specific guidelines..

ICD-9-CM Procedural

81.93 Suture of capsule or ligament of upper extremity

Anesthesia

29806 01630

ICD-9-CM Diagnostic

718.21 Pathological dislocation of shoulder joint
718.31 Recurrent dislocation of shoulder joint
831.00 Closed dislocation of shoulder, unspecified site
831.01 Closed anterior dislocation of humerus
831.02 Closed posterior dislocation of humerus
831.03 Closed inferior dislocation of humerus
831.10 Open unspecified dislocation of shoulder
831.11 Open anterior dislocation of humerus
831.12 Open posterior dislocation of humerus
831.13 Open inferior dislocation of humerus
840.2 Coracohumeral (ligament) sprain and strain
840.4 Rotator cuff (capsule) sprain and strain
840.5 Subscapularis (muscle) sprain and strain

CCI Version 16.3

0213T, 0216T, 0228T, 0230T, 23700, 29805, 29807, 29819-29823, 29825-29826, 36000, 36400-36410, 36420-36430, 36440, 36600, 36640, 37202, 43752, 51701-51703, 62310-62319, 64400-64435, 64445-64450, 64479, 64483, 64490, 64493, 64505-64530, 69990, 76000-76001, 93000-93010, 93040-93042, 93318, 94002, 94200, 94250, 94680-94690, 94770, 95812-95816, 95819, 95822, 95829, 95955, 96360, 96365, 96372, 96374-96376, 99148-99149, 99150

Note: These CCI edits are used for Medicare. Other payers may reimburse on codes listed above.

Medicare Edits

	Fac RVU	Non-Fac RVU	FUD	Assist
29806	31.12	31.12	90	N/A

Medicare References: 100-2,15,260; 100-3,100.2; 100-4,12,30; 100-4,12,90.3; 100-4,14,10

29807

29807 Arthroscopy, shoulder, surgical; repair of SLAP lesion

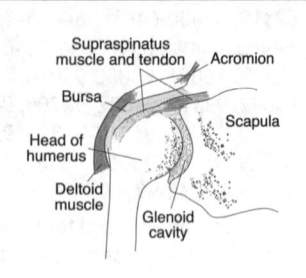

Anterior views of right shoulder

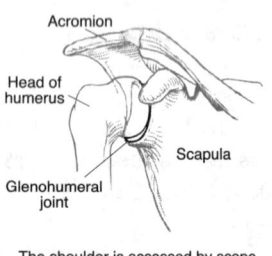

The shoulder is accessed by scope (arthroscopy) for surgical purposes. A slap lesion repair is performed

Explanation

Superior labral anterior posterior (SLAP) lesions are injuries to the labrum that extend from anterior to the biceps tendon to posterior to the biceps tendon. For a SLAP lesion repair, the physician makes three incisions: one for the arthroscope, a second for the suture hook, and a third for a cannula. The surgeon prepares the bony bed with a small ball burr and drills or punches a hole at the cartilage bone junction of the superior labrum. A hook is passed through the anterior superior portal and the inside limb is grasped with a suture retrieval forceps. The physician sets an anchor into the drill hole by mounting the suture anchor on the inserter and sliding it down the suture. The physician closes the loop with a slipknot that is tied and tightened outside the cannula. A knot pusher secures the knot under arthroscopic control. A long acting local anesthetic may be injected into the joint to help with post-operative pain. The joint is irrigated and suture or Steri-strip closes the incisions. The area is covered with a sterile dressing and a sling or shoulder immobilizer is applied.

Coding Tips

This is a unilateral procedure. If performed bilaterally, some payers require that the service be reported twice with modifier 50 appended to the second code, while others require identification of the service only once with modifier 50 appended. Check with individual payers. Modifier 50 identifies a procedure performed identically on the opposite side of the body (mirror image). When 29807 is performed with another separately identifiable procedure, the highest dollar value code is listed as the primary procedure and subsequent procedures are appended with modifier 51. When arthroscopy is performed in conjunction with arthrotomy, add modifier 51. Surgical arthroscopy always includes diagnostic arthroscopy. Local anesthesia is included in this service.

ICD-9-CM Procedural

81.96 Other repair of joint

Anesthesia

29807 01630

ICD-9-CM Diagnostic

718.31 Recurrent dislocation of shoulder joint
840.7 Superior glenoid labrum lesions (SLAP)

Terms To Know

dislocation. Displacement of a bone in relation to its neighboring tissue, especially a joint.

lesion. Area of damaged tissue that has lost continuity or function, due to disease or trauma. Lesions may be located on internal structures such as the brain, nerves, or kidneys, or visible on the skin.

tendon. Fibrous tissue that connects muscle to bone, consisting primarily of collagen and containing little vasculature.

CCI Version 16.3

0213T, 0216T, 0228T, 0230T, 23700, 29805, 36000, 36400-36410, 36420-36430, 36440, 36600, 36640, 37202, 43752, 51701-51703, 62310-62319, 64400-64435, 64445-64450, 64479, 64483, 64490, 64493, 64505-64530, 69990, 76000-76001, 93000-93010, 93040-93042, 93318, 94002, 94200, 94250, 94680-94690, 94770, 95812-95816, 95819, 95822, 95829, 95955, 96360, 96365, 96372, 96374-96376, 99148-99149, 99150

Note: These CCI edits are used for Medicare. Other payers may reimburse on codes listed above.

Medicare Edits

	Fac RVU	Non-Fac RVU	FUD	Assist
29807	30.38	30.38	90	N/A

Medicare References: 100-2,15,260; 100-3,100.2; 100-4,12,30; 100-4,12,90.3; 100-4,14,10

29819

29819 Arthroscopy, shoulder, surgical; with removal of loose body or foreign body

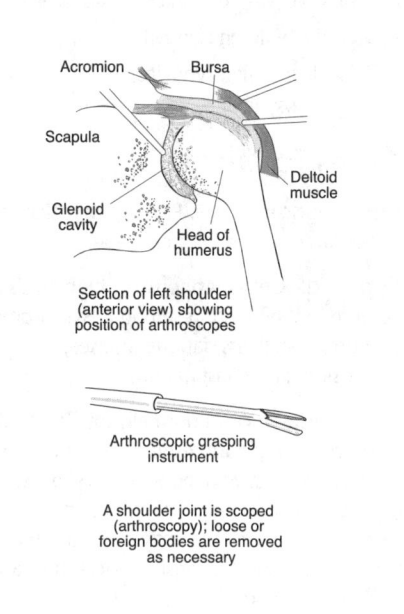

ICD-9-CM Procedural
80.21 Arthroscopy of shoulder

Anesthesia
29819 01630

ICD-9-CM Diagnostic
275.40 Unspecified disorder of calcium metabolism — (Use additional code to identify any associated mental retardation)
275.42 Hypercalcemia — (Use additional code to identify any associated mental retardation)
275.49 Other disorders of calcium metabolism — (Use additional code to identify any associated mental retardation)
718.01 Articular cartilage disorder, shoulder region
718.11 Loose body in shoulder joint
729.6   Residual foreign body in soft tissue — (Use additional code to identify foreign body (V90.01-V90.9))

Terms To Know
foreign body. Any object or substance found in an organ and tissue that does not belong under normal circumstances.

hypercalcemia. Abnormally high levels of calcium in the blood, resulting in symptoms of muscle weakness, fatigue, nausea, depression, and constipation.

soft tissue. Nonepithelial tissues outside of the skeleton that includes subcutaneous adipose tissue, fibrous tissue, fascia, muscles, blood and lymph vessels, and peripheral nervous system tissue.

CCI Version 16.3
0213T, 0216T, 0228T, 0230T, 23700, 29805, 36000, 36400-36410, 36420-36430, 36440, 36600, 36640, 37202, 43752, 51701-51703, 62310-62319, 64400-64435, 64445-64450, 64479, 64483, 64490, 64493, 64505-64530, 69990, 76000-76001, 93000-93010, 93040-93042, 93318, 94002, 94200, 94250, 94680-94690, 94770, 95812-95816, 95819, 95822, 95829, 95955, 96360, 96365, 96372, 96374-96376, 99148-99149, 99150

Note: These CCI edits are used for Medicare. Other payers may reimburse on codes listed above.

Medicare Edits

	Fac RVU	Non-Fac RVU	FUD	Assist
29819	17.12	17.12	90	N/A

Medicare References: 100-2,15,260; 100-3,100.2; 100-4,12,30; 100-4,12,90.3; 100-4,14,10

Explanation
To remove loose bodies, such as floating cartilage, the physician visualizes the foreign bodies and removes them with instruments passed through the portal holes. For a synovectomy, the physician makes several half-inch incisions to allow arthroscopic investigation of any problems associated with the synovium. Through the arthroscope, the physician removes the synovium from inside the shoulder joint using cutting tools and arthroscopic suction equipment. A long acting local anesthetic may be injected into the joint to help with post-operative pain. The joint is irrigated and suture or Steri-strip closes the incisions. The area is covered with a dressing and a sling or shoulder immobilizer is applied.

Coding Tips
When arthroscopy is performed in conjunction with arthrotomy, add modifier 51. Surgical arthroscopy always includes diagnostic arthroscopy. According to CPT guidelines, cast application or strapping (including removal) is only reported as a replacement procedure or when the cast application or strapping is an initial service performed without a restorative treatment or procedure. See "Application of Casts and Strapping" in the CPT book in the Surgery Section, under the Musculoskeletal system. For arthrotomy of the glenohumeral joint, with removal of a loose or foreign body, see 23040 and 23107. For arthrotomy of the acromioclavicular, sternoclavicular joint with removal of a foreign body, see 23044.

29820-29821

29820 Arthroscopy, shoulder, surgical; synovectomy, partial
29821 synovectomy, complete

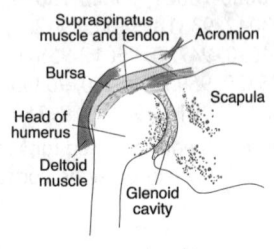

Anterior views of right shoulder

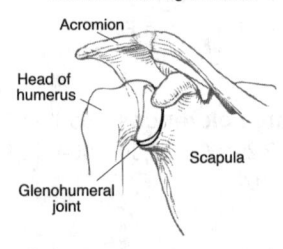

The shoulder is accessed by scope (arthroscopy) for surgical purposes. Synovial tissues are removed. Report 29820 when an entire synovectomy is performed.

Explanation

The patient is positioned side-lying with arm suspended using a weight and a pulley system. An anesthetic is administered. Two to four small poke hole (port) incisions are made around the shoulder joint to allow access to all areas of the shoulder joint. A solution is pumped through one of these incisions and into the joint to expand the joint for better visualization and to cleanse the joint. The arthroscope is inserted through a hole allowing the physician to perform a diagnostic arthroscopic exam by visualizing the shoulder joint. The synovium is removed with a motorized synovial resector inserted through a port. The instruments are removed and a long acting local anesthetic may be injected into the joint to help with post-operative pain. The joint is irrigated and suture or Steri-strip closes the incisions. The area is covered with a dressing and a sling or shoulder immobilizer is applied. Report 29820 for a partial synovectomy and 29821 for a complete synovectomy.

Coding Tips

When arthroscopy is performed in conjunction with arthrotomy, add modifier 51. Surgical arthroscopy always includes diagnostic arthroscopy. According to CPT guidelines, cast application or strapping (including removal) is only reported as a replacement procedure or when the cast application or strapping is an initial service performed without a restorative treatment or procedure. See "Application of Casts and Strapping" in the CPT book in the Surgery Section, under the Musculoskeletal system. For open synovectomy, see 23105.

ICD-9-CM Procedural

80.71 Synovectomy of shoulder

Anesthesia

01630

ICD-9-CM Diagnostic

170.4 Malignant neoplasm of scapula and long bones of upper limb
195.4 Malignant neoplasm of upper limb
213.4 Benign neoplasm of scapula and long bones of upper limb
215.2 Other benign neoplasm of connective and other soft tissue of upper limb, including shoulder
238.0 Neoplasm of uncertain behavior of bone and articular cartilage
239.2 Neoplasms of unspecified nature of bone, soft tissue, and skin
275.41 Hypocalcemia — (Use additional code to identify any associated mental retardation)
275.42 Hypercalcemia — (Use additional code to identify any associated mental retardation)
275.5 Hungry bone syndrome
357.1 Polyneuropathy in collagen vascular disease — (Code first underlying disease: 446.0, 710.0, 714.0)
359.6 Symptomatic inflammatory myopathy in diseases classified elsewhere — (Code first underlying disease: 135, 140.0-208.9, 277.30-277.39, 446.0, 710.0, 710.1, 710.2, 714.0)
446.0 Polyarteritis nodosa
710.0 Systemic lupus erythematosus — (Use additional code to identify manifestation: 424.91, 581.81, 582.81, 583.81)
710.1 Systemic sclerosis — (Use additional code to identify manifestation: 359.6, 517.2)
710.2 Sicca syndrome
712.11 Chondrocalcinosis due to dicalcium phosphate crystals, shoulder region — (Code first underlying disease: 275.4)
712.12 Chondrocalcinosis due to dicalcium phosphate crystals, upper arm — (Code first underlying disease: 275.4)
714.0 Rheumatoid arthritis — (Use additional code to identify manifestation: 357.1, 359.6)
715.11 Primary localized osteoarthrosis, shoulder region
719.21 Villonodular synovitis, shoulder region
726.0 Adhesive capsulitis of shoulder
726.11 Calcifying tendinitis of shoulder
726.12 Bicipital tenosynovitis
727.00 Unspecified synovitis and tenosynovitis

Terms To Know

chondrocalcinosis. Presence of calcium salt deposits within joint cartilage.

hypercalcemia. Abnormally high levels of calcium in the blood, resulting in symptoms of muscle weakness, fatigue, nausea, depression, and constipation.

hypocalcemia. Abnormally low levels of calcium in the blood, resulting in symptoms such as hyperactive deep tendon reflexes, muscle and abdominal cramping, and carpopedal spasm. This may be associated with diseases such as sepsis, pancreatitis, and acute renal failure.

polyarteritis nodosa. Systemic necrotizing vasculitis of small and medium arteries that results in the infarction and scarring within the affected organs.

polyneuropathy. Disease process of severe inflammation of multiple nerves.

CCI Version 16.3

0213T, 0216T, 0228T, 0230T, 23700, 29805, 36000, 36400-36410, 36420-36430, 36440, 36600, 36640, 37202, 43752, 51701-51703, 62310-62319, 64400-64435, 64445-64450, 64479, 64483, 64490, 64493, 64505-64530, 69990, 76000-76001, 93000-93010, 93040-93042, 93318, 94002, 94200, 94250, 94680-94690, 94770, 95812-95816, 95819, 95822, 95829, 95955, 96360, 96365, 96372, 96374-96376, 99148-99149, 99150

Also not with 29820: 11012❖

Also not with 29821: 29820, 29822

Note: These CCI edits are used for Medicare. Other payers may reimburse on codes listed above.

Medicare Edits

	Fac RVU	Non-Fac RVU	FUD	Assist
29820	15.76	15.76	90	80
29821	17.25	17.25	90	80

Medicare References: 100-2,15,260; 100-3,100.2; 100-4,12,30; 100-4,12,90.3; 100-4,14,10

29822-29823

29822 Arthroscopy, shoulder, surgical; debridement, limited
29823 debridement, extensive

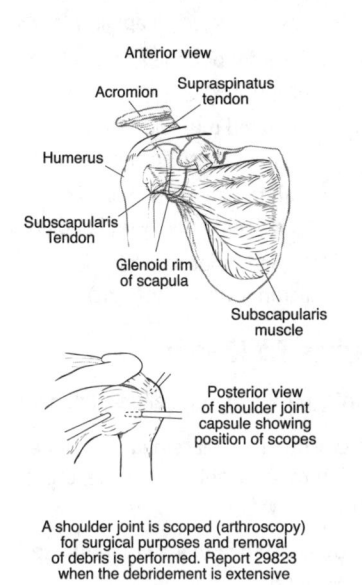

A shoulder joint is scoped (arthroscopy) for surgical purposes and removal of debris is performed. Report 29822 when the debridement is extensive

Explanation

The patient is positioned side-lying with arm suspended using a weight and a pulley system. An anesthetic is administered. Two to four small poke hole (port) incisions are made around the shoulder joint to allow access to all areas of the shoulder joint. A solution is pumped through one of these incisions and into the joint to expand the joint for better visualization and to cleanse the joint. The arthroscope is inserted through a hole allowing the physician to perform a diagnostic arthroscopic exam by visualizing the shoulder joint. A long acting local anesthetic may be injected into the joint to help with post-operative pain. The joint is irrigated and suture or Steri-strip closes the incisions. The area is covered with a dressing and a sling or shoulder immobilizer is applied. Report 29822 if the arthroscopic surgery is performed with limited debridement and 29823 if the procedure includes extensive debridement.

Coding Tips

When arthroscopy is performed in conjunction with arthrotomy, add modifier 51. Surgical arthroscopy always includes diagnostic arthroscopy. According to CPT guidelines, cast application or strapping (including removal) is only reported as a replacement procedure or when the cast application or strapping is an initial service performed without a restorative treatment or procedure. See "Application of Casts and Strapping" in the CPT book in the Surgery Section, under the Musculoskeletal system.

ICD-9-CM Procedural

80.81 Other local excision or destruction of lesion of shoulder joint

Anesthesia
01630

ICD-9-CM Diagnostic

- 357.1 Polyneuropathy in collagen vascular disease — (Code first underlying disease: 446.0, 710.0, 714.0)
- 359.6 Symptomatic inflammatory myopathy in diseases classified elsewhere — (Code first underlying disease: 135, 140.0-208.9, 277.30-277.39, 446.0, 710.0, 710.1, 710.2, 714.0)
- 446.0 Polyarteritis nodosa
- 710.0 Systemic lupus erythematosus — (Use additional code to identify manifestation: 424.91, 581.81, 582.81, 583.81)
- 710.1 Systemic sclerosis — (Use additional code to identify manifestation: 359.6, 517.2)
- 710.2 Sicca syndrome
- 714.0 Rheumatoid arthritis — (Use additional code to identify manifestation: 357.1, 359.6)
- 715.11 Primary localized osteoarthrosis, shoulder region
- 715.31 Localized osteoarthrosis not specified whether primary or secondary, shoulder region
- 715.91 Osteoarthrosis, unspecified whether generalized or localized, shoulder region
- 716.01 Kaschin-Beck disease, shoulder region
- 716.11 Traumatic arthropathy, shoulder region
- 718.01 Articular cartilage disorder, shoulder region
- 718.31 Recurrent dislocation of shoulder joint
- 718.81 Other joint derangement, not elsewhere classified, shoulder region
- 719.01 Effusion of shoulder joint
- 719.21 Villonodular synovitis, shoulder region
- 719.41 Pain in joint, shoulder region
- 726.0 Adhesive capsulitis of shoulder
- 726.10 Unspecified disorders of bursae and tendons in shoulder region
- 726.11 Calcifying tendinitis of shoulder
- 726.12 Bicipital tenosynovitis
- 726.19 Other specified disorders of rotator cuff syndrome of shoulder and allied disorders
- 726.2 Other affections of shoulder region, not elsewhere classified
- 727.00 Unspecified synovitis and tenosynovitis
- 733.90 Disorder of bone and cartilage, unspecified
- 840.0 Acromioclavicular (joint) (ligament) sprain and strain
- 840.4 Rotator cuff (capsule) sprain and strain
- 840.6 Supraspinatus (muscle) (tendon) sprain and strain
- 840.8 Sprain and strain of other specified sites of shoulder and upper arm

CCI Version 16.3

0213T, 0216T, 0228T, 0230T, 23700, 29805, 29819-29820, 36000, 36400-36410, 36420-36430, 36440, 36600, 36640, 37202, 43752, 51701-51703, 62310-62319, 64400-64435, 64445-64450, 64479, 64483, 64490, 64493, 64505-64530, 69990, 76000-76001, 93000-93010, 93040-93042, 93318, 94002, 94200, 94250, 94680-94690, 94770, 95812-95816, 95819, 95822, 95829, 95955, 96360, 96365, 96372, 96374-96376, 99148-99149, 99150

Also not with 29823: 29822, 29825

Note: These CCI edits are used for Medicare. Other payers may reimburse on codes listed above.

Medicare Edits

	Fac RVU	Non-Fac RVU	FUD	Assist
29822	16.76	16.76	90	80
29823	18.31	18.31	90	80

Medicare References: 100-2,15,260; 100-3,100.2; 100-4,12,30; 100-4,12,90.3; 100-4,14,10

29824

29824 Arthroscopy, shoulder, surgical; distal claviculectomy including distal articular surface (Mumford procedure)

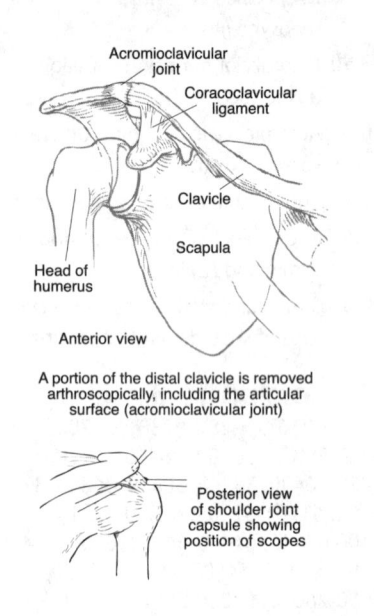

Acromioclavicular joint
Coracoclavicular ligament
Clavicle
Scapula
Head of humerus
Anterior view

A portion of the distal clavicle is removed arthroscopically, including the articular surface (acromioclavicular joint)

Posterior view of shoulder joint capsule showing position of scopes

Explanation

The physician performs two to four small poke hole incisions around the shoulder joint to allow access to all areas of the joint. A sterile solution is pumped through one of these incisions and into the joint to expand the joint for better visualization and to cleanse the joint. The arthroscope is inserted through a hole allowing the physician to perform a diagnostic arthroscopic exam by visualizing the shoulder joint. The physician may shell the entire bone out of its periosteal lining, including the distal articular surface, when using arthroscopic guidance. A long acting local anesthetic may be injected into the joint to help with post-operative pain. The joint is irrigated and suture or Steri-strip closes the incisions. The area is covered with a sterile dressing and a sling or shoulder immobilizer is applied.

Coding Tips

To qualify for reimbursement of distal claviculectomy, documentation should support removal of 8-10 mm from the distal clavicle/joint. This is a unilateral procedure. If performed bilaterally, some payers require that the service be reported twice with modifier 50 appended to the second code, while others require identification of the service only once with modifier 50 appended. Check with individual payers. Modifier 50 identifies a procedure performed identically on the opposite side of the body (mirror image). When 29824 is performed with another separately identifiable procedure, the highest dollar value code is listed as the primary procedure and subsequent procedures are appended with modifier 51. When arthroscopy is performed in conjunction with arthrotomy, add modifier 51. Surgical arthroscopy always includes diagnostic arthroscopy. When arthroscopic decompression (29826) and/or rotator cuff repair (29827) are performed on the same shoulder at the same session, report each (as appropriate) in addition to 29824 and append modifier 51 to the secondary procedure. For an open procedure, see 23120. Local anesthesia is included in this service.

ICD-9-CM Procedural

77.81 Other partial ostectomy of scapula, clavicle, and thorax (ribs and sternum)

Anesthesia

29824   01630

ICD-9-CM Diagnostic

- 170.3 Malignant neoplasm of ribs, sternum, and clavicle
- 196.3 Secondary and unspecified malignant neoplasm of lymph nodes of axilla and upper limb
- 198.5 Secondary malignant neoplasm of bone and bone marrow
- 198.89 Secondary malignant neoplasm of other specified sites
- 213.3 Benign neoplasm of ribs, sternum, and clavicle
- 238.0 Neoplasm of uncertain behavior of bone and articular cartilage
- 239.2 Neoplasms of unspecified nature of bone, soft tissue, and skin
- 715.11 Primary localized osteoarthrosis, shoulder region
- 715.21 Secondary localized osteoarthrosis, shoulder region
- 716.11 Traumatic arthropathy, shoulder region
- 716.61 Unspecified monoarthritis, shoulder region
- 718.01 Articular cartilage disorder, shoulder region
- 718.31 Recurrent dislocation of shoulder joint
- 728.86 Necrotizing fasciitis — (Use additional code to identify infectious organism, 041.00-041.89, 785.4, if applicable)
- 730.11 Chronic osteomyelitis, shoulder region — (Use additional code to identify organism: 041.1. Use additional code to identify major osseous defect, if applicable: 731.3)
- 731.3 Major osseous defects — (Code first underlying disease: 170.0-170.9, 730.00-730.29, 733.00-733.09, 733.40-733.49, 996.45)
- 733.49 Aseptic necrosis of other bone site — (Use additional code to identify major osseous defect, if applicable: 731.3)
- 733.90 Disorder of bone and cartilage, unspecified
- 738.8 Acquired musculoskeletal deformity of other specified site
- 785.4 Gangrene — (Code first any associated underlying condition)
- 831.04 Closed dislocation of acromioclavicular (joint)

Terms To Know

benign. Mild or nonmalignant in nature.

dislocation. Displacement of a bone in relation to its neighboring tissue, especially a joint.

distal. Located farther away from a specified reference point.

malignant. Any condition tending to progress toward death, specifically an invasive tumor with a loss of cellular differentiation that has the ability to spread or metastasize to other areas in the body.

necrosis. Death of cells or tissue within a living organ or structure.

periosteum. Double-layered connective membrane on the outer surface of bone.

CCI Version 16.3

0213T, 0216T, 0228T, 0230T, 23700, 29805, 29820-29823, 29825, 36000, 36400-36410, 36420-36430, 36440, 36600, 36640, 37202, 43752, 51701-51703, 62310-62319, 64400-64435, 64445-64450, 64479, 64483, 64490, 64493, 64505-64530, 69990, 76000-76001, 93000-93010, 93040-93042, 93318, 94002, 94200, 94250, 94680-94690, 94770, 95812-95816, 95819, 95822, 95829, 95955, 96360, 96365, 96372, 96374-96376, 99148-99149, 99150

Note: These CCI edits are used for Medicare. Other payers may reimburse on codes listed above.

Medicare Edits

	Fac RVU	Non-Fac RVU	FUD	Assist
29824	19.68	19.68	90	80

Medicare References: 100-2,15,260; 100-3,100.2; 100-4,12,30; 100-4,12,90.3; 100-4,14,10

29825

29825 Arthroscopy, shoulder, surgical; with lysis and resection of adhesions, with or without manipulation

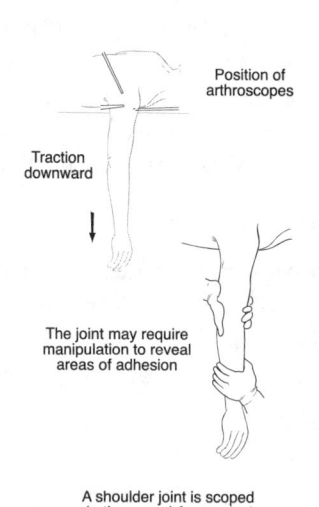

Explanation
The physician makes two to four small poke hole incisions around the shoulder joint to allow access to all areas of the joint. A solution is pumped through one of these incisions and into the joint to expand the joint for better visualization and to cleanse the joint. The arthroscope is inserted through a hole allowing the physician to perform a diagnostic arthroscopic exam by visualizing the shoulder joint. The physician may shell the bone out of its periosteal lining, including the distal articular surface, when using arthroscopic guidance. The physician lyses and resects adhesions, with or without manipulation. A long acting local anesthetic may be injected into the joint to help with postoperative pain. The joint is irrigated and suture or Steri-strip closes the incisions. The area is covered with a dressing and a sling or shoulder immobilizer is applied.

Coding Tips
When arthroscopy is performed in conjunction with arthrotomy, add modifier 51. Surgical arthroscopy always includes diagnostic arthroscopy. According to CPT guidelines, cast application or strapping (including removal) is only reported as a replacement procedure or when the cast application or strapping is an initial service performed without a restorative treatment or procedure. See "Application of Casts and Strapping" in the CPT book in the Surgery Section, under the Musculoskeletal system. For repair of a ruptured musculotendinous cuff (rotator cuff), acute, see 23410; chronic, see 23412.

ICD-9-CM Procedural
- 80.41 Division of joint capsule, ligament, or cartilage of shoulder

Anesthesia
29825 01630

ICD-9-CM Diagnostic
- 357.1 Polyneuropathy in collagen vascular disease — (Code first underlying disease: 446.0, 710.0, 714.0)
- 359.6 Symptomatic inflammatory myopathy in diseases classified elsewhere — (Code first underlying disease: 135, 140.0-208.9, 277.30-277.39, 446.0, 710.0, 710.1, 710.2, 714.0)
- 446.0 Polyarteritis nodosa
- 710.0 Systemic lupus erythematosus — (Use additional code to identify manifestation: 424.91, 581.81, 582.81, 583.81)
- 710.1 Systemic sclerosis — (Use additional code to identify manifestation: 359.6, 517.2)
- 710.2 Sicca syndrome
- 714.0 Rheumatoid arthritis — (Use additional code to identify manifestation: 357.1, 359.6)
- 715.11 Primary localized osteoarthrosis, shoulder region
- 715.31 Localized osteoarthrosis not specified whether primary or secondary, shoulder region
- 715.91 Osteoarthrosis, unspecified whether generalized or localized, shoulder region
- 716.11 Traumatic arthropathy, shoulder region
- 718.31 Recurrent dislocation of shoulder joint
- 718.41 Contracture of shoulder joint
- 718.51 Ankylosis of joint of shoulder region
- 726.0 Adhesive capsulitis of shoulder
- 726.10 Unspecified disorders of bursae and tendons in shoulder region
- 726.11 Calcifying tendinitis of shoulder
- 726.12 Bicipital tenosynovitis
- 726.19 Other specified disorders of rotator cuff syndrome of shoulder and allied disorders
- 726.2 Other affections of shoulder region, not elsewhere classified
- 840.0 Acromioclavicular (joint) (ligament) sprain and strain
- 840.4 Rotator cuff (capsule) sprain and strain
- 840.6 Supraspinatus (muscle) (tendon) sprain and strain
- 840.9 Sprain and strain of unspecified site of shoulder and upper arm

Terms To Know
adhesion. Abnormal fibrous connection between two structures, soft tissue or bony structures, that may occur as the result of surgery, infection, or trauma.

CCI Version 16.3
0213T, 0216T, 0228T, 0230T, 23700, 29805, 29820, 29822, 36000, 36400-36410, 36420-36430, 36440, 36600, 36640, 37202, 43752, 51701-51703, 62310-62319, 64400-64435, 64445-64450, 64479, 64483, 64490, 64493, 64505-64530, 69990, 76000-76001, 93000-93010, 93040-93042, 93318, 94002, 94200, 94250, 94680-94690, 94770, 95812-95816, 95819, 95822, 95829, 95955, 96360, 96365, 96372, 96374-96376, 99148-99149, 99150

Note: These CCI edits are used for Medicare. Other payers may reimburse on codes listed above.

Medicare Edits

	Fac RVU	Non-Fac RVU	FUD	Assist
29825	17.08	17.08	90	80

Medicare References: 100-2,15,260; 100-3,100.2; 100-4,12,30; 100-4,12,90.3; 100-4,14,10

29826

29826 Arthroscopy, shoulder, surgical; decompression of subacromial space with partial acromioplasty, with or without coracoacromial release

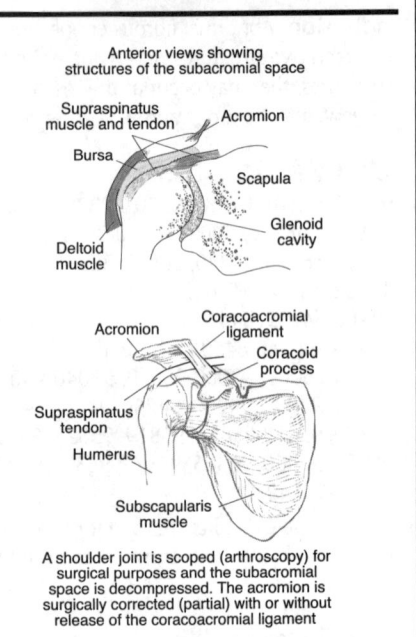

Explanation

The physician makes two to four small poke hole incisions around the shoulder joint to allow access to all areas of the joint. A solution is pumped through one of these incisions and into the joint to expand the joint for better visualization and to cleanse the joint. The subacromial space is decompressed and a partial acromioplasty, with or without coracoacromial release, is performed. The patient is seated with the torso raised and a sheet placed on the medial border of the affected scapula. Anterior, lateral, and posterior arthroscopic portals are established and a cannula is inserted through the anterior and lateral portals to accommodate the inflow and instrumentation. The arthroscope is inserted into the posterior portal, where it is driven into the subacromial space for visualization of the subacromial joint. A limited bursectomy is performed using a full radius shaver and, if necessary, the physician clears the undersurface of the antero-lateral acromion of soft tissue using intra-articular cautery. The acromial ligament may be released. A long acting local anesthetic may be injected into the joint to help with post-operative pain. The joint is irrigated and suture or Steri-strip closes the incisions. The area is covered with a dressing and a sling or shoulder immobilizer is applied.

Coding Tips

When arthroscopy is performed in conjunction with arthrotomy, add modifier 51. Surgical arthroscopy always includes diagnostic arthroscopy. According to CPT guidelines, cast application or strapping (including removal) is only reported as a replacement procedure or when the cast application or strapping is an initial service performed without a restorative treatment or procedure. See "Application of Casts and Strapping" in the CPT book in the Surgery Section, under the Musculoskeletal System. When rotator cuff repair (29827) and/or distal claviculectomy (29824) are performed on the same shoulder at the same session, report each (as appropriate) in addition to 29826 and append modifier 51 to the secondary procedure. For open acromioplasty with decompression, see 23130. For coracoacromial ligament release, with or without acromioplasty, see 23415. For open reconstruction of complete shoulder rotator cuff avulsion, chronic, including acromioplasty, see 23420.

ICD-9-CM Procedural

- 81.82 Repair of recurrent dislocation of shoulder
- 81.83 Other repair of shoulder

Anesthesia

29826 01630

ICD-9-CM Diagnostic

- 353.0 Brachial plexus lesions
- 715.11 Primary localized osteoarthrosis, shoulder region
- 715.21 Secondary localized osteoarthrosis, shoulder region
- 715.31 Localized osteoarthrosis not specified whether primary or secondary, shoulder region
- 715.91 Osteoarthrosis, unspecified whether generalized or localized, shoulder region
- 716.11 Traumatic arthropathy, shoulder region
- 718.01 Articular cartilage disorder, shoulder region
- 718.31 Recurrent dislocation of shoulder joint
- 718.51 Ankylosis of joint of shoulder region
- 718.81 Other joint derangement, not elsewhere classified, shoulder region
- 726.0 Adhesive capsulitis of shoulder
- 726.10 Unspecified disorders of bursae and tendons in shoulder region
- 726.11 Calcifying tendinitis of shoulder
- 726.12 Bicipital tenosynovitis
- 726.19 Other specified disorders of rotator cuff syndrome of shoulder and allied disorders
- 726.2 Other affections of shoulder region, not elsewhere classified
- 727.61 Complete rupture of rotator cuff
- 840.0 Acromioclavicular (joint) (ligament) sprain and strain
- 840.4 Rotator cuff (capsule) sprain and strain
- 840.8 Sprain and strain of other specified sites of shoulder and upper arm

Terms To Know

adhesive capsulitis. Excessive scar tissue in the shoulder, causing stiffness and pain.

ankylosis. Abnormal union or fusion of bones in a joint, which is normally moveable.

bicipital tenosynovitis. Inflammatory condition affecting the bicipital tendon.

calcifying tendinitis. Inflammation and hardening of tissue due to calcium salt deposits, occurring in the tendons and areas of tendonomuscular attachment.

CCI Version 16.3

0213T, 0216T, 0228T, 0230T, 23700, 29805, 29820, 29822, 29825, 36000, 36400-36410, 36420-36430, 36440, 36600, 36640, 37202, 43752, 51701-51703, 62310-62319, 64400-64435, 64445-64450, 64479, 64483, 64490, 64493, 64505-64530, 69990, 76000-76001, 93000-93010, 93040-93042, 93318, 94002, 94200, 94250, 94680-94690, 94770, 95812-95816, 95819, 95822, 95829, 95955, 96360, 96365, 96372, 96374-96376, 99148-99149, 99150

Note: These CCI edits are used for Medicare. Other payers may reimburse on codes listed above.

Medicare Edits

	Fac RVU	Non-Fac RVU	FUD	Assist
29826	19.51	19.51	90	80

Medicare References: 100-2,15,260; 100-3,100.2; 100-4,12,30; 100-4,12,90.3; 100-4,14,10

29827

29827 Arthroscopy, shoulder, surgical; with rotator cuff repair

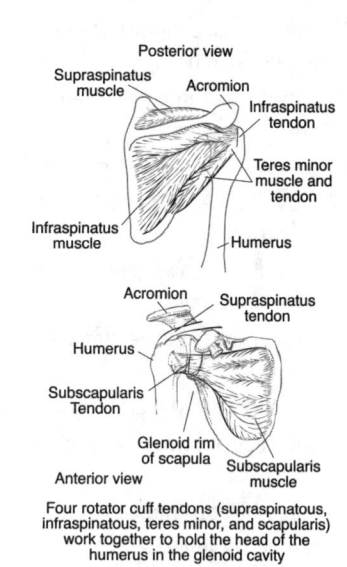

Explanation

The physician performs a surgical arthroscopy of the shoulder to repair a torn rotator cuff. The patient is positioned side-lying with the arm suspended. Small poke hole incisions are made around the shoulder through which the arthroscopic instruments are inserted. A solution is pumped through one of these incisions to cleanse and expand the joint for better visualization. The physician first performs a diagnostic arthroscopic exam to assess the joint. A limited bursectomy may be performed with a subacromial decompression in which the undersurface of the antero-lateral acromion is cleared of soft tissue, if necessary. A small skin incision may be made laterally incorporating one of the portholes to facilitate the arthroscopic repair. The deltoid muscle is split from its acromion attachment about 5 cm and the tendon edge is debrided and mobilized. A transverse bony trough 3 to 4 mm is made and tunnels are drilled through the bone trough to the lateral cortex of the greater tuberosity. The tendon edge is brought into the trough with permanent sutures and anchor sutures are placed. Sutures are placed into the bone and brought through the tendon. A hemostat is placed on the cuff to retract the tendon and take tension off the sutures. The anchor sutures are tied down, followed by the sutures to the bony trough. The free ends of the sutures are passed through the tunnels and tied over a bony bridge. The longitudinal portions of the tear are closed with absorbable suture and a range of motion check is done on the arm. The deltoid splits, subcutaneous tissue, and skin are closed and the arm is placed in a sling to maintain abduction.

Coding Tips

When arthroscopy is performed in conjunction with arthrotomy, add modifier 51. Medicare, as well as some commercial payers, may not allow payment of diagnostic arthroscopy at the same time of an open procedure on the same joint. Since surgical arthroscopy includes any diagnostic arthroscopy, do not report separately. For an open or a mini-open rotator cuff tear, see 23412. When arthroscopic decompression (29826) and/or distal claviculectomy (29824) are performed on the same shoulder at the same session, report each (as appropriate) in addition to 29827 and append modifier 51 to the secondary procedure.

ICD-9-CM Procedural

83.63 Rotator cuff repair

Anesthesia

29827 01630

ICD-9-CM Diagnostic

715.10 Primary localized osteoarthrosis, specified site
715.11 Primary localized osteoarthrosis, shoulder region
715.21 Secondary localized osteoarthrosis, shoulder region
715.31 Localized osteoarthrosis not specified whether primary or secondary, shoulder region
716.11 Traumatic arthropathy, shoulder region
716.61 Unspecified monoarthritis, shoulder region
719.41 Pain in joint, shoulder region
726.10 Unspecified disorders of bursae and tendons in shoulder region
727.61 Complete rupture of rotator cuff
831.00 Closed dislocation of shoulder, unspecified site
831.01 Closed anterior dislocation of humerus
831.02 Closed posterior dislocation of humerus
831.03 Closed inferior dislocation of humerus
840.4 Rotator cuff (capsule) sprain and strain
927.00 Crushing injury of shoulder region — (Use additional code to identify any associated injuries: 800-829, 850.0-854.1, 860.0-869.1)
959.2 Injury, other and unspecified, shoulder and upper arm

Terms To Know

range of motion. Action of a body part throughout its extent of natural movement, measured in degrees of a circle.

soft tissue. Nonepithelial tissues outside of the skeleton that includes subcutaneous adipose tissue, fibrous tissue, fascia, muscles, blood and lymph vessels, and peripheral nervous system tissue.

subcutaneous tissue. Sheet or wide band of adipose (fat) and areolar connective tissue in two layers attached to the dermis.

CCI Version 16.3

0213T, 0216T, 0228T, 0230T, 11010-11012❖, 23700, 29805-29806, 29820, 29822, 29825, 36000, 36400-36410, 36420-36430, 36440, 36600, 36640, 37202, 43752, 51701-51703, 62310-62319, 64400-64435, 64445-64450, 64479, 64483, 64490, 64493, 64505-64530, 69990, 76000-76001, 93000-93010, 93040-93042, 93318, 94002, 94200, 94250, 94680-94690, 94770, 95812-95816, 95819, 95822, 95829, 95955, 96360, 96365, 96372, 96374-96376, 99148-99149, 99150

Note: These CCI edits are used for Medicare. Other payers may reimburse on codes listed above.

Medicare Edits

	Fac RVU	Non-Fac RVU	FUD	Assist
29827	31.69	31.69	90	80

Medicare References: 100-2,15,260; 100-3,100.2; 100-4,12,30; 100-4,12,90.3; 100-4,14,10

29828

29828 Arthroscopy, shoulder, surgical; biceps tenodesis

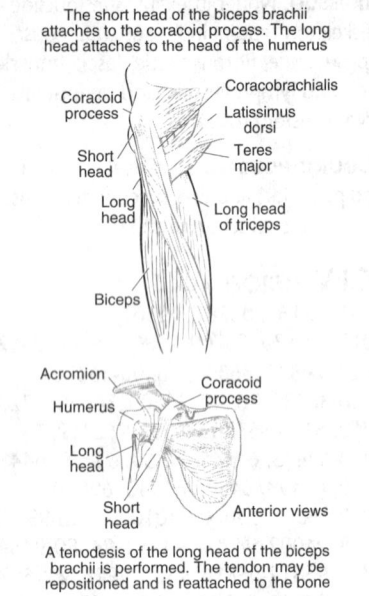

The short head of the biceps brachii attaches to the coracoid process. The long head attaches to the head of the humerus

Anterior views

A tenodesis of the long head of the biceps brachii is performed. The tendon may be repositioned and is reattached to the bone

Explanation
The physician performs arthroscopic biceps tenodesis. With the patient under appropriate anesthesia, standard arthroscopic portals are established. A monofilament suture is passed through an 18-gauge needle placed into the biceps tendon, and an arthroscopic suture instrument is utilized to retrieve the suture. The physician uses an arthroscopic basket to release the tendon from its origin, and the arthroscopic equipment is transferred to the subacromial space. Using the arthroscopic basket, the physician identifies and opens the tendon sheath. Electrocautery may be used to clean the surrounding tissues. A probe is utilized to free the tendon, which is extracted through one of the arthroscopic portals. The tendon is then pulled into a humeral socket that has been drilled at the top of the bicipital groove. Under arthroscopic control, it is fixed using a bioabsorbable interference screw. Instrumentation is removed and the arthroscopic portals are closed with sutures.

Coding Tips
Do not report 29828 in conjunction with 29805, 29820, 29822. For open biceps tenodesis, use 23430.

ICD-9-CM Procedural
- 81.96 Other repair of joint
- 83.01 Exploration of tendon sheath
- 83.13 Other tenotomy
- 83.42 Other tenonectomy
- 83.61 Suture of tendon sheath
- 83.62 Delayed suture of tendon
- 83.64 Other suture of tendon
- 83.71 Advancement of tendon
- 83.72 Recession of tendon
- 83.73 Reattachment of tendon
- 83.75 Tendon transfer or transplantation
- 83.76 Other tendon transposition
- 83.88 Other plastic operations on tendon

Anesthesia
29828 01630

ICD-9-CM Diagnostic
- 170.4 Malignant neoplasm of scapula and long bones of upper limb
- 195.4 Malignant neoplasm of upper limb
- 213.4 Benign neoplasm of scapula and long bones of upper limb
- 446.0 Polyarteritis nodosa
- 714.0 Rheumatoid arthritis — (Use additional code to identify manifestation: 357.1, 359.6)
- 715.11 Primary localized osteoarthrosis, shoulder region
- 715.21 Secondary localized osteoarthrosis, shoulder region
- 715.31 Localized osteoarthrosis not specified whether primary or secondary, shoulder region
- 716.11 Traumatic arthropathy, shoulder region
- 716.61 Unspecified monoarthritis, shoulder region
- 716.91 Unspecified arthropathy, shoulder region
- 718.01 Articular cartilage disorder, shoulder region
- 718.21 Pathological dislocation of shoulder joint
- 718.31 Recurrent dislocation of shoulder joint
- 718.41 Contracture of shoulder joint
- 718.71 Developmental dislocation of joint, shoulder region
- 718.81 Other joint derangement, not elsewhere classified, shoulder region
- 718.91 Unspecified derangement, shoulder region
- 719.01 Effusion of shoulder joint
- 719.11 Hemarthrosis, shoulder region
- 719.41 Pain in joint, shoulder region
- 719.81 Other specified disorders of shoulder joint
- 726.0 Adhesive capsulitis of shoulder
- 726.10 Unspecified disorders of bursae and tendons in shoulder region
- 726.11 Calcifying tendinitis of shoulder
- 726.12 Bicipital tenosynovitis
- 726.2 Other affections of shoulder region, not elsewhere classified
- 727.61 Complete rupture of rotator cuff
- 727.62 Nontraumatic rupture of tendons of biceps (long head)
- 831.00 Closed dislocation of shoulder, unspecified site
- 831.01 Closed anterior dislocation of humerus
- 831.02 Closed posterior dislocation of humerus
- 840.0 Acromioclavicular (joint) (ligament) sprain and strain
- 840.3 Infraspinatus (muscle) (tendon) sprain and strain
- 840.4 Rotator cuff (capsule) sprain and strain
- 840.5 Subscapularis (muscle) sprain and strain
- 840.6 Supraspinatus (muscle) (tendon) sprain and strain
- 840.8 Sprain and strain of other specified sites of shoulder and upper arm
- 880.20 Open wound of shoulder region, with tendon involvement
- 905.2 Late effect of fracture of upper extremities
- 905.6 Late effect of dislocation
- 927.00 Crushing injury of shoulder region — (Use additional code to identify any associated injuries: 800-829, 850.0-854.1, 860.0-869.1)
- 959.2 Injury, other and unspecified, shoulder and upper arm

CCI Version 16.3
0213T, 0216T, 0228T, 0230T, 11010-11012✦, 23700, 29805, 29820, 29822, 29825, 36000, 36400-36410, 36420-36430, 36440, 36600, 36640, 37202, 43752, 62310-62319, 64400-64435, 64445-64450, 64479, 64483, 64490, 64493, 64505-64530, 69990, 76000-76001, 93000-93010, 93040-93042, 93318, 94002, 94200, 94250, 94680-94690, 94770, 95812-95816, 95819, 95822, 95829, 95955, 96360, 96365, 96372, 96374-96376, 99148-99149, 99150

Note: These CCI edits are used for Medicare. Other payers may reimburse on codes listed above.

Medicare Edits

	Fac RVU	Non-Fac RVU	FUD	Assist
29828	26.88	26.88	90	80

Medicare References: None

29830

29830 Arthroscopy, elbow, diagnostic, with or without synovial biopsy (separate procedure)

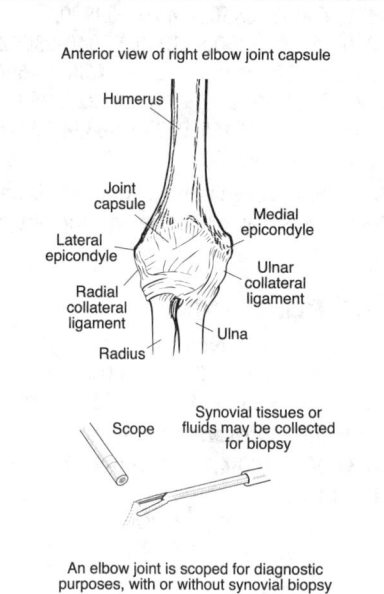

Anterior view of right elbow joint capsule
- Humerus
- Joint capsule
- Lateral epicondyle
- Medial epicondyle
- Radial collateral ligament
- Ulnar collateral ligament
- Radius
- Ulna

Scope — Synovial tissues or fluids may be collected for biopsy

An elbow joint is scoped for diagnostic purposes, with or without synovial biopsy

Explanation
The physician performs elbow arthroscopy with the patient in a supine position. General anesthesia is preferred. The physician makes 1 cm portal incisions to insert the arthroscope into the elbow joint space. The five most commonly used portals are the lateral, anterolateral, anteromedial, posterolateral, and straight positions. The physician places the arthroscope into the elbow joint and examines the humeral-ulnar and radial-ulnar joints. The elbow is flexed and extended, and pronated and supinated to allow visualization and examination of all joint spaces and surfaces. If there is evidence of synovial proliferation or inflammation indicating disease, the physician uses an instrument to obtain a small piece of synovium for biopsy. In 29830, the physician performs a diagnostic arthroscopy. The portal incisions are closed with sutures or Steri-strips.

Coding Tips
When arthroscopy is performed in conjunction with arthrotomy, add modifier 51. Surgical arthroscopy always includes diagnostic arthroscopy. This separate procedure by definition is usually a component of a more complex service and is not identified separately. When performed alone or with other unrelated procedures/services, it may be reported. If performed alone, list the code; if performed with other procedures/services, list the code and append modifier 59. For arthrotomy of the elbow with a synovial biopsy, see 24100. For arthroscopy of the elbow for removal of a loose or foreign body, see 29834. For arthroscopy of the elbow for a partial synovectomy, see 29835; complete synovectomy, see 29836. For arthroscopy of the elbow for limited debridement, see 29837; extensive debridement, see 29838.

ICD-9-CM Procedural
- 80.22 Arthroscopy of elbow
- 80.32 Biopsy of joint structure of elbow

Anesthesia
29830 01732

ICD-9-CM Diagnostic
- 170.4 Malignant neoplasm of scapula and long bones of upper limb
- 195.4 Malignant neoplasm of upper limb
- 213.4 Benign neoplasm of scapula and long bones of upper limb
- 215.2 Other benign neoplasm of connective and other soft tissue of upper limb, including shoulder
- 238.0 Neoplasm of uncertain behavior of bone and articular cartilage
- 239.2 Neoplasms of unspecified nature of bone, soft tissue, and skin
- 275.40 Unspecified disorder of calcium metabolism — (Use additional code to identify any associated mental retardation)
- 275.41 Hypocalcemia — (Use additional code to identify any associated mental retardation)
- 275.42 Hypercalcemia — (Use additional code to identify any associated mental retardation)
- 275.49 Other disorders of calcium metabolism — (Use additional code to identify any associated mental retardation)
- 275.5 Hungry bone syndrome
- 357.1 Polyneuropathy in collagen vascular disease — (Code first underlying disease: 446.0, 710.0, 714.0)
- 359.6 Symptomatic inflammatory myopathy in diseases classified elsewhere — (Code first underlying disease: 135, 140.0-208.9, 277.30-277.39, 446.0, 710.0, 710.1, 710.2, 714.0)
- 446.0 Polyarteritis nodosa
- 710.0 Systemic lupus erythematosus — (Use additional code to identify manifestation: 424.91, 581.81, 582.81, 583.81)
- 710.1 Systemic sclerosis — (Use additional code to identify manifestation: 359.6, 517.2)
- 710.2 Sicca syndrome
- 714.0 Rheumatoid arthritis — (Use additional code to identify manifestation: 357.1, 359.6)
- 715.12 Primary localized osteoarthrosis, upper arm
- 715.22 Secondary localized osteoarthrosis, upper arm
- 716.12 Traumatic arthropathy, upper arm
- 718.02 Articular cartilage disorder, upper arm
- 718.22 Pathological dislocation of upper arm joint
- 718.32 Recurrent dislocation of upper arm joint
- 718.42 Contracture of upper arm joint
- 719.22 Villonodular synovitis, upper arm
- 727.00 Unspecified synovitis and tenosynovitis

CCI Version 16.3
0213T, 0216T, 0228T, 0230T, 11012❖, 24300, 36000, 36400-36410, 36420-36430, 36440, 36600, 36640, 37202, 43752, 51701-51703, 62310-62319, 64400-64435, 64445-64450, 64479, 64483, 64490, 64493, 64505-64530, 69990, 76000-76001, 93000-93010, 93040-93042, 93318, 94002, 94200, 94250, 94680-94690, 94770, 95812-95816, 95819, 95822, 95829, 95955, 96360, 96365, 96372, 96374-96376, 99148-99149, 99150

Note: These CCI edits are used for Medicare. Other payers may reimburse on codes listed above.

Medicare Edits

	Fac RVU	Non-Fac RVU	FUD	Assist
29830	13.23	13.23	90	N/A

Medicare References: 100-2,15,260; 100-3,100.2; 100-4,12,30; 100-4,12,90.3; 100-4,14,10

29834

29834 Arthroscopy, elbow, surgical; with removal of loose body or foreign body

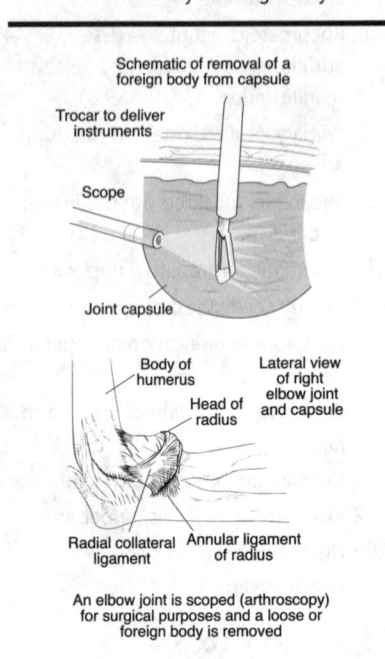

Explanation
The physician performs elbow arthroscopy with the patient in a supine position. General anesthesia is preferred. The physician makes 1 cm portal incisions to insert the arthroscope into the elbow joint space. The five most commonly used portals are the lateral, anterolateral, anteromedial, posterolateral, and straight positions. The physician places the arthroscope into the elbow joint and examines the humeral-ulnar and radial-ulnar joints. The elbow is flexed and extended, and pronated and supinated to allow visualization and examination of all joint spaces and surfaces. In 29834, the physician examines all parts of the elbow joint with the arthroscope. Any loose bodies (e.g., small pieces of cartilage from chondral injuries) or foreign bodies (e.g., bullet or nail) are removed by identifying them through the arthroscope and using another portal incision to remove the object. The portal incisions are closed with sutures or Steri-strips.

Coding Tips
When arthroscopy is performed in conjunction with arthrotomy, add modifier 51. Surgical arthroscopy always includes diagnostic arthroscopy. According to CPT guidelines, cast application or strapping (including removal) is only reported as a replacement procedure or when the cast application or strapping is an initial service performed without a restorative treatment or procedure. See "Application of Casts and Strapping" in the CPT book in the Surgery Section, under the Musculoskeletal system. For arthrotomy of the elbow for removal of a foreign body, see 24000; loose or foreign body, see 24101. For arthroscopy of the elbow, diagnostic or for synovial biopsy, see 29830. For arthroscopy of the elbow for a partial synovectomy, see 29835; complete synovectomy, see 29836. For arthroscopy of the elbow for a limited debridement, see 29837; extensive debridement, see 29838.

ICD-9-CM Procedural
80.22 Arthroscopy of elbow

Anesthesia
29834 01740

ICD-9-CM Diagnostic
718.02 Articular cartilage disorder, upper arm
718.12 Loose body in upper arm joint
729.6 Residual foreign body in soft tissue — (Use additional code to identify foreign body (V90.01-V90.9))

Terms To Know

anterolateral. Situated in the front and off to one side.

anteromedial. Situated in the front and to the side of the central point or midline.

foreign body. Any object or substance found in an organ and tissue that does not belong under normal circumstances.

lateral. To/on the side.

posterolateral. Located in the back and off to the side.

supine. Lying on the back.

CCI Version 16.3
0213T, 0216T, 0228T, 0230T, 11012❖, 24300, 29830, 36000, 36400-36410, 36420-36430, 36440, 36600, 36640, 37202, 43752, 51701-51703, 62310-62319, 64400-64435, 64445-64450, 64479, 64483, 64490, 64493, 64505-64530, 69990, 76000-76001, 93000-93010, 93040-93042, 93318, 94002, 94200, 94250, 94680-94690, 94770, 95812-95816, 95819, 95822, 95829, 95955, 96360, 96365, 96372, 96374-96376, 99148-99149, 99150

Note: These CCI edits are used for Medicare. Other payers may reimburse on codes listed above.

Medicare Edits

	Fac RVU	Non-Fac RVU	FUD	Assist
29834	14.35	14.35	90	80

Medicare References: 100-2,15,260; 100-3,100.2; 100-4,12,30; 100-4,12,90.3; 100-4,14,10

29835-29836

29835 Arthroscopy, elbow, surgical; synovectomy, partial
29836 synovectomy, complete

Schematic of removal of synovial matter from capsule
- Trocar to deliver instruments
- Scope
- Joint capsule

Lateral view of right elbow joint and capsule
- Body of humerus
- Head of radius
- Radial collateral ligament
- Annular ligament of radius

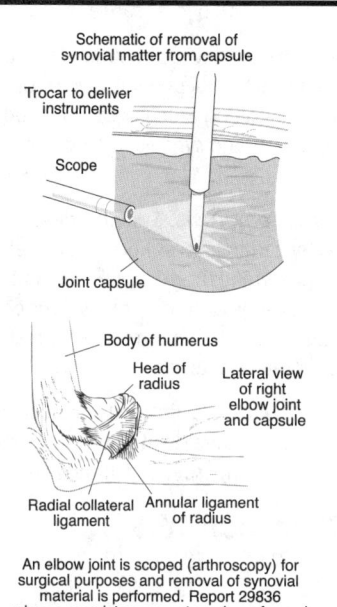

An elbow joint is scoped (arthroscopy) for surgical purposes and removal of synovial material is performed. Report 29836 when a complete synovectomy is performed

Explanation

The physician performs elbow arthroscopy with the patient in a supine position. The physician makes 1.0 cm portal incisions to insert the arthroscope into the elbow joint space. The five most commonly used portals are the lateral, anterolateral, anteromedial, posterolateral, and straight positions. The physician then places the arthroscope into the elbow joint and examines the humeral-ulnar and radial-ulnar joints. The elbow is flexed and extended and pronated and supinated to allow visualization and examination of all joint spaces and surfaces. Proliferative or diseased synovium is identified and removed with a motorized, suction resector. Report 29835 for a partial synovectomy. Report 29836 when a complete synovectomy is performed. The portal incisions are closed with sutures or Steri-strips.

Coding Tips

When arthroscopy is performed in conjunction with arthrotomy, add modifier 51. Surgical arthroscopy always includes diagnostic arthroscopy. According to CPT guidelines, cast application or strapping (including removal) is only reported as a replacement procedure or when the cast application or strapping is an initial service performed without a restorative treatment or procedure. See "Application of Casts and Strapping" in the CPT book in the Surgery Section, under the Musculoskeletal system. For arthrotomy of the elbow with synovectomy, see 24102. For arthroscopy of the elbow, diagnostic or for synovial biopsy, see 29830.

ICD-9-CM Procedural

80.72 Synovectomy of elbow

Anesthesia

01740

ICD-9-CM Diagnostic

- 275.40 Unspecified disorder of calcium metabolism — (Use additional code to identify any associated mental retardation)
- 275.41 Hypocalcemia — (Use additional code to identify any associated mental retardation)
- 275.49 Other disorders of calcium metabolism — (Use additional code to identify any associated mental retardation)
- 275.5 Hungry bone syndrome
- 357.1 Polyneuropathy in collagen vascular disease — (Code first underlying disease: 446.0, 710.0, 714.0)
- 359.6 Symptomatic inflammatory myopathy in diseases classified elsewhere — (Code first underlying disease: 135, 140.0-208.9, 277.30-277.39, 446.0, 710.0, 710.1, 710.2, 714.0)
- 446.0 Polyarteritis nodosa
- 710.0 Systemic lupus erythematosus — (Use additional code to identify manifestation: 424.91, 581.81, 582.81, 583.81)
- 710.1 Systemic sclerosis — (Use additional code to identify manifestation: 359.6, 517.2)
- 710.2 Sicca syndrome
- 712.12 Chondrocalcinosis due to dicalcium phosphate crystals, upper arm — (Code first underlying disease: 275.4)
- 712.22 Chondrocalcinosis due to pyrophosphate crystals, upper arm — (Code first underlying disease: 275.4)
- 714.0 Rheumatoid arthritis — (Use additional code to identify manifestation: 357.1, 359.6)
- 715.12 Primary localized osteoarthrosis, upper arm
- 718.32 Recurrent dislocation of upper arm joint
- 718.82 Other joint derangement, not elsewhere classified, upper arm
- 719.22 Villonodular synovitis, upper arm
- 727.00 Unspecified synovitis and tenosynovitis

Terms To Know

hypocalcemia. Abnormally low levels of calcium in the blood, resulting in symptoms such as hyperactive deep tendon reflexes, muscle and abdominal cramping, and carpopedal spasm. This may be associated with diseases such as sepsis, pancreatitis, and acute renal failure.

polyneuropathy. Disease process of severe inflammation of multiple nerves.

systemic sclerosis. Systemic disease characterized by excess fibrotic collagen build-up, turning the skin thickened and hard. Fibrotic changes also occur in various organs and cause vascular abnormalities and affect more women than men.

villonodular synovitis. Inflammation of the synovial membrane due to excessive synovial tissue formation, especially in the knee.

CCI Version 16.3

0213T, 0216T, 0228T, 0230T, 24300, 29830, 36000, 36400-36410, 36420-36430, 36440, 36600, 36640, 37202, 43752, 51701-51703, 62310-62319, 64400-64435, 64445-64450, 64479, 64483, 64490, 64493, 64505-64530, 69990, 76000-76001, 93000-93010, 93040-93042, 93318, 94002, 94200, 94250, 94680-94690, 94770, 95812-95816, 95819, 95822, 95829, 95955, 96360, 96365, 96372, 96374-96376, 99148-99149, 99150

Also not with 29835: 11012❖

Also not with 29836: 29835, 29837

Note: These CCI edits are used for Medicare. Other payers may reimburse on codes listed above.

Medicare Edits

	Fac RVU	Non-Fac RVU	FUD	Assist
29835	14.76	14.76	90	80
29836	17.02	17.02	90	80

Medicare References: 100-2,15,260; 100-3,100.2; 100-4,12,30; 100-4,12,90.3; 100-4,14,10

29837-29838

29837 Arthroscopy, elbow, surgical; debridement, limited
29838 debridement, extensive

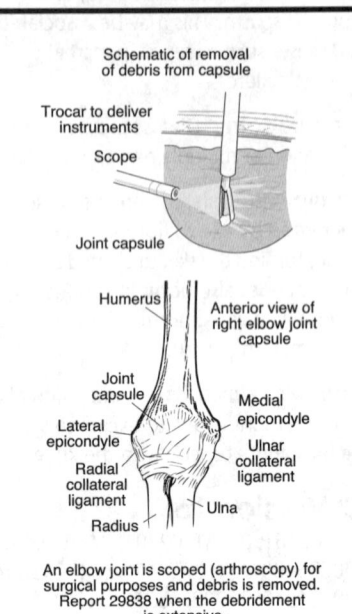

Explanation
The physician performs elbow arthroscopy with the patient in a supine position. The physician makes 1 cm portal incisions to insert the arthroscope into the elbow joint space. The five most commonly used portals are the lateral, anterolateral, anteromedial, posterolateral, and straight positions. The physician places the arthroscope into the elbow joint and examines the humeral-ulnar and radial-ulnar joints. The elbow is flexed and extended and pronated and supinated to allow visualization and examination of all joint spaces and surfaces. Debridement is performed on proliferative cartilage, a degenerative joint, or roughened or frayed articular cartilage. The physician uses instruments through the arthroscope to cut and remove inflamed and proliferated synovium and to clean and smooth the articular joint surfaces of the elbow. In 29837, the physician performs a limited debridement. In 29838, extensive debridement that includes all joints of the elbow is performed. The portal incisions are closed with sutures or Steri-strips.

Coding Tips
When arthroscopy is performed in conjunction with arthrotomy, add modifier 51. Surgical arthroscopy always includes diagnostic arthroscopy. According to CPT guidelines, cast application or strapping (including removal) is only reported as a replacement procedure or when the cast application or strapping is an initial service performed without a restorative treatment or procedure. See "Application of Casts and Strapping" in the CPT book in the Surgery Section, under the Musculoskeletal system. For arthroscopy of the elbow for removal of a loose or foreign body, see 29834. For arthroscopy of the elbow for a partial synovectomy, see 29835; complete synovectomy, see 29836.

ICD-9-CM Procedural
80.82 Other local excision or destruction of lesion of elbow joint

Anesthesia
01740

ICD-9-CM Diagnostic
275.41 Hypocalcemia — (Use additional code to identify any associated mental retardation)
275.42 Hypercalcemia — (Use additional code to identify any associated mental retardation)
275.5 Hungry bone syndrome
357.1 Polyneuropathy in collagen vascular disease — (Code first underlying disease: 446.0, 710.0, 714.0)
359.6 Symptomatic inflammatory myopathy in diseases classified elsewhere — (Code first underlying disease: 135, 140.0-208.9, 277.30-277.39, 446.0, 710.0, 710.1, 710.2, 714.0)
446.0 Polyarteritis nodosa
710.0 Systemic lupus erythematosus — (Use additional code to identify manifestation: 424.91, 581.81, 582.81, 583.81)
710.1 Systemic sclerosis — (Use additional code to identify manifestation: 359.6, 517.2)
710.2 Sicca syndrome
712.12 Chondrocalcinosis due to dicalcium phosphate crystals, upper arm — (Code first underlying disease: 275.4)
712.22 Chondrocalcinosis due to pyrophosphate crystals, upper arm — (Code first underlying disease: 275.4)
714.0 Rheumatoid arthritis — (Use additional code to identify manifestation: 357.1, 359.6)
715.12 Primary localized osteoarthrosis, upper arm
718.32 Recurrent dislocation of upper arm joint
718.82 Other joint derangement, not elsewhere classified, upper arm
719.22 Villonodular synovitis, upper arm
727.00 Unspecified synovitis and tenosynovitis

Terms To Know
chondrocalcinosis. Presence of calcium salt deposits within joint cartilage.

osteoarthrosis. Most common form of a noninflammatory degenerative joint disease with degenerating articular cartilage, bone enlargement, and synovial membrane changes.

systemic sclerosis. Systemic disease characterized by excess fibrotic collagen build-up, turning the skin thickened and hard. Fibrotic changes also occur in various organs and cause vascular abnormalities and affect more women than men.

villonodular synovitis. Inflammation of the synovial membrane due to excessive synovial tissue formation, especially in the knee.

CCI Version 16.3
0213T, 0216T, 0228T, 0230T, 24300, 24357-24358, 29830, 29835, 36000, 36400-36410, 36420-36430, 36440, 36600, 36640, 37202, 43752, 51701-51703, 62310-62319, 64400-64435, 64445-64450, 64479, 64483, 64490, 64493, 64505-64530, 69990, 76000-76001, 93000-93010, 93040-93042, 93318, 94002, 94200, 94250, 94680-94690, 94770, 95812-95816, 95819, 95822, 95829, 95955, 96360, 96365, 96372, 96374-96376, 99148-99149, 99150

Also not with 29837: 11012❖

Also not with 29838: 29837

Note: These CCI edits are used for Medicare. Other payers may reimburse on codes listed above.

Medicare Edits

	Fac RVU	Non-Fac RVU	FUD	Assist
29837	15.44	15.44	90	80
29838	17.26	17.26	90	80

Medicare References: 100-2,15,260; 100-3,100.2; 100-4,12,30; 100-4,12,90.3; 100-4,14,10

29840

29840 Arthroscopy, wrist, diagnostic, with or without synovial biopsy (separate procedure)

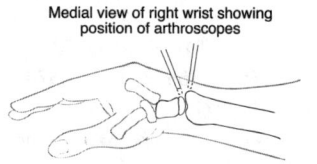

Medial view of right wrist showing position of arthroscopes

A wrist joint is scoped (arthroscopy) for diagnostic purposes, with or without biopsy of synovial material

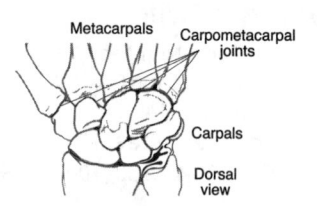

Articular spaces of the wrist. Synovial membranes line these surfaces and synovial fluid lubricates the joint actions

Explanation

The physician performs wrist arthroscopy. The joint is distended using finger traps on the index and long fingers that are attached to a 10 lb weight pulley. Counter traction is applied to the arm with a second 10 lb pulley. The joint is injected with lidocaine and epinephrine to distend the capsule. A sterile wrap is applied to the forearm to prevent extravasation of fluid. Portal incisions are made. The scope is inserted. The physician then inspects the wrist joint. The wrist is manipulated to allow visualization of all joint spaces and surfaces. If there is evidence of synovial proliferation or inflammation, the physician uses an instrument to obtain a small piece of synovium for biopsy. The portal incisions are closed with sutures or Steri-strips.

Coding Tips

When arthroscopy is performed in conjunction with arthrotomy, add modifier 51. Surgical arthroscopy always includes diagnostic arthroscopy. This separate procedure by definition is usually a component of a more complex service and is not identified separately. When performed alone or with other unrelated procedures/services, it may be reported. If performed alone, list the code; if performed with other procedures/services, list the code and append modifier 59. For arthrotomy of the wrist, with biopsy, see 25101. For arthroscopy, wrist, for lavage and drainage, see 29843. For arthroscopy, wrist, for partial synovectomy, see 29844; complete synovectomy, see 29845.

ICD-9-CM Procedural

- 80.23 Arthroscopy of wrist
- 80.33 Biopsy of joint structure of wrist

Anesthesia
29840 01829

ICD-9-CM Diagnostic

- 171.2 Malignant neoplasm of connective and other soft tissue of upper limb, including shoulder
- 198.89 Secondary malignant neoplasm of other specified sites
- 215.2 Other benign neoplasm of connective and other soft tissue of upper limb, including shoulder
- 238.1 Neoplasm of uncertain behavior of connective and other soft tissue
- 239.2 Neoplasms of unspecified nature of bone, soft tissue, and skin
- 275.40 Unspecified disorder of calcium metabolism — (Use additional code to identify any associated mental retardation)
- 275.42 Hypercalcemia — (Use additional code to identify any associated mental retardation)
- 275.49 Other disorders of calcium metabolism — (Use additional code to identify any associated mental retardation)
- 357.1 Polyneuropathy in collagen vascular disease — (Code first underlying disease: 446.0, 710.0, 714.0)
- 359.6 Symptomatic inflammatory myopathy in diseases classified elsewhere — (Code first underlying disease: 135, 140.0-208.9, 277.30-277.39, 446.0, 710.0, 710.1, 710.2, 714.0)
- 446.0 Polyarteritis nodosa
- 710.0 Systemic lupus erythematosus — (Use additional code to identify manifestation: 424.91, 581.81, 582.81, 583.81)
- 710.1 Systemic sclerosis — (Use additional code to identify manifestation: 359.6, 517.2)
- 710.2 Sicca syndrome
- 714.0 Rheumatoid arthritis — (Use additional code to identify manifestation: 357.1, 359.6)
- 715.23 Secondary localized osteoarthrosis, forearm
- 716.13 Traumatic arthropathy, forearm
- 718.03 Articular cartilage disorder, forearm
- 718.23 Pathological dislocation of forearm joint
- 718.33 Recurrent dislocation of forearm joint
- 718.43 Contracture of forearm joint
- 719.23 Villonodular synovitis, forearm
- 727.09 Other synovitis and tenosynovitis

CCI Version 16.3

0213T, 0216T, 0228T, 0230T, 11012❖, 25259, 36000, 36400-36410, 36420-36430, 36440, 36600, 36640, 37202, 43752, 51701-51703, 62310-62319, 64400-64435, 64445-64450, 64479, 64483, 64490, 64493, 64505-64530, 69990, 76000-76001, 93000-93010, 93040-93042, 93318, 94002, 94200, 94250, 94680-94690, 94770, 95812-95816, 95819, 95822, 95829, 95955, 96360, 96365, 96372, 96374-96376, 99148-99149, 99150

Note: These CCI edits are used for Medicare. Other payers may reimburse on codes listed above.

Medicare Edits

	Fac RVU	Non-Fac RVU	FUD	Assist
29840	13.12	13.12	90	80

Medicare References: 100-2,15,260; 100-3,100.2; 100-4,12,30; 100-4,12,90.3; 100-4,14,10

29843

29843 Arthroscopy, wrist, surgical; for infection, lavage and drainage

Medial view of right wrist showing position of arthroscopes

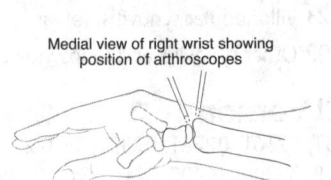

A wrist joint is scoped (arthroscopy) for surgical purposes to treat infection by lavage and drainage

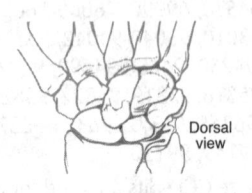

Dorsal view

Affected wrist joint spaces are injected with solution to treat infection; the fluid is then aspirated from the joint

Explanation

The physician performs wrist arthroscopy. The joint is distended using finger traps on the index and long fingers that are attached to a 10 lb weight pulley. Counter traction is applied to the arm with a second 10 lb pulley. The joint is injected with lidocaine and epinephrine to distend the capsule. A sterile wrap is applied to the forearm to prevent extravasation of fluid. Portal incisions are made. The scope is inserted. The physician then inspects the wrist joint. The wrist is manipulated to allow visualization of all joint spaces and surfaces. The infection is treated using lavage and drainage. Irrigation fluid is directed into each compartment of the wrist joint using the arthroscope for visualization. Lavage is continued until the fluid is clear. A motorized suction cutter may be used to remove encrusted fluid (exudate) and any fibrinous clots. Drains are placed as needed. The portal incisions are closed with sutures or Steri-strips.

Coding Tips

When arthroscopy is performed in conjunction with arthrotomy, add modifier 51. Surgical arthroscopy always includes diagnostic arthroscopy. For arthroscopy, wrist, diagnostic or for synovial biopsy, see 29840. For arthroscopy, wrist, for partial synovectomy, see 29844; complete synovectomy, see 29845.

ICD-9-CM Procedural

80.23 Arthroscopy of wrist

Anesthesia

29843 01830

ICD-9-CM Diagnostic

- 711.03 Pyogenic arthritis, forearm — (Use additional code to identify infectious organism: 041.0-041.8)
- 711.43 Arthropathy associated with other bacterial diseases, forearm — (Code first underlying disease, such as diseases classifiable to 010-040 (except 036.82), 090-099 (except 098.50))
- 711.53 Arthropathy associated with other viral diseases, forearm — (Code first underlying disease: 045-049, 050-079, 480, 487)
- 711.63 Arthropathy associated with mycoses, forearm — (Code first underlying disease: 110.0-118)
- 711.83 Arthropathy associated with other infectious and parasitic diseases, forearm — (Code first underlying disease: 080-088, 100-104, 130-136)
- 996.67 Infection and inflammatory reaction due to other internal orthopedic device, implant, and graft — (Use additional code to identify specified infections)
- 996.69 Infection and inflammatory reaction due to other internal prosthetic device, implant, and graft — (Use additional code to identify specified infections)
- 998.51 Infected postoperative seroma — (Use additional code to identify organism)
- 998.59 Other postoperative infection — (Use additional code to identify infection)

Terms To Know

exudate. Fluid or other material, such as debris from cells, that has escaped blood vessel circulation and is deposited in or on tissues and usually occurs due to inflammation.

infected postoperative seroma. Infection within a tumor-like growth of serum following surgery.

infection. Presence of microorganisms in body tissues that may result in cellular damage.

CCI Version 16.3

0213T, 0216T, 0228T, 0230T, 11012✦, 25259, 29840, 29848, 36000, 36400-36410, 36420-36430, 36440, 36600, 36640, 37202, 43752, 51701-51703, 62310-62319, 64400-64435, 64445-64450, 64479, 64483, 64490, 64493, 64505-64530, 69990, 76000-76001, 93000-93010, 93040-93042, 93318, 94002, 94200, 94250, 94680-94690, 94770, 95812-95816, 95819, 95822, 95829, 95955, 96360, 96365, 96372, 96374-96376, 99148-99149, 99150

Note: These CCI edits are used for Medicare. Other payers may reimburse on codes listed above.

Medicare Edits

	Fac RVU	Non-Fac RVU	FUD	Assist
29843	14.05	14.05	90	80

Medicare References: 100-2,15,260; 100-3,100.2; 100-4,12,30; 100-4,12,90.3; 100-4,14,10

29844-29845

29844 Arthroscopy, wrist, surgical; synovectomy, partial
29845 synovectomy, complete

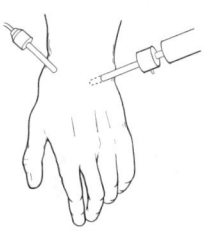

Articular spaces of the wrist (dark) which contain synovial matter

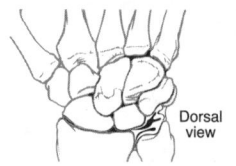

Dorsal view

A wrist joint is scoped for surgical purposes and synovial tissues are removed. Report 29845 when a complete synovectomy is performed

Explanation

The physician performs wrist arthroscopy. The joint is distended using finger traps on the index and long fingers that are attached to a 10 lb weight pulley. Counter traction is applied to the arm with a second 10 lb pulley. The joint is injected with lidocaine and epinephrine to distend the capsule. A sterile wrap is applied to the forearm to prevent extravasation of fluid. Portal incisions are made. The scope is inserted. The physician then inspects the wrist joint. The wrist is manipulated to allow visualization of all joint spaces and surfaces. The synovial membrane lining the joint capsule is partially removed and in 29845 it is completely removed. This is accomplished by use of a motorized, suction resector. The joint is irrigated and all instruments are removed. Drains are placed as needed. The portal incisions are closed with sutures or Steri-strips.

Coding Tips

When arthroscopy is performed in conjunction with arthrotomy, add modifier 51. Surgical arthroscopy always includes diagnostic arthroscopy. According to CPT guidelines, cast application or strapping (including removal) is only reported as a replacement procedure or when the cast application or strapping is an initial service performed without a restorative treatment or procedure. See "Application of Casts and Strapping" in the CPT book in the Surgery Section, under the Musculoskeletal system. For arthrotomy, wrist, with synovectomy, see 25105. For arthroscopy, wrist, diagnostic or for synovial biopsy, see 29840. For arthroscopy, wrist, for lavage and drainage, see 29843.

ICD-9-CM Procedural

80.73 Synovectomy of wrist

Anesthesia

01830

ICD-9-CM Diagnostic

- 171.2 Malignant neoplasm of connective and other soft tissue of upper limb, including shoulder
- 198.89 Secondary malignant neoplasm of other specified sites
- 215.2 Other benign neoplasm of connective and other soft tissue of upper limb, including shoulder
- 238.1 Neoplasm of uncertain behavior of connective and other soft tissue
- 239.2 Neoplasms of unspecified nature of bone, soft tissue, and skin
- 275.40 Unspecified disorder of calcium metabolism — (Use additional code to identify any associated mental retardation)
- 275.41 Hypocalcemia — (Use additional code to identify any associated mental retardation)
- 275.49 Other disorders of calcium metabolism — (Use additional code to identify any associated mental retardation)
- 275.5 Hungry bone syndrome
- 357.1 Polyneuropathy in collagen vascular disease — (Code first underlying disease: 446.0, 710.0, 714.0)
- 359.6 Symptomatic inflammatory myopathy in diseases classified elsewhere — (Code first underlying disease: 135, 140.0-208.9, 277.30-277.39, 446.0, 710.0, 710.1, 710.2, 714.0)
- 446.0 Polyarteritis nodosa
- 710.0 Systemic lupus erythematosus — (Use additional code to identify manifestation: 424.91, 581.81, 582.81, 583.81)
- 710.1 Systemic sclerosis — (Use additional code to identify manifestation: 359.6, 517.2)
- 710.2 Sicca syndrome
- 712.12 Chondrocalcinosis due to dicalcium phosphate crystals, upper arm — (Code first underlying disease: 275.4)
- 712.23 Chondrocalcinosis due to pyrophosphate crystals, forearm — (Code first underlying disease: 275.4)
- 714.0 Rheumatoid arthritis — (Use additional code to identify manifestation: 357.1, 359.6)
- 715.13 Primary localized osteoarthrosis, forearm
- 719.23 Villonodular synovitis, forearm
- 727.00 Unspecified synovitis and tenosynovitis

Terms To Know

tenosynovitis. Inflammation of a tendon sheath due to infection or disease.

villonodular synovitis. Inflammation of the synovial membrane due to excessive synovial tissue formation, especially in the knee.

CCI Version 16.3

0213T, 0216T, 0228T, 0230T, 25259, 36000, 36400-36410, 36420-36430, 36440, 36600, 36640, 37202, 43752, 51701-51703, 62310-62319, 64400-64435, 64445-64450, 64479, 64483, 64490, 64493, 64505-64530, 69990, 76000-76001, 93000-93010, 93040-93042, 93318, 94002, 94200, 94250, 94680-94690, 94770, 95812-95816, 95819, 95822, 95829, 95955, 96360, 96365, 96372, 96374-96376, 99148-99149, 99150

Also not with 29844: 11012❖, 29840-29843

Also not with 29845: 29840-29844, 29846-29847

Note: These CCI edits are used for Medicare. Other payers may reimburse on codes listed above.

Medicare Edits

	Fac RVU	Non-Fac RVU	FUD	Assist
29844	14.49	14.49	90	80
29845	16.73	16.73	90	80

Medicare References: 100-2,15,260; 100-3,100.2; 100-4,12,30; 100-4,12,90.3; 100-4,14,10

29846

29846 Arthroscopy, wrist, surgical; excision and/or repair of triangular fibrocartilage and/or joint debridement

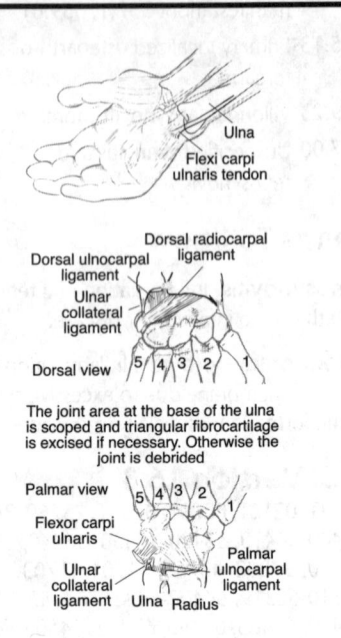

Explanation

The physician performs wrist arthroscopy. The joint is distended using finger traps on the index and long fingers that are attached to a 10 lb weight pulley. Counter traction is applied to the arm with a second 10 lb pulley. The joint is injected with lidocaine and epinephrine to distend the capsule. A sterile wrap is applied to the forearm to prevent extravasation of fluid. Portal incisions are made. The scope is inserted. The physician then inspects the wrist joint. The wrist is manipulated to allow visualization of all joint spaces and surfaces. The joint is debrided, which involves removing any inflamed or devitalized tissue. The articular surfaces are cleaned and smoothed. If tears are present in the triangular fibrocartilage, the physician uses instruments through the arthroscope to suture the tears. The joint is irrigated and all instruments are removed. The portal incisions are closed with sutures or Steri-strips.

Coding Tips

When arthroscopy is performed in conjunction with arthrotomy, add modifier 51. Surgical arthroscopy always includes diagnostic arthroscopy. According to CPT guidelines, cast application or strapping (including removal) is only reported as a replacement procedure or when the cast application or strapping is an initial service performed without a restorative treatment or procedure. See "Application of Casts and Strapping" in the CPT book in the Surgery Section, under the Musculoskeletal system. For arthrotomy, distal radioulnar joint, with repair of cartilage, see 25107. For arthroscopy, wrist, for lavage and drainage, see 29843. For arthroscopy, wrist, for a partial synovectomy, see 29844; complete synovectomy, see 29845.

ICD-9-CM Procedural

80.83 Other local excision or destruction of lesion of wrist joint
81.96 Other repair of joint

Anesthesia

29846 01830

ICD-9-CM Diagnostic

718.03 Articular cartilage disorder, forearm
718.83 Other joint derangement, not elsewhere classified, forearm

Terms To Know

extravasation. Escape of fluid from a vessel into the surrounding tissue.

lesion. Area of damaged tissue that has lost continuity or function, due to disease or trauma. Lesions may be located on internal structures such as the brain, nerves, or kidneys, or visible on the skin.

CCI Version 16.3

0213T, 0216T, 0228T, 0230T, 11012❖, 25259, 29840-29844, 36000, 36400-36410, 36420-36430, 36440, 36600, 36640, 37202, 43752, 51701-51703, 62310-62319, 64400-64435, 64445-64450, 64479, 64483, 64490, 64493, 64505-64530, 69990, 76000-76001, 93000-93010, 93040-93042, 93318, 94002, 94200, 94250, 94680-94690, 94770, 95812-95816, 95819, 95822, 95829, 95955, 96360, 96365, 96372, 96374-96376, 99148-99149, 99150

Note: These CCI edits are used for Medicare. Other payers may reimburse on codes listed above.

Medicare Edits

	Fac RVU	Non-Fac RVU	FUD	Assist
29846	15.2	15.2	90	80

Medicare References: 100-2,15,260; 100-3,100.2; 100-4,12,30; 100-4,12,90.3; 100-4,14,10

29847

29847 Arthroscopy, wrist, surgical; internal fixation for fracture or instability

Arthroscopic equipment in place at the wrist

Trans-scaphoperilunar fracture with wire fixation

A wrist joint is scoped for surgical purposes and internal fixation of a fracture or instability is placed

Explanation
The physician performs surgical wrist arthroscopy with internal fixation for a fracture or joint instability. The joint is distended using finger traps on the index and long fingers that are attached to a 10 pound weight pulley. Counter traction is applied to the arm with a second 10 lb pulley. The joint is injected with lidocaine and epinephrine to distend the capsule. A wrap is applied to the forearm to prevent extravasation of fluid. Portal incisions are made. The scope is inserted. The physician inspects the wrist joint. The wrist is manipulated to allow visualization of all joint spaces and surfaces. The site of the fracture or instability is identified. The physician uses instruments placed through the arthroscope to manipulate the fracture or unstable area into proper alignment. Internal fixation, consisting of wires, pins, and/or screws, is applied. The joint is irrigated and all instruments are removed. The portal incisions are closed with sutures or Steri-strips.

Coding Tips
When arthroscopy is performed in conjunction with arthrotomy, add modifier 51. Surgical arthroscopy always includes diagnostic arthroscopy. According to CPT guidelines, cast application or strapping (including removal) is only reported as a replacement procedure or when the cast application or strapping is an initial service performed without a restorative treatment or procedure. See "Application of Casts and Strapping" in the CPT book in the Surgery Section, under the Musculoskeletal system.

ICD-9-CM Procedural
78.59 Internal fixation of other bone, except facial bones, without fracture reduction

Anesthesia
29847 01830

ICD-9-CM Diagnostic
718.83 Other joint derangement, not elsewhere classified, forearm
718.93 Unspecified derangement, forearm joint
733.12 Pathologic fracture of distal radius and ulna
733.81 Malunion of fracture
733.82 Nonunion of fracture
813.40 Unspecified closed fracture of lower end of forearm
813.41 Closed Colles' fracture
813.42 Other closed fractures of distal end of radius (alone)
813.43 Closed fracture of distal end of ulna (alone)
813.44 Closed fracture of lower end of radius with ulna
813.45 Torus fracture of radius (alone)
813.46 Torus fracture of ulna (alone)
813.47 Torus fracture of radius and ulna
V54.12 Aftercare for healing traumatic fracture of lower arm
V54.22 Aftercare for healing pathologic fracture of lower arm

Terms To Know
closed fracture. Break in a bone without a concomitant opening in the skin. A closed fracture is coded when the type of fracture is not specified.

fracture. Break in bone or cartilage.

nonunion. Failure of two ends of a fracture to mend or completely heal.

CCI Version 16.3
0213T, 0216T, 0228T, 0230T, 25259, 29840-29844, 29846, 29848, 36000, 36400-36410, 36420-36430, 36440, 36600, 36640, 37202, 43752, 51701-51703, 62310-62319, 64400-64435, 64445-64450, 64479, 64483, 64490, 64493, 64505-64530, 69990, 76000-76001, 93000-93010, 93040-93042, 93318, 94002, 94200, 94250, 94680-94690, 94770, 95812-95816, 95819, 95822, 95829, 95955, 96360, 96365, 96372, 96374-96376, 99148-99149, 99150

Note: These CCI edits are used for Medicare. Other payers may reimburse on codes listed above.

Medicare Edits

	Fac RVU	Non-Fac RVU	FUD	Assist
29847	15.84	15.84	90	80

Medicare References: 100-2,15,260; 100-3,100.2; 100-4,12,30; 100-4,12,90.3; 100-4,14,10

29848

29848 Endoscopy, wrist, surgical, with release of transverse carpal ligament

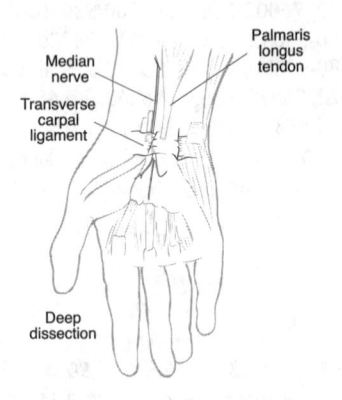

Explanation
The patient is placed supine with the arm positioned on a hand table. Endoscopic release may be accomplished by a one or two portal technique. In a single portal technique, a small, 1 1/2 cm, horizontal incision is made at the wrist. Using a two portal technique, two small incisions are made, one in the palm and one at the wrist. The palmar skin, underlying cushioning fat, protective fascia, and muscle are not cut. The endoscope is introduced underneath the transverse carpal ligament. The endoscope allows the physician to view the procedure on a monitor. A blade attached to the arthroscope is used to incise the transverse carpal ligament from the inside of the carpal tunnel. The instruments are removed and the portal(s) closed with sutures or Steri-strips. A splint may be applied.

Coding Tips
Surgical arthroscopy always includes diagnostic arthroscopy. According to CPT guidelines, cast application or strapping (including removal) is only reported as a replacement procedure or when the cast application or strapping is an initial service performed without a restorative treatment or procedure. See "Application of Casts and Strapping" in the CPT book in the Surgery Section, under the Musculoskeletal system. For open carpel tunnel release, see 64721.

ICD-9-CM Procedural
04.43 Release of carpal tunnel

Anesthesia
29848 01810, 01830

ICD-9-CM Diagnostic
354.0 Carpal tunnel syndrome

Terms To Know

carpal tunnel syndrome. Swelling and inflammation in the tendons or bursa surrounding the median nerve caused by repetitive activity. The resulting compression on the nerve causes pain, numbness, and tingling especially to the palm, index, middle finger, and thumb.

fascia. Fibrous sheet or band of tissue that envelops organs, muscles, and groupings of muscles.

ligament. Band or sheet of fibrous tissue that connects the articular surfaces of bones or supports visceral organs.

supine. Lying on the back.

CCI Version 16.3
0213T, 0216T, 0228T, 0230T, 11012❖, 25259, 26055, 29840, 36000, 36400-36410, 36420-36430, 36440, 36600, 36640, 37202, 43752, 51701-51703, 62310-62319, 64400-64435, 64445-64450, 64479, 64483, 64490, 64493, 64505-64530, 69990, 76000-76001, 93000-93010, 93040-93042, 93318, 94002, 94200, 94250, 94680-94690, 94770, 95812-95816, 95819, 95822, 95829, 95955, 96360, 96365, 96372, 96374-96376, 99148-99149, 99150

Note: These CCI edits are used for Medicare. Other payers may reimburse on codes listed above.

Medicare Edits

	Fac RVU	Non-Fac RVU	FUD	Assist
29848	14.75	14.75	90	N/A

Medicare References: 100-2,15,260; 100-3,100.2; 100-4,12,30; 100-4,12,90.3; 100-4,14,10

29900

29900 Arthroscopy, metacarpophalangeal joint, diagnostic, includes synovial biopsy

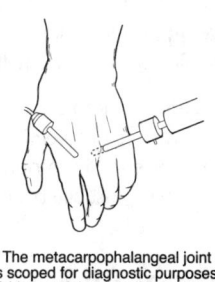

The metacarpophalangeal joint is scoped for diagnostic purposes. A biopsy of the synovium may be collected

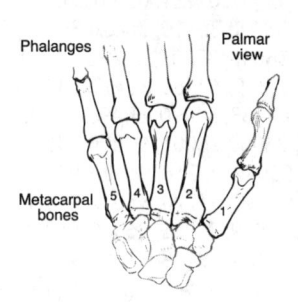

Phalanges / Palmar view / Metacarpal bones

Explanation

The metacarpophalangeal joints consist of the convex heads of the metacarpals articulating with the concave bases of the proximal phalanges. The metacarpophalangeal joint of interest is placed for easy access and an injection of local anesthetic is administered. Incisions for portals are made in the respective metacarpal to allow the arthroscope and surgical instruments to be introduced into the joint. The arthroscope is inserted through a portal into the joint, and the surgical equipment is passed through a second portal. A third portal may have been made for pumping fluid in to expand the joint space for clearer visualization. A needle is inserted through the trocar and twisted to cut out the tissue segment for biopsy. The biopsy needle, trocar, and arthroscope are removed. The site is cleansed and a pressure bandage is applied.

Coding Tips

When 29900 is performed with another separately identifiable procedure, the highest dollar value code is listed as the primary procedure and subsequent procedures are appended with modifier 51. When arthroscopy is performed in conjunction with arthrotomy, add modifier 51. Surgical arthroscopy always includes diagnostic arthroscopy. Local anesthesia is included in this service. Do no report 29900 with 29901 or 29902. Some payers may require the use of HCPCS Level II modifiers FA–F9 to identify the specific finger involved.

ICD-9-CM Procedural
- 80.24 Arthroscopy of hand and finger
- 80.34 Biopsy of joint structure of hand and finger

Anesthesia
29900 01820, 01829

ICD-9-CM Diagnostic
- 357.1 Polyneuropathy in collagen vascular disease — (Code first underlying disease: 446.0, 710.0, 714.0)
- 359.6 Symptomatic inflammatory myopathy in diseases classified elsewhere — (Code first underlying disease: 135, 140.0-208.9, 277.30-277.39, 446.0, 710.0, 710.1, 710.2, 714.0)
- 682.4 Cellulitis and abscess of hand, except fingers and thumb — (Use additional code to identify organism, such as 041.1, etc.)
- 709.4 Foreign body granuloma of skin and subcutaneous tissue — (Use additional code to identify foreign body (V90.01-V90.9))
- 710.0 Systemic lupus erythematosus — (Use additional code to identify manifestation: 424.91, 581.81, 582.81, 583.81)
- 710.1 Systemic sclerosis — (Use additional code to identify manifestation: 359.6, 517.2)
- 710.2 Sicca syndrome
- 711.04 Pyogenic arthritis, hand — (Use additional code to identify infectious organism: 041.0-041.8)
- 714.0 Rheumatoid arthritis — (Use additional code to identify manifestation: 357.1, 359.6)
- 714.30 Polyarticular juvenile rheumatoid arthritis, chronic or unspecified
- 714.31 Polyarticular juvenile rheumatoid arthritis, acute
- 714.9 Unspecified inflammatory polyarthropathy
- 716.04 Kaschin-Beck disease, hand
- 716.14 Traumatic arthropathy, hand
- 716.64 Unspecified monoarthritis, hand
- 718.74 Developmental dislocation of joint, hand
- 719.24 Villonodular synovitis, hand
- 727.00 Unspecified synovitis and tenosynovitis
- 727.01 Synovitis and tenosynovitis in diseases classified elsewhere — (Code first underlying disease: 015.0-015.9)
- 727.05 Other tenosynovitis of hand and wrist
- 728.0 Infective myositis
- 728.82 Foreign body granuloma of muscle — (Use additional code to identify foreign body (V90.01-V90.9))
- 729.4 Unspecified fasciitis
- 729.6 Residual foreign body in soft tissue — (Use additional code to identify foreign body (V90.01-V90.9))
- 730.04 Acute osteomyelitis, hand — (Use additional code to identify organism: 041.1. Use additional code to identify major osseous defect, if applicable: 731.3)
- 730.14 Chronic osteomyelitis, hand — (Use additional code to identify organism: 041.1. Use additional code to identify major osseous defect, if applicable: 731.3)
- 730.24 Unspecified osteomyelitis, hand — (Use additional code to identify organism: 041.1. Use additional code to identify major osseous defect, if applicable: 731.3)
- 730.34 Periostitis, without mention of osteomyelitis, hand — (Use additional code to identify organism: 041.1)
- 730.84 Other infections involving diseases classified elsewhere, hand bone — (Use additional code to identify organism: 041.1. Code first underlying disease: 002.0, 015.0-015.9)
- 882.1 Open wound of hand except finger(s) alone, complicated
- 883.1 Open wound of finger(s), complicated

CCI Version 16.3

0213T, 0216T, 0228T, 0230T, 26340, 36000, 36400-36410, 36420-36430, 36440, 36600, 36640, 37202, 43752, 51701-51703, 62310-62319, 64400-64435, 64445-64450, 64479, 64483, 64490, 64493, 64505-64530, 69990, 76000-76001, 93000-93010, 93040-93042, 93318, 94002, 94200, 94250, 94680-94690, 94770, 95812-95816, 95819, 95822, 95829, 95955, 96360, 96365, 96372, 96374-96376, 99148-99149, 99150

Note: These CCI edits are used for Medicare. Other payers may reimburse on codes listed above.

Medicare Edits

	Fac RVU	Non-Fac RVU	FUD	Assist
29900	13.15	13.15	90	80

Medicare References: 100-2,15,260; 100-3,100.2; 100-4,12,30; 100-4,12,90.3; 100-4,14,10

29901

29901 Arthroscopy, metacarpophalangeal joint, surgical; with debridement

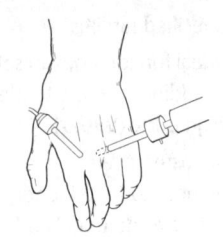

The metacarpophalangeal joint is scoped and debris is removed

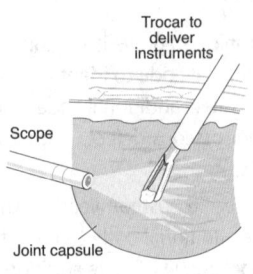

Trocar to deliver instruments

Scope

Joint capsule

Schematic of removal of debris from the MP joint

Explanation
The metacarpophalangeal joints consist of the convex heads of the metacarpals articulating with the concave bases of the proximal phalanges. The metacarpophalangeal joint of interest is placed for easy access and an injection of local anesthetic is administered. Incisions for portals are made in the respective metacarpal to allow the arthroscope and surgical instruments to be introduced into the joint. The arthroscope is inserted through a portal into the joint, and the surgical equipment is passed through a second portal. A third portal may have been made for pumping fluid in to expand the joint space for clearer visualization. Arthroscopic debridement is carried out over the surface of the lesion. The physician must avoid debridement of the adjacent joint surface, so as to avoid possible ankylosis. Closure of the wound includes a re-approximation of the attachment of adductor tendon to the dorsal extensor hood.

Coding Tips
When 29901 is performed with another separately identifiable procedure, the highest dollar value code is listed as the primary procedure and subsequent procedures are appended with modifier 51. Local anesthesia is included in this service. When arthroscopy is performed in conjunction with arthrotomy, add modifier 51. Surgical arthroscopy always includes diagnostic arthroscopy. Some payers may require the use of HCPCS Level II modifiers FA–F9 to identify the specific finger involved.

ICD-9-CM Procedural
80.84 Other local excision or destruction of lesion of joint of hand and finger

Anesthesia
29901 01830

ICD-9-CM Diagnostic
682.4 Cellulitis and abscess of hand, except fingers and thumb — (Use additional code to identify organism, such as 041.1, etc.)
709.4 Foreign body granuloma of skin and subcutaneous tissue — (Use additional code to identify foreign body (V90.01-V90.9))
711.04 Pyogenic arthritis, hand — (Use additional code to identify infectious organism: 041.0-041.8)
728.0 Infective myositis
728.82 Foreign body granuloma of muscle — (Use additional code to identify foreign body (V90.01-V90.9))
729.4 Unspecified fasciitis
729.6 Residual foreign body in soft tissue — (Use additional code to identify foreign body (V90.01-V90.9))
730.04 Acute osteomyelitis, hand — (Use additional code to identify organism: 041.1. Use additional code to identify major osseous defect, if applicable: 731.3)
730.14 Chronic osteomyelitis, hand — (Use additional code to identify organism: 041.1. Use additional code to identify major osseous defect, if applicable: 731.3)
730.24 Unspecified osteomyelitis, hand — (Use additional code to identify organism: 041.1. Use additional code to identify major osseous defect, if applicable: 731.3)
730.34 Periostitis, without mention of osteomyelitis, hand — (Use additional code to identify organism: 041.1)
730.84 Other infections involving diseases classified elsewhere, hand bone — (Use additional code to identify organism: 041.1. Code first underlying disease: 002.0, 015.0-015.9)
731.3 Major osseous defects — (Code first underlying disease: 170.0-170.9, 730.00-730.29, 733.00-733.09, 733.40-733.49, 996.45)
882.1 Open wound of hand except finger(s) alone, complicated
883.1 Open wound of finger(s), complicated

Terms To Know
ankylosis. Abnormal union or fusion of bones in a joint, which is normally moveable.

osteomyelitis. Inflammation of bone that may remain localized or spread to the marrow, cortex, or periosteum, in response to an infecting organism, usually bacterial and pyogenic.

CCI Version 16.3
0213T, 0216T, 0228T, 0230T, 26340, 29900, 36000, 36400-36410, 36420-36430, 36440, 36600, 36640, 37202, 43752, 51701-51703, 62310-62319, 64400-64435, 64445-64450, 64479, 64483, 64490, 64493, 64505-64530, 69990, 76000-76001, 93000-93010, 93040-93042, 93318, 94002, 94200, 94250, 94680-94690, 94770, 95812-95816, 95819, 95822, 95829, 95955, 96360, 96365, 96372, 96374-96376, 99148-99149, 99150

Note: These CCI edits are used for Medicare. Other payers may reimburse on codes listed above.

Medicare Edits

	Fac RVU	Non-Fac RVU	FUD	Assist
29901	15.08	15.08	90	80

Medicare References: 100-2,15,260; 100-3,100.2; 100-4,12,30; 100-4,12,90.3; 100-4,14,10

29902

29902 Arthroscopy, metacarpophalangeal joint, surgical; with reduction of displaced ulnar collateral ligament (eg, Stenar lesion)

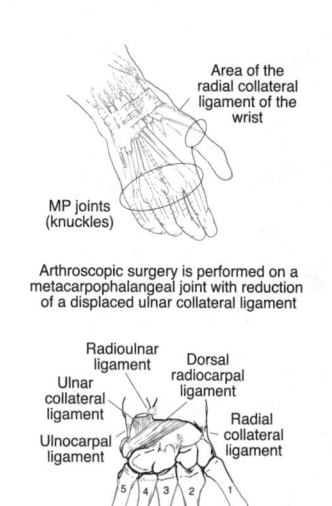

Explanation

The physician makes an incision along the midlateral aspect of the thumb, curves the incision over the MP joint, and extends the incision to the EPL tendon. The Stener lesion can be seen as a mass of tissue proximal to the adductor aponeurosis. A Stener lesion occurs when a torn distal edge of ulnar collateral ligament displaces superficially and proximally to the adductor aponeurosis. The ruptured end of ligament is no longer in contact with its area of insertion of the phalanx. A longitudinal incision is made through the aponeurosis volar to the edge of the EPL, leaving a rim of tissue on the tendon to be used for later closure. The adductor tendon is retracted volarly and the dorsal capsule is reflected to permit a clear view of the joint and the inside portion of the collateral ligament. The physician assesses the injury (i.e., ligament rupture at the insertion into the phalanx). The ulnar collateral ligament flap is partially dissected and mobilized off the metacarpal and the volar edge of the proximal phalange is debrided of soft tissue. The physician drills two parallel holes distally and dorsally to exit on the far side of the cortex. Sutures are passed through the distal ligament and pulled through the drill holes and tied over a padded button. Closure of the wound includes a re-approximation of the attachment of adductor tendon to the dorsal extensor hood.

Coding Tips

When 29002 is performed with another separately identifiable procedure, the highest dollar value code is listed as the primary procedure and subsequent procedures are appended with modifier 51. When arthroscopy is performed in conjunction with arthrotomy, add modifier 51. Surgical arthroscopy always includes diagnostic arthroscopy. Some payers may require the use of HCPCS Level II modifiers FA–F9 to identify the specific finger involved.

ICD-9-CM Procedural

81.96 Other repair of joint

Anesthesia

29902 01830

ICD-9-CM Diagnostic

815.01 Closed fracture of base of thumb (first) metacarpal bone(s)
815.11 Open fracture of base of thumb (first) metacarpal bone(s)
834.01 Closed dislocation of metacarpophalangeal (joint)
834.11 Open dislocation of metacarpophalangeal (joint)
841.1 Ulnar collateral ligament sprain and strain
842.12 Sprain and strain of metacarpophalangeal (joint) of hand
883.2 Open wound of finger(s), with tendon involvement
927.20 Crushing injury of hand(s) — (Use additional code to identify any associated injuries: 800-829, 850.0-854.1, 860.0-869.1)
927.3 Crushing injury of finger(s) — (Use additional code to identify any associated injuries: 800-829, 850.0-854.1, 860.0-869.1)

Terms To Know

dorsal. Pertaining to the back or posterior aspect.

extensor. Any muscle that extends a joint.

ligament. Band or sheet of fibrous tissue that connects the articular surfaces of bones or supports visceral organs.

volar. Palm of the hand (palmar) or sole of the foot (plantar).

CCI Version 16.3

0213T, 0216T, 0228T, 0230T, 26340, 29900, 36000, 36400-36410, 36420-36430, 36440, 36600, 36640, 37202, 43752, 51701-51703, 62310-62319, 64400-64435, 64445-64450, 64479, 64483, 64490, 64493, 64505-64530, 69990, 76000-76001, 93000-93010, 93040-93042, 93318, 94002, 94200, 94250, 94680-94690, 94770, 95812-95816, 95819, 95822, 95829, 95955, 96360, 96365, 96372, 96374-96376, 99148-99149, 99150

Note: These CCI edits are used for Medicare. Other payers may reimburse on codes listed above.

Medicare Edits

	Fac RVU	Non-Fac RVU	FUD	Assist
29902	16.0	16.0	90	80

Medicare References: 100-2,15,260; 100-3,100.2; 100-4,12,30; 100-4,12,90.3; 100-4,14,10

38220

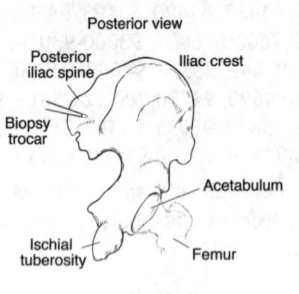

38220 Bone marrow; aspiration only

Posterior view
Posterior iliac spine
Iliac crest
Biopsy trocar
Acetabulum
Ischial tuberosity
Femur

Collection is frequently performed on the posterior iliac spine

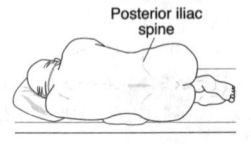

Posterior iliac spine

Bone marrow is aspirated

Explanation

Bone marrow samples are usually taken from the pelvic bone or sternum. The skin over the bone is first cleaned with an antiseptic solution. A local anesthetic is injected and the physician inserts a needle, known as a University of Illinois needle, beneath the skin and rotates it until the needle penetrates the cortex. At least half a teaspoon of marrow is sucked out of the bone by a syringe attached to the needle. If more marrow is needed, the needle is repositioned slightly, a new syringe is attached, and a second sample is taken. The samples are transferred from the syringes to slides and sent to a laboratory for analysis.

Coding Tips

For interpretation of bone marrow smear, see 85097. For special stains, report 88312, or 88313.

ICD-9-CM Procedural

41.31 Biopsy of bone marrow

Anesthesia

38220 01112

ICD-9-CM Diagnostic

The application of this code is too broad to adequately present ICD-9-CM diagnostic code links here. Refer to your ICD-9-CM book.

Terms To Know

aspiration. Drawing fluid out by suction.

bone marrow. Soft tissue found filling the cavities of bones. Red bone marrow is a hematopoietic tissue that manufactures various cellular components of blood, such as platelets and red and white blood cells. Yellow marrow consists mostly of fat cells and is found in the medullary cavities of large bones. It may be harvested and transplanted for its progenitor or stem cells in cases of leukemia and other diseases biopsied to help diagnose many diseases of the blood.

CCI Version 16.3

01112, 01120, 0213T, 0216T, 36000, 36410, 37202, 62318-62319, 64415-64417, 64450, 64490, 64493, 80500-80502, 96360, 96365, 96372, 96374-96376, G0364✦, J0670, J2001

Note: These CCI edits are used for Medicare. Other payers may reimburse on codes listed above.

Medicare Edits

	Fac RVU	Non-Fac RVU	FUD	Assist
38220	1.81	4.47	N/A	80

Medicare References: 100-1,5,90.2; 100-2,15,80; 100-4,12,30

38221

38221 Bone marrow; biopsy, needle or trocar

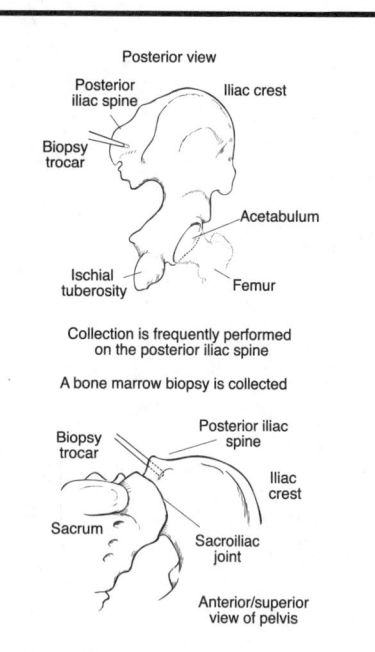

Explanation

Bone marrow samples are usually taken from the pelvic bone or sternum. The skin over the bone is first cleaned with an antiseptic solution. A local anesthetic is injected and the needle is inserted, rotated to the right, then to the left, withdrawn, and reinserted at a different angle. This procedure is repeated until a small chip is separated from the bone marrow. The needle is again removed, and a piece of fine wire threaded through its tip transfers the specimen onto sterile gauze. Samples contain bone marrow of which the structure has not been disturbed or destroyed. The bone must be decalcified overnight before it can be properly stained and examined.

Coding Tips

For bone marrow biopsy interpretation, see 88305.

ICD-9-CM Procedural

41.31 Biopsy of bone marrow

Anesthesia

38221 01112

ICD-9-CM Diagnostic

The application of this code is too broad to adequately present ICD-9-CM diagnostic code links here. Refer to your ICD-9-CM book.

Terms To Know

biopsy. Tissue or fluid removed for diagnostic purposes through analysis of the cells in the biopsy material.

bone marrow. Soft tissue found filling the cavities of bones. Red bone marrow is a hematopoietic tissue that manufactures various cellular components of blood, such as platelets and red and white blood cells. Yellow marrow consists mostly of fat cells and is found in the medullary cavities of large bones. It may be harvested and transplanted for its progenitor or stem cells in cases of leukemia and other diseases biopsied to help diagnose many diseases of the blood.

trocar. Cannula or a sharp pointed instrument used to puncture and aspirate fluid from cavities.

CCI Version 16.3

01112, 01120, 0213T, 0216T, 20220, 36000, 36410, 37202, 38220, 62318-62319, 64415-64417, 64450, 64490, 64493, 80500-80502, 96360, 96365, 96372, 96374-96376, J0670, J2001

Note: These CCI edits are used for Medicare. Other payers may reimburse on codes listed above.

Medicare Edits

	Fac RVU	Non-Fac RVU	FUD	Assist
38221	2.23	4.82	N/A	80

Medicare References: 100-1,5,90.2; 100-2,15,80; 100-4,12,30

38500-38505

38500 Biopsy or excision of lymph node(s); open, superficial
38505 by needle, superficial (eg, cervical, inguinal, axillary)

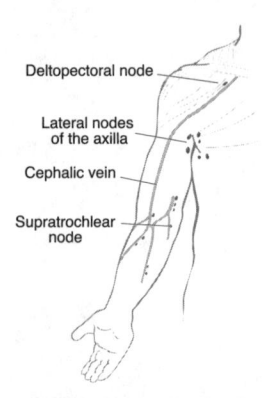

Select superficial lymph nodes of the upper extremity

An incisional biopsy or excision of a superficial lymph node of the upper extremity, or elsewhere, is performed. Report 38505 for superficial lymph node biopsy by needle

Explanation

The physician performs an excisional (38500) or percutaneous (38505) needle biopsy on one or more superficial lymph nodes. When an excisional biopsy is performed, the physician makes a small incision through the skin overlying the lymph node. The tissue is dissected to the node. A small piece of the node and surrounding tissue are removed or the entire node may be removed. The incision is repaired with layered closure. When a percutaneous needle biopsy is performed, the physician may locate the node by palpation. A biopsy needle is inserted percutaneously through the skin over the site of the suspicious node and advanced to the node. The node is entered and a biopsy is taken and the needle is withdrawn. A band-aid or a small gauze dressing is applied to the puncture site.

Coding Tips

Local anesthesia is included in these services. If specimen is transported to an outside laboratory, report 99000 for handling or conveyance. Surgical trays, A4550, are not separately reimbursed by Medicare; however, other third-party payers may cover them. Check with the specific payer to determine coverage.

ICD-9-CM Procedural

40.11 Biopsy of lymphatic structure
40.23 Excision of axillary lymph node
40.24 Excision of inguinal lymph node
40.29 Simple excision of other lymphatic structure

Anesthesia

38500 00320, 00400, 01610
38505 N/A

ICD-9-CM Diagnostic

The application of this code is too broad to adequately present ICD-9-CM diagnostic code links here. Refer to your ICD-9-CM book.

Terms To Know

biopsy. Tissue or fluid removed for diagnostic purposes through analysis of the cells in the biopsy material.

dissection. Separating by cutting tissue or body structures apart.

excision. Surgical removal of an organ or tissue.

lymph nodes. Bean-shaped structures along the lymphatic vessels that intercept and destroy foreign materials in the tissue and bloodstream.

percutaneous. Through the skin.

superficial. On the skin surface or near the surface of any involved structure or field of interest.

CCI Version 16.3

0213T, 0216T, 0228T, 0230T, 10021-10022, 36000, 36400-36410, 36420-36430, 36440, 36600, 36640, 37202, 43752, 51701-51703, 62310-62319, 64400-64435, 64445-64450, 64479, 64483, 64490, 64493, 64505-64530, 69990, 93000-93010, 93040-93042, 93318, 94002, 94200, 94250, 94680-94690, 94770, 95812-95816, 95819, 95822, 95829, 95955, 96360, 96365, 96372, 96374-96376, 99148-99149, 99150, J2001

Also not with 38500: 12001-12007, 12020-12047, 13100-13101, 13120-13121, 13131-13132, 38505❖, J0670

Also not with 38505: 77002

Note: These CCI edits are used for Medicare. Other payers may reimburse on codes listed above.

Medicare Edits

	Fac RVU	Non-Fac RVU	FUD	Assist
38500	7.33	9.44	10	N/A
38505	2.15	3.71	0	N/A

Medicare References: 100-2,15,260; 100-4,3,20.2.1; 100-4,12,30; 100-4,12,90.3; 100-4,14,10

62263-62264

62263 Percutaneous lysis of epidural adhesions using solution injection (eg, hypertonic saline, enzyme) or mechanical means (eg, catheter) including radiologic localization (includes contrast when administered), multiple adhesiolysis sessions; 2 or more days

62264 1 day

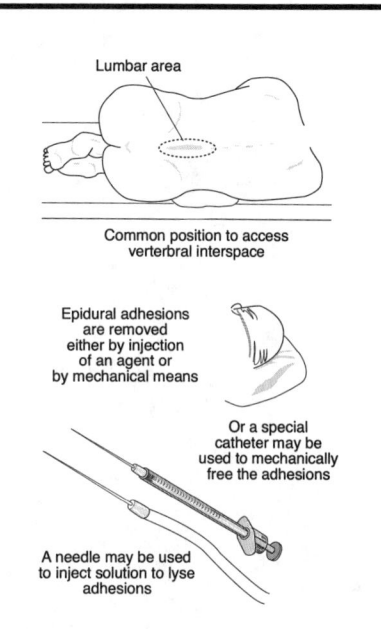

Explanation

Epidural adhesions are lysed percutaneously by an injection, such as hypertonic saline or an enzyme solution, or by mechanical means. The patient is placed in the sitting or lateral decubitus position for insertion of a needle into a vertebral interspace. The site to be entered is sterilized, local anesthesia is administered, and the needle is inserted. Contrast media with fluoroscopy may be injected to confirm proper needle placement and to identify epidural adhesions. The physician injects the adhesiolytic solution or performs mechanical adhesion destruction, such as with a catheter, to lyse epidural adhesions. With the procedure completed, the needle and/or catheter is removed and the wound is dressed. Report 62263 for multiple adhesiolysis sessions on two or more days and 62264 for multiple adhesiolysis sessions occurring only on one day.

Coding Tips

Injection of contrast for epidurography (72275) and fluoroscopic guidance and localization (77003) are included in 62263 and 62264 and should not be reported separately. Percutaneous lysis of epidural adhesions includes insertion and removal of the epidural catheter. Both 62263 and 62264 include lysis of scarring or adhesions performed mechanically using the percutaneously deployed catheter. Code 62263 refers to injections in a series occurring over two or more days and should be reported only once per series. Do not report 62264 with 62263. For endoscopic lysis of epidural adhesions, see 64999.

ICD-9-CM Procedural

- 03.6 Lysis of adhesions of spinal cord and nerve roots
- 03.90 Insertion of catheter into spinal canal for infusion of therapeutic or palliative substances
- 03.91 Injection of anesthetic into spinal canal for analgesia
- 03.92 Injection of other agent into spinal canal
- 03.96 Percutaneous denervation of facet
- 86.09 Other incision of skin and subcutaneous tissue

Anesthesia

N/A

ICD-9-CM Diagnostic

- 349.2 Disorders of meninges, not elsewhere classified
- 742.59 Other specified congenital anomaly of spinal cord

Terms To Know

adhesion. Abnormal fibrous connection between two structures, soft tissue or bony structures, that may occur as the result of surgery, infection, or trauma.

anomaly. Irregularity in the structure or position of an organ or tissue.

congenital. Present at birth, occurring through heredity or an influence during gestation up to the moment of birth.

subcutaneous tissue. Sheet or wide band of adipose (fat) and areolar connective tissue in two layers attached to the dermis.

CCI Version 16.3

00600-00604, 00620, 00625-00626, 00630, 00670, 01935-01936, 0230T, 36000, 36400-36410, 36420-36430, 36440, 36600, 36640, 37202, 43752, 51701-51703, 62282-62284, 62311, 62319, 64400-64435, 64445-64450, 64483, 64505-64530, 64722, 69990, 72265, 72275, 76000-76001, 77002-77003, 93000-93010, 93040-93042, 93318, 94002, 94200, 94250, 94680-94690, 94770, 95812-95816, 95819, 95822, 95829, 95955, 96360, 96365, 96372, 96374-96376, 99148-99149, 99150

Also not with 62263: 62264, J2001

Note: These CCI edits are used for Medicare. Other payers may reimburse on codes listed above.

Medicare Edits

	Fac RVU	Non-Fac RVU	FUD	Assist
62263	11.78	20.91	10	N/A
62264	6.84	12.17	10	N/A

Medicare References: 100-2,15,260; 100-4,12,30; 100-4,12,90.3; 100-4,14,10

62267

62267 Percutaneous aspiration within the nucleus pulposus, intervertebral disc, or paravertebral tissue for diagnostic purposes

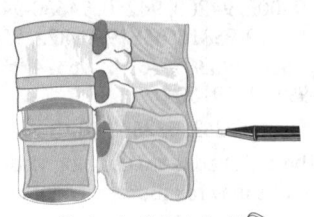

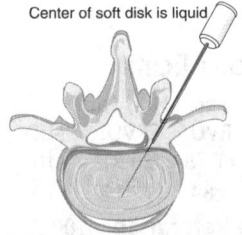

Explanation
The physician removes contents within the intervertebral disc, nucleus pulposus, or paravertebral tissue with a needle for diagnostic purposes. Separately reportable computed tomography or fluoroscopic guidance verifies placement of the needle. A spinal needle is inserted, the contents of the targeted location are aspirated, and the needle is removed. The wound is dressed. If this procedure is performed under fluoroscopic guidance, injection of the contrast is an inclusive component and is not reported separately.

Coding Tips
For imaging guidance of needle placement, see 77003. Do not report 62267 with 1022, 20225, 62287, 62290 or 62291.

ICD-9-CM Procedural
03.39 Other diagnostic procedures on spinal cord and spinal canal structures

Anesthesia
62267 01935

ICD-9-CM Diagnostic
- 192.2 Malignant neoplasm of spinal cord
- 192.8 Malignant neoplasm of other specified sites of nervous system
- 198.3 Secondary malignant neoplasm of brain and spinal cord
- 198.4 Secondary malignant neoplasm of other parts of nervous system
- 225.3 Benign neoplasm of spinal cord
- 225.8 Benign neoplasm of other specified sites of nervous system
- 237.5 Neoplasm of uncertain behavior of brain and spinal cord
- 237.9 Neoplasm of uncertain behavior of other and unspecified parts of nervous system
- 324.1 Intraspinal abscess
- 336.0 Syringomyelia and syringobulbia
- 340 Multiple sclerosis

Terms To Know
intervertebral disc. Fibrocartilaginous cushion found between the vertebral bodies of the spine and composed of the annulus fibrosus, or the outer fibrous ring, surrounding a soft, central elastic area called the nucleus pulposus.

nucleus pulposus. Semi-gelatinous mass of fine white and elastic fibers forming the central portion of the intervertebral disk, contained within the annulus fibrosus, preventing it from protruding out of the disk space.

syringomyelia. Progressive condition that may be from developmental origin or caused by trauma, tumor, hemorrhage, or infarction. An abnormal cavity (syrinx) forms in the spinal cord and enlarges over time, resulting in symptoms of muscle weakness; stiffness in the back, shoulders, arms, or legs; atrophy; headaches; dissociated memory loss; loss of sensory ability to feel pain; and extremes of hot or cold temperatures.

CCI Version 16.3
01935-01936, 0213T, 0216T, 0228T, 0230T, 10021-10022, 20220-20225, 20240-20245, 20250-20251, 36000, 36410, 37202, 51701-51703, 62291, 62311-62319, 64415-64417, 64450, 64479, 64483, 64490, 64493, 69990, 76000-76001, 77002, 96360, 96365, 96372, 96374-96376, 99148-99149, 99150

Note: These CCI edits are used for Medicare. Other payers may reimburse on codes listed above.

Medicare Edits

	Fac RVU	Non-Fac RVU	FUD	Assist
62267	4.69	7.28	0	80

Medicare References: None

62270

62270 Spinal puncture, lumbar, diagnostic

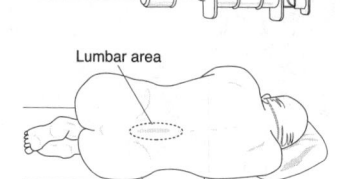

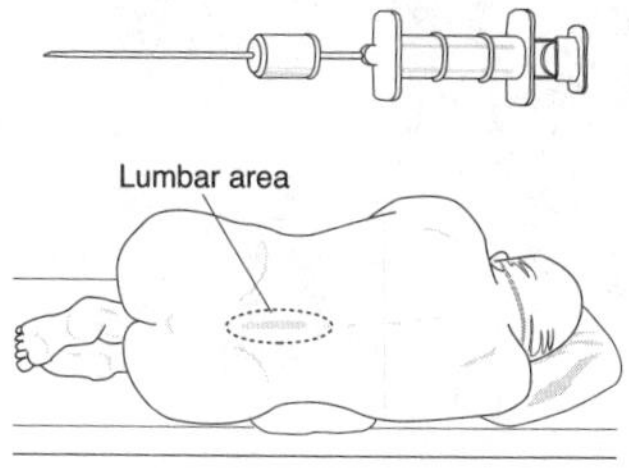

Spinal fluid is drained from the lumbar area for diagnostic purposes

Lumbar area

Spinal tap position

Explanation

The patient is placed in a spinal tap position. The biopsy needle is inserted. Fluid is drawn through the needle for separately reportable testing. When the procedure is complete, the needle is removed and the wound is dressed.

Coding Tips

Injection of contrast is included in 62270 and should not be reported separately. For fluoroscopic guidance and localization, see 77003.

ICD-9-CM Procedural

03.31 Spinal tap

Anesthesia

62270 00635

ICD-9-CM Diagnostic

- 170.2 Malignant neoplasm of vertebral column, excluding sacrum and coccyx
- 192.2 Malignant neoplasm of spinal cord
- 192.3 Malignant neoplasm of spinal meninges
- 198.3 Secondary malignant neoplasm of brain and spinal cord
- 198.4 Secondary malignant neoplasm of other parts of nervous system
- 198.5 Secondary malignant neoplasm of bone and bone marrow
- 199.0 Disseminated malignant neoplasm
- 225.3 Benign neoplasm of spinal cord
- 225.4 Benign neoplasm of spinal meninges
- 320.0 Hemophilus meningitis
- 320.1 Pneumococcal meningitis
- 320.2 Streptococcal meningitis
- 320.3 Staphylococcal meningitis
- 320.7 Meningitis in other bacterial diseases classified elsewhere — (Code first underlying disease: 002.0, 027.0, 033.0-033.9, 039.8)
- 320.81 Anaerobic meningitis
- 320.82 Meningitis due to gram-negative bacteria, not elsewhere classified
- 320.89 Meningitis due to other specified bacteria
- 321.0 Cryptococcal meningitis — (Code first underlying disease: 117.5)
- 321.1 Meningitis in other fungal diseases — (Code first underlying disease: 110.0-118)
- 321.2 Meningitis due to viruses not elsewhere classified — (Code first underlying disease: 060.0-066.9)
- 321.3 Meningitis due to trypanosomiasis — (Code first underlying disease: 086.0-086.9)
- 321.4 Meningitis in sarcoidosis — (Code first underlying disease: 135)
- 321.8 Meningitis due to other nonbacterial organisms classified elsewhere — (Code first underlying disease)
- 322.0 Nonpyogenic meningitis
- 322.1 Eosinophilic meningitis
- 322.2 Chronic meningitis
- 323.01 Encephalitis and encephalomyelitis in viral diseases classified elsewhere — (Code first underlying disease: 073.7, 075, 078.3)
- 323.1 Encephalitis, myelitis, and encephalomyelitis in rickettsial diseases classified elsewhere — (Code first underlying disease: 080-083.9)
- 323.2 Encephalitis, myelitis, and encephalomyelitis in protozoal diseases classified elsewhere — (Code first underlying disease: 084.0-084.9, 086.0-086.9)
- 323.41 Other encephalitis and encephalomyelitis due to infection classified elsewhere — (Code first underlying disease)
- 323.63 Postinfectious myelitis — (Code first underlying disease)
- 324.0 Intracranial abscess
- 324.1 Intraspinal abscess
- 334.1 Hereditary spastic paraplegia
- 334.8 Other spinocerebellar diseases
- 335.10 Unspecified spinal muscular atrophy
- 335.19 Other spinal muscular atrophy
- 335.20 Amyotrophic lateral sclerosis
- 335.21 Progressive muscular atrophy
- 335.24 Primary lateral sclerosis
- 336.2 Subacute combined degeneration of spinal cord in diseases classified elsewhere — (Code first underlying disease: 266.2, 281.0, 281.1)
- 336.3 Myelopathy in other diseases classified elsewhere — (Code first underlying disease: 140.0-239.9)
- 336.8 Other myelopathy — (Use additional E code to identify cause)
- 340   Multiple sclerosis
- 341.8 Other demyelinating diseases of central nervous system
- 344.30 Monoplegia of lower limb affecting unspecified side
- 344.31 Monoplegia of lower limb affecting dominant side
- 344.32 Monoplegia of lower limb affecting nondominant side
- 724.2 Lumbago
- 724.5 Unspecified backache

CCI Version 16.3

00635, 01935-01936, 0213T, 0216T, 0228T, 0230T, 36000, 36400-36410, 36420-36430, 36440, 36600, 36640, 37202, 43752, 51701-51703, 62273, 62310-62311, 64400-64435, 64445-64450, 64479, 64483, 64490, 64493, 64505-64530, 69990, 76000-76001, 77002, 93000-93010, 93040-93042, 93318, 94002, 94200, 94250, 94680-94690, 94770, 95812-95816, 95819, 95822, 95829, 95955, 96360, 96365, 96372, 96374-96376, 99148-99149, 99150

Note: These CCI edits are used for Medicare. Other payers may reimburse on codes listed above.

Medicare Edits

	Fac RVU	Non-Fac RVU	FUD	Assist
62270	2.32	4.58	0	N/A

Medicare References: 100-2,15,260; 100-4,12,30; 100-4,12,90.3; 100-4,14,10

62273

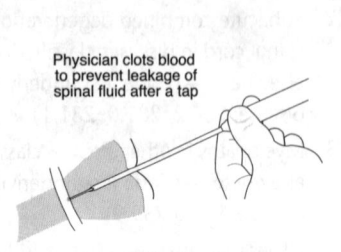

62273 Injection, epidural, of blood or clot patch

Physician clots blood to prevent leakage of spinal fluid after a tap

Lateral cutaway schematic

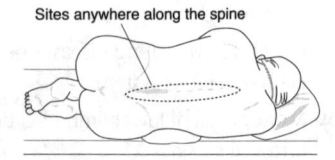

Sites anywhere along the spine

Explanation

This procedure is performed following a lumbar puncture to prevent spinal fluid leakage. The patient remains in a spinal tap position. The patient's blood is injected outside the dura to clot and plug the wound, preventing spinal fluid leakage. The wound is dressed and monitored.

Coding Tips

Injection of contrast is included in 62273 and should not be reported separately. For fluoroscopic guidance and localization, see 77003. For injection of a diagnostic or therapeutic substance, see 62310, 62311, 62318, and 62319.

ICD-9-CM Procedural

03.95 Spinal blood patch

Anesthesia

62273 N/A

ICD-9-CM Diagnostic

349.0 Reaction to spinal or lumbar puncture
784.0 Headache
997.09 Other nervous system complications — (Use additional code to identify complications)

Terms To Know

dura mater. Outermost, hard, fibrous layer or membrane that surrounds the brain and spinal cord.

epidural. Anesthesia commonly used during labor and delivery achieved by the injection of anesthetic agent between the vertebral spines into the extradural space.

CCI Version 16.3

01935-01936, 0213T, 0216T, 0228T, 0230T, 36000, 36140, 36400-36410, 36420-36430, 36440, 36600, 36640, 37202, 43752, 51701-51703, 62310-62311, 64400-64435, 64445-64450, 64479, 64483, 64490, 64493, 64505-64530, 69990, 76000-76001, 77002, 93000-93010, 93040-93042, 93318, 94002, 94200, 94250, 94680-94690, 94770, 95812-95816, 95819, 95822, 95829, 95955, 96360, 96365, 96372, 96374-96376, 99148-99149, 99150, J0670, J2001

Note: These CCI edits are used for Medicare. Other payers may reimburse on codes listed above.

Medicare Edits

	Fac RVU	Non-Fac RVU	FUD	Assist
62273	3.28	4.94	0	N/A

Medicare References: 100-2,15,260; 100-3,10.5; 100-4,12,30; 100-4,12,90.3; 100-4,14,10

62284

62284 Injection procedure for myelography and/or computed tomography, spinal (other than C1-C2 and posterior fossa)

Physician injects contrast material into spine

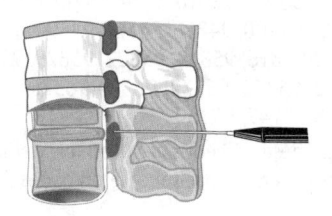

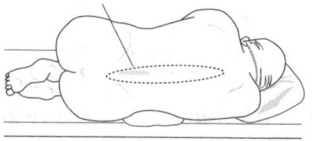

Sites other than cervical

Lateral cutaway view

Explanation
The physician injects dye into the epidural or intrathecal space for myelography and/or computed tomography (CT scan), reported separately. The patient is placed in a spinal tap position. The site is sterilized and the needle is inserted. The needle is placed to the proper level and the dye is administered. The needle is removed and the wound dressed.

Coding Tips
For an injection procedure at C1-C2, see 61055. For radiological supervision and interpretation, see 72240, 72255, 72265, and 72270. Surgical trays, A4550, are not separately reimbursed by Medicare; however, other third-party payers may cover them. Check with the specific payer to determine coverage.

ICD-9-CM Procedural
- 03.92 Injection of other agent into spinal canal
- 87.21 Contrast myelogram
- 88.38 Other computerized axial tomography

Anesthesia
62284 01935

ICD-9-CM Diagnostic
- 170.2 Malignant neoplasm of vertebral column, excluding sacrum and coccyx
- 192.2 Malignant neoplasm of spinal cord
- 192.3 Malignant neoplasm of spinal meninges
- 198.3 Secondary malignant neoplasm of brain and spinal cord
- 198.5 Secondary malignant neoplasm of bone and bone marrow
- 209.73 Secondary neuroendocrine tumor of bone
- 213.2 Benign neoplasm of vertebral column, excluding sacrum and coccyx
- 225.3 Benign neoplasm of spinal cord
- 225.4 Benign neoplasm of spinal meninges
- 237.70 Neurofibromatosis, unspecified
- 237.71 Neurofibromatosis, Type 1 (von Recklinghausen's disease)
- 237.72 Neurofibromatosis, Type 2 (acoustic neurofibromatosis)
- 237.73 Schwannomatosis
- 237.79 Other neurofibromatosis
- 324.1 Intraspinal abscess
- 344.1 Paraplegia
- 353.1 Lumbosacral plexus lesions
- 359.1 Hereditary progressive muscular dystrophy
- 721.0 Cervical spondylosis without myelopathy
- 721.1 Cervical spondylosis with myelopathy
- 721.2 Thoracic spondylosis without myelopathy
- 721.3 Lumbosacral spondylosis without myelopathy
- 721.41 Spondylosis with myelopathy, thoracic region
- 721.42 Spondylosis with myelopathy, lumbar region
- 721.5 Kissing spine
- 721.6 Ankylosing vertebral hyperostosis
- 721.7 Traumatic spondylopathy
- 722.0 Displacement of cervical intervertebral disc without myelopathy
- 722.10 Displacement of lumbar intervertebral disc without myelopathy
- 722.11 Displacement of thoracic intervertebral disc without myelopathy
- 722.4 Degeneration of cervical intervertebral disc
- 722.51 Degeneration of thoracic or thoracolumbar intervertebral disc
- 722.52 Degeneration of lumbar or lumbosacral intervertebral disc
- 722.71 Intervertebral cervical disc disorder with myelopathy, cervical region
- 722.72 Intervertebral thoracic disc disorder with myelopathy, thoracic region
- 722.73 Intervertebral lumbar disc disorder with myelopathy, lumbar region
- 722.81 Postlaminectomy syndrome, cervical region
- 722.82 Postlaminectomy syndrome, thoracic region
- 722.83 Postlaminectomy syndrome, lumbar region
- 723.0 Spinal stenosis in cervical region
- 724.02 Spinal stenosis of lumbar region, without neurogenic claudication
- 724.4 Thoracic or lumbosacral neuritis or radiculitis, unspecified
- 733.13 Pathologic fracture of vertebrae
- 738.4 Acquired spondylolisthesis
- 756.11 Congenital spondylolysis, lumbosacral region
- 756.12 Congenital spondylolisthesis
- 756.14 Hemivertebra
- 756.15 Congenital fusion of spine (vertebra)

CCI Version 16.3
01935-01936, 0213T, 0216T, 0228T, 0230T, 36000, 36400-36410, 36420-36430, 36440, 36600, 36640, 37202, 43752, 51701-51703, 62270-62273, 62282, 64400-64435, 64445-64450, 64479, 64483, 64490, 64493, 64505-64530, 69990, 76000-76001, 77002-77003, 93000-93010, 93040-93042, 93318, 94002, 94200, 94250, 94680-94690, 94770, 95812-95816, 95819, 95822, 95829, 95955, 96360, 96365, 96372, 96374-96376, 99148-99149, 99150

Note: These CCI edits are used for Medicare. Other payers may reimburse on codes listed above.

Medicare Edits

	Fac RVU	Non-Fac RVU	FUD	Assist
62284	2.58	6.3	0	N/A

Medicare References: 100-3,220.1

62287

62287 Decompression procedure, percutaneous, of nucleus pulposus of intervertebral disc, any method, single or multiple levels, lumbar (eg, manual or automated percutaneous discectomy, percutaneous laser discectomy)

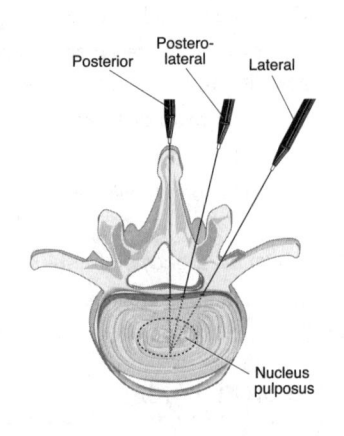

Posterior *Posterolateral* *Lateral*

Nucleus pulposus

Physician aspirates intervertebral disk

Explanation

This decompression procedure corrects a bulge in an intervertebral disc. It is commonly referred to as percutaneous discectomy and may be accomplished by several techniques including nonautomated (manual), automated, or laser. For all techniques, the patient is placed in a spinal tap position on the left side. In a separately reportable procedure, a C-arm x-ray verifies placement of the needle in the disc. Once the disc is located, local anesthesia is injected and a small stab wound is made. A spinal needle is inserted with additional monitoring of placement and injection of anesthesia. Using a manual technique, the physician inserts one or two needles into the disc without puncturing the dura. The patient is placed on pure oxygen, and the nucleus pulposus is suctioned out until the desired decompression is accomplished. The needle(s) are removed, and the wound is dressed. The automated technique makes use of a probe that can simultaneously dissect the disc and suck it into the probe. Laser discectomy accomplishes the decompression by vaporizing the protruding disc.

Coding Tips

Do not report 62287 in conjunction with 62267. For injection of a non-neurolytic diagnostic or therapeutic substance, see 62310 and 62311. For laminotomy with excision of the herniated intervertebral disc, see 63020–63044. For transpedicular approach for posterolateral extradural exploration/decompression of the spinal cord, equina, and/or nerve roots (e.g., herniated intervertebral disc), see 63055–63057. For fluoroscopic guidance, see 77003.

ICD-9-CM Procedural

80.59 Other destruction of intervertebral disc

Anesthesia

62287 01936

ICD-9-CM Diagnostic

722.10 Displacement of lumbar intervertebral disc without myelopathy
722.73 Intervertebral lumbar disc disorder with myelopathy, lumbar region
722.93 Other and unspecified disc disorder of lumbar region
724.2 Lumbago
724.4 Thoracic or lumbosacral neuritis or radiculitis, unspecified
724.5 Unspecified backache

Terms To Know

lumbago. Low back pain.

myelopathy. Pathological or functional changes in the spinal cord, often resulting from nonspecific and noninflammatory lesions.

neuritis. Inflammation of a nerve or group of nerves, often manifested by loss of function and reflexes, pain, and numbness or tingling.

posterior. Located in the back part or caudal end of the body.

posterolateral. Located in the back and off to the side.

radiculitis. Pain along an inflamed nerve, with inflammation of the root of the associated spinal nerve.

CCI Version 16.3

01935-01936, 0195T❖, 0216T, 0228T, 0230T, 22224❖, 22558❖, 36000, 36400-36410, 36420-36430, 36440, 36600, 36640, 37202, 43752, 51701-51703, 62267, 62290, 62311, 62319, 63005❖, 63017❖, 63030❖, 63042❖, 63056❖, 64400-64435, 64445-64450, 64479, 64483, 64493, 64505-64530, 69990, 72295, 76000-76001, 77002, 93000-93010, 93040-93042, 93318, 94002, 94200, 94250, 94680-94690, 94770, 95812-95816, 95819, 95822, 95829, 95955, 96360, 96365, 96372, 96374-96376, 99148-99149, 99150

Note: These CCI edits are used for Medicare. Other payers may reimburse on codes listed above.

Medicare Edits

	Fac RVU	Non-Fac RVU	FUD	Assist
62287	16.19	16.19	90	N/A

Medicare References: 100-2,15,260; 100-4,12,30; 100-4,12,90.3; 100-4,14,10

62290-62291

62290 Injection procedure for discography, each level; lumbar
62291 cervical or thoracic

Under radiological guidance, physician injects contrast medium into lumbar disc (62290) or into cervical or thoracic disc (62291)

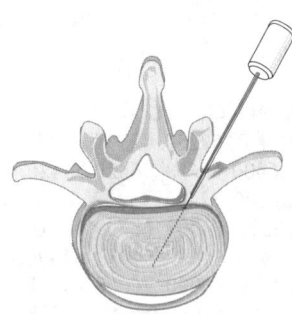

Explanation
This procedure is performed to gauge the amount of damage suffered by an intervertebral disc. The patient is placed on an image intensification table in a left lateral decubitus position with hips and knees are flexed. The injection site is determined and marked on the sterilized surface, and local anesthesia is injected. A small stab wound is made in the tissue overlying the vertebrae. For code 62290, the physician directs a needle at a 45 degree angle to the center line toward the spine. For code 62291, the physician directs a needle at a 35 degree angle to the sagittal plane toward the spine. In a separately reported procedure, the needle is monitored radiographically. A small needle is inserted through original needle once the needle reaches the lamina. The physician pushes this needle to the disc and injects 1 ml to 2 ml of contrast medium. In separately reported procedures, radiographs are made and the procedure may be performed again on another level. The wound is dressed.

Coding Tips
For radiological supervision and interpretation, see 72285 and 72295. Surgical trays, A4550, are not separately reimbursed by Medicare; however, other third-party payers may cover them. Check with the specific payer to determine coverage.

ICD-9-CM Procedural
- 03.92 Injection of other agent into spinal canal
- 87.22 Other x-ray of cervical spine
- 87.24 Other x-ray of lumbosacral spine

Anesthesia
01935

ICD-9-CM Diagnostic
- 719.48 Pain in joint, other specified sites
- 721.0 Cervical spondylosis without myelopathy
- 721.1 Cervical spondylosis with myelopathy
- 721.2 Thoracic spondylosis without myelopathy
- 721.3 Lumbosacral spondylosis without myelopathy
- 721.41 Spondylosis with myelopathy, thoracic region
- 721.42 Spondylosis with myelopathy, lumbar region
- 722.0 Displacement of cervical intervertebral disc without myelopathy
- 722.10 Displacement of lumbar intervertebral disc without myelopathy
- 722.11 Displacement of thoracic intervertebral disc without myelopathy
- 722.31 Schmorl's nodes, thoracic region
- 722.32 Schmorl's nodes, lumbar region
- 722.4 Degeneration of cervical intervertebral disc
- 722.51 Degeneration of thoracic or thoracolumbar intervertebral disc
- 722.52 Degeneration of lumbar or lumbosacral intervertebral disc
- 722.71 Intervertebral cervical disc disorder with myelopathy, cervical region
- 722.72 Intervertebral thoracic disc disorder with myelopathy, thoracic region
- 722.73 Intervertebral lumbar disc disorder with myelopathy, lumbar region
- 722.82 Postlaminectomy syndrome, thoracic region
- 722.83 Postlaminectomy syndrome, lumbar region
- 722.91 Other and unspecified disc disorder of cervical region
- 722.92 Other and unspecified disc disorder of thoracic region
- 722.93 Other and unspecified disc disorder of lumbar region
- 723.1 Cervicalgia
- 723.4 Brachial neuritis or radiculitis nos.
- 724.01 Spinal stenosis of thoracic region
- 724.02 Spinal stenosis of lumbar region, without neurogenic claudication
- 724.1 Pain in thoracic spine
- 724.2 Lumbago
- 724.4 Thoracic or lumbosacral neuritis or radiculitis, unspecified
- 724.5 Unspecified backache
- 724.9 Other unspecified back disorder
- 729.5 Pain in soft tissues of limb
- 756.10 Congenital anomaly of spine, unspecified
- 756.19 Other congenital anomaly of spine

CCI Version 16.3
01935-01936, 0228T, 36000, 36400-36410, 36420-36430, 36440, 36600, 36640, 37202, 43752, 51701-51703, 62310-62319, 64400-64435, 64445-64450, 64479, 64505-64530, 69990, 76000-76001, 76942, 77002-77003, 93000-93010, 93040-93042, 93318, 94002, 94200, 94250, 94680-94690, 94770, 95812-95816, 95819, 95822, 95829, 95955, 96360, 96365, 96372, 96374-96376, 99148-99149, 99150

Also not with 62290: 62267

Also not with 62291: 0213T, 0216T, 0230T, 64483, 64490, 64493

Note: These CCI edits are used for Medicare. Other payers may reimburse on codes listed above.

Medicare Edits

	Fac RVU	Non-Fac RVU	FUD	Assist
62290	5.03	9.79	0	N/A
62291	4.85	9.24	0	N/A

Medicare References: None

63001-63011

63001 Laminectomy with exploration and/or decompression of spinal cord and/or cauda equina, without facetectomy, foraminotomy or discectomy (eg, spinal stenosis), 1 or 2 vertebral segments; cervical
63003 thoracic
63005 lumbar, except for spondylolisthesis
63011 sacral

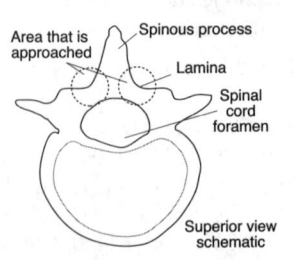

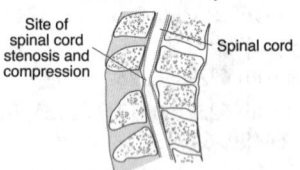

Explanation

The physician makes a posterior midline incision overlying the vertebrae. The paravertebral muscles are retracted. The physician removes the appropriate spinous process and interspinous ligament with a rongeur. The physician excises the lamina and the attached ligamentum flavum may be removed. Decompression is continued by removal of bony overgrowths or tissue until the dural sac and nerve roots are free from any compression. Free-fat grafts or Gelfoam may be placed over the exposed nerve roots. If the ligamentum flavum has not been removed or if only portions of it were removed, it may be closed over the fat graft. A drain is placed superficial to the fat graft; the fascia, subcutaneous tissue, and skin are closed in layers. Report 63003 if vertebrae are thoracic; report 63005 if vertebrae are lumbar, except in the case of spondylolisthesis; and report 63011 if vertebrae are sacral.

Coding Tips

Arthrodesis is reported separately; see 22590-22614. Note that 63001-63011 are used to report the procedure when performed on one or two vertebral segments. For more than two vertebral segments, see 63015-63017. For laminectomy for lumbar spondylolisthesis (Gill type procedure), see 63012. When decompression includes partial excision of the lamina (laminotomy, hemilaminectomy), with partial facetectomy, foraminotomy, and/or excision of the herniated intervertebral disc, see 63020-63035. For re-exploration laminotomy (hemilaminectomy), with partial facetectomy, foraminotomy, and/or excision of the herniated intervertebral disc, see 63040-63044.

ICD-9-CM Procedural

03.09 Other exploration and decompression of spinal canal

Anesthesia

63001 00600, 00604, 00670
63003 00620, 00670
63005 00630, 00670
63011 00630, 00670

ICD-9-CM Diagnostic

344.60 Cauda equina syndrome without mention of neurogenic bladder
721.0 Cervical spondylosis without myelopathy
721.1 Cervical spondylosis with myelopathy
721.2 Thoracic spondylosis without myelopathy
721.3 Lumbosacral spondylosis without myelopathy
721.41 Spondylosis with myelopathy, thoracic region
721.42 Spondylosis with myelopathy, lumbar region
722.0 Displacement of cervical intervertebral disc without myelopathy
722.10 Displacement of lumbar intervertebral disc without myelopathy
722.52 Degeneration of lumbar or lumbosacral intervertebral disc
722.71 Intervertebral cervical disc disorder with myelopathy, cervical region
722.73 Intervertebral lumbar disc disorder with myelopathy, lumbar region
722.83 Postlaminectomy syndrome, lumbar region
723.0 Spinal stenosis in cervical region
724.01 Spinal stenosis of thoracic region
724.02 Spinal stenosis of lumbar region, without neurogenic claudication
724.09 Spinal stenosis, other region other than cervical
738.4 Acquired spondylolisthesis
756.11 Congenital spondylolysis, lumbosacral region
806.4 Closed fracture of lumbar spine with spinal cord injury
806.5 Open fracture of lumbar spine with spinal cord injury
907.2 Late effect of spinal cord injury
952.2 Lumbar spinal cord injury without spinal bone injury
952.3 Sacral spinal cord injury without spinal bone injury
953.3 Injury to sacral nerve root
953.5 Injury to lumbosacral plexus

CCI Version 16.3

0213T, 0216T, 0228T, 0230T, 20926, 22505, 36000, 36400-36410, 36420-36430, 36440, 36600, 36640, 37202, 43752, 51701-51703, 62310-62319, 63707, 63709, 64400-64435, 64445-64450, 64479, 64483, 64490, 64493, 64505-64530, 69990, 76000-76001, 92585, 93000-93010, 93040-93042, 93318, 94002, 94200, 94250, 94680-94690, 94770, 95812-95816, 95819, 95822, 95829, 95860-95861, 95867-95868, 95870, 95900, 95904, 95920, 95925-95934, 95936-95937, 95955, 96360, 96365, 96372, 96374-96376, 99148-99149, 99150

Also not with 63001: 20660, 22100, 62291, 63020, 63030, 72285

Also not with 63003: 20650, 62291, 72285

Also not with 63005: 0171T❖, 0202T, 20660, 22102, 62267❖, 62284, 62290, 63020, 63030, 64722, 64831, 64834-64836, 64840-64858, 64861-64870, 64885-64898, 64905-64907, 72295

Also not with 63011: 20660, 64714

Note: These CCI edits are used for Medicare. Other payers may reimburse on codes listed above.

Medicare Edits

	Fac RVU	Non-Fac RVU	FUD	Assist
63001	36.25	36.25	90	80
63003	36.41	36.41	90	80
63005	34.58	34.58	90	80
63011	31.85	31.85	90	80

Medicare References: None

63012

63012 Laminectomy with removal of abnormal facets and/or pars inter-articularis with decompression of cauda equina and nerve roots for spondylolisthesis, lumbar (Gill type procedure)

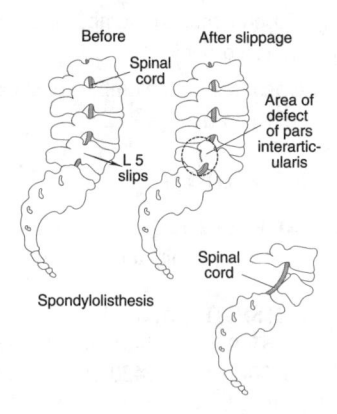

Gill procedure involves removal of spinous processes of L4, L5 and S1; much of the lamina of L5 and sometimes affected discs of L4 and L5; the procedure relieves pain without fusion

Physician corrects spondylolisthesis, or slippage of the bottom lumbar vertebra forward, using the Gill procedure

Explanation

The physician performs the laminectomy to correct spondylolisthesis, the slipping of the lumbar vertebrae forward where they join the sacral vertebrae. The patient is placed prone. The physician makes a midline incision overlying the lumbar vertebrae to facilitate repair of the spondylolisthesis. The fascia are incised and the paravertebral muscles are retracted. The physician resects the spinous processes of all three vertebrae and the middle part of the loose fifth lumbar neural arch. The ligamentum flavum is freed or excised at various levels of vertebrae. The fifth lumbar nerve root is carefully retracted. Decompression is carried out to include the facets as well as other bony or soft tissue structures that may be applying pressure to the spinal cord, nerve roots, or cauda equina. The procedure is then repeated on the opposite side. The incision is closed with layered sutures.

Coding Tips

Arthrodesis is reported separately; see 22590–22614. Report 63012 only when a laminectomy is performed for lumbar spondylolisthesis. For laminectomy one or two vertebral segments for spinal stenosis, lumbar, see 63005. For partial excision of the lamina (laminotomy, hemilaminectomy), with facetectomy, foraminotomy, and/or excision of the herniated intervertebral disc, see 63030–63035. For re-exploration laminotomy (hemilaminectomy), with partial facetectomy, foraminotomy, and/or excision of the herniated intervertebral disc, see 63042. For laminectomy (complete excision of the lamina), unilateral or bilateral, with facetectomy and foraminotomy, see 63047–63048.

ICD-9-CM Procedural

03.09 Other exploration and decompression of spinal canal

Anesthesia
63012 00630, 00670

ICD-9-CM Diagnostic

721.3 Lumbosacral spondylosis without myelopathy
721.42 Spondylosis with myelopathy, lumbar region
724.2 Lumbago
724.4 Thoracic or lumbosacral neuritis or radiculitis, unspecified
724.5 Unspecified backache
738.4 Acquired spondylolisthesis
756.11 Congenital spondylolysis, lumbosacral region
756.12 Congenital spondylolisthesis

Terms To Know

cauda equina. Spinal roots occupying the lower end of the vertebral canal and descending from the distal end of the spinal cord, named for their appearance resembling that of the tail of a horse.

congenital. Present at birth, occurring through heredity or an influence during gestation up to the moment of birth.

neuritis. Inflammation of a nerve or group of nerves, often manifested by loss of function and reflexes, pain, and numbness or tingling.

radiculitis. Pain along an inflamed nerve, with inflammation of the root of the associated spinal nerve.

spondylolisthesis. Forward displacement of one vertebra slipping over another, usually in the fourth or fifth lumbar area.

CCI Version 16.3

0171T❖, 0202T, 0213T, 0216T, 0228T, 0230T, 20660, 20926, 22102, 22505, 36000, 36400-36410, 36420-36430, 36440, 36600, 36640, 37202, 43752, 51701-51703, 62310-62319, 63005❖, 63030, 63042, 63045-63046, 63275, 63707, 63709, 64400-64435, 64445-64450, 64479, 64483, 64490, 64493, 64505-64530, 64714, 64722, 64831, 64834-64836, 64840-64858, 64861-64870, 64885-64898, 64905-64907, 69990, 76000-76001, 92585, 93000-93010, 93040-93042, 93318, 94002, 94200, 94250, 94680-94690, 94770, 95812-95816, 95819, 95822, 95829, 95860-95861, 95867-95868, 95870, 95900, 95904, 95920, 95925-95934, 95936-95937, 95955, 96360, 96365, 96372, 96374-96376, 99148-99149, 99150

Note: These CCI edits are used for Medicare. Other payers may reimburse on codes listed above.

Medicare Edits

	Fac RVU	Non-Fac RVU	FUD	Assist
63012	34.9	34.9	90	80

Medicare References: None

63015-63017

63015 Laminectomy with exploration and/or decompression of spinal cord and/or cauda equina, without facetectomy, foraminotomy or discectomy (eg, spinal stenosis), more than 2 vertebral segments; cervical
63016 thoracic
63017 lumbar

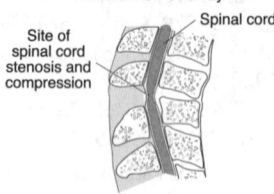

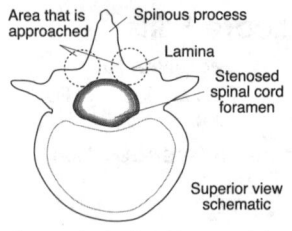

Explanation
The patient is face down and the physician makes a posterior midline incision overlying the vertebrae. The paravertebral muscles are retracted. A rongeur removes the appropriate spinous processes and interspinous ligaments. The physician excises the affected laminae and the attached ligamentum flavum may be removed. Decompression is continued by removal of bony overgrowths or tissue until the dural sac and nerve roots are free from compression. Free-fat grafts or Gelfoam may be placed over the exposed nerve roots. If the ligamentum flavum has not been removed or if only portions of it were removed it may be closed over the fat graft. A drain is placed superficial to the fat graft; the fascia, subcutaneous tissue, and skin are closed in layers. Report 63015 if vertebrae are cervical; report 63016 if the laminae are thoracic; report 63017 if lumbar.

Coding Tips
Arthrodesis is reported separately; see 22590–22614. Note that 63015–63017 report laminectomy with exploration and/or decompression of more than two vertebral segments. For laminectomy of one or two segments, see 63001–63011. For laminectomy for lumbar spondylolisthesis (Gill type procedure), see 63012. For partial excision of the lamina (laminotomy, hemilaminectomy), with partial facetectomy, foraminotomy, and/or excision of the herniated intervertebral disc, see 63020–63035. For re-exploration laminotomy, with partial facetectomy, foraminotomy, and/or excision of the herniated intervertebral disc, see 63040–63044. For laminectomy (complete excision of the lamina), unilateral or bilateral, with facetectomy and foraminotomy, see 63045–63048.

ICD-9-CM Procedural
03.09 Other exploration and decompression of spinal canal

Anesthesia
63015 00600, 00604, 00670
63016 00620, 00670
63017 00630, 00670

ICD-9-CM Diagnostic
721.0 Cervical spondylosis without myelopathy
721.1 Cervical spondylosis with myelopathy
721.2 Thoracic spondylosis without myelopathy
721.3 Lumbosacral spondylosis without myelopathy
722.10 Displacement of lumbar intervertebral disc without myelopathy
722.83 Postlaminectomy syndrome, lumbar region
723.0 Spinal stenosis in cervical region
723.4 Brachial neuritis or radiculitis nos.
723.7 Ossification of posterior longitudinal ligament in cervical region
724.01 Spinal stenosis of thoracic region
724.02 Spinal stenosis of lumbar region, without neurogenic claudication
756.11 Congenital spondylolysis, lumbosacral region
756.12 Congenital spondylolisthesis
756.19 Other congenital anomaly of spine
805.10 Open fracture of cervical vertebra, unspecified level without mention of spinal cord injury
805.2 Closed fracture of dorsal (thoracic) vertebra without mention of spinal cord injury
805.3 Open fracture of dorsal (thoracic) vertebra without mention of spinal cord injury
805.4 Closed fracture of lumbar vertebra without mention of spinal cord injury
805.5 Open fracture of lumbar vertebra without mention of spinal cord injury
806.19 Open fracture of C5-C7 level with other specified spinal cord injury
806.20 Closed fracture of T1-T6 level with unspecified spinal cord injury
806.30 Open fracture of T1-T6 level with unspecified spinal cord injury
806.4 Closed fracture of lumbar spine with spinal cord injury
806.5 Open fracture of lumbar spine with spinal cord injury

Terms To Know
foramina. Passage in the body that is naturally formed, usually through a bone.

CCI Version 16.3
0213T, 0216T, 0228T, 0230T, 20926, 22505, 36000, 36400-36410, 36420-36430, 36440, 36600, 36640, 37202, 43752, 51701-51703, 62310-62319, 63707, 63709, 64400-64435, 64445-64450, 64479, 64483, 64490, 64493, 64505-64530, 69990, 76000-76001, 92585, 93000-93010, 93040-93042, 93318, 94002, 94200, 94250, 94680-94690, 94770, 95812-95816, 95819, 95822, 95829, 95860-95861, 95867-95868, 95870, 95900, 95904, 95920, 95925-95934, 95936-95937, 95955, 96360, 96365, 96372, 96374-96376, 99148-99149, 99150

Also not with 63015: 20660, 62291, 63001, 63020, 63030, 72285

Also not with 63016: 62291, 63003, 72285

Also not with 63017: 0171T❖, 0202T, 62267❖, 62290, 63005, 63012, 63020, 63030, 64712, 64722, 64831, 64834-64836, 64840-64858, 64861-64870, 64885-64898, 64905-64907, 72295

Note: These CCI edits are used for Medicare. Other payers may reimburse on codes listed above.

Medicare Edits

	Fac RVU	Non-Fac RVU	FUD	Assist
63015	43.53	43.53	90	80
63016	44.52	44.52	90	80
63017	36.59	36.59	90	80

Medicare References: None

63020-63035

63020 Laminotomy (hemilaminectomy), with decompression of nerve root(s), including partial facetectomy, foraminotomy and/or excision of herniated intervertebral disc, including open and endoscopically-assisted approaches; 1 interspace, cervical
63030 1 interspace, lumbar
63035 each additional interspace, cervical or lumbar (List separately in addition to code for primary procedure)

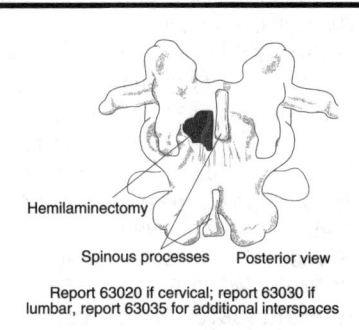

Hemilaminectomy
Spinous processes Posterior view

Report 63020 if cervical; report 63030 if lumbar, report 63035 for additional interspaces

Physician performs hemilaminectomy to decompress specific nerve roots; facets, foramen, and disc may also be removed

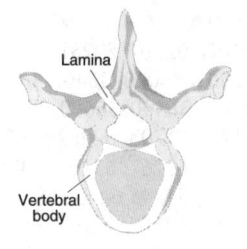

Lamina
Vertebral body

Explanation

In one method, a midline incision is made through a posterior (back) approach overlying the vertebrae. The incision is carried down through the tissue to the paravertebral muscles, which are retracted. The ligamentum flavum, which attaches the lamina from one vertebra to the lamina of another may be partially or completely removed. Part of the lamina is removed on one side to allow access to the spinal cord. If a disc has ruptured, fragments or the part of the disc compressing the nerves are removed. A partial removal of a facet (facetectomy) or removal of bone around the foramen (foraminotomy) may also be performed to relieve pressure on the nerve. When decompression is complete, a free-fat graft may be placed to protect the nerve root. If the ligamentum flavum was not removed, it is placed over the fat graft. Paravertebral muscles are repositioned and the tissue is closed in layers. Report 63020 if the discs are cervical. Report 63030 if lumbar. Note that approaches may be open as described above or endoscopically assisted. In an endoscopically assisted approach, a small guide probe is inserted under fluoroscopic guidance. Using magnified video as well as fluoroscopic guidance, the endoscope is manipulated through the foramen and into the spinal canal. Once the guide probe has been advanced to the surgical site, a slightly larger tube is manipulated over the guide probe. Surgical instruments are advanced through the hollow center of the tube. Herniated disc fragments are removed, and the disc is reconfigured to eliminate pressure on the nerve root(s). The endoscope is withdrawn. The incision is sutured or simply dressed with an adhesive bandage. Report 63035 for additional interspaces, cervical or lumbar.

Coding Tips

As an "add-on" code, 63035 is not subject to multiple procedure rules. No reimbursement reduction or modifier 51 is applied. Add-on codes describe additional intra-service work associated with the primary procedure. They are performed by the same physician on the same date of service as the primary service/procedure, and must never be reported as a stand-alone code. Use 63035 in conjunction with 63020–63030. Arthrodesis is reported separately; see 22590–22632. For re-exploration laminotomy, with partial facetectomy, foraminotomy, and/or excision of the herniated intervertebral disc, see 63040–63044. For laminectomy (complete excision of the lamina), unilateral or bilateral, with facetectomy and foraminotomy, see 63045–63048. For laminectomy performed on one or two vertebral segments, without facetectomy, foraminotomy, or excision of the herniated lumbar disc, see 63001–63011. Hemilaminectomy codes are unilateral by definition. If performed on both sides of the spine (bilaterally), append modifier 50.

ICD-9-CM Procedural

80.51 Excision of intervertebral disc

Anesthesia

63020 00600, 00604, 00670
63030 00630, 00670
63035 N/A

ICD-9-CM Diagnostic

721.0 Cervical spondylosis without myelopathy
721.1 Cervical spondylosis with myelopathy
721.3 Lumbosacral spondylosis without myelopathy
721.42 Spondylosis with myelopathy, lumbar region
722.0 Displacement of cervical intervertebral disc without myelopathy
722.10 Displacement of lumbar intervertebral disc without myelopathy
722.51 Degeneration of thoracic or thoracolumbar intervertebral disc
722.52 Degeneration of lumbar or lumbosacral intervertebral disc
722.71 Intervertebral cervical disc disorder with myelopathy, cervical region
722.73 Intervertebral lumbar disc disorder with myelopathy, lumbar region
723.0 Spinal stenosis in cervical region
723.1 Cervicalgia
723.4 Brachial neuritis or radiculitis nos.
724.02 Spinal stenosis of lumbar region, without neurogenic claudication
756.11 Congenital spondylolysis, lumbosacral region
756.12 Congenital spondylolisthesis

CCI Version 16.3

92585, 95822, 95860-95861, 95867-95868, 95900, 95904, 95920, 95936-95937

Also not with 63020: 0213T, 0216T, 0228T, 0230T, 20251, 20926, 22100, 22102, 22505, 36000, 36400-36410, 36420-36430, 36440, 36600, 36640, 37202, 43752, 51701-51703, 62291, 62310-62319, 63042❖, 63707, 63709, 64400-64435, 64445-64450, 64479, 64483, 64490, 64493, 64505-64530, 64722, 69990, 72285, 76000-76001, 93000-93010, 93040-93042, 93318, 94002, 94200, 94250, 94680-94690, 94770, 95812-95816, 95819, 95829, 95870, 95925-95934, 95955, 96360, 96365, 96372, 96374-96376, 99148-99149, 99150

Also not with 63030: 0171T❖, 0202T, 0213T, 0216T, 0228T, 0230T, 20251, 20926, 22102, 22505, 36000, 36400-36410, 36420-36430, 36440, 36600, 36640, 37202, 43752, 51701-51703, 62267❖, 62284, 62290, 62310-62319, 63042❖, 63707, 63709, 64400-64435, 64445-64450, 64479, 64483, 64490, 64493, 64505-64530, 64722, 69990, 72295, 76000-76001, 93000-93010, 93040-93042, 93318, 94002, 94200, 94250, 94680-94690, 94770, 95812-95816, 95819, 95829, 95870, 95925-95934, 95955, 96360, 96365, 96372, 96374-96376, 99148-99149, 99150

Also not with 63035: 95925-95927, 95930-95934

Note: These CCI edits are used for Medicare. Other payers may reimburse on codes listed above.

Medicare Edits

	Fac RVU	Non-Fac RVU	FUD	Assist
63020	34.23	34.23	90	80
63030	28.34	28.34	90	80
63035	5.77	5.77	N/A	80

Medicare References: None

63040-63044

63040 Laminotomy (hemilaminectomy), with decompression of nerve root(s), including partial facetectomy, foraminotomy and/or excision of herniated intervertebral disc, reexploration, single interspace; cervical
63042 lumbar
63043 each additional cervical interspace (List separately in addition to code for primary procedure)
63044 each additional lumbar interspace (List separately in addition to code for primary procedure)

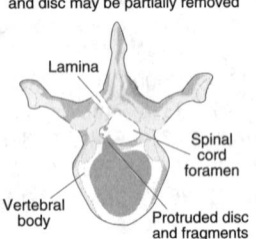

Explanation

Through a posterior approach, a midline incision is made overlying the vertebrae. The incision is carried through the tissue to the paravertebral muscles, which are retracted. If the ligamentum flavum (which attaches lamina from one vertebrae to the lamina of another) is still present, it may be partially or completely removed. The lamina may be removed on the opposite side or more of the lamina may be removed from the previous site to allow access to the spinal cord. If ruptured intervertebral disc fragments or part of the disc continues to compress the nerve, they are removed. A partial removal of a facet or removal of bone around the foramen may also be performed if they are causing pressure on the nerve. When decompression is complete, a previously placed free-fat graft may be replaced over the nerve root. If the ligamentum flavum was not removed in the first surgery or in the exploration it is placed over the fat graft. Paravertebral muscles are repositioned and the tissue is closed in layers. Report 63040 if performed on a single cervical interspace; report 63042 if performed on a single lumbar interspace; report 63043 for each additional cervical interspace; report 63044 for each additional lumbar interspace.

Coding Tips

As "add-on" codes, 63043 and 63044 are not subject to multiple procedure rules. No reimbursement reduction or modifier 51 is applied. Add-on codes describe additional intra-service work associated with the primary procedure. They are performed by the same physician on the same date of service as the primary service/procedure, and must never be reported as a stand-alone code. Use 63043 in conjunction with 63040. Use 63044 in conjunction with 63042. Due to the nature of re-exploration, higher relative values are assigned to these procedures to take into account difficult dissection associated with revisiting a previous surgical site. Modifier 22 should not be reported with these codes when the unusual circumstance is difficult dissection associated with re-exploration. Hemilaminectomy codes are unilateral by definition. If performed on both sides of the spine (bilaterally), append modifier 50. Arthrodesis is reported separately; see 22590–22632. Note that 63040–63044 are for re-exploration laminotomy/hemilaminectomy (partial excision of the lamina) only. For an initial laminotomy/hemilaminectomy, with partial facetectomy, foraminotomy, and/or excision of the herniated intervertebral disc, see 63020–63035.

ICD-9-CM Procedural

03.02   Reopening of laminectomy site
80.51   Excision of intervertebral disc

Anesthesia

63040   00600, 00604, 00670
63042   00630, 00670
63043   N/A
63044   N/A

ICD-9-CM Diagnostic

721.1   Cervical spondylosis with myelopathy
721.42 Spondylosis with myelopathy, lumbar region
722.0   Displacement of cervical intervertebral disc without myelopathy
722.10 Displacement of lumbar intervertebral disc without myelopathy
722.52 Degeneration of lumbar or lumbosacral intervertebral disc
722.71 Intervertebral cervical disc disorder with myelopathy, cervical region
722.73 Intervertebral lumbar disc disorder with myelopathy, lumbar region
756.11 Congenital spondylolysis, lumbosacral region
756.12 Congenital spondylolisthesis
806.4   Closed fracture of lumbar spine with spinal cord injury
806.5   Open fracture of lumbar spine with spinal cord injury
953.2   Injury to lumbar nerve root
953.5   Injury to lumbosacral plexus

CCI Version 16.3

92585, 95822, 95860-95861, 95867-95868, 95900, 95904, 95920, 95936-95937

Also not with 63040: 0213T, 0216T, 0228T, 0230T, 20251, 20926, 22100, 22505, 36000, 36400-36410, 36420-36430, 36440, 36600, 36640, 37202, 43752, 51701-51703, 62291, 62310-62319, 63707, 63709, 64400-64435, 64445-64450, 64479, 64483, 64490, 64493, 64505-64530, 64722, 69990, 72285, 76000-76001, 93000-93010, 93040-93042, 93318, 94002, 94200, 94250, 94680-94690, 94770, 95812-95816, 95819, 95829, 95870, 95925-95934, 95955, 96360, 96365, 96372, 96374-96376, 99148-99149, 99150

Also not with 63042: 0171T❖, 0202T, 0213T, 0216T, 0228T, 0230T, 20251, 20926, 22102, 22114, 22505, 36000, 36400-36410, 36420-36430, 36440, 36600, 36640, 37202, 43752, 51701-51703, 62267❖, 62290, 62310-62319, 63267, 63707, 63709, 64400-64435, 64445-64450, 64479, 64483, 64490, 64493, 64505-64530, 64714, 64722, 64831, 64834-64836, 64840-64858, 64861-64870, 64885-64898, 64905-64907, 69990, 72295, 76000-76001, 93000-93010, 93040-93042, 93318, 94002, 94200, 94250, 94680-94690, 94770, 95812-95816, 95819, 95829, 95870, 95925-95934, 95955, 96360, 96365, 96372, 96374-96376, 99148-99149, 99150

Also not with 63043: 95925-95927, 95930-95934

Also not with 63044: 95925-95927, 95930-95934

Note: These CCI edits are used for Medicare. Other payers may reimburse on codes listed above.

Medicare Edits

	Fac RVU	Non-Fac RVU	FUD	Assist
63040	41.3	41.3	90	80
63042	38.22	38.22	90	80
63043	0.0	0.0	N/A	80
63044	0.0	0.0	N/A	80

Medicare References: None

63045-63048

63045 Laminectomy, facetectomy and foraminotomy (unilateral or bilateral with decompression of spinal cord, cauda equina and/or nerve root[s], [eg, spinal or lateral recess stenosis]), single vertebral segment; cervical
63046 thoracic
63047 lumbar
63048 each additional segment, cervical, thoracic, or lumbar (List separately in addition to code for primary procedure)

Report 63045 if cervical; report 63046 if thoracic; report 63047 if lumbar; report 63048 for each additional segment

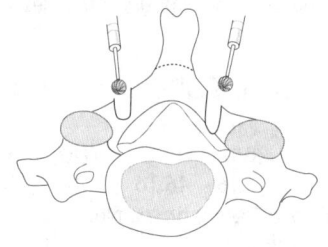

To relieve stenosis, the physician trims the facets and cuts the cervical lamina free with burrs and chisels

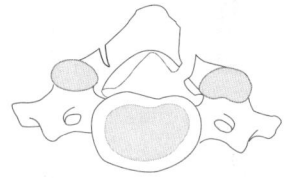

With some techniques the lamina remains partially connected and "floats" on the dura

Explanation

The patient is face down. Magnification may be used during the procedure. The physician makes a midline incision overlying the affected vertebrae. Fascia is incised. Paravertebral muscles are retracted. The physician removes the spinous processes with rongeurs. If the stenosis is central, the physician removes the lamina out to the articular facets using a burr. If the compression is in the lateral recess, only half of the lamina is removed. A Penfield elevator peels the ligamentum flavum away from the dura. Nerve root canals are freed by additional resection of the facet, and compression is relieved by removal of any bony or tissue overgrowth around the foramen. Removal of the lamina, facets, and bony tissue or overgrowths may be performed bilaterally when indicated. The rongeur, retractor, and microscope are removed. A free-fat graft may be placed over the nerve root(s) for protection. If the ligamentum flavum was spared, it is placed over the free-fat graft. Paravertebral muscles are repositioned and the deeper tissues and skin are closed with layered sutures. Report 63046 if the procedure affects a thoracic vertebra; report 63047 if the procedure affects a lumbar vertebra; and 63048 for procedures affecting each additional vertebra.

Coding Tips

Use 63048 in conjunction with 63045–63047. As an "add-on" code, 63048 is not subject to multiple procedure rules. No reimbursement reduction or modifier 51 is applied. Add-on codes describe additional intra-service work associated with the primary procedure. They are performed by the same physician on the same date of service as the primary service/procedure, and must never be reported as a stand-alone code. Arthrodesis is reported separately; see 22590–22614. Codes 63045–63048 report laminectomy (complete excision of the lamina), with facetectomy and foraminotomy. For laminectomy, without facetectomy, foraminotomy, or discectomy, one or two segments, see 63001–63011; more than two segments, see 63015–63017.

ICD-9-CM Procedural

03.09 Other exploration and decompression of spinal canal

Anesthesia

63045 00600, 00670
63046 00620, 00670
63047 00630, 00670
63048 N/A

ICD-9-CM Diagnostic

722.10 Displacement of lumbar intervertebral disc without myelopathy
722.51 Degeneration of thoracic or thoracolumbar intervertebral disc
722.52 Degeneration of lumbar or lumbosacral intervertebral disc
722.71 Intervertebral cervical disc disorder with myelopathy, cervical region
722.72 Intervertebral thoracic disc disorder with myelopathy, thoracic region
722.73 Intervertebral lumbar disc disorder with myelopathy, lumbar region
805.3   Open fracture of dorsal (thoracic) vertebra without mention of spinal cord injury
805.5   Open fracture of lumbar vertebra without mention of spinal cord injury
806.4   Closed fracture of lumbar spine with spinal cord injury
806.5   Open fracture of lumbar spine with spinal cord injury
839.21 Closed dislocation, thoracic vertebra
839.31 Open dislocation, thoracic vertebra

CCI Version 16.3

92585, 95822, 95860-95861, 95867-95868, 95900, 95904, 95920, 95936-95937

Also not with 63045: 0213T, 0216T, 0228T, 0230T, 20660, 20926, 22505, 36000, 36400-36410, 36420-36430, 36440, 36600, 36640, 37202, 43752, 51701-51703, 62310-62319, 63015❖, 63017-63020, 63040❖, 63046, 63707, 63709, 64400-64435, 64445-64450, 64479, 64483, 64490, 64493, 64505-64530, 69990, 76000-76001, 93000-93010, 93040-93042, 93318, 94002, 94200, 94250, 94680-94690, 94770, 95812-95816, 95819, 95829, 95870, 95925-95934, 95955, 96360, 96365, 96372, 96374-96376, 99148-99149, 99150

Also not with 63046: 0213T, 0216T, 0228T, 0230T, 20926, 22212, 22505, 36000, 36400-36410, 36420-36430, 36440, 36600, 36640, 37202, 43752, 51701-51703, 62310-62319, 63015❖, 63017❖, 63047, 63707, 63709, 64400-64435, 64445-64450, 64479, 64483, 64490, 64493, 64505-64530, 69990, 76000-76001, 93000-93010, 93040-93042, 93318, 94002, 94200, 94250, 94680-94690, 94770, 95812-95816, 95819, 95829, 95870, 95925-95934, 95955, 96360, 96365, 96372, 96374-96376, 99148-99149, 99150

Also not with 63047: 0171T❖, 0202T, 0213T, 0216T, 0228T, 0230T, 20926, 22102, 22325, 22505, 22852, 32100, 36000, 36400-36410, 36420-36430, 36440, 36600, 36640, 37202, 43752, 51701-51703, 62284, 62310-62319, 63005❖, 63012-63015❖, 63017-63020, 63030, 63042, 63707, 63709-63710, 64400-64435, 64445-64450, 64479, 64483, 64490, 64493, 64505-64530, 64722, 64831, 64834-64836, 64840-64858, 64861-64870, 64885-64898, 64905-64907, 69990, 76000-76001, 93000-93010, 93040-93042, 93318, 94002, 94200, 94250, 94680-94690, 94770, 95812-95816, 95819, 95829, 95870, 95925-95934, 95955, 96360, 96365, 96372, 96374-96376, 99148-99149, 99150

Also not with 63048: 95925-95927, 95930-95934

Note: These CCI edits are used for Medicare. Other payers may reimburse on codes listed above.

Medicare Edits

	Fac RVU	Non-Fac RVU	FUD	Assist
63045	37.32	37.32	90	80
63046	35.54	35.54	90	80
63047	32.27	32.27	90	80
63048	6.37	6.37	N/A	80

Medicare References: None

63050

63050 Laminoplasty, cervical, with decompression of the spinal cord, 2 or more vertebral segments;

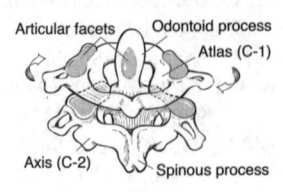

Explanation

Cervical laminoplasty with decompression of the spinal cord is performed to treat cases of myelopathy related to severe spinal stenosis that will not respond to conservative treatment. Intraoperative neurologic monitoring is used during the procedure. The head is immobilized. The surgeon makes an incision in the back of the neck over the target spinal area and dissects down through the soft tissues to access the spine. The spinous processes are exposed. A subperiosteal dissection is done to mobilize the muscles, taking care to preserve the ligaments. Foraminotomies may be done when foraminal stenosis or lateral disc herniation is present. A high-speed drill burr is used to create a gutter in the lamina on both an opening and closing side so the spinous processes may be opened like a door on a hinge. The cancellous bone and outer cortex are removed. An osteotomy is then performed by lifting up on the opening side with a hook while displacing the processes to the opposite side. The laminae are opened like a door on a hinge to the side that displays the worst compression or signs of myeloradiculopathy. This opens the restriction and decompresses the previously pinched spinal cord. The hinge is held in place by small pieces of bone struts.

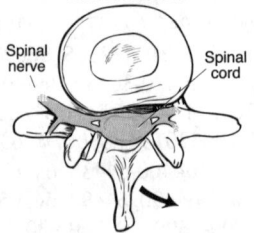

Coding Tips

Do not report 63050 in conjunction with 22600, 22614, 22840–22842, 63001, 63015, 63045, 63048, 63295 for the same vertebral segment(s).

ICD-9-CM Procedural

- 03.09 Other exploration and decompression of spinal canal
- 03.59 Other repair and plastic operations on spinal cord structures

Anesthesia

63050 00600, 00670

ICD-9-CM Diagnostic

- 720.0 Ankylosing spondylitis
- 721.1 Cervical spondylosis with myelopathy
- 722.71 Intervertebral cervical disc disorder with myelopathy, cervical region
- 723.0 Spinal stenosis in cervical region
- 723.1 Cervicalgia
- 723.4 Brachial neuritis or radiculitis nos.
- 756.10 Congenital anomaly of spine, unspecified
- 756.19 Other congenital anomaly of spine
- 905.1 Late effect of fracture of spine and trunk without mention of spinal cord lesion

Terms To Know

decompression. Release of pressure.

dissection. Separating by cutting tissue or body structures apart.

incision. Act of cutting into tissue or an organ.

lamina. Thin, flat plate or layer of membrane or other tissue; generally refers to the lamina of the vertebra.

neuritis. Inflammation of a nerve or group of nerves, often manifested by loss of function and reflexes, pain, and numbness or tingling.

radiculitis. Pain along an inflamed nerve, with inflammation of the root of the associated spinal nerve.

soft tissue. Nonepithelial tissues outside of the skeleton that includes subcutaneous adipose tissue, fibrous tissue, fascia, muscles, blood and lymph vessels, and peripheral nervous system tissue.

stenosis. Narrowing or constriction of a passage.

CCI Version 16.3

0213T, 0216T, 0228T, 0230T, 20926, 22505, 22600, 22614, 36000, 36400-36410, 36420-36430, 36440, 36600, 36640, 37202, 43752, 51701-51703, 62310-62319, 63001, 63015, 63020✦, 63040✦, 63045, 63048, 63295, 63707, 63709, 64400-64435, 64445-64450, 64479, 64483, 64490, 64493, 64505-64530, 69990, 76000-76001, 92585, 93000-93010, 93040-93042, 93318, 94002, 94200, 94250, 94680-94690, 94770, 95812-95816, 95819, 95822, 95829, 95860-95861, 95867-95868, 95870, 95900, 95904, 95920, 95925-95934, 95936-95937, 95955, 96360, 96365, 96372, 96374-96376, 99148-99149, 99150

Note: These CCI edits are used for Medicare. Other payers may reimburse on codes listed above.

Medicare Edits

	Fac RVU	Non-Fac RVU	FUD	Assist
63050	46.16	46.16	90	80

Medicare References: None

63051

63051 Laminoplasty, cervical, with decompression of the spinal cord, 2 or more vertebral segments; with reconstruction of the posterior bony elements (including the application of bridging bone graft and non-segmental fixation devices (eg, wire, suture, mini-plates), when performed)

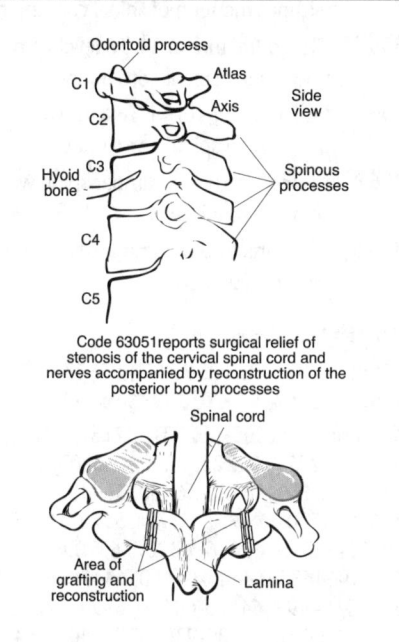

Explanation

Cervical laminoplasty with decompression of the spinal cord is performed to treat cases of myelopathy related to severe spinal stenosis that will not respond to conservative treatment. Intraoperative neurologic monitoring is used during the procedure. The head is immobilized. The surgeon makes an incision in the back of the neck over the target spinal area and dissects down through the soft tissues to access the spine. The spinous processes are exposed. A subperiosteal dissection is done to mobilize the muscles, taking care to preserve the ligaments. Foraminotomies may be done when foraminal stenosis or lateral disc herniation is present. A high-speed drill burr is used to create a gutter in the lamina on both an opening and closing side so the spinous processes may be opened like a door on a hinge. The cancellous bone and outer cortex are removed. An osteotomy is then performed by lifting up on the opening side with a hook while displacing the processes to the opposite side. The laminae are opened like a door on a hinge to the side that displays the worst compression or signs of myeloradiculopathy. This opens the restriction and decompresses the previously pinched spinal cord. The hinge is held in place by small pieces of bone struts. Reconstruction of the posterior bony elements is then performed. Fibular or tricortical iliac crest allografts are used. The prepared graft is notched and fitted into place in the "open door" position of the lamina. Titanium miniplates (or other fixation device) may be used to stabilize each level. The tissues are sutured back into place and a suction drain is placed.

Coding Tips

Do not report 63051 in conjunction with 22600, 22614, 22840–22842, 63001, 63015, 63045, 63048, 63295 for the same vertebral segment(s).

ICD-9-CM Procedural

- 03.09 Other exploration and decompression of spinal canal
- 03.59 Other repair and plastic operations on spinal cord structures

Anesthesia

63051 00600

ICD-9-CM Diagnostic

- 720.0 Ankylosing spondylitis
- 721.1 Cervical spondylosis with myelopathy
- 722.71 Intervertebral cervical disc disorder with myelopathy, cervical region
- 723.0 Spinal stenosis in cervical region
- 723.1 Cervicalgia
- 723.4 Brachial neuritis or radiculitis nos.
- 756.10 Congenital anomaly of spine, unspecified
- 756.19 Other congenital anomaly of spine
- 905.1 Late effect of fracture of spine and trunk without mention of spinal cord lesion

Terms To Know

decompression. Release of pressure.

dissection. Separating by cutting tissue or body structures apart.

lamina. Thin, flat plate or layer of membrane or other tissue; generally refers to the lamina of the vertebra.

soft tissue. Nonepithelial tissues outside of the skeleton that includes subcutaneous adipose tissue, fibrous tissue, fascia, muscles, blood and lymph vessels, and peripheral nervous system tissue.

stenosis. Narrowing or constriction of a passage.

CCI Version 16.3

0213T, 0216T, 0228T, 0230T, 20926, 22505, 22600, 22614, 36000, 36400-36410, 36420-36430, 36440, 36600, 36640, 37202, 43752, 51701-51703, 62310-62319, 63001, 63015, 63020❖, 63040❖, 63045, 63048-63050, 63265❖, 63295, 63707, 63709, 64400-64435, 64445-64450, 64479, 64483, 64490, 64493, 64505-64530, 69990, 76000-76001, 92585, 93000-93010, 93040-93042, 93318, 94002, 94200, 94250, 94680-94690, 94770, 95812-95816, 95819, 95822, 95829, 95860-95861, 95867-95868, 95870, 95900, 95904, 95920, 95925-95934, 95936-95937, 95955, 96360, 96365, 96372, 96374-96376, 99148-99149, 99150

Note: These CCI edits are used for Medicare. Other payers may reimburse on codes listed above.

Medicare Edits

	Fac RVU	Non-Fac RVU	FUD	Assist
63051	50.49	50.49	90	80

Medicare References: None

63055-63057

63055 Transpedicular approach with decompression of spinal cord, equina and/or nerve root(s) (eg, herniated intervertebral disc), single segment; thoracic

63056 lumbar (including transfacet, or lateral extraforaminal approach) (eg, far lateral herniated intervertebral disc)

63057 each additional segment, thoracic or lumbar (List separately in addition to code for primary procedure)

Explanation

This procedure is performed to relieve pressure on the spinal cord, equina, and nerve roots caused by a herniated disc. The physician approaches the herniated disc through the pedicle on the side of the disc's bulge. Additional exposure is made by removing the lamina and facet joint. The physician removes the disc fragments and closes the wound in layers. Report 63055 if the segment is thoracic. Report 63056 if the segment is lumbar. A far lateral herniated lumbar intervertebral disc may require an alternative approach through the facet joint (transfacet) or foramina (transforaminal). Report 63057 for each additional segment, thoracic or lumbar.

Coding Tips

Use 63057 in conjunction with 63055–63056. As an "add-on" code, 63057 is not subject to multiple procedure rules. No reimbursement reduction or modifier 51 is applied. Add-on codes describe additional intra-service work associated with the primary procedure. They are performed by the same physician on the same date of service as the primary service/procedure, and must never be reported as a stand-alone code. The removal of a rib in the course of dissection is not reported separately. When an anterior approach to the thoracic cavity is performed, the negative pressure is lost and a thoracotomy tube is routinely inserted to help re-establish the normal negative pressure and re-inflate the lung(s) after closure. This is a life-sustaining measure that must be performed in order to complete the procedure and, as such, tube thoracostomy (32551) should not be reported separately. When an anterior approach to the spine is achieved using the skills of two surgeons of different specialties (e.g., a thoracic or general surgeon provides exposure and the neurosurgeon provides the definitive procedure), this is a co-surgery scenario. Both surgeons report the primary procedure with modifier 62 and submit the claim with operative notes attached.

ICD-9-CM Procedural

03.09 Other exploration and decompression of spinal canal

Anesthesia

63055 00620, 00670
63056 00630, 00670
63057 N/A

ICD-9-CM Diagnostic

722.10 Displacement of lumbar intervertebral disc without myelopathy
722.11 Displacement of thoracic intervertebral disc without myelopathy
722.51 Degeneration of thoracic or thoracolumbar intervertebral disc
722.52 Degeneration of lumbar or lumbosacral intervertebral disc
722.72 Intervertebral thoracic disc disorder with myelopathy, thoracic region
722.73 Intervertebral lumbar disc disorder with myelopathy, lumbar region
724.01 Spinal stenosis of thoracic region
724.02 Spinal stenosis of lumbar region, without neurogenic claudication
724.03 Spinal stenosis of lumbar region, with neurogenic claudication
724.3 Sciatica
724.4 Thoracic or lumbosacral neuritis or radiculitis, unspecified
729.2 Unspecified neuralgia, neuritis, and radiculitis
729.5 Pain in soft tissues of limb
733.13 Pathologic fracture of vertebrae
805.2 Closed fracture of dorsal (thoracic) vertebra without mention of spinal cord injury
805.3 Open fracture of dorsal (thoracic) vertebra without mention of spinal cord injury
805.4 Closed fracture of lumbar vertebra without mention of spinal cord injury
805.5 Open fracture of lumbar vertebra without mention of spinal cord injury
806.20 Closed fracture of T1-T6 level with unspecified spinal cord injury
806.30 Open fracture of T1-T6 level with unspecified spinal cord injury
806.4 Closed fracture of lumbar spine with spinal cord injury
806.5 Open fracture of lumbar spine with spinal cord injury

CCI Version 16.3

92585, 95822, 95860-95861, 95867-95868, 95900, 95904, 95920, 95936-95937

Also not with 63055: 0213T, 0216T, 0228T, 0230T, 22212, 22222, 22505, 36000, 36400-36410, 36420-36430, 36440, 36600, 36640, 37202, 43752, 51701-51703, 62291, 62310-62319, 63056, 63707, 63709, 64400-64435, 64445-64450, 64479, 64483, 64490, 64493, 64505-64530, 69990, 72285, 76000-76001, 93000-93010, 93040-93042, 93318, 94002, 94200, 94250, 94680-94690, 94770, 95812-95816, 95819, 95829, 95870, 95925-95934, 95955, 96360, 96365, 96372, 96374-96376, 99148-99149, 99150

Also not with 63056: 0171T✦, 0202T, 0213T, 0216T, 0228T, 0230T, 22214, 22224, 22505, 36000, 36400-36410, 36420-36430, 36440, 36600, 36640, 37202, 43752, 51701-51703, 62267✦, 62290, 62310-62319, 63087✦, 63090✦, 63707, 63709, 64400-64435, 64445-64450, 64479, 64483, 64490, 64493, 64505-64530, 69990, 72295, 76000-76001, 93000-93010, 93040-93042, 93318, 94002, 94200, 94250, 94680-94690, 94770, 95812-95816, 95819, 95829, 95870, 95925-95934, 95955, 96360, 96365, 96372, 96374-96376, 99148-99149, 99150

Also not with 63057: 95925-95927, 95930-95934

Note: These CCI edits are used for Medicare. Other payers may reimburse on codes listed above.

Medicare Edits

	Fac RVU	Non-Fac RVU	FUD	Assist
63055	47.94	47.94	90	80
63056	43.56	43.56	90	80
63057	9.64	9.64	N/A	80

Medicare References: None

63064-63066

63064 Costovertebral approach with decompression of spinal cord or nerve root(s) (eg, herniated intervertebral disc), thoracic; single segment

63066 each additional segment (List separately in addition to code for primary procedure)

Physician approaches spinal cord with costovertebral approach, allowing access to impingements on nerve roots

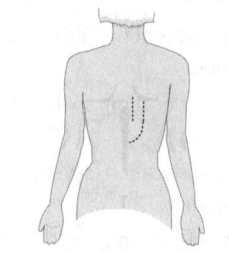

Report 63064 if single segment thoracic; report 63066 for additional segments

Transverse costal facet
Area of approach
Superior costal facet
Superior articular process
Disc (usually herniated)

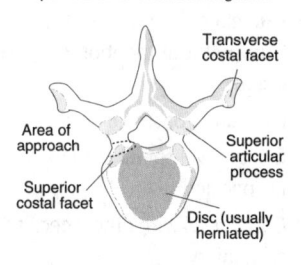

Explanation

The physician makes an incision two inches to three inches lateral to the spine through fascia, muscles, and a section of a rib. The physician enters anterior to the transverse process and the pedicle using a Kerrington rongeur or burr. Exposure may be increased by removal of the transverse process. The spinal cord or nerve root is decompressed by removing the herniated disc. The wound is filled with saline and radiographs (separately reported) are made to assure no air is leading into the lungs. The muscles fall over a drain and the tissue is closed with layered sutures. Report 63064 if a single segment is repaired. Report 63066 for additional segments.

Coding Tips

Use 63066 in conjunction with 63064. As an "add-on" code, 63066 is not subject to multiple procedure rules. No reimbursement reduction or modifier 51 is applied. Add-on codes describe additional intra-service work associated with the primary procedure. They are performed by the same physician on the same date of service as the primary service/procedure, and must never be reported as a stand-alone code. The removal of a rib in the course of dissection is not reported separately. When an anterior approach to the thoracic cavity is performed, the negative pressure is lost and a thoracotomy tube is routinely inserted to help re-establish the normal negative pressure and re-inflate the lung(s) after closure. This is a life-sustaining measure that must be performed in order to complete the procedure and, as such, tube thoracostomy (32551) should not be reported separately. When an anterior approach to the spine is achieved using the skills of two surgeons of different specialties (e.g., a thoracic or general surgeon provides exposure and the neurosurgeon provides the definitive procedure), this is a co-surgery scenario. Both surgeons report the primary procedure with modifier 62 and submit the claim with operative notes attached.

ICD-9-CM Procedural

03.09 Other exploration and decompression of spinal canal

Anesthesia

63064 00620, 00625, 00626, 00670
63066 N/A

ICD-9-CM Diagnostic

722.11 Displacement of thoracic intervertebral disc without myelopathy
722.51 Degeneration of thoracic or thoracolumbar intervertebral disc
722.72 Intervertebral thoracic disc disorder with myelopathy, thoracic region
722.92 Other and unspecified disc disorder of thoracic region
724.01 Spinal stenosis of thoracic region
738.4 Acquired spondylolisthesis
756.12 Congenital spondylolisthesis
805.2 Closed fracture of dorsal (thoracic) vertebra without mention of spinal cord injury
805.3 Open fracture of dorsal (thoracic) vertebra without mention of spinal cord injury
806.20 Closed fracture of T1-T6 level with unspecified spinal cord injury
806.21 Closed fracture of T1-T6 level with complete lesion of cord
806.30 Open fracture of T1-T6 level with unspecified spinal cord injury
952.19 T7-T12 level with other specified spinal cord injury

Terms To Know

anterior. Situated in the front area or toward the belly surface of the body; an anatomical reference point used to show the position and relationship of one body structure to another.

fascia. Fibrous sheet or band of tissue that envelops organs, muscles, and groupings of muscles.

fracture. Break in bone or cartilage.

injury. Harm or damage sustained by the body.

lesion. Area of damaged tissue that has lost continuity or function, due to disease or trauma. Lesions may be located on internal structures such as the brain, nerves, or kidneys, or visible on the skin.

spinal stenosis. Narrowing of the canal (vertebral or nerve root) or intervertebral foramina of the lumbar spine.

spondylolisthesis. Forward displacement of one vertebra slipping over another, usually in the fourth or fifth lumbar area.

CCI Version 16.3

92585, 95822, 95860-95861, 95867-95868, 95900, 95904, 95920, 95936-95937

Also not with 63064: 0213T, 0216T, 0228T, 0230T, 22505, 36000, 36400-36410, 36420-36430, 36440, 36600, 36640, 37202, 43752, 51701-51703, 62291, 62310-62319, 63707, 63709, 64400-64435, 64445-64450, 64479, 64483, 64490, 64493, 64505-64530, 69990, 72285, 76000-76001, 93000-93010, 93040-93042, 93318, 94002, 94200, 94250, 94680-94690, 94770, 95812-95816, 95819, 95829, 95870, 95925-95934, 95955, 96360, 96365, 96372, 96374-96376, 99148-99149, 99150

Also not with 63066: 95925-95927, 95930-95934

Note: These CCI edits are used for Medicare. Other payers may reimburse on codes listed above.

Medicare Edits

	Fac RVU	Non-Fac RVU	FUD	Assist
63064	52.07	52.07	90	80
63066	6.2	6.2	N/A	80

Medicare References: None

63075-63076

63075 Discectomy, anterior, with decompression of spinal cord and/or nerve root(s), including osteophytectomy; cervical, single interspace

63076 cervical, each additional interspace (List separately in addition to code for primary procedure)

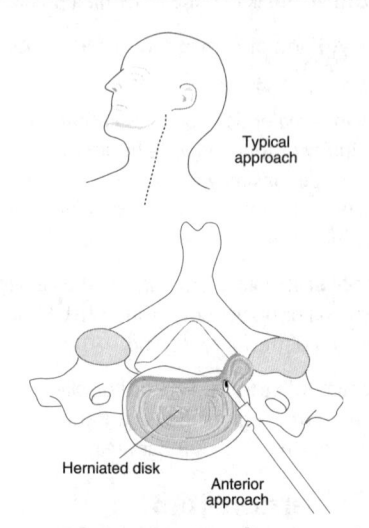

Typical approach

Herniated disk
Anterior approach

Physician removes herniated cervical disc

Report 63075 if cervical, single interspace; report 63076 for each additional cervical interspace

Explanation

The physician performs a cervical discectomy to remove all or part of a herniated intervertebral disc. The patient is placed supine with a head halter on the jawbone (mandible). The physician makes a transverse incision overlying the intervertebral disc. The sternocleidomastoid muscle and the carotid artery are retracted. The physician excises the anterior anulus of the disc and uses pituitary forceps to remove as much disc material as possible. A spreader and microscope are used to enhance the evacuation. A drill is used to remove the transverse bar above and below. Graft material is obtained from the ilium and fashioned into a T-shape. The graft is placed into the disc space and traction is released. The muscles fall back into place and the incision is closed with layered sutures. Report 63075 if the discectomy is in a single interspace. Report 63076 for each additional cervical interspace.

Coding Tips

Use 63076 in conjunction with 63075. As an "add-on" code, 63076 is not subject to multiple procedure rules. No reimbursement reduction or modifier 51 is applied. Add-on codes describe additional intra-service work associated with the primary procedure. They are performed by the same physician on the same date of service as the primary service/procedure, and must never be reported as a stand-alone code. Do not report tube thoracostomy (32551) separately, as it is integral to an anterior approach. If the services of two primary surgeons performing separate and distinct components of the procedure are required, a co-surgery scenario exists. Both surgeons should report the primary procedure with modifier 62 and submit the claim with operative notes attached. Arthrodesis is reported separately; see 22554-22585. Any bone graft is reported separately; see 20930-20938.

ICD-9-CM Procedural

80.51 Excision of intervertebral disc

Anesthesia

63075 00600, 00670
63076 N/A

ICD-9-CM Diagnostic

721.0 Cervical spondylosis without myelopathy
721.1 Cervical spondylosis with myelopathy
721.8 Other allied disorders of spine
722.0 Displacement of cervical intervertebral disc without myelopathy
722.4 Degeneration of cervical intervertebral disc
722.71 Intervertebral cervical disc disorder with myelopathy, cervical region
722.91 Other and unspecified disc disorder of cervical region
723.0 Spinal stenosis in cervical region
723.1 Cervicalgia
723.2 Cervicocranial syndrome
723.3 Cervicobrachial syndrome (diffuse)
723.4 Brachial neuritis or radiculitis nos.
723.7 Ossification of posterior longitudinal ligament in cervical region
729.5 Pain in soft tissues of limb
738.4 Acquired spondylolisthesis
738.5 Other acquired deformity of back or spine
756.10 Congenital anomaly of spine, unspecified
756.19 Other congenital anomaly of spine
839.03 Closed dislocation, third cervical vertebra
839.04 Closed dislocation, fourth cervical vertebra
839.05 Closed dislocation, fifth cervical vertebra
839.06 Closed dislocation, sixth cervical vertebra
839.07 Closed dislocation, seventh cervical vertebra
839.08 Closed dislocation, multiple cervical vertebrae
839.11 Open dislocation, first cervical vertebra
839.12 Open dislocation, second cervical vertebra
839.13 Open dislocation, third cervical vertebra
839.14 Open dislocation, fourth cervical vertebra
839.15 Open dislocation, fifth cervical vertebra
839.16 Open dislocation, sixth cervical vertebra
839.17 Open dislocation, seventh cervical vertebra
839.18 Open dislocation, multiple cervical vertebrae
905.1 Late effect of fracture of spine and trunk without mention of spinal cord lesion
907.2 Late effect of spinal cord injury
952.00 C1-C4 level spinal cord injury, unspecified
952.09 C5-C7 level with other specified spinal cord injury

CCI Version 16.3

69990, 92585, 95822, 95860-95861, 95867-95868, 95900, 95904, 95920, 95936-95937

Also not with 63075: 0213T, 0216T, 0228T, 0230T, 22505, 36000, 36400-36410, 36420-36430, 36440, 36600, 36640, 37202, 43752, 51701-51703, 62291, 62310-62319, 63077, 63707, 63709, 64400-64435, 64445-64450, 64479, 64483, 64490, 64493, 64505-64530, 72285, 76000-76001, 93000-93010, 93040-93042, 93318, 94002, 94200, 94250, 94680-94690, 94770, 95812-95816, 95819, 95829, 95870, 95925-95934, 95955, 96360, 96365, 96372, 96374-96376, 99148-99149, 99150

Also not with 63076: 95925-95927, 95930-95934

Note: These CCI edits are used for Medicare. Other payers may reimburse on codes listed above.

Medicare Edits

	Fac RVU	Non-Fac RVU	FUD	Assist
63075	40.48	40.48	90	80
63076	7.5	7.5	N/A	80

Medicare References: None

63077-63078

63077 Discectomy, anterior, with decompression of spinal cord and/or nerve root(s), including osteophytectomy; thoracic, single interspace

63078 thoracic, each additional interspace (List separately in addition to code for primary procedure)

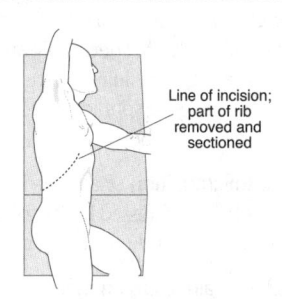

Report 63077 for thoracic, single interspace; report 63078 for thoracic, each additional interspace

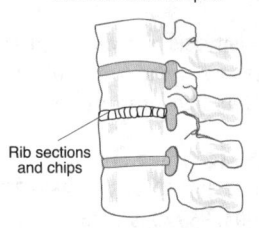

Physician removes herniated thoracic intervertebral disk

Explanation

The physician makes an incision along the rib corresponding to the second thoracic vertebra above the involved intervertebral disc, except in cases involving the top five discs. The rib is removed for access and eventually used in the graft, which is obtained through an extrapleural or transpleural approach. Vessels are tied away from the spine. The disc is removed to the posterior ligament using a microscope and nibbling instruments. The end plates are stripped of their cartilage. The physician makes a slot in one vertebral body and a hole in the other to accept the graft, which is made of several sections of rib. The physician ties the grafts together with heavy suture material and closes the tissue with layered sutures. A chest drain may be inserted. Report 63077 for a single thoracic interspace. Report 63078 for each additional thoracic interspace.

Coding Tips

Use 63078 in conjunction with 63077. As an "add-on" code, 63078 is not subject to multiple procedure rules. No reimbursement reduction or modifier 51 is applied. Add-on codes describe additional intra-service work associated with the primary procedure. They are performed by the same physician on the same date of service as the primary service/procedure, and must never be reported as a stand-alone code. When an anterior approach to the thoracic cavity is performed, the negative pressure is lost and a thoracotomy tube is routinely inserted to help re-establish the normal negative pressure and re-inflate the lung(s) after closure. This is a life-sustaining measure that must be performed in order to complete the procedure and, as such, tube thoracostomy (32551) should not be reported separately. When an anterior approach to the spine is achieved using the skills of two surgeons of different specialties (e.g., a thoracic or general surgeon provides exposure and the neurosurgeon provides the definitive procedure), this is a co-surgery scenario. Both surgeons report the primary procedure with modifier 62 and submit the claim with operative notes attached. Arthrodesis is reported separately; see 22554–22585. Any bone graft is also reported separately; see 20930–20938. For anterior cervical discectomy, see 63075–63076.

ICD-9-CM Procedural

80.51 Excision of intervertebral disc

Anesthesia

63077 00620, 00625, 00626
63078 N/A

ICD-9-CM Diagnostic

- 721.2 Thoracic spondylosis without myelopathy
- 721.41 Spondylosis with myelopathy, thoracic region
- 721.8 Other allied disorders of spine
- 722.11 Displacement of thoracic intervertebral disc without myelopathy
- 722.51 Degeneration of thoracic or thoracolumbar intervertebral disc
- 722.72 Intervertebral thoracic disc disorder with myelopathy, thoracic region
- 722.92 Other and unspecified disc disorder of thoracic region
- 724.01 Spinal stenosis of thoracic region
- 724.1 Pain in thoracic spine
- 729.2 Unspecified neuralgia, neuritis, and radiculitis
- 754.2 Congenital musculoskeletal deformity of spine
- 952.10 T1-T6 level spinal cord injury, unspecified

Terms To Know

congenital. Present at birth, occurring through heredity or an influence during gestation up to the moment of birth.

ligament. Band or sheet of fibrous tissue that connects the articular surfaces of bones or supports visceral organs.

spinal stenosis. Narrowing of the canal (vertebral or nerve root) or intervertebral foramina of the lumbar spine.

CCI Version 16.3

69990, 92585, 95822, 95860-95861, 95867-95868, 95900, 95904, 95920, 95936-95937

Also not with 63077: 0213T, 0216T, 0228T, 0230T, 22505, 32100, 36000, 36400-36410, 36420-36430, 36440, 36600, 36640, 37202, 43752, 51701-51703, 62291, 62310-62319, 63707, 63709, 64400-64435, 64445-64450, 64479, 64483, 64490, 64493, 64505-64530, 72285, 76000-76001, 93000-93010, 93040-93042, 93318, 94002, 94200, 94250, 94680-94690, 94770, 95812-95816, 95819, 95829, 95870, 95925-95934, 95955, 96360, 96365, 96372, 96374-96376, 99148-99149, 99150

Also not with 63078: 95925-95927, 95930-95934

Note: These CCI edits are used for Medicare. Other payers may reimburse on codes listed above.

Medicare Edits

	Fac RVU	Non-Fac RVU	FUD	Assist
63077	44.23	44.23	90	80
63078	5.81	5.81	N/A	80

Medicare References: None

63081-63082

63081 Vertebral corpectomy (vertebral body resection), partial or complete, anterior approach with decompression of spinal cord and/or nerve root(s); cervical, single segment

63082 cervical, each additional segment (List separately in addition to code for primary procedure)

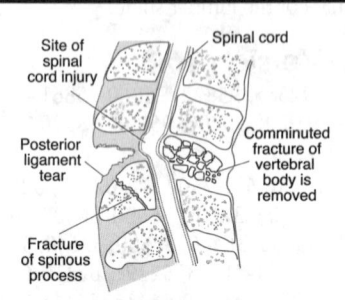

Lateral cutaway view of spinal fracture

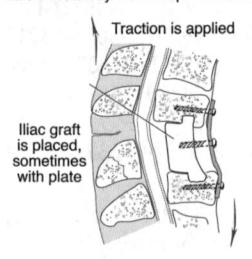

Report 63081 for single segment; report 63082 for each additional segment

Explanation
The patient is placed supine with traction-producing tongs. The physician makes a right transverse incision at mid-position of the planned surgical procedure, and longitudinally between the thyroid gland and the carotid sheath. The discs above and below the vertebrae are excised using a curette. Cartilaginous endplates are removed using a high-speed burr. The crushed part of the vertebral body is partially or completely removed, and the section is prepared for the graft. The anterior surfaces of the vertebrae above and below the fusion are debrided. The physician prepares a separately reportable, tricortical iliac graft and inserts it into the site, tapping it into place with a Moe impacter. Traction is released. Bone chips are packed in and, if needed, a metal plate is screwed to the spine over the graft. The muscles fall back into place and the wound is closed with layered sutures. Report 63081 if one segment is involved; report 63082 for each additional cervical segment.

Coding Tips
Use 63082 in conjunction with 63081. As an "add-on" code, 63082 is not subject to multiple procedure rules. No reimbursement reduction or modifier 51 is applied. Add-on codes describe additional intra-service work associated with the primary procedure. They are performed by the same physician on the same date of service as the primary service/procedure, and must never be reported as a stand-alone code. Diskectomy above and below the vertebral segment is included and should not be reported separately. Do not report tube thoracostomy (32551) separately, as it is integral to an anterior approach. If the services of two primary surgeons performing separate and distinct components of the procedure are required, a co-surgery scenario exists. Both surgeons should report the primary procedure with modifier 62 and submit the claim with operative notes attached. Arthrodesis is reported separately; see 22554–22585. Any bone graft is also reported separately; see 20930–20938. Spinal instrumentation is reported separately; see 22840–22855. If the procedure is completed through an operating microscope, list 69990 in addition to 63081.

ICD-9-CM Procedural
- 03.09 Other exploration and decompression of spinal canal
- 03.59 Other repair and plastic operations on spinal cord structures

Anesthesia
- **63081** 00600, 00670
- **63082** N/A

ICD-9-CM Diagnostic
- 170.2 Malignant neoplasm of vertebral column, excluding sacrum and coccyx
- 721.0 Cervical spondylosis without myelopathy
- 721.1 Cervical spondylosis with myelopathy
- 722.0 Displacement of cervical intervertebral disc without myelopathy
- 722.4 Degeneration of cervical intervertebral disc
- 722.71 Intervertebral cervical disc disorder with myelopathy, cervical region
- 722.91 Other and unspecified disc disorder of cervical region
- 723.0 Spinal stenosis in cervical region
- 723.1 Cervicalgia
- 723.4 Brachial neuritis or radiculitis nos.
- 730.28 Unspecified osteomyelitis, other specified sites — (Use additional code to identify organism: 041.1. Use additional code to identify major osseous defect, if applicable: 731.3)
- 756.10 Congenital anomaly of spine, unspecified
- 756.12 Congenital spondylolisthesis
- 806.00 Closed fracture of C1-C4 level with unspecified spinal cord injury
- 806.10 Open fracture of C1-C4 level with unspecified spinal cord injury

Terms To Know
cervicalgia. Pain localized to the cervical region, generally referring to the posterior or lateral regions of the neck.

malignant. Any condition tending to progress toward death, specifically an invasive tumor with a loss of cellular differentiation that has the ability to spread or metastasize to other areas in the body.

neuritis. Inflammation of a nerve or group of nerves, often manifested by loss of function and reflexes, pain, and numbness or tingling.

radiculitis. Pain along an inflamed nerve, with inflammation of the root of the associated spinal nerve.

spondylolisthesis. Forward displacement of one vertebra slipping over another, usually in the fourth or fifth lumbar area.

CCI Version 16.3
92585, 95822, 95860-95861, 95867-95868, 95900, 95904, 95920, 95936-95937

Also not with 63081: 0213T, 0216T, 0228T, 0230T, 22100-22102, 22110, 22112, 22114, 22505, 36000, 36400-36410, 36420-36430, 36440, 36600, 36640, 37202, 43752, 51701-51703, 62310-62319, 63075, 63707, 63709, 64400-64435, 64445-64450, 64479, 64483, 64490, 64493, 64505-64530, 76000-76001, 93000-93010, 93040-93042, 93318, 94002, 94200, 94250, 94680-94690, 94770, 95812-95816, 95819, 95829, 95870, 95925-95934, 95955, 96360, 96365, 96372, 96374-96376, 99148-99149, 99150

Also not with 63082: 95925-95927, 95930-95934

Note: These CCI edits are used for Medicare. Other payers may reimburse on codes listed above.

Medicare Edits

	Fac RVU	Non-Fac RVU	FUD	Assist
63081	52.23	52.23	90	80
63082	8.05	8.05	N/A	80

Medicare References: None

63085-63088

63085 Vertebral corpectomy (vertebral body resection), partial or complete, transthoracic approach with decompression of spinal cord and/or nerve root(s); thoracic, single segment

63086 thoracic, each additional segment (List separately in addition to code for primary procedure)

63087 Vertebral corpectomy (vertebral body resection), partial or complete, combined thoracolumbar approach with decompression of spinal cord, cauda equina or nerve root(s), lower thoracic or lumbar; single segment

63088 each additional segment (List separately in addition to code for primary procedure)

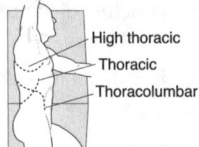

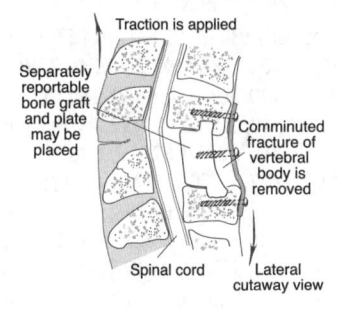

Explanation

This procedure corrects compression on the spinal cord resulting from an anterior fracture of the vertebra. The patient is placed in a swimmer's position. The physician makes an incision through the fascia, muscles, and moves aside any organs. The discs above and below the vertebrae are excised using a curette. Cartilaginous endplates are removed using a high-speed burr. The crushed part of the vertebral body is partially or completely removed, and the section is prepared for the graft. The anterior surfaces of adjacent vertebrae are debrided. The physician prepares a tricortical iliac graft and inserts it into the site, tapping it into place with a Moe impacter. Traction is released. Bone chips are packed in and, if needed, a metal plate is screwed to the spine over the graft. The muscles fall back into place and the wound is closed with layered sutures. Report 63085 if one thoracic segment is involved; report 63086 if more than one is involved; report 63087 if caudal equina, lower thoracic, or lumbar, single segment is involved; report 63088 for each additional segment.

Coding Tips

Use 63086 in conjunction with 63085. Use 63088 in conjunction with 63087. As "add-on" codes, 63086 and 63088 are not subject to multiple procedure rules. No reimbursement reduction or modifier 51 is applied. Add-on codes describe additional intra-service work associated with the primary procedure. They are performed by the same physician on the same date of service as the primary service/procedure, and must never be reported as a stand-alone code. Diskectomy above and below the vertebral segment is included and should not be reported separately. Arthrodesis is reported separately; see 22554–22585. Any bone graft is also reported separately; see 20930–20938. Spinal instrumentation is reported separately; see 22840–22855. If the procedure is completed through an operating microscope, list 69990 in addition to 63085–63088.

ICD-9-CM Procedural

03.09 Other exploration and decompression of spinal canal

03.59 Other repair and plastic operations on spinal cord structures

Anesthesia

63085 00620, 00625, 00626, 00670
63086 N/A
63087 00620, 00625, 00626, 00630, 00670
63088 N/A

ICD-9-CM Diagnostic

722.10 Displacement of lumbar intervertebral disc without myelopathy

722.11 Displacement of thoracic intervertebral disc without myelopathy

722.51 Degeneration of thoracic or thoracolumbar intervertebral disc

722.52 Degeneration of lumbar or lumbosacral intervertebral disc

722.72 Intervertebral thoracic disc disorder with myelopathy, thoracic region

722.73 Intervertebral lumbar disc disorder with myelopathy, lumbar region

722.93 Other and unspecified disc disorder of lumbar region

805.3 Open fracture of dorsal (thoracic) vertebra without mention of spinal cord injury

805.5 Open fracture of lumbar vertebra without mention of spinal cord injury

806.35 Open fracture of T7-T12 level with unspecified spinal cord injury

806.5 Open fracture of lumbar spine with spinal cord injury

CCI Version 16.3

92585, 95822, 95860-95861, 95867-95868, 95900, 95904, 95920, 95936-95937

Also not with 63085: 0213T, 0216T, 0228T, 0230T, 22100-22102, 22110, 22112, 22114, 22505, 32100, 36000, 36400-36410, 36420-36430, 36440, 36600, 36640, 37202, 43752, 51701-51703, 62310-62319, 63075, 63077, 63707, 63709, 64400-64435, 64445-64450, 64479, 64483, 64490, 64493, 64505-64530, 76000-76001, 93000-93010, 93040-93042, 93318, 94002, 94200, 94250, 94680-94690, 94770, 95812-95816, 95819, 95829, 95870, 95925-95934, 95955, 96360, 96365, 96372, 96374-96376, 99148-99149, 99150

Also not with 63086: 95925-95927, 95930-95934

Also not with 63087: 0213T, 0216T, 0228T, 0230T, 22100-22102, 22110, 22112, 22114, 22505, 22857❖, 22862❖, 22865❖, 32095-32100, 36000, 36400-36410, 36420-36430, 36440, 36600, 36640, 37202, 39530, 43752, 49000-49010, 51701-51703, 62310-62319, 63075, 63077, 63101-63102❖, 63707, 63709, 64400-64435, 64445-64450, 64479, 64483, 64490, 64493, 64505-64530, 76000-76001, 93000-93010, 93040-93042, 93318, 94002, 94200, 94250, 94680-94690, 94770, 95812-95816, 95819, 95829, 95870, 95925-95934, 95955, 96360, 96365, 96372, 96374-96376, 99148-99149, 99150

Also not with 63088: 95925-95927, 95930-95934

Note: These CCI edits are used for Medicare. Other payers may reimburse on codes listed above.

Medicare Edits

	Fac RVU	Non-Fac RVU	FUD	Assist
63085	56.03	56.03	90	80
63086	5.74	5.74	N/A	80
63087	70.68	70.68	90	80
63088	7.76	7.76	N/A	80

Medicare References: None

63090-63091

63090 Vertebral corpectomy (vertebral body resection), partial or complete, transperitoneal or retroperitoneal approach with decompression of spinal cord, cauda equina or nerve root(s), lower thoracic, lumbar, or sacral; single segment

63091 each additional segment (List separately in addition to code for primary procedure)

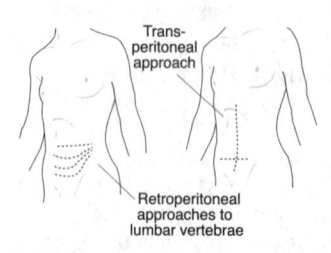

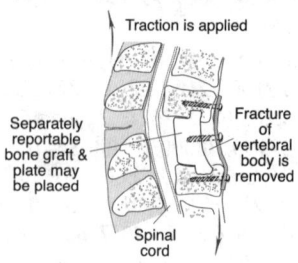

Explanation

The physician makes a transperitoneal or retroperitoneal approach through skin, fascia, muscles, and ligaments. The physician incises the anterior longitudinal ligament above and below the vertebral body. Using magnification, the physician removes the disc to the posterior longitudinal ligament using nipper instruments. The physician may use dowel or tricortical iliac grafts and prepares the site as appropriate using an osteotome. Usually three grafts can be inserted. They are tapped into place and surrounded with bone chips. The physician sutures the anterior longitudinal ligament. The peritoneum and abdomen are closed in the usual manner. Report 63090 for a single segment. Report 63091 for each additional segment.

Coding Tips

Use 63091 in conjunction with 63090. As an "add-on" code, 63091 is not subject to multiple procedure rules. No reimbursement reduction or modifier 51 is applied. Add-on codes describe additional intra-service work associated with the primary procedure. They are performed by the same physician on the same date of service as the primary service/procedure, and must never be reported as a stand-alone code. Diskectomy above and below the vertebral segment is included and should not be reported separately. Arthrodesis is reported separately; see 22554–22585. Any bone graft is also reported separately; see 20930–20938. Spinal instrumentation is reported separately; see 22840–22855. Report 69990 if the procedure is completed through an operating microscope. When two primary surgeons are required, a co-surgery scenario exists. Both surgeons report the primary procedure with modifier 62 and submit supporting documentation.

ICD-9-CM Procedural

- 03.09 Other exploration and decompression of spinal canal
- 03.59 Other repair and plastic operations on spinal cord structures

Anesthesia

63090 00620, 00630, 00670
63091 N/A

ICD-9-CM Diagnostic

- 170.2 Malignant neoplasm of vertebral column, excluding sacrum and coccyx
- 170.6 Malignant neoplasm of pelvic bones, sacrum, and coccyx
- 721.2 Thoracic spondylosis without myelopathy
- 721.3 Lumbosacral spondylosis without myelopathy
- 721.41 Spondylosis with myelopathy, thoracic region
- 722.10 Displacement of lumbar intervertebral disc without myelopathy
- 722.11 Displacement of thoracic intervertebral disc without myelopathy
- 722.51 Degeneration of thoracic or thoracolumbar intervertebral disc
- 722.52 Degeneration of lumbar or lumbosacral intervertebral disc
- 722.72 Intervertebral thoracic disc disorder with myelopathy, thoracic region
- 722.73 Intervertebral lumbar disc disorder with myelopathy, lumbar region
- 722.93 Other and unspecified disc disorder of lumbar region
- 724.02 Spinal stenosis of lumbar region, without neurogenic claudication
- 724.03 Spinal stenosis of lumbar region, with neurogenic claudication
- 724.4 Thoracic or lumbosacral neuritis or radiculitis, unspecified
- 724.6 Disorders of sacrum
- 730.28 Unspecified osteomyelitis, other specified sites — (Use additional code to identify organism: 041.1. Use additional code to identify major osseous defect, if applicable: 731.3)
- 738.4 Acquired spondylolisthesis
- 805.2 Closed fracture of dorsal (thoracic) vertebra without mention of spinal cord injury
- 805.3 Open fracture of dorsal (thoracic) vertebra without mention of spinal cord injury
- 805.4 Closed fracture of lumbar vertebra without mention of spinal cord injury
- 805.5 Open fracture of lumbar vertebra without mention of spinal cord injury
- 806.25 Closed fracture of T7-T12 level with unspecified spinal cord injury
- 806.35 Open fracture of T7-T12 level with unspecified spinal cord injury
- 806.4 Closed fracture of lumbar spine with spinal cord injury
- 806.5 Open fracture of lumbar spine with spinal cord injury

CCI Version 16.3

92585, 95822, 95860-95861, 95867-95868, 95900, 95904, 95920, 95936-95937

Also not with 63090: 0213T, 0216T, 0228T, 0230T, 22505, 22857❖, 22862❖, 22865❖, 36000, 36400-36410, 36420-36430, 36440, 36600, 36640, 37202, 43752, 49000-49002, 51701-51703, 62310-62319, 63075, 63077, 63170, 63707, 63709, 64400-64435, 64445-64450, 64479, 64483, 64490, 64493, 64505-64530, 76000-76001, 93000-93010, 93040-93042, 93318, 94002, 94200, 94250, 94680-94690, 94770, 95812-95816, 95819, 95829, 95870, 95925-95934, 95955, 96360, 96365, 96372, 96374-96376, 99148-99149, 99150

Also not with 63091: 95925-95927, 95930-95934

Note: These CCI edits are used for Medicare. Other payers may reimburse on codes listed above.

Medicare Edits

	Fac RVU	Non-Fac RVU	FUD	Assist
63090	58.07	58.07	90	80
63091	5.34	5.34	N/A	80

Medicare References: None

63101-63103

63101 Vertebral corpectomy (vertebral body resection), partial or complete, lateral extracavitary approach with decompression of spinal cord and/or nerve root(s) (eg, for tumor or retropulsed bone fragments); thoracic, single segment

63102 lumbar, single segment

63103 thoracic or lumbar, each additional segment (List separately in addition to code for primary procedure)

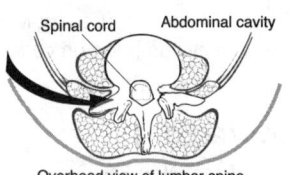

Overhead view of lumbar spine and surrounding muscles showing surgical approach

A vertebral body is resected, either in whole or in part, via a lateral extracavitary approach. The spinal cord is decompressed as part of the surgery. Report according to general area of the spine (thoracic or lumbar). Report 63103 for each additional segment

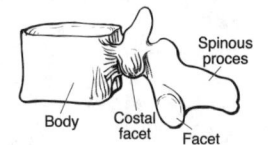

Lateral view of thoracic vertebra

Explanation

A vertebral corpectomy with correction of spinal cord or nerve root compression is done for fractures or tumors of the vertebrae. The body of the vertebra may be partially or completely resected. The lateral extracavitary approach is done with a midline incision made in the area of the fractured segment and inferiorly curved out to the lateral plane. The paraspinous muscles are exposed, lifted off the spinous processes, then divided and lifted off the ribs. The targeted vertebral body is identified. The corresponding ribs are dissected from the intercostal muscles and the pleura and resected in one piece from the posterior curve to the costovertebral connection. The appropriate transverse process and part of the facet and pedicle are removed with a drill from the lateral aspect. The dura and the vertebral body are now exposed from the dorsolateral view. Further posterior and lateral access to the vertebral body is gained by gently retracting the nerve root and surrounding structures. The central portion of the vertebral body is removed with a drill, exposing more area, and any bone fragments or tumor masses are carefully removed away from the spinal cord or nerve roots. Curettes and rongeurs are used to remove disc material. At this point, any necessary fusion, intervertebral reconstruction, or grafting is undertaken and reported separately. Cartilage is scraped, bone is decorticated, and an arthrodesis or reconstruction is accomplished by tapping bone graft material into the vertebral endplates. A drain is placed and closure is done in layers. Report 63101 for vertebral corpectomy by lateral extracavitary approach on a single thoracic segment, 63102 for a single lumbar segment, and 63103 for each additional thoracic or lumbar segment.

Coding Tips

Any vertebral corpectomy, bone graft, arthrodesis, or spinal instrumentation is reported separately.

ICD-9-CM Procedural

- **03.09** Other exploration and decompression of spinal canal
- **03.59** Other repair and plastic operations on spinal cord structures

Anesthesia
- **63101** 00620, 00670
- **63102** 00630, 00670
- **63103** N/A

ICD-9-CM Diagnostic

- **721.41** Spondylosis with myelopathy, thoracic region
- **722.10** Displacement of lumbar intervertebral disc without myelopathy
- **722.11** Displacement of thoracic intervertebral disc without myelopathy
- **722.51** Degeneration of thoracic or thoracolumbar intervertebral disc
- **722.52** Degeneration of lumbar or lumbosacral intervertebral disc
- **722.72** Intervertebral thoracic disc disorder with myelopathy, thoracic region
- **722.73** Intervertebral lumbar disc disorder with myelopathy, lumbar region
- **724.02** Spinal stenosis of lumbar region, without neurogenic claudication
- **724.03** Spinal stenosis of lumbar region, with neurogenic claudication
- **805.2** Closed fracture of dorsal (thoracic) vertebra without mention of spinal cord injury
- **805.3** Open fracture of dorsal (thoracic) vertebra without mention of spinal cord injury
- **805.4** Closed fracture of lumbar vertebra without mention of spinal cord injury
- **805.5** Open fracture of lumbar vertebra without mention of spinal cord injury
- **806.20** Closed fracture of T1-T6 level with unspecified spinal cord injury
- **806.25** Closed fracture of T7-T12 level with unspecified spinal cord injury
- **806.30** Open fracture of T1-T6 level with unspecified spinal cord injury
- **806.35** Open fracture of T7-T12 level with unspecified spinal cord injury
- **806.4** Closed fracture of lumbar spine with spinal cord injury
- **806.5** Open fracture of lumbar spine with spinal cord injury

CCI Version 16.3

92585, 95822, 95860-95861, 95867-95868, 95900, 95904, 95920, 95936-95937

Also not with 63101: 0213T, 0216T, 0228T, 0230T, 22112, 22505, 36000, 36400-36410, 36420-36430, 36440, 36600, 36640, 37202, 43752, 51701-51703, 62310-62319, 63055, 63085❖, 63090❖, 63301-63302❖, 63707, 63709, 64400-64435, 64445-64450, 64479, 64483, 64490, 64493, 64505-64530, 76000-76001, 93000-93010, 93040-93042, 93318, 94002, 94200, 94250, 94680-94690, 94770, 95812-95816, 95819, 95829, 95870, 95925-95934, 95955, 96360, 96365, 96372, 96374-96376, 99148-99149, 99150

Also not with 63102: 0213T, 0216T, 0228T, 0230T, 22114, 22505, 22630, 36000, 36400-36410, 36420-36430, 36440, 36600, 36640, 37202, 43752, 51701-51703, 62310-62319, 63056, 63090❖, 63303❖, 63307❖, 63707, 63709, 64400-64435, 64445-64450, 64479, 64483, 64490, 64493, 64505-64530, 76000-76001, 93000-93010, 93040-93042, 93318, 94002, 94200, 94250, 94680-94690, 94770, 95812-95816, 95819, 95829, 95870, 95925-95934, 95955, 96360, 96365, 96372, 96374-96376, 99148-99149, 99150

Also not with 63103: 95925-95927, 95930-95934

Note: These CCI edits are used for Medicare. Other payers may reimburse on codes listed above.

Medicare Edits

	Fac RVU	Non-Fac RVU	FUD	Assist
63101	68.44	68.44	90	80
63102	66.08	66.08	90	80
63103	8.78	8.78	N/A	80

Medicare References: None

63170

63170 Laminectomy with myelotomy (eg, Bischof or DREZ type), cervical, thoracic, or thoracolumbar

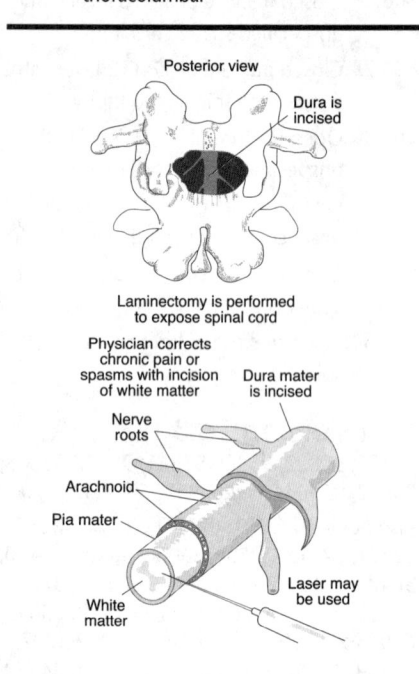

Explanation

This procedure is performed to alleviate peripheral pain caused by avulsion of parts of the spinal cord's white matter. The patient is placed prone. The physician makes an incision. The fascia are incised. The paravertebral muscles and ligaments are retracted. Following a laminectomy, the physician incises the dura to gain access to the spinal cord. Without disturbing the central gray matter, the physician incises the outer white matter of the spinal cord, using a laser or a radio frequency electrode to thermally coagulate the white matter. Fascia, muscles, and ligaments are allowed to fall back into place. The physician closes the incision with layered sutures.

Coding Tips

If the procedure is completed through an operating microscope, list 69990 in addition to 63170.

ICD-9-CM Procedural

- 03.09 Other exploration and decompression of spinal canal
- 03.29 Other chordotomy

Anesthesia

63170 00600, 00604, 00620, 00630, 00670

ICD-9-CM Diagnostic

- 336.0 Syringomyelia and syringobulbia
- 353.6 Phantom limb (syndrome)
- 724.1 Pain in thoracic spine
- 724.2 Lumbago
- 724.4 Thoracic or lumbosacral neuritis or radiculitis, unspecified
- 724.5 Unspecified backache
- 741.01 Spina bifida with hydrocephalus, cervical region
- 741.02 Spina bifida with hydrocephalus, dorsal (thoracic) region
- 741.03 Spina bifida with hydrocephalus, lumbar region
- 741.91 Spina bifida without mention of hydrocephalus, cervical region
- 741.92 Spina bifida without mention of hydrocephalus, dorsal (thoracic) region
- 741.93 Spina bifida without mention of hydrocephalus, lumbar region

Terms To Know

gray matter. Gray nervous tissue, made up of demyelinated nerve fibers, supportive tissue, and nerve cell bodies.

lumbago. Low back pain.

neuritis. Inflammation of a nerve or group of nerves, often manifested by loss of function and reflexes, pain, and numbness or tingling.

peripheral. Outside of a structure or organ.

phantom limb syndrome. Itching, dull ache, or sharp, shooting pains mimicking the nerves of amputated limb.

prone. Lying face downward.

spina bifida cystica. Defective closure of the spinal column during early fetal development with a protrusion or herniation of the cord and meninges through the defect.

CCI Version 16.3

0171T❖, 0213T, 0216T, 0228T, 0230T, 20926, 22505, 36000, 36400-36410, 36420-36430, 36440, 36600, 36640, 37202, 43752, 49000-49002, 51701-51703, 62310-62319, 63707, 63709, 64400-64435, 64445-64450, 64479, 64483, 64490, 64493, 64505-64530, 76000-76001, 92585, 93000-93010, 93040-93042, 93318, 94002, 94200, 94250, 94680-94690, 94770, 95812-95816, 95819, 95822, 95829, 95860-95861, 95867-95868, 95870, 95900, 95904, 95920, 95925-95934, 95936-95937, 95955, 96360, 96365, 96372, 96374-96376, 99148-99149, 99150

Note: These CCI edits are used for Medicare. Other payers may reimburse on codes listed above.

Medicare Edits

	Fac RVU	Non-Fac RVU	FUD	Assist
63170	46.42	46.42	90	80

Medicare References: None

63172-63173

63172 Laminectomy with drainage of intramedullary cyst/syrinx; to subarachnoid space
63173 to peritoneal or pleural space

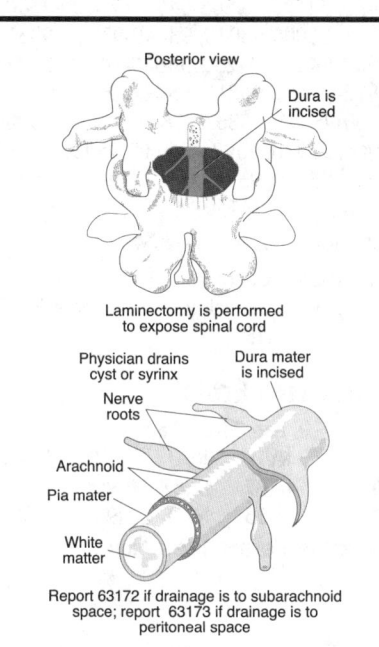

Report 63172 if drainage is to subarachnoid space; report 63173 if drainage is to peritoneal space

Explanation

This procedure is performed to alleviate the effects of a spinal cyst or syrinx. The patient is face down. The physician makes a midline incision overlying the affected vertebrae. The fascia are incised. The paravertebral muscles are retracted. Laminectomy is performed. The spinal needle is placed in the intramedullary cyst or syrinx, and the cyst or syrinx is drained to the subarachnoid space. Fascia, muscles, and ligaments are allowed to fall back into place. The incision is closed with layered sutures. Report 63172 if the drainage is to the subarachnoid space. Report 63173 if the drainage is to the peritoneal or pleural space.

Coding Tips

If the procedure is completed through an operating microscope, list 69990 in addition to 63172 or 63173. For percutaneous aspiration, spinal cord cyst or syrinx, see 62268.

ICD-9-CM Procedural

- 03.09 Other exploration and decompression of spinal canal
- 03.79 Other shunt of spinal theca

Anesthesia
00670

ICD-9-CM Diagnostic

- 336.0 Syringomyelia and syringobulbia
- 349.2 Disorders of meninges, not elsewhere classified

Terms To Know

cyst. Elevated encapsulated mass containing fluid, semisolid, or solid material with a membranous lining.

decompression. Release of pressure.

drain. Device that creates a channel to allow fluid from a cavity, wound, or infected area to exit the body.

dura mater. Outermost, hard, fibrous layer or membrane that surrounds the brain and spinal cord.

fascia. Fibrous sheet or band of tissue that envelops organs, muscles, and groupings of muscles.

laminectomy. Removal or excision of the posterior arch of a vertebra to provide additional space for the nerves and widen the spinal canal.

ligament. Band or sheet of fibrous tissue that connects the articular surfaces of bones or supports visceral organs.

meninges. Tough membranous protectors of the central nervous system that cover the brain and spinal cord comprising three layers: the dura mater, arachnoid mater, and pia mater.

peritoneal cavity. Space between the lining of the abdominal wall, or parietal peritoneum, and the surface layer of the abdominal organs, or visceral peritoneum. It contains a thin, watery fluid that keeps the peritoneal surfaces moist.

prone. Lying face downward.

subarachnoid. Located below the arachnoid meningeal layer.

CCI Version 16.3

0213T, 0216T, 0228T, 0230T, 20926, 22505, 36000, 36400-36410, 36420-36430, 36440, 36600, 36640, 37202, 43752, 49000-49002, 51701-51703, 62310-62319, 63707, 63709, 64400-64435, 64445-64450, 64479, 64483, 64490, 64493, 64505-64530, 76000-76001, 92585, 93000-93010, 93040-93042, 93318, 94002, 94200, 94250, 94680-94690, 94770, 95812-95816, 95819, 95822, 95829, 95860-95861, 95867-95868, 95870, 95900, 95904, 95920, 95925-95934, 95936-95937, 95955, 96360, 96365, 96372, 96374-96376, 99148-99149, 99150

Also not with 63172: 63173❖

Also not with 63173: 32095-32100, 32421-32422, 32551

Note: These CCI edits are used for Medicare. Other payers may reimburse on codes listed above.

Medicare Edits

	Fac RVU	Non-Fac RVU	FUD	Assist
63172	41.32	41.32	90	80
63173	50.77	50.77	90	80

Medicare References: None

63180-63182

63180 Laminectomy and section of dentate ligaments, with or without dural graft, cervical; 1 or 2 segments
63182 more than 2 segments

Explanation
The patient is face down. The physician makes a midline incision overlying the affected vertebrae. The fascia are incised. The paravertebral muscles are retracted. The physician incises the dura and locates the dentate ligaments. With the aid of magnification, the physician sections the affected ligaments. The dura is closed with sutures or a graft to assure competency. The incision is closed with layered sutures. Report 63180 if the one or two vertebra is affected; report 63182 if more than two vertebrae are affected.

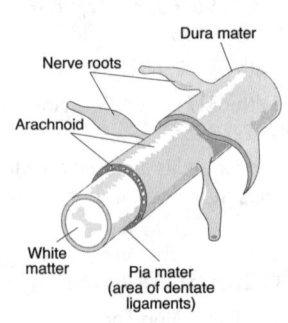

Coding Tips
If the procedure is completed through an operating microscope, list 69990 in addition to 63180 or 63182. For spinal dural graft, without laminectomy and section of the dentate ligaments, see 63710.

ICD-9-CM Procedural
03.09 Other exploration and decompression of spinal canal

Anesthesia
63180 00600, 00604, 00670
63182 00600

ICD-9-CM Diagnostic
353.2 Cervical root lesions, not elsewhere classified
354.5 Mononeuritis multiplex
723.1 Cervicalgia
723.4 Brachial neuritis or radiculitis nos.

Terms To Know

cervicalgia. Pain localized to the cervical region, generally referring to the posterior or lateral regions of the neck.

dura mater. Outermost, hard, fibrous layer or membrane that surrounds the brain and spinal cord.

fascia. Fibrous sheet or band of tissue that envelops organs, muscles, and groupings of muscles.

laminectomy. Removal or excision of the posterior arch of a vertebra to provide additional space for the nerves and widen the spinal canal.

lesion. Area of damaged tissue that has lost continuity or function, due to disease or trauma. Lesions may be located on internal structures such as the brain, nerves, or kidneys, or visible on the skin.

ligament. Band or sheet of fibrous tissue that connects the articular surfaces of bones or supports visceral organs.

mononeuritis multiplex. Peripheral neuropathy involving isolated damage to at least two separate nerves.

neuritis. Inflammation of a nerve or group of nerves, often manifested by loss of function and reflexes, pain, and numbness or tingling.

operating microscope. Compound microscope with two or more lens systems or several grouped lenses in one unit that provides magnifying power to the surgeon up to 40X.

prone. Lying face downward.

radiculitis. Pain along an inflamed nerve, with inflammation of the root of the associated spinal nerve.

CCI Version 16.3
0213T, 0216T, 0228T, 0230T, 20926, 22505, 36000, 36400-36410, 36420-36430, 36440, 36600, 36640, 37202, 43752, 51701-51703, 62310-62319, 63707, 63709-63710, 64400-64435, 64445-64450, 64479, 64483, 64490, 64493, 64505-64530, 76000-76001, 92585, 93000-93010, 93040-93042, 93318, 94002, 94200, 94250, 94680-94690, 94770, 95812-95816, 95819, 95822, 95829, 95860-95861, 95867-95868, 95870, 95900, 95904, 95920, 95925-95934, 95936-95937, 95955, 96360, 96365, 96372, 96374-96376, 99148-99149, 99150

Also not with 63180: 63182❖

Note: These CCI edits are used for Medicare. Other payers may reimburse on codes listed above.

Medicare Edits

	Fac RVU	Non-Fac RVU	FUD	Assist
63180	42.87	42.87	90	80
63182	46.15	46.15	90	80

Medicare References: None

63185-63190

63185 Laminectomy with rhizotomy; 1 or 2 segments
63190 more than 2 segments

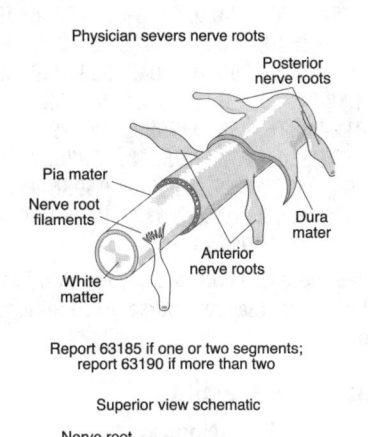

Explanation
A rhizotomy is performed on the anterior nerve roots to stop involuntary spasmodic movements associated with paraplegia or torticollis. It is also performed on the posterior nerve roots to eliminate pain in a restricted area. The patient is face down. The physician makes a midline incision overlying the affected vertebrae. The fascia are incised. The paravertebral muscles are retracted. Laminectomy is performed. The physician identifies the anterior or posterior nerve roots to be divided. Each is lifted with a nerve hook and severed. Fascia, muscles, and ligaments are allowed to fall back into place. The incision is closed with layered sutures. Report 63185 if the procedure includes one or two segments; report 63190 if the procedure includes two or more segments.

Coding Tips
If the procedure is completed through an operating microscope, list 69990 in addition to 63185 or 63190.

ICD-9-CM Procedural
03.09 Other exploration and decompression of spinal canal
03.1   Division of intraspinal nerve root

Anesthesia
00620, 00630, 00670

ICD-9-CM Diagnostic
343.9   Unspecified infantile cerebral palsy
720.2   Sacroiliitis, not elsewhere classified
723.1   Cervicalgia
723.4   Brachial neuritis or radiculitis nos.
724.1   Pain in thoracic spine
724.2   Lumbago
724.3   Sciatica
724.4   Thoracic or lumbosacral neuritis or radiculitis, unspecified
724.6   Disorders of sacrum
729.1   Unspecified myalgia and myositis
729.2   Unspecified neuralgia, neuritis, and radiculitis
729.5   Pain in soft tissues of limb
786.52 Painful respiration

Terms To Know

anterior. Situated in the front area or toward the belly surface of the body; an anatomical reference point used to show the position and relationship of one body structure to another.

cerebral palsy. Brain damage occurring before, during, or shortly after birth that impedes muscle control and tone.

cervicalgia. Pain localized to the cervical region, generally referring to the posterior or lateral regions of the neck.

fascia. Fibrous sheet or band of tissue that envelops organs, muscles, and groupings of muscles.

lumbago. Low back pain.

neuritis. Inflammation of a nerve or group of nerves, often manifested by loss of function and reflexes, pain, and numbness or tingling.

prone. Lying face downward.

radiculitis. Pain along an inflamed nerve, with inflammation of the root of the associated spinal nerve.

torticollis. Twisted, unnatural position of the neck due to contracted cervical muscles that pull the head to one side.

CCI Version 16.3
0171T❖, 0213T, 0216T, 0228T, 0230T, 20926, 22505, 36000, 36400-36410, 36420-36430, 36440, 36600, 36640, 37202, 43752, 49000-49002, 51701-51703, 62310-62319, 63707, 63709, 64400-64435, 64445-64450, 64479, 64483, 64490, 64493, 64505-64530, 76000-76001, 92585, 93000-93010, 93040-93042, 93318, 94002, 94200, 94250, 94680-94690, 94770, 95812-95816, 95819, 95822, 95829, 95860-95861, 95867-95868, 95870, 95900, 95904, 95920, 95925-95934, 95936-95937, 95955, 96360, 96365, 96372, 96374-96376, 99148-99149, 99150

Also not with 63185: 63190❖

Note: These CCI edits are used for Medicare. Other payers may reimburse on codes listed above.

Medicare Edits

	Fac RVU	Non-Fac RVU	FUD	Assist
63185	34.86	34.86	90	80
63190	37.28	37.28	90	80

Medicare References: None

63191

63191 Laminectomy with section of spinal accessory nerve

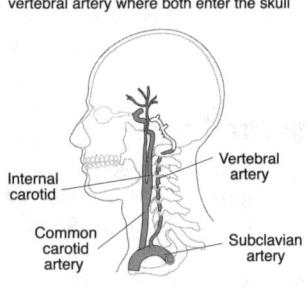

Explanation
This procedure is performed to alleviate chronic pain. The patient is face down. The physician makes a midline incision overlying the affected vertebrae. The fascia are incised. The paravertebral muscles are retracted. The physician removes the lamina. The physician identifies and incises the spinal accessory nerve. The lesion is removed and sutures are placed in the perineurium of the nerves. The sutures are approximated and tied. Fascia, muscles, and ligaments are allowed to fall back into place. The incision is closed with layered sutures.

Coding Tips
If the procedure is completed through an operating microscope, list 69990 in addition to 63191. This is a unilateral procedure. If performed bilaterally, some payers require that the service be reported twice with modifier 50 appended to the second code, while others require identification of the service only once with modifier 50 appended. Check with individual payers. Modifier 50 identifies a procedure performed identically on the opposite side of the body (mirror image). For resection of the sternocleidomastoid muscle, see 21720.

ICD-9-CM Procedural
- 03.09 Other exploration and decompression of spinal canal
- 03.59 Other repair and plastic operations on spinal cord structures
- 04.04 Other incision of cranial and peripheral nerves

Anesthesia
63191 00600, 00670

ICD-9-CM Diagnostic
- 334.1 Hereditary spastic paraplegia
- 343.0 Diplegic infantile cerebral palsy
- 343.8 Other specified infantile cerebral palsy
- 343.9 Unspecified infantile cerebral palsy
- 724.1 Pain in thoracic spine
- 724.3 Sciatica
- 724.4 Thoracic or lumbosacral neuritis or radiculitis, unspecified
- 724.6 Disorders of sacrum
- 729.1 Unspecified myalgia and myositis
- 729.2 Unspecified neuralgia, neuritis, and radiculitis
- 739.4 Nonallopathic lesion of sacral region, not elsewhere classified
- 781.0 Abnormal involuntary movements
- 786.52 Painful respiration

Terms To Know
cerebral palsy. Brain damage occurring before, during, or shortly after birth that impedes muscle control and tone.

fascia. Fibrous sheet or band of tissue that envelops organs, muscles, and groupings of muscles.

lesion. Area of damaged tissue that has lost continuity or function, due to disease or trauma. Lesions may be located on internal structures such as the brain, nerves, or kidneys, or visible on the skin.

neuritis. Inflammation of a nerve or group of nerves, often manifested by loss of function and reflexes, pain, and numbness or tingling.

prone. Lying face downward.

radiculitis. Pain along an inflamed nerve, with inflammation of the root of the associated spinal nerve.

spasmodic torticollis. Neck muscle spasms and cervical dystonia, resulting in the head becoming inclined toward the affected side and the face toward the opposite side.

CCI Version 16.3
0171T✢, 0213T, 0216T, 0228T, 0230T, 20926, 22505, 36000, 36400-36410, 36420-36430, 36440, 36600, 36640, 37202, 43752, 49000-49002, 51701-51703, 62310-62319, 63707, 63709, 64400-64435, 64445-64450, 64479, 64483, 64490, 64493, 64505-64530, 76000-76001, 92585, 93000-93010, 93040-93042, 93318, 94002, 94200, 94250, 94680-94690, 94770, 95812-95816, 95819, 95822, 95829, 95860-95861, 95867-95868, 95870, 95900, 95904, 95920, 95925-95934, 95936-95937, 95955, 96360, 96365, 96372, 96374-96376, 99148-99149, 99150

Note: These CCI edits are used for Medicare. Other payers may reimburse on codes listed above.

Medicare Edits

	Fac RVU	Non-Fac RVU	FUD	Assist
63191	34.88	34.88	90	80

Medicare References: None

63194-63195

63194 Laminectomy with cordotomy, with section of 1 spinothalamic tract, 1 stage; cervical
63195 thoracic

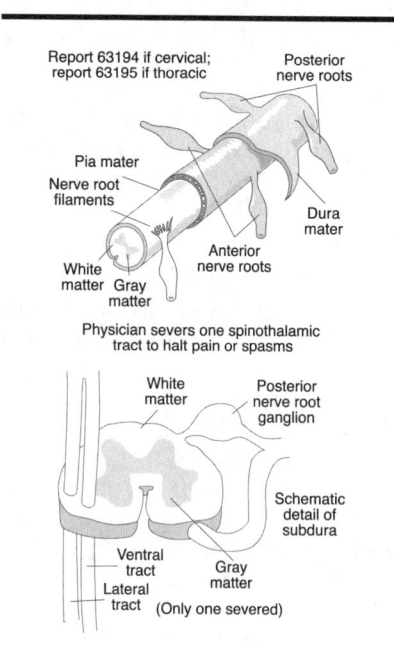

ICD-9-CM Procedural
- 03.09 Other exploration and decompression of spinal canal
- 03.29 Other chordotomy

Anesthesia
- **63194** 00600, 00604, 00670
- **63195** 00620, 00670

ICD-9-CM Diagnostic
- 334.1 Hereditary spastic paraplegia
- 343.0 Diplegic infantile cerebral palsy
- 343.8 Other specified infantile cerebral palsy
- 343.9 Unspecified infantile cerebral palsy
- 724.1 Pain in thoracic spine
- 724.4 Thoracic or lumbosacral neuritis or radiculitis, unspecified
- 729.1 Unspecified myalgia and myositis
- 729.2 Unspecified neuralgia, neuritis, and radiculitis
- 781.0 Abnormal involuntary movements
- 781.7 Tetany

CCI Version 16.3
0213T, 0216T, 0228T, 0230T, 20926, 22505, 36000, 36400-36410, 36420-36430, 36440, 36600, 36640, 37202, 43752, 51701-51703, 62310-62319, 63707, 63709, 64400-64435, 64445-64450, 64479, 64483, 64490, 64493, 64505-64530, 76000-76001, 92585, 93000-93010, 93040-93042, 93318, 94002, 94200, 94250, 94680-94690, 94770, 95812-95816, 95819, 95822, 95829, 95860-95861, 95867-95868, 95870, 95900, 95904, 95920, 95925-95934, 95936-95937, 95955, 96360, 96365, 96372, 96374-96376, 99148-99149, 99150

Note: These CCI edits are used for Medicare. Other payers may reimburse on codes listed above.

Medicare Edits

	Fac RVU	Non-Fac RVU	FUD	Assist
63194	40.37	40.37	90	80
63195	44.93	44.93	90	80

Medicare References: None

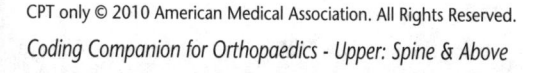

Explanation
This procedure is performed to alleviate pain. The patient is face down. The physician makes a midline incision overlying the affected vertebrae. The fascia are incised. The paravertebral muscles are retracted. A laminectomy is performed. The physician identifies the anterolateral tracts in the appropriate level on the side opposite the pain. The dentate ligament is divided at the level of the cordotomy. The ligament is drawn posteriorly toward the midline to expose the anterolateral part of the cord. A cordotomy knife is introduced into the spinal cord anterior to the dentate ligament and directed toward the anterior spinal artery. The tissue in front of this artery is divided with the knife. The incision is closed with layered sutures. Report 63194 if the affected vertebrae are cervical; report 63195 if the affected vertebrae are thoracic.

Coding Tips
If the procedure is completed through an operating microscope, list 69990 in addition to 63194 or 63195. For laminectomy with cordotomy, with section of both spinothalamic tracts, one stage, cervical, see 63196; thoracic, see 63197. For laminectomy with cordotomy, with section of both spinothalamic tracts, two stages within 14 days, cervical, see 63198; thoracic, see 63199.

Terms To Know
anterior. Situated in the front area or toward the belly surface of the body; an anatomical reference point used to show the position and relationship of one body structure to another.

cerebral palsy. Brain damage occurring before, during, or shortly after birth that impedes muscle control and tone.

fascia. Fibrous sheet or band of tissue that envelops organs, muscles, and groupings of muscles.

ligament. Band or sheet of fibrous tissue that connects the articular surfaces of bones or supports visceral organs.

neuralgia. Sharp, shooting pains extending along one or more nerve pathways. Underlying causes may include nerve injury, diabetes, or viral complications.

neuritis. Inflammation of a nerve or group of nerves, often manifested by loss of function and reflexes, pain, and numbness or tingling.

prone. Lying face downward.

radiculitis. Pain along an inflamed nerve, with inflammation of the root of the associated spinal nerve.

spasmodic torticollis. Neck muscle spasms and cervical dystonia, resulting in the head becoming inclined toward the affected side and the face toward the opposite side.

63196-63197

63196 Laminectomy with cordotomy, with section of both spinothalamic tracts, 1 stage; cervical
63197 thoracic

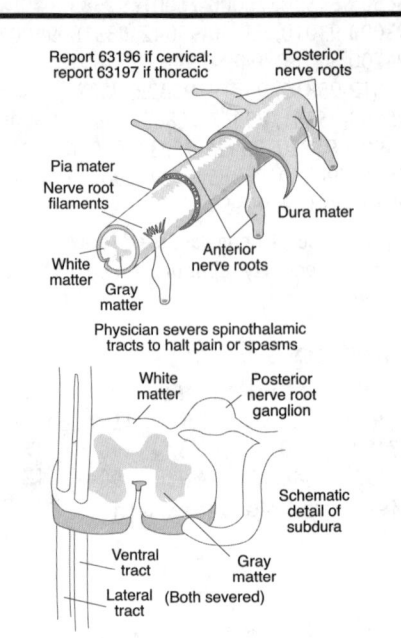

Explanation

This procedure is performed to alleviate pain. The patient is face down. The physician makes a midline incision overlying the site of the cordotomy. The fascia are incised. The paravertebral muscles are retracted. A laminectomy is performed. The physician identifies the spinothalamic tracts in the appropriate levels. The dentate ligament is divided at the level of the cordotomy. The ligament is drawn posteriorly toward the midline to expose the anterolateral part of the cord. A cordotomy knife is introduced into the spinal cord anterior to the dentate ligament and directed toward the anterior spinal artery. The tissue in front of this artery is divided with the knife. The incision is closed with layered sutures. Report 63196 if the affected vertebrae are cervical; report 63197 if the affected vertebrae are thoracic.

Coding Tips

If the procedure is completed through an operating microscope, list 69990 in addition to 63196 or 63197. For laminectomy with cordotomy, with section of one spinothalamic tract, one stage, cervical, see 63194; thoracic, see 63195. For laminectomy with cordotomy, with section of both spinothalamic tracts, two stages within 14 days, cervical, see 63198; thoracic, see 63199.

ICD-9-CM Procedural
- 03.09 Other exploration and decompression of spinal canal
- 03.29 Other chordotomy

Anesthesia
63196 00600, 00604, 00670
63197 00620, 00670

ICD-9-CM Diagnostic
- 334.1 Hereditary spastic paraplegia
- 343.0 Diplegic infantile cerebral palsy
- 343.8 Other specified infantile cerebral palsy
- 343.9 Unspecified infantile cerebral palsy
- 724.1 Pain in thoracic spine
- 724.4 Thoracic or lumbosacral neuritis or radiculitis, unspecified
- 729.1 Unspecified myalgia and myositis
- 729.2 Unspecified neuralgia, neuritis, and radiculitis
- 781.0 Abnormal involuntary movements
- 781.7 Tetany

Terms To Know

cerebral palsy. Brain damage occurring before, during, or shortly after birth that impedes muscle control and tone.

fascia. Fibrous sheet or band of tissue that envelops organs, muscles, and groupings of muscles.

neuralgia. Sharp, shooting pains extending along one or more nerve pathways. Underlying causes may include nerve injury, diabetes, or viral complications.

neuritis. Inflammation of a nerve or group of nerves, often manifested by loss of function and reflexes, pain, and numbness or tingling.

prone. Lying face downward.

radiculitis. Pain along an inflamed nerve, with inflammation of the root of the associated spinal nerve.

spasmodic torticollis. Neck muscle spasms and cervical dystonia, resulting in the head becoming inclined toward the affected side and the face toward the opposite side.

CCI Version 16.3

0213T, 0216T, 0228T, 0230T, 20926, 22505, 36000, 36400-36410, 36420-36430, 36440, 36600, 36640, 37202, 43752, 51701-51703, 62310-62319, 63707, 63709, 64400-64435, 64445-64450, 64479, 64483, 64490, 64493, 64505-64530, 76000-76001, 92585, 93000-93010, 93040-93042, 93318, 94002, 94200, 94250, 94680-94690, 94770, 95812-95816, 95819, 95822, 95829, 95860-95861, 95867-95868, 95870, 95900, 95904, 95920, 95925-95934, 95936-95937, 95955, 96360, 96365, 96372, 96374-96376, 99148-99149, 99150

Also not with 63196: 63194
Also not with 63197: 63195

Note: These CCI edits are used for Medicare. Other payers may reimburse on codes listed above.

Medicare Edits

	Fac RVU	Non-Fac RVU	FUD	Assist
63196	42.36	42.36	90	80
63197	50.25	50.25	90	80

Medicare References: None

63198-63199

63198 Laminectomy with cordotomy with section of both spinothalamic tracts, 2 stages within 14 days; cervical
63199 thoracic

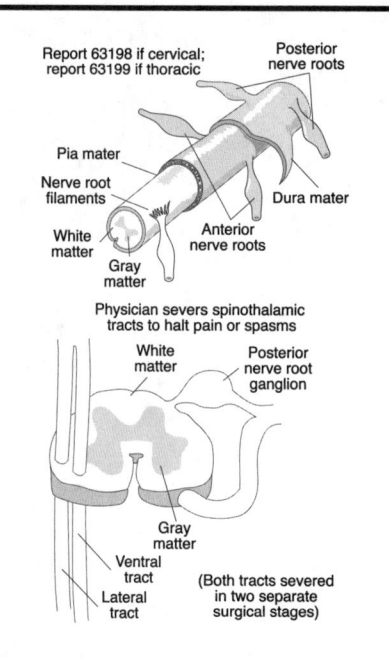

Explanation
This procedure is performed to stop chronic pain or spasms. The patient is face down. The physician makes a midline incision overlying the affected vertebrae. The fascia are incised. The paravertebral muscles are retracted. The physician identifies the spinothalamic tracts in the appropriate level. The dentate ligament is divided at the level of the cordotomy. The ligament is drawn posteriorly toward the midline to expose the anterolateral part of the cord. A cordotomy knife is introduced into the spinal cord anterior to the dentate ligament and directed toward the anterior spinal artery. The tissue in front of this artery is divided with the knife. Muscles, fascia, and ligaments are allowed to fall back into place. The incision is closed with layered sutures. The procedure is performed on the opposite side of the spinal cord within 14 days. Report 63198 if the cervical vertebrae are affected; report 63199 if the thoracic vertebrae are affected.

Coding Tips
If the procedure is completed through an operating microscope, list 69990 in addition to 63198 or 63199. For laminectomy with cordotomy, with section of spinothalamic tract, one stage, cervical, see 63194; with section of both spinothalamic tract, cervical, see 63196. For laminectomy with cordotomy, with section of one spinothalamic tract, one stage, thoracic, see 63195; with section of both spinothalamic tracts, see 63197.

ICD-9-CM Procedural
03.09 Other exploration and decompression of spinal canal
03.29 Other chordotomy

Anesthesia
63198 00600, 00604, 00670
63199 00620, 00670

ICD-9-CM Diagnostic
334.1 Hereditary spastic paraplegia
343.0 Diplegic infantile cerebral palsy
343.8 Other specified infantile cerebral palsy
343.9 Unspecified infantile cerebral palsy
724.1 Pain in thoracic spine
724.4 Thoracic or lumbosacral neuritis or radiculitis, unspecified
729.1 Unspecified myalgia and myositis
729.2 Unspecified neuralgia, neuritis, and radiculitis
781.0 Abnormal involuntary movements
781.7 Tetany

Terms To Know
cerebral palsy. Brain damage occurring before, during, or shortly after birth that impedes muscle control and tone.

chronic. Persistent, continuing, or recurring.

fascia. Fibrous sheet or band of tissue that envelops organs, muscles, and groupings of muscles.

myositis. Inflammation of a muscle with voluntary movement.

neuralgia. Sharp, shooting pains extending along one or more nerve pathways. Underlying causes may include nerve injury, diabetes, or viral complications.

neuritis. Inflammation of a nerve or group of nerves, often manifested by loss of function and reflexes, pain, and numbness or tingling.

radiculitis. Pain along an inflamed nerve, with inflammation of the root of the associated spinal nerve.

spasm. Involuntary muscle contraction.

spasmodic torticollis. Neck muscle spasms and cervical dystonia, resulting in the head becoming inclined toward the affected side and the face toward the opposite side.

CCI Version 16.3
0213T, 0216T, 0228T, 0230T, 20926, 22505, 36000, 36400-36410, 36420-36430, 36440, 36600, 36640, 37202, 43752, 51701-51703, 62310-62319, 63707, 63709, 64400-64435, 64445-64450, 64479, 64483, 64490, 64493, 64505-64530, 76000-76001, 92585, 93000-93010, 93040-93042, 93318, 94002, 94200, 94250, 94680-94690, 94770, 95812-95816, 95819, 95822, 95829, 95860-95861, 95867-95868, 95870, 95900, 95904, 95920, 95925-95934, 95936-95937, 95955, 96360, 96365, 96372, 96374-96376, 99148-99149, 99150

Also not with 63198: 63194, 63196
Also not with 63199: 63195, 63197

Note: These CCI edits are used for Medicare. Other payers may reimburse on codes listed above.

Medicare Edits

	Fac RVU	Non-Fac RVU	FUD	Assist
63198	46.86	46.86	90	80
63199	51.66	51.66	90	80

Medicare References: None

63295

63295 Osteoplastic reconstruction of dorsal spinal elements, following primary intraspinal procedure (List separately in addition to code for primary procedure)

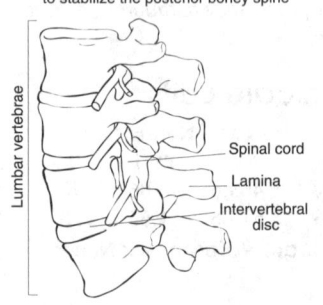

Explanation

The physician performs an osteoplastic reconstruction of the dorsal spine elements at the time of a separate intraspinal procedure. Osteoplastic reconstruction is performed to stabilize elements in the spine that have been damaged by benign or malignant lesions or by disease processes. Following the intraspinal procedure, the dura is closed. Dorsal spinal elements including laminae, spinous processes and supporting ligaments are replaced in anatomic position in the spine. Holes are drilled into the lateral aspect of each lamina and the dorsal spine elements are secured in place using sutures, wires, or miniplates.

Coding Tips

As an "add-on" code, 63295 is not subject to multiple procedure rules. No reimbursement reduction or modifier 51 is applied. Add-on codes describe additional intra-service work associated with the primary procedure. They are performed by the same physician on the same date of service as the primary service/procedure, and must never be reported as a stand-alone code. Use 63295 in conjunction with 63172, 63173, 63185, 63190, 63200–63290. Do not report 63295 in conjunction with 22590–22614, 22840–22844, 63050, 63051 for the same vertebral segment(s).

ICD-9-CM Procedural

03.59 Other repair and plastic operations on spinal cord structures

Anesthesia

63295 N/A

ICD-9-CM Diagnostic

This is an add-on code. Refer to the corresponding primary procedure code for ICD-9-CM diagnosis code links.

Terms To Know

benign. Mild or nonmalignant in nature.

malignant. Any condition tending to progress toward death, specifically an invasive tumor with a loss of cellular differentiation that has the ability to spread or metastasize to other areas in the body.

reconstruction. Recreating, restoring, or rebuilding a body part or organ.

CCI Version 16.3

No CCI Edits apply to this code.

Medicare Edits

	Fac RVU	Non-Fac RVU	FUD	Assist
63295	9.86	9.86	N/A	80

Medicare References: None

63300

63300 Vertebral corpectomy (vertebral body resection), partial or complete, for excision of intraspinal lesion, single segment; extradural, cervical

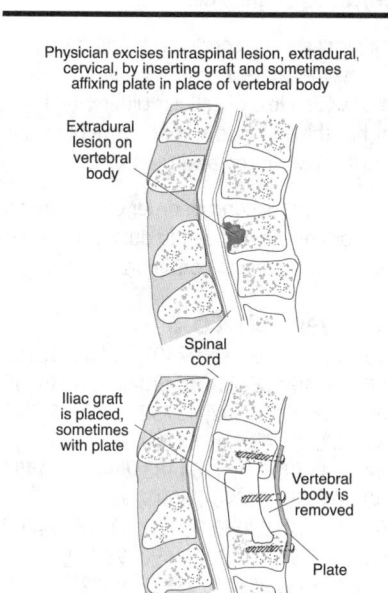

Physician excises intraspinal lesion, extradural, cervical, by inserting graft and sometimes affixing plate in place of vertebral body

Lateral cutaway views

Explanation

This procedure is performed to remove an intraspinal lesion in the extradural space of the spinal canal. The patient is placed supine with the head extended by tongs and traction. Either a right transverse incision or right vertical incision is made in the lateral neck. The muscles and fascia are incised and retracted. Entering between the trachea and the carotid sheath, the physician resects the vertebral body and the intraspinal lesion is excised by the physician. After repair of the muscles, fascia, and ligaments, the wound is closed with layered sutures.

Coding Tips

Note that 63300 reports anterior or anterolateral vertebral corpectomy, extradural, cervical, for excision of an intraspinal lesion of one vertebral segment. Report 63308 for each additional segment. If the procedure is completed through an operating microscope, list 69990 in addition to 63300. Arthrodesis is reported separately; see 22554–22585. Bone graft is reported separately; see 20930–20938. For vertebral corpectomy for decompression, see 63085–63091.

ICD-9-CM Procedural

- 03.39 Other diagnostic procedures on spinal cord and spinal canal structures
- 03.4 Excision or destruction of lesion of spinal cord or spinal meninges
- 03.6 Lysis of adhesions of spinal cord and nerve roots

Anesthesia

63300 00600, 00670

ICD-9-CM Diagnostic

- 192.2 Malignant neoplasm of spinal cord
- 192.3 Malignant neoplasm of spinal meninges
- 198.3 Secondary malignant neoplasm of brain and spinal cord
- 199.0 Disseminated malignant neoplasm
- 225.3 Benign neoplasm of spinal cord
- 225.4 Benign neoplasm of spinal meninges
- 237.5 Neoplasm of uncertain behavior of brain and spinal cord
- 237.6 Neoplasm of uncertain behavior of meninges
- 239.7 Neoplasm of unspecified nature of endocrine glands and other parts of nervous system
- 324.1 Intraspinal abscess
- 336.1 Vascular myelopathies

Terms To Know

abscess. Circumscribed collection of pus resulting from bacteria, frequently associated with swelling and other signs of inflammation.

adhesion. Abnormal fibrous connection between two structures, soft tissue or bony structures, that may occur as the result of surgery, infection, or trauma.

benign. Mild or nonmalignant in nature.

disseminated. Spread over an extensive area.

fascia. Fibrous sheet or band of tissue that envelops organs, muscles, and groupings of muscles.

lesion. Area of damaged tissue that has lost continuity or function, due to disease or trauma. Lesions may be located on internal structures such as the brain, nerves, or kidneys, or visible on the skin.

malignant. Any condition tending to progress toward death, specifically an invasive tumor with a loss of cellular differentiation that has the ability to spread or metastasize to other areas in the body.

secondary. Second in order of occurrence or importance, or appearing during the course of another disease or condition.

supine. Lying on the back.

CCI Version 16.3

0213T, 0216T, 0228T, 0230T, 22505, 36000, 36400-36410, 36420-36430, 36440, 36600, 36640, 37202, 43752, 51701-51703, 62310-62319, 63707, 63709, 64400-64435, 64445-64450, 64479, 64483, 64490, 64493, 64505-64530, 76000-76001, 92585, 93000-93010, 93040-93042, 93318, 94002, 94200, 94250, 94680-94690, 94770, 95812-95816, 95819, 95822, 95829, 95860-95861, 95867-95868, 95870, 95900, 95904, 95920, 95925-95934, 95936-95937, 95955, 96360, 96365, 96372, 96374-96376, 99148-99149, 99150

Note: These CCI edits are used for Medicare. Other payers may reimburse on codes listed above.

Medicare Edits

	Fac RVU	Non-Fac RVU	FUD	Assist
63300	53.97	53.97	90	80

Medicare References: None

63301

63301 Vertebral corpectomy (vertebral body resection), partial or complete, for excision of intraspinal lesion, single segment; extradural, thoracic by transthoracic approach

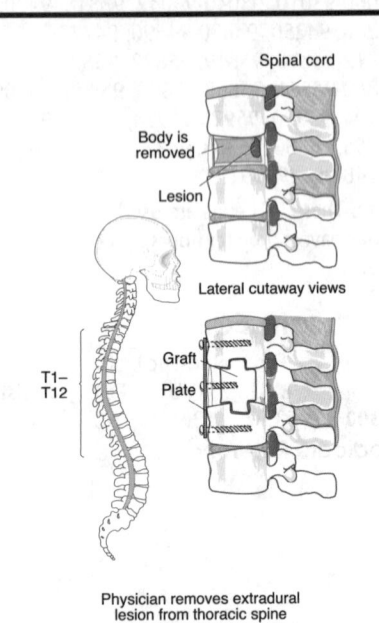

Physician removes extradural lesion from thoracic spine

Explanation

This procedure is performed to remove a lesion from a vertebra. The patient is placed in a lateral decubitus position and the physician makes a transthoracic approach overlying the rib corresponding to the affected vertebrae. The physician removes the rib and retracts muscles, fascia, and organs to expose the spine. The tumor mass is completely excised. Following repair of the muscles, fascia, and ligaments, the wound is closed in a routine fashion over suction drains.

Coding Tips

Note that 63301 reports transthoracic vertebral corpectomy, extradural, thoracic, for excision of an intraspinal lesion of one vertebral segment. Report 63308 for each additional segment. If the procedure is completed through an operating microscope, list 69990 in addition to 63301. When an anterior approach to the thoracic cavity is performed, the negative pressure is lost and a thoracotomy tube is routinely inserted to help re-establish the normal negative pressure and re-inflate the lung(s) after closure. This is a life-sustaining measure that must be performed in order to complete the procedure and, as such, tube thoracostomy (32551) should not be reported separately. When an anterior approach to the spine is achieved using the skills of two surgeons of different specialties (e.g., a thoracic or general surgeon provides exposure and the neurosurgeon provides the definitive procedure), this is a co-surgery scenario. Both surgeons report the primary procedure with modifier 62 and submit the claim with operative notes attached. Arthrodesis is reported separately; see 22554–22585. Bone graft is reported separately; see 20930–20938. For vertebral corpectomy for decompression, see 63085–63091.

ICD-9-CM Procedural

- 03.39 Other diagnostic procedures on spinal cord and spinal canal structures
- 03.4 Excision or destruction of lesion of spinal cord or spinal meninges
- 03.6 Lysis of adhesions of spinal cord and nerve roots

Anesthesia

63301 00620, 00625, 00626

ICD-9-CM Diagnostic

- 192.2 Malignant neoplasm of spinal cord
- 192.3 Malignant neoplasm of spinal meninges
- 198.3 Secondary malignant neoplasm of brain and spinal cord
- 199.0 Disseminated malignant neoplasm
- 225.3 Benign neoplasm of spinal cord
- 225.4 Benign neoplasm of spinal meninges
- 237.5 Neoplasm of uncertain behavior of brain and spinal cord
- 237.6 Neoplasm of uncertain behavior of meninges
- 239.7 Neoplasm of unspecified nature of endocrine glands and other parts of nervous system
- 324.1 Intraspinal abscess
- 336.1 Vascular myelopathies

Terms To Know

abscess. Circumscribed collection of pus resulting from bacteria, frequently associated with swelling and other signs of inflammation.

adhesion. Abnormal fibrous connection between two structures, soft tissue or bony structures, that may occur as the result of surgery, infection, or trauma.

benign. Mild or nonmalignant in nature.

decubitus ulcer. Progressively eroding skin lesion produced by inflamed necrotic tissue as it sloughs off caused by continual pressure to a localized area, especially over bony areas, where blood circulation is cut off when a patient lies still for too long without changing position.

disseminated. Spread over an extensive area.

fascia. Fibrous sheet or band of tissue that envelops organs, muscles, and groupings of muscles.

lateral. To/on the side.

malignant. Any condition tending to progress toward death, specifically an invasive tumor with a loss of cellular differentiation that has the ability to spread or metastasize to other areas in the body.

secondary. Second in order of occurrence or importance, or appearing during the course of another disease or condition.

CCI Version 16.3

0213T, 0216T, 0228T, 0230T, 22505, 32100, 36000, 36400-36410, 36420-36430, 36440, 36600, 36640, 37202, 43752, 51701-51703, 62310-62319, 63707, 63709, 64400-64435, 64445-64450, 64479, 64483, 64490, 64493, 64505-64530, 76000-76001, 92585, 93000-93010, 93040-93042, 93318, 94002, 94200, 94250, 94680-94690, 94770, 95812-95816, 95819, 95822, 95829, 95860-95861, 95867-95868, 95870, 95900, 95904, 95920, 95925-95934, 95936-95937, 95955, 96360, 96365, 96372, 96374-96376, 99148-99149, 99150

Note: These CCI edits are used for Medicare. Other payers may reimburse on codes listed above.

Medicare Edits

	Fac RVU	Non-Fac RVU	FUD	Assist
63301	63.95	63.95	90	80

Medicare References: None

63302

63302 Vertebral corpectomy (vertebral body resection), partial or complete, for excision of intraspinal lesion, single segment; extradural, thoracic by thoracolumbar approach

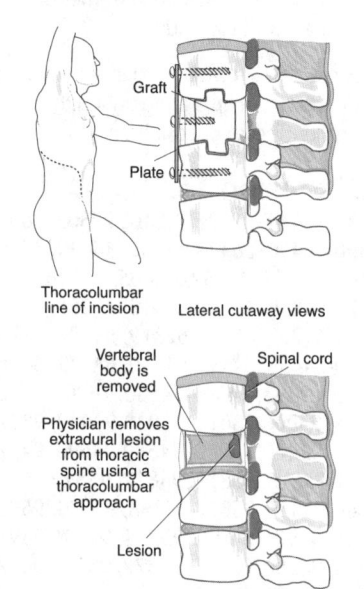

Explanation

This procedure is performed to remove a lesion of the vertebral body, which compresses the spinal cord. The patient is placed in a lateral decubitus position with supports under the buttocks and shoulder, and the muscle, fascia, ribs, and organs are incised or retracted. An incision is made in the diaphragm to purchase access to the spine. The tumor mass is completely excised. After muscles, fascia, and ligaments are repaired, the wound is closed in a routine fashion over suction drains.

Coding Tips

Note that 63302 reports thoracolumbar vertebral corpectomy, extradural, thoracic, for excision of an intraspinal lesion of one vertebral segment. Report 63308 for each additional segment. When an anterior approach to the thoracic cavity is performed, the negative pressure is lost and a thoracotomy tube is routinely inserted to help re-establish the normal negative pressure and re-inflate the lung(s) after closure. This is a life-sustaining measure that must be performed in order to complete the procedure and, as such, tube thoracostomy (32551) should not be reported separately. When an anterior approach to the spine is achieved using the skills of two surgeons of different specialties (e.g., a thoracic or general surgeon provides exposure and the neurosurgeon provides the definitive procedure), this is a co-surgery scenario. Both surgeons report the primary procedure with modifier 62 and submit the claim with operative notes attached. If the procedure is completed through an operating microscope, list 69990 in addition to 63302. Arthrodesis is reported separately; see 22554–22585. Bone graft is reported separately; see 20930–20938. For vertebral corpectomy for decompression, see 63085–63091.

ICD-9-CM Procedural

- 03.39 Other diagnostic procedures on spinal cord and spinal canal structures
- 03.4 Excision or destruction of lesion of spinal cord or spinal meninges
- 03.6 Lysis of adhesions of spinal cord and nerve roots

Anesthesia

63302 00620, 00625, 00626

ICD-9-CM Diagnostic

- 192.2 Malignant neoplasm of spinal cord
- 192.3 Malignant neoplasm of spinal meninges
- 198.3 Secondary malignant neoplasm of brain and spinal cord
- 199.0 Disseminated malignant neoplasm
- 225.3 Benign neoplasm of spinal cord
- 225.4 Benign neoplasm of spinal meninges
- 237.5 Neoplasm of uncertain behavior of brain and spinal cord
- 237.6 Neoplasm of uncertain behavior of meninges
- 239.7 Neoplasm of unspecified nature of endocrine glands and other parts of nervous system
- 324.1 Intraspinal abscess
- 336.1 Vascular myelopathies

Terms To Know

abscess. Circumscribed collection of pus resulting from bacteria, frequently associated with swelling and other signs of inflammation.

benign. Mild or nonmalignant in nature.

decubitus ulcer. Progressively eroding skin lesion produced by inflamed necrotic tissue as it sloughs off caused by continual pressure to a localized area, especially over bony areas, where blood circulation is cut off when a patient lies still for too long without changing position.

disseminated. Spread over an extensive area.

fascia. Fibrous sheet or band of tissue that envelops organs, muscles, and groupings of muscles.

lateral. To/on the side.

lesion. Area of damaged tissue that has lost continuity or function, due to disease or trauma. Lesions may be located on internal structures such as the brain, nerves, or kidneys, or visible on the skin.

malignant. Any condition tending to progress toward death, specifically an invasive tumor with a loss of cellular differentiation that has the ability to spread or metastasize to other areas in the body.

secondary. Second in order of occurrence or importance, or appearing during the course of another disease or condition.

CCI Version 16.3

0213T, 0216T, 0228T, 0230T, 22505, 32100, 36000, 36400-36410, 36420-36430, 36440, 36600, 36640, 37202, 43752, 49000-49010, 51701-51703, 62310-62319, 63707, 63709, 64400-64435, 64445-64450, 64479, 64483, 64490, 64493, 64505-64530, 76000-76001, 92585, 93000-93010, 93040-93042, 93318, 94002, 94200, 94250, 94680-94690, 94770, 95812-95816, 95819, 95822, 95829, 95860-95861, 95867-95868, 95870, 95900, 95904, 95920, 95925-95934, 95936-95937, 95955, 96360, 96365, 96372, 96374-96376, 99148-99149, 99150

Note: These CCI edits are used for Medicare. Other payers may reimburse on codes listed above.

Medicare Edits

	Fac RVU	Non-Fac RVU	FUD	Assist
63302	63.26	63.26	90	80

Medicare References: None

63303

63303 Vertebral corpectomy (vertebral body resection), partial or complete, for excision of intraspinal lesion, single segment; extradural, lumbar or sacral by transperitoneal or retroperitoneal approach

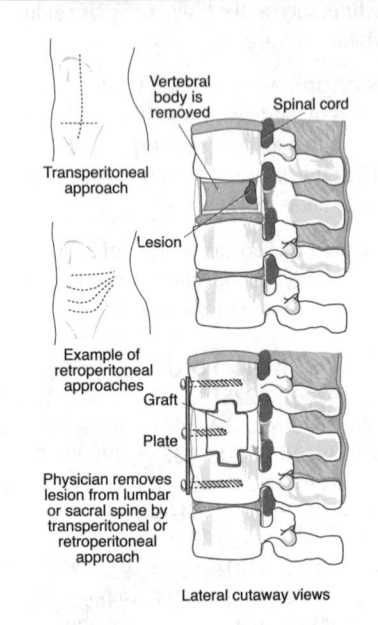

Explanation

This procedure is performed to remove a lesion of the vertebral body, which compresses the spinal cord. The patient is placed in a lateral decubitus position with approach from the left side, and the muscle, fascia, ribs, and organs are incised or retracted. The physician makes a groove in the vertebral bodies above and below the crushed vertebra and removes the discs above and below. Tricortical iliac crest grafts are obtained, prepared, and tapped into the grooves with a Moe impactor. An AO plate is screwed to the vertebra above and below the injured level to maintain fusion. A separately reported radiograph is obtained to assure proper placement, and the wound closed with layered sutures.

Coding Tips

Note that 63303 reports transperitoneal or retroperitoneal vertebral corpectomy, extradural, lumbar or sacral, for excision of an intraspinal lesion of one vertebral segment. Report 63308 for each additional segment. When an anterior approach to the spine is achieved using the skills of two surgeons of different specialties (e.g., a thoracic or general surgeon provides exposure and the neurosurgeon provides the definitive procedure), this is a co-surgery scenario. Both surgeons report the primary procedure with modifier 62 and submit the claim with operative notes attached. If the procedure is completed through an operating microscope, list 69990 in addition to 63303. Arthrodesis is reported separately; see 22554–22585. Bone graft is reported separately; see 20930–20938. For vertebral corpectomy for decompression, see 63085–63091.

ICD-9-CM Procedural

- 03.39 Other diagnostic procedures on spinal cord and spinal canal structures
- 03.4 Excision or destruction of lesion of spinal cord or spinal meninges
- 03.6 Lysis of adhesions of spinal cord and nerve roots

Anesthesia

63303 00630, 00670

ICD-9-CM Diagnostic

- 192.2 Malignant neoplasm of spinal cord
- 192.3 Malignant neoplasm of spinal meninges
- 198.3 Secondary malignant neoplasm of brain and spinal cord
- 199.0 Disseminated malignant neoplasm
- 225.3 Benign neoplasm of spinal cord
- 225.4 Benign neoplasm of spinal meninges
- 237.5 Neoplasm of uncertain behavior of brain and spinal cord
- 237.6 Neoplasm of uncertain behavior of meninges
- 239.7 Neoplasm of unspecified nature of endocrine glands and other parts of nervous system
- 324.1 Intraspinal abscess
- 336.1 Vascular myelopathies

Terms To Know

abscess. Circumscribed collection of pus resulting from bacteria, frequently associated with swelling and other signs of inflammation.

adhesion. Abnormal fibrous connection between two structures, soft tissue or bony structures, that may occur as the result of surgery, infection, or trauma.

benign. Mild or nonmalignant in nature.

decubitus ulcer. Progressively eroding skin lesion produced by inflamed necrotic tissue as it sloughs off caused by continual pressure to a localized area, especially over bony areas, where blood circulation is cut off when a patient lies still for too long without changing position.

disseminated. Spread over an extensive area.

fascia. Fibrous sheet or band of tissue that envelops organs, muscles, and groupings of muscles.

lateral. To/on the side.

malignant. Any condition tending to progress toward death, specifically an invasive tumor with a loss of cellular differentiation that has the ability to spread or metastasize to other areas in the body.

secondary. Second in order of occurrence or importance, or appearing during the course of another disease or condition.

CCI Version 16.3

0213T, 0216T, 0228T, 0230T, 22505, 36000, 36400-36410, 36420-36430, 36440, 36600, 36640, 37202, 43752, 44005, 44180, 44820-44850, 49000-49010, 49255, 51701-51703, 62310-62319, 63707, 63709, 64400-64435, 64445-64450, 64479, 64483, 64490, 64493, 64505-64530, 76000-76001, 92585, 93000-93010, 93040-93042, 93318, 94002, 94200, 94250, 94680-94690, 94770, 95812-95816, 95819, 95822, 95829, 95860-95861, 95867-95868, 95870, 95900, 95904, 95920, 95925-95934, 95936-95937, 95955, 96360, 96365, 96372, 96374-96376, 99148-99149, 99150

Note: These CCI edits are used for Medicare. Other payers may reimburse on codes listed above.

Medicare Edits

	Fac RVU	Non-Fac RVU	FUD	Assist
63303	67.21	67.21	90	80

Medicare References: None

63304

63304 Vertebral corpectomy (vertebral body resection), partial or complete, for excision of intraspinal lesion, single segment; intradural, cervical

Physician excises intraspinal lesion, intradural, cervical, by inserting graft and sometimes affixing plate in place of vertebral body

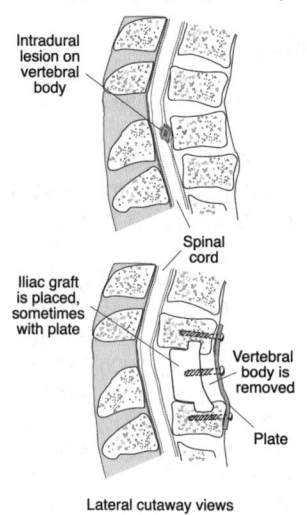

Lateral cutaway views

Explanation
This procedure is performed to correct a fracture or growth of the vertebral body, which compresses the spinal cord. The patient is placed supine with the head extended by tongs and traction. A right transverse incision or right vertical incision is made in the lateral neck. The muscles and fascia are incised and retracted. The dura may be incised. Entering between the trachea and the carotid sheath, the physician makes a groove in the vertebral bodies above and below the crushed vertebra and removes the discs above and below. Tricortical iliac crest grafts are obtained, prepared, and tapped into the grooves with a Moe impactor. Traction is removed. An AO plate is screwed to the vertebra above and below the injured level to maintain fusion. A separately reported radiograph is obtained to assure proper placement, and the wound closed with layered sutures.

Coding Tips
Note that 63304 reports anterior or anterolateral vertebral corpectomy, intradural, cervical, for excision of an intraspinal lesion of one vertebral segment. Report 63308 for each additional segment. If the procedure is completed through an operating microscope, list 69990 in addition to 63304. Arthrodesis is reported separately; see 22554–22585. Bone graft is reported separately; see 20930–20938.

For vertebral corpectomy for decompression, see 63085–63091.

ICD-9-CM Procedural
- 03.39 Other diagnostic procedures on spinal cord and spinal canal structures
- 03.4 Excision or destruction of lesion of spinal cord or spinal meninges
- 03.6 Lysis of adhesions of spinal cord and nerve roots

Anesthesia
63304 00600, 00670

ICD-9-CM Diagnostic
- 192.2 Malignant neoplasm of spinal cord
- 192.3 Malignant neoplasm of spinal meninges
- 198.3 Secondary malignant neoplasm of brain and spinal cord
- 199.0 Disseminated malignant neoplasm
- 225.3 Benign neoplasm of spinal cord
- 225.4 Benign neoplasm of spinal meninges
- 237.5 Neoplasm of uncertain behavior of brain and spinal cord
- 237.6 Neoplasm of uncertain behavior of meninges
- 239.7 Neoplasm of unspecified nature of endocrine glands and other parts of nervous system
- 324.1 Intraspinal abscess
- 336.1 Vascular myelopathies

Terms To Know

abscess. Circumscribed collection of pus resulting from bacteria, frequently associated with swelling and other signs of inflammation.

benign. Mild or nonmalignant in nature.

disseminated. Spread over an extensive area.

dura mater. Outermost, hard, fibrous layer or membrane that surrounds the brain and spinal cord.

lesion. Area of damaged tissue that has lost continuity or function, due to disease or trauma. Lesions may be located on internal structures such as the brain, nerves, or kidneys, or visible on the skin.

malignant. Any condition tending to progress toward death, specifically an invasive tumor with a loss of cellular differentiation that has the ability to spread or metastasize to other areas in the body.

secondary. Second in order of occurrence or importance, or appearing during the course of another disease or condition.

CCI Version 16.3
0213T, 0216T, 0228T, 0230T, 22505, 36000, 36400-36410, 36420-36430, 36440, 36600, 36640, 37202, 43752, 51701-51703, 62310-62319, 63300, 63707, 63709, 64400-64435, 64445-64450, 64479, 64483, 64490, 64493, 64505-64530, 76000-76001, 92585, 93000-93010, 93040-93042, 93318, 94002, 94200, 94250, 94680-94690, 94770, 95812-95816, 95819, 95822, 95829, 95860-95861, 95867-95868, 95870, 95900, 95904, 95920, 95925-95934, 95936-95937, 95955, 96360, 96365, 96372, 96374-96376, 99148-99149, 99150

Note: These CCI edits are used for Medicare. Other payers may reimburse on codes listed above.

Medicare Edits

	Fac RVU	Non-Fac RVU	FUD	Assist
63304	69.03	69.03	90	80

Medicare References: None

63305

63305 Vertebral corpectomy (vertebral body resection), partial or complete, for excision of intraspinal lesion, single segment; intradural, thoracic by transthoracic approach

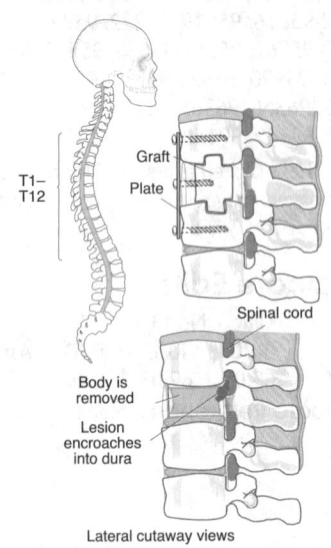

T1–T12
Graft
Plate
Spinal cord
Body is removed
Lesion encroaches into dura

Lateral cutaway views
Physician removes intradural lesion from thoracic spine by transthoracic approach

Explanation

This procedure is performed to correct a fracture or growth of the vertebral body, which compresses the spinal cord. The patient is placed in a lateral decubitus position and the muscle, fascia, ribs, and organs are incised or retracted. The dura may be incised. The physician makes a groove in the vertebral bodies above and below the crushed vertebra and removes the discs above and below. Tricortical iliac crest grafts are obtained, prepared, and tapped into the grooves with a Moe impactor. An AO plate is screwed to the vertebra above and below the injured level to maintain fusion. A separately reported radiograph is obtained to assure proper placement, and the wound closed with layered sutures.

Coding Tips

Note that 63305 reports transthoracic vertebral corpectomy, intradural, thoracic, for excision of an intraspinal lesion of one vertebral segment. Report 63308 for each additional segment. When an anterior approach to the thoracic cavity is performed, the negative pressure is lost and a thoracotomy tube is routinely inserted to help re-establish the normal negative pressure and re-inflate the lung(s) after closure. This is a life-sustaining measure that must be performed in order to complete the procedure

and, as such, tube thoracostomy (32551) should not be reported separately. When an anterior approach to the spine is achieved using the skills of two surgeons of different specialties (e.g., a thoracic or general surgeon provides exposure and the neurosurgeon provides the definitive procedure), this is a co-surgery scenario. Both surgeons report the primary procedure with modifier 62 and submit the claim with operative notes attached. If the procedure is completed through an operating microscope, list 69990 in addition to 63305. Arthrodesis is reported separately; see 22554–22585. Bone graft is reported separately; see 20930–20938. For vertebral corpectomy for decompression, see 63085–63091.

ICD-9-CM Procedural

- 03.39 Other diagnostic procedures on spinal cord and spinal canal structures
- 03.4 Excision or destruction of lesion of spinal cord or spinal meninges
- 03.6 Lysis of adhesions of spinal cord and nerve roots

Anesthesia

63305 00620, 00625, 00626

ICD-9-CM Diagnostic

- 192.2 Malignant neoplasm of spinal cord
- 192.3 Malignant neoplasm of spinal meninges
- 198.3 Secondary malignant neoplasm of brain and spinal cord
- 199.0 Disseminated malignant neoplasm
- 225.3 Benign neoplasm of spinal cord
- 225.4 Benign neoplasm of spinal meninges
- 237.5 Neoplasm of uncertain behavior of brain and spinal cord
- 237.6 Neoplasm of uncertain behavior of meninges
- 239.7 Neoplasm of unspecified nature of endocrine glands and other parts of nervous system
- 324.1 Intraspinal abscess
- 336.1 Vascular myelopathies

Terms To Know

abscess. Circumscribed collection of pus resulting from bacteria, frequently associated with swelling and other signs of inflammation.

benign. Mild or nonmalignant in nature.

fascia. Fibrous sheet or band of tissue that envelops organs, muscles, and groupings of muscles.

lesion. Area of damaged tissue that has lost continuity or function, due to disease or trauma. Lesions may be located on internal structures such as the brain, nerves, or kidneys, or visible on the skin.

malignant. Any condition tending to progress toward death, specifically an invasive tumor with a loss of cellular differentiation that has the ability to spread or metastasize to other areas in the body.

secondary. Second in order of occurrence or importance, or appearing during the course of another disease or condition.

CCI Version 16.3

0213T, 0216T, 0228T, 0230T, 22505, 32100, 36000, 36400-36410, 36420-36430, 36440, 36600, 36640, 37202, 43752, 51701-51703, 62310-62319, 63101✦, 63301, 63707, 63709, 64400-64435, 64445-64450, 64479, 64483, 64490, 64493, 64505-64530, 76000-76001, 92585, 93000-93010, 93040-93042, 93318, 94002, 94200, 94250, 94680-94690, 94770, 95812-95816, 95819, 95822, 95829, 95860-95861, 95867-95868, 95870, 95900, 95904, 95920, 95925-95934, 95936-95937, 95955, 96360, 96365, 96372, 96374-96376, 99148-99149, 99150

Note: These CCI edits are used for Medicare. Other payers may reimburse on codes listed above.

Medicare Edits

	Fac RVU	Non-Fac RVU	FUD	Assist
63305	72.43	72.43	90	80

Medicare References: None

63306

63306 Vertebral corpectomy (vertebral body resection), partial or complete, for excision of intraspinal lesion, single segment; intradural, thoracic by thoracolumbar approach

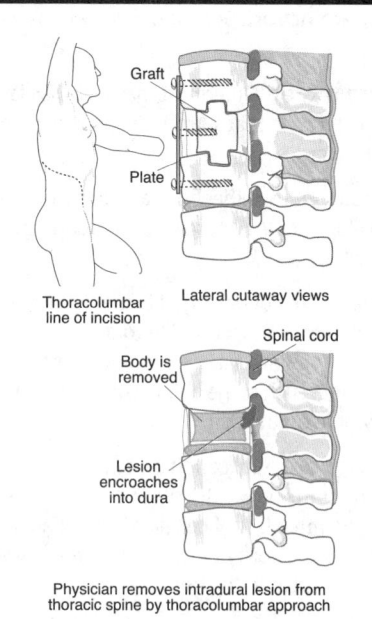

Explanation
This procedure is performed to remove a lesion of the vertebral body, which compresses the spinal cord. The patient is placed in a lateral decubitus position with supports under the buttocks and shoulder, and the muscle, fascia, ribs, and organs are incised or retracted. The dura may be incised. An incision is made in the diaphragm to purchase access to the spine. The physician makes a groove in the vertebral bodies above and below the crushed vertebra and removes the discs above and below. Tricortical iliac crest grafts are obtained, prepared, and tapped into the grooves with a Moe impactor. An AO plate is screwed to the vertebra above and below the injured level to maintain fusion. A separately reported radiograph is obtained to assure proper placement, and the wound closed with layered sutures.

Coding Tips
Note that 63306 reports thoracolumbar vertebral corpectomy, intradural, thoracic, for excision of an intraspinal lesion of one vertebral segment. Report 63308 for each additional segment. When an anterior approach to the thoracic cavity is performed, the negative pressure is lost and a thoracotomy tube is routinely inserted to help re-establish the normal negative pressure and re-inflate the lung(s) after closure. This is a life-sustaining measure that must be performed in order to complete the procedure and, as such, a tube thoracostomy (32551) should not be reported separately. When an anterior approach to the spine is achieved using the skills of two surgeons of different specialties (e.g., a thoracic or general surgeon provides exposure and the neurosurgeon provides the definitive procedure), this is a co-surgery scenario. Both surgeons report the primary procedure with modifier 62 and submit the claim with operative notes attached. If the procedure is completed through an operating microscope, list 69990 in addition to 63306. Arthrodesis is reported separately; see 22554–22585. Bone graft is reported separately; see 20930–20938.

ICD-9-CM Procedural
- 03.39 Other diagnostic procedures on spinal cord and spinal canal structures
- 03.4 Excision or destruction of lesion of spinal cord or spinal meninges
- 03.6 Lysis of adhesions of spinal cord and nerve roots

Anesthesia
63306 00620, 00625, 00626

ICD-9-CM Diagnostic
- 192.2 Malignant neoplasm of spinal cord
- 192.3 Malignant neoplasm of spinal meninges
- 198.3 Secondary malignant neoplasm of brain and spinal cord
- 199.0 Disseminated malignant neoplasm
- 225.3 Benign neoplasm of spinal cord
- 225.4 Benign neoplasm of spinal meninges
- 237.5 Neoplasm of uncertain behavior of brain and spinal cord
- 237.6 Neoplasm of uncertain behavior of meninges
- 239.7 Neoplasm of unspecified nature of endocrine glands and other parts of nervous system
- 324.1 Intraspinal abscess
- 336.1 Vascular myelopathies

Terms To Know
benign. Mild or nonmalignant in nature.

disseminated. Spread over an extensive area.

dura mater. Outermost, hard, fibrous layer or membrane that surrounds the brain and spinal cord.

fascia. Fibrous sheet or band of tissue that envelops organs, muscles, and groupings of muscles.

lateral. To/on the side.

malignant. Any condition tending to progress toward death, specifically an invasive tumor with a loss of cellular differentiation that has the ability to spread or metastasize to other areas in the body.

secondary. Second in order of occurrence or importance, or appearing during the course of another disease or condition.

CCI Version 16.3
0213T, 0216T, 0228T, 0230T, 22206❖, 22505, 32100, 36000, 36400-36410, 36420-36430, 36440, 36600, 36640, 37202, 43752, 49000-49010, 51701-51703, 62310-62319, 63101❖, 63302, 63707, 63709, 64400-64435, 64445-64450, 64479, 64483, 64490, 64493, 64505-64530, 76000-76001, 92585, 93000-93010, 93040-93042, 93318, 94002, 94200, 94250, 94680-94690, 94770, 95812-95816, 95819, 95822, 95829, 95860-95861, 95867-95868, 95870, 95900, 95904, 95920, 95925-95934, 95936-95937, 95955, 96360, 96365, 96372, 96374-96376, 99148-99149, 99150

Note: These CCI edits are used for Medicare. Other payers may reimburse on codes listed above.

Medicare Edits

	Fac RVU	Non-Fac RVU	FUD	Assist
63306	67.59	67.59	90	80

Medicare References: None

63307-63308

63307 Vertebral corpectomy (vertebral body resection), partial or complete, for excision of intraspinal lesion, single segment; intradural, lumbar or sacral by transperitoneal or retroperitoneal approach

63308 each additional segment (List separately in addition to codes for single segment)

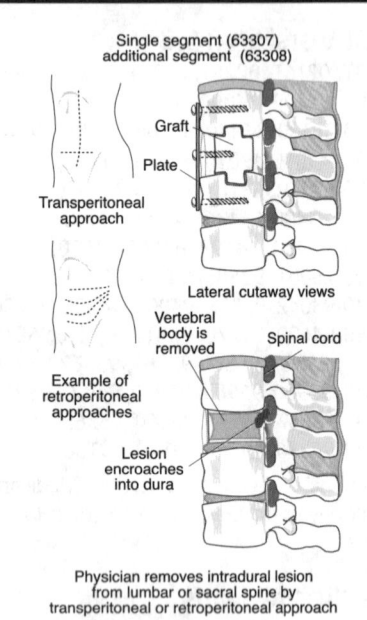

Single segment (63307) additional segment (63308)

Transperitoneal approach

Lateral cutaway views

Vertebral body is removed

Spinal cord

Example of retroperitoneal approaches

Lesion encroaches into dura

Physician removes intradural lesion from lumbar or sacral spine by transperitoneal or retroperitoneal approach

Explanation

Code 63307 is performed to remove a lesion of the vertebral body, which compresses the spinal cord. The patient is placed in a lateral decubitus position with approach from the left side, and the muscle, fascia, ribs, and organs are incised or retracted. The dura may be incised. The physician makes a groove in the vertebral bodies above and below the crushed vertebra and removes the discs above and below. Tricortical iliac crest grafts are obtained, prepared, and tapped into the grooves with a Moe impactor. An AO plate is screwed to the vertebra above and below the injured level to maintain fusion. A separately reported radiograph is obtained to assure proper placement, and the wound closed with layered sutures. Code 63308 is performed to remove a lesion of the vertebral body, which compresses the spinal cord. The patient is placed in a lateral decubitus position with approach from the left side, and the muscle, fascia, ribs, and organs are incised or retracted. The physician makes a groove in the vertebral bodies above and below the crushed vertebra and removes the discs above and below. Tricortical iliac crest grafts are obtained, prepared, and tapped into the grooves with a Moe impactor. An AO plate is screwed to the vertebra above and below the injured level to maintain fusion. A separately reported radiograph is obtained to assure proper placement, and the wound closed with layered sutures.

Coding Tips

Note that 63307 reports transperitoneal or retroperitoneal vertebral corpectomy, intradural, lumbar or sacral, for excision of an intraspinal lesion of one vertebral segment. Use 63308 in conjunction with 63300–63307. As an "add-on" code, 63308 is not subject to multiple procedure rules. No reimbursement reduction or modifier 51 is applied. Add-on codes describe additional intra-service work associated with the primary procedure. They are performed by the same physician on the same date of service as the primary service/procedure, and must never be reported as stand-alone codes. When an anterior approach to the spine is achieved using the skills of two surgeons of different specialties (e.g., a thoracic or general surgeon provides exposure and the neurosurgeon provides the definitive procedure), this is a co-surgery scenario. Both surgeons report the primary procedure with modifier 62 and submit the claim with operative notes attached. If the procedure is completed through an operating microscope, list 69990 in addition to 63307. Arthrodesis is reported separately; see 22554–22585. Bone graft is reported separately; see 20930–20938. For vertebral corpectomy for decompression, see 63085–63091.

ICD-9-CM Procedural

- 03.39 Other diagnostic procedures on spinal cord and spinal canal structures
- 03.4 Excision or destruction of lesion of spinal cord or spinal meninges
- 03.6 Lysis of adhesions of spinal cord and nerve roots

Anesthesia

63307 00630, 00670
63308 N/A

ICD-9-CM Diagnostic

- 192.2 Malignant neoplasm of spinal cord
- 192.3 Malignant neoplasm of spinal meninges
- 198.3 Secondary malignant neoplasm of brain and spinal cord
- 199.0 Disseminated malignant neoplasm
- 225.3 Benign neoplasm of spinal cord
- 225.4 Benign neoplasm of spinal meninges
- 237.5 Neoplasm of uncertain behavior of brain and spinal cord
- 237.6 Neoplasm of uncertain behavior of meninges
- 239.7 Neoplasm of unspecified nature of endocrine glands and other parts of nervous system
- 324.1 Intraspinal abscess
- 336.1 Vascular myelopathies

Terms To Know

disseminated. Spread over an extensive area.

dura mater. Outermost, hard, fibrous layer or membrane that surrounds the brain and spinal cord.

fascia. Fibrous sheet or band of tissue that envelops organs, muscles, and groupings of muscles.

lesion. Area of damaged tissue that has lost continuity or function, due to disease or trauma. Lesions may be located on internal structures such as the brain, nerves, or kidneys, or visible on the skin.

malignant. Any condition tending to progress toward death, specifically an invasive tumor with a loss of cellular differentiation that has the ability to spread or metastasize to other areas in the body.

secondary. Second in order of occurrence or importance, or appearing during the course of another disease or condition.

CCI Version 16.3

92585, 95822, 95860-95861, 95867-95868, 95900, 95904, 95920, 95936-95937

Also not with 63307: 0213T, 0216T, 0228T, 0230T, 22505, 36000, 36400-36410, 36420-36430, 36440, 36600, 36640, 37202, 43752, 44005, 44180, 44820-44850, 49000-49010, 49255, 51701-51703, 62310-62319, 63303, 63707, 63709, 64400-64435, 64445-64450, 64479, 64483, 64490, 64493, 64505-64530, 76000-76001, 93000-93010, 93040-93042, 93318, 94002, 94200, 94250, 94680-94690, 94770, 95812-95816, 95819, 95829, 95870, 95925-95934, 95955, 96360, 96365, 96372, 96374-96376, 99148-99149, 99150

Also not with 63308: 95925-95927, 95930-95934

Note: These CCI edits are used for Medicare. Other payers may reimburse on codes listed above.

Medicare Edits

	Fac RVU	Non-Fac RVU	FUD	Assist
63307	70.56	70.56	90	80
63308	9.62	9.62	N/A	80

Medicare References: None

63710

63710 Dural graft, spinal

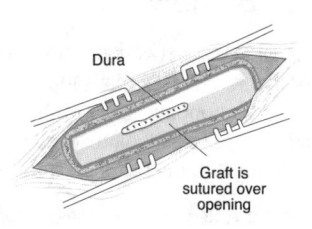

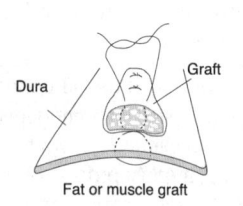

Explanation

At the end of a procedure where the dura has been incised, the physician sometimes prepares a graft of subcutaneous fat, freeze-dried dura, fascia, or muscle. Suction is used to keep the incision free of cerebral spinal fluid. Single dural stitches are used to achieve closure. A second needle is attached to the free suture ends and the needles are passed through the graft, which is tied down outside of the repaired tear to achieve watertight closure. If the dural defect is small and difficult to access, the graft can be placed inside the dura. After verifying that the repair is watertight, the physician proceeds with closure.

Coding Tips

If the procedure is completed through an operating microscope, list 69990 in addition to 63710. For repair of dural/CSF leak, not requiring laminectomy, see 63707; requiring laminectomy, see 63709. For laminectomy and section of dentate ligaments, with or without dural graft, cervical, see 63180 and 63182.

ICD-9-CM Procedural

02.12 Other repair of cerebral meninges

Anesthesia

63710 00630

ICD-9-CM Diagnostic

225.2 Benign neoplasm of cerebral meninges
237.5 Neoplasm of uncertain behavior of brain and spinal cord
349.31 Accidental puncture or laceration of dura during a procedure
349.39 Other dural tear
996.75 Other complications due to nervous system device, implant, and graft — (Use additional code to identify complication: 338.18-338.19, 338.28-338.29)
998.31 Disruption of internal operation (surgical) wound

Terms To Know

benign. Mild or nonmalignant in nature.

cerebrospinal fluid. Thin, clear fluid circulating in the cranial cavity and spinal column that bathes the brain and spinal cord.

dura mater. Outermost, hard, fibrous layer or membrane that surrounds the brain and spinal cord.

fascia. Fibrous sheet or band of tissue that envelops organs, muscles, and groupings of muscles.

graft. Tissue implant from another part of the body or another person.

meninges. Tough membranous protectors of the central nervous system that cover the brain and spinal cord comprising three layers: the dura mater, arachnoid mater, and pia mater.

suction. Vacuum evacuation of fluid or tissue.

CCI Version 16.3

0213T, 0216T, 0228T, 0230T, 22505, 36000, 36400-36410, 36420-36430, 36440, 36600, 36640, 37202, 43752, 51701-51703, 62310-62319, 64400-64435, 64445-64450, 64479, 64483, 64490, 64493, 64505-64530, 76000-76001, 92585, 93000-93010, 93040-93042, 93318, 94002, 94200, 94250, 94680-94690, 94770, 95812-95816, 95819, 95822, 95829, 95860-95861, 95867-95868, 95870, 95900, 95904, 95920, 95925-95934, 95936-95937, 95955, 96360, 96365, 96372, 96374-96376, 99148-99149, 99150

Note: These CCI edits are used for Medicare. Other payers may reimburse on codes listed above.

Medicare Edits

	Fac RVU	Non-Fac RVU	FUD	Assist
63710	32.38	32.38	90	80

Medicare References: None

64449

64449 Injection, anesthetic agent; lumbar plexus, posterior approach, continuous infusion by catheter (including catheter placement)

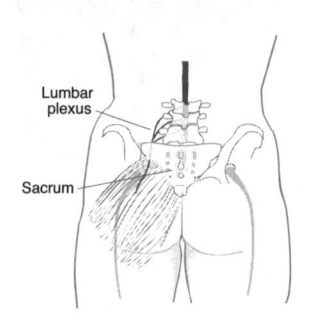

Lumbar plexus
Sacrum

The nerves of the lumbar plexus are injected with an anesthetic agent by continuous catheter infusion

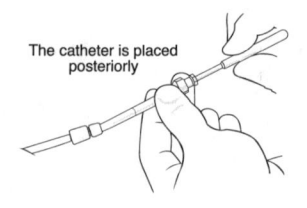

The catheter is placed posteriorly

Explanation

The physician performs a nerve block, posterior approach, on the lumbar plexus by infusing an anesthetic agent through a catheter placed for daily management of pain and administration of anesthesia. The lumbar plexus is formed from the nerve branches in the psoas major muscle: the ilioinguinal, obturator, iliohypogastric, lateral femoral cutaneous, genito-femoral, and the femoral nerve. IV sedatives and analgesics are set up. With the patient in the right lateral decubitus position, the insertion point for the needle is marked. Local anesthetic is also given. The needle is advanced toward the lumbar plexus, avoiding any transverse processes of the lumbar vertebrae until it is in proper position within the compartment of the psoas muscle, and stimulation of the plexus is seen by the contraction of certain muscles. Blood and cerebral spinal fluid is aspirated. After determining that the needle is in the right position and that the injection will not go intravenously or intrathecally, local anesthesia is injected through the needle and an infusion catheter is fed through the needle past the tip. Catheter placement is also checked, the catheter is secured in place, and continuous infusion is begun.

Coding Tips

Do not report 64449 in conjunction with 01996. For destruction by neurolytic agent, see 64622–64623.

ICD-9-CM Procedural

04.81 Injection of anesthetic into peripheral nerve for analgesia

Anesthesia

64449 N/A

ICD-9-CM Diagnostic

- 353.1 Lumbosacral plexus lesions
- 353.4 Lumbosacral root lesions, not elsewhere classified
- 353.6 Phantom limb (syndrome)
- 353.8 Other nerve root and plexus disorders
- 355.0 Lesion of sciatic nerve
- 355.79 Other mononeuritis of lower limb
- 719.45 Pain in joint, pelvic region and thigh
- 719.48 Pain in joint, other specified sites
- 720.0 Ankylosing spondylitis
- 720.1 Spinal enthesopathy
- 721.3 Lumbosacral spondylosis without myelopathy
- 721.42 Spondylosis with myelopathy, lumbar region
- 721.6 Ankylosing vertebral hyperostosis
- 721.7 Traumatic spondylopathy
- 722.10 Displacement of lumbar intervertebral disc without myelopathy
- 722.32 Schmorl's nodes, lumbar region
- 722.52 Degeneration of lumbar or lumbosacral intervertebral disc
- 722.73 Intervertebral lumbar disc disorder with myelopathy, lumbar region
- 722.83 Postlaminectomy syndrome, lumbar region
- 722.93 Other and unspecified disc disorder of lumbar region
- 724.02 Spinal stenosis of lumbar region, without neurogenic claudication
- 724.03 Spinal stenosis of lumbar region, with neurogenic claudication
- 724.2 Lumbago
- 724.3 Sciatica
- 724.4 Thoracic or lumbosacral neuritis or radiculitis, unspecified
- 724.5 Unspecified backache
- 724.6 Disorders of sacrum
- 724.8 Other symptoms referable to back
- 724.9 Other unspecified back disorder
- 729.2 Unspecified neuralgia, neuritis, and radiculitis
- 739.3 Nonallopathic lesion of lumbar region, not elsewhere classified
- 739.4 Nonallopathic lesion of sacral region, not elsewhere classified
- 756.12 Congenital spondylolisthesis
- 847.2 Lumbar sprain and strain
- 847.3 Sprain and strain of sacrum

Terms To Know

lumbar plexus. Network of spinal nerves from lumbar levels L1-L4 that supplies motor, sensory, and autonomic fibers to the lower extremity, as well as the gluteal and inguinal regions along with the sacral plexus.

nerve block. Regional anesthesia/analgesia administered by injection that prevents sensory nerve impulses from reaching the central nervous system.

vertebra. Any one of the 33 bones composing the spinal column, generally having a disc-shaped body, two transverse processes, and a spinal process centered posteriorly. Vertebrae are connected by the laminae between them and are attached to the body by pedicles, forming an enclosed, protective ring around the vertebral foramen through which the spinal cord runs.

CCI Version 16.3

0178T-0179T, 0180T, 01991-01992, 01996, 20550-20553, 36000, 36400-36410, 36420-36430, 36440, 36600, 51701-51703, 69990, 76000-76001, 76998, 77002, 90862, 92585, 93000-93010, 93040-93042, 93318, 94002, 94200, 94250, 94680-94690, 94770, 95812-95816, 95819, 95822, 95829, 95860-95861, 95867-95868, 95870, 95900, 95904, 95920, 95925-95934, 95936-95937, 95955, 96360, 96365, 96372, 96374-96376, 97033❖, 99148-99149, 99150, J2001

Note: These CCI edits are used for Medicare. Other payers may reimburse on codes listed above.

Medicare Edits

	Fac RVU	Non-Fac RVU	FUD	Assist
64449	2.48	2.48	0	N/A

Medicare References: None

64614

64614 Chemodenervation of muscle(s); extremity(s) and/or trunk muscle(s) (eg, for dystonia, cerebral palsy, multiple sclerosis)

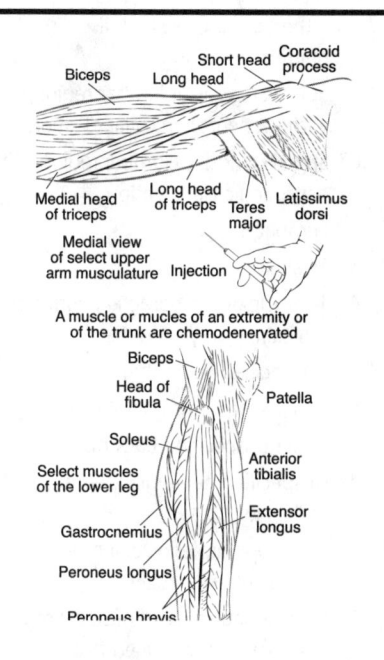

Explanation

The physician administers a neurotoxin to paralyze dysfunctional muscle tissue in the extremities or trunk. Chemodenervation works by introducing a substance used to block the transfer of chemicals at the presynaptic membrane. Botulinum toxin type A (BTX-A, Botox®), phenol (sometimes combined with botulinum toxin type A), and/or ethyl alcohol may be used. The physician identifies the nerve(s) or muscle endplate(s) by direct surgical exposure or through the insertion of an electromyographic needle into the muscle. A small amount of the selected agent is injected into nerve(s) or muscle endplate(s), inducing muscle paralysis. The duration of the effect is variable, usually one to 12 months when phenol or alcohol is used, and three to four months when BTX-A is used. BTX-A is dose-dependent and reversible secondary to the regeneration process. Gradually, blocked nerves form new neuromuscular junctions resulting in the return of muscle function.

Coding Tips

For chemodenervation of the cervical spinal muscles, see 64613. Surgical trays, A4550, are not separately reimbursed by Medicare; however, other third-party payers may cover them. Check with the specific payer to determine coverage.

ICD-9-CM Procedural
04.2 Destruction of cranial and peripheral nerves

Anesthesia
64614 N/A

ICD-9-CM Diagnostic
- 333.0 Other degenerative diseases of the basal ganglia
- 333.1 Essential and other specified forms of tremor — (Use additional E code to identify drug, if drug-induced)
- 333.2 Myoclonus — (Use additional E code to identify drug, if drug-induced)
- 333.3 Tics of organic origin — (Use additional E code to identify drug, if drug-induced)
- 333.4 Huntington's chorea
- 333.5 Other choreas — (Use additional E code to identify drug, if drug-induced)
- 333.6 Genetic torsion dystonia
- 333.71 Athetoid cerebral palsy
- 333.72 Acute dystonia due to drugs — (Use additional E code to identify drug)
- 333.79 Other acquired torsion dystonia
- 333.84 Organic writers' cramp — (Use additional E code to identify drug, if drug-induced)
- 333.89 Other fragments of torsion dystonia — (Use additional E code to identify drug, if drug-induced)
- 333.90 Unspecified extrapyramidal disease and abnormal movement disorder — (Use additional E code to identify drug, if drug-induced)
- 333.91 Stiff-man syndrome
- 333.92 Neuroleptic malignant syndrome — (Use additional E code to identify drug)
- 333.93 Benign shuddering attacks
- 333.99 Other extrapyramidal disease and abnormal movement disorder — (Use additional E code to identify drug, if drug-induced)
- 340 Multiple sclerosis
- 341.1 Schilder's disease
- 341.8 Other demyelinating diseases of central nervous system
- 341.9 Unspecified demyelinating disease of central nervous system
- 342.10 Spastic hemiplegia affecting unspecified side
- 342.11 Spastic hemiplegia affecting dominant side
- 342.12 Spastic hemiplegia affecting nondominant side
- 343.0 Diplegic infantile cerebral palsy
- 343.1 Hemiplegic infantile cerebral palsy
- 343.2 Quadriplegic infantile cerebral palsy
- 343.3 Monoplegic infantile cerebral palsy
- 343.4 Infantile hemiplegia
- 343.8 Other specified infantile cerebral palsy
- 343.9 Unspecified infantile cerebral palsy
- 344.89 Other specified paralytic syndrome
- 781.0 Abnormal involuntary movements

Terms To Know

cerebral palsy. Brain damage occurring before, during, or shortly after birth that impedes muscle control and tone.

CCI Version 16.3

0213T, 0216T, 0228T, 0230T, 36000, 36400-36410, 36420-36430, 36440, 36600, 36640, 37202, 43752, 51701-51703, 62310-62319, 64400-64435, 64445-64450, 64479, 64483, 64490, 64493, 64505-64530, 69990, 92585, 93000-93010, 93040-93042, 93318, 94002, 94200, 94250, 94680-94690, 94770, 95812-95816, 95819, 95822, 95829, 95860-95864, 95866-95870, 95900, 95904, 95920, 95925-95934, 95936-95937, 95955, 96360, 96365, 96372, 96374-96376, 99148-99149, 99150

Note: These CCI edits are used for Medicare. Other payers may reimburse on codes listed above.

Medicare Edits

	Fac RVU	Non-Fac RVU	FUD	Assist
64614	4.48	5.16	10	N/A

Medicare References: 100-3,160.20

64622-64623

64622 Destruction by neurolytic agent, paravertebral facet joint nerve; lumbar or sacral, single level

64623 lumbar or sacral, each additional level (List separately in addition to code for primary procedure)

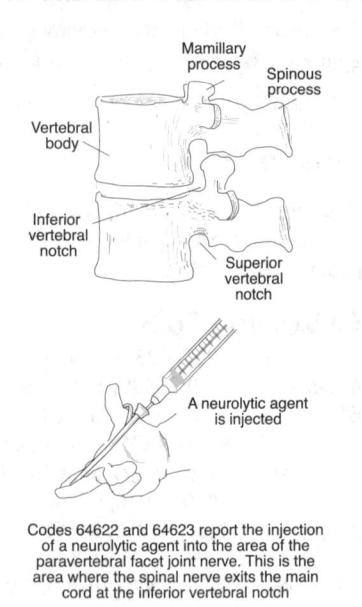

Codes 64622 and 64623 report the injection of a neurolytic agent into the area of the paravertebral facet joint nerve. This is the area where the spinal nerve exits the main cord at the inferior vertebral notch

Explanation

These procedures are performed to treat chronic pain. The affected nerve is destroyed using chemical, thermal, electrical, or radiofrequency techniques. These techniques may be used singley or in combination. These procedures are designed to destroy the specific site(s) in the nerve root that produce(s) the pain while leaving sensation intact. Generally intravenous conscious sedation is utilized during the initial phase of the procedure so that the patient can assist the physician in identifying the site of pain and the correct placement of the neurolytic agent and local anesthesia is administered during the destruction phase of the procedure. Using separately reportable fluoroscopic guidance, a needle is inserted into the affected nerve root. An electrode is then inserted through the needle and a mild electrical current is passed through the electrode. The current produces a tingling sensation at a site on the nerve. The electrode is manipulated until the tingling sensation is felt at the same site as the pain. Once the physician has determined that the electrode is positioned at the site responsible for the pain, a local anesthetic is adminstered and a neurolytic agent applied. Chemical destruction involves injection of a neurolytic substance (eg, alcohol, phenol, glycerol) into the affected nerve root. Thermal techniques utilize heat. Electrical techniques utilize an electrical current. Radiofrequency, also referred to as radiofrequency rhizotomy, utilizes a solar or microwave current. Report 64622–64623 when one or more lumbar/sacral paravertebral facet joint nerve are treated.

Coding Tips

Use 64623 in conjunction with 64622. As an "add-on" code, 64623 is not subject to multiple procedure rules. No reimbursement reduction or modifier 51 is applied. Add-on codes describe additional intra-service work associated with the primary procedure. They are performed by the same physician on the same date of service as the primary service/procedure, and must never be reported as a stand-alone code. These are unilateral procedures. If performed bilaterally, some payers require that the service be reported twice with modifier 50 appended to the second code, while others require identification of the service only once with modifier 50 appended. Check with individual payers. Modifier 50 identifies a procedure performed identically on the opposite side of the body (mirror image). Fluoroscopic guidance is reported separately; see 77003.

ICD-9-CM Procedural

04.2 Destruction of cranial and peripheral nerves

Anesthesia

N/A

ICD-9-CM Diagnostic

- 353.1 Lumbosacral plexus lesions
- 353.4 Lumbosacral root lesions, not elsewhere classified
- 353.6 Phantom limb (syndrome)
- 353.8 Other nerve root and plexus disorders
- 355.0 Lesion of sciatic nerve
- 355.79 Other mononeuritis of lower limb
- 719.45 Pain in joint, pelvic region and thigh
- 719.48 Pain in joint, other specified sites
- 720.0 Ankylosing spondylitis
- 720.1 Spinal enthesopathy
- 721.3 Lumbosacral spondylosis without myelopathy
- 721.42 Spondylosis with myelopathy, lumbar region
- 721.6 Ankylosing vertebral hyperostosis
- 721.7 Traumatic spondylopathy
- 722.10 Displacement of lumbar intervertebral disc without myelopathy
- 722.32 Schmorl's nodes, lumbar region
- 722.52 Degeneration of lumbar or lumbosacral intervertebral disc
- 722.73 Intervertebral lumbar disc disorder with myelopathy, lumbar region
- 722.83 Postlaminectomy syndrome, lumbar region
- 722.93 Other and unspecified disc disorder of lumbar region
- 724.02 Spinal stenosis of lumbar region, without neurogenic claudication
- 724.03 Spinal stenosis of lumbar region, with neurogenic claudication
- 724.2 Lumbago
- 724.3 Sciatica
- 724.4 Thoracic or lumbosacral neuritis or radiculitis, unspecified
- 724.5 Unspecified backache
- 724.8 Other symptoms referable to back
- 724.9 Other unspecified back disorder
- 729.2 Unspecified neuralgia, neuritis, and radiculitis
- 739.3 Nonallopathic lesion of lumbar region, not elsewhere classified
- 739.4 Nonallopathic lesion of sacral region, not elsewhere classified
- 756.12 Congenital spondylolisthesis

CCI Version 16.3

0230T, 62311, 64483, 92585, 95822, 95860-95861, 95867-95868, 95900, 95904, 95920, 95936-95937

Also not with 64622: 0216T, 0228T, 36000, 36400-36410, 36420-36430, 36440, 36600, 36640, 37202, 43752, 51701-51703, 62319, 64400-64413, 64418-64435, 64445-64450, 64479, 64493, 64505-64530, 69990, 76000-76001, 77002, 93000-93010, 93040-93042, 93318, 94002, 94200, 94250, 94680-94690, 94770, 95812-95816, 95819, 95829, 95870, 95925-95934, 95955, 96360, 96365, 96372, 96374-96376, 99148-99149, 99150, J2001

Also not with 64623: 95925-95927, 95930-95934

Note: These CCI edits are used for Medicare. Other payers may reimburse on codes listed above.

Medicare Edits

	Fac RVU	Non-Fac RVU	FUD	Assist
64622	5.39	9.88	10	N/A
64623	1.47	3.68	N/A	N/A

Medicare References: 100-2,15,260; 100-3,160.1; 100-4,12,30; 100-4,12,90.3; 100-4,14,10

64626-64627

64626 Destruction by neurolytic agent, paravertebral facet joint nerve; cervical or thoracic, single level

64627 cervical or thoracic, each additional level (List separately in addition to code for primary procedure)

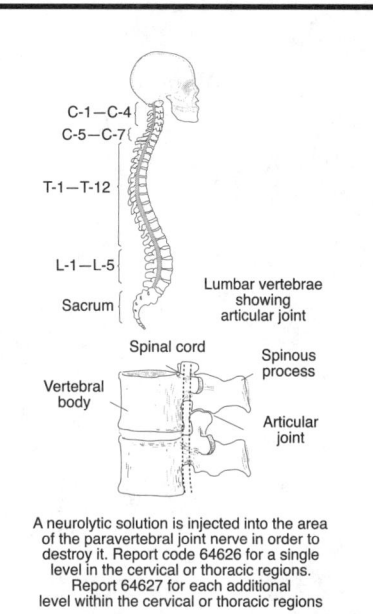

A neurolytic solution is injected into the area of the paravertebral joint nerve in order to destroy it. Report code 64626 for a single level in the cervical or thoracic regions. Report 64627 for each additional level within the cervical or thoracic regions

Explanation

These procedures are performed to treat chronic pain by destroying specific sites in the nerve root that produce pain while leaving sensation intact. A cervical or thoracic paravertebral facet nerve is destroyed using chemical, thermal, electrical, or radiofrequency techniques, either singly or in combination. Intravenous conscious sedation is utilized during the initial phase of the procedure, allowing the patient to assist the physician in identifying the site of pain and correct placement of the neurolytic agent. Local anesthesia is administered during the destruction phase of the procedure. Using fluoroscopic guidance (reported separately), a needle is inserted into the affected nerve root. An electrode is then inserted through the needle and a mild electrical current is passed through the electrode. The current produces a tingling sensation at a site on the nerve. The electrode is manipulated until the tingling sensation is felt at the same site as the pain. Once the physician has determined that the electrode is positioned at the site responsible for the pain, a local anesthetic is administered and a neurolytic agent applied. Chemical destruction involves injection of a neurolytic substance (e.g., alcohol, phenol, glycerol) into the affected nerve root. Thermal techniques utilize heat. Electrical techniques utilize an electrical current. Radiofrequency, also referred to as radiofrequency rhizotomy, utilizes a solar or microwave current. Report 64626 when one cervical/thoracic paravertebral facet joint nerve is treated and 64627 for each additional paravertebral facet joint nerve.

Coding Tips

Use 64627 in conjunction with 64626. As an "add-on" code, 64627 is not subject to multiple procedure rules. No reimbursement reduction or modifier 51 is applied. Add-on codes describe additional intra-service work associated with the primary procedure. They are performed by the same physician on the same date of service as the primary service/procedure, and must never be reported as a stand-alone code. These are unilateral procedures. If performed bilaterally, some payers require that the service be reported twice with modifier 50 appended to the second code, while others require identification of the service only once with modifier 50 appended. Check with individual payers. Modifier 50 identifies a procedure performed identically on the opposite side of the body (mirror image). Fluoroscopic guidance is reported separately; see 77003.

ICD-9-CM Procedural

04.2 Destruction of cranial and peripheral nerves

Anesthesia
N/A

ICD-9-CM Diagnostic

353.2 Cervical root lesions, not elsewhere classified
353.3 Thoracic root lesions, not elsewhere classified
353.8 Other nerve root and plexus disorders
720.0 Ankylosing spondylitis
720.1 Spinal enthesopathy
721.1 Cervical spondylosis with myelopathy
721.6 Ankylosing vertebral hyperostosis
721.7 Traumatic spondylopathy
722.0 Displacement of cervical intervertebral disc without myelopathy
722.11 Displacement of thoracic intervertebral disc without myelopathy
722.4 Degeneration of cervical intervertebral disc
722.51 Degeneration of thoracic or thoracolumbar intervertebral disc
722.71 Intervertebral cervical disc disorder with myelopathy, cervical region
722.72 Intervertebral thoracic disc disorder with myelopathy, thoracic region
722.81 Postlaminectomy syndrome, cervical region
722.82 Postlaminectomy syndrome, thoracic region
723.0 Spinal stenosis in cervical region
723.2 Cervicocranial syndrome
723.3 Cervicobrachial syndrome (diffuse)
723.4 Brachial neuritis or radiculitis nos.
723.6 Panniculitis specified as affecting neck
724.01 Spinal stenosis of thoracic region
724.4 Thoracic or lumbosacral neuritis or radiculitis, unspecified

CCI Version 16.3

62310, 92585, 95822, 95860-95861, 95867-95868, 95900, 95904, 95920, 95936-95937

Also not with 64626: 0213T, 0228T, 0230T, 36000, 36400-36410, 36420-36430, 36440, 36600, 36640, 37202, 43752, 51701-51703, 62318, 64400-64435, 64445-64449, 64479, 64483, 64490, 64505-64530, 69990, 76000-76001, 77002, 93000-93010, 93040-93042, 93318, 94002, 94200, 94250, 94680-94690, 94770, 95812-95816, 95819, 95829, 95870, 95925-95934, 95955, 96360, 96365, 96372, 96374-96376, 99148-99149, 99150, J2001

Also not with 64627: 95925-95927, 95930-95934

Note: These CCI edits are used for Medicare. Other payers may reimburse on codes listed above.

Medicare Edits

	Fac RVU	Non-Fac RVU	FUD	Assist
64626	7.3	11.75	10	N/A
64627	1.73	5.04	N/A	N/A

Medicare References: 100-2,15,260; 100-3,160.1; 100-4,12,30; 100-4,12,90.3; 100-4,14,10

64640

64640 Destruction by neurolytic agent; other peripheral nerve or branch

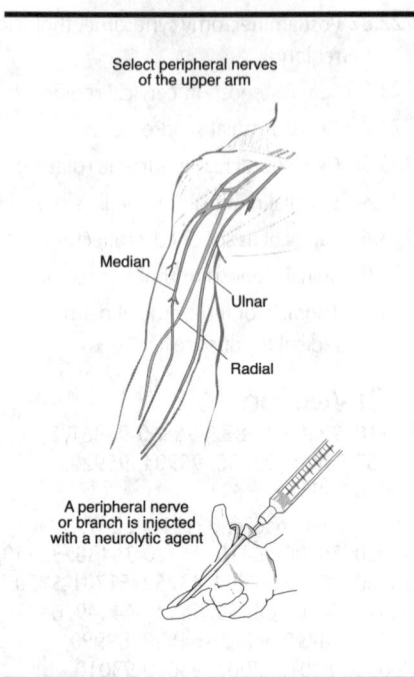

Explanation

This procedure is performed to treat chronic pain. The affected nerve is destroyed using chemical, thermal, electrical, or radiofrequency techniques. These techniques may be used singly or in combination. These procedures are designed to destroy the specific site in the nerve root that produce the pain while leaving sensation intact. Generally intravenous conscious sedation is utilized during the initial phase of the procedure so that the patient can assist the physician in identifying the site of pain and the correct placement of the neurolytic agent. Local anesthesia is administered during the destruction phase of the procedure. Using separately reportable fluoroscopic guidance, a needle is inserted into the affected nerve root. An electrode is then inserted through the needle and a mild electrical current is passed through the electrode. The current produces a tingling sensation at a site on the nerve. The electrode is manipulated until the tingling sensation is felt at the same site as the pain. Once the physician has determined that the electrode is positioned at the site responsible for the pain, a local anesthetic is administered and a neurolytic agent applied. Chemical destruction involves injection of a neurolytic substance (e.g., alcohol, phenol, glycerol) into the affected nerve root. Thermal techniques utilize heat. Electrical techniques utilize an electrical current. Radiofrequency, also referred to as radiofrequency rhizotomy, utilizes a solar or microwave current.

Coding Tips

For fluoroscopic guidance for this procedure, see 77003.

ICD-9-CM Procedural

04.2 Destruction of cranial and peripheral nerves

Anesthesia

64640 N/A

ICD-9-CM Diagnostic

The application of this code is too broad to adequately present ICD-9-CM diagnostic code links here. Refer to your ICD-9-CM book.

Terms To Know

chronic. Persistent, continuing, or recurring.

destruction. Ablation or eradication of a structure or tissue.

fluoroscopy. Radiology technique that allows visual examination of part of the body or a function of an organ using a device that projects an x-ray image on a fluorescent screen.

lesion. Area of damaged tissue that has lost continuity or function, due to disease or trauma. Lesions may be located on internal structures such as the brain, nerves, or kidneys, or visible on the skin.

neurolytic. Destruction of nerve tissue.

peripheral. Outside of a structure or organ.

CCI Version 16.3

0213T, 0216T, 0228T, 0230T, 36000, 36400-36410, 36420-36430, 36440, 36600, 36640, 37202, 43752, 51701-51703, 62310-62319, 64400-64435, 64445-64455, 64479, 64483, 64490, 64493, 64505-64530, 64632❖, 69990, 92585, 93000-93010, 93040-93042, 93318, 94002, 94200, 94250, 94680-94690, 94770, 95812-95816, 95819, 95822, 95829, 95860-95870, 95900, 95904, 95920, 95925-95934, 95936-95937, 95955, 96360, 96365, 96372, 96374-96376, 99148-99149, 99150, J2001

Note: These CCI edits are used for Medicare. Other payers may reimburse on codes listed above.

Medicare Edits

	Fac RVU	Non-Fac RVU	FUD	Assist
64640	4.95	6.42	10	N/A

Medicare References: 100-3,160.1

64702-64704

64702 Neuroplasty; digital, 1 or both, same digit
64704 nerve of hand or foot

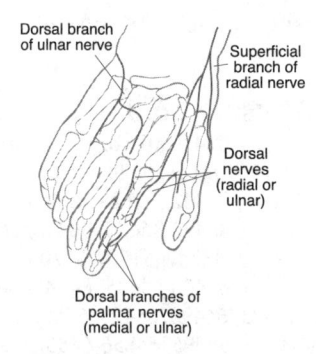

Either a dorsal or palmar digital nerve (or both) is decompressed or freed of scar tissue. Report 64704 when any nerve of the hand undergoes neuroplasty

Explanation
In 64702, the physician releases a compressed nerve in a digit of the hand or foot. The physician makes an incision overlying the nerve. Surrounding tissues are dissected from the nerve freeing it from scar tissue or adhesions. The incision is repaired in layers. One or both of the digital nerves in a single finger or toe are decompressed. In 64704, a nerve in the hand or foot is decompressed.

Coding Tips
Report 64702 only once for one or both digital nerves per finger or hand. Neuroplasty includes external neurolysis and transposition. For internal neurolysis requiring the use of an operating microscope, report 64727 in addition to the code for the primary procedure. Surgical trays, A4550, are not separately reimbursed by Medicare; however, other third-party payers may cover them. Check with the specific payer to determine coverage.

ICD-9-CM Procedural
04.49 Other peripheral nerve or ganglion decompression or lysis of adhesions
04.79 Other neuroplasty

Anesthesia
01810

ICD-9-CM Diagnostic
354.2 Lesion of ulnar nerve
354.3 Lesion of radial nerve
354.4 Causalgia of upper limb
355.4 Lesion of medial popliteal nerve
355.5 Tarsal tunnel syndrome
709.2 Scar condition and fibrosis of skin
711.44 Arthropathy, associated with other bacterial diseases, hand — (Code first underlying disease, such as diseases classifiable to 010-040 (except 036.82), 090-099 (except 098.50))
718.54 Ankylosis of hand joint
719.44 Pain in joint, hand
719.64 Other symptoms referable to hand joint
727.03 Trigger finger (acquired)
727.05 Other tenosynovitis of hand and wrist
727.42 Ganglion of tendon sheath
727.81 Contracture of tendon (sheath)
728.6 Contracture of palmar fascia
729.2 Unspecified neuralgia, neuritis, and radiculitis
729.5 Pain in soft tissues of limb
736.21 Boutonniere deformity
736.22 Swan-neck deformity
755.12 Syndactyly of fingers with fusion of bone
782.0 Disturbance of skin sensation
906.1 Late effect of open wound of extremities without mention of tendon injury
907.4 Late effect of injury to peripheral nerve of shoulder girdle and upper limb
907.9 Late effect of injury to other and unspecified nerve
908.6 Late effect of certain complications of trauma
908.9 Late effect of unspecified injury
909.3 Late effect of complications of surgical and medical care
955.6 Injury to digital nerve, upper limb
955.7 Injury to other specified nerve(s) of shoulder girdle and upper limb
955.8 Injury to multiple nerves of shoulder girdle and upper limb
955.9 Injury to unspecified nerve of shoulder girdle and upper limb
957.8 Injury to multiple nerves in several parts

Terms To Know
contracture. Shortening of muscle or connective tissue.

ganglion. Fluid-filled, benign cyst appearing on a tendon sheath or aponeurosis, frequently found in the hand, wrist, or foot and connecting to an underlying joint.

lesion. Area of damaged tissue that has lost continuity or function, due to disease or trauma. Lesions may be located on internal structures such as the brain, nerves, or kidneys, or visible on the skin.

wound repair. Surgical closure of a wound is divided into three categories: simple, intermediate, and complex. *simple repair:* Surgical closure of a superficial wound, requiring single layer suturing of the skin epidermis, dermis, or subcutaneous tissue. *intermediate repair:* Surgical closure of a wound requiring closure of one or more of the deeper subcutaneous tissue and non-muscle fascia layers in addition to suturing the skin; contaminated wounds with single layer closure that need extensive cleaning or foreign body removal. *complex repair:* Repair of wounds requiring more than layered closure (debridement, scar revision, stents, retention sutures).

CCI Version 16.3
01250, 01320, 01470, 01610, 01710, 01782, 01810, 0213T, 0216T, 0228T, 0230T, 11040-11042, 36000, 36400-36410, 36420-36430, 36440, 36600, 36640, 37202, 43752, 51701-51703, 62310-62319, 64400-64435, 64445-64450, 64479, 64483, 64490, 64493, 64505-64530, 64795, 69990, 92585, 93000-93010, 93040-93042, 93318, 94002, 94200, 94250, 94680-94690, 94770, 95812-95816, 95819, 95822, 95829, 95860-95861, 95867-95868, 95870, 95900, 95904, 95920, 95925-95934, 95936-95937, 95955, 96360, 96365, 96372, 96374-96376, 97597-97598, 97602-97606, 99148-99149, 99150

Also not with 64702: 13132, 29125, 64722-64726

Also not with 64704: 20526-20553, 29085, 29515, 29580-29581, 64721-64726

Note: These CCI edits are used for Medicare. Other payers may reimburse on codes listed above.

Medicare Edits

	Fac RVU	Non-Fac RVU	FUD	Assist
64702	14.12	14.12	90	N/A
64704	9.48	9.48	90	80

Medicare References: 100-2,15,260; 100-4,12,30; 100-4,12,90.3; 100-4,14,10

64708

64708 Neuroplasty, major peripheral nerve, arm or leg, open; other than specified

Major nerves of the upper extremity
- Musculocutaneous
- Median
- Ulnar
- Radial

A major peripheral nerve is decompressed or freed of scar tissues (neuroplasty)

Explanation

The physician performs an open surgical decompression of a compressed major peripheral nerve in the arm. The physician makes an incision in the area of nerve tension and locates the nerve. Surrounding soft tissue or scar tissue is dissected from the nerve to release pressure and the intact nerve is freed. External neurolysis or nerve transposition may also be performed to restore or repair the nerve.

Coding Tips

This code has been revised for 2011 in the official CPT description. Neuroplasty includes external neurolysis and transposition. For internal neurolysis requiring the use of an operating microscope, report 64727. For neuroplasty of a major peripheral nerve, brachial plexus, see 64713.

ICD-9-CM Procedural

- 04.49 Other peripheral nerve or ganglion decompression or lysis of adhesions
- 04.79 Other neuroplasty

Anesthesia

64708 01710, 01810

ICD-9-CM Diagnostic

- 353.9 Unspecified nerve root and plexus disorder
- 354.3 Lesion of radial nerve
- 354.4 Causalgia of upper limb
- 354.9 Unspecified mononeuritis of upper limb
- 355.0 Lesion of sciatic nerve
- 729.5 Pain in soft tissues of limb
- 782.0 Disturbance of skin sensation
- 906.1 Late effect of open wound of extremities without mention of tendon injury
- 907.4 Late effect of injury to peripheral nerve of shoulder girdle and upper limb
- 907.5 Late effect of injury to peripheral nerve of pelvic girdle and lower limb
- 907.9 Late effect of injury to other and unspecified nerve
- 908.6 Late effect of certain complications of trauma
- 908.9 Late effect of unspecified injury
- 909.3 Late effect of complications of surgical and medical care
- 955.0 Injury to axillary nerve
- 955.1 Injury to median nerve
- 955.2 Injury to ulnar nerve
- 955.3 Injury to radial nerve
- 955.4 Injury to musculocutaneous nerve
- 955.7 Injury to other specified nerve(s) of shoulder girdle and upper limb
- 955.8 Injury to multiple nerves of shoulder girdle and upper limb
- 955.9 Injury to unspecified nerve of shoulder girdle and upper limb
- 956.0 Injury to sciatic nerve
- 957.8 Injury to multiple nerves in several parts
- 996.75 Other complications due to nervous system device, implant, and graft — (Use additional code to identify complication: 338.18-338.19, 338.28-338.29)
- 998.2 Accidental puncture or laceration during procedure

Terms To Know

causalgia. Condition due to an injury of a peripheral nerve causing burning pain and possible trophic skin changes.

decompression. Release of pressure.

dissection. Separating by cutting tissue or body structures apart.

late effect. Abnormality, dysfunction, or other residual condition produced after the acute phase of an illness, injury, or disease is over. There is no time limit on when late effects can appear.

lesion. Area of damaged tissue that has lost continuity or function, due to disease or trauma. Lesions may be located on internal structures such as the brain, nerves, or kidneys, or visible on the skin.

mononeuritis. Inflammation of one nerve.

neurolysis. Dissection of a nerve.

soft tissue. Nonepithelial tissues outside of the skeleton.

CCI Version 16.3

01250, 01320, 01470, 01610, 01710, 01782, 01810, 0213T, 0216T, 0228T, 0230T, 11040-11042, 24332, 29125, 36000, 36400-36410, 36420-36430, 36440, 36600, 36640, 37202, 43752, 51701-51703, 62310-62319, 64400-64435, 64445-64450, 64479, 64483, 64490, 64493, 64505-64530, 64718-64722, 64795, 64856-64857, 69990, 92585, 93000-93010, 93040-93042, 93318, 94002, 94200, 94250, 94680-94690, 94770, 95812-95816, 95819, 95822, 95829, 95860-95861, 95867-95868, 95870, 95900, 95904, 95920, 95925-95934, 95936-95937, 95955, 96360, 96365, 96372, 96374-96376, 97597-97598, 97602-97606, 99148-99149, 99150

Note: These CCI edits are used for Medicare. Other payers may reimburse on codes listed above.

Medicare Edits

	Fac RVU	Non-Fac RVU	FUD	Assist
64708	14.14	14.14	90	80

Medicare References: 100-2,15,260; 100-4,12,30; 100-4,12,90.3; 100-4,14,10

64713

64713 Neuroplasty, major peripheral nerve, arm or leg, open; brachial plexus

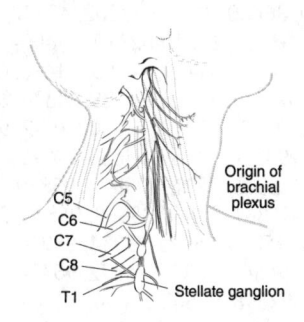

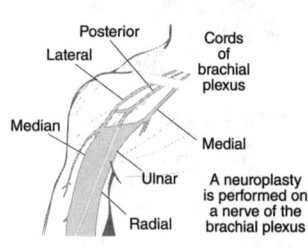

Explanation
The physician performs an open surgical decompression of a compressed brachial plexus nerve. The physician makes an incision in the area of nerve tension and locates the nerve. Surrounding soft tissue or scar tissue is dissected from the nerve to release pressure and the intact nerve is freed. External neurolysis or nerve transposition may also be performed to restore or repair the nerve; this is included in the codes for the decompression procedure.

Coding Tips
This code has been revised for 2011 in the official CPT description. Neuroplasty includes external neurolysis and transposition. For internal neurolysis requiring use of an operating microscope, report 64727 in addition to the code for the primary procedure.

ICD-9-CM Procedural
04.79 Other neuroplasty

Anesthesia
64713 01610

ICD-9-CM Diagnostic
353.0 Brachial plexus lesions
723.4 Brachial neuritis or radiculitis nos.
953.4 Injury to brachial plexus

996.75 Other complications due to nervous system device, implant, and graft — (Use additional code to identify complication: 338.18-338.19, 338.28-338.29)

Terms To Know

lesion. Area of damaged tissue that has lost continuity or function, due to disease or trauma. Lesions may be located on internal structures such as the brain, nerves, or kidneys, or visible on the skin.

neuritis. Inflammation of a nerve or group of nerves, often manifested by loss of function and reflexes, pain, and numbness or tingling.

peripheral. Outside of a structure or organ.

radiculitis. Pain along an inflamed nerve, with inflammation of the root of the associated spinal nerve.

CCI Version 16.3
0213T, 0216T, 0228T, 0230T, 11040-11042, 21700-21705, 36000, 36400-36410, 36420-36430, 36440, 36600, 36640, 37202, 43752, 51701-51703, 62310-62319, 64400-64435, 64445-64450, 64479, 64483, 64490, 64493, 64505-64530, 64722, 64795, 64861, 69990, 92585, 93000-93010, 93040-93042, 93318, 94002, 94200, 94250, 94680-94690, 94770, 95812-95816, 95819, 95822, 95829, 95860-95861, 95867-95868, 95870, 95900, 95904, 95920, 95925-95934, 95936-95937, 95955, 96360, 96365, 96372, 96374-96376, 97597-97598, 97602-97606, 99148-99149, 99150

Note: These CCI edits are used for Medicare. Other payers may reimburse on codes listed above.

Medicare Edits

	Fac RVU	Non-Fac RVU	FUD	Assist
64713	22.29	22.29	90	80

Medicare References: 100-2,15,260; 100-4,12,30; 100-4,12,90.3; 100-4,14,10

64718

64718 Neuroplasty and/or transposition; ulnar nerve at elbow

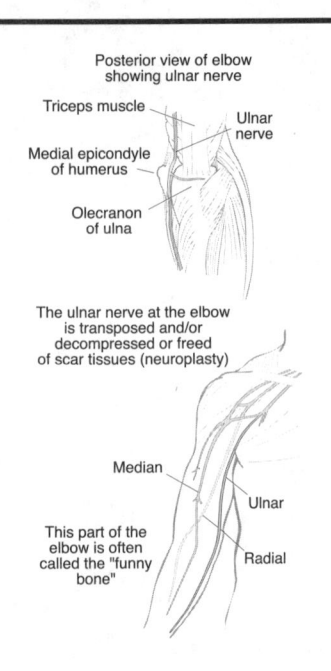

Posterior view of elbow showing ulnar nerve
- Triceps muscle
- Ulnar nerve
- Medial epicondyle of humerus
- Olecranon of ulna

The ulnar nerve at the elbow is transposed and/or decompressed or freed of scar tissues (neuroplasty)
- Median
- Ulnar
- Radial
- This part of the elbow is often called the "funny bone"

Explanation

The physician decompresses a stressed ulnar nerve by freeing the nerve and the tissue surrounding the nerve. The physician makes an incision at the medial epicondyle and locates the nerve. Surrounding tissues are dissected from the nerve and the nerve is freed from the underlying bed. The nerve is moved over the epicondyle and stabilized with sutures in the surrounding tissue. The incision is sutured in layers.

Coding Tips

Neuroplasty includes external neurolysis and transposition. For internal neurolysis requiring the use of an operating microscope, report 64727 in addition to the code for the primary procedure. According to CPT guidelines, cast application or strapping (including removal) is only reported as a replacement procedure or when the cast application or strapping is an initial service performed without a restorative treatment or procedure. See "Application of Casts and Strapping" in the CPT book in the Surgery Section, under the Musculoskeletal system.

ICD-9-CM Procedural

- 04.49 Other peripheral nerve or ganglion decompression or lysis of adhesions
- 04.6 Transposition of cranial and peripheral nerves
- 04.79 Other neuroplasty

Anesthesia

64718 01710

ICD-9-CM Diagnostic

- 354.2 Lesion of ulnar nerve
- 354.5 Mononeuritis multiplex
- 356.8 Other specified idiopathic peripheral neuropathy
- 718.42 Contracture of upper arm joint
- 719.42 Pain in joint, upper arm
- 723.4 Brachial neuritis or radiculitis nos.
- 727.41 Ganglion of joint
- 729.5 Pain in soft tissues of limb
- 782.0 Disturbance of skin sensation
- 906.1 Late effect of open wound of extremities without mention of tendon injury
- 907.4 Late effect of injury to peripheral nerve of shoulder girdle and upper limb
- 908.9 Late effect of unspecified injury
- 909.3 Late effect of complications of surgical and medical care
- 955.2 Injury to ulnar nerve
- 955.9 Injury to unspecified nerve of shoulder girdle and upper limb
- 996.75 Other complications due to nervous system device, implant, and graft — (Use additional code to identify complication: 338.18-338.19, 338.28-338.29)

Terms To Know

contracture. Shortening of muscle or connective tissue.

epicondyle. Bony protrusion at the distal end of the humerus (elbow).

ganglion. Fluid-filled, benign cyst appearing on a tendon sheath or aponeurosis, frequently found in the hand, wrist, or foot and connecting to an underlying joint.

lesion. Area of damaged tissue that has lost continuity or function, due to disease or trauma. Lesions may be located on internal structures such as the brain, nerves, or kidneys, or visible on the skin.

mononeuritis multiplex. Peripheral neuropathy involving isolated damage to at least two separate nerves.

neuritis. Inflammation of a nerve or group of nerves, often manifested by loss of function and reflexes, pain, and numbness or tingling.

radiculitis. Pain along an inflamed nerve, with inflammation of the root of the associated spinal nerve.

CCI Version 16.3

01250, 01320, 01470, 01610, 01710, 01782, 01810, 0213T, 0216T, 0228T, 0230T, 11040-11042, 24310, 24332, 24358, 25290, 29105, 36000, 36400-36410, 36420-36430, 36440, 36600, 36640, 37202, 43752, 51701-51703, 62310-62319, 64400-64435, 64445-64450, 64479, 64483, 64490, 64493, 64505-64530, 64722, 64795, 64836, 69990, 92585, 93000-93010, 93040-93042, 93318, 94002, 94200, 94250, 94680-94690, 94770, 95812-95816, 95819, 95822, 95829, 95860-95861, 95867-95868, 95870, 95900, 95904, 95920, 95925-95934, 95936-95937, 95955, 96360, 96365, 96372, 96374-96376, 97597-97598, 97602-97606, 99148-99149, 99150

Note: These CCI edits are used for Medicare. Other payers may reimburse on codes listed above.

Medicare Edits

	Fac RVU	Non-Fac RVU	FUD	Assist
64718	17.03	17.03	90	80

Medicare References: 100-2,15,260; 100-4,12,30; 100-4,12,90.3; 100-4,14,10

64719-64721

64719 Neuroplasty and/or transposition; ulnar nerve at wrist
64721 median nerve at carpal tunnel

Neuroplasty and/or transposition is performed on the ulnar nerve at the wrist

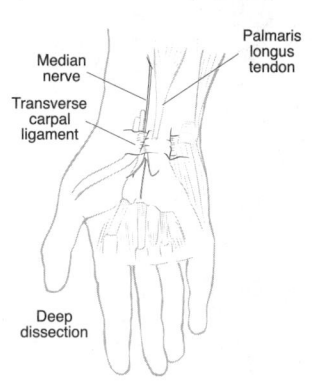

Median nerve
Transverse carpal ligament
Palmaris longus tendon
Deep dissection

Surgery is performed on the median nerve at the carpal tunnel. Ordinarily, the transverse ligament is cut to decrease pressure on the median nerve. Or the position of the nerve may be changed

Explanation

The physician decompresses or transposes a portion of the ulnar or median nerve to restore feeling to the hand. The physician makes a horizontal incision in the wrist at the metacarpal joints and locates the nerve. In 64719, the ulnar nerve is located and freed. In 64721, the median nerve is decompressed by freeing the nerve inside the carpal tunnel. Soft tissues are resected and the nerve is freed from the underlying bed. Care is taken to ensure tension is released and the incision is closed in sutured layers.

Coding Tips

Neuroplasty includes external neurolysis and transposition. For internal neurolysis requiring the use of an operating microscope, report 64727 in addition to the code for the primary procedure. According to CPT guidelines, cast application or strapping (including removal) is only reported as a replacement procedure or when the cast application or strapping is an initial service performed without a restorative treatment or procedure. See "Application of Casts and Strapping" in the CPT book in the Surgery Section, under the Musculoskeletal system. For carpel tunnel release performed endoscopically, see 29848.

ICD-9-CM Procedural

04.43 Release of carpal tunnel
04.49 Other peripheral nerve or ganglion decompression or lysis of adhesions
04.6 Transposition of cranial and peripheral nerves
04.79 Other neuroplasty

Anesthesia
01810

ICD-9-CM Diagnostic

354.0 Carpal tunnel syndrome
354.2 Lesion of ulnar nerve
354.5 Mononeuritis multiplex
357.1 Polyneuropathy in collagen vascular disease — (Code first underlying disease: 446.0, 710.0, 714.0)
359.6 Symptomatic inflammatory myopathy in diseases classified elsewhere — (Code first underlying disease: 135, 140.0-208.9, 277.30-277.39, 446.0, 710.0, 710.1, 710.2, 714.0)
714.0 Rheumatoid arthritis — (Use additional code to identify manifestation: 357.1, 359.6)
715.94 Osteoarthrosis, unspecified whether generalized or localized, hand
716.14 Traumatic arthropathy, hand
719.44 Pain in joint, hand
723.4 Brachial neuritis or radiculitis nos.
726.4 Enthesopathy of wrist and carpus
727.04 Radial styloid tenosynovitis
727.41 Ganglion of joint
728.6 Contracture of palmar fascia
729.5 Pain in soft tissues of limb
782.0 Disturbance of skin sensation
794.17 Nonspecific abnormal electromyogram (EMG)
906.1 Late effect of open wound of extremities without mention of tendon injury
907.4 Late effect of injury to peripheral nerve of shoulder girdle and upper limb
908.9 Late effect of unspecified injury
909.3 Late effect of complications of surgical and medical care
955.1 Injury to median nerve
955.2 Injury to ulnar nerve

Terms To Know

ganglion. Fluid-filled, benign cyst appearing on a tendon sheath or aponeurosis, frequently found in the hand, wrist, or foot and connecting to an underlying joint.

lesion. Area of damaged tissue that has lost continuity or function, due to disease or trauma. Lesions may be located on internal structures such as the brain, nerves, or kidneys, or visible on the skin.

mononeuritis. Inflammation of one nerve.

tenosynovitis. Inflammation of a tendon sheath due to infection or disease.

CCI Version 16.3

01250, 01320, 01470, 01610, 01710, 01782, 01810, 0213T, 0216T, 0228T, 0230T, 25000-25001, 29125, 36000, 36400-36410, 36420-36430, 36440, 36600, 36640, 37202, 43752, 51701-51703, 62310-62319, 64400-64435, 64445-64450, 64479, 64483, 64490, 64493, 64505-64530, 64722, 69990, 92585, 93000-93010, 93040-93042, 93318, 94002, 94200, 94250, 94680-94690, 94770, 95812-95816, 95819, 95822, 95829, 95860-95861, 95867-95868, 95870, 95900, 95904, 95920, 95925-95934, 95936-95937, 95955, 96360, 96365, 96372, 96374-96376, 97597-97598, 97602-97606, 99148-99149, 99150

Also not with 64719: 11040-11042, 25020, 25024-25025, 25110-25111, 35761, 64795, 64836

Also not with 64721: 11900, 20526-20553, 25071, 25110, 25295, 29075, 29843-29845, 29848, 64712

Note: These CCI edits are used for Medicare. Other payers may reimburse on codes listed above.

Medicare Edits

	Fac RVU	Non-Fac RVU	FUD	Assist
64719	11.53	11.53	90	N/A
64721	12.29	12.35	90	N/A

Medicare References: 100-2,15,260; 100-4,12,30; 100-4,12,90.3; 100-4,14,10

64727

64727 Internal neurolysis, requiring use of operating microscope (List separately in addition to code for neuroplasty)
(Neuroplasty includes external neurolysis)

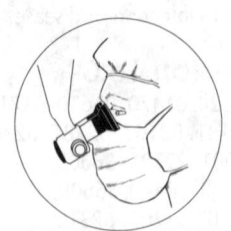

Microsurgical techniques are employed

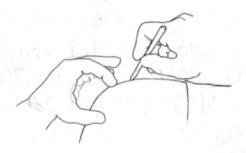

The nerve is surgically accessed

Neurolysis requiring the use of an operating microscope is performed

Explanation

The physician makes an incision over the affected nerve and locates the nerve. The physician resects the nerve sheath parallel to the fibers and releases scar tissue within the nerve.

Coding Tips

As an "add-on" code, 64727 is not subject to multiple procedure rules. No reimbursement reduction or modifier 51 is applied. Add-on codes describe additional intra-service work associated with the primary procedure. They are performed by the same physician on the same date of service as the primary service/procedure, and must never be reported as a stand-alone code. Neuroplasty includes external neurolysis. Report 64727 in addition to a procedure for neuroplasty.

ICD-9-CM Procedural

04.41	Decompression of trigeminal nerve root
04.42	Other cranial nerve decompression
04.43	Release of carpal tunnel
04.49	Other peripheral nerve or ganglion decompression or lysis of adhesions
04.6	Transposition of cranial and peripheral nerves
04.79	Other neuroplasty

Anesthesia

64727 N/A

ICD-9-CM Diagnostic

This is an add-on code. Refer to the corresponding primary procedure code for ICD-9-CM diagnosis code links.

Terms To Know

decompression. Release of pressure.

neurolysis. Dissection of a nerve.

transposition. Removal or exchange from one side to another; change of position from one place to another.

CCI Version 16.3

62310-62311, 69990, 92585, 95822, 95860-95861, 95867-95868, 95870, 95900, 95904, 95920, 95925-95934, 95936-95937

Note: These CCI edits are used for Medicare. Other payers may reimburse on codes listed above.

Medicare Edits

	Fac RVU	Non-Fac RVU	FUD	Assist
64727	5.47	5.47	N/A	N/A

Medicare References: 100-2,15,260; 100-4,12,30; 100-4,12,90.3; 100-4,14,10

64772

64772 Transection or avulsion of other spinal nerve, extradural

Extradural spinal nerves not previously delineated are transected or avulsed

Explanation
The physician cuts or avulses another spinal nerve, such as branch nerves of major nerves not listed in other codes. The physician incises the skin overlying the nerve from C1 to S4. The tissues are dissected and the nerve is exposed. The nerve is destroyed. The incision is sutured in layers.

Coding Tips
For section of spinal accessory nerve requiring laminectomy, see 63191. For injection, anesthetic agent, spinal accessory nerve, see 64412.

ICD-9-CM Procedural
- 03.1 Division of intraspinal nerve root
- 04.07 Other excision or avulsion of cranial and peripheral nerves
- 07.42 Division of nerves to adrenal glands

Anesthesia
64772 00600, 00620, 00630

ICD-9-CM Diagnostic
- 237.70 Neurofibromatosis, unspecified
- 237.71 Neurofibromatosis, Type 1 (von Recklinghausen's disease)
- 237.72 Neurofibromatosis, Type 2 (acoustic neurofibromatosis)
- 237.73 Schwannomatosis
- 237.79 Other neurofibromatosis
- 353.6 Phantom limb (syndrome)
- 354.4 Causalgia of upper limb
- 355.1 Meralgia paresthetica
- 716.15 Traumatic arthropathy, pelvic region and thigh
- 729.2 Unspecified neuralgia, neuritis, and radiculitis
- 879.4 Open wound of abdominal wall, lateral, without mention of complication
- 926.11 Crushing injury of back — (Use additional code to identify any associated injuries: 800-829, 850.0-854.1, 860.0-869.1)
- 953.4 Injury to brachial plexus
- 954.1 Injury to other sympathetic nerve, excluding shoulder and pelvic girdles
- 955.3 Injury to radial nerve

Terms To Know

avulsion. Forcible tearing away of a part, by surgical means or traumatic injury.

causalgia. Condition due to an injury of a peripheral nerve causing burning pain and possible trophic skin changes.

dissection. Separating by cutting tissue or body structures apart.

meralgia paresthetica. Neurologic disorder due to constriction of the lateral femoral cutaneous nerve as it exits the pelvis, manifested by tingling, lack of sensation, and burning pain of the outer thigh. It is often associated with obesity, diabetes, pregnancy, or restrictive clothing.

neuralgia. Sharp, shooting pains extending along one or more nerve pathways. Underlying causes may include nerve injury, diabetes, or viral complications.

neurofibromatosis. Autosomal dominant inherited condition with developmental changes in the nervous system, muscles, bones, and skin, producing coffee colored spots of pigmented skin (café au lait spots) and multiple soft tumor neurofibromas distributed over the entire body.

phantom limb syndrome. Itching, dull ache, or sharp, shooting pains mimicking the nerves of amputated limb.

radiculitis. Pain along an inflamed nerve, with inflammation of the root of the associated spinal nerve.

CCI Version 16.3
0213T, 0216T, 0228T, 0230T, 36000, 36400-36410, 36420-36430, 36440, 36600, 36640, 37202, 43752, 51701-51703, 62310-62319, 64400-64435, 64445-64450, 64479, 64483, 64490, 64493, 64505-64530, 69990, 92585, 93000-93010, 93040-93042, 93318, 94002, 94200, 94250, 94680-94690, 94770, 95812-95816, 95819, 95822, 95829, 95860-95861, 95867-95868, 95870, 95900, 95904, 95920, 95925-95934, 95936-95937, 95955, 96360, 96365, 96372, 96374-96376, 99148-99149, 99150

Note: These CCI edits are used for Medicare. Other payers may reimburse on codes listed above.

Medicare Edits

	Fac RVU	Non-Fac RVU	FUD	Assist
64772	16.83	16.83	90	80

Medicare References: 100-2,15,260; 100-4,12,30; 100-4,12,90.3; 100-4,14,10

64774

64774 Excision of neuroma; cutaneous nerve, surgically identifiable

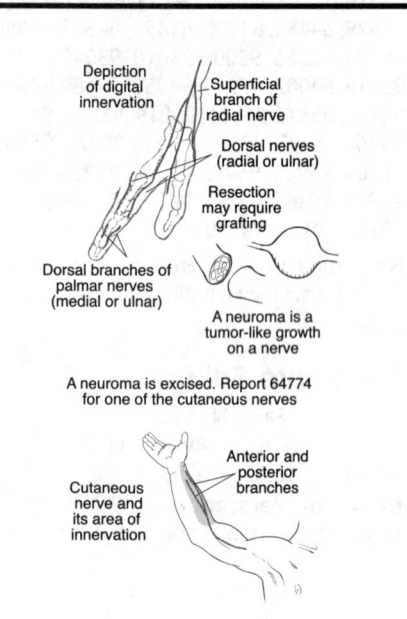

Explanation

The physician excises a neuroma of a peripheral nerve. A neuroma is a benign tumor formed secondarily by trauma to the nerve. The physician incises the skin and locates and excises the neuroma in the subcutaneous tissue.

Coding Tips

When nerve end is implanted into bone or muscle, report 64787 in addition to the neuroma excision. For excision of a Morton neuroma, see 28080. For excision of a tender scar, skin and subcutaneous tissue, with or without a tiny neuroma, see 11400–11446 for the excision and 13100–13153 if complex repair is required.

ICD-9-CM Procedural

04.07 Other excision or avulsion of cranial and peripheral nerves

Anesthesia

64774 00300, 00400, 00402, 00404, 00406, 00410

ICD-9-CM Diagnostic

The application of this code is too broad to adequately present ICD-9-CM diagnostic code links here. Refer to your ICD-9-CM book.

Terms To Know

benign. Mild or nonmalignant in nature.

neuroma. Any type of tumor growing from a nerve or comprised of nerve cells and fibers.

subcutaneous tissue. Sheet or wide band of adipose (fat) and areolar connective tissue in two layers attached to the dermis.

CCI Version 16.3

01250, 01320, 01470, 01610, 01710, 01782, 01810, 0213T, 0216T, 0228T, 0230T, 36000, 36400-36410, 36420-36430, 36440, 36600, 36640, 37202, 43752, 51701-51703, 62310-62319, 64400-64435, 64445-64455, 64479, 64483, 64490, 64493, 64505-64530, 64702-64708, 64722-64726, 64795, 69990, 92585, 93000-93010, 93040-93042, 93318, 94002, 94200, 94250, 94680-94690, 94770, 95812-95816, 95819, 95822, 95829, 95860-95861, 95867-95868, 95870, 95900, 95904, 95920, 95925-95934, 95936-95937, 95955, 96360, 96365, 96372, 96374-96376, 99148-99149, 99150

Note: These CCI edits are used for Medicare. Other payers may reimburse on codes listed above.

Medicare Edits

	Fac RVU	Non-Fac RVU	FUD	Assist
64774	12.12	12.12	90	N/A

Medicare References: 100-2,15,260; 100-4,12,30; 100-4,12,90.3; 100-4,14,10

64776-64778

64776 Excision of neuroma; digital nerve, 1 or both, same digit

64778 digital nerve, each additional digit (List separately in addition to code for primary procedure)

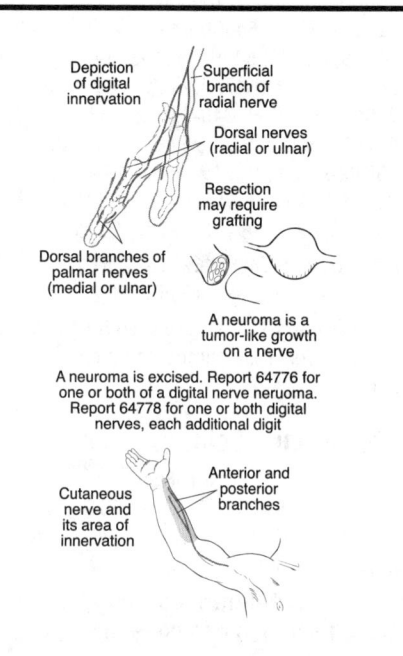

Explanation

The physician excises a neuroma of a peripheral nerve. A neuroma is a tumor formed secondarily by trauma to the nerve. In 64776, the physician incises the skin over the digital nerve and excises the neuroma. Report 64778 for each additional neuroma of a separate digit.

Coding Tips

Use 64778 in conjunction with 64776. As an "add-on" code, 64778 is not subject to multiple procedure rules. No reimbursement reduction or modifier 51 is applied. Add-on codes describe additional intra-service work associated with the primary procedure. They are performed by the same physician on the same date of service as the primary service/procedure, and must never be reported as a stand-alone code. When nerve end is implanted into bone or muscle, report 64787 in addition to the neuroma excision. For excision of a Morton neuroma, see 28080.

ICD-9-CM Procedural

04.07 Other excision or avulsion of cranial and peripheral nerves

Anesthesia

64776 01810
64778 N/A

ICD-9-CM Diagnostic

237.70 Neurofibromatosis, unspecified
237.71 Neurofibromatosis, Type 1 (von Recklinghausen's disease)
237.72 Neurofibromatosis, Type 2 (acoustic neurofibromatosis)
237.73 Schwannomatosis
237.79 Other neurofibromatosis
354.9 Unspecified mononeuritis of upper limb
355.6 Lesion of plantar nerve
356.4 Idiopathic progressive polyneuropathy
782.2 Localized superficial swelling, mass, or lump

Terms To Know

benign. Mild or nonmalignant in nature.

excision. Surgical removal of an organ or tissue.

idiopathic progressive polyneuropathy. Pathological change in multiple peripheral nerves of unknown cause.

innervation. Nerve distribution to a body part.

lesion. Area of damaged tissue that has lost continuity or function, due to disease or trauma. Lesions may be located on internal structures such as the brain, nerves, or kidneys, or visible on the skin.

mononeuritis. Inflammation of one nerve.

neurofibromatosis. Autosomal dominant inherited condition with developmental changes in the nervous system, muscles, bones, and skin, producing coffee colored spots of pigmented skin (café au lait spots) and multiple soft tumor neurofibromas distributed over the entire body.

neuroma. Any type of tumor growing from a nerve or comprised of nerve cells and fibers.

peripheral. Outside of a structure or organ.

superficial. On the skin surface or near the surface of any involved structure or field of interest.

CCI Version 16.3

92585, 95822, 95860-95861, 95867-95868, 95900, 95904, 95920, 95936-95937

Also not with 64776: 01250, 01320, 01470, 01610, 01710, 01782, 01810, 0213T, 0216T, 0228T, 0230T, 36000, 36400-36410, 36420-36430, 36440, 36600, 36640, 37202, 43752, 51701-51703, 62310-62319, 64400-64435, 64445-64455, 64479, 64483, 64490, 64493, 64505-64530, 64702-64722, 64795, 69990, 93000-93010, 93040-93042, 93318, 94002, 94200, 94250, 94680-94690, 94770, 95812-95816, 95819, 95829, 95870, 95925-95934, 95955, 96360, 96365, 96372, 96374-96376, 99148-99149, 99150

Also not with 64778: 62310-62311, 95925-95927, 95930-95934

Note: These CCI edits are used for Medicare. Other payers may reimburse on codes listed above.

Medicare Edits

	Fac RVU	Non-Fac RVU	FUD	Assist
64776	11.4	11.4	90	80
64778	5.65	5.65	N/A	N/A

Medicare References: 100-2,15,260; 100-4,12,30; 100-4,12,90.3; 100-4,14,10

64782-64783

64782 Excision of neuroma; hand or foot, except digital nerve
64783 hand or foot, each additional nerve, except same digit (List separately in addition to code for primary procedure)

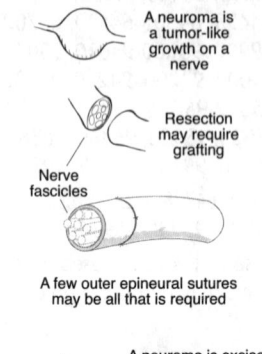

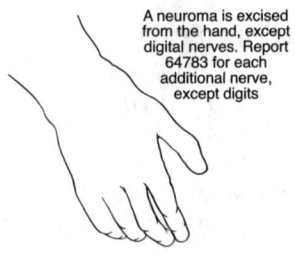

Explanation
The physician excises a neuroma of a peripheral nerve (except digital nerve) of the hand or foot. A neuroma is a benign tumor formed secondarily by trauma to the nerve. The physician incises the affected area in a hand or foot. After locating the nerve with the symptomatic neuroma, the physician excises the tumor. The incision is sutured in layers. Report 64783 for additional neuromas of the hand or foot.

Coding Tips
Use 64783 in conjunction with 64782. As an "add-on" code, 64783 is not subject to multiple procedure rules. No reimbursement reduction or modifier 51 is applied. Add-on codes describe additional intra-service work associated with the primary procedure. They are performed by the same physician on the same date of service as the primary service/procedure, and must never be reported as a stand-alone code. Local anesthesia is included in these services. However, these procedures may be performed under general anesthesia, depending on the age and/or condition of the patient. For implantation of nerve end into bone or muscle after neuroma excision, see 64787. Surgical trays, A4550, are not separately reimbursed by Medicare; however, other third-party payers may cover them. Check with the specific payer to determine coverage.

ICD-9-CM Procedural
04.07 Other excision or avulsion of cranial and peripheral nerves

Anesthesia
64782 01810
64783 N/A

ICD-9-CM Diagnostic
215.2 Other benign neoplasm of connective and other soft tissue of upper limb, including shoulder
354.8 Other mononeuritis of upper limb
729.2 Unspecified neuralgia, neuritis, and radiculitis
729.5 Pain in soft tissues of limb
782.0 Disturbance of skin sensation
782.2 Localized superficial swelling, mass, or lump
955.7 Injury to other specified nerve(s) of shoulder girdle and upper limb
955.8 Injury to multiple nerves of shoulder girdle and upper limb
955.9 Injury to unspecified nerve of shoulder girdle and upper limb

Terms To Know
benign. Mild or nonmalignant in nature.

excision. Surgical removal of an organ or tissue.

incision. Act of cutting into tissue or an organ.

mononeuritis. Inflammation of one nerve.

neuralgia. Sharp, shooting pains extending along one or more nerve pathways. Underlying causes may include nerve injury, diabetes, or viral complications.

neuritis. Inflammation of a nerve or group of nerves, often manifested by loss of function and reflexes, pain, and numbness or tingling.

radiculitis. Pain along an inflamed nerve, with inflammation of the root of the associated spinal nerve.

soft tissue. Nonepithelial tissues outside of the skeleton that includes subcutaneous adipose tissue, fibrous tissue, fascia, muscles, blood and lymph vessels, and peripheral nervous system tissue.

CCI Version 16.3
92585, 95822, 95860-95861, 95867-95868, 95900, 95904, 95920, 95936-95937

Also not with 64782: 01250, 01320, 01470, 01610, 01710, 01782, 01810, 0213T, 0216T, 0228T, 0230T, 12020, 20526-20553, 29515, 36000, 36400-36410, 36420-36430, 36440, 36600, 36640, 37202, 43752, 51701-51703, 62310-62319, 64400-64435, 64445-64455, 64479, 64483, 64490, 64493, 64505-64530, 64702-64726, 64774, 64795, 69990, 93000-93010, 93040-93042, 93318, 94002, 94200, 94250, 94680-94690, 94770, 95812-95816, 95819, 95829, 95870, 95925-95934, 95955, 96360, 96365, 96372, 96374-96376, 99148-99149, 99150

Also not with 64783: 62310-62311, 95925-95927, 95930-95934

Note: These CCI edits are used for Medicare. Other payers may reimburse on codes listed above.

Medicare Edits

	Fac RVU	Non-Fac RVU	FUD	Assist
64782	13.22	13.22	90	N/A
64783	6.44	6.44	N/A	N/A

Medicare References: 100-2,15,260; 100-4,12,30; 100-4,12,90.3; 100-4,14,10

64784

64784 Excision of neuroma; major peripheral nerve, except sciatic

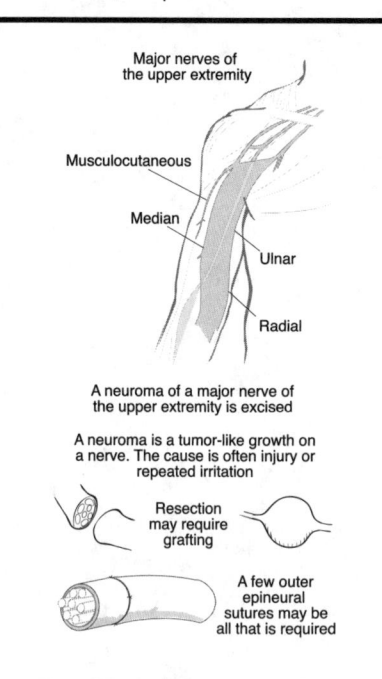

Major nerves of the upper extremity
- Musculocutaneous
- Median
- Ulnar
- Radial

A neuroma of a major nerve of the upper extremity is excised

A neuroma is a tumor-like growth on a nerve. The cause is often injury or repeated irritation

Resection may require grafting

A few outer epineural sutures may be all that is required

Explanation

The physician excises a neuroma of a peripheral nerve. A neuroma is a benign tumor formed secondarily by trauma to the nerve. The physician incises the area over the affected major peripheral nerve. After locating the nerve with the symptomatic neuroma, the physician excises the tumor. The incision is closed in sutured layers.

Coding Tips

This procedure involves major peripheral nerves excluding cutaneous, digital, sciatic, and nerves of the hands or feet. To report excision of a neuroma of the cutaneous nerve, see 64774. For excision of a digital neuroma, see 64776–64778. For excision of a neuroma of the hand or foot, see 64782–64783. When nerve end is implanted into bone or muscle, report 64787 in addition to the neuroma excision.

ICD-9-CM Procedural

- 04.06 Other cranial or peripheral ganglionectomy
- 04.07 Other excision or avulsion of cranial and peripheral nerves

Anesthesia

64784 01610, 01710, 01810

ICD-9-CM Diagnostic

- 215.2 Other benign neoplasm of connective and other soft tissue of upper limb, including shoulder
- 353.6 Phantom limb (syndrome)
- 729.5 Pain in soft tissues of limb

Terms To Know

benign. Mild or nonmalignant in nature.

neuroma. Any type of tumor growing from a nerve or comprised of nerve cells and fibers.

peripheral. Outside of a structure or organ.

phantom limb syndrome. Itching, dull ache, or sharp, shooting pains mimicking the nerves of amputated limb.

soft tissue. Nonepithelial tissues outside of the skeleton that includes subcutaneous adipose tissue, fibrous tissue, fascia, muscles, blood and lymph vessels, and peripheral nervous system tissue.

tumor. Pathological swelling or enlargement; a neoplastic growth of uncontrolled, abnormal multiplication of cells.

CCI Version 16.3

01250, 01320, 01470, 01610, 01710, 01782, 01810, 0213T, 0216T, 0228T, 0230T, 36000, 36400-36410, 36420-36430, 36440, 36600, 36640, 37202, 43752, 51701-51703, 62310-62319, 64400-64435, 64445-64450, 64479, 64483, 64490, 64493, 64505-64530, 64702-64726, 64795, 64856-64857, 69990, 92585, 93000-93010, 93040-93042, 93318, 94002, 94200, 94250, 94680-94690, 94770, 95812-95816, 95819, 95822, 95829, 95860-95861, 95867-95868, 95870, 95900, 95904, 95920, 95925-95934, 95936-95937, 95955, 96360, 96365, 96372, 96374-96376, 99148-99149, 99150

Note: These CCI edits are used for Medicare. Other payers may reimburse on codes listed above.

Medicare Edits

	Fac RVU	Non-Fac RVU	FUD	Assist
64784	21.38	21.38	90	80

Medicare References: 100-2,15,260; 100-4,12,30; 100-4,12,90.3; 100-4,14,10

64786

64786 Excision of neuroma; sciatic nerve

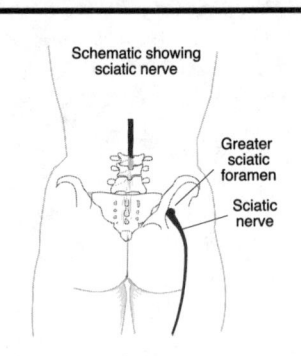

Schematic showing sciatic nerve

Greater sciatic foramen

Sciatic nerve

The sciatic nerve enters the buttock through the greater sciatic foramen. It lies under the gluteus maximus and enters the thigh where it descends the middle back of the leg

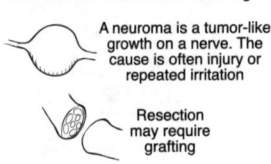

A neuroma is a tumor-like growth on a nerve. The cause is often injury or repeated irritation

Resection may require grafting

A neuroma of the sciatic nerve is excised

Explanation

The physician excises a neuroma of the sciatic nerve. A neuroma is a benign tumor formed secondarily by trauma to the nerve. The physician incises the affected area in the buttocks or back of the upper leg over the sciatic nerve. After locating the site of the symptomatic neuroma, the physician excises the tumor. The incision is closed in sutured layers.

Coding Tips

When nerve end is implanted into bone or muscle, report 64787 in addition to the neuroma excision.

ICD-9-CM Procedural

- 04.06 Other cranial or peripheral ganglionectomy
- 04.07 Other excision or avulsion of cranial and peripheral nerves

Anesthesia

64786   01250

ICD-9-CM Diagnostic

- 237.70 Neurofibromatosis, unspecified
- 237.79 Other neurofibromatosis
- 355.0 Lesion of sciatic nerve
- 724.3 Sciatica
- 729.5 Pain in soft tissues of limb

Terms To Know

benign. Mild or nonmalignant in nature.

causalgia. Condition due to an injury of a peripheral nerve causing burning pain and possible trophic skin changes.

excision. Surgical removal of an organ or tissue.

lesion. Area of damaged tissue that has lost continuity or function, due to disease or trauma. Lesions may be located on internal structures such as the brain, nerves, or kidneys, or visible on the skin.

neurofibromatosis. Autosomal dominant inherited condition with developmental changes in the nervous system, muscles, bones, and skin, producing coffee colored spots of pigmented skin (café au lait spots) and multiple soft tumor neurofibromas distributed over the entire body.

neuroma. Any type of tumor growing from a nerve or comprised of nerve cells and fibers.

secondary. Second in order of occurrence or importance, or appearing during the course of another disease or condition.

tumor. Pathological swelling or enlargement; a neoplastic growth of uncontrolled, abnormal multiplication of cells.

CCI Version 16.3

0213T, 0216T, 0228T, 0230T, 36000, 36400-36410, 36420-36430, 36440, 36600, 36640, 37202, 43752, 51701-51703, 62310-62319, 64400-64435, 64445-64450, 64479, 64483, 64490, 64493, 64505-64530, 64702-64726, 64795, 64858, 69990, 92585, 93000-93010, 93040-93042, 93318, 94002, 94200, 94250, 94680-94690, 94770, 95812-95816, 95819, 95822, 95829, 95860-95861, 95867-95868, 95870, 95900, 95904, 95920, 95925-95934, 95936-95937, 95955, 96360, 96365, 96372, 96374-96376, 99148-99149, 99150

Note: These CCI edits are used for Medicare. Other payers may reimburse on codes listed above.

Medicare Edits

	Fac RVU	Non-Fac RVU	FUD	Assist
64786	31.55	31.55	90	80

Medicare References: 100-2,15,260; 100-4,12,30; 100-4,12,90.3; 100-4,14,10

64787

64787 Implantation of nerve end into bone or muscle (List separately in addition to neuroma excision)

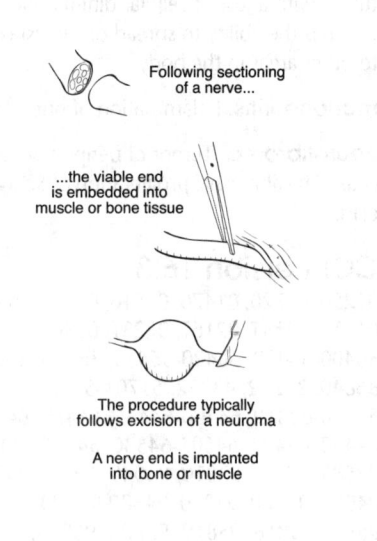

Following sectioning of a nerve...

...the viable end is embedded into muscle or bone tissue

The procedure typically follows excision of a neuroma

A nerve end is implanted into bone or muscle

Explanation

The physician implants a nerve into a bone or muscle to prevent neuroma formation after excision of a neuroma. In bony implantation, the physician drills a small hole in the bone to implant the nerve. The surrounding tissue is brought together around the nerve to secure the nerve to the bone. In muscle implantation, the nerve is sutured into muscle bed. The surrounding tissue is brought together and sutured to secure the nerve in the muscle.

Coding Tips

Use 64787 in conjunction with 64774–64786. As an "add-on" code, 64787 is not subject to multiple procedure rules. No reimbursement reduction or modifier 51 is applied. Add-on codes describe additional intra-service work associated with the primary procedure. They are performed by the same physician on the same date of service as the primary service/procedure, and must never be reported as a stand-alone code.

ICD-9-CM Procedural

04.07 Other excision or avulsion of cranial and peripheral nerves

Anesthesia

64787 N/A

ICD-9-CM Diagnostic

This is an add-on code. Refer to the corresponding primary procedure code for ICD-9-CM diagnosis code links.

Terms To Know

avulsion. Forcible tearing away of a part, by surgical means or traumatic injury.

excision. Surgical removal of an organ or tissue.

neuroma. Any type of tumor growing from a nerve or comprised of nerve cells and fibers.

CCI Version 16.3

62310-62311, 92585, 95822, 95860-95861, 95867-95868, 95900, 95904, 95920, 95925-95927, 95930-95934, 95936-95937

Note: These CCI edits are used for Medicare. Other payers may reimburse on codes listed above.

Medicare Edits

	Fac RVU	Non-Fac RVU	FUD	Assist
64787	7.23	7.23	N/A	80

Medicare References: 100-2,15,260; 100-4,12,30; 100-4,12,90.3; 100-4,14,10

64788-64792

64788 Excision of neurofibroma or neurolemmoma; cutaneous nerve
64790 major peripheral nerve
64792 extensive (including malignant type)

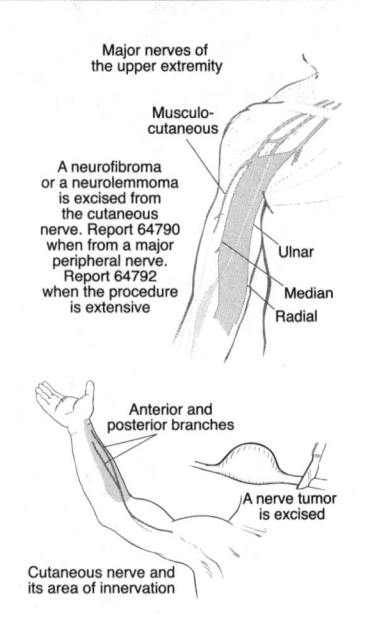

A neurofibroma or a neurolemmoma is excised from the cutaneous nerve. Report 64790 when from a major peripheral nerve. Report 64792 when the procedure is extensive

Explanation
The physician excises a neurofibroma or a neurolemmoma. A neurofibroma is a tumor of peripheral nerves caused by abnormal proliferation of Schwann cells. A neurolemmoma is a tumor of a peripheral nerve sheath. To remove the tumor, the physician incises the skin over the tumor and dissects the surrounding tissue. The tumor is freed and excised from the nerve, without damaging the nerve when possible. The incision is sutured in layers. In 64788, the tumor is located on a cutaneous nerve. In 64790, the tumor lies on a major peripheral nerve. In 64792, an extensive excision is required due to size or malignancy.

Coding Tips
For biopsy of nerve, see 64795. For excision of a neuroma of cutaneous nerve, see 64774. For excision of a neuroma of the digital nerve, see 64776 and 64778. For excision of a neuroma of the hand, see 64782 and 64783.

ICD-9-CM Procedural
04.07 Other excision or avulsion of cranial and peripheral nerves

Anesthesia
00300, 01610, 01710, 01810

ICD-9-CM Diagnostic
171.0 Malignant neoplasm of connective and other soft tissue of head, face, and neck
171.2 Malignant neoplasm of connective and other soft tissue of upper limb, including shoulder
171.4 Malignant neoplasm of connective and other soft tissue of thorax
171.5 Malignant neoplasm of connective and other soft tissue of abdomen
171.7 Malignant neoplasm of connective and other soft tissue of trunk, unspecified site
171.9 Malignant neoplasm of connective and other soft tissue, site unspecified
215.0 Other benign neoplasm of connective and other soft tissue of head, face, and neck
215.2 Other benign neoplasm of connective and other soft tissue of upper limb, including shoulder
215.4 Other benign neoplasm of connective and other soft tissue of thorax
215.5 Other benign neoplasm of connective and other soft tissue of abdomen
215.7 Other benign neoplasm of connective and other soft tissue of trunk, unspecified
215.9 Other benign neoplasm of connective and other soft tissue of unspecified site
237.70 Neurofibromatosis, unspecified
237.71 Neurofibromatosis, Type 1 (von Recklinghausen's disease)
237.72 Neurofibromatosis, Type 2 (acoustic neurofibromatosis)
237.73 Schwannomatosis
237.79 Other neurofibromatosis
238.1 Neoplasm of uncertain behavior of connective and other soft tissue
353.9 Unspecified nerve root and plexus disorder
354.3 Lesion of radial nerve
354.8 Other mononeuritis of upper limb
354.9 Unspecified mononeuritis of upper limb
355.9 Mononeuritis of unspecified site
729.5 Pain in soft tissues of limb

Terms To Know
excision. Surgical removal of an organ or tissue.

incision. Act of cutting into tissue or an organ.

lesion. Area of damaged tissue that has lost continuity or function, due to disease or trauma. Lesions may be located on internal structures such as the brain, nerves, or kidneys, or visible on the skin.

malignant. Any condition tending to progress toward death, specifically an invasive tumor with a loss of cellular differentiation that has the ability to spread or metastasize to other areas in the body.

mononeuritis. Inflammation of one nerve.

neurofibroma. Tumor of peripheral nerves caused by abnormal proliferation of Schwann cells.

CCI Version 16.3
01250, 01320, 01470, 01610, 01710, 01782, 01810, 0213T, 0216T, 0228T, 0230T, 36000, 36400-36410, 36420-36430, 36440, 36600, 36640, 37202, 43752, 51701-51703, 62310-62319, 64400-64435, 64479, 64483, 64490, 64493, 64505-64530, 64795, 69990, 92585, 93000-93010, 93040-93042, 93318, 94002, 94200, 94250, 94680-94690, 94770, 95812-95816, 95819, 95822, 95829, 95860-95861, 95867-95868, 95870, 95900, 95904, 95920, 95925-95934, 95936-95937, 95955, 96360, 96365, 96372, 96374-96376, 99148-99149, 99150

Also not with 64788: 64445-64455, 64702-64704, 64722-64726

Also not with 64790: 29125, 64445-64450, 64702-64726

Also not with 64792: 64445-64450, 64702-64726

Note: These CCI edits are used for Medicare. Other payers may reimburse on codes listed above.

Medicare Edits

	Fac RVU	Non-Fac RVU	FUD	Assist
64788	11.57	11.57	90	N/A
64790	24.39	24.39	90	80
64792	33.31	33.31	90	80

Medicare References: 100-2,15,260; 100-4,12,30; 100-4,12,90.3; 100-4,14,10

64795

64795 Biopsy of nerve

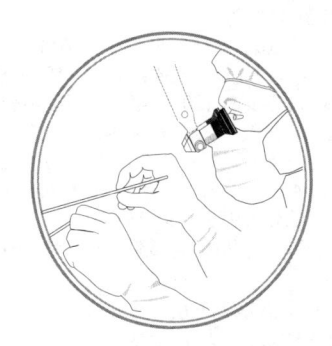

A surgical microscope and/or microsurgical instruments can be used for a biopsy of an upper extremity nerve

Explanation

The physician biopsies a nerve. The physician makes an incision overlying the suspect nerve. The tissues are dissected to locate the nerve and a biopsy specimen is obtained. The incision is closed in sutured layers.

Coding Tips

Local anesthesia is included in this service. For excision of a neurofibroma or neurolemmoma, see 64788–64792. For neurorrhaphy, see 69990 and 64864–64876. For neurorrhaphy with a nerve graft, see 64885–64886 and 64901–64907.

ICD-9-CM Procedural

- 04.12 Open biopsy of cranial or peripheral nerve or ganglion
- 04.19 Other diagnostic procedures on cranial and peripheral nerves and ganglia
- 05.11 Biopsy of sympathetic nerve or ganglion

Anesthesia

64795 00300

ICD-9-CM Diagnostic

- 171.0 Malignant neoplasm of connective and other soft tissue of head, face, and neck
- 195.0 Malignant neoplasm of head, face, and neck
- 198.4 Secondary malignant neoplasm of other parts of nervous system
- 215.0 Other benign neoplasm of connective and other soft tissue of head, face, and neck
- 234.8 Carcinoma in situ of other specified sites
- 237.70 Neurofibromatosis, unspecified
- 237.71 Neurofibromatosis, Type 1 (von Recklinghausen's disease)
- 237.72 Neurofibromatosis, Type 2 (acoustic neurofibromatosis)
- 237.73 Schwannomatosis
- 237.79 Other neurofibromatosis
- 238.1 Neoplasm of uncertain behavior of connective and other soft tissue
- 239.2 Neoplasms of unspecified nature of bone, soft tissue, and skin
- 277.30 Amyloidosis, unspecified — (Use additional code to identify any associated mental retardation)
- 277.31 Familial Mediterranean fever — (Use additional code to identify any associated mental retardation)
- 277.39 Other amyloidosis — (Use additional code to identify any associated mental retardation)
- 350.8 Other specified trigeminal nerve disorders

Terms To Know

benign. Mild or nonmalignant in nature.

biopsy. Tissue or fluid removed for diagnostic purposes through analysis of the cells in the biopsy material.

malignant. Any condition tending to progress toward death, specifically an invasive tumor with a loss of cellular differentiation that has the ability to spread or metastasize to other areas in the body.

neurofibromatosis. Autosomal dominant inherited condition with developmental changes in the nervous system, muscles, bones, and skin, producing coffee colored spots of pigmented skin (café au lait spots) and multiple soft tumor neurofibromas distributed over the entire body.

secondary. Second in order of occurrence or importance, or appearing during the course of another disease or condition.

soft tissue. Nonepithelial tissues outside of the skeleton that includes subcutaneous adipose tissue, fibrous tissue, fascia, muscles, blood and lymph vessels, and peripheral nervous system tissue.

CCI Version 16.3

01250, 01320, 01470, 01610, 01710, 01782, 01810, 0213T, 0216T, 0228T, 0230T, 10021-10022, 20205, 36000, 36400-36410, 36420-36430, 36440, 36600, 36640, 37202, 43752, 51701-51703, 62310-62319, 64400-64435, 64445-64455, 64479, 64483, 64490, 64493, 64505-64530, 64721, 64726, 69990, 92585, 93000-93010, 93040-93042, 93318, 94002, 94200, 94250, 94680-94690, 94770, 95812-95816, 95819, 95822, 95829, 95860-95861, 95867-95868, 95870, 95900, 95904, 95920, 95925-95934, 95936-95937, 95955, 96360, 96365, 96372, 96374-96376, 99148-99149, 99150

Note: These CCI edits are used for Medicare. Other payers may reimburse on codes listed above.

Medicare Edits

	Fac RVU	Non-Fac RVU	FUD	Assist
64795	5.82	5.82	0	N/A

Medicare References: 100-2,15,260; 100-4,12,30; 100-4,12,90.3; 100-4,14,10

64831-64832

64831 Suture of digital nerve, hand or foot; 1 nerve
64832 each additional digital nerve (List separately in addition to code for primary procedure)

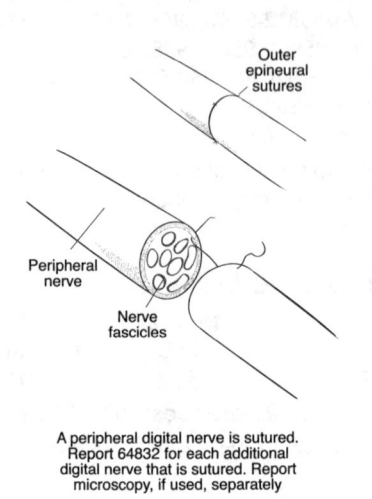

A peripheral digital nerve is sutured. Report 64832 for each additional digital nerve that is sutured. Report microscopy, if used, separately

Explanation
The physician repairs a digital nerve. The physician locates the damaged nerve in a previously opened incision or wound of a finger. The nerve is sutured to restore sensory or motor function. Report 64831 for a single nerve; 64832 for each additional nerve repaired.

Coding Tips
If the procedure is completed through an operating microscope, report 69990 in addition to the primary procedure. However, head gear (e.g., loupes or binoculars) is considered an integral part of this procedure. Use 64832 in conjunction with 64831. As an "add-on" code, 64832 is not subject to multiple procedure rules. No reimbursement reduction or modifier 51 is applied. Add-on codes describe additional intra-service work associated with the primary procedure. They are performed by the same physician on the same date of service as the primary service/procedure, and must never be reported as a stand-alone code. Surgical trays, A4550, are not separately reimbursed by Medicare; however, other third-party payers may cover them. Check with the specific payer to determine coverage.

ICD-9-CM Procedural
04.3 Suture of cranial and peripheral nerves

Anesthesia
64831 01810
64832 N/A

ICD-9-CM Diagnostic
816.11 Open fracture of middle or proximal phalanx or phalanges of hand
882.2 Open wound of hand except finger(s) alone, with tendon involvement
883.0 Open wound of finger(s), without mention of complication
883.2 Open wound of finger(s), with tendon involvement
927.20 Crushing injury of hand(s) — (Use additional code to identify any associated injuries: 800-829, 850.0-854.1, 860.0-869.1)
927.3 Crushing injury of finger(s) — (Use additional code to identify any associated injuries: 800-829, 850.0-854.1, 860.0-869.1)
955.6 Injury to digital nerve, upper limb
959.5 Injury, other and unspecified, finger

Terms To Know
fracture. Break in bone or cartilage.

incision. Act of cutting into tissue or an organ.

injury. Harm or damage sustained by the body.

open fracture. Exposed break in a bone, always considered compound due to its high risk of infection from the open wound leading to the fracture. Broken bone ends may protrude through the skin and contaminants or foreign bodies are often embedded in the tissues.

open wound. Opening or break of the skin.

tendon. Fibrous tissue that connects muscle to bone, consisting primarily of collagen and containing little vasculature.

wound repair. Surgical closure of a wound is divided into three categories: simple, intermediate, and complex. **simple repair:** Surgical closure of a superficial wound, requiring single layer suturing of the skin epidermis, dermis, or subcutaneous tissue. **intermediate repair:** Surgical closure of a wound requiring closure of one or more of the deeper subcutaneous tissue and non-muscle fascia layers in addition to suturing the skin; contaminated wounds with single layer closure that need extensive cleaning or foreign body removal. **complex repair:** Repair of wounds requiring more than layered closure (debridement, scar revision, stents, retention sutures).

CCI Version 16.3
92585, 95822, 95860-95861, 95867-95868, 95900, 95904, 95920, 95936-95937

Also not with 64831: 01250, 01320, 01470, 01610, 01710, 01782, 01810, 0213T, 0216T, 0228T, 0230T, 12002, 12045, 13132, 20526-20553, 29125, 29130, 35761, 36000, 36400-36410, 36420-36430, 36440, 36600, 36640, 37202, 43752, 51701-51703, 62310-62319, 64400-64435, 64445-64455, 64479, 64483, 64490, 64493, 64505-64530, 64702, 76000-76001, 93000-93010, 93040-93042, 93318, 94002, 94200, 94250, 94680-94690, 94770, 95812-95816, 95819, 95829, 95870, 95925-95934, 95955, 96360, 96365, 96372, 96374-96376, 99148-99149, 99150

Also not with 64832: 62310-62311, 95925-95927, 95930-95934

Note: These CCI edits are used for Medicare. Other payers may reimburse on codes listed above.

Medicare Edits

	Fac RVU	Non-Fac RVU	FUD	Assist
64831	19.92	19.92	90	N/A
64832	10.09	10.09	N/A	80

Medicare References: 100-2,15,260; 100-4,12,30; 100-4,12,90.3; 100-4,14,10

64834-64837

64834 Suture of 1 nerve; hand or foot, common sensory nerve
64835 median motor thenar
64836 ulnar motor
64837 Suture of each additional nerve, hand or foot (List separately in addition to code for primary procedure)

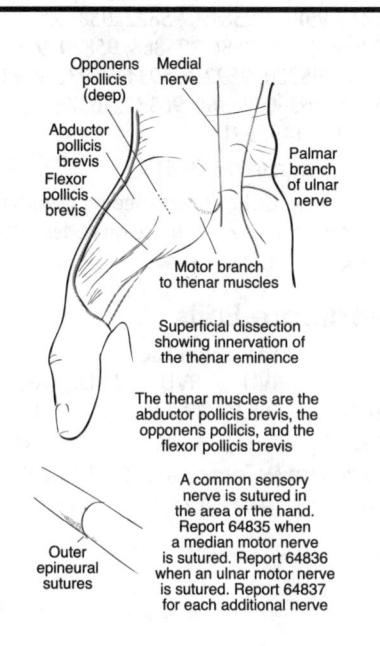

Explanation

The physician repairs a sensory or motor nerve in the hand. The physician locates the damaged nerve in a previously opened incision or wound of the hand. The nerve is sutured to restore sensory function. In 64834, a common sensory nerve is repaired. In 64835, the median motor thenar nerve is repaired. This nerve supplies motor innervation to the thenar eminence (proximal thumb). In 64836, the ulnar motor nerve is repaired. This nerve supplies motor innervation to the extensor muscles of the forearm and hand. Report 64837 for repair of additional nerves in the hand. Closure or reconstruction is separately reported.

Coding Tips

If the procedure is completed through an operating microscope, report 69990 in addition to the primary procedure. However, head gear (e.g., loupes or binoculars) is considered an integral part of this procedure. Use 64837 in conjunction with 64834–64836. As an "add-on" code, 64837 is not subject to multiple procedure rules. No reimbursement reduction or modifier 51 is applied. Add-on codes describe additional intra-service work associated with the primary procedure. They are performed by the same physician on the same date of service as the primary service/procedure, and must never be reported as a stand-alone code. Local anesthesia is included in these services. However, these procedures may be performed under general anesthesia, depending on the age and/or condition of the patient.

ICD-9-CM Procedural

04.3 Suture of cranial and peripheral nerves

Anesthesia

64834 01810
64835 01810
64836 01810
64837 N/A

ICD-9-CM Diagnostic

881.02 Open wound of wrist, without mention of complication
881.22 Open wound of wrist, with tendon involvement
882.0 Open wound of hand except finger(s) alone, without mention of complication
883.0 Open wound of finger(s), without mention of complication
927.21 Crushing injury of wrist — (Use additional code to identify any associated injuries: 800-829, 850.0-854.1, 860.0-869.1)
955.1 Injury to median nerve
955.2 Injury to ulnar nerve
955.5 Injury to cutaneous sensory nerve, upper limb
959.4 Injury, other and unspecified, hand, except finger

Terms To Know

innervation. Nerve distribution to a body part.

open wound. Opening or break of the skin.

tendon. Fibrous tissue that connects muscle to bone, consisting primarily of collagen and containing little vasculature.

CCI Version 16.3

92585, 95822, 95860-95861, 95867-95868, 95900, 95904, 95920, 95936-95937

Also not with 64834: 01250, 01320, 01470, 01610, 01710, 01782, 01810, 0213T, 0216T, 0228T, 0230T, 20526-20553, 36000, 36400-36410, 36420-36430, 36440, 36600, 36640, 37202, 43752, 51701-51703, 62310-62319, 64400-64435, 64445-64455, 64479, 64483, 64490, 64493, 64505-64530, 64704, 93000-93010, 93040-93042, 93318, 94002, 94200, 94250, 94680-94690, 94770, 95812-95816, 95819, 95829, 95870, 95925-95934, 95955, 96360, 96365, 96372, 96374-96376, 99148-99149, 99150

Also not with 64835: 01250, 01320, 01470, 01610, 01710, 01782, 01810, 0213T, 0216T, 0228T, 0230T, 20526-20553, 36000, 36400-36410, 36420-36430, 36440, 36600, 36640, 37202, 43752, 51701-51703, 62310-62319, 64400-64435, 64445-64450, 64479, 64483, 64490, 64493, 64505-64530, 64721, 93000-93010, 93040-93042, 93318, 94002, 94200, 94250, 94680-94690, 94770, 95812-95816, 95819, 95829, 95870, 95925-95934, 95955, 96360, 96365, 96372, 96374-96376, 99148-99149, 99150

Also not with 64836: 01250, 01320, 01470, 01610, 01710, 01782, 01810, 0213T, 0216T, 0228T, 0230T, 20526-20553, 36000, 36400-36410, 36420-36430, 36440, 36600, 36640, 37202, 43752, 51701-51703, 62310-62319, 64400-64435, 64445-64450, 64479, 64483, 64490, 64493, 64505-64530, 93000-93010, 93040-93042, 93318, 94002, 94200, 94250, 94680-94690, 94770, 95812-95816, 95819, 95829, 95870, 95925-95934, 95955, 96360, 96365, 96372, 96374-96376, 99148-99149, 99150

Also not with 64837: 62310-62311, 95925-95927, 95930-95934

Note: These CCI edits are used for Medicare. Other payers may reimburse on codes listed above.

Medicare Edits

	Fac RVU	Non-Fac RVU	FUD	Assist
64834	21.77	21.77	90	80
64835	23.75	23.75	90	80
64836	23.77	23.77	90	80
64837	10.64	10.64	N/A	80

Medicare References: 100-2,15,260; 100-4,12,30; 100-4,12,90.3; 100-4,14,10

64856-64857

64856 Suture of major peripheral nerve, arm or leg, except sciatic; including transposition
64857 without transposition

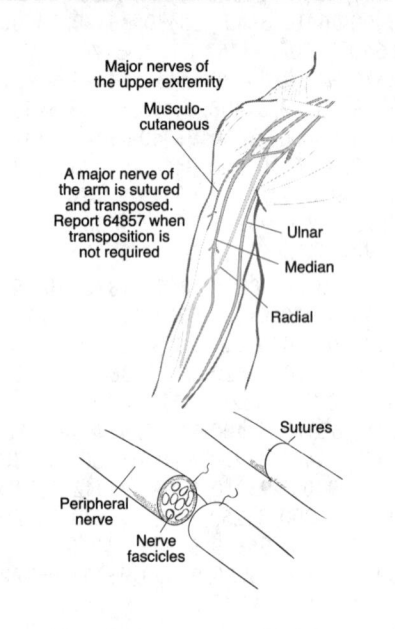

Major nerves of the upper extremity
Musculocutaneous
A major nerve of the arm is sutured and transposed. Report 64857 when transposition is not required
Ulnar
Median
Radial
Sutures
Peripheral nerve
Nerve fascicles

Explanation

The physician repairs a major peripheral of the arm nerve. The physician locates the damaged nerve in a previously opened incision or wound. The nerve is sutured to restore sensory function. Complex closure or plastic reconstruction of overlying tissues is separately reported.

Coding Tips

If the procedure is completed through an operating microscope, report 69990 in addition to the primary procedure. However, head gear (e.g., loupes or binoculars) is considered an integral part of this procedure.

ICD-9-CM Procedural

04.3 Suture of cranial and peripheral nerves
04.6 Transposition of cranial and peripheral nerves

Anesthesia
01710, 01810

ICD-9-CM Diagnostic

880.03 Open wound of upper arm, without mention of complication
880.23 Open wound of upper arm, with tendon involvement
881.02 Open wound of wrist, without mention of complication
881.22 Open wound of wrist, with tendon involvement
884.0 Multiple and unspecified open wound of upper limb, without mention of complication
927.8 Crushing injury of multiple sites of upper limb — (Use additional code to identify any associated injuries: 800-829, 850.0-854.1, 860.0-869.1)
955.0 Injury to axillary nerve
955.1 Injury to median nerve
955.2 Injury to ulnar nerve
955.3 Injury to radial nerve
955.7 Injury to other specified nerve(s) of shoulder girdle and upper limb

Terms To Know

incision. Act of cutting into tissue or an organ.

injury. Harm or damage sustained by the body.

innervation. Nerve distribution to a body part.

suture. Numerous stitching techniques employed in wound closure.

buried suture. Continuous or interrupted suture placed under the skin for a layered closure.

continuous suture. Running stitch with tension evenly distributed across a single strand to provide a leakproof closure line.

interrupted suture. Series of single stitches with tension isolated at each stitch, in which all stitches are not affected if one becomes loose, and the isolated sutures cannot act as a wick to transport an infection.

purse-string suture. Continuous suture placed around a tubular structure and tightened, to reduce or close the lumen.

retention suture. Secondary stitching that bridges the primary suture, providing support for the primary repair; a plastic or rubber bolster may be placed over the primary repair and under the retention sutures.

tendon. Fibrous tissue that connects muscle to bone, consisting primarily of collagen and containing little vasculature.

transposition. Removal or exchange from one side to another; change of position from one place to another.

CCI Version 16.3

01250, 01320, 01470, 01610, 01710, 01782, 01810, 0213T, 0216T, 0228T, 0230T, 20526-20553, 36000, 36400-36410, 36420-36430, 36440, 36600, 36640, 37202, 43752, 51701-51703, 62310-62319, 64400-64435, 64445-64450, 64479, 64483, 64490, 64493, 64505-64530, 92585, 93000-93010, 93040-93042, 93318, 94002, 94200, 94250, 94680-94690, 94770, 95812-95816, 95819, 95822, 95829, 95860-95861, 95867-95868, 95870, 95900, 95904, 95920, 95925-95934, 95936-95937, 95955, 96360, 96365, 96372, 96374-96376, 99148-99149, 99150

Also not with 64856: 37618

Note: These CCI edits are used for Medicare. Other payers may reimburse on codes listed above.

Medicare Edits

	Fac RVU	Non-Fac RVU	FUD	Assist
64856	29.82	29.82	90	N/A
64857	31.04	31.04	90	80

Medicare References: 100-2,15,260; 100-4,12,30; 100-4,12,90.3; 100-4,14,10

64859

64859 Suture of each additional major peripheral nerve (List separately in addition to code for primary procedure)

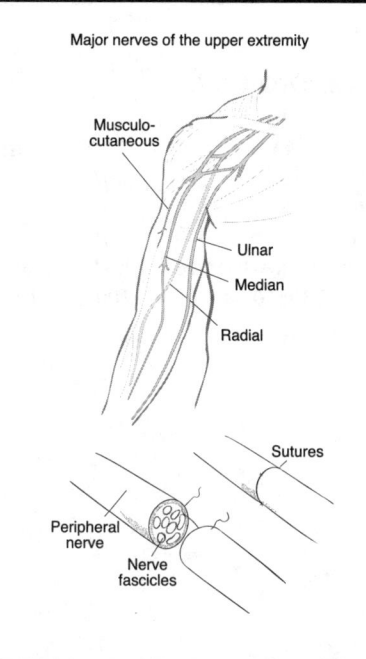

Explanation

The physician repairs second or multiple major peripheral nerves in the arm, except for the sciatic nerve. The physician locates the damaged nerve in a previously opened incision or wound of the arm. The nerve is sutured to restore sensory and/or motor innervation. The nerve may be moved (transposed) to decrease tension on the nerve. Report 64859 for each additional nerve. Complex closure or plastic reconstruction of overlying tissues is reported separately.

Coding Tips

Use 64859 in conjunction with 64856–64857. As an "add-on" code, 64859 is not subject to multiple procedure rules. No reimbursement reduction or modifier 51 is applied. Add-on codes describe additional intra-service work associated with the primary procedure. They are performed by the same physician on the same date of service as the primary service/procedure, and must never be reported as a stand-alone code.

ICD-9-CM Procedural

- 04.3 Suture of cranial and peripheral nerves
- 04.6 Transposition of cranial and peripheral nerves

Anesthesia

64859 N/A

ICD-9-CM Diagnostic

- 880.03 Open wound of upper arm, without mention of complication
- 880.23 Open wound of upper arm, with tendon involvement
- 881.02 Open wound of wrist, without mention of complication
- 881.22 Open wound of wrist, with tendon involvement
- 884.0 Multiple and unspecified open wound of upper limb, without mention of complication
- 927.8 Crushing injury of multiple sites of upper limb — (Use additional code to identify any associated injuries: 800-829, 850.0-854.1, 860.0-869.1)
- 955.0 Injury to axillary nerve
- 955.1 Injury to median nerve
- 955.2 Injury to ulnar nerve
- 955.3 Injury to radial nerve
- 955.7 Injury to other specified nerve(s) of shoulder girdle and upper limb

Terms To Know

innervation. Nerve distribution to a body part.

CCI Version 16.3

62310-62311, 92585, 95822, 95860-95861, 95867-95868, 95900, 95904, 95920, 95925-95927, 95930-95934, 95936-95937

Note: These CCI edits are used for Medicare. Other payers may reimburse on codes listed above.

Medicare Edits

	Fac RVU	Non-Fac RVU	FUD	Assist
64859	7.8	7.8	N/A	80

Medicare References: 100-2,15,260; 100-4,12,30; 100-4,12,90.3; 100-4,14,10

64872-64876

64872 Suture of nerve; requiring secondary or delayed suture (List separately in addition to code for primary neurorrhaphy)

64874 requiring extensive mobilization, or transposition of nerve (List separately in addition to code for nerve suture)

64876 requiring shortening of bone of extremity (List separately in addition to code for nerve suture)

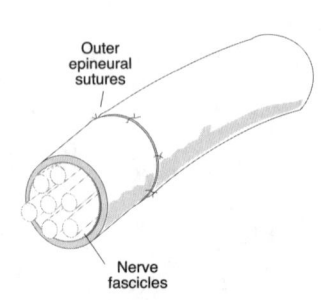

A nerve in the upper extremity area requires a secondary or delayed suture (64872). Code 64874 when extensive mobilization or transposition is required during the procedure. Report 64876 when nerve suture of the upper extremity requires shortening of a bone. These codes are listed in addition to the primary nerve repair code

Explanation

The physician repairs a nerve where repair was delayed because the initial wound was contaminated. The wound is explored to locate the distal portion of the nerve. In 64872, the proximal and distal nerves are sutured together to restore innervation. In 64874, the nerve was shortened during damage. To reanastomose the nerve, the distal and proximal portions of the nerve are freed from surrounding tissues, approximated, and sutured to restore innervation. Report 64876 if excessive trauma caused loss of a significant section of a major nerve. For this procedure, a portion of the parallel bone is resected in order to approximate the distal and proximal ends of the nerve.

Coding Tips

Use 64872–64876 in conjunction with 64831–64865. As "add-on" codes, 64872–64876 are not subject to multiple procedure rules. No reimbursement reduction or modifier 51 is applied. Add-on codes describe additional intra-service work associated with the primary procedure. They are performed by the same physician on the same date of service as the primary service/procedure, and must never be reported as a stand-alone code. Surgical trays, A4550, are not separately reimbursed by Medicare; however, other third-party payers may cover them. Check with the specific payer to determine coverage.

ICD-9-CM Procedural

04.3	Suture of cranial and peripheral nerves
04.6	Transposition of cranial and peripheral nerves
04.76	Repair of old traumatic injury of cranial and peripheral nerves
05.81	Repair of sympathetic nerve or ganglion
78.29	Limb shortening procedures, other

Anesthesia
N/A

ICD-9-CM Diagnostic

This is an add-on code. Refer to the corresponding primary procedure code for ICD-9-CM diagnosis code links.

Terms To Know

distal. Located farther away from a specified reference point.

ganglion. Fluid-filled, benign cyst appearing on a tendon sheath or aponeurosis, frequently found in the hand, wrist, or foot and connecting to an underlying joint.

innervation. Nerve distribution to a body part.

proximal. Located closest to a specified reference point, usually the midline.

resection. Surgical removal of a part or all of an organ or body part.

wound repair. Surgical closure of a wound is divided into three categories: simple, intermediate, and complex. *simple repair:* Surgical closure of a superficial wound, requiring single layer suturing of the skin epidermis, dermis, or subcutaneous tissue. *intermediate repair:* Surgical closure of a wound requiring closure of one or more of the deeper subcutaneous tissue and non-muscle fascia layers in addition to suturing the skin; contaminated wounds with single layer closure that need extensive cleaning or foreign body removal. *complex repair:* Repair of wounds requiring more than layered closure (debridement, scar revision, stents, retention sutures).

CCI Version 16.3

62310-62311, 92585, 95822, 95860-95861, 95867-95868, 95900, 95904, 95920, 95925-95927, 95930-95934, 95936-95937

Note: These CCI edits are used for Medicare. Other payers may reimburse on codes listed above.

Medicare Edits

	Fac RVU	Non-Fac RVU	FUD	Assist
64872	3.41	3.41	N/A	80
64874	5.19	5.19	N/A	80
64876	5.76	5.76	N/A	80

Medicare References: 100-2,15,260; 100-4,12,30; 100-4,12,90.3; 100-4,14,10

64890-64891

64890 Nerve graft (includes obtaining graft), single strand, hand or foot; up to 4 cm length
64891 more than 4 cm length

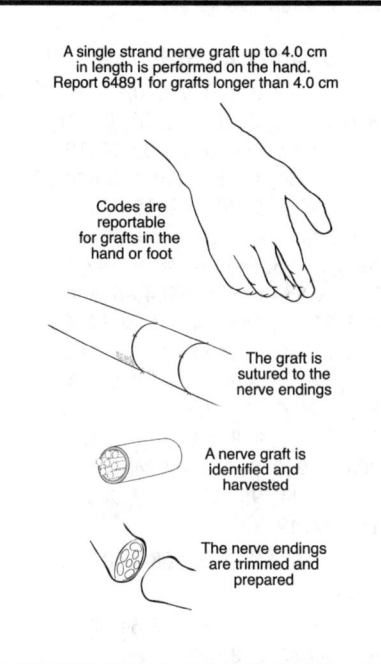

A single strand nerve graft up to 4.0 cm in length is performed on the hand. Report 64891 for grafts longer than 4.0 cm

Codes are reportable for grafts in the hand or foot

The graft is sutured to the nerve endings

A nerve graft is identified and harvested

The nerve endings are trimmed and prepared

Explanation

The physician obtains and places a nerve graft to restore innervation to the hand. In 64890, the graft is less than 4 cm long. In 64891, the graft is greater than 4 cm. A typical graft harvest is obtained from the sural nerve. To harvest the graft, the physician makes a lateral incision of the lateral malleolus of the ankle. The nerve is identified and freed. The physician cuts the nerve to obtain the length needed for the graft, elongating the incision as necessary. The proximal and distal sural nerve endings are anastomosed. The physician makes an incision over the damaged nerve and dissects the tissues to locate the nerve. The damaged area of the nerve is resected and removed. Innervation is restored by suturing the graft to the proximal and distal ends of the damaged nerve.

Coding Tips

Any nerve graft harvest is not reported separately. If the procedure is completed through an operating microscope, report 69990 in addition to the primary procedure. However, head gear (e.g., loupes or binoculars) is considered an integral part of these procedures.

ICD-9-CM Procedural

04.5 Cranial or peripheral nerve graft

Anesthesia

01810

ICD-9-CM Diagnostic

171.2 Malignant neoplasm of connective and other soft tissue of upper limb, including shoulder
215.2 Other benign neoplasm of connective and other soft tissue of upper limb, including shoulder
238.1 Neoplasm of uncertain behavior of connective and other soft tissue
239.2 Neoplasms of unspecified nature of bone, soft tissue, and skin
277.30 Amyloidosis, unspecified — (Use additional code to identify any associated mental retardation)
277.31 Familial Mediterranean fever — (Use additional code to identify any associated mental retardation)
277.39 Other amyloidosis — (Use additional code to identify any associated mental retardation)
354.0 Carpal tunnel syndrome
354.5 Mononeuritis multiplex
356.0 Hereditary peripheral neuropathy
356.4 Idiopathic progressive polyneuropathy
357.81 Chronic inflammatory demyelinating polyneuritis
357.82 Critical illness polyneuropathy
357.89 Other inflammatory and toxic neuropathy
359.6 Symptomatic inflammatory myopathy in diseases classified elsewhere — (Code first underlying disease: 135, 140.0-208.9, 277.30-277.39, 446.0, 710.0, 710.1, 710.2, 714.0)
446.0 Polyarteritis nodosa
710.0 Systemic lupus erythematosus — (Use additional code to identify manifestation: 424.91, 581.81, 582.81, 583.81)
710.1 Systemic sclerosis — (Use additional code to identify manifestation: 359.6, 517.2)
710.2 Sicca syndrome
714.0 Rheumatoid arthritis — (Use additional code to identify manifestation: 357.1, 359.6)
882.1 Open wound of hand except finger(s) alone, complicated
883.1 Open wound of finger(s), complicated
927.20 Crushing injury of hand(s) — (Use additional code to identify any associated injuries: 800-829, 850.0-854.1, 860.0-869.1)
927.3 Crushing injury of finger(s) — (Use additional code to identify any associated injuries: 800-829, 850.0-854.1, 860.0-869.1)

Terms To Know

amyloidosis. Condition in which insoluble, fibril-like proteins (amyloid) build up in one or more organs and tissues within the body.

anastomosis. Surgically created connection between ducts, blood vessels, or bowel segments to allow flow from one to the other.

graft. Tissue implant from another part of the body or another person.

incision. Act of cutting into tissue or an organ.

resection. Surgical removal of a part or all of an organ or body part.

CCI Version 16.3

01250, 01320, 01470, 01610, 01710, 01782, 01810, 0213T, 0216T, 0228T, 0230T, 20526-20553, 36000, 36400-36410, 36420-36430, 36440, 36600, 36640, 37202, 43752, 51701-51703, 62310-62319, 64400-64435, 64445-64455, 64479, 64483, 64490, 64493, 64505-64530, 64722-64726, 64831, 64834-64836, 64840-64858, 64861-64870, 64874-64886, 64907-64911❖, 92585, 93000-93010, 93040-93042, 93318, 94002, 94200, 94250, 94680-94690, 94770, 95812-95816, 95819, 95822, 95829, 95860-95861, 95867-95868, 95870, 95900, 95904, 95920, 95925-95934, 95936-95937, 95955, 96360, 96365, 96372, 96374-96376, 99148-99149, 99150

Also not with 64890: 64702-64708, 64891❖, 64893❖

Also not with 64891: 64702-64704

Note: These CCI edits are used for Medicare. Other payers may reimburse on codes listed above.

Medicare Edits

	Fac RVU	Non-Fac RVU	FUD	Assist
64890	31.88	31.88	90	80
64891	34.62	34.62	90	80

Medicare References: 100-2,15,260; 100-4,12,30; 100-4,12,90.3; 100-4,14,10

64892-64893

64892 Nerve graft (includes obtaining graft), single strand, arm or leg; up to 4 cm length

64893 more than 4 cm length

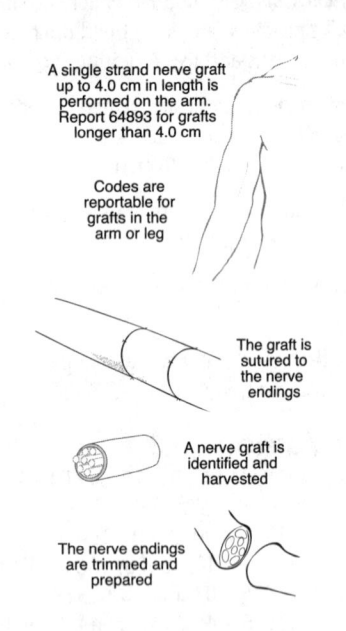

Explanation

The physician obtains and places a nerve graft to restore innervation to the arm. In 64892, the graft is less than 4 cm long. In 64893, the graft is greater than 4 cm. A typical graft harvest is obtained from the sural nerve. To harvest the graft, the physician makes a lateral incision of the lateral malleolus of the ankle. The nerve is identified and freed. The physician cuts the nerve to obtain the length needed for the graft, elongating the incision as necessary. The proximal and distal sural nerve endings are anastomosed. The physician makes an incision over the damaged nerve and dissects the tissues to locate the nerve. The damaged area of the nerve is resected and removed. Innervation is restored by suturing the graft to the proximal and distal ends of the damaged nerve.

Coding Tips

Any nerve graft harvest is not reported separately. If the procedure is completed through an operating microscope, report 69990 in addition to the primary procedure. However, head gear (e.g., loupes or binoculars) is considered an integral part of these procedures.

ICD-9-CM Procedural

04.5 Cranial or peripheral nerve graft

Anesthesia
01610, 01710, 01810

ICD-9-CM Diagnostic

- 171.2 Malignant neoplasm of connective and other soft tissue of upper limb, including shoulder
- 215.2 Other benign neoplasm of connective and other soft tissue of upper limb, including shoulder
- 238.1 Neoplasm of uncertain behavior of connective and other soft tissue
- 239.2 Neoplasms of unspecified nature of bone, soft tissue, and skin
- 354.3 Lesion of radial nerve
- 355.0 Lesion of sciatic nerve
- 880.13 Open wound of upper arm, complicated
- 881.10 Open wound of forearm, complicated
- 927.03 Crushing injury of upper arm — (Use additional code to identify any associated injuries: 800-829, 850.0-854.1, 860.0-869.1)
- 927.10 Crushing injury of forearm — (Use additional code to identify any associated injuries: 800-829, 850.0-854.1, 860.0-869.1)
- 956.0 Injury to sciatic nerve

Terms To Know

anastomosis. Surgically created connection between ducts, blood vessels, or bowel segments to allow flow from one to the other.

benign. Mild or nonmalignant in nature.

distal. Located farther away from a specified reference point.

graft. Tissue implant from another part of the body or another person.

incision. Act of cutting into tissue or an organ.

injury. Harm or damage sustained by the body.

innervation. Nerve distribution to a body part.

lesion. Area of damaged tissue that has lost continuity or function, due to disease or trauma. Lesions may be located on internal structures such as the brain, nerves, or kidneys, or visible on the skin.

malignant. Any condition tending to progress toward death, specifically an invasive tumor with a loss of cellular differentiation that has the ability to spread or metastasize to other areas in the body.

open wound. Opening or break of the skin.

proximal. Located closest to a specified reference point, usually the midline.

soft tissue. Nonepithelial tissues outside of the skeleton that includes subcutaneous adipose tissue, fibrous tissue, fascia, muscles, blood and lymph vessels, and peripheral nervous system tissue.

CCI Version 16.3

01250, 01320, 01470, 01610, 01710, 01782, 01810, 0213T, 0216T, 0228T, 0230T, 20526-20553, 36000, 36400-36410, 36420-36430, 36440, 36600, 36640, 37202, 43752, 51701-51703, 62310-62319, 64400-64435, 64445-64450, 64479, 64483, 64490, 64493, 64505-64530, 64718-64726, 64831, 64834-64836, 64840-64858, 64861-64870, 64907-64911❖, 92585, 93000-93010, 93040-93042, 93318, 94002, 94200, 94250, 94680-94690, 94770, 95812-95816, 95819, 95822, 95829, 95860-95861, 95867-95868, 95870, 95900, 95904, 95920, 95925-95934, 95936-95937, 95955, 96360, 96365, 96372, 96374-96376, 99148-99149, 99150

Also not with 64892: 64708, 64874-64891❖, 64893❖

Also not with 64893: 64702-64708, 64874-64886, 64891❖

Note: These CCI edits are used for Medicare. Other payers may reimburse on codes listed above.

Medicare Edits

	Fac RVU	Non-Fac RVU	FUD	Assist
64892	30.93	30.93	90	80
64893	33.11	33.11	90	80

Medicare References: 100-2,15,260; 100-4,12,30; 100-4,12,90.3; 100-4,14,10

64895-64896

64895 Nerve graft (includes obtaining graft), multiple strands (cable), hand or foot; up to 4 cm length

64896 more than 4 cm length

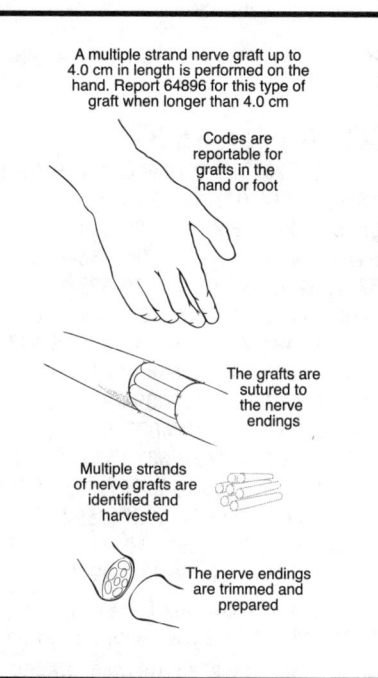

Explanation

The physician obtains and places a nerve graft to restore innervation where a cable nerve of the hand is damaged. In 64895, the graft is less than 4 cm long. In 64896, the graft is greater than 4 cm. A typical graft harvest is obtained by taking multiple sections of the sural nerve. To harvest the graft, the physician makes an incision near the lateral malleolus of the ankle. The nerve is identified and freed. The physician cuts the nerve to obtain the length needed for the graft, elongating the incision as necessary. The proximal and distal sural nerve endings are anastomosed. The physician makes an incision over the damaged nerve and dissects the tissues to locate the nerve. The damaged area of the nerve is resected and removed. Innervation is restored by suturing graft strands to multiple proximal and distal ends of the damaged nerve cable.

Coding Tips

Any nerve graft harvest is not reported separately. If the procedure is completed through an operating microscope, report 69990 in addition to the primary procedure. However, head gear (e.g., loupes or binoculars) is considered an integral part of these procedures.

ICD-9-CM Procedural

04.5 Cranial or peripheral nerve graft

Anesthesia

01810

ICD-9-CM Diagnostic

- 171.2 Malignant neoplasm of connective and other soft tissue of upper limb, including shoulder
- 215.2 Other benign neoplasm of connective and other soft tissue of upper limb, including shoulder
- 238.1 Neoplasm of uncertain behavior of connective and other soft tissue
- 239.2 Neoplasms of unspecified nature of bone, soft tissue, and skin
- 277.30 Amyloidosis, unspecified — (Use additional code to identify any associated mental retardation)
- 277.31 Familial Mediterranean fever — (Use additional code to identify any associated mental retardation)
- 277.39 Other amyloidosis — (Use additional code to identify any associated mental retardation)
- 354.5 Mononeuritis multiplex
- 356.0 Hereditary peripheral neuropathy
- 356.4 Idiopathic progressive polyneuropathy
- 357.81 Chronic inflammatory demyelinating polyneuritis
- 357.82 Critical illness polyneuropathy
- 357.89 Other inflammatory and toxic neuropathy
- 359.6 Symptomatic inflammatory myopathy in diseases classified elsewhere — (Code first underlying disease: 135, 140.0-208.9, 277.30-277.39, 446.0, 710.0, 710.1, 710.2, 714.0)
- 446.0 Polyarteritis nodosa
- 710.0 Systemic lupus erythematosus — (Use additional code to identify manifestation: 424.91, 581.81, 582.81, 583.81)
- 710.1 Systemic sclerosis — (Use additional code to identify manifestation: 359.6, 517.2)
- 710.2 Sicca syndrome
- 714.0 Rheumatoid arthritis — (Use additional code to identify manifestation: 357.1, 359.6)
- 882.1 Open wound of hand except finger(s) alone, complicated
- 883.1 Open wound of finger(s), complicated
- 927.20 Crushing injury of hand(s) — (Use additional code to identify any associated injuries: 800-829, 850.0-854.1, 860.0-869.1)
- 927.3 Crushing injury of finger(s) — (Use additional code to identify any associated injuries: 800-829, 850.0-854.1, 860.0-869.1)
- 955.8 Injury to multiple nerves of shoulder girdle and upper limb

Terms To Know

anastomosis. Surgically created connection between ducts, blood vessels, or bowel segments to allow flow from one to the other.

dissection. Separating by cutting tissue or body structures apart.

graft. Tissue implant from another part of the body or another person.

CCI Version 16.3

01250, 01320, 01470, 01610, 01710, 01782, 01810, 0213T, 0216T, 0228T, 0230T, 20526-20553, 36000, 36400-36410, 36420-36430, 36440, 36600, 36640, 37202, 43752, 51701-51703, 62310-62319, 64400-64435, 64445-64455, 64479, 64483, 64490, 64493, 64505-64530, 64702-64704, 64722, 64831, 64834-64836, 64840-64858, 64861-64870, 64874-64893, 64910-64911❖, 92585, 93000-93010, 93040-93042, 93318, 94002, 94200, 94250, 94680-94690, 94770, 95812-95816, 95819, 95822, 95829, 95860-95861, 95867-95868, 95870, 95900, 95904, 95920, 95925-95934, 95936-95937, 95955, 96360, 96365, 96372, 96374-96376, 99148-99149, 99150

Also not with 64895: 64896❖, 64898❖

Note: These CCI edits are used for Medicare. Other payers may reimburse on codes listed above.

Medicare Edits

	Fac RVU	Non-Fac RVU	FUD	Assist
64895	39.93	39.93	90	80
64896	45.33	45.33	90	80

Medicare References: 100-2,15,260; 100-4,12,30; 100-4,12,90.3; 100-4,14,10

64897-64898

64897 Nerve graft (includes obtaining graft), multiple strands (cable), arm or leg; up to 4 cm length

64898 more than 4 cm length

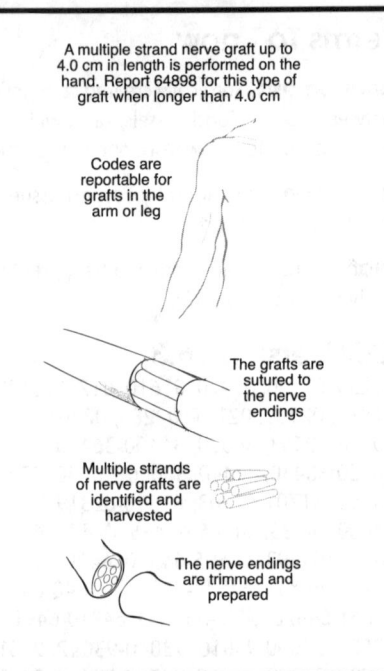

A multiple strand nerve graft up to 4.0 cm in length is performed on the hand. Report 64898 for this type of graft when longer than 4.0 cm

Codes are reportable for grafts in the arm or leg

The grafts are sutured to the nerve endings

Multiple strands of nerve grafts are identified and harvested

The nerve endings are trimmed and prepared

Explanation

The physician obtains and places a nerve graft to restore innervation where a cable nerve of the arm is damaged (e.g., sciatic nerve or lumbar plexus nerve). In 64897, the graft is less than 4 cm long. In 64898, the graft is greater than 4 cm. A typical graft harvest is obtained by taking multiple sections of the sural nerve. To harvest the graft, the physician makes an incision near the lateral malleolus of the ankle. The nerve is identified and freed. The physician cuts the nerve to obtain the length needed for the graft, elongating the incision as necessary. The proximal and distal sural nerve endings are anastomosed. The physician makes an incision over the damaged nerve and dissects the tissues to locate the nerve. The damaged area of the nerve is resected and removed. Innervation is restored by suturing graft strands to multiple proximal and distal ends of the damaged nerve cable.

Coding Tips

Any nerve graft harvest is not reported separately. If the procedure is completed through an operating microscope, report 69990 in addition to the primary procedure. However, head gear (e.g., loupes or binoculars) is considered an integral part of these procedures.

ICD-9-CM Procedural

04.5 Cranial or peripheral nerve graft

Anesthesia

01610, 01710, 01810

ICD-9-CM Diagnostic

171.2   Malignant neoplasm of connective and other soft tissue of upper limb, including shoulder
215.2   Other benign neoplasm of connective and other soft tissue of upper limb, including shoulder
238.1   Neoplasm of uncertain behavior of connective and other soft tissue
239.2   Neoplasms of unspecified nature of bone, soft tissue, and skin
277.30 Amyloidosis, unspecified — (Use additional code to identify any associated mental retardation)
277.31 Familial Mediterranean fever — (Use additional code to identify any associated mental retardation)
277.39 Other amyloidosis — (Use additional code to identify any associated mental retardation)
354.5   Mononeuritis multiplex
356.0   Hereditary peripheral neuropathy
356.4   Idiopathic progressive polyneuropathy
357.81 Chronic inflammatory demyelinating polyneuritis
357.82 Critical illness polyneuropathy
357.89 Other inflammatory and toxic neuropathy
359.6   Symptomatic inflammatory myopathy in diseases classified elsewhere — (Code first underlying disease: 135, 140.0-208.9, 277.30-277.39, 446.0, 710.0, 710.1, 710.2, 714.0)
446.0   Polyarteritis nodosa
710.0   Systemic lupus erythematosus — (Use additional code to identify manifestation: 424.91, 581.81, 582.81, 583.81)
710.1   Systemic sclerosis — (Use additional code to identify manifestation: 359.6, 517.2)
710.2   Sicca syndrome
714.0   Rheumatoid arthritis — (Use additional code to identify manifestation: 357.1, 359.6)
881.10 Open wound of forearm, complicated
927.03 Crushing injury of upper arm — (Use additional code to identify any associated injuries: 800-829, 850.0-854.1, 860.0-869.1)
955.7   Injury to other specified nerve(s) of shoulder girdle and upper limb

Terms To Know

anastomosis. Surgically created connection between ducts, blood vessels, or bowel segments to allow flow from one to the other.

graft. Tissue implant from another part of the body or another person.

incision. Act of cutting into tissue or an organ.

CCI Version 16.3

01250, 01320, 01470, 01610, 01710, 01782, 01810, 0213T, 0216T, 0228T, 0230T, 20526-20553, 36000, 36400-36410, 36420-36430, 36440, 36600, 36640, 37202, 43752, 51701-51703, 62310-62319, 64400-64435, 64445-64450, 64479, 64483, 64490, 64493, 64505-64530, 64718-64726, 64831, 64834-64836, 64840-64858, 64861-64870, 92585, 93000-93010, 93040-93042, 93318, 94002, 94200, 94250, 94680-94690, 94770, 95812-95816, 95819, 95822, 95829, 95860-95861, 95867-95868, 95870, 95900, 95904, 95920, 95925-95934, 95936-95937, 95955, 96360, 96365, 96372, 96374-96376, 99148-99149, 99150

Also not with 64897: 64702-64708, 64874-64896❖, 64898❖, 64907-64911❖

Also not with 64898: 64708, 64874-64893, 64896❖, 64910-64911❖

Note: These CCI edits are used for Medicare. Other payers may reimburse on codes listed above.

Medicare Edits

	Fac RVU	Non-Fac RVU	FUD	Assist
64897	37.61	37.61	90	80
64898	40.59	40.59	90	80

Medicare References: 100-2,15,260; 100-4,12,30; 100-4,12,90.3; 100-4,14,10

64901-64902

64901 Nerve graft, each additional nerve; single strand (List separately in addition to code for primary procedure)

64902 multiple strands (cable) (List separately in addition to code for primary procedure)

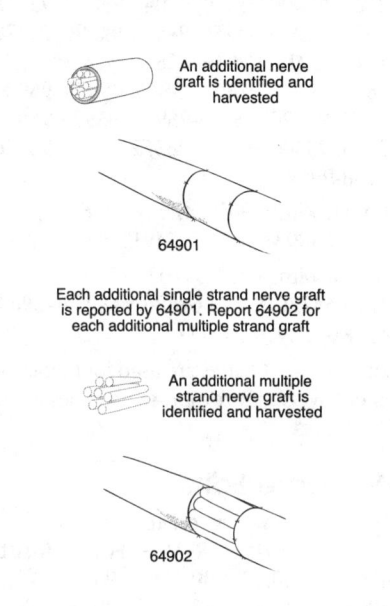

An additional nerve graft is identified and harvested

64901

Each additional single strand nerve graft is reported by 64901. Report 64902 for each additional multiple strand graft

An additional multiple strand nerve graft is identified and harvested

64902

Explanation

The physician grafts additional nerves. These codes are used in addition to initial nerve graft codes, and include graft harvest. Report 64901 for each additional single strand graft; 64902 for each additional multiple strand graft.

Coding Tips

Any nerve graft harvest is not reported separately. Use 64901 in conjunction with 64885–64893. Use 64902 in conjunction with 64885, 64886, and 64895–64898. As "add-on" codes, 64901 and 64902 are not subject to multiple procedure rules. No reimbursement reduction or modifier 51 is applied. Add-on codes describe additional intra-service work associated with the primary procedure. They are performed by the same physician on the same date of service as the primary service/procedure, and must never be reported as a stand-alone code.

ICD-9-CM Procedural

04.5 Cranial or peripheral nerve graft

Anesthesia

N/A

ICD-9-CM Diagnostic

This is an add-on code. Refer to the corresponding primary procedure code for ICD-9-CM diagnosis code links.

Terms To Know

graft. Tissue implant from another part of the body or another person.

CCI Version 16.3

20550-20553, 62310-62311, 92585, 95822, 95860-95861, 95867-95868, 95900, 95904, 95920, 95925-95927, 95930-95934, 95936-95937

Note: These CCI edits are used for Medicare. Other payers may reimburse on codes listed above.

Medicare Edits

	Fac RVU	Non-Fac RVU	FUD	Assist
64901	18.61	18.61	N/A	80
64902	21.47	21.47	N/A	80

Medicare References: 100-2,15,260; 100-4,12,30; 100-4,12,90.3; 100-4,14,10

64905-64907

64905 Nerve pedicle transfer; first stage
64907 second stage

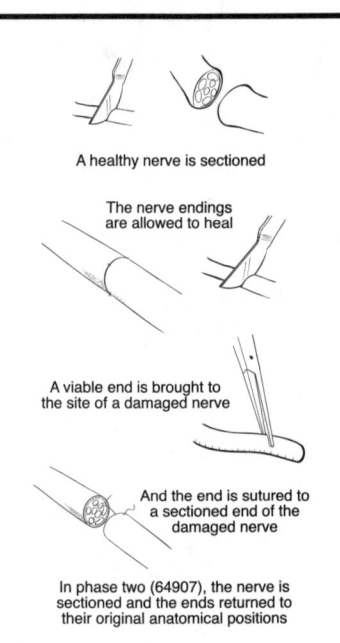

Explanation
The physician transfers a nerve pedicle from an intact nerve to a damaged nerve. A pedicle is an intact nerve used as a donor for regeneration of axons in the damaged nerve. In 64905, the first stage is completed. The physician makes an incision over the donor nerve site and locates the nerve. The nerve is freed from surrounding tissues and cut. The proximal portion of the donor nerve is transferred to the distal portion of the recipient nerve. The incision is closed in sutured layers. In 64907, the second stage is completed. The physician reopens the surgical incision and locates the donor and recipient nerves. The donor nerve is resected from the recipient nerve and primarily reanastomosed to its distal end. The distal end of the recipient nerve is reanastomosed to its proximal end. The nerves may be freed from surrounding tissues if necessary to complete anastomosis. The incision is closed in sutured layers.

Coding Tips
If the procedure is completed through an operating microscope, report 69990 in addition to the primary procedure. However, head gear (e.g., loupes or binoculars) is considered an integral part of these procedures.

ICD-9-CM Procedural
04.5 Cranial or peripheral nerve graft

Anesthesia
01610, 01710, 01810

ICD-9-CM Diagnostic
The application of this code is too broad to adequately present ICD-9-CM diagnostic code links here. Refer to your ICD-9-CM book.

Terms To Know
anastomosis. Surgically created connection between ducts, blood vessels, or bowel segments to allow flow from one to the other.

axon. Extension from a neuron that carries impulses to receiving terminal branches.

distal. Located farther away from a specified reference point.

incision. Act of cutting into tissue or an organ.

proximal. Located closest to a specified reference point, usually the midline.

resection. Surgical removal of a part or all of an organ or body part.

suture. Numerous stitching techniques employed in wound closure.

buried suture. Continuous or interrupted suture placed under the skin for a layered closure.

continuous suture. Running stitch with tension evenly distributed across a single strand to provide a leakproof closure line.

interrupted suture. Series of single stitches with tension isolated at each stitch, in which all stitches are not affected if one becomes loose, and the isolated sutures cannot act as a wick to transport an infection.

purse-string suture. Continuous suture placed around a tubular structure and tightened, to reduce or close the lumen.

retention suture. Secondary stitching that bridges the primary suture, providing support for the primary repair; a plastic or rubber bolster may be placed over the primary repair and under the retention sutures.

CCI Version 16.3
01250, 01320, 01470, 01610, 01710, 01782, 01810, 0213T, 0216T, 0228T, 0230T, 20526-20553, 36000, 36400-36410, 36420-36430, 36440, 36600, 36640, 37202, 43752, 51701-51703, 62310-62319, 64400-64435, 64445-64455, 64479, 64483, 64490, 64493, 64505-64530, 64831, 64834-64836, 64840-64858, 64861-64870, 92585, 93000-93010, 93040-93042, 93318, 94002, 94200, 94250, 94680-94690, 94770, 95812-95816, 95819, 95822, 95829, 95860-95861, 95867-95868, 95870, 95900, 95904, 95920, 95925-95934, 95936-95937, 95955, 96360, 96365, 96372, 96374-96376, 99148-99149, 99150

Also not with 64905: 64702-64726, 64874-64898✦, 64907-64911✦

Also not with 64907: 64702-64714, 64718-64726, 64874-64886, 64895-64896✦, 64898✦, 64910-64911✦

Note: These CCI edits are used for Medicare. Other payers may reimburse on codes listed above.

Medicare Edits

	Fac RVU	Non-Fac RVU	FUD	Assist
64905	30.17	30.17	90	80
64907	33.88	33.88	90	80

Medicare References: 100-2,15,260; 100-4,12,30; 100-4,12,90.3; 100-4,14,10

64910

64910 Nerve repair; with synthetic conduit or vein allograft (eg, nerve tube), each nerve

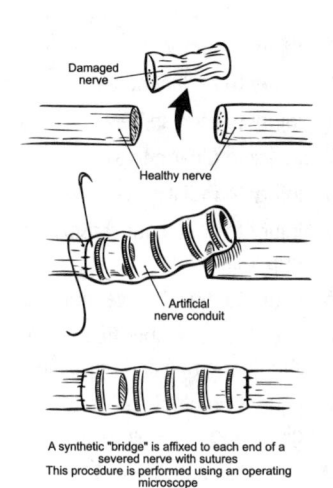

A synthetic "bridge" is affixed to each end of a severed nerve with sutures. This procedure is performed using an operating microscope.

Explanation

The physician repairs a nerve and uses a graft to restore innervation. The physician makes an incision over the damaged nerve and dissects tissues to locate the nerve. The damaged area of the nerve is resected and removed. Innervation is restored by building a bridge to each end of the resected nerve and suturing the proximal and distal ends of the bridge into place around each severed nerve end. This technique is usually limited to nerve gaps of 3 cm or less. The bridge is usually 1 cm longer than the defect so that it covers the distal and proximal ends of the resected nerve. The bridge is composed of a bioabsorbable, corrugated synthetic conduit of polyglycolic acid. Once the bridge is sutured into place, the artificial nerve conduit is infused with a solution of heparin and saline to prevent clot formation. The operative wound is repaired in layers. Over time, the nerve conduit is restored and the tube is resorbed by surrounding tissue.

Coding Tips

For nerve repair with autogenous vein graft, see 64911. Do not report 69990 with 64910.

ICD-9-CM Procedural

- 04.3 Suture of cranial and peripheral nerves
- 04.5 Cranial or peripheral nerve graft
- 04.6 Transposition of cranial and peripheral nerves
- 04.75 Revision of previous repair of cranial and peripheral nerves
- 04.76 Repair of old traumatic injury of cranial and peripheral nerves
- 04.79 Other neuroplasty

Anesthesia

64910 01610, 01710, 01810

ICD-9-CM Diagnostic

- 816.11 Open fracture of middle or proximal phalanx or phalanges of hand
- 876.0 Open wound of back, without mention of complication
- 876.1 Open wound of back, complicated
- 880.03 Open wound of upper arm, without mention of complication
- 880.23 Open wound of upper arm, with tendon involvement
- 881.02 Open wound of wrist, without mention of complication
- 881.22 Open wound of wrist, with tendon involvement
- 882.0 Open wound of hand except finger(s) alone, without mention of complication
- 882.1 Open wound of hand except finger(s) alone, complicated
- 882.2 Open wound of hand except finger(s) alone, with tendon involvement
- 883.0 Open wound of finger(s), without mention of complication
- 883.1 Open wound of finger(s), complicated
- 883.2 Open wound of finger(s), with tendon involvement
- 884.0 Multiple and unspecified open wound of upper limb, without mention of complication
- 926.11 Crushing injury of back — (Use additional code to identify any associated injuries: 800-829, 850.0-854.1, 860.0-869.1)
- 927.00 Crushing injury of shoulder region — (Use additional code to identify any associated injuries: 800-829, 850.0-854.1, 860.0-869.1)
- 927.20 Crushing injury of hand(s) — (Use additional code to identify any associated injuries: 800-829, 850.0-854.1, 860.0-869.1)
- 927.21 Crushing injury of wrist — (Use additional code to identify any associated injuries: 800-829, 850.0-854.1, 860.0-869.1)
- 927.3 Crushing injury of finger(s) — (Use additional code to identify any associated injuries: 800-829, 850.0-854.1, 860.0-869.1)
- 927.8 Crushing injury of multiple sites of upper limb — (Use additional code to identify any associated injuries: 800-829, 850.0-854.1, 860.0-869.1)
- 953.4 Injury to brachial plexus
- 953.5 Injury to lumbosacral plexus
- 955.0 Injury to axillary nerve
- 955.1 Injury to median nerve
- 955.2 Injury to ulnar nerve
- 955.3 Injury to radial nerve
- 955.5 Injury to cutaneous sensory nerve, upper limb
- 955.6 Injury to digital nerve, upper limb
- 955.7 Injury to other specified nerve(s) of shoulder girdle and upper limb
- 955.8 Injury to multiple nerves of shoulder girdle and upper limb
- 956.0 Injury to sciatic nerve
- 959.4 Injury, other and unspecified, hand, except finger
- 959.5 Injury, other and unspecified, finger

CCI Version 16.3

01250, 01320, 01470, 01610, 01710, 01810, 0213T, 0216T, 0228T, 0230T, 20926, 36000, 36400-36410, 36420-36430, 36440, 36600, 36640, 37202, 43752, 51701-51703, 62310-62319, 64400-64435, 64445-64455, 64479, 64483, 64490, 64493, 64505-64530, 64702-64726, 64831, 64834-64836, 64840-64858, 64861-64870, 69990, 92585, 93000-93010, 93040-93042, 93318, 94002, 94200, 94250, 94680-94690, 94770, 95812-95816, 95819, 95822, 95829, 95860-95861, 95867-95868, 95870, 95900, 95904, 95920, 95925-95934, 95936-95937, 95955, 96360, 96365, 96372, 96374-96376, 99148-99149, 99150

Note: These CCI edits are used for Medicare. Other payers may reimburse on codes listed above.

Medicare Edits

	Fac RVU	Non-Fac RVU	FUD	Assist
64910	24.06	24.06	90	80

Medicare References: None

64911

64911 Nerve repair; with autogenous vein graft (includes harvest of vein graft), each nerve

A venous "bridge" is affixed to each end of a severed nerve with sutures. This procedure is performed using an operating microscope

Explanation
The physician repairs a nerve and uses a vein graft to restore innervation. The physician obtains the venous graft by making an incision over the donor site and locating the vein. The vein is freed from surrounding tissues and excised, and vessels are tied or cauterized. The incision is sutured in layers. The physician makes an incision over the damaged nerve and dissects tissues to locate the nerve. The damaged area of the nerve is resected and removed. Innervation is restored by building a bridge of vein to each end of the resected nerve and suturing the proximal and distal ends of the bridge into place around each severed nerve end. This technique is usually limited to nerve gaps of 3 cm or less. The bridge is usually 1 cm longer than the defect so that it covers the distal and proximal ends of the resected nerve. Once the bridge is sutured into place, it is infused with a solution of heparin and saline to prevent clot formation. The operative wound is repaired in layers. Over time, the nerve conduit is restored.

Coding Tips
For nerve repair with synthetic conduit or vein allograft, see 64910. Do not report 69990 with 64911.

ICD-9-CM Procedural
- 04.3 Suture of cranial and peripheral nerves
- 04.5 Cranial or peripheral nerve graft
- 04.6 Transposition of cranial and peripheral nerves
- 04.75 Revision of previous repair of cranial and peripheral nerves
- 04.76 Repair of old traumatic injury of cranial and peripheral nerves
- 04.79 Other neuroplasty

Anesthesia
64911 01610, 01710, 01810

ICD-9-CM Diagnostic
- 816.11 Open fracture of middle or proximal phalanx or phalanges of hand
- 876.0 Open wound of back, without mention of complication
- 876.1 Open wound of back, complicated
- 880.03 Open wound of upper arm, without mention of complication
- 880.23 Open wound of upper arm, with tendon involvement
- 881.02 Open wound of wrist, without mention of complication
- 881.22 Open wound of wrist, with tendon involvement
- 882.0 Open wound of hand except finger(s) alone, without mention of complication
- 882.1 Open wound of hand except finger(s) alone, complicated
- 883.0 Open wound of finger(s), without mention of complication
- 883.1 Open wound of finger(s), complicated
- 883.2 Open wound of finger(s), with tendon involvement
- 884.0 Multiple and unspecified open wound of upper limb, without mention of complication
- 926.11 Crushing injury of back — (Use additional code to identify any associated injuries: 800-829, 850.0-854.1, 860.0-869.1)
- 927.00 Crushing injury of shoulder region — (Use additional code to identify any associated injuries: 800-829, 850.0-854.1, 860.0-869.1)
- 927.20 Crushing injury of hand(s) — (Use additional code to identify any associated injuries: 800-829, 850.0-854.1, 860.0-869.1)
- 927.21 Crushing injury of wrist — (Use additional code to identify any associated injuries: 800-829, 850.0-854.1, 860.0-869.1)
- 927.3 Crushing injury of finger(s) — (Use additional code to identify any associated injuries: 800-829, 850.0-854.1, 860.0-869.1)
- 927.8 Crushing injury of multiple sites of upper limb — (Use additional code to identify any associated injuries: 800-829, 850.0-854.1, 860.0-869.1)
- 953.4 Injury to brachial plexus
- 953.5 Injury to lumbosacral plexus
- 955.0 Injury to axillary nerve
- 955.1 Injury to median nerve
- 955.2 Injury to ulnar nerve
- 955.3 Injury to radial nerve
- 955.5 Injury to cutaneous sensory nerve, upper limb
- 955.6 Injury to digital nerve, upper limb
- 955.7 Injury to other specified nerve(s) of shoulder girdle and upper limb
- 955.8 Injury to multiple nerves of shoulder girdle and upper limb
- 956.0 Injury to sciatic nerve
- 959.4 Injury, other and unspecified, hand, except finger
- 959.5 Injury, other and unspecified, finger

CCI Version 16.3
01250, 01320, 01470, 01610, 01710, 01810, 0213T, 0216T, 0228T, 0230T, 20926, 36000, 36400-36410, 36420-36430, 36440, 36600, 36640, 37202, 43752, 51701-51703, 62310-62319, 64400-64435, 64445-64455, 64479, 64483, 64490, 64493, 64505-64530, 64702-64726, 64831, 64834-64836, 64840-64858, 64861-64870, 64910❖, 69990, 92585, 93000-93010, 93040-93042, 93318, 94002, 94200, 94250, 94680-94690, 94770, 95812-95816, 95819, 95822, 95829, 95860-95861, 95867-95868, 95870, 95900, 95904, 95920, 95925-95934, 95936-95937, 95955, 96360, 96365, 96372, 96374-96376, 99148-99149, 99150

Note: These CCI edits are used for Medicare. Other payers may reimburse on codes listed above.

Medicare Edits

	Fac RVU	Non-Fac RVU	FUD	Assist
64911	30.02	30.02	90	80

Medicare References: None

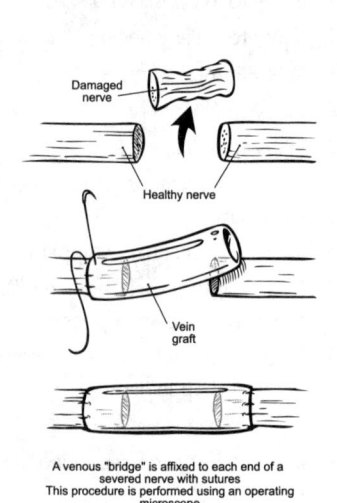

69990

69990 Microsurgical techniques, requiring use of operating microscope (List separately in addition to code for primary procedure)

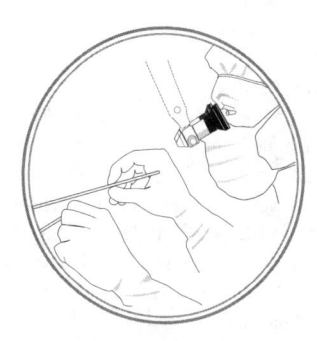

Code 69990 reports the use of an operating microscope for procedures performed with microsurgery techniques. The code is reported in addition to a primary procedure in which use of an operating microscope is not an inclusive component

Anesthesia
69990 N/A

ICD-9-CM Diagnostic
This is an add-on code. Refer to the corresponding primary procedure code for ICD-9-CM diagnosis code links.

CCI Version 16.3
No CCI Edits apply to this code.

Medicare Edits

	Fac RVU	Non-Fac RVU	FUD	Assist
69990	6.48	6.48	N/A	80

Medicare References: None

Explanation
The physician uses a surgical microscope when the services are performed using the techniques of microsurgery, except when the microscopy is part of the procedure (such as in 15756). This code is reported in addition to the primary procedure.

Coding Tips
This code is used when surgical services are performed using the techniques of microsurgery. Do not use 69990 for visualization with magnifying loupes or to correct vision. Do not use this code when an operating microscope is considered an inclusive component of these upper extremity and neurosurgery procedures: 15756–15758, 26551–26554, 26556, 63075–63078, and 64727. As an "add-on" code, 69990 is not subject to multiple procedure rules. No reimbursement reduction or modifier 51 is applied. Add-on codes describe additional intra-service work associated with the primary procedure. They are performed by the same physician on the same date of service as the primary service/procedure, and must never be reported as a stand-alone code.

ICD-9-CM Procedural
The ICD-9-CM procedural code(s) would be the same as the actual procedure performed because these are in-addition-to codes.

70010

70010 Myelography, posterior fossa, radiological supervision and interpretation

Explanation
A radiographic study using fluoroscopy is performed on the posterior fossa when a lesion is suspected, or to detect cerebrospinal fluid (CSF) leaks or normal pressure hydrocephalus (NPH). Contrast medium, usually barium sulfate, may be used to enhance visibility and is instilled in the patient through a lumbar area puncture into the subarachnoid space. The radiologist takes a series of pictures by sending an x-ray beam through the body, using fluoroscopy to view the enhanced structure on a television camera. The patient is angled from an erect position through a recumbent position with the body tilted so as to maintain feet higher than the head to help the flow of contrast into the study area.

70360

70360 Radiologic examination; neck, soft tissue

Explanation
The technologist uses x-rays to obtain soft tissue images of the patient's neck rather than bone. The radiologist obtains two views, typically front to back (AP), and side to side (lateral). This procedure is performed to visualize abnormal air patterns or suspected foreign bodies or obstructions within the throat or neck.

70490-70492

70490 Computed tomography, soft tissue neck; without contrast material
70491 with contrast material(s)
70492 without contrast material followed by contrast material(s) and further sections

Explanation
Computerized axial tomography directs multiple narrow beams of x-rays around the body structure being studied and uses computer imaging to produce thin cross-sectional views of various layers (or slices) of the body. It is useful for the evaluation of trauma, tumor, and foreign bodies as CT is able to visualize soft tissue as well as bones. Patients are required to remain motionless during the study and sedation may need to be administered as well as a contrast medium for image enhancement. These codes report an exam of the soft tissue of the neck. Report 70490 if no contrast is used. Report 70491 if performed with contrast and 70492 if performed first without contrast and then again following the injection of contrast.

70496-70498

70496 Computed tomographic angiography, head, with contrast material(s), including noncontrast images, if performed, and image postprocessing
70498 Computed tomographic angiography, neck, with contrast material(s), including noncontrast images, if performed, and image postprocessing

Explanation
Computed tomographic angiography (CTA) is a procedure used for the imaging of vessels to detect aneurysms, blood clots, and other vascular irregularities. Contrast medium is rapidly infused intravenously, at intervals, usually with an automatic injector, and the patient is scanned with thin section axial or spiral mode x-ray beams. The images obtained are acquired with narrower collimation and reconstructed at shorter intervals than standard CT images. Three-dimensional images are generated and postprocessing reconstruction is done at a workstation on the scanner. CTA also provides information unavailable with conventional angiography, such as vessel wall thickness (mural thrombus) and the venous anatomy of a target organ and/or associated organs within the scan range. Report 70496 for an exam of the head and 70498 for an exam of the neck. These codes report exams with contrast materials and image postprocessing. Noncontrast images, if performed, are also included in these procedures.

70540-70543

70540 Magnetic resonance (eg, proton) imaging, orbit, face, and/or neck; without contrast material(s)
70542 with contrast material(s)
70543 without contrast material(s), followed by contrast material(s) and further sequences

Explanation
Magnetic resonance imaging (MRI) is a radiation-free, noninvasive, technique to produce high quality sectional images of the inside of the body in multiple planes. MRI uses the natural magnetic properties of the hydrogen atoms in our bodies that emit radiofrequency signals when exposed to radio waves within a strong electro-magnetic field. These signals are then processed and converted by the computer into high-resolution, three-dimensional, tomographic images. Patients with metallic or electronic implants or foreign bodies cannot be exposed to MRI. The patient must remain still while lying on a motorized table within the large, circular MRI tunnel. A sedative may be administered as well as contrast material for image enhancement. These codes report an exam of the orbit, face, and neck. Report 70540 if no contrast is used. Report 70542 if performed with contrast and 70543 if performed first without contrast and then again following the injection of contrast.

70547-70549

70547 Magnetic resonance angiography, neck; without contrast material(s)
70548 with contrast material(s)
70549 without contrast material(s), followed by contrast material(s) and further sequences

Explanation
Magnetic Resonance Angiography (MRA) is a special type of magnetic resonance imaging (MRI) that specifically visualizes blood vessels and blood flow to evaluate vascular disorders within the structure being studied. Unlike CT, it does not rely on the absorption of x-ray energy. Magnetic resonance imaging uses the natural magnetic properties of the hydrogen atoms in our bodies that emit radiofrequency signals when exposed to radio waves within a strong electro-magnetic field. These signals are then processed and converted by the computer into high-resolution, three-dimensional tomographic images. Patients with metallic or electronic implants or foreign bodies cannot be exposed to MRI. The patient must remain still while lying on a motorized table within the large, circular MRI tunnel. A sedative may be administered as well as contrast material for image enhancement. These codes report and exam of the neck. Report 70547 if no contrast is used. Report 70548 if performed with contrast and 70549 if performed first without contrast and then again following the injection of contrast.

72010

72010 Radiologic examination, spine, entire, survey study, anteroposterior and lateral

Explanation
The entire spine is surveyed in a radiologic exam that includes anteroposterior views, with the patient supine, knees flexed, and feet flat on the table; and lateral views, either recumbent or erect. Right and left posterior obliques may be performed with the patient in the semi-supine position with the spine at a 45 degree angle to the table.

72020

72020 Radiologic examination, spine, single view, specify level

Explanation
One film is taken of the spine that requires specification of the level examined.

72040-72052

72040 Radiologic examination, spine, cervical; 2 or 3 views
72050 minimum of 4 views
72052 complete, including oblique and flexion and/or extension studies

Explanation
A radiologic examination of the cervical spine is performed that includes a minimum of two views in 72040, a minimum of four views in 72050, and a complete study in 72052. The complete study includes films taken in oblique (angled) positions and in flexion and/or extension positioning.

72069
72069 Radiologic examination, spine, thoracolumbar, standing (scoliosis)

Explanation
Typically a film is taken of the thoracolumbar spine from front to back (AP) while the patient is standing erect. This film is used to detect any curvature of the spine when scoliosis or other pathology may be present.

72070-72074
72070 Radiologic examination, spine; thoracic, 2 views
72072 thoracic, 3 views
72074 thoracic, minimum of 4 views

Explanation
A radiologic examination of the thoracic spine is performed that includes two views in 72070, three views in 72072, and a minimum of four views in 72074. These procedures do not specify that a certain view must be performed.

72080
72080 Radiologic examination, spine; thoracolumbar, 2 views

Explanation
Films are taken of the thoracolumbar area of the spine in two views not specifically stated.

72090
72090 Radiologic examination, spine; scoliosis study, including supine and erect studies

Explanation
A typical scoliosis series consists of four views of the thoracic and lumbar spine: one from front to back (AP) with the patient standing; one from front to back (AP) with the patient supine, or lying down; and finally, two views with alternate right and left flexion in the supine position. In addition, a lateral, or side to side projection made with the patient standing to show spondylolisthesis or to demonstrate exaggerated degrees of kyphosis or lordosis is often recommended. The key element to this code is that it includes supine and erect studies. The number of films allowed is not specified.

72100-72110
72100 Radiologic examination, spine, lumbosacral; 2 or 3 views
72110 minimum of 4 views

Explanation
A radiologic examination of the lumbosacral spine is performed that includes two or three views in 72100, and a minimum of four views in 72110. These procedures do not specify that a certain view must be performed.

72114
72114 Radiologic examination, spine, lumbosacral; complete, including bending views

Explanation
Films are taken of the lumbosacral spine, or lower back, for a complete radiologic study. A complete lumbar spine series typically includes x-rays taken from front to back (AP), side to side (lateral), and oblique, or angled right and left views. In addition, this code includes bending views, films taken with the patient bending to the left and right to demonstrate mobility of the intervertebral joints, and/or films taken with the patient in both flexion and extension, typically in cases of disc protrusion to localize the involved joint.

72120
72120 Radiologic examination, spine, lumbosacral, bending views only, minimum of 4 views

Explanation
Films are taken of the lumbar spine, or lower back, with the patient bending to the left and right to demonstrate the mobility of the intervertebral joints and/or films with the patient in both flexion and extension, typically in cases of disc protrusion to localize the involved joint. The key element to this code is that a minimum of four films in bending views only are taken.

72125-72127
72125 Computed tomography, cervical spine; without contrast material
72126 with contrast material
72127 without contrast material, followed by contrast material(s) and further sections

Explanation
Computerized axial tomography directs multiple narrow beams of x-rays around the body structure being studied and uses computer imaging to produce thin cross-sectional views of various layers (or slices) of the body. It is useful for the evaluation of trauma, tumor, and foreign bodies as CT is able to visualize soft tissue as well as bones. Patients are required to remain motionless during the study and sedation may need to be administered. These codes report an exam of the cervical spine. For CT of the spine, contrast material may be administered either intravenously (part of the procedure) or intrathecally (reported separately). These codes report and exam of the cervical spine. Report 72125 if no contrast is used. Report 72126 if performed with contrast and 72127 if performed first without contrast and then again following the injection of contrast.

72128-72130
72128 Computed tomography, thoracic spine; without contrast material
72129 with contrast material
72130 without contrast material, followed by contrast material(s) and further sections

Explanation
Computerized axial tomography directs multiple narrow beams of x-rays around the body structure being studied and uses computer imaging to produce thin cross-sectional views of various layers (or slices) of the body. It is useful for the evaluation of trauma, tumor, and foreign bodies as CT is able to visualize soft tissue as well as bones. Patients are required to remain motionless during the study and sedation may need to be administered. These codes report an exam of the thoracic spine. For CT of the spine, contrast material may be administered either intravenously (part of the procedure) or intrathecally (reported separately). These codes report an exam of the thoracic spine. Report 72128 if no contrast is used. Report 72129 if performed with contrast and 72130 if performed first without contrast and then again following the injection of contrast.

72131-72133
72131 Computed tomography, lumbar spine; without contrast material
72132 with contrast material
72133 without contrast material, followed by contrast material(s) and further sections

Explanation
Computerized axial tomography directs multiple thin beams of x-rays at the body structure being studied and uses computer imaging to produce thin cross-sectional views of various layers (or slices) of the body. It is useful for the evaluation of trauma, tumor, and foreign bodies as CT is able to visualize soft tissue as well as bones. Patients are required to remain motionless during the study and sedation may need to be administered. These codes report an exam of the lumbar spine. For CT of the spine, contrast material may be administered either intravenously (part of the procedure) or intrathecally (reported separately). These codes report an exam of the lumbar spine. Report 72131 if no contrast is used. Report 72132 if performed with contrast and 72133 if performed first without contrast and then again following the injection of contrast.

72141-72142, 72156

72141 Magnetic resonance (eg, proton) imaging, spinal canal and contents, cervical; without contrast material

72142 with contrast material(s)

72156 Magnetic resonance (eg, proton) imaging, spinal canal and contents, without contrast material, followed by contrast material(s) and further sequences; cervical

Explanation

Magnetic resonance imaging (MRI) is a radiation-free, noninvasive, technique to produce high quality sectional images of the inside of the body in multiple planes. MRI uses the natural magnetic properties of the hydrogen atoms in our bodies that emit radiofrequency signals when exposed to radio waves within a strong electro-magnetic field. These signals are then processed and converted by the computer into high-resolution, three-dimensional, tomographic images. Patients with metallic or electronic implants or foreign bodies cannot be exposed to MRI. The patient must remain still while lying on a motorized table within the large, circular MRI tunnel. A sedative may be administered as well as contrast material for image enhancement. For cervical spinal canal and contents, report 72141 if no contrast is used; report 72142 if performed with contrast and 72156 if performed first without contrast and then again following the injection of contrast.

72146-72147, 72157

72146 Magnetic resonance (eg, proton) imaging, spinal canal and contents, thoracic; without contrast material

72147 with contrast material(s)

72157 Magnetic resonance (eg, proton) imaging, spinal canal and contents, without contrast material, followed by contrast material(s) and further sequences; thoracic

Explanation

Magnetic resonance imaging (MRI) is a radiation-free, noninvasive, technique to produce high quality sectional images of the inside of the body in multiple planes. MRI uses the natural magnetic properties of the hydrogen atoms in our bodies that emit radiofrequency signals when exposed to radio waves within a strong electro-magnetic field. These signals are then processed and converted by the computer into high-resolution, three-dimensional, tomographic images. Patients with metallic or electronic implants or foreign bodies cannot be exposed to MRI. The patient must remain still while lying on a motorized table within the large, circular MRI tunnel. A sedative may be administered as well as contrast material for image enhancement. For thoracic spinal canal and contents, report 72146 if no contrast is used; report 72147 if performed with contrast and 72157 if performed first without contrast and then again following the injection of contrast.

72148-72149, 72158

72148 Magnetic resonance (eg, proton) imaging, spinal canal and contents, lumbar; without contrast material

72149 with contrast material(s)

72158 Magnetic resonance (eg, proton) imaging, spinal canal and contents, without contrast material, followed by contrast material(s) and further sequences; lumbar

Explanation

Magnetic resonance imaging (MRI) is a radiation-free, noninvasive, technique to produce high quality sectional images of the inside of the body in multiple planes. MRI uses the natural magnetic properties of the hydrogen atoms in our bodies that emit radiofrequency signals when exposed to radio waves within a strong electro-magnetic field. These signals are then processed and converted by the computer into high-resolution, three-dimensional, tomographic images. Patients with metallic or electronic implants or foreign bodies cannot be exposed to MRI. The patient must remain still while lying on a motorized table within the large, circular MRI tunnel. A sedative may be administered as well as contrast material for image enhancement. For lumbar spinal canal and contents, report 72148 if no contrast is used; report 72149 if performed with contrast and 72158 if performed first without contrast and then again following the injection of contrast.

72220

72220 Radiologic examination, sacrum and coccyx, minimum of 2 views

Explanation

Films are taken (minimum of two views) of the sacrum and the coccyx. The sacrum is a triangular bone located between the fifth lumbar vertebra and the coccyx. It is formed by five connected vertebrae and is wedged between the two innominate bones. The coccyx is the small bone at the very base of the spinal column, and is formed by the fusion of four vertebrae. The sacrum and the coccyx form the posterior (back) boundary of the pelvis. While anteroposterior (AP; front to back) and lateral (side) views are the most common views taken, this procedure is used for any two or more views reported.

72240-72270

72240 Myelography, cervical, radiological supervision and interpretation

72255 Myelography, thoracic, radiological supervision and interpretation

72265 Myelography, lumbosacral, radiological supervision and interpretation

72270 Myelography, 2 or more regions (eg, lumbar/thoracic, cervical/thoracic, lumbar/cervical, lumbar/thoracic/cervical), radiological supervision and interpretation

Explanation

In myelography, a radiographic study using fluoroscopy is performed on the spinal cord and nerve root branches when a lesion is suspected. Contrast medium, usually barium sulfate, is used to enhance visibility and is instilled in the patient through a lumbar or cervical area puncture into the subarachnoid space. The radiologist takes a series of pictures by sending an x-ray beam through the body, using fluoroscopy to view the enhanced structure on a television camera. The patient is angled from an erect position through a recumbent position with the body tilted so as to maintain feet higher than the head to help the flow of contrast into the study area. Code 72240 reports a cervical myelogram; 72255 reports a thoracic myelogram; 72265 reports lumbosacral myelogram; and 72270 reports a myelogram of the entire spinal canal.

72285, 72295

72285 Discography, cervical or thoracic, radiological supervision and interpretation

72295 Discography, lumbar, radiological supervision and interpretation

Explanation

Individual intervertebral discs are imaged and examined in discography, also known as nucleography. Iodinated contrast medium is injected into the center of the disc. A series of images is taken by the radiologist and interpreted and reported. This technique is used to determine the extent of the target disc(s) disease. Report 72285 for the cervical or thoracic discs and 72295 for the lumbar discs.

72291-72292

72291 Radiological supervision and interpretation, percutaneous vertebroplasty, vertebral augmentation, or sacral augmentation (sacroplasty), including cavity creation, per vertebral body or sacrum; under fluoroscopic guidance

72292 under CT guidance

Explanation

These codes report the radiological supervision and interpretation for percutaneous vertebroplasty, vertebral augmentation, or sacroplasty (sacral augmentation), per vertebral body or sacrum. Percutaneous vertebroplasty is the injection of polymethyl methacrylate into collapsed or diseased vertebra. The polymethyl methacrylate acts as a bone cement to relieve debilitating pain resulting from osteoporosis, bone metastases, and hemangiomas. Vertebral augmentation is a similar procedure that, in addition, involves the introduction of inflatable balloon catheters (tamps) into the vertebral body to restore height and to create a cavity into which the polymethyl methacrylate can be injected. In a sacroplasty procedure, the polymethyl methacrylate cement is injected into the sacrum and the sacral defect or insufficiency fracture rather than the vertebral body, using CT or fluoroscopic guidance. Report 72291 if fluoroscopic guidance was provided and 72292 if CT guidance was provided.

73000

73000 Radiologic examination; clavicle, complete

Explanation
Films are taken of the clavicle for a complete radiologic examination. The number of films is not specified. The patient is placed supine for a front to back (AP) view and the x-ray is directed to the midpoint and perpendicular to the clavicle.

73010

73010 Radiologic examination; scapula, complete

Explanation
Films are taken of the scapula for a complete examination. The number of films is not specified. Anteroposterior (AP) and lateral views may be taken. The patient is placed supine for a front to back (AP) view and may be erect or recumbent for a lateral view. The arm is abducted to make a 90 degree angle to the body with the elbow flexed.

73020-73030

73020 Radiologic examination, shoulder; 1 view
73030 complete, minimum of 2 views

Explanation
Films are taken of the shoulder. The patient is supine with the arm extended to a 90 degree angle from the body and externally rotated while the head is turned to face opposite the affected side. Code 73020 is for reporting one view only and 73030 specifies a minimum of two views.

73040

73040 Radiologic examination, shoulder, arthrography, radiological supervision and interpretation

Explanation
The synovial joint of the shoulder is visualized internally through arthrography, the direct injection of air and/or contrast material into the joint for radiological examination. Local anesthesia in injected into the joint followed by the contrast material and/or air. A series of images are taken and interpreted. Fluoroscopic films and guidance for needle localization is included. Arthrography helps diagnose conditions of cartilage abnormalities, arthritis and bursitis, rotator cuff tear, and frozen joint. AP (front to back) views are taken with the affected arm rotated externally and internally and with the arm in a neutral, flexed position lying over the abdomen.

73050

73050 Radiologic examination; acromioclavicular joints, bilateral, with or without weighted distraction

Explanation
A radiologic examination is made of the acromioclavicular joints bilaterally, with no specified amount of views. The patient is placed in a sitting or standing upright position with arms at the side for an anteroposterior view. The patient may also be given weights to hold in each hand for weighted distraction radiographs of each joint.

73060

73060 Radiologic examination; humerus, minimum of 2 views

Explanation
Two or more films are taken of the humerus with the x-ray beam aimed midshaft. The patient is supine with the hand also supinated for an AP view and with the hand rotated internally for an oblique view.

73070-73080

73070 Radiologic examination, elbow; 2 views
73080 complete, minimum of 3 views

Explanation
A radiologic examination of the elbow joint is made. Films of the elbow may be taken in the AP position with the hand supinated, oblique positioning with the hand pronated and/or externally rotated, and in the lateral position with the wrist lateral and the elbow flexed at 90 degrees. Code 73070 reports two views and 73080 reports a complete exam with a minimum of three views.

73085

73085 Radiologic examination, elbow, arthrography, radiological supervision and interpretation

Explanation
The synovial joint of the elbow is visualized internally through arthrography, the direct injection of air and/or contrast material into the joint for radiological examination. Local anesthesia in injected into the joint followed by the contrast material and/or air. A series of images are taken by the radiologist and interpreted. Fluoroscopic films and guidance for needle localization is included. Arthrography helps diagnose conditions of cartilage abnormalities, arthritis and bursitis, and frozen joint.

73090

73090 Radiologic examination; forearm, 2 views

Explanation
Two films of the forearm are taken with the x-ray beam aimed at the midforearm. Films may be taken in the AP position with the hand supinated, in the true lateral position and in oblique positioning.

73092

73092 Radiologic examination; upper extremity, infant, minimum of 2 views

Explanation
A minimum of two films of an infant's forearm are taken with the x-ray beam aimed at the midforearm. The infant or child must first be immobilized to prevent movement during the film taking. Films may be taken in the AP position with the hand supinated, in the true lateral position and in oblique positioning.

73100-73110

73100 Radiologic examination, wrist; 2 views
73110 complete, minimum of 3 views

Explanation
A radiologic examination of the wrist is made in either posteroanterior, oblique, or lateral views. Code 73100 reports two views only and code 73110 reports three or more views.

73115

73115 Radiologic examination, wrist, arthrography, radiological supervision and interpretation

Explanation
The wrist is visualized internally through arthrography, the direct injection of air and/or contrast material into the joint for radiological examination. Local anesthesia in injected into the joint followed by the contrast material and/or air. A series of images are taken and interpreted. Fluoroscopic films and guidance for needle localization is included. Arthrography helps diagnose conditions of cartilage abnormalities, arthritis and bursitis, and frozen joint. The hand and wrist is placed in the posteroanterior (PA) position with the hand rotated outward and the x-ray beam aimed vertically at the wrist or with the hand and wrist in PA position with the beam aimed at the wrist from a few degrees below the elbow.

73120-73130

73120 Radiologic examination, hand; 2 views
73130 minimum of 3 views

Explanation
A radiologic exam of the hand is made with films being taken in either the PA (posteroanterior), internal or external oblique, or lateral positions. Code 73120 reports two views only. Code 73130 reports three or more views.

73140
73140 Radiologic examination, finger(s), minimum of 2 views

Explanation
Two or more views of the fingers (second through fifth digits, not thumb) are taken. The x-ray beam is aimed at the proximal interphalangeal joint for all positions, either back to front, external or internal oblique, or lateral views.

73200-73202
73200 Computed tomography, upper extremity; without contrast material
73201 with contrast material(s)
73202 without contrast material, followed by contrast material(s) and further sections

Explanation
Computerized axial tomography directs multiple narrow beams of x-rays around the body structure being studied and uses computer imaging to produce thin cross-sectional views of various layers (or slices) of the body. It is useful for the evaluation of trauma, tumor, and foreign bodies as CT is able to visualize soft tissue as well as bones. Patients are required to remain motionless during the study and sedation may need to be administered as well as a contrast medium for image enhancement. These codes report an exam of the upper extremity. Report 73200 if no contrast is used. Report 73201 if performed with contrast and 73202 if performed first without contrast and then again following the injection of contrast.

73206
73206 Computed tomographic angiography, upper extremity, with contrast material(s), including noncontrast images, if performed, and image postprocessing

Explanation
Computed tomographic angiography (CTA) is a procedure used for the imaging of vessels to detect aneurysms, blood clots, and other vascular irregularities. Contrast medium is rapidly infused intravenously, at intervals, usually with an automatic injector, and the patient is scanned with thin section axial or spiral mode x-ray beams. The images obtained are acquired with narrower collimation and reconstructed at shorter intervals than standard CT images. Three-dimensional images are generated and postprocessing reconstruction is done at a workstation on the scanner. CTA also provides information unavailable with conventional angiography, such as vessel wall thickness (mural thrombus) and the venous anatomy of a target organ and/or associated organs within the scan range. This code reports an exam of the upper extremity with contrast materials and image postprocessing. Noncontrast images, if performed, are also included in this procedure.

73218-73220
73218 Magnetic resonance (eg, proton) imaging, upper extremity, other than joint; without contrast material(s)
73219 with contrast material(s)
73220 without contrast material(s), followed by contrast material(s) and further sequences

Explanation
Magnetic resonance imaging (MRI) is a radiation-free, noninvasive, technique to produce high quality sectional images of the inside of the body in multiple planes. MRI uses the natural magnetic properties of the hydrogen atoms in our bodies that emit radiofrequency signals when exposed to radio waves within a strong electro-magnetic field. These signals are then processed and converted by the computer into high-resolution, three-dimensional, tomographic images. Patients with metallic or electronic implants or foreign bodies cannot be exposed to MRI. The patient must remain still while lying on a motorized table within the large, circular MRI tunnel. A sedative may be administered as well as contrast material for image enhancement. For upper extremity other than joint, report 73218 if no contrast is used; 73219 if performed with contrast; and 73220 if performed first without contrast and then again following the injection of contrast.

73221-73223
73221 Magnetic resonance (eg, proton) imaging, any joint of upper extremity; without contrast material(s)
73222 with contrast material(s)
73223 without contrast material(s), followed by contrast material(s) and further sequences

Explanation
Magnetic resonance imaging (MRI) is a radiation-free, noninvasive, technique to produce high quality sectional images of the inside of the body in multiple planes. MRI uses the natural magnetic properties of the hydrogen atoms in our bodies that emit radiofrequency signals when exposed to radio waves within a strong electro-magnetic field. These signals are then processed and converted by the computer into high-resolution, three-dimensional, tomographic images. Patients with metallic or electronic implants or foreign bodies cannot be exposed to MRI. The patient must remain still while lying on a motorized table within the large, circular MRI tunnel. A sedative may be administered as well as contrast material for image enhancement. For any joint of the upper extremity. Report 73221 if no contrast is used; 73222 if performed with contrast; and 73223 if performed first without contrast and then again following the injection of contrast.

73225
73225 Magnetic resonance angiography, upper extremity, with or without contrast material(s)

Explanation
Magnetic Resonance Angiography (MRA) is a special type of magnetic resonance imaging (MRI) that specifically visualizes blood vessels and blood flow to evaluate vascular disorders within the structure being studied. Unlike CT, it does not rely on the absorption of x-ray energy. Magnetic resonance imaging uses the natural magnetic properties of the hydrogen atoms in our bodies that emit radiofrequency signals when exposed to radio waves within a strong electro-magnetic field. These signals are then processed and converted by the computer into high-resolution, three-dimensional tomographic images. Patients with metallic or electronic implants or foreign bodies cannot be exposed to MRI. The patient must remain still while lying on a motorized table within the large, circular MRI tunnel. A sedative may be administered as well as contrast material for image enhancement. This code reports an exam of the upper extremity.

76000
76000 Fluoroscopy (separate procedure), up to 1 hour physician time, other than 71023 or 71034 (eg, cardiac fluoroscopy)

Explanation
A radiologist provides separate fluoroscopic monitoring of the body for up to one hour for procedures that do not always include fluoroscopy as an integral component of the procedure. This is reported separately to describe the physician work entailed in providing fluoroscopic monitoring. If formal contrast x-ray studies are done and included as a part of the procedure to produce films with written interpretation and report, then fluoroscopy is already included and can not be separately reported.

76001
76001 Fluoroscopy, physician time more than 1 hour, assisting a nonradiologic physician (eg, nephrostolithotomy, ERCP, bronchoscopy, transbronchial biopsy)

Explanation
A radiologist provides fluoroscopic monitoring of the body for more than one hour while assisting a non-radiologic physician (e.g., nephrologist, pulmonologist). This is reported to describe the physician work entailed in providing fluoroscopic during procedures such as nephrostolithotomy and

bronchoscopy. If formal contrast x-ray studies are done and included as a part of the procedure to produce films with written interpretation and report, then fluoroscopy is already included and can not be separately reported.

76380

76380 Computed tomography, limited or localized follow-up study

Explanation

Computerized axial tomography (CT) scanning directs multiple narrow beams of x-rays around the body structure(s) being studied and uses computer imaging to produce thin cross-sectional views of various layers (or slices) of the body. It is able to visualize soft tissue as well as bones. This code reports a limited or a localized follow-up study.

76881-76882

76881 Ultrasound, extremity, nonvascular, real-time with image documentation; complete

76882 limited, anatomic specific

Explanation

Diagnostic ultrasound is an imaging technique bouncing sound waves far above the level of human perception through interior body structures. The sound waves pass through different densities of tissue and reflect back to a receiving unit at varying speeds. The unit converts the waves to electrical pulses that are immediately displayed in picture form on screen. Real time scanning displays structure images and movement with time. These codes include image documentation and report ultrasonography of structures other than veins and arteries of an arm, leg, hand, or foot. Report 76881 for a complete study and 76882 for a limited study that is anatomy specific.

Coding Tips

These codes are new for 2011.

76942

76942 Ultrasonic guidance for needle placement (eg, biopsy, aspiration, injection, localization device), imaging supervision and interpretation

Explanation

Ultrasonic guidance is used for guiding needle placement required for procedures such as breast biopsies, needle aspirations, injections, or placing localizing devices. Ultrasound is the process of bouncing sound waves far above the level of human perception through interior body structures. The sound waves pass through different densities of tissue and reflect back to a receiving unit at varying speeds. The unit then converts the waves to electrical pulses that are immediately displayed in picture form on screen. Once the exact needle entry site is determined along with the depth of the lesion, the optimal route from the skin to the lesion is decided. The needle is inserted and advanced to the lesion under ultrasonic guidance. This code reports the imaging supervision and interpretation only for this procedure.

76977

76977 Ultrasound bone density measurement and interpretation, peripheral site(s), any method

Explanation

Bone mineral density studies are used to evaluate diseases of bone and/or the responses of bone disease to treatment. Densities are measured at the wrist, hip, spine, or calcaneous. The studies assess bone mass or density associated with such diseases as osteoporosis, osteomalacia, and renal osteodystrophy. This code reports using low level ultrasound for measuring bone density instead of ionizing radiation.

76998

76998 Ultrasonic guidance, intraoperative

Explanation

Ultrasonography is used during a procedure to guide the physician in successfully accomplishing the surgery. Ultrasonic guidance may be used by the physician intraoperatively during many different types of operations on various areas of the body. Examples of intraoperative ultrasonic guidance include evaluating tissue removal in anatomical structures such as the breast, brain, abdominal organs, etc. This procedure may also be used to determine the location and depth of incisions to be made. This code is not to be used for ultrasound guidance for open or laparoscopic radiofrequency tissue ablation.

77002

77002 Fluoroscopic guidance for needle placement (eg, biopsy, aspiration, injection, localization device)

Explanation

Needle biopsy or fine needle aspiration is guided by fluoroscopic visualization. A cutting biopsy or fine needle is inserted into the target area and the position reaffirmed by fluoroscopy. This is done for an internal mass or lesion that has been positively identified by other diagnostic imaging performed earlier.

77003

77003 Fluoroscopic guidance and localization of needle or catheter tip for spine or paraspinous diagnostic or therapeutic injection procedures (epidural, subarachnoid, or sacroiliac joint), including neurolytic agent destruction

Explanation

Spinal and certain paraspinal diagnostic or therapeutic nerve injection procedures (e.g., epidural, subarachnoid, or sacroiliac joint injections) are guided by fluoroscopy before and during catheter or needle insertion. The target structure is localized, the needle is placed and advanced, and the contrast injection is visualized under fluoroscopic monitoring.

Coding Tips

This code has been revised for 2011 in the official CPT description.

77011

77011 Computed tomography guidance for stereotactic localization

Explanation

For stereotactic localization, a movable arm holding a needle is guided by computerized tomography (CT) to locate the lesion from different angles at different fixed points. The CT images tell the computer where the coordinates are to correctly align the needle.

77012

77012 Computed tomography guidance for needle placement (eg, biopsy, aspiration, injection, localization device), radiological supervision and interpretation

Explanation

Computed tomography (CT) is used for guiding needle biopsies. CT scanning directs multiple narrow beams of x-rays around the body structure being studied and uses computer imaging to produce thin cross-sectional views of various layers (or slices) of the body. It is able to visualize soft tissue, as well as bones. Patients are required to remain motionless during the study. Once the exact needle entry site is determined, along with the depth of the lesion, the optimal route from the skin to the lesion is decided. The needle is inserted and advanced to the lesion and another CT scan image is done to confirm placement for the biopsy. This code reports the radiological supervision and interpretation only for this procedure.

77013

77013 Computed tomography guidance for, and monitoring of, parenchymal tissue ablation

Explanation

Computed tomographic guidance is used for the ablation of parenchymal (vital organ) tissue. The patient receives intravenous pain medication and sedation. Grounding pads are placed on the patient's thigh. A needle-electrode with an insulated shaft and a noninsulated distal tip is inserted through the skin and directly into the tissue to be ablated. Computed tomography (CT) is used to guide the needle to the correct spot and to monitor treatment. Each treatment session has about 10 to 15 minutes of active ablation. The energy at the needle tip causes ionic agitation and frictional heat in the surrounding tissue, which leads to cell death and coagulative necrosis. This results in a 3 to 5 cm sphere of dead tissue per treatment session. In large tumors, the physician may create more than one sphere next to each other to try to turn the tumor edges in three dimensions. A small margin of normal tissue next to tumors is also burned. The dead tumor cells are not removed, but are gradually replaced by fibrosis and scar tissue. This code reports the CT guidance and monitoring of the ablation procedure.

77021

77021 Magnetic resonance guidance for needle placement (eg, for biopsy, needle aspiration, injection, or placement of localization device) radiological supervision and interpretation

Explanation
Magnetic resonance is used for guiding needle placement required for procedures such as breast biopsies, needle aspirations, injections, or placing localizing devices. Magnetic resonance imaging (MRI) is a radiation-free, noninvasive technique that produces high-quality images. MRI uses the natural magnetic properties of the hydrogen atoms in our bodies that emit radiofrequency signals when exposed to radio waves within a strong electromagnetic field. These signals are processed and converted by the computer into high-resolution, three-dimensional, tomographic images. Some methods for magnetic resonance needle placement include coating the needle with contrast material, placing metallic ringlets along the needle, or using a receiving coil in the tip of the needle. This code reports the radiological supervision and interpretation only for this procedure.

77071

77071 Manual application of stress performed by physician for joint radiography, including contralateral joint if indicated

Explanation
Joint radiography is done under manual stress application conditions performed by the physician to visualize characteristics of the joint that would not normally be seen on films taken in routine positioning. The physician puts on lead-lined gloves and forcibly holds the body part in the desired position to maintain stress on the joint while x-rays are taken. This code includes radiography of the contralateral joint, if indicated.

77075

77075 Radiologic examination, osseous survey; complete (axial and appendicular skeleton)

Explanation
A radiologic exam is performed in which the axial (head and trunk) and appendicular (extremities) skeleton is surveyed for evidence of metastatic disease. It may also be performed on children to identify current and/or old healed fractures in the case of suspected child abuse. This procedure is rarely performed for metastatic disease, having been replaced by nuclear bone scanning, a more precise study for diagnosing metastases.

77076

77076 Radiologic examination, osseous survey, infant

Explanation
A radiologic exam is performed in which an infant's axial (head and trunk) and appendicular (extremities) skeleton is surveyed for evidence of current and/or old healed fractures in the case of suspected child abuse or to identify signs of lesions due to leukemic infiltrates.

77077

77077 Joint survey, single view, 2 or more joints (specify)

Explanation
A radiologic exam is done in which two or more joints are surveyed. A single view only is taken of the joints being examined. The joints surveyed require specification and are not delineated in the code.

77078-77079

77078 Computed tomography, bone mineral density study, 1 or more sites; axial skeleton (eg, hips, pelvis, spine)
77079 appendicular skeleton (peripheral) (eg, radius, wrist, heel)

Explanation
A CT density study is performed to measure the patient's bone mass. Bone mineral density is evaluated as a screening test for osteoporosis, to evaluate diseases of bone, and to review the responses of bone disease to treatment. Densities can be measured at the wrist, hip, spine, or calcaneus. The studies assess bone mass or density associated with such diseases as osteoporosis, osteomalacia, and renal osteodystrophy. This particular bone density study uses computerized tomography (CT) for the imaging modality. CT directs multiple, narrow beams of x-rays around the body structure being studied and uses computer imaging to produce thin cross-sectional views of various layers (or slices) of the body. Report 77078 for a bone density study by CT of the hips, pelvis, or spine (axial skeleton) and 77079 for a bone density study by CT of peripheral bones, such as the wrist or heel bone (appendicular skeleton).

77080-77082

77080 Dual-energy X-ray absorptiometry (DXA), bone density study, 1 or more sites; axial skeleton (eg, hips, pelvis, spine)
77081 appendicular skeleton (peripheral) (eg, radius, wrist, heel)
77082 vertebral fracture assessment

Explanation
An x-ray density study is performed to measure the patient's bone mass. Bone mineral density is evaluated as a screening test for osteoporosis, to evaluate diseases of bone, and to review the responses of bone disease to treatment. Densities can be measured at the wrist, radius, hip, pelvis, spine, or heel. Dual energy x-ray absorptiometry (DEXA) is a two-dimensional projection system that involves two x-ray beams with different levels of energy being pulsed alternately. The results are given in two scores reported as standard deviations from bone density of a person 30 years of age, which is the age of peak bone mass. Report 77080 for DEXA of the hips, pelvis, or spine (axial skeleton); 77081 for DEXA of peripheral bones, such as the wrist or heel bone (appendicular skeleton); and 77082 for one or more vertebral sites to assess a fracture.

77083

77083 Radiographic absorptiometry (eg, photodensitometry, radiogrammetry), 1 or more sites

Explanation
Bone mineral density studies are used to evaluate diseases of bone and/or the responses of bone disease to treatment. Densities are measured at the wrist, hip, spine, or calcaneus. The studies assess bone mass or density associated with such diseases as osteoporosis, osteomalacia, and renal osteodystrophy. Photodensitometry, or radiographic absorptiometry, provides a quantitative measurement of the bone mineral density of the cortical bone (outer layer) by taking two radiographs with direct exposure film at different settings. This procedure is done to monitor for gross bone changes as occurs with osteoporosis.

78300-78315

78300 Bone and/or joint imaging; limited area
78305 multiple areas
78306 whole body
78315 3 phase study

Explanation
Various radiopharmaceutical agents are used for diagnostic nuclear imaging of bones and/or joints. Gallium, a calcium analogue, is the radiopharmaceutical of choice when scanning for an inflammatory process because it accumulates in areas of bone mineral turnover, such as fractures, and localizes to infected or inflamed areas like

inflammatory arthritis. Combining gallium with radiolabeled white blood cells, which also localize at infection sites, adds more diagnostic specificity when searching for acute osteomyelitis or osteoarthropathy. Radioactive diphosphonates are used for bony metastatic disease screening. A special camera scans the area of study and detects the gamma radiation from the radiotracer introduced into the patient to detect and localize the disease process. Report 78300 for bone and/or joint imaging of a limited area; 78305 for multiple areas; 78306 for a whole body scan; and 78315 for a three-phase scan.

78320

78320 Bone and/or joint imaging; tomographic (SPECT)

Explanation

Tomographic SPECT (single photon emission computed tomography) imaging permits an in-depth evaluation of complex anatomy within body structures such as the bones and joints by introducing a special radionuclide and then detecting the distribution of gamma radiation emitted from the radiotracer with a single or multiple-head camera mounted on a gantry to rotate around the patient. SPECT images give three-dimensional computer reconstructed views of cross-sectional slices of the body. Gallium, a calcium analogue, is the radiopharmaceutical of choice when scanning for an inflammatory process in the bones or joints because it accumulates in areas of bone mineral turnover, such as fractures, and localizes to infected or inflamed areas like inflammatory arthritis. Combining gallium with radiolabeled white blood cells, which also localize at infection sites, adds more diagnostic specificity when searching for acute osteomyelitis or osteoarthropathy. Radioactive diphosphonates are used for bony metastatic disease screening.

78350-78351

78350 Bone density (bone mineral content) study, 1 or more sites; single photon absorptiometry

78351 dual photon absorptiometry, 1 or more sites

Explanation

Single and dual photon absorptiometry are both noninvasive techniques to measure the absorption of the mono or dichromatic photon beam by bone material. The painless study device is placed directly on the patient and uses a small amount of radionuclide to measure the bone mass absorption efficiency of the energy used. This provides a quantitative measurement of the bone mineral density of cortical bone in diseases like osteoporosis and can be used to assess an individual's response to treatment at different intervals. Report 78350 for single photon energy and 78351 for dual photon energy.

80047

80047 Basic metabolic panel (Calcium, ionized)

Explanation

A basic metabolic panel with ionized calcium includes the following tests: calcium (ionized) (82330), carbon dioxide (82374), chloride (82435), creatinine (82565), glucose (82947), potassium (84132), sodium (84295), and urea nitrogen (BUN) (84520). Blood specimen is obtained by venipuncture. See the specific codes for additional information about the listed tests.

80048

80048 Basic metabolic panel (Calcium, total)

Explanation

A basic metabolic panel with total calcium includes the following tests: calcium (82310), carbon dioxide (82374), chloride (82435), creatinine (82565), glucose (82947), potassium (84132), sodium (84295), and urea nitrogen (BUN) (84520). Blood specimen is obtained by venipuncture. See the specific codes for additional information about the listed tests.

80050

80050 General health panel

Explanation

A general health panel includes the following tests: albumin (82040), total bilirubin (82247), calcium (82310), carbon dioxide (bicarbonate) (82374), chloride (82435), creatinine (82565), glucose (82947), alkaline phosphatase (84075), potassium (84132), total protein (84155), sodium (84295), aspartate amino transferase (AST) (SGOT) (84450), urea nitrogen (BUN) (84520), and thyroid stimulating hormone (84443). In addition, this panel includes a hemogram as described by either 85022 or 85025. Blood specimen is obtained by venipuncture. See specific codes for additional information about the listed tests.

80051

80051 Electrolyte panel

Explanation

An electrolyte panel includes the following tests: carbon dioxide (82374), chloride (82435), potassium (84132), and sodium (84295). Blood specimen is obtained by venipuncture. See specific codes for additional information about the listed tests.

80053

80053 Comprehensive metabolic panel

Explanation

A comprehensive metabolic panel includes the following tests: albumin (82040), total bilirubin (82247), total calcium (82310), carbon dioxide (bicarbonate) (82374), chloride (82435), creatinine (82565), glucose (82947), alkaline phosphatase (84075), potassium (84132), total protein (84155), sodium (84295), alanine amino transferase (ALT) (SGPT) (84460), aspartate amino transferase (AST) (SGOT) (84450), and urea nitrogen (BUN) (84520). Blood specimen is obtained by venipuncture. See the specific codes for additional information about the listed tests.

80061

80061 Lipid panel

Explanation

A lipid panel includes the following tests: total serum cholesterol (82465), high-density cholesterol (HDL cholesterol) by direct measurement (83718), and triglycerides (84478). Blood specimen is obtained by venipuncture. See specific codes for additional information about the listed tests.

80076

80076 Hepatic function panel

Explanation

A hepatic function panel includes the following tests: albumin (82040), total bilirubin (82247), direct bilirubin (82248), alkaline phosphatase (84075), protein, total (84155), alanine amino transferase (ALT) (SGPT) (84460), and aspartate amino transferase (AST) (SGOT) (84450). Blood specimen is obtained by venipuncture. See the specific codes for additional information about the listed tests.

80150

80150 Amikacin

Explanation

Amikacin is a type of antibiotic. Test specimens are frequently collected at peak and trough periods, which is shortly after administration of amikacin and again just before the next administration when serum concentration is at its lowest. This is an effective approach to determine a therapeutic level of drug. Method is radioimmunoassay (RIA) or high performance liquid chromatography (HPLC).

80170

80170 Gentamicin

Explanation

This drug is classified as an aminoglycoside, an antibiotic. In its injectable form, the drug may be prescribed for gram-negative infections, septicemia, and other serious infections, as well as unknown causative organisms. Common trade names include Garamycin and Gentacidin. A typical course will run seven to 10 days. Monitoring may be initiated to measure drug clearance via the kidneys. Patients with impaired renal function may accumulate the drug. Peak serum concentrations can be expected about 30 to 60 minutes following an intramuscular injection. Trough concentrations occur just before the next dose. Dosage is highly dependent on the severity of infection. Methodology may include radioimmunoassay (RIA) and microbiological assay.

80172

80172 Gold

Explanation
This test may include the abbreviation for gold, Au, or the name Myochrysine. Gold salts are sometimes used in the treatment of rheumatoid arthritis. Therapeutic levels may be difficult to determine. Method is atomic absorption spectrophotometry (AAS).

80196

80196 Salicylate

Explanation
This drug is known universally as aspirin and may also be referred to as a nonsteroidal antiinflammatory drug (NSAID). Specimen collection is at trough, which is the time just before the next dose of the drug when blood concentration is at its lowest. Overdose may also prompt this test. Methodology may include high performance liquid chromatography (HPLC) or gas liquid chromatography (GLC). Colorimetry and fluorometry may also be used.

80200

80200 Tobramycin

Explanation
This drug is also known as Nebcin. This drug has bactericidal properties and is usually injected. Specimen collection is at peak and trough. Peak will occur about one hour after an intramuscular injection and trough will occur about 12 hours after that. Method will often be by radioimmunoassay (RIA), microbiological assay, or high performance liquid chromatography (HPLC).

80202

80202 Vancomycin

Explanation
This drug may also be known as Vancocin. Specimen collection may be drawn during the trough period. This occurs around 30 minutes prior to the next dose. It is sometimes also drawn at peak. Toxic and therapeutic dosages for vancomycin can be difficult to determine due to the way the drug is metabolized. Methods include radioimmunoassay (RIA), high performance liquid chromatography (HPLC), and microbiological assay.

80428

80428 Growth hormone stimulation panel (eg, arginine infusion, l-dopa administration)

Explanation
This panel may be ordered as a GH provocation test, insulin tolerance test (ITT), and as the Arginine test. Baseline blood work is typically drawn. Stimulation of growth hormone is often achieved through an intravenous infusion of arginine hydrochloride, L-dopa, or clonidine. This may be administered over about 30 minutes. Blood specimens are then collected at 15 minutes, 30 minutes, and 45 minutes. These samples will be tested for HCG as specified in 83003.

80430

80430 Growth hormone suppression panel (glucose administration)

Explanation
This panel may be ordered as a GH suppression test. Blood work is typically drawn before the test as a baseline. Glucose is the suppression agent for GH and administration may be orally. Blood is again drawn, often at 60 and 120 minutes for glucose, with one more specimen drawn for HCG.

80435

80435 Insulin tolerance panel; for growth hormone deficiency This panel must include the following: Glucose (82947 x 5) Human growth hormone (HGH) (83003 x 5)

Explanation
The insulin tolerance panel for growth hormone insufficiency typically involves baseline blood work before testing. The insulin is administered following a fasting period, typically orally. The panel is specifically for growth hormone or human growth hormone (GH or HGH). Glucose is administered, typically by IV bolus, and specimens are drawn at regular intervals following dosage. Note the number of times each component is drawn.

80500-80502

80500 Clinical pathology consultation; limited, without review of patient's history and medical records
80502 comprehensive, for a complex diagnostic problem, with review of patient's history and medical records

Explanation
A clinical pathology consultation is a service performed by a physician (pathologist) in response to a request from the attending physician regarding test results requiring additional medical interpretive judgment. Pharmacokinetic consultations regarding therapeutic drug levels may be reported with this code. Code 80500 reports a limited consultation not requiring review of the patient's history and medical records. Code 80502 reports a comprehensive consultation related to more complex diagnostic problems and requires review of the patient's history and medical records.

81000

81000 Urinalysis, by dip stick or tablet reagent for bilirubin, glucose, hemoglobin, ketones, leukocytes, nitrite, pH, protein, specific gravity, urobilinogen, any number of these constituents; non-automated, with microscopy

Explanation
This type of test may be ordered by the brand name product and the analytes tested. Although screens are considered to show the presence of an analyte (qualitative), some newer products are semi-quantitative. Many are plastic strips that contain sites impregnated with chemicals that react with urine when the strip is dipped into a specimen. The result is a color change that is compared against a standardized chart. Most strips will test for numerous analytes, as well as for pH and specific gravity. Tablets work in a similar fashion. A drop of urine is placed on the tablet and a chemical reaction causes a color change that is compared to a standard chart. Usually only a single analyte is under consideration, per tablet. Code 81000 involves a manual (nonautomated) test and includes a microscopic examination. Microscopy involves examination of the urine sediments or solids. The urine is first centrifuged in a graduated tube to concentrate the sediments. Samples (either wet or dry) are examined, usually under both high and low power, and abnormal constituents are noted. These may include a wide range of biological abnormalities, such as blood cells, casts, and bacteria, as well as chemical anomalies, such as crystals.

81001

81001 Urinalysis, by dip stick or tablet reagent for bilirubin, glucose, hemoglobin, ketones, leukocytes, nitrite, pH, protein, specific gravity, urobilinogen, any number of these constituents; automated, with microscopy

Explanation
This type of test may be ordered by the type of processor used and the analytes tested. The testing methodology is similar to the manual strips, except that the color change caused by the chemical reaction with urine is processed and read mechanically. The strip is exposed to the urine sample and is mechanically fed through a processor that reads the colors emitted by the reaction. The unit will be calibrated according to international standards and readings have a high degree of accuracy. The result may be displayed on a monitor, but is always printed or recorded in some form. Code 81001 also includes a microscopy. Microscopy involves examination of the urine sediments or solids. The urine is first centrifuged in a graduated tube to concentrate the sediments. Samples (either wet or dry) are examined, usually under both high and low power, and abnormal constituents are noted. These may include a wide range of biological

abnormalities, such as blood cells, casts, and bacteria, as well as chemical anomalies, such as crystals.

81002

81002 Urinalysis, by dip stick or tablet reagent for bilirubin, glucose, hemoglobin, ketones, leukocytes, nitrite, pH, protein, specific gravity, urobilinogen, any number of these constituents; non-automated, without microscopy

Explanation
This type of test may be ordered by the brand name product and the analytes tested. Although usually considered screens to show the presence of an analyte (qualitative), some newer products are semi-quantitative. Many are plastic strips that contain sites impregnated with chemicals that react with urine when the strip is dipped into a specimen. The result is a color change that is compared against a standardized chart. Most strips will test for numerous analytes, as well as for pH and specific gravity. Tablets work in a similar fashion. A drop of urine is placed on the tablet and a chemical reaction causes a color change that is compared to a standard chart. Usually only a single analyte is under consideration per tablet, however. Code 81002 does not include a microscopic examination of the urine sample or its components.

81003

81003 Urinalysis, by dip stick or tablet reagent for bilirubin, glucose, hemoglobin, ketones, leukocytes, nitrite, pH, protein, specific gravity, urobilinogen, any number of these constituents; automated, without microscopy

Explanation
This type of test may be ordered by the type of processor used and the analytes tested. The testing methodology is similar to the manual strips, except that the color change caused by the chemical reaction with urine is processed and read mechanically. The strip is exposed to the urine sample and is mechanically fed through a processor that reads the colors emitted by the reaction. The unit will be calibrated according to international standards and readings have a high degree of accuracy. The result may be displayed on a monitor, but is always printed or recorded in some form. Code 81003 does not include a microscopic examination of the urine sample or its components.

81005

81005 Urinalysis; qualitative or semiquantitative, except immunoassays

Explanation
This test may be ordered by the type of processor used and the analytes under examination. The method will be any type of automated analyzer, usually colorimetry. The results of a semi-quantitative test indicate the presence or absence of an analyte and may be expressed as simply positive or negative. A qualitative result may be indicated as trace, 1+, 2+, etc.

81007

81007 Urinalysis; bacteriuria screen, except by culture or dipstick

Explanation
This type of test may be ordered by the brand name of the commercial kit used and the bacteria that the kit screens for. Human urine is normally almost entirely free of bacteria. However, bacteria can easily be introduced upon voiding. In addition, specimens containing any amount of pathological bacteria can have the organisms rapidly multiply after collection. For this reason, specimens are often examined shortly after collection. Method includes any method except culture or dipstick. The test is often performed by commercial kit. The type of kit used should be specified in the report.

81015

81015 Urinalysis; microscopic only

Explanation
This test may be ordered as a microscopic analysis. Human urine is normally almost entirely free of bacteria. However, bacteria can easily be introduced upon voiding. In addition, specimens containing any amount of pathological bacteria can have the organisms rapidly multiply after collection. For this reason, specimens are often examined shortly after collection. The sample may first be centrifuged into a graduated tube to concentrate the sediments, or solid matter, held in suspension. Bacteria cells are comparatively small and a combination of stains and high power microscopy is usually employed. The concentration of bacteria will be noted.

81020

81020 Urinalysis; 2 or 3 glass test

Explanation
This test may be ordered as a two-glass or three-glass test, a MacConkey-blood agar test, an MC-blood agar test, or any of the previous with a gram-positive plate. This is a culture for bacteria and will typically involve a culture plate of 5 percent sheep's blood agar and a MacConkey plate (a medium containing differentiate for lactose and nonlactose fermenters). A third plate of gram-positive media may offer further discrimination of bacteria cultured. The test is useful in determining the types and prevalence of bacteria in the urine.

81025

81025 Urine pregnancy test, by visual color comparison methods

Explanation
This test may be ordered by any of the brand name kits available. The tests typically involve a dipstick impregnated with reagents that chemically react upon contact with urine. A change in color indicates positive or negative for the presence of hormones found in the urine of women in early pregnancy.

82040

82040 Albumin; serum, plasma or whole blood

Explanation
This test measures the concentration of albumin in serum, plasma, or whole blood. It is often used to determine nutritional status, renal disease, and other chronic diseases, particularly those involving the kidneys or liver. A blood sample is typically drawn from a vein in the hand or forearm. The skin over the vein is cleaned with an antiseptic, and a tourniquet is wrapped around the upper arm to enlarge the lower arm veins by restricting the blood flow. A thin needle is inserted into the vein, the tourniquet is removed, and blood flows from the vein through the needle and is collected into a vial or syringe. The needle is withdrawn and the puncture site covered to prevent bleeding. The blood sample is sent to the laboratory for testing.

82042

82042 Albumin; urine or other source, quantitative, each specimen

Explanation
This code reports quantitative analysis for albumin on urine, CSF, or amniotic fluid. Urine tests are usually performed on a 24-hour urine specimen to measure protein loss of patients with hypoalbuminemia. Patients typically perform specimen collection over a 24-hour period. Method is colorimetry. CSF analysis requires separately reportable spinal puncture and the test is performed using nephelometry. Amniotic fluid analysis requires separately reportable ultrasound guidance and amniocentesis and test is usually performed by autoanalyzer.

82085

82085 Aldolase

Explanation
This test may also be requested as aldolase (ALD) or fructose biphosphate aldolase. Specimen collection is by venipuncture. Methods may include ultraviolet, kinetic, coupled enzymatic and colorimetric. This test can be useful in the identification of a variety of degenerative diseases, myopathies, and inflammations.

82127-82128

82127 Amino acids; single, qualitative, each specimen
82128   multiple, qualitative, each specimen

Explanation
These tests may also be referred to as a metabolic screen for amino acids. Blood specimen is obtained by venipuncture. A random urine sample is obtained. Several methods may be used including thin layer chromatography (TLC), gas chromatography (GC), and ion-exchange chromatography. These tests determine whether an amino acid is or is not present (qualitative analysis). Code 82127 tests for the presence of single amino acids, while 82128 tests for the presence of multiple amino acids.

82131
82131 Amino acids; single, quantitative, each specimen

Explanation
This test may be requested as specific amino acid (e.g., cystine, tyrosine, methionine, propionic acid). Blood specimen is obtained by venipuncture. A 24-hour urine specimen is used. The patient flushes the first urine of the day and discards it. All voided urine for the next 24 hours is collected and refrigerated. Method is ion-exchange chromatography. This test measures (quantifies) amounts of single specified amino acids.

82136-82139
82136 Amino acids, 2 to 5 amino acids, quantitative, each specimen
82139 Amino acids, 6 or more amino acids, quantitative, each specimen

Explanation
These tests may be requested as specific amino acids (e.g., cystine, tyrosine, methionine, propionic acid). Blood specimen is obtained by venipuncture. A 24-hour urine specimen is required. The patient flushes the first urine of the day and discards it. All voided urine for the next 24 hours is collected and refrigerated. Method is ion-exchange chromatography. This test measures (quantifies) amounts of multiple specified amino acids. Report 82136 for two to five amino acids. Report 82139 for six or more.

82140
82140 Ammonia

Explanation
This test may be requested as NH3. Elevated levels may indicate that the liver is not able to detoxify ammonia from the blood due to severe liver disease. Blood is obtained by venipuncture or arterial puncture. A 24-hour urine specimen is required. The patient flushes the first urine of the day and discards it. All voided urine for the next 24 hours is collected and refrigerated. A number of methods are used including enzymatic, resin enzymatic, and ion-selective electrode (ISE).

82190
82190 Atomic absorption spectroscopy, each analyte

Explanation
AAS is a method for detecting the absorption of specific wavelengths of light by analyte that have been vaporized in a flame. The analysis is performed using a specialized instrument known as an atomic absorption spectrometer. Analytes are typically pure elements, since each element has a specific absorption spectrum.

82286
82286 Bradykinin

Explanation
Bradykinin is a biologically active peptide, found in plasma and many other tissues and fluids, important in the inflammatory response. A pathogenic role for Bradykinin has been suggested in diseases ranging from asthma to hereditary angioedema, as well as other kinds of swelling disorders and allergic-type diseases. It is measured in body fluids by techniques including immunoassay, capillary electrophoresis, chromatography and mass-spectrometry.

82306 (82652)
82306 Vitamin D; 25 hydroxy, includes fraction(s), if performed
82652 1, 25 dihydroxy, includes fraction(s), if performed

Explanation
Code 82306 may be requested as 25-OHD3, 25(OH) Calciferol, Vitamin D 25-Hydroxy, Vitamin D3 25-OH, or Calciferol 25-Hydroxy. Methodology is high performance liquid chromatography (HPLC), competitive protein binding (CPB), or radioimmunoassay (RIA). Code 82652 may be requested as 1,25 (OH) Vitamin D, 1,25-Dihydroxy Vitamin D, 1,25-Dihydroxycholecalciferal, and Vitamin D, 1,25-Dihydroxy. This is the most active form of Vitamin D. It is formed by the renal cells and is essential for calcium absorption. Methodology is radioimmunoassay (RIA) or column chromatography. These codes are for serum or plasma specimens and include fractions, if performed.

82308
82308 Calcitonin

Explanation
This test may be requested as thyrocalcitonin. This test may be used to screen for specific malignant neoplasms. Blood specimen is obtained by venipuncture. A fasting specimen should be taken. The specimen is collected in a chilled tube and the test performed within 10 minutes of collection. Serum (plasma) is separated in a refrigerated centrifuge and frozen. The test is performed by assay or radioimmunoassay (RIA).

82310
82310 Calcium; total

Explanation
May be abbreviated Ca. Blood is obtained by venipuncture or heel stick. Specimen is obtained in the morning and a fasting sample is preferable. Postural changes and venous stasis may provide misleading results. Accurate diagnosis may require obtaining additional specimens on subsequent days. Method is spectrophotometry or atomic absorption spectroscopy (AAS). The test may be used to assess thyroid and parathyroid function.

82330
82330 Calcium; ionized

Explanation
This test may also be referred to as free calcium. It may be abbreviated Ca++ or Ca+2. Ionized or free calcium refers to calcium that is not bound to proteins in the blood. It is the metabolically active portion of the calcium in the blood. Blood is obtained by venipuncture and collected anaerobically. Method is by ion-selective electrode (ISE). The test may be used to assess thyroid and parathyroid function.

82331
82331 Calcium; after calcium infusion test

Explanation
The calcium infusion test is a provocative test for evaluation of medullary thyroid carcinoma (MTC). Calcitonin levels are measured following an IV infusion of calcium solution, and sometimes calcium levels are also measured to evaluate calcium incorporation or monitor hypercalcemia.

82340
82340 Calcium; urine quantitative, timed specimen

Explanation
This test may be abbreviated Ca++ or Ca+2. A 24-hour urine specimen is required. The patient flushes the first urine of the day and discards it. All voided urine for the next 24 hours is collected and refrigerated. Method is spectrophotometry or atomic absorption spectrometry (AAS).

82374
82374 Carbon dioxide (bicarbonate)

Explanation
This test may be requested as HCO3 or bicarbonate. Bicarbonate (carbon dioxide) is an indicator of electrolyte and acid-base status (alkalosis, acidosis). It is elevated in metabolic alkalosis, compensated

respiratory acidosis, and hypokalemia. It is decreased in metabolic acidosis, compensated respiratory alkalosis, and in diabetic ketoacidosis. Blood specimen is normally obtained by arterial puncture, but venipuncture may also be used. Bicarbonate is usually calculated using the Henderson-Hasselbalch equation (HCO3 = Total CO2-H2CO3). However, it can also be determined by titration.

82397
82397 Chemiluminescent assay

Explanation
Chemiluminescent assay refers to a detection method, whereby a chemiluminogenic substrate is converted to a chemiluminescent (light emitting) product.

82415
82415 Chloramphenicol

Explanation
This test may be requested as a chloramphenicol, Chloromycetin, or Mychel-S level. Chloramphenicol is a broad spectrum antibiotic. This test is used to monitor therapeutic and toxic levels. Blood specimen is obtained by venipuncture. Several methods may be used, including high performance liquid chromatography (HPLC), gas-liquid chromatography (GLC), microbiological assay (MB), colorimetry, or enzymatic immunoassay (EIA).

82435
82435 Chloride; blood

Explanation
This test may be requested as Cl, blood. Chloride is a salt of hydrochloric acid and is important in maintaining electrolyte balance. Blood specimen is obtained by venipuncture. Methods include colorimetry, coulometry, and ion-selective electrode (ISE).

82436
82436 Chloride; urine

Explanation
This test may be requested as Cl, urine. Chloride is a salt of hydrochloric acid, the most common being sodium chloride (table salt). It is important in maintaining proper electrolyte balance. A 24-hour urine test is preferred, but shorter timed collections and random specimens may also be used. If a timed specimen is used, the patient flushes the first urine of the day and discards it. All voided urine for the next 24 hours (or shorter time increment) is collected and refrigerated. Methods include colorimetry, coulometry, and ion-selective electrode (ISE).

82441
82441 Chlorinated hydrocarbons, screen

Explanation
Chlorinated hydrocarbons are contained in solvents and are absorbed cutaneously and by inhalation. While they vary in toxicity, all are CNS depressants and can cause liver and kidney damage with prolonged exposure. This test is used to screen for toxic levels. Levels of one or more of the following substances are screened: carbon tetrachloride, chloroform, dichloromethane, trichloroethylene, and tetrachloroethylene. Testing methods include gas chromatography flame ionization detection (GC-FID) and gas chromatography electron capture detector (GC-ECD). Colorimetry measurement of metabolites may also be used but is nonspecific.

82465
82465 Cholesterol, serum or whole blood, total

Explanation
Cholesterol level is a risk indicator for atherosclerosis and myocardial infarction. Blood specimen is obtained by venipuncture. Method is enzymatic. This test reports total cholesterol in serum or whole blood.

82495
82495 Chromium

Explanation
Blood specimen is obtained by venipuncture. A 24-hour urine specimen is required. The patient flushes the first urine of the day and discards it. All voided urine for the next 24 hours is collected and refrigerated. Hair samples must be cut close to the scalp. Methods used include atomic absorption spectrometry (AAS) and neutron activation analysis (NAA).

82523
82523 Collagen cross links, any method

Explanation
This test may be ordered as collagen crosslink N-telopeptide or pyridinium collagen crosslinks. Pyridinium includes pyrinoline and deoxypyridinoline. Collagen cross-links are markers for bone resorption and are useful in evaluating and managing osteoporosis. A timed urine specimen is required. When testing for N-telopeptide, a two-hour specimen is usually obtained. Pyridinium, including pyrinoline and deoxypyridinoline, requires a 24-hour specimen. When a timed specimen is used, the patient flushes the first urine of the day and discards it. All voided urine for the next 24 hours (or shorter time increment) is collected and refrigerated. Method is enzyme-linked immunosorbent assay (ELISA) for N-telopeptide and high performance liquid chromatography (HPLC) for pyridinium.

82528
82528 Corticosterone

Explanation
This test may be requested as Compound B. Corticosterone is a natural corticosteroid, similar to cortisol except that it does not possess anti-inflammatory qualities. Blood specimen is obtained by venipuncture. Method is radioimmunoassay.

82530
82530 Cortisol; free

Explanation
Cortisol is a naturally occurring glucocorticoid responsible for metabolism of glucose, protein, and fats and is important in immune system function. Urinary free cortisol is used in initial screening for Cushing's syndrome. A 24-hour urine specimen is required. The patient flushes the first urine of the day and discards it. All voided urine for the next 24 hours is collected and refrigerated. Amniotic fluid levels of free cortisol are useful in evaluating fetal lung maturation. To obtain an amniotic fluid specimen, an ultrasound is performed to determine the exact location of the fetus. Methods include high performance liquid chromatography (HPLC) for urine and radioimmunoassay (RIA) for amniotic fluid. This test measures free (unbound) cortisol only.

82533
82533 Cortisol; total

Explanation
Cortisol is a naturally occurring glucocorticoid responsible for metabolism of glucose, protein, and fats and is important in immune system function. Blood specimen is obtained by venipuncture. To obtain an amniotic fluid specimen, an ultrasound is performed to determine the exact location of the fetus. The fluid is sent to the lab for analysis. Method is radioimmunoassay (RIA), competitive protein binding (CPB), or fluorescent assay. This test measures total cortisol (both free and bound).

82540
82540 Creatine

Explanation
Creatine is measured in urine or serum to evaluate certain conditions involving increased muscle tissue breakdown. It has been measured in erythrocytes as an indicator of erythrocyte survival time in the evaluation of hemolytic disorders. Blood specimen is obtained by venipuncture. It can be measured by colorimetric or enzymatic/spectrophotometric methods.

82585
82585 Cryofibrinogen

Explanation
Fibrinogen with an abnormal physical property causing it to precipitate in the cold (4? C) and

dissolve again when warmed to 37? C is known as cryofibrinogen. This test is performed to evaluate cold intolerance. Blood specimen is obtained by venipuncture in a prewarmed tube and must be kept warmed. Method is cold precipitation.

82595

82595 Cryoglobulin, qualitative or semi-quantitative (eg, cryocrit)

Explanation
Cryoglobulin is a serum globulin with an abnormal physical property causing it to precipitate at cold temperatures (4 degrees C) and dissolve again when warmed to 37 degrees C. It is indicative of lymphoproliferative disorders, collagen vascular disease, and a variety of infections and other diseases. Blood specimen is obtained by venipuncture in a prewarmed tube and must be kept warmed. Method is cold precipitation.

82615

82615 Cystine and homocystine, urine, qualitative

Explanation
Cystine and homocystine are amino acids indicative of disease when found in the urine. A 24-hour urine specimen is preferred but random urine may also be used. If a timed urine specimen is requested, the patient flushes the first urine of the day and discards it. All voided urine for the next 24 hours is collected and refrigerated. Method is ion exchange chromatography or spectrophotometry.

82657-82658

82657 Enzyme activity in blood cells, cultured cells, or tissue, not elsewhere specified; nonradioactive substrate, each specimen
82658 radioactive substrate, each specimen

Explanation
These codes report enzyme assays using a variety of different methods, some established and some relatively new. Code 82657 reports enzyme assay with nonradioactive substrate (substance upon which an enzyme acts), while 82658 reports enzyme assay with radioactive substrate.

82800

82800 Gases, blood, pH only

Explanation
This test may be requested as blood pH. Blood pH is tested to identify acidemia or alkalemia. Arterial puncture is preferred, but venipuncture may also be performed. Method is glass pH electrode or potentiometry.

82803-82805

82803 Gases, blood, any combination of pH, pCO2, pO2, CO2, HCO3 (including calculated O2 saturation);
82805 with O2 saturation, by direct measurement, except pulse oximetry

Explanation
These tests may be requested as arterial blood gases (ABGs). Blood gases are usually requested to evaluate disturbances of acid-base balance, which may be caused by respiratory or metabolic disorders. Blood specimen is obtained by arterial puncture. Code 82803 reports any combination of pH, pCO2, pO2, CO2, and HCO3, including calculated O2 saturation. Code 82805 reports any combination of the same gases, but O2 saturation is performed by direct measurement. Method is selective electrode, potentiometry, or spectrophotometry (O2 saturation).

82810

82810 Gases, blood, O2 saturation only, by direct measurement, except pulse oximetry

Explanation
This test may be requested as O2. Oxygen saturation is the percent of the oxygen in the blood that combines with hemoglobin. Blood specimen is obtained by arterial puncture. Method is spectrophotometry.

82820

82820 Hemoglobin-oxygen affinity (pO2 for 50% hemoglobin saturation with oxygen)

Explanation
This test may be requested as oxygen, P50 or as pO2, P50. This test is performed to measure the affinity of hemoglobin for oxygen, which allows evaluation of oxygen delivery to body tissues. Blood specimen is obtained by arterial puncture. Method is spectrophotometry or potentiometry.

82945

82945 Glucose, body fluid, other than blood

Explanation
Glucose is the end product of carbohydrate metabolism, providing energy for living organisms. It is found in body fluids including joint fluid and CSF. Both elevated and decreased levels of glucose may be indicative of disease processes. Joint fluid specimen is obtained by separately reportable arthrocentesis. CSF specimen is obtained by separately reportable spinal puncture. Method is enzymatic.

82946

82946 Glucagon tolerance test

Explanation
Glucagon is a hormone secreted by the pancreas. It stimulates the conversion of glycogen stored in the liver to glucose. Glucagon tolerance test may be requested to evaluate suspected diabetes mellitus or glucagonoma. Blood specimen is obtained by venipuncture. A fasting glucagon level is obtained. A high carbohydrate meal or an oral dose of glucose is given. Glucagon levels are then tested at 30, 60, and 120-minute intervals. Method is radioimmunoassay (RIA).

82947

82947 Glucose; quantitative, blood (except reagent strip)

Explanation
This test may be requested as a fasting blood sugar (FBS). This quantitative test is used to evaluate disorders of carbohydrate metabolism. The patient has ordinarily fasted for eight hours. Blood specimen is obtained by venipuncture. Method is enzymatic.

82948

82948 Glucose; blood, reagent strip

Explanation
This test is used to monitor disorders of carbohydrate metabolism. Blood specimen is obtained by finger stick. A drop of blood is placed on the reagent strip for a specified amount of time. When the prescribed amount of time has elapsed, the strip is blotted and the reagent strip is compared to a color chart. Method is reagent strip with visual comparison.

82975

82975 Glutamine (glutamic acid amide)

Explanation
This test may be abbreviated as Gln. Glutamine is an amino acid and is the most abundant amino acid found in CSF. This test may used to evaluate hepatic encephalopathy, Reye's syndrome, meningitis, rheumatoid arthritis, and other conditions. Blood specimen is obtained by venipuncture. A 24-hour urine specimen is required. The patient flushes the first urine of the day and discards it. All urine for the next 24-hours is collected and refrigerated. CSF is obtained by spinal puncture, which is reported separately. Method is ion-exchange chromatography or colorimetry.

83003

83003 Growth hormone, human (HGH) (somatotropin)

Explanation
This test may be requested as GH, HGH, or somatotropin. This test may be used to evaluate pituitary gigantism or dwarfism, acromegaly, hypopituitarism, adrenocortical hyperfunction, fetal anencephaly (amniotic fluid analysis), as well as

other conditions. Blood specimen is obtained by venipuncture. Amniotic fluid sample is obtained by amniocentesis, which is reported separately. Method is radioimmunoassay.

83008

83008 Guanosine monophosphate (GMP), cyclic

Explanation
Cyclic guanosine monophosphate (cGMP) is a so-called "messenger" nucleotide, important in cell function. Levels have been measured in the evaluation of calcium metabolism disorders, including pseudohypoparathyroidism, and in certain other endocrine disorders. The most common method reported in the literature is radioimmunoassay.

83516-83518

83516 Immunoassay for analyte other than infectious agent antibody or infectious agent antigen; qualitative or semiquantitative, multiple step method

83518 qualitative or semiquantitative, single step method (eg, reagent strip)

Explanation
Immunoassay uses highly specific antigen to antibody binding to identify specific chemical substances. This code reports a number of immunoassay techniques for identifying analytes (chemical substances) that are not specifically identified elsewhere, excluding infectious agent antibody or infectious agent antigen. More specific methods reported with these codes include enzyme immunoassay (EIA) and fluoroimmunoassay (FIA). This test identifies (qualitative analysis) the substance or roughly measures (semi-quantitative analysis) the amount of the substance. Code 83516 reports multiple step method, while 83518 reports single step method.

83519

83519 Immunoassay for analyte other than infectious agent antibody or infectious agent antigen; quantitative, by radioimmunoassay (eg, RIA)

Explanation
Immunoassay uses highly specific antigen to antibody binding to identify specific chemical substances. This code reports measurement (quantitative analysis) using radioimmunoassay (RIA) technique for identifying analytes (chemical substances) that are not specifically identified elsewhere, excluding infectious agent antibody or infectious agent antigen.

83520

83520 Immunoassay for analyte other than infectious agent antibody or infectious agent antigen; quantitative, not otherwise specified

Explanation
Immunoassay uses highly specific antigen to antibody binding to identify specific chemical substances. This code reports measurement (quantitative analysis) using a technique other than radioimmunoassay (RIA) for identifying analytes (chemical substances) that are not specifically identified elsewhere, excluding infectious agent antibody or infectious agent antigen.

83605

83605 Lactate (lactic acid)

Explanation
This test is used to assess lactic blood levels to document the presence of tissue hypoxia, determine the degree of hypoxia, and monitor the effect of therapy in blood, plasma, or cerebrospinal fluid (CSF). Specimen collection is either CSF from a spinal puncture or arterial or venous blood. Hand clenching and the use of a tourniquet should be avoided to prevent the build-up of potassium and lactic acid. Method is enzymatic or gas chromatography (GS). This test may be used to determine lactic acidosis when unaccountable anion gap metabolic acidosis is detected.

83615

83615 Lactate dehydrogenase (LD), (LDH);

Explanation
This test may also be ordered as LD or LDH. The test is a measure of LD or LDH, which is found in many body tissues, particularly the heart, liver, red blood cells, and kidneys. Specimen collection is by spinal puncture for cerebral spinal fluid (CSF), venous blood, or other body fluid, such as urine. Methods used are lactate to pyruvate or pyruvate to lactate. This test may be ordered for a wide variety of disorders, including renal diseases and congestive heart failure.

83625

83625 Lactate dehydrogenase (LD), (LDH); isoenzymes, separation and quantitation

Explanation
This test may be ordered as LDH isoenzymes or LD isoenzymes. Specimen collection is collected in a series of three venipunctures: one initially and two more at six to eight-hour intervals. This differs from a total LDH (83615) in that several isoenzymes are individually identified (e.g., LDH1, LDH2). Method is by electrophoresis or immunochemical methods, including immunoprecipitation. This test may be ordered for a wide variety of reasons, and results may point to numerous diagnoses.

83655

83655 Lead

Explanation
This test may be ordered using Pb, the chemical abbreviation for lead. A whole blood test may used to identify more recent lead exposures; the urine test is used to determine lead body burden, rather than to diagnose lead poisoning. In some instances, serum, hair samples, or bronchoalveolar lavage fluids may be tested. Specimen collection for urine is usually a 24-hour collection. Method used is source dependent, but commonly electrothermal atomic absorption spectrometry (AAS). Bronchoalveolar lavage specimens may be tested by x-ray fluorescence spectrometry.

83718

83718 Lipoprotein, direct measurement; high density cholesterol (HDL cholesterol)

Explanation
This test may be requested as HDL, HDLC, or HDL cholesterol. Lipoproteins are compounds composed of lipids bound to proteins, which are transported through the blood. High-density lipoprotein (HDL) is frequently referred to as "good cholesterol," or "friendly lipid," as it is responsible for decreasing plaque deposits in blood vessels. High levels of HDL decrease the risk of premature coronary artery disease. Blood specimen is post-fasting venipuncture. This code reports direct measurement only, normally performed using either an enzymatic or precipitation method.

83719

83719 Lipoprotein, direct measurement; VLDL cholesterol

Explanation
This test measures the amount of VLDLs, the lipoprotein that carries triglycerides in the blood. The test is useful to determine a patient's risk of arteriosclerotic occlusive disease, as well as other cholesterol-related disorders. Specimen collection is post-fasting venipuncture. The method used is electrophoresis and may first involve ultracentrifugation.

83721

83721 Lipoprotein, direct measurement; LDL cholesterol

Explanation
This test may also be referred to as LDL-C. It measures the amount of low-density lipoproteins (LDLs), also known as "bad cholesterol." The test is useful to determine the patient's risk of coronary heart disease (CHD), among other disorders. Specimen collection is post-fasting venipuncture.

Method may be by precipitation procedure with results derived by the Friedewald formula.

83735
83735 Magnesium

Explanation
This test is used to determine magnesium levels and the chemical abbreviation Mg may be used. Specimen collection is post-fasting venipuncture or 24-urine collection. Cerebrospinal fluid (CSF) would be collected by a spinal puncture. Methods are atomic absorption spectrophotometry (blood and urine) and colorimetry (CSF). Other methods may also be employed. The test may be ordered for a wide variety of reasons.

83788
83788 Mass spectrometry and tandem mass spectrometry (MS, MS/MS), analyte not elsewhere specified; qualitative, each specimen

Explanation
This test identifies the presence (qualitative) of specific analytes in protein. The specimen varies. Method is mass spectrometry. The test is used for identifying the chemical makeup and structure of a substance. Tandem MS (MS/MS) is a method using sequential analysis to provide structural information by establishing relationships between substances. This test assists in analyzing viruses, sequencing and analyzing peptides and proteins, and providing information on such life-threatening diseases as AIDS and various types of skin cancers.

83789
83789 Mass spectrometry and tandem mass spectrometry (MS, MS/MS), analyte not elsewhere specified; quantitative, each specimen

Explanation
This test is used for identifying the chemical makeup and structure of a substance. The specimen type varies. Method is mass spectometry (MS). This test is used to analyze viruses, sequence and analyze peptides and proteins, and to provide information on such life-threatening diseases as AIDS and various types of skin cancers. This test quantifies (measures) the amount of analyte in the specimen.

83825
83825 Mercury, quantitative

Explanation
This test may also be ordered as Hg. The specimen is whole blood, a 24 hour urine sample or hair cut close to the scalp. Methods are electrothermal atomic absorption, gold electrode deposition, or gas chromatography. Mercury toxicity may cause neurological defects, pneumonitis, and other problems depending on mode of entry into the body (e.g., vapor, ingestion) and which form it enters as: elemental, inorganic, and organic.

83835
83835 Metanephrines

Explanation
The test is performed to determine metanephrine or normetanephrine concentrations. The specimen is urine collected over a 24-hour period. Method is high performance liquid chromatography (HPLC). Metanephrine or normetanephrine concentrations may be associated with neuroendocrine tumors or even associated with intense physical activity, life threatening illness and drug interferences.

83858
83858 Methsuximide

Explanation
This test is also known as methsuximide/normethsuximide and celontin. The specimen is serum or plasma. Methods may include gas-liquid chromatography and high-performance liquid chromatography. This test may be ordered to measure the amount of methsuximide, which is an anticonvulsant used in treating petit mal and psychomotor epilepsy.

83872
83872 Mucin, synovial fluid (Ropes test)

Explanation
This test may also be referred to as a mucin coagulation test or joint fluid test, in addition to Rope's test. This test analyzes the hyaluronic acid in synovial fluid. Specimen collection is by arthrocentesis. Method involves adding a few drops of synovial fluid into a weak solution of acetic acid. The mixture is evaluated for clumping and change of fluid opacity. Test results may be a general guide to numerous rheumatological disorders.

83873
83873 Myelin basic protein, cerebrospinal fluid

Explanation
This test may be ordered as an MBP assay. The specimen is spinal fluid. . In rare instances, serum may be tested for myelin basic protein from patients with recent head injuries. Ordinarily, the CSF sample is taken when a patient is experiencing certain symptoms characteristic of disease activity, typically multiple sclerosis. Test methods include radial immunodiffusion (RIA), electroimmunodiffusion, immunofluorometry, immunoprecipitation, or immunonephelometry. This test is typically used as an evaluation of disease activity, rather than for diagnostic purposes.

83874
83874 Myoglobin

Explanation
Myoglobin is a principle protein of skeletal and cardiac muscle tissue. Elevated serum levels may be found in severe muscle conditions, such as polymyositis and crushing traumas to muscle and bone. This test may be used in association with other disorders as well, such as acute myocardial infarct and infections. The specimen is serum (preferred method) or random urine sample. Methods include radioimmunoassay (RIA), fluorometric immunoassay, and immunoturbidimetry for blood. Urine specimens may be processed by antigen-antibody reaction nephelometry.

83883
83883 Nephelometry, each analyte not elsewhere specified

Explanation
Nephelometry is a method to measure the concentration of a suspension using an instrument (nephelometer) for assessing turbidity of a solution. For example, this code can be used to measure the concentration of albumin in body fluid. Albumins make up about 60 percent of plasma proteins, and exert considerable pressure in maintaining water balance between blood and tissues. Report this nephelometry test when the analyte is not specifically cited elsewhere in this section.

83915
83915 Nucleotidase 5'-

Explanation
This test is also known as 5'-N'TASE, and 5'-NT. The specimen is serum or synovial fluid. Methods vary greatly, and may include molybdate color reaction, high performance liquid chromatography, and colorimetry. The test may be ordered to assist in identifying the cause of increased 5'-nucleotidase, a liver-related enzyme.

83916
83916 Oligoclonal immune (oligoclonal bands)

Explanation
The specimen is cerebrospinal fluid (CFS) and serum. Methods may include thin-gel agarose high-resolution electrophoresis and isoelectric focusing. This test may be used to identify diagnoses of inflammatory and autoimmune diseases of the CNS and other degenerative states.

83930
83930 Osmolality; blood

Explanation
This test is also known as osmolal gap and serum osmolality. The specimen is serum or plasma. Methodology may involve freezing point depression or vapor pressure techniques. The test measures the amount of molecules or ions (particles) in a solution

of water or the presence of osmotically active molecules in serum. The test may be used to determine liver disease and disorders, electrolyte and water balance.

83935
83935 Osmolality; urine

Explanation
This test may also be known as osmolal gap. The specimen is a random urine sample. Method may be by freezing point depression. The test may be used to determine renal disease and disorders, electrolyte and water balance. The results may be high or low urine osmolality, depending on the differential diagnosis.

83937
83937 Osteocalcin (bone g1a protein)

Explanation
Osteocalcin is a test developed to measure bone formation and for monitoring therapy of preexisting bone conditions. An imbalance between the two (formation and reabsorption) may account for many of the metabolic bone diseases, such as Paget's disease and osteomalacia. The specimen is serum or plasma. Methods may include enzyme-linked immunosorbent assay (ELISA).

84060
84060 Phosphatase, acid; total

Explanation
This is also known as phosphoric monoester phosphohydrolase and PAP. This test is often performed on individuals with diagnoses such as skeletal metastasis, myelocytic leukemia, and is useful in staging prostatic cancer rather than initial diagnosis of prostate cancer. The specimen is post-fasting serum. Methods may include radioimmunoassay (RIA), enzyme immunoassay (EIA), thymolphthalein monophosphate, and titrate inhibition.

84075
84075 Phosphatase, alkaline;

Explanation
This test may be requested as ALP or AP-EC. ALP is an enzyme. It is an indicator of liver cell damage. Amniotic fluid ALP may be screened for cystic fibrosis in mothers who have had a child affected with the disease. Blood specimen is serum. Methods include a number of kinetic spectrophotometry and fluorescent techniques, as well as 4-nitrylphenophosphate (4-NPP) and diethanolamine (DEA).

84078
84078 Phosphatase, alkaline; heat stable (total not included)

Explanation
This may also be known as ALP and AP. This test may be performed to identify general liver and bone diseases. The specimen is post-fasting serum. Methodology may involve heat inhibition at 56!C.

84080
84080 Phosphatase, alkaline; isoenzymes

Explanation
This test may also be known as ALP isoenzymes and AP. This test may be ordered for patients with increased serum total alkaline phosphatase, or to compare total alkaline phosphatase to placental, liver, bone, and Regan isoenzymes. The specimen is post-fasting serum. Methods may include King-Armstrong phenyl phosphate, Bowers and McComb, and Kodak.

84100
84100 Phosphorus inorganic (phosphate);

Explanation
This test may be ordered as PO4. The specimen is post-fasting serum or plasma. Methods may include phosphomolybdatecolorimetric and modified molybdateenzymatic, and colorimetric. The testing may be performed to measure high or low levels of phosphorus to determine a variety of differential diagnoses. Potassium supplements increase phosphate levels. Also, phosphate levels may increase during the last trimester of pregnancy.

84105
84105 Phosphorus inorganic (phosphate); urine

Explanation
This test is performed to identify the calcium/phosphorus balance. High values may be associated with primary hyperparathyroidism, vitamin D deficiency, and renal tubular acidosis; low values may be due to hypoparathyroidism, pseudohypoparathyroidism, and vitamin D toxicity. The test may also be used for nephrolithiasis assessment.

84106
84106 Porphobilinogen, urine; qualitative

Explanation
This test may also be known as Watson-Schwartz and Hoesch tests. The specimen is random urine which requires special handling. Methods are the Watson-Schwartz and Hoesch tests, and Ehrlich's reagent. The Hoesch test does not respond to urobilinogen. The test may be used to screen for acute intermittent porphyria and for acute attacks of abdominal and extremity pain.

84110
84110 Porphobilinogen, urine; quantitative

Explanation
This test may also be known as Porphobilinogen (PBG), urine. The specimen is a 24-hour or a random urine sample, requiring special handling. Urine colored amber-red or burgundy, which darkens in light, indicates the presence of abnormally high levels. This test may be used to detect levels of porphobilinogen associated in the diagnosis of genetic or drug-induced abnormal porphyrin metabolism. Methods may involve gas chromatography, colorimetry, and spectrophotometry. This test measures (quantifies) porphobilinogen present in the specimen.

84132
84132 Potassium; serum, plasma or whole blood

Explanation
This test may be requested as K or K+. Potassium is the major electrolyte found in intracellular fluids. Potassium influences skeletal and cardiac muscle activity. Very small fluctuations outside the normal range may cause significant health risk, including muscle weakness and cardiac arrhythmias. Blood specimen is serum, plasma, or whole blood. Methods include atomic absorption spectrometry (AAS), ion-selective electrode (ISE), and flame emission spectroscopy (FES).

84133
84133 Potassium; urine

Explanation
This test may be ordered as urine K+. The specimen is collected by the patient over a 24-hour period or is random urine sample. Methods may include flame emission photometry and ion-selective electrode (ISE). The test may be ordered to determine elevated levels for the differential diagnoses of chronic renal failure, renal tubular acidosis, and for diuretic therapy.

84155
84155 Protein, total, except by refractometry; serum, plasma or whole blood

Explanation
A total protein test may be performed to assess nutritional status. Serum, plasma, or whole blood is tested for protein in 84155. Aspiration of other body fluids (CSF, bronchial fluid, exudates) may also require separately reportable procedures. The method is biuret for blood (serum). For other body fluids, the method is turbidimetry or biuret.

84160
84160 Protein, total, by refractometry, any source

Explanation
A total protein test may be performed to assess nutritional status. This code reports any source of specimenserum, blood, urine, amniotic fluid, cerebral spinal fluid, or synovial fluid.

Collection/aspiration of other body fluids (CSF, amniotic fluid, exudates) may require separately reportable procedures. Blood is collected by venipuncture for adults and heel stick for the specimen in children. A 24-hour urine specimen is required for urine testing. This code reports protein tested for by refractometry. The method determines the velocity of light through a refractive material (plasma).

84165

84165 Protein; electrophoretic fractionation and quantitation, serum

Explanation
Specimen collection is by venipuncture for adults; heel stick for children. Methods may be cellulose acetate and agarose electrophoresis. The test is performed for the quantitation of albumin, alpha1, alpha2 beta, and gammaglobulins. CSF electrophoresis may be useful in the diagnosis of tumors in the central nervous system or neurological illnesses.

84181-84182

84181 Protein; Western Blot, with interpretation and report, blood or other body fluid

84182 Western Blot, with interpretation and report, blood or other body fluid, immunological probe for band identification, each

Explanation
Specimen collection is by venipuncture for blood; separately reportable lumbar puncture for cerebrospinal fluid (CSF). Methods may include enzyme immunoassay (EIA), enzyme-linked immunosorbent assay (ELISA), and indirect fluorescent (IFA) for screening; Western blot for confirmation. For Western blot test, report 84181; for Western blot with immunological probe for band identification, report 84182. This test identifies serological response to the causative organism Borrelia burgdorferi and may be performed to assist in diagnosing Lyme disease.

84210

84210 Pyruvate

Explanation
This test is also known as pyruvic acid test. The specimen is blood. Methods are usually enzymatic and colorimetry. This test measures the level of pyruvate in whole blood for possible diagnosis of an inherited disorder of metabolism. The abnormal breakdown of red blood cells and subsequent release of hemoglobin characterize a congenital deficiency of pyruvate.

84228

84228 Quinine

Explanation
Quinine is used in the treatment of malaria, atrial fibrillation, and other disorders of muscular tissues. Urine is collected by a patient over a 24-hour period. Method is thin-layer chromatography.

84244

84244 Renin

Explanation
This test may be ordered as plasma renin activity, or PRA. The specimen is plasma. Certain medications such as beta-blockers, may affect testing outcome. Methodology may include radioimmunoassay.

84295

84295 Sodium; serum, plasma or whole blood

Explanation
This test may be requested as Na. Sodium is an electrolyte found in extracellular fluid. Blood specimen is obtained by venipuncture. Methods include atomic absorption spectrometry (AAS), flame emission photometry, and ion-selective electrode (ISE).

84300

84300 Sodium; urine

Explanation
This test may also be ordered as urine Na. Specimen collection is often by the patient over a 24-hour period or by random urine sample. For a 24-hour urine specimen, the patient flushes the first urine of the day. All voided urine for the next 24 hours is collected. Methods may include flame emission photometry and ion selective electrode (ISE). Sodium is an electrolyte found in extracellular fluid. This test is used to identify increased (hypernatremia), and decreased (hyponatremia) levels of sodium due to various conditions or disease states.

84305

84305 Somatomedin

Explanation
Somatomedin is a protein mainly produced in the liver. It is a peptide dependent on growth hormone for its actions. This test may be used to diagnose and evaluate response to therapy for a variety of growth disorders. The test may be performed to diagnose acromegaly, dwarfism, pituitary disease and disorders, nutritional deficiencies, and to monitor response to therapies. The specimen is plasma, which requires special handling. . Methodology may use a process of dissociation from binding protein and chromatography, followed by radioimmunoassay (RIA).

84311

84311 Spectrophotometry, analyte not elsewhere specified

Explanation
Specimen types include blood, random urine, or a 24-hour timed urine collection. Method is typically spectrophotometry, which provides a quantitative measure of the amount of a material in a solution absorbing applied light. Report this test for an analyte not elsewhere specified. Measuring the absorption of visible, ultraviolet or infrared light makes quantitative measurements of concentrations of reagents. 4315 The specimen is by the bodily fluid chosen as a sample (e.g., gastric secretions). Method is by specific gravity, which measures the concentration or the weight of a substance as compared to an equal volume of water. For laboratory testing, specific gravity shows the density of a specific material.

84315

84315 Specific gravity (except urine)

Explanation
Specimen collection is by the bodily fluid chosen as a sample (e.g., gastric secretions). Method is by specific gravity, which measures the concentration-or the weight of a substance-as compared to an equal volume of water. For laboratory testing, specific gravity shows the density of a specific material.

84436

84436 Thyroxine; total

Explanation
This test may be ordered as a T4. The specimen is serum. Methods may include radioimmunoassay (RIA), enzyme-linked immunosorbent assay (ELISA), fluorescence polarization immunoassay (FPIA), and chemiluminescence assay (CIA). The test is performed to determine thyroid function screening test; total thyroxine makes up approximately 99 percent of the thyroid hormone.

84437

84437 Thyroxine; requiring elution (eg, neonatal)

Explanation
This test may be ordered as a neonatal T4. The specimen is whole blood. The specimen may be taken at the same time as a PKU (Phenylalanine) test. Method is typically radioimmunoassay (RIA). The test may be performed to determine hypothyroidism in newborns (performed in all 50 states) to prevent mental retardation and to monitor suppressive and replacement therapy.

84439

84439 Thyroxine; free

Explanation
This test may be ordered as a FT4, free T4, FTI or FT4 index. The specimen is serum, requiring special handling. Methods may include radioimmunoassay and equilibrium dialysis for reference method. Free thyroxine is a minimal amount of the total T4 level (approximately one percent). This test is not influenced by thyroid-binding abnormalities and perhaps correlates more closely with the true hormonal status. It may be effective in the diagnosis of hyperthyroidism and hypothyroidism.

84442
84442 Thyroxine binding globulin (TBG)

Explanation
The specimen is serum. Methods may include chemiluminescent immunoassay, equilibrium dialysis, ultrafiltration, and solid phase enzyme immunoassay (EIA) technology. Thyroxin binding globulin is a plasma protein that binds with thyroxine and transports it in the blood. Elevated levels may be associated with pregnancy and newborn states, hepatitis, and other disorders. Decreased levels may be associated with liver diseases and acromegaly, among other disorders.

84443
84443 Thyroid stimulating hormone (TSH)

Explanation
TSH is produced in the pituitary gland and stimulates the secretion of thyrotropin (T3) and thyroxine (T4); these secretory products monitor TSH. The specimen is serum, requiring special handling. Heel stick or umbilical cord sample is drawn from newborns and may be collected on a special paper. Methods may include radioimmunoassay (RIA), sandwich immunoradiometric assay (IRMA), fluorometric enzyme immunoassay with use of monoclonal antibodies, or microparticle enzyme immunoassay on IMx (MEIA). This test may be performed to determine thyroid function, to differentiate from various types of hypothyroidism (e.g., primary, and pituitary/hypothalamic), or to diagnose hyperthyroidism. The test may be ordered to evaluate therapy in patients receiving hypothyroid treatment, and to detect congenital hypothyroidism.

84445
84445 Thyroid stimulating immune globulins (TSI)

Explanation
This test may also be ordered as TSI. This serum test measures the amount of thyroid stimulating antibody, which stimulates the thyroid to produce excessive amounts of thyroid hormone. The specimen is serum. Methods may include vitro bioassay and radioimmunoassay. The test may be useful in diagnosis of Grave's disease (hyperthyroidism).

84450
84450 Transferase; aspartate amino (AST) (SGOT)

Explanation
This test is usually referred to as aspartate aminotransferase (AST) or as serum glutamic oxaloacetic transaminase (SGOT). AST is an enzyme found primarily in heart muscle and the liver. Serum levels are low unless there is cellular damage, at which time large amounts are released into circulation. AST levels are increased following acute myocardial infarction (MI). Liver disease may also cause elevated levels of AST. Blood specimen is serum or plasma. Method is spectrophotometry, kinetic assay, and enzymatic.

84460
84460 Transferase; alanine amino (ALT) (SGPT)

Explanation
This test is usually referred to as alanine aminotransferase (ALT) or as serum glutamic pyruvic transaminase (SGPT). ALT is an enzyme found primarily in liver cells and elevations may be indicative of liver disease. Blood specimen is serum or plasma. Method is spectrophotometry or enzymatic.

84466
84466 Transferrin

Explanation
This test may also be called a TRF, Tf, siderophilin, and pertains to a transferrin index or receptor. The specimen is serum, plasma. or a 24-hour urine specimen. Methods may include radial immunodiffusion (RID), and electro-immunodiffusion for urine, and rate nephelometry for serum. The test is performed to determine a patient's nutritional status, differentiate between iron deficiency anemia, acquired liver disorders and diseases, and kidney diseases.

84478
84478 Triglycerides

Explanation
This test may be requested as TG. Triglycerides are blood lipids that are transported through the circulatory system by lipoproteins. Triglycerides contribute to atherosclerosis and other arterial diseases. Blood specimen is serum or plasma. Method is enzymatic or colorimetry.

84479
84479 Thyroid hormone (T3 or T4) uptake or thyroid hormone binding ratio (THBR)

Explanation
This test may be requested as T3 uptake and T4 uptake or THBR. The specimen is serum. Method is chemiluminescent immunoassay.

84520
84520 Urea nitrogen; quantitative

Explanation
This test may be requested as blood urea nitrogen (BUN). Urea is an end product of protein metabolism. BUN may be requested to evaluate dehydration or renal function. Blood specimen is serum or plasma. Method is colorimetry, enzymatic, or rate conductivity. This test measures (quantitates) the amount of urea in the blood.

84525
84525 Urea nitrogen; semiquantitative (eg, reagent strip test)

Explanation
This test may also be ordered as a BUN. This test may provide useful information regarding carbohydrate metabolism (diabetes), kidney function, and acid-base balance. The specimen is by random urine sample. Method is reagent strip.

84540
84540 Urea nitrogen, urine

Explanation
This test may provide useful information regarding carbohydrate metabolism (diabetes), kidney function, and acid-base balance, in addition to dietary protein. Urea is a measure of protein breakdown in the body. Urine urea excretion can be measured to obtain a ratio between the plasma (blood) urea and the urine urea; this ratio is an indicator of kidney function. Urine collection over a 24-hour period. Methods may include enzymatic assay, colorimetry, and conductometric.

84545
84545 Urea nitrogen, clearance

Explanation
This test is also known as BUNblood urea nitrogen. The specimen is taken over a 24-hour period. Urea nitrogen is formed in the liver as an end product of protein metabolism. Increased or decreased levels of urea nitrogen can indicate renal disease, dehydration, congestive heart failure, and gastrointestinal bleeding, starvation, shock or urinary tract obstruction (by tumor or prostate gland).

84550
84550 Uric acid; blood

Explanation
This test may be requested as urate. Uric acid may be ordered to evaluate gout, renal function and a number of other disorders. Blood specimen is serum or plasma. Method is enzymatic or high performance liquid chromatography (HPLC).

84560
84560 Uric acid; other source

Explanation
Uric acid is also known as urate. The specimen may be over a 24-hour period. Cerebrospinal fluid (CSF) is obtained by separately reportable lumbar puncture. Methods may include high performance liquid chromatography, uricase, and phosphotungstate. The test may be ordered to determine the possible occurrence of calculus formation, evaluate uric acid in gout, and to identify genetic defects and some malignancies.

84588
84588 Vasopressin (antidiuretic hormone, ADH)

Explanation
This test is also known as Arginine Vasopressin Hormone and Antidiuretic Hormone (ADH). The specimen is plasma. Method is radioimmunoassay. Vasopressin, secreted by the hypothalamus and stored and released by the posterior pituitary gland, increases blood pressure and the rate at which the kidneys absorb water.

84590
84590 Vitamin A

Explanation
This vitamin may is also known as retinol. The specimen is post-fasting serum, and requires special handling. Methods are electrochemical, high performance liquid chromatography (HPLC), and fluorescence or UV/VIS spectroscopy. Serum levels of vitamin A can be increased in specific diseases and toxic states, and decreased levels are seen in other conditions, such as, nutritional deficiency.

84597
84597 Vitamin K

Explanation
This test is used to analyze vitamin K, a fat-soluble vitamin that plays an important role in blood clotting. The specimen is post-fasting serum which requires special handling. Method is high-performance liquid chromatography A. A deficiency in vitamin K is characterized by the increased tendency to bleed, including internal bleeding. Such bleeding episodes may be severe in newborn infants.

84630
84630 Zinc

Explanation
This test is also known as Serum Zn. The specimen is serum or whole blood or a 24-hour urine sample. Methods may include atomic absorption spectrometry (AAS). Zinc is a trace mineral in the body, linked to thyroid hormone function and blood clotting. The test may be performed to determine nutrient levels for patients on total parenteral nutrition (TPN) and for burn victims and critically ill patients. The test may also be ordered to evaluate possible zinc toxicity.

85002
85002 Bleeding time

Explanation
This test may be ordered as a bleeding time or as an Ivy bleeding time. A small, superficial wound is nicked in the patient's forearm. Essentially, the amount of time it takes for the wound to stop bleeding is recorded at bedside. The Ivy bleeding time test is one standardized method. All methods are manual or point of care. A bleeding time is a rough measure of platelet (thrombocyte) function. The test is often performed on a pre-operative patient.

85007
85007 Blood count; blood smear, microscopic examination with manual differential WBC count

Explanation
This test may be ordered as a blood count with manual differential. Specimen collection is venipuncture, finger stick, or heel stick in infants. Method is manual testing. A blood count typically includes measurement of white blood cells or leukocytes, hemoglobin, and hematocrit (volume of packed red cells or VPRC). In addition, this test includes a manual differential of white blood cells or "diff." The following leukocytes will be differentiated: neutrophils or granulocytes, lymphocytes, monocytes, eosinophils, and basophils. The platelet count will be estimated and red cell morphology will be commented on if abnormal.

85008
85008 Blood count; blood smear, microscopic examination without manual differential WBC count

Explanation
This test may be ordered as a manual blood smear examination without differential parameters, RBC smear, peripheral blood smear, or RBC morphology. Method is manual testing. A blood smear is prepared and examined for the presence of normal cell constituents, including white blood cells, red blood cells, and platelets. The white blood cell and platelet or thrombocyte counts are estimated and red cell morphology will be commented on if abnormal.

85009
85009 Blood count; manual differential WBC count, buffy coat

Explanation
This test may be ordered as a buffy coat differential or as a differential WBC count, buffy coat. Blood is whole blood. Other collection types (e.g., finger stick or heel stick) do not yield the volume of blood required for this test. Method is manual testing. The whole blood is centrifuged to concentrate the white blood cells, and a manual WBC differential is performed in which the following leukocytes are differentiated: neutrophils or granulocytes, lymphocytes, monocytes, eosinophils, and basophils. This test is usually performed when the number of WBCs or leukocytes is abnormally low and the presence of abnormal white cells (e.g., blasts or cancer cells) is suspected clinically.

85013
85013 Blood count; spun microhematocrit

Explanation
This test may be ordered as a microhematocrit, a spun microhematocrit, or a "spun crit." The specimen (whole blood) is by finger stick or heel stick in infants. The sample is placed in a tube and into a microcentrifuge device. The vials can be read manually against a chart for the volume of packed red cells or a digital reader in the centrifuge device. A spun microhematocrit only reports the volume of packed red cells. It is typically performed at sites where limited testing is available, the patient is a very difficult blood draw, or on infants.

85014
85014 Blood count; hematocrit (Hct)

Explanation
This test may be ordered as a hematocrit, Hmt, or Hct. The specimen is whole blood. Method is automated cell counter. The hematocrit or volume of packed red cells (VPRC) in the blood sample is calculated by multiplying the red blood cell count or RBC times the mean corpuscular volume or MCV.

85018
85018 Blood count; hemoglobin (Hgb)

Explanation
This test may be ordered as hemoglobin, Hgb, or hemoglobin concentration. The specimen is whole blood. Method is usually automated cell counter but a manual method is seen in labs with a limited test menu and blood bank drawing stations. Hemoglobin is an index of the oxygen-carrying capacity of the blood.

85025

85025 Blood count; complete (CBC), automated (Hgb, Hct, RBC, WBC and platelet count) and automated differential WBC count

Explanation

This test may be ordered as a complete blood count (CBC) with platelets and automated differential. Specimen collection is venipuncture, finger stick, or heel stick in infants. Method is automated cell counter. The hemogram in this code includes measurement of erythrocytes (red blood cells or RBC), leukocytes (white blood cells or WBC), hemoglobin, hematocrit (volume of packed red blood cells or VPRC), platelet or thrombocyte count, and indices (mean corpuscular hemoglobin or MCH, mean corpuscular hemoglobin concentration or MCHC, mean corpuscular volume or MCV, and red cell distribution width or RDW). In addition, this test includes an automated differential of white blood cells or "diff." The following leukocytes will be differentiated: neutrophils or granulocytes, lymphocytes, monocytes, eosinophils and basophils.

85027

85027 Blood count; complete (CBC), automated (Hgb, Hct, RBC, WBC and platelet count)

Explanation

Specimen collection is venipuncture, finger stick, or heel stick in infants. Method is automated cell counter. The hemogram in this code includes measurement of erythrocytes (red blood cells or RBC), leukocytes (white blood cells or WBC), hemoglobin, hematocrit (volume of packed red blood cells or VPRC), platelet or thrombocyte count, and indices (mean corpuscular hemoglobin or MCH, mean corpuscular hemoglobin concentration or MCHC, mean corpuscular volume or MCV, and red cell distribution width or RDW).

85041

85041 Blood count; red blood cell (RBC), automated

Explanation

This test may be ordered as red blood cell count or RBC. The specimen is by whole blood Method is automated cell counter.

85044

85044 Blood count; reticulocyte, manual

Explanation

This test may be ordered as a manual reticulocyte count or as a manual "retic." The specimen is whole. Method is manual. A blood smear is prepared and stained with a dye that highlights the reticulum in the immature red blood cells, or the reticulocytes. The reticulocytes reported as a percentage of total red blood cells.

85045

85045 Blood count; reticulocyte, automated

Explanation

This test may be ordered as an automated reticulocyte count, an "auto retic," or a reticulocyte by flow cytometry. The specimen is whole blood. Method is automated cell counter or flow cytometer. Reticulocytes are immature red blood cells that still contain mitochondria and ribosomes. The reticulocytes are reported as a percentage of total red blood cells.

85046

85046 Blood count; reticulocytes, automated, including 1 or more cellular parameters (eg, reticulocyte hemoglobin content [CHr], immature reticulocyte fraction [IRF], reticulocyte volume [MRV], RNA content), direct measurement

Explanation

This test may be ordered as a reticulocyte count and hemoglobin concentration, "retics" and Hgb, or as an "auto retic" and hemoglobin. The specimen is whole blood. Method is automated cell counter. The blood is stained with a dye that marks the reticulum in immature red blood cells, or reticulocytes. The reticulocytes are reported as a percentage of total red blood cells. The automated reticulocyte blood count also includes one or more cellular parameters, such as the hemoglobin content of the reticulocytes (CHr), the fraction of immature reticulocytes (IRF), the RNA content, or the volume of reticulocytes.

85048

85048 Blood count; leukocyte (WBC), automated

Explanation

This test may be ordered as a white blood cell or WBC count, white cell count, or leukocyte count. Specimen collection is venipuncture, finger stick, or heel stick in infants. Method is usually automated cell count but this test may also be performed manually. The number of white blood cells or leukocytes are measured and reported.

85060

85060 Blood smear, peripheral, interpretation by physician with written report

Explanation

This test may be ordered as a peripheral blood smear with interpretation by a physician, with a written report. It would more usually be ordered following a hemogram with WBC differential where the technologist noted the presence of significant abnormalities and requested a pathology review. Although lacking specificity, peripheral smears also provide a quick and cost-effective screening for the presence of bacteremia. The specimen is whole blood. The method is manual. A blood smear is prepared and reviewed by a physician/pathologist, who submits a written interpretation of the findings.

85097

85097 Bone marrow, smear interpretation

Explanation

This test may be ordered as a bone marrow smear interpretation with or without differential cell count. The specimen is by aspiration with a syringe. The bone marrow aspirate may be collected from a variety of sites, including the posterior iliac crest (preferred) and the sternum. The method is manual. Slides or smears are prepared from the aspirate and stained. The slides are reviewed by a physician/pathologist and a written interpretation of the findings is submitted. This report may include a differential count of the white blood cells present.

85345

85345 Coagulation time; Lee and White

Explanation

This test may be ordered as a clotting time, a whole blood clotting time, or a Lee-White clotting time. The specimen is whole blood. The method is manual. The Lee-White clotting time measures the ability of blood to clot and is performed at the patient's bedside to monitor anti-coagulant therapy such as heparin, warfarin, or coumadin.

85520

85520 Heparin assay

Explanation

This test may be ordered as a heparin assay, a quantitative heparin analysis, or as a heparin level. The specimen is plasma. The method is chromogenic assay. This test measures the amount of heparin in a patient's blood and is usually ordered when the patient is on low-dose heparin therapy.

85525

85525 Heparin neutralization

Explanation

This test may be ordered as a heparin neutralization test, a heparin-thrombin coagulation time test, or as protamine neutralization test. The specimen plasma. The method is manual. This test is used to determine the dose of protamine needed to neutralize heparin-induced bleeding.

85530

85530 Heparin-protamine tolerance test

Explanation

This test may be ordered as a heparin-protamine tolerance test. Protamine is given as an antidote to heparin overdose. However, some patients develop hypersensitivity to protamine and may go into anaphylactic shock if they receive a dosage. Method is point of care testing. This test is used to assess hypersensitivity to protamine and measures the amount of protamine that can be safely administered.

85540

85540 Leukocyte alkaline phosphatase with count

Explanation

This test may be ordered as a leukocyte alkaline phosphatase test (LAP), LAP score, or as a tartrate-inhibited acid phosphatase. The specimen is whole blood or finger stick in adults, or heel stick in infants. The method is enzyme reaction with leukocyte alkaline phosphatase liberating naphthol, which is manually stained. Smears from freshly collected whole blood are prepared, stained, and examined microscopically. One hundred cells are counted and phosphatase activity scores (0 to 4+) totalled. The amount of leukocyte alkaline phosphatase present aids in the differential diagnosis of various leukemias.

85576

85576 Platelet, aggregation (in vitro), each agent

Explanation

This test may be ordered as a platelet aggregation study, or as an in vitro platelet aggregation study. Specimen is collected plasma. The method may be platelet aggregometer. Platelet function is measured by observing the amount of platelet clumping that occurs when certain chemicals are added to a solution of platelets. The test is an in vitro enactment of the platelet aggregation that occurs naturally at the site of vascular injury. The test may be used to detect von Willebrand's disease or other inherited platelet disjunction diseases.

85597-85598

85597 Phospholipid neutralization; platelet
85598 hexagonal phospholipid

Explanation

These are confirmatory tests for lupus anticoagulants (or other autoimmune diseases) using phospholipids derived from platelets (85597) or "hexagonal phase" phospholipids (85598). Some patients with systemic lupus develop an anticoagulant that reacts with platelet or hexagonal phase phospholipids. This test is very sensitive to this anticoagulant. The specimen is by venipuncture.

Coding Tips

Code 85597 has been revised for 2011 in the official CPT description. Code 85598 is new for 2011.

85610

85610 Prothrombin time;

Explanation

This test may be ordered as a prothrombin time (PT), a prothrombin, or as simply PT. The specimen is plasma. Method is one-stage using an automated device. The prothrombin time is prolonged when deficiencies of coagulation factors II, V, VII, or X are present. More commonly, this test monitors the effectiveness of the anticoagulant drug Coumadin or warfarin, prescribed to patients who have had blood clots or myocardial infarction.

85611

85611 Prothrombin time; substitution, plasma fractions, each

Explanation

This test may be ordered as a diluted prothrombin time (PT), a prothrombin 1:1, or as plasma diluted PT. The specimen is plasma. Addition or dilution with normal plasma differentiates between a clotting factor deficiency and a circulating anticoagulant. Prolonged prothrombin times due to a clotting factor deficiency will shorten to normal with the addition of normal plasma while a prolonged prothrombin time due to a circulating anticoagulant may increase with the addition of normal plasma.

85635

85635 Reptilase test

Explanation

This test may be ordered as a reptilase test or, more commonly, reptilase time (RT). The specimen is plasma. Method involves adding venom of pit viper to a sample of the patient's plasma and recording the clotting time. This test is most often used to monitor the effectiveness of thrombolytic or clot-lysing drugs such as streptokinase or urokinase. It may also be used to detect the presence of coagulation disorders such as dysfibrinogenemias (non-functional or abnormal fibrinogen) and clotting disorders such as disseminated intravascular coagulation (DIC).

85651

85651 Sedimentation rate, erythrocyte; non-automated

Explanation

This test may be ordered as an erythrocyte sedimentation rate (ESR), a Westergren sedimentation rate, Wintrobe sedimentation rate, or simply as a "sed rate." The specimen is whole blood. This test is a non-specific screening test for a number of diseases including anemia, disorders of protein production such as multiple myeloma, other conditions that alter the size and/or shape of red cells or erythrocytes, and to screen diseases that cause an increase or decrease in the amount of protein in the plasma. Further studies are often launched by ESR results. The method is manual. A variety of procedures have been used over time to study sedimentation rate. A common one performed manually is the Westergren tube. 85652 This test may be ordered as a Zeta sedimentation rate or as a Zeta sed rate. The specimen is whole blood. Method is an automated test, by centrifugation. This test is a non-specific screening test for a number of diseases including anemia, disorders of protein production such as multiple myeloma

85652

85652 Sedimentation rate, erythrocyte; automated

Explanation

This test may be ordered as a Zeta sedimentation rate or as a Zeta sed rate. Specimen collection is by venipuncture. Method is centrifugation; this is an automated test. This test is a non-specific screening test for a number of diseases including anemia, disorders of protein production such as multiple myeloma, and other conditions that alter the size and/or shape of red cells or erythrocytes. This test may also be used to screen diseases that cause an increase or decrease in the amount of protein in the plasma or liquid portion of the blood.

85730

85730 Thromboplastin time, partial (PTT); plasma or whole blood

Explanation

This test may be ordered as a partial thromboplastin time or PTT, or as an activated partial thromboplastin time or APTT. The specimen is plasma. Finger stick or heel stick is unacceptable. The method is automated coagulation instrument. The partial thromboplastin time is prolonged when deficiencies of coagulation factors VIII, IX, XI, and XII are present. This test is used to monitor the effectiveness of the anticoagulant drug heparin, which is prescribed for patients who have had blood clots or heart attacks.

85732

85732 Thromboplastin time, partial (PTT); substitution, plasma fractions, each

Explanation

This test may be ordered as a diluted partial thromboplastin time, a PTT or APTT 1:1, or as a plasma diluted PTT or APTT. The specimen is plasma. Finger stick or heel stick is not acceptable. The method is automated coagulation instrument. Addition of or dilution with normal plasma differentiates between a clotting factor deficiency and a circulating anticoagulant. Prolonged partial thromboplastin times due to a clotting factor deficiency will shorten to normal with the addition of normal plasma while a prolonged PTT due to a circulating anticoagulant may increase with the addition of normal plasma.

86148

86148 Anti-phosphatidylserine (phospholipid) antibody

Explanation
Test may also be ordered as apoptotic cell assay or necrotic cell assay. The specimen is serum or finger stick in adults, or heel stick in infants. Various autoimmune diseases appear to be a consequence of a defective regulatory mechanism of apoptosis (cell death). Detection method may be by light scatter.

86200
86200 Cyclic citrullinated peptide (CCP), antibody

Explanation
This test may also be known as anti-CCP or CCP antibodies. The test is used to diagnose rheumatoid arthritis (RA) in the earliest stages. The specimen is serum and the method of testing is by enzyme linked immunosorbent assay. (ELISA).

86277
86277 Growth hormone, human (HGH), antibody

Explanation
This test may also be ordered as somatotropin antibody, GH antibody test, or IGF (insulin-like growth factor) antibody. Portions of the pituitary gland secrete growth hormone. Serum levels normally rise and fall throughout the day. The literature is unclear about methodology for an antibody assay. However, radioimmunoassay (RIA) is probably method of choice.

86317
86317 Immunoassay for infectious agent antibody, quantitative, not otherwise specified

Explanation
This code is may be requested to measure the amount of specific infectious disease antibodies in the blood that are not otherwise specified. It would normally be obtained subsequent to qualitative or semi-quantitative immunoassays (86318, 86602-86804), which identify the presence of specific antibodies but do not measure the amount of antibody present. Blood is obtained by venipuncture. Method is immunoassay.

86318
86318 Immunoassay for infectious agent antibody, qualitative or semiquantitative, single step method (eg, reagent strip)

Explanation
This code is may be requested as single step qualitative or semi-quantitative immunoassay to identify the presence of a specific infectious agent antibodies. Blood is serum. Method is immunoassay. Single step methods frequently use a reagent strip for the specific antibody.

86320
86320 Immunoelectrophoresis; serum

Explanation
This code may be abbreviated as serum IEP. Blood specimen is obtained serum. This code is used to report a technique most often used to identify monoclonal gammopathy or lymphoproliferative processes, specifically myelomas. It combines electrophoresis and immunodiffusion. This test is qualitative only.

86325
86325 Immunoelectrophoresis; other fluids (eg, urine, cerebrospinal fluid) with concentration

Explanation
This code may be abbreviated as IEP. A random urine specimen is obtained. CSF is obtained by separately reportable spinal puncture. This code is used to report a technique most often used to identify monoclonal gammopathy or lymphoproliferative processes, specifically myelomas. It combines electrophoresis and immunodiffusion. This test is qualitative only.

86327
86327 Immunoelectrophoresis; crossed (2-dimensional assay)

Explanation
Two-dimensional or crossed immunoelectrophoresis (IEP) is similar to standard IEP as described in 86320 and 86325; however, following immunodiffusion, electrophoresis is performed a second time at right angles to the original separation.

86334-86335
86334 Immunofixation electrophoresis; serum
86335 other fluids with concentration (eg, urine, CSF)

Explanation
Immunofixation electrophoresis (IFE) is a method or technique used to detect the presence of aberrant proteins, especially monoclonal proteins, and to identify when certain protein groups are being increased or decreased in blood serum or urine, particularly. This test can help diagnose and monitor the progression of diseases like multiple myeloma, monoclonal gammopathies, and kidney-damaging diseases. The specimen is serum. For urine testing, a 24-hour urine specimen is required. IFE involves high-resolution electrophoresis combined with immunoprecipitation The value in performing immunofixation electrophoresis is identifying the presence of a particular type of protein, or immunoglobulin. Report 86334 for a serum test and 86335 for another fluid, such as urine or cerebral spinal fluid.

86430
86430 Rheumatoid factor; qualitative

Explanation
This test may be ordered as rheumatoid antibody (RA), arthritis screen, or rheumatoid factor (RF). The specimen is serum,. The test is most significantly used as a qualitative measurement in evaluating patients with inflammatory polyarthritis. The presence of RF is not by itself usually considered sufficient to establish a diagnosis of rheumatoid arthritis, but as a contributing factor or a prognostic marker to a diagnosis. Testing methodology is by latex agglutination, ELISA, or nephelometry.

86431
86431 Rheumatoid factor; quantitative

Explanation
This test may be ordered as rheumatoid antibody (RA) titer, arthritis screen, or rheumatoid factor (RF) titer. The specimen is serum. The test is most significantly used as a quantitative measurement in evaluating patients with inflammatory polyarthritis. The presence or quantity of RF is not by itself usually considered sufficient to establish a diagnosis of rheumatoid arthritis, but as a contributing factor or a prognostic marker to a diagnosis. Testing methodology is by latex agglutination, ELISA, or nephelometry.

87015
87015 Concentration (any type), for infectious agents

Explanation
Concentration may also be referred to as thick smear preparation. The source samples are treated to concentrate the presence of suspect organisms, usually through sedimentation or flotation. There are two common methods of concentration for ova and parasite exams: formalin concentration and zinc sulfate flotation. The two most common concentration methods for AFB stains or cultures are the N-acetyl-L cysteine method and the Zephiran-trisodium phosphate method. Do not report 87015 in conjunction with 87177.

87040
87040 Culture, bacterial; blood, aerobic, with isolation and presumptive identification of isolates (includes anaerobic culture, if appropriate)

Explanation
Samples for bacterial blood culture are drawn by venipuncture and usually consist of a set of bottles, an aerobic and an anaerobic bottle. Drawing at least two sets of cultures increases the effectiveness of the test. This code includes anaerobic culture along with aerobic, if appropriate. Presumptive identification of aerobic pathogens or

microorganisms in the blood sample is by means of identifying colony morphology. The test includes gram staining and subculturing to selective media for the detection of bacterial growth. There are several automated systems that detect the presence of bacteria using colorimetric, radiometric, or spectrophotometric means. The purpose of blood culture tests is to detect the presence of aerobic and anaerobic bacteria in blood and to identify the bacteria, but not to the specific level of genus or species requiring additional testing, such as slide cultures.

87070

87070 Culture, bacterial; any other source except urine, blood or stool, aerobic, with isolation and presumptive identification of isolates

Explanation
Common names for this test are numerous and may include routine culture, aerobic culture, or, using a body or source site, they may be referred to as vaginal culture, CSF culture, etc. The methodology is by bacterial culture and includes various identification procedures for the presumptive identification of any and multiple pathogens. The collection and transport of specimen is varied and specimen dependent.

87071

87071 Culture, bacterial; quantitative, aerobic with isolation and presumptive identification of isolates, any source except urine, blood or stool

Explanation
Common names for this test are numerous and may include routine culture, aerobic culture, or, using a body or source site, they may be referred to as vaginal culture, CSF culture, etc. The methodology is by bacterial culture and includes various identification procedures for the quantitation and presumptive identification of any and multiple pathogens. The collection and transport of specimen is varied and specimen dependent.

87073

87073 Culture, bacterial; quantitative, anaerobic with isolation and presumptive identification of isolates, any source except urine, blood or stool

Explanation
The most common name for this procedure is anaerobic culture. Presumptive identification of anaerobic pathogens or microorganisms in the sample is by means of identifying colony morphology. The test includes gram staining and subculturing to selective media for the detection of bacterial growth. There are several automated systems that detect the presence of bacteria using colorimetric, radiometric, or spectrophotometric

means. This culture test detects the presence of anaerobic bacteria in a body site or source, except blood, urine, or stool, and identifies the micro-organism(s), but not to the specific level of genus or species requiring additional testing, such as slide cultures. The isolate(s) identified is quantified in growth numbers. Tissues, fluids, and aspirations, except from blood, urine, or stool samples, are collected in anaerobic vials or with anaerobic transport swabs and transported immediately. Anaerobic bacteria are sensitive to oxygen and cold.

87075

87075 Culture, bacterial; any source, except blood, anaerobic with isolation and presumptive identification of isolates

Explanation
The most common name for this procedure is anaerobic culture. Presumptive identification of anaerobic pathogens or microorganisms in the sample is by means of identifying colony morphology. The test includes gram staining and subculturing to selective media for the detection of bacterial growth. There are several automated systems that detect the presence of bacteria using colorimetric, radiometric, or spectrophotometric means. The purpose of this culture test is to detect the presence of any or multiple anaerobic bacteria from any body source or site, except blood, and to identify the micro-organism(s), but not to the specific level of genus or species requiring additional testing, such as slide cultures. Tissues, fluids, and aspirations, except blood samples, are collected in anaerobic vials or with anaerobic transport swabs and transported immediately. Anaerobic bacteria are sensitive to oxygen and cold.

87076

87076 Culture, bacterial; anaerobic isolate, additional methods required for definitive identification, each isolate

Explanation
Anaerobic organism identification is for definitive identification of an already-isolated anaerobic bacterium. It involves the use of traditional special media and biochemicals for the identification of anaerobic bacteria.

87077

87077 Culture, bacterial; aerobic isolate, additional methods required for definitive identification, each isolate

Explanation
Aerobic organism identification is for definitive identification of an already-isolated aerobic bacterium. It involves the use of traditional special media and biochemicals for the identification of aerobic bacteria.

87081

87081 Culture, presumptive, pathogenic organisms, screening only;

Explanation
This is a presumptive screening culture for one or more pathogenic organisms. The methodology is by culture and the culture should be identified by type (e.g., anaerobic, aerobic) and specimen source (e.g., pleural, peritoneal, bronchial aspirates). If a specific organism is suspected, the client will typically use common names, such as strep screen, staph screen, etc., to specify the organism for screening.

87084

87084 Culture, presumptive, pathogenic organisms, screening only; with colony estimation from density chart

Explanation
This is a presumptive screening culture for one or more pathogenic organisms, which includes an estimation of the number of organisms based on a density chart. The methodology is by culture and the culture should be identified by type (e.g., anaerobic, aerobic) and specimen source (e.g., pleural, peritoneal, bronchial aspirates). If a specific organism is suspected, the client will typically use common names, such as strep screen, staph screen, etc., to specify the organism for screening.

87101

87101 Culture, fungi (mold or yeast) isolation, with presumptive identification of isolates; skin, hair, or nail

Explanation
Dermatophyte culture and fungal culture are common names for this test. Fungi are divided into two broad categories, yeasts and molds. Skin, hair or nail scrapings from infected site are transferred to appropriate agar. Growth and confirmation by microscopic methods identify, or confirm, a presumptive identification of fungus isolated. Alternately, the scrapings are dropped onto dermatophyte test media (DMT) at the time of collection. The media changes color to indicate dermatophyte growth.

87102

87102 Culture, fungi (mold or yeast) isolation, with presumptive identification of isolates; other source (except blood)

Explanation
Fungal culture, yeast culture, and mold culture are common names for this procedure. Collection is as varied as the sources and the same specimen may be used for other tests. This test is to culture and isolate fungi (yeast or mold) with presumptive identification. Presumptive identification may

include fungi (yeast or mold) present or a genus name with no species (e.g., Aspergillus sp.).

87106

87106 Culture, fungi, definitive identification, each organism; yeast

Explanation
This test is commonly known as a fungal yeast identification. Yeast isolates from fungal cultures are further tested for definitive identification. This code reports testing only for yeast pathogens. Various identification procedures, including growth patterns, and macroscopic and microscopic characteristics, are employed. Examples of fungal yeast pathogens that might require definitive identification include: Histoplasma, Coccidioides and Blastomyces.

87116

87116 Culture, tubercle or other acid-fast bacilli (eg, TB, AFB, mycobacteria) any source, with isolation and presumptive identification of isolates

Explanation
Common names include AFB culture, TB culture, mycobacterium culture, and acid-fast culture. Collection methods are source dependent. The methodology is by culture for the isolation and presumptive identification of mycobacterium. An acid-fast smear should be done at the time the specimen is cultured. Media for isolation should include both solid and liquid types.

87181

87181 Susceptibility studies, antimicrobial agent; agar dilution method, per agent (eg, antibiotic gradient strip)

Explanation
A susceptibility study is performed to determine the susceptibility of a bacterium to an antibiotic. The methodology is agar diffusion (the E test is a method of agar diffusion). The specific antibiotics could be chosen and limited. The test is reported per antibiotic tested. The agar dilution is reported as minimum inhibitory concentration (MIC), which is a method of measuring the exact amount of antibiotic needed to inhibit an organism.

87184

87184 Susceptibility studies, antimicrobial agent; disk method, per plate (12 or fewer agents)

Explanation
This is commonly called a Kirby-Bauer or Bauer-Kirby sensitivity test. It is a sensitivity test to determine the susceptibility of a bacterium to an antibiotic. The methodology is disk diffusion and results are reported as sensitive, intermediate, or resistant. As many as 12 antibiotic disks may be used per plate and the procedure is billed per plate not per antibiotic disk.

87185

87185 Susceptibility studies, antimicrobial agent; enzyme detection (eg, beta lactamase), per enzyme

Explanation
Bacteria produce enzymes that can inactivate some types of antibiotics. This susceptibility test identifies those bacteria that will be resistant to certain types of antibiotics by detecting the presence of these enzymes. 87186 This procedure may be called an MIC, or a sensitivity test. It is a sensitivity test to determine the susceptibility of a bacterium to an antibiotic. The methodology is microtiter dilution (several commercial panels use this method). Results are given as a minimum inhibitory concentration (MIC) with an interpretation of sensitive, intermediate, or resistant. The antibiotics on commercial plates are numerous, but predetermined. The procedure is charged by plate not by antibiotic.

87186

87186 Susceptibility studies, antimicrobial agent; microdilution or agar dilution (minimum inhibitory concentration [MIC] or breakpoint), each multi-antimicrobial, per plate

Explanation
This procedure may be called an MIC, or a sensitivity test. It is a sensitivity test to determine the susceptibility of a bacterium to an antibiotic. The methodology is microtiter dilution (several commercial panels use this method). Results are given as a minimum inhibitory concentration (MIC) with an interpretation of sensitive, intermediate, or resistant. The antibiotics on commercial plates are numerous, but predetermined. The procedure is charged by plate not by antibiotic.

87187

87187 Susceptibility studies, antimicrobial agent; microdilution or agar dilution, minimum lethal concentration (MLC), each plate (List separately in addition to code for primary procedure)

Explanation
This test may be called an MBC (minimum bactericidal concentration). MBC is the dilution of antibiotic needed to kill the bacteria. MICs are tube dilutions read visually. Tubes that may visually appear to have no growth are cultured to solid media to detect a concentration of antibiotic where no organisms grow (MBC).

87188

87188 Susceptibility studies, antimicrobial agent; macrobroth dilution method, each agent

Explanation
This test may be referred to as an MIC (minimum inhibitory concentration). It is a susceptibility test to determine the sensitivity of a bacterium to an antibiotic. The methodology is macrobroth dilution. Results are given as a minimum inhibitory concentration (MIC) with an interpretation of sensitive, intermediate, or resistant. The procedure is charged per antibiotic tested.

87205

87205 Smear, primary source with interpretation; Gram or Giemsa stain for bacteria, fungi, or cell types

Explanation
Any smear done on a primary source (e.g., sputum, CSF, etc.) to identify bacteria, fungi, and cell types. An interpretation of findings is provided. Bacteria, fungi, WBCs, and epithelial cells may be estimated in quantity with an interpretation as to the possibility of contamination by normal flora. A gram stain may be the most commonly performed smear of this type.

87206

87206 Smear, primary source with interpretation; fluorescent and/or acid fast stain for bacteria, fungi, parasites, viruses or cell types

Explanation
A fluorescent or acid-fast stain for bacteria, fungi, parasites, viruses or cell types. These are stains usually for specific groups of organisms (e.g., mycobacterium and Nocardia). Identification of Cryptosporidium and related parasites are examples of parasites that can be identified by fluorescent or acid fast stain. An interpretation is included.

87207

87207 Smear, primary source with interpretation; special stain for inclusion bodies or parasites (eg, malaria, coccidia, microsporidia, trypanosomes, herpes viruses)

Explanation
This is a stain to look for inclusion bodies or parasites (e.g., malaria inside red cells). Its use to detect herpes has been outdated by amplification and immunological methods. An interpretation is included.

87210

87210 Smear, primary source with interpretation; wet mount for infectious agents (eg, saline, India ink, KOH preps)

Explanation
This test may be requested as a KOH prep. A wet mount is prepared from a primary source to detect bacteria, fungi, or ova and parasites. Motility of organisms is visible on wet mounts and the addition of a simple stain, such as iodine, India ink, or simple dyes, may aid detection of bacteria, fungi, and parasites. An interpretation of findings is included.

87802

87802 Infectious agent antigen detection by immunoassay with direct optical observation; Streptococcus, group B

Explanation
Enzyme immunoassays (EIA) are methods for identifying organisms, extracellular toxins, and viral agents using protein and polysaccharide antigens. The test may my performed directly on clinical samples or after growth on agar plates or in viral cell cultures. The basis of detection is antigen-antibody binding. Cultures and impression smears for both aerobic and anaerobic infectious agents are commonly taken from involved lymph nodes, sputum, pleural fluid, cerebrospinal fluid (CSF), and spleen. Direct optical microscopic observation allows for continuous direct observation of low-light or low-contrast samples in the presence of fluorescence. This code reports the detection of Streptococcus, group B.

88304-88309

88304 Level III - Surgical pathology, gross and microscopic examination
88305 Level IV - Surgical pathology, gross and microscopic examination
88307 Level V - Surgical pathology, gross and microscopic examination
88309 Level VI - Surgical pathology, gross and microscopic examination

Explanation
These examinations would be ordered as a gross and microscopic pathology exam or a gross and microscopic tissue exam. Tissue is submitted in a container labeled with the tissue source, preoperative diagnosis, and patient identification information. Specimens from separate sites must be submitted in separate containers, each labeled with the tissue source. Codes 88304-88309 describe levels of service for specimens requiring additional levels of work due to a presumed presence of disease. Code 88304 describes the lowest level of complexity for diseased or abnormal tissue with each subsequent code (88305, 88307, and 88309) describing in ascending order higher levels of complexity and physician work. Specific types of disease and tissue sites are listed for each code in the CPT(r) description.

88312-88314

88312 Special stains; Group I for microorganisms (eg, Gridley, acid fast, methenamine silver), including interpretation and report, each
88313 Group II, all other (eg, iron, trichrome), except immunocytochemistry and immunoperoxidase stains, including interpretation and report, each
88314 histochemical staining with frozen section(s), including interpretation and report (List separately in addition to code for primary procedure)

Explanation
These codes report stains used in the evaluation of some tissue specimens. Depending on the type of specimen and the reason for the pathology examination, different stains may be required to highlight or outline cells for identification. Code 88312 reports Group I stains for microorganisms; 88313 reports Group II stains for all other conditions excluding immunocytochemistry and immunoperoxidase. Examples of Group II stains include Ziehl-Neelsen, acid phosphatase stain with and without tartrate, alpha-naphthyl esterase stain with and without fluoride, amyloid, ASD chloroacetate esterase stain, nonspecific esterase, PAS stain, and Sudan black stain. Code 88314 reports histochemical staining with frozen sections, and is reported in addition to the code for the primary procedure. All codes within this range include interpretation and report.

88362

88362 Nerve teasing preparations

Explanation
Teased fiber evaluation is a technique used in specialty neuropathology labs. Peripheral nerves are often encased in a myelin sheath. This lipid-like substance is important to nerve function and can be an element in diagnostic evaluation. The technique involves biopsy collection, usually under local anesthetic. Light and electron microscopy are usually employed. Individual nerve fibers are "teased" from surrounding tissues to analyze myelinated nerve fiber size, distribution, and density.

88380

88380 Microdissection (ie, sample preparation of microscopically identified target); laser capture

Explanation
Laser capture microdissection (LCM) is a method for procuring pure cells from specific microscopic regions of tissue sections to study developing disease lesions in actual tissue. A transfer film is applied to the surface of the tissue section. Under the microscope, the diagnostic pathologist or researcher views the thin tissue section and chooses microscopic clusters of cells to study. When the cells of choice are in the center of the field of view, a pulsed laser beam activates a spot on the transfer film immediately above the cells of interest. At this location the film melts and fuses with the underlying cells. When the film is removed, the chosen cells are held, while the rest of the tissue is left behind. This allows multiple homogeneous samples within the tissue section to be targeted for analysis. Under the microscope, tissues are heterogeneous structures with hundreds of different cell types locked in units that adhere to adjacent cells, connective stroma, blood vessels, glandular and muscle co

89050-89051

89050 Cell count, miscellaneous body fluids (eg, cerebrospinal fluid, joint fluid), except blood;
89051 with differential count

Explanation
CSF cell count may also be referred to as a CSF analysis or spinal fluid analysis; joint fluid cell count may also be referred to as synovial fluid analysis. In 89050, a manual nucleated blood cell count using a hemacytometer is performed on fluids obtained during a separately reportable spinal puncture or arthrocentesis. In 89051, a differential cell study using manually prepared smears or a cytocentrifuge is performed in addition to the cell count. Depending on the suspected condition, a number of separately reportable additional tests may be performed.

89060

89060 Crystal identification by light microscopy with or without polarizing lens analysis, tissue or any body fluid (except urine)

Explanation
A fluid sample is obtained. A variety of different methods may be used to process the specimen depending on the source. The fluid is analyzed for the presence of crystals using direct light or polarized light microscopy. A newer technique using atomic force microscopy (AFM) may be available in some laboratories.

93922-93923

93922 Limited bilateral noninvasive physiologic studies of upper or lower extremity arteries (eg, for lower extremity: ankle/brachial indices at distal posterior tibial and anterior tibial/dorsalis pedis arteries plus bidirectional, Doppler waveform recording and analysis at 1-2 levels, or ankle/brachial indices at distal posterior tibial and anterior tibial/dorsalis pedis arteries plus volume plethysmography at 1-2 levels, or ankle/brachial indices at distal posterior tibial and anterior tibial/dorsalis pedis arteries with transcutaneous oxygen tension measurements at 1-2 levels)

93923 Complete bilateral noninvasive physiologic studies of upper or lower extremity arteries, 3 or more levels (eg, for lower extremity: ankle/brachial indices at distal posterior tibial and anterior tibial/dorsalis pedis arteries plus segmental blood pressure measurements with bidirectional Doppler waveform recording and analysis, at 3 or more levels, or ankle/brachial indices at distal posterior tibial and anterior tibial/dorsalis pedis arteries plus segmental volume plethysmography at 3 or more levels, or ankle/brachial indices at distal posterior tibial and anterior tibial/dorsalis pedis arteries plus segmental transcutaneous oxygen tension measurements at 3 or more level(s), or single level study with provocative functional maneuvers (eg, measurements with postural provocative tests, or measurements with reactive hyperemia)

Explanation
The physician or assistant evaluates the arteries of the arms or legs to check blood flow in relation to blockage. In one example, the physician places a transducer on each leg at a prescribed level and measures the change in blood-handling characteristics during constriction by pneumatic cuffs. Technique is similar to constriction and measuring of tension in the vascular system, but the medium may change. Code 93922 applies to ultrasound, plethysmography, and oxygen tension measurements in a bilateral evaluation limited to one or two levels. Code 93923 includes three or more levels or a single-level study with provocative functional maneuvers.

Coding Tips
These codes have been revised for 2011 in the official CPT description.

93930

93930 Duplex scan of upper extremity arteries or arterial bypass grafts; complete bilateral study

Explanation
A diagnostic study is performed on the upper extremity arteries or arterial bypass grafts. A duplex scan involves a two-dimensional ultrasonic scan, which provides a two-dimensional display of the structure. This procedure is a complete bilateral study and is not intended to report unilateral procedures.

93931

93931 Duplex scan of upper extremity arteries or arterial bypass grafts; unilateral or limited study

Explanation
A diagnostic study is performed on a specific site or area of the upper extremity arteries. A duplex scan involves a two-dimensional ultrasonic scan, which provides a two-dimensional display of the structure. This reports limited or follow-up ultrasounds.

93965

93965 Noninvasive physiologic studies of extremity veins, complete bilateral study (eg, Doppler waveform analysis with responses to compression and other maneuvers, phleborheography, impedance plethysmography)

Explanation
The physician or assistant evaluates the veins in the arms and legs. This code applies to a complete bilateral evaluation including blood flow, plethysmography, and ultrasound.

93970

93970 Duplex scan of extremity veins including responses to compression and other maneuvers; complete bilateral study

Explanation
The physician or assistant performs a Duplex ultrasound scan, which is a combination of real-time and Doppler studies, of the veins in the arms or legs to evaluate vascular blood flow in relation to blockage. This code applies to complete responses to compression and other tests and includes both sides.

93971

93971 Duplex scan of extremity veins including responses to compression and other maneuvers; unilateral or limited study

Explanation
The physician or assistant performs a Duplex ultrasound scan, which is a combination of real-time and Doppler studies, of the veins in the arms or legs to evaluate vascular blood flow in relation to blockage. This code applies to complete responses to compression and other tests and includes one side or limited areas of both sides.

95831

95831 Muscle testing, manual (separate procedure) with report; extremity (excluding hand) or trunk

Explanation
Muscles or muscle groups are tested for strength. This code applies to manually testing the arm, leg, or trunk.

95832

95832 Muscle testing, manual (separate procedure) with report; hand, with or without comparison with normal side

Explanation
Muscles or muscle groups are tested for strength. This code applies to manually testing the hands.

95833

95833 Muscle testing, manual (separate procedure) with report; total evaluation of body, excluding hands

Explanation
Muscles or muscle groups are tested for strength. This code applies to manually testing the body exclusive of the hands.

95834

95834 Muscle testing, manual (separate procedure) with report; total evaluation of body, including hands

Explanation
Muscles or muscle groups are tested for strength. This code applies to manually testing the body inclusive of the hands.

95851

95851 Range of motion measurements and report (separate procedure); each extremity (excluding hand) or each trunk section (spine)

Explanation
Testing determines active and passive range of motion for extremities and joints. This code applies to manually testing each arm or leg or sections of the spinal muscles in a separately reported procedure.

95852

95852 Range of motion measurements and report (separate procedure); hand, with or without comparison with normal side

Explanation
Testing determines active and passive range of motion for extremities and joints. This code applies to manually testing the hands.

95860-95864

95860 Needle electromyography; 1 extremity with or without related paraspinal areas
95861 2 extremities with or without related paraspinal areas
95863 3 extremities with or without related paraspinal areas
95864 4 extremities with or without related paraspinal areas

Explanation
Needle electromyography (EMG) records the electrical properties of muscle using an oscilloscope. Recordings, which may be amplified and heard through a loudspeaker, are made during needle insertion, with the muscle at rest, and during contraction. Report 95860 when one extremity (arm or leg) is tested; 95861 for tests of two extremities; 95863 for tests of three extremities; and 95864 for tests of four extremities.

95869-95870

95869 Needle electromyography; thoracic paraspinal muscles (excluding T1 or T12)
95870 limited study of muscles in 1 extremity or non-limb (axial) muscles (unilateral or bilateral), other than thoracic paraspinal, cranial nerve supplied muscles, or sphincters

Explanation
Needle electromyography (EMG) records the electrical properties of thoracic paraspinal muscles (95869) using an oscilloscope. Recordings, which may be amplified and heard through a loudspeaker, are made during needle insertion, with the muscle at rest, and during contraction. Report 95870 for a limited study of muscles in one extremity or non-limb (axial) muscles other than thoracic paraspinal or cranial supplied muscles or sphincters.

95872

95872 Needle electromyography using single fiber electrode, with quantitative measurement of jitter, blocking and/or fiber density, any/all sites of each muscle studied

Explanation
Needle electromyography (EMG) records the electrical properties of muscle using an oscilloscope. Recordings, which may be amplified and heard through a loudspeaker, are made during needle insertion, with the muscle at rest, and during contraction. This procedure uses a single fiber electrode to obtain additional information on specific muscles, including quantitative measurement of jitter, blocking, and/or fiber density.

95875

95875 Ischemic limb exercise test with serial specimen(s) acquisition for muscle(s) metabolite(s)

Explanation
Needle electromyography (EMG) records the electrical properties of muscle using an oscilloscope. Recordings, which may be amplified and heard through a loudspeaker, are made during needle insertion, with the muscle at rest, and during contraction. This procedure tests electrical properties of ischemic limb during exercise and includes lactic acid determination.

95900-95904

95900 Nerve conduction, amplitude and latency/velocity study, each nerve; motor, without F-wave study
95903 motor, with F-wave study
95904 sensory

Explanation
Nerve testing uses sensors to measure and record nerve functions including conduction, amplitude, and latency/velocity. Nerves are stimulated with electric shocks along the course of the muscle. The time required to initiate contraction is measured and recorded. Measurements of distal latency, the time required to traverse the segment nearest the muscle, and conduction velocity, the time required for an impulse to travel a measured length of nerve, are also recorded. Report 95900 for motor testing without F-wave studies; 95903 for motor testing with F-wave studies; and 95904 if the test is of sensory response.

95905

95905 Motor and/or sensory nerve conduction, using preconfigured electrode array(s), amplitude and latency/velocity study, each limb, includes F-wave study when performed, with interpretation and report

Explanation
Nerve testing uses sensors to measure and record nerve functions including conduction, amplitude, and latency/velocity. Nerves are stimulated with electric shocks along the course of the muscle. The time required to initiate contraction is measured and recorded. Measurements of distal latency (the time required to traverse the segment nearest the muscle) and conduction velocity (the time required for an impulse to travel a measured length of nerve) are also recorded. Code 95905 reports motor and/or sensory nerve conduction tests performed using preconfigured electrode arrays. It includes F-wave study, when performed, as well as interpretation and report. Report 95905 only once for each limb studied.

95920

95920 Intraoperative neurophysiology testing, per hour (List separately in addition to code for primary procedure)

Explanation
This code is used when an evoked potential study is required during surgery. This is often necessary to determine what effect a surgery is having on specific nerve functions. In some cases, continuous monitoring is necessary. Report this code per hour.

95925-95927

95925 Short-latency somatosensory evoked potential study, stimulation of any/all peripheral nerves or skin sites, recording from the central nervous system; in upper limbs
95926 in lower limbs
95927 in the trunk or head

Explanation
The physician uses somatosensory-evoked potential to provide information about the integrity of the peripheral nerves, spinal cord, brain stem, and the cortex. Evoked potentials require low voltages and the placement of electrodes on the scalp near the parts of the nervous system where the signals are generated. The physician may place electrical stimulation at the median nerve of the wrist or the posterior tibial nerve at the ankle, or the physician may stimulate points between these and the central nervous system. Many applications may be necessary to screen background noise to measure the interval between stimulation and generated response. Report 95925 if the upper limbs are being tested; 95926 for tests of the lower limbs; and 95927 for tests of the trunk or head.

95934

95934 H-reflex, amplitude and latency study; record gastrocnemius/soleus muscle

Explanation
The physician uses sensors to measure and record nerve functions such as conduction and amplitude. This code applies to testing the amplitude and latency (H-reflex) of the lower leg muscles.

95936

95936 H-reflex, amplitude and latency study; record muscle other than gastrocnemius/soleus muscle

Explanation
The physician uses sensors to measure and record nerve functions such as conduction and amplitude. This code applies to testing the amplitude and latency (H-reflex) of muscles other than the lower leg muscles.

95937
95937 Neuromuscular junction testing (repetitive stimulation, paired stimuli), each nerve, any 1 method

Explanation
The physician uses sensors to measure and record nerve functions such as conduction and amplitude. This code applies to measure the junction between nerves and muscles for one nerve.

95965-95967
95965 Magnetoencephalography (MEG), recording and analysis; for spontaneous brain magnetic activity (eg, epileptic cerebral cortex localization)
95966 for evoked magnetic fields, single modality (eg, sensory, motor, language, or visual cortex localization)
95967 for evoked magnetic fields, each additional modality (eg, sensory, motor, language, or visual cortex localization) (List separately in addition to code for primary procedure)

Explanation
Magnetoencephalography (MEG) provides functional mapping information about how the brain processes sensory stimulation by measuring the associated magnetic fields emanating from the outer surface of the brain. MEG can be used both as a tool for fundamental study of the brain and for assessing patients with specific neurological disorders. The biomagnetometer is commonly housed in a shielded room; the recording device contains magnetic detection coils continuously bathed in liquid helium to superconducting temperatures of -269 degrees Celsius. The spontaneous (95965) or evoked (95966-95967) magnetic fields emanating from the brain induce a current in these coils, which in turn produce a magnetic field in a device called a superconducting quantum interference device (SQUID), which makes images every 1/1000 of a second. MEG identifies where in the brain the electrical current is flowing in response to the stimulus. For example, MEG can be used to determine the millimeters of the brain responsible for fingertip sensation and movement, which can be crucial in surgeries involving neuroresection.

95970
95970 Electronic analysis of implanted neurostimulator pulse generator system (eg, rate, pulse amplitude and duration, configuration of wave form, battery status, electrode selectability, output modulation, cycling, impedance and patient compliance measurements); simple or complex brain, spinal cord, or peripheral (ie, cranial nerve, peripheral nerve, autonomic nerve, neuromuscular) neurostimulator pulse generator/transmitter, without reprogramming

Explanation
A previously placed neurostimulator pulse generator is tested to verify that is it functioning properly. The neurostimulator may be either a simple or complex brain, spinal cord, or peripheral device. Functions that may be tested include rate, pulse amplitude and duration, configuration of waveform, battery status, electrode selectability, output modulation, cycling, impedance, and patient compliance. This code reports testing without reprogramming of the device.

95971
95971 Electronic analysis of implanted neurostimulator pulse generator system (eg, rate, pulse amplitude and duration, configuration of wave form, battery status, electrode selectability, output modulation, cycling, impedance and patient compliance measurements); simple spinal cord, or peripheral (ie, peripheral nerve, autonomic nerve, neuromuscular) neurostimulator pulse generator/transmitter, with intraoperative or subsequent programming

Explanation
A previously placed neurostimulator pulse generator is tested to verify that is it functioning properly. In this case, a simple brain, spinal cord, or peripheral device is tested. A simple device affects only three or fewer of the following: pulse amplitude, pulse duration, pulse frequency, eight or more electrode contacts, cycling, stimulation train duration, train spacing, number of programs, number of channels, phase angle, alternating electrode polarities, configuration of wave form, or more than one clinical feature. All of the functions that apply may be tested intraoperatively or on subsequent occasions. This code reports testing with reprogramming of the device.

95972-95973
95972 Electronic analysis of implanted neurostimulator pulse generator system (eg, rate, pulse amplitude and duration, configuration of wave form, battery status, electrode selectability, output modulation, cycling, impedance and patient compliance measurements); complex spinal cord, or peripheral (except cranial nerve) neurostimulator pulse generator/transmitter, with intraoperative or subsequent programming, first hour
95973 complex spinal cord, or peripheral (except cranial nerve) neurostimulator pulse generator/transmitter, with intraoperative or subsequent programming, each additional 30 minutes after first hour (List separately in addition to code for primary procedure)

Explanation
A previously placed neurostimulator pulse generator is tested to verify that is it functioning properly. In this case, a complex brain, spinal cord or peripheral device is tested. A complex device affects more than three of the following: pulse amplitude, pulse duration, pulse frequency, eight or more electrode contacts, cycling, stimulation train duration, train spacing, number of programs, number of channels, phase angle, alternating electrode polarities, configuration of wave form, or more than one clinical feature. All of the functions that apply may be tested intraoperatively or on subsequent occasions. Report 95972 for the first hour of testing and reprogramming of the device. Report 95973 for each additional 30 minutes of testing and reprogramming.

95990-95991
95990 Refilling and maintenance of implantable pump or reservoir for drug delivery, spinal (intrathecal, epidural) or brain (intraventricular);
95991 administered by physician

Explanation
Refilling and maintenance of an implantable spinal (intrathecal, epidural) or intraventricular (brain) pump or reservoir is done. Implantable pumps or reservoirs are placed in subcutaneous pockets at appropriate sites on the body and hold a long-term supply of the drug or medication being infused into the patient. They are refilled through the skin by a needle placed into the pump device. The patient's specific pump is identified and the required volume amount is checked. The site of the implant is prepped. The refill kit is assembled in a sterile procedure and a template is positioned over the site. A needle is inserted through the template center hole and into the pump/reservoir, which is

then filled with more drug infusate. Report 95991 when a physician administers the drug refill.

96002

96002 Dynamic surface electromyography, during walking or other functional activities, 1-12 muscles

Explanation

Electrodes placed on the muscle belly, parallel to the grain of the muscle fiber, detects an electrical signal that comes from active muscles (the patient is in motion during the test). The strength and pattern of the signal is seen on a computer screen and the data is collected in a software program that is able to run various analyses of the data to create useful reports regarding muscle function. For example, gait analysis allows the clinician to analyze time normal activation patterns separately for stance and swing phases between conditions or against data base values. Report 96002 for a study of one to 12 muscles. Report 96004 in addition to this code for physician review and interpretation of results, which includes the physician's written report.

96003

96003 Dynamic fine wire electromyography, during walking or other functional activities, 1 muscle

Explanation

Electrodes placed on the muscle belly, parallel to the grain of the muscle fiber, detect an electrical signal that comes from active muscles (the patient is in motion during the test). The strength and pattern of the signal is seen on a computer screen and the data is collected in a software program that is able to run various analyses of the data to create useful reports regarding muscle function. For example, gait analysis allows the clinician to analyze time normal activation patterns separately for stance and swing phases between conditions or against database values. Use 96003 to report dynamic fine wire electromyography for one muscle. Report 96004 in addition to this code for physician review and interpretation of results, which includes the physician's written report.

96004

96004 Physician review and interpretation of comprehensive computer-based motion analysis, dynamic plantar pressure measurements, dynamic surface electromyography during walking or other functional activities, and dynamic fine wire electromyography, with written report

Explanation

The physician reviews and interprets computer-based motion analysis, dynamic plantar pressure measurements, dynamic surface electromyography during walking or other functional activities, and dynamic fine wire electromyography performed using codes 96000, 96001, 96002, and 96003 to report the service.

96365-96368

96365 Intravenous infusion, for therapy, prophylaxis, or diagnosis (specify substance or drug); initial, up to 1 hour
96366 each additional hour (List separately in addition to code for primary procedure)
96367 additional sequential infusion, up to 1 hour (List separately in addition to code for primary procedure)
96368 concurrent infusion (List separately in addition to code for primary procedure)

Explanation

A physician or an assistant under direct physician supervision injects or infuses a therapeutic, prophylactic (preventive), or diagnostic medication other than chemotherapy or other highly complex drugs or biologic agents via intravenous route. Infusions are administered through an intravenous catheter inserted by needle into a patient's vein or by injection or infusion through an existing indwelling intravascular access catheter or port. Report 96365 for the initial hour and 96366 for each additional hour. Report 96367 for each additional sequential infusion, up to one hour, and 96368 for each concurrent infusion of substances other than chemotherapy or other highly complex drugs or biologic agents.

96372-96376

96372 Therapeutic, prophylactic, or diagnostic injection (specify substance or drug); subcutaneous or intramuscular
96373 intra-arterial
96374 intravenous push, single or initial substance/drug
96375 each additional sequential intravenous push of a new substance/drug (List separately in addition to code for primary procedure)
96376 each additional sequential intravenous push of the same substance/drug provided in a facility (List separately in addition to code for primary procedure)

Explanation

The physician or an assistant under direct physician supervision administers a therapeutic, prophylactic, or diagnostic substance by subcutaneous or intramuscular injection (96372), intra-arterial injection (96373), or by push into an intravenous catheter or intravascular access device (96374 for a single or initial substance, 96375 for each additional sequential IV push of a new substance, and 96376 for each additional sequential IV push of the same substance after 30 minutes have elapsed). The push technique involves an infusion of less than 15 minutes. Code 96376 may be reported only by facilities.

96450

96450 Chemotherapy administration, into CNS (eg, intrathecal), requiring and including spinal puncture

Explanation

The physician or supervised assistant prepares and administers medication to combat diseases such as malignant neoplasms or microorganisms. This code applies to medication injected into the spinal cord through a catheter placed through the space between the lower back bones (lumbar puncture).

97001

97001 Physical therapy evaluation

Explanation

The physical therapist (PT) examines the patient/client. This includes taking a comprehensive history, systems review, and tests and measures. Tests and measures may include but are not limited to tests of range of motion, motor function, muscle performance, joint integrity, neuromuscular status, and review of orthotic or prosthetic devices. The PT formulates an assessment, prognosis, and notes an anticipated intervention.

97002

97002 Physical therapy re-evaluation

Explanation

The physical therapist (PT) re-examines the patient/client to obtain objective measures of progress toward stated goals. Tests and measures include but are not limited to those noted in 97001. The PT modifies the treatment plan as is indicated to support medical necessity of skilled intervention.

97003

97003 Occupational therapy evaluation

Explanation

The occupational therapist evaluates the patient. Various movements required for activities of daily living are examined. Dexterity, range of movement, and other elements may also be studied.

97004

97004 Occupational therapy re-evaluation

Explanation

The occupational therapist re-evaluates the patient to gauge progress of therapy. Various movements required for activities of daily living are examined. Dexterity, range of movement, and other elements may also be studied.

97005

97005 Athletic training evaluation

Explanation
The health care provider examines the patient, which includes taking a comprehensive history, systems review, and obtaining tests of range of motion, motor function, muscle performance, joint integrity, and neuromuscular status. The physical therapist formulates an assessment, prognosis, and notes the anticipated intervention.

97006
97006 Athletic training re-evaluation

Explanation
The health care provider re-examines the patient to obtain objective measures of progress toward stated goals. Tests include, but are not limited to, range of motion, motor function, muscle performance, joint integrity, and neuromuscular status. The physical therapist modifies the treatment plan as is indicated to support medical necessity of skilled intervention.

97010
97010 Application of a modality to 1 or more areas; hot or cold packs

Explanation
The clinician applies heat (dry or moist) or cold to one or more body parts with appropriate padding to prevent skin irritation. The patient is given necessary safety instructions. The treatment requires supervision only and one unit may be billed per day.

97012
97012 Application of a modality to 1 or more areas; traction, mechanical

Explanation
The clinician applies sustained or intermittent mechanical traction to the cervical and/or lumbar spine. The mechanical force produces distraction between the vertebrae thereby relieving pain and increasing tissue flexibility. Once applied, the treatment requires supervision and one unit may be billed per day.

97014
97014 Application of a modality to 1 or more areas; electrical stimulation (unattended)

Explanation
The clinician applies electrical stimulation to one or more areas in order to stimulate muscle function, enhance healing, and alleviate pain and/or edema. The clinician chooses which type of electrical stimulation is appropriate. The treatment is supervised after the electrodes are applied and only one unit may be billed per day.

97016
97016 Application of a modality to 1 or more areas; vasopneumatic devices

Explanation
The clinician applies a vasopneumatic device to treat extremity edema (usually lymphedema). A pressurized sleeve is applied. Girth measurements are taken pre- and posttreatment. This code can only be billed one unit per day.

97018
97018 Application of a modality to 1 or more areas; paraffin bath

Explanation
A clinician uses a paraffin bath to apply superficial heat to a hand or foot. The part is repeatedly dipped into the paraffin forming a glove. Use of paraffin facilitates treatment of arthritis and other conditions that cause limitations in joint flexibility. Once the paraffin is applied and the patient instruction provided, the procedure requires supervision. This code can only be billed one unit per day.

97022
97022 Application of a modality to 1 or more areas; whirlpool

Explanation
The clinician uses a whirlpool to provide superficial heat in an environment that facilitates tissue debridement, wound cleaning, and/or exercise. The clinician decides the appropriate water temperature, provides safety instruction, and supervises the treatment. This code can only be billed one unit per day.

97024
97024 Application of a modality to 1 or more areas; diathermy (eg, microwave)

Explanation
The clinician uses diathermy or microwave as a form of superficial heat for one or more body areas. After application and safety instructions have been provided, the clinician supervises the treatment.

97026
97026 Application of a modality to 1 or more areas; infrared

Explanation
The clinician uses infrared light as a form of superficial heat that will increase circulation to one or more localized areas. Once applied and safety instructions have been provided, the treatment is supervised. This code can only be billed one unit per day.

97028
97028 Application of a modality to 1 or more areas; ultraviolet

Explanation
The clinician applies ultraviolet light to treat dermatological problems. Once applied and safety instructions have been provided, the treatment is supervised. This code can only be billed one unit per day.

97032
97032 Application of a modality to 1 or more areas; electrical stimulation (manual), each 15 minutes

Explanation
The clinician applies electrical stimulation to one or more areas to promote muscle function, wound healing edema, and/or pain control. This treatment requires direct contact by the provider and can be billed in multiple 15-minute units.

97033
97033 Application of a modality to 1 or more areas; iontophoresis, each 15 minutes

Explanation
The clinician uses electrical current to administer medication to one or more areas. Iontophoresis is usually prescribed for soft tissue inflammatory conditions and pain control. This code requires constant attendance by the clinician and can be billed in 15-minute units.

97034
97034 Application of a modality to 1 or more areas; contrast baths, each 15 minutes

Explanation
The clinician uses hot and cold baths in a repeated, alternating fashion to stimulate the vasomotor response of a localized body part. This code requires constant attendance and can be billed in 15-minute units.

97035
97035 Application of a modality to 1 or more areas; ultrasound, each 15 minutes

Explanation
The clinician applies ultrasound to increase circulation to one or more areas. A water bath or some form of ultrasound lotion must be used as a coupling agent to facilitate the procedure. The delivery of corticosteroid medication via ultrasound is called phonophoresis. Ultrasound or phonophoresis requires constant attendance and can be billed in 15-minute units.

97036
97036 Application of a modality to 1 or more areas; Hubbard tank, each 15 minutes

Explanation
Hubbard tank is used when it is necessary to immerse the full body into water. Care of wounds and burns my require use of the Hubbard tank to facilitate tissue cleansing and debridement. This code requires constant attendance and can be billed in 15-minute units.

97110
97110 Therapeutic procedure, 1 or more areas, each 15 minutes; therapeutic exercises to develop strength and endurance, range of motion and flexibility

Explanation
The clinician and/or patient perform therapeutic exercises to one or more body areas to develop strength, endurance, and flexibility. This code requires direct contact and may be billed in 15-minute units.

97112
97112 Therapeutic procedure, 1 or more areas, each 15 minutes; neuromuscular reeducation of movement, balance, coordination, kinesthetic sense, posture, and/or proprioception for sitting and/or standing activities

Explanation
The clinician and/or patient perform activities to one or more body areas that facilitate reeducation of movement, balance, coordination, kinesthetic sense, posture, and proprioception. This code requires direct contact and may be billed in 15-minute units.

97113
97113 Therapeutic procedure, 1 or more areas, each 15 minutes; aquatic therapy with therapeutic exercises

Explanation
The clinician directs and/or performs therapeutic exercises with the patient/client in the aquatic environment. This code requires skilled intervention by the clinician and documentation must support medical necessity of the aquatic environment. This code can be billed in 15-minute units.

97116
97116 Therapeutic procedure, 1 or more areas, each 15 minutes; gait training (includes stair climbing)

Explanation
The clinician instructs the patient in specific activities that will facilitate ambulation and stair climbing with or without an assistive device. Proper sequencing and safety instructions are included when appropriate. This code requires direct contact and may be billed in 15-minute units.

97124
97124 Therapeutic procedure, 1 or more areas, each 15 minutes; massage, including effleurage, petrissage and/or tapotement (stroking, compression, percussion)

Explanation
The clinician uses massage to provide muscle relaxation, increase localized circulation, soften scar tissue, or mobilize mucous secretions in the lung via tapotement and/or percussion. This code requires direct contact and can be billed in 15-minute units, regardless of number of body parts treated.

97139
97139 Unlisted therapeutic procedure (specify)

Explanation
This code may be used if the clinician performs a therapeutic procedure to one or more body areas that is not listed under the current codes. A narrative descriptor should be noted on the claim. This code is reported for each 15-minute unit.

97140
97140 Manual therapy techniques (eg, mobilization/ manipulation, manual lymphatic drainage, manual traction), 1 or more regions, each 15 minutes

Explanation
The clinician performs manual therapy techniques including soft tissue and joint mobilization, manipulation, manual traction, and/or manual lymphatic drainage to one or more areas. This code requires direct contact with the patient and can be billed in 15-minute units.

97150
97150 Therapeutic procedure(s), group (2 or more individuals)

Explanation
The clinician supervises group activities (two or more patients/clients) of therapeutic procedures on land or the aquatic environment. The patients/clients do not have to be performing the same activity simultaneously, however, the need for skilled intervention must be documented. This code can be billed in 15-minute units.

97530
97530 Therapeutic activities, direct (one-on-one) patient contact by the provider (use of dynamic activities to improve functional performance), each 15 minutes

Explanation
The clinician uses dynamic therapeutic activities designed to achieve improved functional performance (e.g., lifting, pulling, bending). This code requires direct contact and can be billed in 15-minute units.

97533
97533 Sensory integrative techniques to enhance sensory processing and promote adaptive responses to environmental demands, direct (one-on-one) patient contact by the provider, each 15 minutes

Explanation
Sensory experiences include touch, movement, body awareness, sight, sound, and the pull of gravity. The process of the brain organizing and interpreting this information is called sensory integration. Sensory integration provides a crucial foundation for later, more complex learning and behavior. An occupational therapist or rehabilitation specialist works one-on-one with individuals with sensory integration disorders to provide techniques for enhancing sensory processing and adapting to environmental demands. Sensory integration disorders may be the result of a learning disability, illness, or brain injury.

97535
97535 Self-care/home management training (eg, activities of daily living (ADL) and compensatory training, meal preparation, safety procedures, and instructions in use of assistive technology devices/adaptive equipment) direct one-on-one contact by provider, each 15 minutes

Explanation
The clinician instructs and trains the patients in self-care and home management activities (e.g., ADL and use of adaptive equipment in the kitchen, bath, and/or car). Direct contact is required. This code can be billed in 15-minute units.

97537
97537 Community/work reintegration training (eg, shopping, transportation, money management, avocational activities and/or work environment/modification analysis, work task analysis, use of assistive technology device/adaptive equipment), direct one-on-one contact by provider, each 15 minutes

Explanation
The clinician instructs and trains the patient/client in community re-integration activities (e.g., work task analysis and modification, safe accessing of transportation). This requires direct supervision and can be billed in 15-minute units.

97542
97542 Wheelchair management (eg, assessment, fitting, training), each 15 minutes

Explanation
The clinician assesses the patient for the type and size of a wheelchair or trains the patient in the proper wheelchair skills (e.g., propulsion, safety techniques).

97545-97546

97545 Work hardening/conditioning; initial 2 hours

97546 each additional hour (List separately in addition to code for primary procedure)

Explanation
This code is used for a procedure where the injured worker is put through a series of conditioning exercises and job simulation tasks in preparation for return to work. Endurance, strength, and proper body mechanics are emphasized. The patient is also educated in problem solving skills related to job task performance and employing correct lifting and positioning techniques. Report 97546 for each additional hour after the initial two hours.

97597-97598

97597 Debridement (eg, high pressure waterjet with/without suction, sharp selective debridement with scissors, scalpel and forceps), open wound, (eg, fibrin, devitalized epidermis and/or dermis, exudate, debris, biofilm), including topical application(s), wound assessment, use of a whirlpool, when performed and instruction(s) for ongoing care, per session, total wound(s) surface area; first 20 sq cm or less

97598 each additional 20 sq cm, or part thereof (List separately in addition to code for primary procedure)

Explanation
A health care provider performs wound care management by using selective debridement techniques to remove devitalized or necrotic tissue from an open wound. Selective techniques are those in which the provider has complete control over which tissue is removed and which is left behind, and include high-pressure waterjet with or without suction and sharp debridement using scissors, a scalpel, or forceps. Autolytic debridement is accomplished using occlusive or semi-occlusive dressings that keep wound fluid in contact with the necrotic tissue. Types of dressing applications used in autolytic debridement include hydrocolloids, hydrogels, and transparent films. Wound assessment, topical applications, instructions regarding ongoing care of the wound, and the possible use of a whirlpool for treatment are included in these codes. Report 97597 for a total wound surface area less than or equal to 20 sq cm and 97598 for each additional 20 sq cm or part thereof.

Coding Tips
These codes have been revised for 2011 in the official CPT description.

97602

97602 Removal of devitalized tissue from wound(s), non-selective debridement, without anesthesia (eg, wet-to-moist dressings, enzymatic, abrasion), including topical application(s), wound assessment, and instruction(s) for ongoing care, per session

Explanation
The physician performs wound care management to promote healing using either selective or non-selective debridement techniques to remove devitalized tissue. Selective techniques are those in which the physician has complete control over which tissue is removed and which is left behind. Selective techniques include high-pressure waterjet and sharp debridement techniques using scissors, a scalpel, or tweezers. Another newer method of selective debridement is autolysis, which uses the body's own enzymes and moisture to re-hydrate, soften, and finally liquefy hard eschar and slough. Autolytic debridement is accomplished using occlusive or semi-occlusive dressings that keep wound fluid in contact with the necrotic tissue. Types of dressings used in autolytic debridement include hydrocolloids, hydrogels, and transparent films. Non-selective debridement techniques are those in which both necrotic and healthy tissue are removed. Non-selective techniques, sometimes referred to as mechanical debridement, include wet-to-moist dressings, enzymatic chemicals, and abrasion. Wet-to-moist debridement involves allowing a dressing to proceed from moist to wet, then manually removing the dressing, which removes both the necrotic and healthy tissue. Chemical enzymes are fast acting products that produce slough of necrotic tissue.

97605-97606

97605 Negative pressure wound therapy (eg, vacuum assisted drainage collection), including topical application(s), wound assessment, and instruction(s) for ongoing care, per session; total wound(s) surface area less than or equal to 50 square centimeters

97606 total wound(s) surface area greater than 50 square centimeters

Explanation
The physician prescribes negative pressure wound therapy (NPWT) with vacuum assisted drainage collection to promote healing of a chronic non-healing wound, including diabetic or pressure (decubitus) ulcer. This procedure includes topical applications to the wound, wound assessment, and patient or caregiver instruction related to on-going care per session. Negative pressure wound therapy uses controlled application of subatmospheric pressure to a wound. The subatmospheric pressure is generated using an electrical pump. The electrical pump conveys intermittent or continuous subatmospheric pressure through connecting tubing to a specialized wound dressing. The specialized wound dressing includes a porous foam dressing that covers the entire wound surface and an airtight adhesive dressing that seals the wound and contains the subatmospheric pressure at the wound site. Negative pressure wound therapy promotes healing by increasing local vascularity and oxygenation of the wound bed, evacuating wound fluid thereby reducing edema, and removing exudates and bacteria. Drainage from the wound is collected in a canister. Report 97605 for a wound(s) with a total surface area less than or equal to 50.0 sq. cm. Report 97606 for a wound(s) with a total surface area greater than 50.0 sq. cm.

97750

97750 Physical performance test or measurement (eg, musculoskeletal, functional capacity), with written report, each 15 minutes

Explanation
The clinician performs a test of physical performance evaluating function of one or more body areas and evaluates functional capacity. A written report is included. This is in addition to a routine evaluation or re-evaluation (97001-97004). This code can be billed in 15-minute increments.

97760

97760 Orthotic(s) management and training (including assessment and fitting when not otherwise reported), upper extremity(s), lower extremity(s) and/or trunk, each 15 minutes

Explanation
The clinician fits and/or trains the patient in the use of an orthotic device for one or more body parts. This includes assessment as to type of orthotic when appropriate. This does not include fabrication time, if appropriate, or cost of materials.

97761

97761 Prosthetic training, upper and/or lower extremity(s), each 15 minutes

Explanation
The clinician fits and/or trains the patient in the use of a prosthetic device for one or more body parts. This includes assessment for the appropriate type of prosthetic device. This does not include fabrication time, if applicable, or cost of materials.

97762

97762 Checkout for orthotic/prosthetic use, established patient, each 15 minutes

Explanation

The clinician evaluates the effectiveness of an existing orthotic or prosthetic device and makes recommendations for changes, as appropriate.

97810-97811

97810 Acupuncture, 1 or more needles; without electrical stimulation, initial 15 minutes of personal one-on-one contact with the patient

97811 without electrical stimulation, each additional 15 minutes of personal one-on-one contact with the patient, with re-insertion of needle(s) (List separately in addition to code for primary procedure)

Explanation

The physician applies acupuncture therapy by inserting one or more fine needles into the patient as dictated by acupuncture meridians for the relief of pain. The needles are then twirled or manipulated by hand to generate therapeutic stimulation. Report 97810 for the initial 15 minutes of personal one-on-one contact with the patient and 97811 for each additional 15 minutes of personal one-on-one contact with re-insertion of the needle.

97813-97814

97813 Acupuncture, 1 or more needles; with electrical stimulation, initial 15 minutes of personal one-on-one contact with the patient

97814 with electrical stimulation, each additional 15 minutes of personal one-on-one contact with the patient, with re-insertion of needle(s) (List separately in addition to code for primary procedure)

Explanation

The physician applies acupuncture therapy by inserting one or more fine needles into the patient as dictated by acupuncture meridians for the relief of pain. The needles are then energized by employing a micro-current for electrical stimulation. Report 97813 for the initial 15 minutes of personal one-on-one contact with the patient and 97814 for each additional 15 minutes of personal one-on-one contact with re-insertion of the needle.

98925-98929

98925 Osteopathic manipulative treatment (OMT); 1-2 body regions involved
98926 3-4 body regions involved
98927 5-6 body regions involved
98928 7-8 body regions involved
98929 9-10 body regions involved

Explanation

The physician uses these codes to report osteopathic manipulation, unique manual treatments that are used to treat somatic dysfunction and related disorders. Several techniques exist. Body regions included are head, cervical thoracic, lumbar, sacral, pelvic, extremities, rib cage, abdomen, and viscera. Report 98925 if one to two body regions are involved; 98926 if three to four body regions are involved; 98927 if five to six body regions are involved; 98928 if seven to eight body regions are involved; and 98929 if nine body regions are involved.

99051

99051 Service(s) provided in the office during regularly scheduled evening, weekend, or holiday office hours, in addition to basic service

Explanation

This code is adjunct to basic services rendered. The physician reports this code to indicate services provided during posted evening, weekend, or holiday office hours in addition to basic services.

99053

99053 Service(s) provided between 10:00 PM and 8:00 AM at 24-hour facility, in addition to basic service

Explanation

This code is adjunct to basic services rendered. The physician reports this code to indicate services provided between 10 p.m. and 8 a.m. at a 24-hour facility in addition to basic services.

99060

99060 Service(s) provided on an emergency basis, out of the office, which disrupts other scheduled office services, in addition to basic service

Explanation

This code is adjunct to basic services rendered. The physician reports this code to indicate services provided on an emergency basis in a location other than the physician's office that disrupt other scheduled office services.

99506

99506 Home visit for intramuscular injections

Explanation

The home health provider visits a patient's home to perform an intermuscular injection of medication per a physician's or another valid order. The home health provider brings supplies and medications that are necessary to accomplish the injection to the patient's home, including a syringe, needle, liquid disinfectant, cotton ball, and adhesive tape. The procedure involves inserting the needle, aspiration and slow injection, and at the end of the procedure a cotton ball is placed over the injection site. Adhesive tape is applied over the cotton ball.

99601-99602

99601 Home infusion/specialty drug administration, per visit (up to 2 hours);
99602 each additional hour (List separately in addition to code for primary procedure)

Explanation

A home health professional visits the patient at home to perform the infusion of a specialty drug per a physician's order. The home health provider brings the supplies and medication required and administers and oversees the infusion. Each infusion takes up to two hours per visit for 99601. Report 99602 for each additional hour.

0019T

0019T Extracorporeal shock wave involving musculoskeletal system, not otherwise specified, low energy

Explanation

Low energy extracorporeal shock wave delivery involves the application of pressure waves that travel through fluid and soft tissue, with effects of the shock wave occurring at sites where there is a change in impedance, such as the bone-soft tissue interface. The clinician can deliver this therapy in various ways: piezoelectric, electromagnetic, and electrohydraulic. The piezoelectric system utilizes a crystalline material, which when stimulated with high-voltage electricity can expand or contract to initiate a pressure wave in the surrounding fluid. The electromagnetic mechanism has coils that create opposing magnetic fields when an electric current is applied to them, causing a submerged membrane to move, and starting a pressure wave within the fluid. The electrohydraulic method uses a high voltage spark gap. The spark generates a plasma bubble that compresses the liquid, initiating the pressure wave. Each mechanism creates a characteristic waveform and energy density. Extracorporeal shock wave therapy is used in Europe to treat common orthopedic conditions (i.e., plantar calcaneal spurs, epicondylopathic humeri radialis) because of the therapy's stimulatory effect on bone formation. The Food and Drug Administration (FDA) is currently studying the feasibility for similar use in the United States. Other potential uses of extracorporeal shock wave therapy include treating bone marrow hypoxia and subperiosteal hemorrhage, increasing regional blood flow, and activating osteogenic factors such as bone morphogenic protein, direct cellular effects, and mechanical effects as a result of strain gradients.

0054T-0055T

0054T Computer-assisted musculoskeletal surgical navigational orthopedic procedure, with image-guidance based on fluoroscopic images (List separately in addition to code for primary procedure)

0055T Computer-assisted musculoskeletal surgical navigational orthopedic procedure, with image-guidance based on CT/MRI images (List separately in addition to code for primary procedure)

Explanation

Computer-assisted musculoskeletal navigation techniques are used with many orthopedic procedures, especially for accurate placement of the acetabular component during hip replacement surgery. Preoperative images of patient-specific bone geometry are first obtained for the surgical plan in whatever imaging modality is to be used. The patient-specific surgical plan and images are used during surgery to guide the surgeon by combining these with intraoperative navigation capabilities. Optical targets, or trackers, such as digitizing or LED-equipped probes, are attached to points on the bone anatomy or to surgical tools. An optical camera tracks the position of these for accurate navigation and measurement in relation to any bone or instrument movement as the surgery is performed. The software in these navigational systems matches or "registers" the position of the patient on the operating table to the geometric description of the bony surface derived from the images already used to plan the surgery. Multiple images are simultaneously displayed on the monitor. The "virtual" tool trajectory that corresponds to the tracked tool movements is displayed over the previously saved views in real-time as the surgeon operates. These are add-on codes to be used in addition to the primary procedure. Report 0054T for image-guidance based on fluoroscopic imaging and 0055T for CT/MRI imaging. If CT and MRI are both performed, 0055T is reported only once.

0092T

0092T Total disc arthroplasty (artificial disc), anterior approach, including discectomy with end plate preparation (includes osteophytectomy for nerve root or spinal cord decompression and microdissection), each additional interspace, cervical (List separately in addition to code for primary procedure)

Explanation

Total disc arthroplasty is done to replace a severely damaged or diseased intervertebral cervical disc, most often caused by degenerative disc disease. The physician uses an anterior approach to reach multiple damaged cervical vertebrae by making an incision through the neck, avoiding the esophagus, trachea, and thyroid. Retractors separate the intervertebral muscles. The affected intervertebral location is confirmed by separately reportable x-ray. The physician cleans out the intervertebral disc space with a rongeur, removing the cartilaginous material to be replaced in preparation for inserting the implants. This may include osteophytectomy for nerve root or spinal cord decompression, as well as microdissection. One type of implant for total disc replacement has two endplates made of a metal alloy and a convex weight-bearing surface made of ultra high molecular weight polyethylene. The endplates are inserted in a collapsed form and seated into the vertebral bodies above and below the interspaces. Minimal distraction is applied to open the intervertebral spaces, and the polyethylene disc material is snap-fit into the lower endplates. With the disc assemblies complete, the wound is closed and a drain may be placed. Report 0092T for each additional cervical interspace treated with total disc arthroplasty in conjunction with 22856.

0095T

0095T Removal of total disc arthroplasty (artificial disc), anterior approach, each additional interspace, cervical (List separately in addition to code for primary procedure)

Explanation

The physician removes an artificial disc prosthesis placed during a previous disc arthroplasty by anterior approach. The physician approaches the cervical vertebrae by making an incision through the neck, avoiding the esophagus, trachea, and thyroid. Retractors separate the intervertebral muscles. The implant is located and any adhesions are freed. Distraction is applied to open the intervertebral space and the implant is removed. The area is explored and debrided. When the procedure is complete, the fascia and vertebral muscles are repaired and returned to their anatomical positions, drains are placed, and the wound is closed. Code 0095T must be reported in conjunction with 22864; assign once for each additional cervical interspace.

0098T

0098T Revision including replacement of total disc arthroplasty (artificial disc), anterior approach, each additional interspace, cervical (List separately in addition to code for primary procedure)

Explanation

The physician revises an artificial disc prosthesis placed during a previous disc arthroplasty through anterior approach. The prosthesis may be migrating from a lack of fixation and require components to be replaced or adjusted. The physician approaches the cervical vertebrae by making an incision through the neck, avoiding the esophagus, trachea, and thyroid. Retractors separate the intervertebral muscles. The implant is located, the area is explored, and any adhesions are freed. Distraction is applied to open the intervertebral space. The arthroplastic disc is removed, and the endplates of the vertebral body are reshaped and prepped for reinsertion. New height, depth, and width dimensions may also be taken with the vertebral body distracted in cases where another, more appropriately sized disc prosthesis is required. The components are reinserted, and the fascia and vertebral muscles are repaired and returned to their anatomical positions. The incision is closed. Code 0098T must be reported in conjunction with 22861; assign once for each additional cervical interspace.

0101T-0102T

0101T Extracorporeal shock wave involving musculoskeletal system, not otherwise specified, high energy

0102T Extracorporeal shock wave, high energy, performed by a physician, requiring anesthesia other than local, involving lateral humeral epicondyle

Explanation

High-energy extracorporeal shock wave delivery involves the application of pressure waves that travel through fluid and soft tissue, with effects of the shock wave occurring at sites where there is a change in impedance, such as the bone-soft tissue interface. The clinician can deliver this therapy in various ways: piezoelectric, electromagnetic, and electrohydraulic. The piezoelectric system utilizes a crystalline material, which when stimulated with high-voltage electricity can expand or contract to initiate a pressure wave in the surrounding fluid. The electromagnetic mechanism has coils that create opposing magnetic fields when an electric current is applied to them, causing a submerged membrane to move, and starting a pressure wave within the fluid. The electrohydraulic method uses a high-voltage spark gap. The spark generates a plasma bubble that compresses the liquid, initiating the pressure wave. Each mechanism creates a characteristic waveform and energy density. Extracorporeal shock wave therapy is used in Europe to treat common orthopedic conditions (i.e., plantar calcaneal spurs, epicondylopathic humeri radialis) because of the therapy's stimulatory effect on bone formation. The Food and Drug Administration (FDA) is currently studying the feasibility for similar use in the United States. Other potential uses of extracorporeal shock wave therapy include treating bone marrow hypoxia and subperiosteal hemorrhage, increasing regional blood flow, and activating osteogenic factors such as bone morphogenic protein, direct cellular effects, and mechanical effects as a result of strain gradients. Code 0101T reports high energy extracorporeal shock wave application to the musculoskeletal system, not otherwise specified, and 0102T requires anesthesia other than local for high energy shock wave application performed by a physician on the lateral humeral epicondyle.

0163T

0163T Total disc arthroplasty (artificial disc), anterior approach, including discectomy to prepare interspace (other than for decompression), each additional interspace, lumbar (List separately in addition to code for primary procedure)

Explanation

Total disc arthroplasty is done to replace a severely damaged or diseased intervertebral disc, most often caused by degenerative disc disease. The physician uses an anterior approach to reach damaged lumbar vertebrae by making an incision through the abdomen. Some implants require only minimal access, approximately 7 cm long, for a mini-retroperitoneal approach. Retractors separate the intervertebral muscles. The affected intervertebral disc locations are confirmed by separately reportable x-ray. The physician cleans out the intervertebral disc spaces with a rongeur, removing the cartilaginous material to be replaced in preparation for inserting implants. One type of implant for total disc replacement has two endplates made of a metal alloy and a convex weight-bearing surface made of ultra high molecular weight polyethylene. The endplates are inserted in a collapsed form and seated into the vertebral bodies above and below the interspace. Minimal distraction is applied to open the intervertebral spaces, and the polyethylene disc material is snap-fit into the lower endplate. With the disc assemblies complete, the wound is closed and a drain may be placed. Report this code for each additional lumbar disc replacement after the first, which is reported with 22857.

0164T

0164T Removal of total disc arthroplasty, (artificial disc), anterior approach, each additional interspace, lumbar (List separately in addition to code for primary procedure)

Explanation

The physician removes an artificial disc prosthesis placed during a previous disc arthroplasty by anterior approach. The physician uses an anterior approach to reach the implant in the lumbar vertebrae by making an incision through the abdomen. Some implants require only minimal access, approximately 7 cm long, for a mini-retroperitoneal approach. Retractors separate the intervertebral muscles. The affected intervertebral implant location is confirmed by separately reportable x-ray. The physician cleans out the intervertebral disc space with a rongeur, removing the cartilaginous material to be replaced in preparation for removing an implant, and removes the implant. With the disc assembly removal complete, the wound is closed and a drain may be placed. Report 0164T for each additional lumbar artificial disc removal after the first, which is reported with 22865.

0165T

0165T Revision including replacement of total disc arthroplasty (artificial disc), anterior approach, each additional interspace, lumbar (List separately in addition to code for primary procedure)

Explanation

The physician revises an artificial disc prosthesis placed during a previous disc arthroplasty through an anterior approach. The prosthesis may be migrating from a lack of fixation and require components to be replaced or adjusted. The lumbar vertebrae are approached by making an incision through the abdomen. Retractors separate the intervertebral muscles. The implant is located, the area is explored, and any adhesions are freed. Distraction is applied to open the intervertebral space. The arthroplastic disc is removed, and the endplates of the vertebral body are reshaped and prepped for reinsertion. New height, depth, and width dimensions may also be taken with the vertebral body distracted in cases where another, more appropriately sized disc prosthesis is required. The components are reinserted, and the fascia and vertebral muscles are repaired and returned to their anatomical positions. The incision is closed. This code reports each additional lumbar interspace and must be reported in conjunction with 22862.

0171T-0172T

0171T Insertion of posterior spinous process distraction device (including necessary removal of bone or ligament for insertion and imaging guidance), lumbar; single level

0172T each additional level (List separately in addition to code for primary procedure)

Explanation

The physician inserts spinous process distraction devices, also known as interspinous process decompression devices (IPD), in the posterior column of the lumbar spine to enable spinal stabilization without the restrictions in motion that are created by spinal fusion. With the patient under appropriate anesthesia (often local anesthesia with light IV sedation) and in the lateral decubitus position (on the side), the physician makes a posterior 2 to 4 inch midline incision. Removal of bone or ligament may be necessary for device insertion. The spinous processes are exposed at the appropriate level and confirmed radiographically. While preserving the supraspinous ligament, the physician dilates the interspinous ligament and inserts and secures the IPD implant. Report 0171T if the device is inserted at a single level and 0172T for each additional level.

0195T-0196T

0195T Arthrodesis, pre-sacral interbody technique, including instrumentation, imaging (when performed), and discectomy to prepare interspace, lumbar; single interspace

0196T each additional interspace (List separately in addition to code for primary procedure)

Explanation

The physician performs lumbar spinal fusion using a presacral interbody technique. In one method, the intervertebral space is accessed over the presacral fat pad, typically under fluoroscopic guidance. The physician makes a small incision in the midline over the tail bone (coccyx), incises the adjacent fascia, and enters the presacral space. A blunt instrument is advanced along the sacrum's anterior surface to a point at which the center of the disc can be accessed. When the correct position is confirmed, a 3 mm sharp wire is advanced up to the disc space. Dilator tubes are inserted over this wire in order to create an opening in the sacrum that will accommodate a 10 mm working channel. The disc space is cleared through this channel using appropriate surgical instruments, the bone plates are scraped clean, and a mixture of bone, bone substitute, and bone marrow is inserted into the disc space. A hole is then created in the fifth lumbar vertebra, and the working channel is exchanged to allow for passage of the larger instrumentation rod. Report 0195T for a single lumbar interspace and 0196T for each additional interspace.

0200T-0201T

0200T Percutaneous sacral augmentation (sacroplasty), unilateral injection(s), including the use of a balloon or mechanical device, when used, 1 or more needles

0201T Percutaneous sacral augmentation (sacroplasty), bilateral injections, including the use of a balloon or mechanical device, when used, 2 or more needles

Explanation

Percutaneous sacroplasty (sacral augmentation) is performed by a one- or two-sided injection into a sacral insufficiency fracture. A local anesthetic is administered. In a separately reportable procedure, the radiologist uses imaging techniques, such as CT scanning and fluoroscopy, to guide percutaneous placement of the needle during the procedure and to monitor the injection procedure. Sterile biomaterial such as polymethyl methacrylate is injected from one side or both sides into the sacrum and sacral insufficiency fracture and acts as bone cement. Report 0200T for unilateral percutaneous sacroplasty using one or more needles and 0201T for a bilateral procedure using two or more needles.

These codes include the use of a balloon or mechanical device, if utilized.

Coding Tips
These codes have been revised for 2011 in the official CPT description.

0202T

0202T Posterior vertebral joint(s) arthroplasty (eg, facet joint[s] replacement), including facetectomy, laminectomy, foraminotomy, and vertebral column fixation, injection of bone cement, when performed, including fluoroscopy, single level, lumbar spine

Explanation
The physician performs facet joint replacement (facet arthroplasty) of a posterior vertebral joint at a single level of the lumbar spine using fluoroscopic guidance. The paravertebral facet joint consists of the bony surfaces between the vertebrae that articulate with each other. A facet replacement device is inserted in the posterior column of the lumbar spine to restore structure and function. The device replaces all or a portion of a facet joint on a vertebral body. In one method, the physician removes, by partial resection, a posterior vertebral component (facet) and inserts a facet prosthesis. The patient is placed prone and an incision is made overlying the affected vertebra and taken down to the level of the fascia. The fascia is incised and the paravertebral muscles are retracted. The physician removes the affected facet and replaces it with the prosthesis. Facetectomy, laminectomy, foraminotomy, and vertebral column fixation (with or without bone cement injection) may also be performed and are included in this code. Paravertebral muscles are repositioned and the tissue and skin are closed with layered sutures.

0213T-0215T

0213T Injection(s), diagnostic or therapeutic agent, paravertebral facet (zygapophyseal) joint (or nerves innervating that joint) with ultrasound guidance, cervical or thoracic; single level
0214T second level (List separately in addition to code for primary procedure)
0215T third and any additional level(s) (List separately in addition to code for primary procedure)

Explanation
The physician injects a diagnostic or therapeutic agent into a cervical or thoracic paravertebral facet joint or into the nerves that innervate the joint. Using ultrasound guidance, the physician places a needle in the facet joint and injects the indicated substance, often a long-acting local anesthetic agent that may or may not contain a steroid. The paravertebral facet joints, also called zygapophyseal or "Z" joints, consist of the bony surfaces between the vertebrae that articulate with each other. The injection may be performed on a single level or on multiple levels. Report 0213T for a single level, 0214T for a second level, and 0215T for the third and any additional levels.

Coding Tips
These codes are new for 2011 and were implemented at an earlier date by the AMA.

0216T-0218T

0216T Injection(s), diagnostic or therapeutic agent, paravertebral facet (zygapophyseal) joint (or nerves innervating that joint) with ultrasound guidance, lumbar or sacral; single level
0217T second level (List separately in addition to code for primary procedure)
0218T third and any additional level(s) (List separately in addition to code for primary procedure)

Explanation
The physician injects a diagnostic or therapeutic agent into a lumbar or sacral paravertebral facet joint or into the nerves that innervate the joint. Using ultrasound guidance, the physician places a needle in the facet joint and injects the indicated substance, often a long-acting local anesthetic agent that may or may not contain a steroid. The paravertebral facet joints, also called zygapophyseal "Z" joints, consist of the bony surfaces between the vertebrae that articulate with each other. The injection may be performed on a single level or on multiple levels. Report 0216T for a single level, 0217T for a second level, and 0218T for the third and any additional levels.

Coding Tips
These codes are new for 2011 and were implemented at an earlier date by the AMA.

0219T-0222T

0219T Placement of a posterior intrafacet implant(s), unilateral or bilateral, including imaging and placement of bone graft(s) or synthetic device(s), single level; cervical
0220T thoracic
0221T lumbar
0222T each additional vertebral segment (List separately in addition to code for primary procedure)

Explanation
The physician treats facet joint pain caused by degenerative changes or trauma by placing unilateral or bilateral posterior intrafacet implants in the cervical (0219T), thoracic (0220T), or lumbar (0221T) vertebral segments. An alternative to surgical fusion, one operative technique uses an allograft made from bone obtained from both the femur and thigh. Using an open surgical approach or a minimally invasive technique aided by fluoroscopic guidance, the surgeon preps the affected facet surfaces. An allograft dowel with instrumentation is inserted, resulting in expansion and stabilization of the facet joint space. Any bone grafts or synthetic devices used are included in these codes. Report 0222T for each additional vertebral segment.

Coding Tips
These codes are new for 2011 and were implemented at an earlier date by the AMA.

0228T-0229T

0228T Injection(s), anesthetic agent and/or steroid, transforaminal epidural, with ultrasound guidance, cervical or thoracic; single level
0229T each additional level (List separately in addition to code for primary procedure)

Explanation
The physician injects an anesthetic agent and/or a long-acting corticosteroid into the area between the protective covering of the spinal cord (dura) and the bony vertebrae of the cervical or thoracic spine. Nerve roots enter the body after exiting the spinal canal through tiny openings between the vertebrae (foraminae). Using ultrasound guidance, the physician injects the appropriate substance between the foraminae into the area around a selected nerve root. This minimally invasive procedure is frequently used to treat pain caused by herniated discs or spinal stenosis. Report 0228T for an injection to a single level and 0229T for each additional level injected.

Coding Tips
These codes are new for 2011.

0230T-0231T

0230T Injection(s), anesthetic agent and/or steroid, transforaminal epidural, with ultrasound guidance, lumbar or sacral; single level
0231T each additional level (List separately in addition to code for primary procedure)

Explanation
The physician injects an anesthetic agent and/or a long-acting corticosteroid into the area between the protective covering of the spinal cord (dura) and the bony vertebrae of the lumbar or sacral spine. Nerve roots enter the body after exiting the spinal canal through tiny openings between the vertebrae (foraminae). Using ultrasound guidance, the physician injects the appropriate substance between the foraminae into the area around a selected nerve root. This minimally invasive procedure is frequently used to treat pain caused by herniated discs or spinal stenosis. Report 0230T for an injection to a single level and 0231T for each additional level injected.

Coding Tips
These codes are new for 2011.

0232T
0232T Injection(s), platelet rich plasma, any site, including image guidance, harvesting and preparation when performed

Explanation
The physician injects platelet rich plasma (PRP) into a targeted site. Harvesting and preparation may also be performed using a variety of techniques. In one, venous blood is drawn from the region of the arm in front of the elbow (antecubital vein) using a butterfly needle. The blood is placed into an appropriate container, centrifuged, and separated into platelet poor plasma (PPP), RBC, and PRP. The PPP is extracted and discarded and the PRP is withdrawn for use. The injection site is marked in order to localize the PRP injection; image guidance may be used. Under sterile conditions, the physician injects the PRP directly into the target area, sometimes using lidocaine or Marcaine. If administered to a joint space, calcium chloride and thrombin may also be added in order to provide a gel matrix for the PRP to adhere to. PRP has many indications, including wound care for the treatment of diabetic and venous stasis ulcers, chronic nonhealing tendon injuries, plantar fasciitis, and augmentation and fusion of bone. Studies suggest that PRP can aid in wound and soft tissue healing and can affect narcotic requirements, bone production (osteogenesis), postoperative blood loss, and inflammation.

Coding Tips
This code is new for 2011.

0245T-0248T
0245T Open treatment of rib fracture requiring internal fixation, unilateral; 1-2 ribs
0246T 3-4 ribs
0247T 5-6 ribs
0248T 7 or more ribs

Explanation
The physician performs surgery on one or more unilateral rib fractures requiring internal fixation. With the patient under anesthesia, the physician makes an incision overlying the fractured rib. This is carried deep to the bone. The fracture is found, the pieces are identified, and dead tissue is debrided as needed. The physician manipulates and aligns the fracture fragments into an acceptable position and stabilizes the fragments using devices such as pins, rods, screws, or wires. The wound is irrigated and closed in layers. Report 0245T for treatment of one to two ribs; 0246T for three to four ribs; 0247T for five to six ribs; and 0248T for seven or more ribs.

Coding Tips
These codes are new for 2011.

11010-11012

CCI

0183T, 0213T, 0216T, 0228T, 0230T, 10060, 10120-10121, 10160-10180, 11055, 11100, 12001-12007, 15002, 15004, 15851-15852, 16000, 20000-20005, 20200-20206, 20220-20225, 20240-20245, 20250-20251, 20520-20525, 20551-20553, 20955-20957❖, 20962-20970❖, 20972-20973❖, 21010❖, 21034❖, 21044-21045❖, 21050❖, 21060❖, 21070❖, 21076-21088❖, 21145-21199❖, 21206❖, 21240-21249❖, 21550, 21742-21750❖, 22100-22102❖, 22110❖, 22112❖, 22114❖, 22548❖, 22554❖, 22556-22558❖, 22800❖, 22802❖, 22804-22812❖, 22830-22840❖, 23020-23030, 23035❖, 23040❖, 23180❖, 23182❖, 23184❖, 23331-23332❖, 23395-23491❖, 24340-24346❖, 24360-24498❖, 25065-25066, 25390-25393❖, 25400-25426❖, 25440-25492❖, 26010-26011, 26121❖, 26123❖, 26580❖, 26587-26590❖, 26862❖, 27041❖, 27158-27187❖, 27280❖, 27282-27295❖, 27445-27448❖, 27450❖, 27454-27457❖, 27607❖, 27610❖, 27635-27638❖, 27709-27725❖, 28003❖, 28005❖, 28130❖, 28238❖, 29086, 29897-29898❖, 29900-29902❖, 36000, 36400-36410, 36420-36430, 36440, 36600, 36640, 37202, 43752, 51701-51703, 62310-62319, 64400-64435, 64445-64450, 64479, 64483, 64490, 64493, 64505-64530, 69990, 93000-93010, 93040-93042, 93318, 94002, 94200, 94250, 94680-94690, 94770, 95812-95816, 95819, 95822, 95829, 95955, 96360, 96365, 96372, 96374-96376, 97597-97598❖, 97602-97606❖, 99148-99149, 99150, G0168, J0670, J2001

Also not with 11010: 11450-11470, 12011-12016, 12020-12021, 16020-16030, 20100-20102, 20150❖, 20661-20663❖, 20692-20693❖, 20802❖, 20805❖, 20808❖, 20816❖, 20822❖, 20824❖, 20827❖, 20838❖, 20900-20926❖, 21025-21030❖, 21110❖, 21120-21143❖, 21208-21235❖, 21255-21280❖, 21501, 21600-21632❖, 21700-21740❖, 21925❖, 22210-22226❖, 22585-22600❖, 22610-22614❖, 22630-22632❖, 22842-22855❖, 23044❖, 23100-23106❖, 23120-23155❖, 23170❖, 23172❖, 23190-23195❖, 23800-23921❖, 23930-23931, 24066❖, 24100-24102❖, 24110-24134❖, 24136❖, 24138❖, 24140❖, 24145❖, 24147❖, 24149❖, 24155-24164❖, 24201❖, 24300-24331❖, 24800-24940❖, 25031, 25085❖, 25105-25107❖, 25112❖, 25116❖, 25119-25145❖, 25150-25151❖, 25210-25240❖, 25800-25810❖, 25820-25931❖, 26025-26030❖, 26034-26037❖, 26045❖, 26125❖, 26130-26145❖, 26412-26416❖, 26433-26449❖, 26471-26498❖, 26500-26502❖, 26508-26525❖, 26530-26551❖, 26553-26556❖, 26560-26568❖, 26593-26596❖, 26820-26860❖, 26910-26952❖, 27052-27054❖, 27060-27066❖, 27138-27156❖, 27301-27303❖, 27324❖, 27305-27310❖, 27330-27335❖, 27345-27360❖, 27372-27409❖, 27418-27443❖, 27465-27498❖, 27580-27598❖, 27600-27604❖, 27612❖, 27614❖, 27620-27630❖, 27650-27691❖, 27695-27705❖, 27727-27745❖, 27870-27894❖, 28008, 28020-28022❖, 28035❖, 28055-28072❖, 28086❖, 28090❖, 28100-28107❖, 28111-28120❖, 28122❖, 28124❖, 28140❖, 28192-28202❖, 28210-28222❖, 28226❖, 28250-28270❖, 28280-28341❖, 28345-28360❖, 28705-28810❖, 29800-29807❖, 29819-29826❖, 29830-29856❖, 29870-29871❖, 29873-29889❖, 29894-29895❖

Also not with 11011: 11010, 11450-11471, 11720-11721, 12011-12016, 12020-12021, 15781-15783, 16020-16035, 20101-20102, 21025❖, 21029-21030❖, 21110❖, 21121-21143❖, 21208-21235❖, 21255-21280❖, 21501, 21600-21632❖, 21700-21740❖, 22210-22226❖, 22585-22600❖, 22610-22614❖, 22630-22632❖, 22842-22855❖, 23044❖, 23100-23106❖, 23120-23155❖, 23170❖, 23172❖, 23190-23195❖, 23800-23921❖, 23930-23931, 24066❖, 24101-24102❖, 24300, 24331❖, 25028-25031, 25085❖, 25101-25107❖, 25115-25116❖, 25119-25145❖, 25150-25151❖, 25210-25215❖, 25929-25931❖, 26030❖, 26034-26037❖, 26045❖, 26130-26135❖, 26554-26556❖, 26560-26568❖, 26596❖, 26820-26852❖, 26910❖, 26952❖, 27052-27054❖, 27065-27071❖, 27080❖, 27087❖, 27090-27091❖, 27097-27111❖, 27120-27125❖, 27130❖, 27132-27134❖, 27137-27156❖, 27301-27303❖, 27305❖, 27307-27310❖, 27326❖, 27331-27335❖, 27345-27357❖, 27360❖, 27380-27386❖, 27391-27409❖, 27418-27443❖, 27465-27495❖, 27497-27498❖, 27580-27598❖, 27600-27602❖, 27612❖, 27614❖, 27620-27626❖, 27650-27654❖, 27659❖, 27665-27691❖, 27695-27705❖, 27727-27745❖, 27870-27894❖, 28055-28062❖, 28100-28103❖, 28106-28107❖, 28114-28119❖, 28122❖, 28140❖, 28193❖, 28202❖, 28210❖, 28222❖, 28250-28264❖, 28289-28310❖, 28320-28341❖, 28345-28360❖, 28705-28750❖, 28760-28810❖, 29800-29807❖, 29819-29826❖, 29830-29856❖, 29871❖, 29873-29888❖, 29894-29895❖

Also not with 11012: 11010-11011, 11450-11471, 11720-11721, 12011-12021, 15780-15783, 15950, 16020-16035, 20101-20103, 21025❖, 21029❖, 21121-21143❖, 21208❖, 21210-21230❖, 21255-21275❖, 21501-21510, 21610-21616❖, 21630-21632❖, 21705❖, 21740❖, 22210-22214❖, 22220-22224❖, 22590-22600❖, 22610-22612❖, 22630❖, 22842-22847❖, 22849-22850❖, 22852-22855❖, 23105❖, 23125-23130❖, 23145-23155❖, 23195❖, 23800-23920❖, 23930-23935, 24000, 24102❖, 24300, 24331❖, 25020, 25028-25035, 25040, 25101, 25109❖, 25115❖, 25125-25126❖, 25215, 25929-25931❖, 26035❖, 26554-26556❖, 26561-26562❖, 26568❖, 26596❖, 26820❖, 26842-26844❖, 26852❖, 26910, 26990-26991, 27000-27001, 27003, 27054❖, 27066-27071❖, 27087❖, 27090-27091❖, 27097-27111❖, 27120-27125❖, 27130❖, 27132-27134❖, 27137-27156❖, 27303❖, 27310❖, 27325-27326❖, 27332, 27334-27335❖, 27350-27357❖, 27360❖, 27381-27386❖, 27392❖, 27394-27409❖, 27418-27424❖, 27427-27437❖, 27440-27443❖, 27465-27495❖, 27580-27592❖, 27596-27598❖, 27625-27626❖, 27650-27654❖, 27676❖, 27686❖, 27690-27691❖, 27696-27702❖, 27704-27705❖, 27727-27730❖, 27734-27745❖, 27870-27889❖, 27894❖, 28055❖, 28102❖, 28114-28116❖, 28260-28264❖, 28289❖, 28293-28305❖, 28309❖, 28320-28322❖, 28341❖, 28360❖, 28705-28750❖, 28760-28805❖, 29804❖, 29806-29807❖, 29819❖, 29821-29826❖, 29836❖, 29838❖, 29845❖, 29847❖, 29850-29856❖, 29873❖, 29876-29889❖, 29894❖

Evaluation and Management

This section provides an overview of evaluation and management (E/M) services, tables that identify the documentation elements associated with each code, and the federal documentation guidelines with emphasis on the 1997 exam guidelines. This set of guidelines represent the most complete discussion of the elements of the currently accepted versions. The 1997 version identifies both general multi-system physical examinations and single-system examinations, but providers may also use the original 1995 version of the E/M guidelines; both are currently supported by the Centers for Medicare and Medicaid Services (CMS) for audit purposes.

Although some of the most commonly used codes by physicians of all specialties, the E/M service codes are among the least understood. These codes, introduced in the 1992 CPT® manual, were designed to increase accuracy and consistency of use in the reporting of levels of non-procedural encounters. This was accomplished by defining the E/M codes based on the degree that certain common elements are addressed or performed and reflected in the medical documentation.

The Office of the Inspector General (OIG) Work Plan for physicians consistently lists these codes as an area of continued investigative review. This is primarily because Medicare payments for these services total approximately $29 billion per year and are responsible for close to half of Medicare payments for physician services.

The levels of E/M services define the wide variations in skill, effort, and time and are required for preventing and/or diagnosing and treating illness or injury, and promoting optimal health. These codes are intended to represent physician work, and because much of this work involves the amount of training, experience, expertise, and knowledge that a provider may bring to bear on a given patient presentation, the true indications of the level of this work may be difficult to recognize without some explanation.

At first glance, selecting an E/M code may appear to be difficult, but the system of coding clinical visits may be mastered once the requirements for code selection are learned and used.

Types of E/M Services

When approaching E/M, the first choice that a provider must make is what type of code to use. The following tables outline the E/M codes for different levels of care for:

- Office or other outpatient services—new patient
- Office or other outpatient services—established patient
- Hospital observation services—initial care, subsequent, and discharge
- Hospital inpatient services—initial care, subsequent, and discharge
- Observation or inpatient care (including admission and discharge services)
- Consultations—office or other outpatient
- Consultations—inpatient

The specifics of the code components that determine code selection are listed in the table and discussed in the next section. Before a level of service is decided upon, the correct type of service is identified.

Office or other outpatient services are E/M services provided in the physician's office, the outpatient area, or other ambulatory facility. Until the patient is admitted to a health care facility, he/she is considered to be an outpatient.

A new patient is a patient who has not received any face-to-face professional services from the physician within the past three years. An established patient is a patient who has received face-to-face professional services from the physician within the past three years. In the case of group practices, if a physician of the same specialty has seen the patient within three years, the patient is considered established.

If a physician is on call or covering for another physician, the patient's encounter is classified as it would have been by the physician who is not available. Thus, a locum tenens physician who sees a patient on behalf of the patient's attending physician may not bill a new patient code unless the attending physician has not seen the patient for any problem within three years.

Hospital observation services are E/M services provided to patients who are designated or admitted as "observation status" in a hospital.

Codes 99218-99220 are used to indicate initial observation care. These codes include the initiation of the observation status, supervision of patient care including writing orders, and the performance of periodic reassessments. These codes are used only by the physician "admitting" the patient for observation.

Codes 99234-99236 are used to indicate evaluation and management services to a patient who is admitted to and discharged from observation status or hospital inpatient on the same day. If the patient is admitted as an inpatient from observation on the same day, use the appropriate level of Initial Hospital Care (99221-99223).

Code 99217 indicates discharge from observation status. It includes the final physical examination of the patient, instructions, and preparation of the discharge records. It should not be used when admission and discharge are on the same date of service. As mentioned above, report codes 99234-99236 to appropriately describe same day observation services.

If a patient is in observation longer than one day, subsequent observation care codes 99224-99226 should be reported. If the patient is discharged on the second day, observation discharge code 99217 should be reported. If the patient status is changed to inpatient on a subsequent date, the appropriate inpatient code, 99221-99233, should be reported.

Initial hospital care is defined as E/M services provided during the first hospital inpatient encounter with the patient by the admitting physician. (If a physician other than the admitting physician performs the initial inpatient encounter, refer to consultations or subsequent hospital care in the CPT book.) Subsequent hospital care includes all follow-up encounters with the patient by all physicians.

A consultation is the provision of a physician's opinion or advice about a patient for a specific problem at the request of another physician or other appropriate source. CPT also states that a consultation may be performed when a physician is determining whether to accept the transfer of patient care at the request of another physician or appropriate source. An office or other outpatient consultation is a consultation provided in the consultant's office, in the emergency department, or in an outpatient or other ambulatory facility including hospital observation services, home services, domiciliary, rest home, or custodial care. An inpatient consultation is a consultation provided in the hospital or partial hospital nursing facility setting. Report only one inpatient consultation by a consultant for each admission to the hospital or nursing facility.

If a consultant participates in the patient's management after the opinion or advice is provided, use codes for subsequent hospital observation care or for office or other outpatient services (established patient), as appropriate.

CMS adopted new policies regarding the use of consultation codes beginning in 2010. Under these guidelines the inpatient and office/outpatient consultation codes contained in the CPT manual will not be a covered service for CMS. However, Medicare will cover telehealth consultations when reported with the appropriate HCPCS Level II G code.

Additional changes regarding inpatient services were initiated in 2010 by CMS. All outpatient services will be reported using the appropriate new or established evaluation and management (E/M) codes. Inpatient services for the first initial encounter should be reported by the physician providing the service using initial hospital care codes 99221–99223, and subsequent inpatient care codes 99231–99233. As there may only be one admitting physician, CMS has added HCPCS Level II modifier AI, Principal physician of record, which may be appended to the initial hospital care code by the attending physician.

Office or Other Outpatient Services—New Patient

E/M Code	History[1]	Exam[1]	Medical Decision Making[1]	Problem Severity	Coordination of Care; Counseling	Time Spent Face-to-Face (avg.)
99201	Problem-focused	Problem-focused	Straight-forward	Minor or self-limited	Consistent with problem(s) and patient's needs	10 min.
99202	Expanded problem-focused	Expanded problem-focused	Straight-forward	Low to moderate	Consistent with problem(s) and patient's needs	20 min.
99203	Detailed	Detailed	Low complexity	Moderate	Consistent with problem(s) and patient's needs	30 min.
99204	Comprehensive	Comprehensive	Moderate complexity	Moderate to high	Consistent with problem(s) and patient's needs	45 min.
99205	Comprehensive	Comprehensive	High complexity	Moderate to high	Consistent with problem(s) and patient's needs	60 min.

1 Key component. For new patients, all three components (history, exam, and medical decision making) are crucial for selecting the correct code.

Office or Other Outpatient Services—Established Patient[1]

E/M Code	History[2]	Exam[2]	Medical Decision Making[2]	Problem Severity	Coordination of Care; Counseling	Time Spent Face-to-Face (avg.)
99211	—	—	Physician supervision, but presence not required	Minimal	Consistent with problem(s) and patient's needs	5 min.
99212	Problem-focused	Problem-focused	Straight-forward	Minor or self-limited	Consistent with problem(s) and patient's needs	10 min.
99213	Expanded problem-focused	Expanded problem-focused	Low complexity	Low to moderate	Consistent with problem(s) and patient's needs	15 min.
99214	Detailed	Detailed	Moderate complexity	Moderate to high	Consistent with problem(s) and patient's needs	25 min.

E/M Code	History[2]	Exam[2]	Medical Decision Making[2]	Problem Severity	Coordination of Care; Counseling	Time Spent Face-to-Face (avg.)
99215	Comprehensive	Comprehensive	High complexity	Moderate to high	Consistent with problem(s) and patient's needs	40 min.

1 Includes follow-up, periodic reevaluation, and evaluation and management of new problems.
2 Key component. For established patients, at least two of the three components (history, exam, and medical decision making) are needed to select the correct code.

Hospital Observation Services

E/M Code	History[1]	Exam[1]	Medical Decision Making[1]	Problem Severity	Coordination of Care; Counseling	Time[2]
99217	Observation care discharge day management					
99218	Detailed or comprehensive	Detailed or comprehensive	Straight-forward or low complexity	Low	Consistent with problem(s) and patient's needs	N/A
99219	Comprehensive	Comprehensive	Moderate complexity	Moderate	Consistent with problem(s) and patient's needs	N/A
99220	Comprehensive	Comprehensive	High complexity	High	Consistent with problem(s) and patient's needs	N/A

1 Key component. All three components (history, exam, and medical decision making) are crucial for selecting the correct code.
2 Typical times have not been established for this category of services.

Subsequent Hospital Observation Services[1]

E/M Code[2]	History[3]	Exam[3]	Medical Decision Making[3]	Problem Severity	Coordination of Care; Counseling	Time Spent Bedside and on Unit/Floor (avg.)
99224	Problem-focused interval	Problem-focused	Straight-forward or low complexity	Stable, recovering, or improving	Consistent with problem(s) and patient's needs	15
99225	Expanded problem-focused interval	Expanded problem-focused	Moderate complexity	Inadequate response to treatment; minor complications	Consistent with problem(s) and patient's needs	25
99226	Detailed interval	Detailed	High complexity	Unstable; significant new problem or significant complication	Consistent with problem(s) and patient's needs	35

1 All subsequent levels of service include reviewing the medical record, diagnostic studies, and changes in the patient's status, such as history, physical condition, and response to treatment since the last assessment.
2 These codes are resequenced in CPT and printed following codes 99217-99220.
3 Key component. For subsequent care, at least two of the three components (history, exam, and medical decision making) are needed to select the correct code.

Hospital Inpatient Services—Initial Care[1]

E/M Code	History[2]	Exam[2]	Medical Decision Making[2]	Problem Severity	Coordination of Care; Counseling	Time Spent Bedside and on Unit/Floor (avg.)
99221	Detailed or comprehensive	Detailed or comprehensive	Straight-forward or low complexity	Low	Consistent with problem(s) and patient's needs	30 min.
99222	Comprehensive	Comprehensive	Moderate complexity	Moderate	Consistent with problem(s) and patient's needs	50 min.
99223	Comprehensive	Comprehensive	High complexity	High	Consistent with problem(s) and patient's needs	70 min.

1 The admitting physician should append modifier AI, Principal physician of record, for Medicare patients
2 Key component. For initial care, all three components (history, exam, and medical decision making) are crucial for selecting the correct code.

Hospital Inpatient Services—Subsequent Care[1]

E/M Code	History[2]	Exam[2]	Medical Decision Making[2]	Problem Severity	Coordination of Care; Counseling	Time Spent Bedside and on Unit/Floor (avg.)
99231	Problem-focused interval	Problem-focused	Straight-forward or low complexity	Stable, recovering or Improving	Consistent with problem(s) and patient's needs	15 min.
99232	Expanded problem-focused interval	Expanded problem-focused	Moderate complexity	Inadequate response to treatment; minor complications	Consistent with problem(s) and patient's needs	25 min.
99233	Detailed interval	Detailed	High complexity	Unstable; significant new problem or significant complication	Consistent with problem(s) and patient's needs	35 min.
99238	Hospital discharge day management					30 min. or less
99239	Hospital discharge day management					> 30 min.

1 All subsequent levels of service include reviewing the medical record, diagnostic studies, and changes in the patient's status, such as history, physical condition, and response to treatment since the last assessment.
2 Key component. For subsequent care, at least two of the three components (history, exam, and medical decision making) are needed to select the correct code.

Observation or Inpatient Care Services (Including Admission and Discharge Services)

E/M Code	History[1]	Exam[1]	Medical Decision Making[1]	Problem Severity	Coordination of Care; Counseling	Time[2]
99234	Detailed or comprehensive	Detailed or comprehensive	Straight-forward or low complexity	Low	Consistent with problem(s) and patient's needs	N/A
99235	Comprehensive	Comprehensive	Moderate	Moderate	Consistent with problem(s) and patient's needs	N/A
99236	Comprehensive	Comprehensive	High	High	Consistent with problem(s) and patient's needs	N/A

1 Key component. All three components (history, exam, and medical decision making) are crucial for selecting the correct code.
2 Typical times have not been established for this category of services.

Consultations—Office or Other Outpatient

E/M Code	History[1]	Exam[1]	Medical Decision Making[1]	Problem Severity	Coordination of Care; Counseling	Time Spent Face-to-Face (avg.)
99241	Problem-focused	Problem-focused	Straight-forward	Minor or self-limited	Consistent with problem(s) and patient's needs	15 min.
99242	Expanded problem-focused	Expanded problem-focused	Straight-forward	Low	Consistent with problem(s) and patient's needs	30 min.
99243	Detailed	Detailed	Low complexity	Moderate	Consistent with problem(s) and patient's needs	40 min.
99244	Comprehensive	Comprehensive	Moderate complexity	Moderate to high	Consistent with problem(s) and patient's needs	60 min.
99245	Comprehensive	Comprehensive	High complexity	Moderate to high	Consistent with problem(s) and patient's needs	80 min.

1 Key component. For office or other outpatient consultations, all three components (history, exam, and medical decision making) are crucial for selecting the correct code.

Consultations—Inpatient[1]

E/M Code	History[2]	Exam[2]	Medical Decision Making[2]	Problem Severity	Coordination of Care; Counseling	Time Spent Bedside and on Unit/Floor (avg.)
99251	Problem-focused	Problem-focused	Straight-forward	Minor or self-limited	Consistent with problem(s) and patient's needs	20 min.
99252	Expanded problem-focused	Expanded problem-focused	Straight-forward	Low	Consistent with problem(s) and patient's needs	40 min.
99253	Detailed	Detailed	Low complexity	Moderate	Consistent with problem(s) and patient's needs	55 min.
99254	Comprehensive	Comprehensive	Moderate complexity	Moderate to high	Consistent with problem(s) and patient's needs	80 min.
99255	Comprehensive	Comprehensive	High complexity	Moderate to high	Consistent with problem(s) and patient's needs	110 min.

1 These codes are used for hospital inpatients, residents of nursing facilities or patients in a partial hospital setting.
2 Key component. For initial inpatient consultations, all three components (history, exam, and medical decision making) are crucial for selecting the correct code.

Emergency Department Services, New or Established Patient

E/M Code	History[1]	Exam[1]	Medical Decision Making[1]	Problem Severity[3]	Coordination of Care; Counseling	Time Spent[2] Face-to-Face (avg.)
99281	Problem-focused	Problem-focused	Straight-forward	Minor or self-limited	Consistent with problem(s) and patient's needs	N/A
99282	Expanded problem-focused	Expanded problem-focused	Low complexity	Low to moderate	Consistent with problem(s) and patient's needs	N/A
99283	Expanded problem-focused	Expanded problem-focused	Moderate complexity	Moderate	Consistent with problem(s) and patient's needs	N/A
99284	Detailed	Detailed	Moderate complexity	High; requires urgent evaluation	Consistent with problem(s) and patient's needs	N/A
99285	Comprehensive	Comprehensive	High complexity	High; poses immediate/significant threat to life or physiologic function	Consistent with problem(s) and patient's needs	N/A
99288[4]			High complexity			N/A

1 Key component. For emergency department services, all three components (history, exam, and medical decision making) are crucial for selecting the correct code and must be adequately documented in the medical record to substantiate the level of service reported.
2 Typical times have not been established for this category of services.
3 NOTE: The severity of the patient's problem, while taken into consideration when evaluating and treating the patient, does not automatically determine the level of E/M service unless the medical record documentation reflects the severity of the patient's illness, injury, or condition in the details of the history, physical examination, and medical decision making process. Federal auditors will "downcode" the level of E/M service despite the nature of the patient's problem when the documentation does not support the E/M code reported.
4 Code 99288 is used to report two-way communication with emergency medical services personnel in the field.

Critical Care

E/M Code	Patient Status	Physician Attendance	Time[1]
99291	Critically ill or critically injured	Constant	First 30–74 minutes
99292	Critically ill or critically injured	Constant	Each additional 30 minutes beyond the first 74 minutes

1 Per the guidelines for time in *CPT 2011*, "A unit of time is attained when the mid-point is passed. For example, an hour is attained when 31 minutes have elapsed (more than midway between zero and 60 minutes)."

Nursing Facility Services—Initial Nursing Facility Care

E/M Code	History[1]	Exam[1]	Medical Decision Making[1]	Problem Severity	Coordination of Care; Counseling
99304	Detailed or comprehensive	Detailed or comprehensive	Straight-forward or low complexity	Low	25 min.
99305	Comprehensive	Comprehensive	Moderate complexity	Moderate	35 min.
99306	Comprehensive	Comprehensive	High complexity	High	45 min.

1 Key component. For new patients, all three components (history, exam, and medical decision making) are crucial for selecting the correct code.

Nursing Facility Services—Subsequent Nursing Facility Care

E/M Code	History[1]	Exam[1]	Medical Decision Making[2]	Problem Severity	Coordination of Care; Counseling
99307	Problem-focused interval	Problem-focused	Straight-forward	Stable, recovering or improving	10 min.
99308	Expanded problem-focused interval	Expanded problem-focused	Low complexity	Responding inadequately or has developed a minor complication	15 min.
99309	Detailed interval	Detailed	Moderate complexity	Significant complication or a significant new problem	25 min.
99310	Comprehensive interval	Comprehensive	High complexity	Developed a significant new problem requiring immediate attention	35 min.

1 Key component. For established patients, at least two of the three components (history, exam, and medical decision making) are needed for selecting the correct code.

Nursing Facility Discharge and Annual Assessment

E/M Code	History[1]	Exam[1]	Medical Decision Making[1]	Problem Severity	Coordination of Care; Counseling
99315	Nursing facility discharge day management; 30 minutes or less				
99316	Nursing facility discharge day management; more than 30 minutes				
99318	Detailed interval	Comprehensive	Low to moderate complexity	Stable, recovering or improving	30 min.

1 Key component. For annual nursing facility assessment, all three components (history, exam, and medical decision making) are crucial for selecting the correct code.

Domiciliary, Rest Home (e.g., Boarding Home) or Custodial Care Services—New Patient

E/M Code	History[1]	Exam[1]	Medical Decision Making[1]	Problem Severity	Coordination of Care; Counseling	Time Spent Face-to-Face (avg.)
99324	Problem-focused	Problem-focused	Straight-forward	Low	Consistent with problem(s) and patient's needs	20 min.
99325	Expanded problem-focused	Expanded problem-focused	Low complexity	Moderate	Consistent with problem(s) and patient's needs	30 min.
99326	Detailed	Detailed	Moderate complexity	Moderate to high	Consistent with problem(s) and patient's needs	45 min.
99327	Comprehensive	Comprehensive	Moderate complexity	High	Consistent with problem(s) and patient's needs	60 min.
99328	Comprehensive	Comprehensive	High complexity	Unstable or developed a new problem requiring immediate physician attention	Consistent with problem(s) and patient's needs	75 min.

1 Key component. For new patients, all three components (history, exam, and medical decision making) are crucial for selecting the correct code and must be adequately documented in the medical record to substantiate the level of service reported.

Domiciliary, Rest Home (e.g., Boarding Home) or Custodial Care Services—Established Patient

E/M Code	History[1]	Exam[1]	Medical Decision Making[1]	Problem Severity	Coordination of Care; Counseling	Time Spent Face-to-Face (avg.)
99334	Problem-focused interval	Problem-focused	Straight-forward	Self-limited or minor	Consistent with problem(s) and patient's needs	15 min.
99335	Expanded problem-focused interval	Expanded problem-focused	Low complexity	Low to moderate	Consistent with problem(s) and patient's needs	25 min.
99336	Detailed interval	Detailed	Moderate complexity	Moderate to high	Consistent with problem(s) and patient's needs	40 min.
99337	Comprehensive interval	Comprehensive	Moderate to high complexity	Moderate to high	Consistent with problem(s) and patient's needs	60 min.

1 Key component. For established patients, at least two of the three components (history, exam, and medical decision making) are needed for selecting the correct code.

Domiciliary, Rest Home (e.g., Assisted Living Facility), or Home Care Plan Oversight Services

E/M Code	Intent of Service	Presence of Patient	Time
99339	Individual physician supervision of a patient (patient not present) in home, domiciliary or rest home (e.g., assisted living facility) requiring complex and multidisciplinary care modalities involving regular physician development and/or revision of care plans, review of subsequent reports of patient status, review of related laboratory and other studies, communication (including telephone calls) for purposes of assessment or care decisions with health care professional(s), family member(s), surrogate decision maker(s) (e.g., legal guardian) and/or key caregiver(s) involved in patient's care, integration of new information into the medical treatment plan and/or adjustment of medical therapy, within a calendar month	Patient not present	15–29 min.
99340	Same as 99339	Patient not present	30 min. or more

Home Services—New Patient

E/M Code	History[1]	Exam[1]	Medical Decision Making[1]	Problem Severity	Coordination of Care; Counseling	Time Spent Face-to-Face (avg.)
99341	Problem-focused	Problem-focused	Straight-forward complexity	Low	Consistent with problem(s) and patient's needs	20 min.
99342	Expanded problem-focused	Expanded problem-focused	Low complexity	Moderate	Consistent with problem(s) and patient's needs	30 min.
99343	Detailed	Detailed	Moderate complexity	Moderate to high	Consistent with problem(s) and patient's needs	45 min.
99344	Comprehensive	Comprehensive	Moderate complexity	High	Consistent with problem(s) and patient's needs	60 min.
99345	Comprehensive	Comprehensive	High complexity	Usually the patient has developed a significant new problem requiring immediate physician attention	Consistent with problem(s) and patient's needs	75 min.

1 Key component. For new patients, all three components (history, exam, and medical decision making) are crucial for selecting the correct code and must be adequately documented in the medical record to substantiate the level of service reported.

Home Services—Established Patient

E/M Code	History[1]	Exam[1]	Medical Decision Making[1]	Problem Severity	Coordination of Care; Counseling	Time Spent Face-to-Face (avg.)
99347	Problem-focused interval	Problem-focused	Straight-forward	Self-limited or minor	Consistent with problem(s) and patient's needs	15 min.
99348	Expanded problem-focused interval	Expanded problem-focused	Low complexity	Low to moderate	Consistent with problem(s) and patient's needs	25 min.
99349	Detailed interval	Detailed	Moderate complexity	Moderate to high	Consistent with problem(s) and patient's needs	40 min.
99350	Comprehensive interval	Comprehensive	Moderate to high complexity	Moderate to high Usually the patient has developed a significant new problem requiring immediate physician attention	Consistent with problem(s) and patient's needs	60 min.

1 Key component. For established patients, at least two of the three components (history, exam, and medical decision making) are needed to select the correct code and must be adequately documented in the medical record to substantiate the level of service reported.

Newborn Care Services

E/M Code	Patient Status	Type of Visit
99460	Normal newborn	Inpatient initial inpatient hospital or birthing center
99461	Normal newborn	Inpatient initial treatment not in hospital or birthing center
99462	Normal newborn	Inpatient subsequent
99463	Normal newborn	Inpatient initial inpatient and discharge in hospital or birthing center
99464	Unstable newborn	Attendance at delivery
99465	High-risk newborn at delivery	Resuscitation, ventilation, and cardiac treatment

Inpatient Neonatal and Pediatric Critical Care

E/M Code	Patient Status	Type of Visit
99468	Critically ill neonate, aged 28 days or less	Inpatient initial
99469	Critically ill neonate, aged 28 days or less	Inpatient subsequent
99471	Critically ill infant or young child, aged 29 days to 24 months	Inpatient initial
99472	Critically ill infant or young child, aged 29 days to 24 months	Inpatient subsequent
99475	Critically ill infant or young child, 2 to 5 years	Inpatient initial
99476	Critically ill infant or young child, 2 to 5 years	Inpatient subsequent

Initial and Continuing Intensive Care Services

E/M Code	Patient Status	Type of Visit
99477	Neonate, aged 28 days or less	Inpatient initial
99478	Infant with present body weight of less than 1500 grams, no longer critically ill	Inpatient subsequent
99479	Infant with present body weight of 1501-2500 grams, no longer critically ill	Inpatient subsequent
99480	Infant with present body weight of 2501-5000 grams, no longer critically ill	Inpatient subsequent

Levels of E/M Services

Confusion may be experienced when first approaching E/M due to the way that each description of a code component or element seems to have another layer of description beneath. The three key components—history, exam, and decision making—are each comprised of elements that combine to create varying levels of that component.

For example, an expanded problem-focused history includes the chief complaint, a brief history of the present illness, and a system review focusing on the patient's problems. The level of exam is not made up of different elements but rather distinguished by the extent of exam across body areas or organ systems.

The single largest source of confusion are the "labels" or names applied to the varying degrees of history, exam, and decision-making. Terms such as expanded problem-focused, detailed, and comprehensive are somewhat meaningless unless they are defined. The lack of definition in CPT guidelines relative to these terms is precisely what caused the first set of federal guidelines to be developed in 1995 and again in 1997.

Documentation Guidelines for Evaluation and Management Services

Both versions of the federal guidelines go well beyond CPT guidelines in defining specific code requirements. The current version of the CPT guidelines does not explain the number of history of present illness (HPI) elements or the specific number of organ systems or body areas to be examined as they are in the federal guidelines. Adherence to some version of the guidelines is required when billing E/M to federal payers, but at this time, the CPT guidelines do not incorporate this level of detail into the code definitions. Although that could be interpreted to mean that non-governmental payers have a lesser documentation standard, it is best to adopt one set of the federal versions for all payer types for both consistency and ease of use.

The 1997 guidelines supply a great amount of detail relative to history and exam and will give the provider clear direction to following documentation elements. With that stated, the 1995 guidelines are equally valid and place a lesser documentation burden on the provider in regards to the physical exam.

The 1995 guidelines ask only for a notation of "normal" on systems with normal findings. The only narrative required is for abnormal findings. The 1997 version calls for much greater detail, or an "elemental" or "bullet-point" approach to organ systems, although a notation of normal is sufficient when addressing the elements within a system. The 1997 version works well in a template format for recording E/M services.

The 1997 version did produce the single system specialty exam guidelines. When reviewing the complete guidelines listed below, note the differences between exam requirements in the 1995 and 1997 versions.

A Comparison of 1995 and 1997 Exam Guidelines

There are four types of exams indicated in the levels of E/M codes. Although the descriptors or labels are the same under 1995 and 1997 guidelines, the degree of detail required is different. The remaining content on this topic references the 1997 general multi-system speciality examination, at the end of this chapter.

The levels under each set of guidelines are:

1995 Exam Guidelines:

Problem focused:	One body area or system
Expanded problem focused:	Two to seven body areas or organ systems
Detailed:	Two to seven body areas or organ systems
Comprehensive:	Eight or more organ systems or a complete single-system examination

1997 Exam Guidelines:

Problem-focused:	Perform and document examination of one to five bullet point elements in one or more organ systems/body areas from the general multi-system examination
OR	
	Perform or document examination of one to five bullet point elements from one of the 10 single-organ-system examinations, shaded or unshaded boxes
Expanded problem-focused:	Perform and document examination of at least six bullet point elements in one or more organ systems from the general multi-system examination
OR	
	Perform and document examination of at least six bullet point elements from one of the 10 single-organ-system examinations, shaded or unshaded boxes
Detailed:	Perform and document examination of at least six organ systems or body areas, including at least two bullet point elements for each organ system or body area from the general multi-system examination
OR	
	Perform and document examination of at least 12 bullet point elements in two or more organ systems or body areas from the general multisystem examination
OR	

	Perform and document examination of at least 12 bullet elements from one of the single-organ-system examinations, shaded or unshaded boxes
Comprehensive:	Perform and document examination of at least nine organ systems or body areas, with all bullet elements for each organ system or body area (unless specific instructions are expected to limit examination content with at least two bullet elements for each organ system or body area) from the general multi-system examination
OR	
	Perform and document examination of all bullet point elements from one of the 10 single-organ system examinations with documentation of every element in shaded boxes and at least one element in each unshaded box from the single-organ-system examination.

The Documentation Guidelines

The following guidelines were developed jointly by the American Medical Association (AMA) and the Centers for Medicare and Medicaid Services (CMS). Their mutual goal was to provide physicians and claims reviewers with advice about preparing or reviewing documentation for Evaluation and Management (E/M) services.

I. Introduction

What is Documentation and Why Is It Important?

Medical record documentation is required to record pertinent facts, findings, and observations about an individual's health history, including past and present illnesses, examinations, tests, treatments, and outcomes. The medical record chronologically documents the care of the patient and is an important element contributing to high quality care. The medical record facilitates:

- The ability of the physician and other health care professionals to evaluate and plan the patient's immediate treatment and to monitor his/her health care over time
- Communication and continuity of care among physicians and other health care professionals involved in the patient's care
- Accurate and timely claims review and payment
- Appropriate utilization review and quality of care evaluations
- Collection of data that may be useful for research and education

An appropriately documented medical record can reduce many of the problems associated with claims processing and may serve as a legal document to verify the care provided, if necessary.

What Do Payers Want and Why?

Because payers have a contractual obligation to enrollees, they may require reasonable documentation that services are consistent with the insurance coverage provided. They may request information to validate:

- The site of service
- The medical necessity and appropriateness of the diagnostic and/or therapeutic services provided
- Services provided have been accurately reported

II. General Principles of Medical Record Documentation

The principles of documentation listed below are applicable to all types of medical and surgical services in all settings. For Evaluation and Management (E/M) services, the nature and amount of physician work and documentation varies by type of service, place of service, and the patient's status. The general principles listed below may be modified to account for these variable circumstances in providing E/M services.

- The medical record should be complete and legible
- The documentation of each patient encounter should include:
  - A reason for the encounter and relevant history, physical examination findings, and prior diagnostic test results
  - Assessment, clinical impression, or diagnosis
  - Plan for care
  - Date and legible identity of the practitioner
- If not documented, the rationale for ordering diagnostic and other ancillary services should be easily inferred
- Past and present diagnoses should be accessible to the treating and/or consulting physician
- Appropriate health risk factors should be identified
- The patient's progress, response to, and changes in treatment and revision of diagnosis should be documented
- The CPT and ICD-9-CM codes reported on the health insurance claim form or billing statement should be supported by the documentation in the medical record

III. Documentation of E/M Services 1995 and 1997

The following information provides definitions and documentation guidelines for the three key components of E/M services and for visits that consist predominately of counseling or coordination of care. The three key components—history, examination, and medical decision making—appear in the descriptors for office and other outpatient services, hospital observation services, hospital inpatient services, consultations, emergency department services, nursing facility services, domiciliary care services, and home services. While some of the text of the CPT guidelines has been repeated in this document, the reader should refer to CMS or CPT for the complete descriptors for E/M services and instructions for selecting a level of service. Documentation guidelines are identified by the symbol DG.

The descriptors for the levels of E/M services recognize seven components that are used in defining the levels of E/M services. These components are:

- History
- Examination
- Medical decision making
- Counseling
- Coordination of care

- Nature of presenting problem
- Time

The first three of these components (i.e., history, examination, and medical decision making) are the key components in selecting the level of E/M services. In the case of visits that consist predominately of counseling or coordination of care, time is the key or controlling factor to qualify for a particular level of E/M service.

Because the level of E/M service is dependent on two or three key components, performance and documentation of one component (e.g., examination) at the highest level does not necessarily mean that the encounter in its entirety qualifies for the highest level of E/M service.

These Documentation Guidelines for E/M services reflect the needs of the typical adult population. For certain groups of patients, the recorded information may vary slightly from that described here. Specifically, the medical records of infants, children, adolescents, and pregnant women may have additional or modified information, as appropriate, recorded in each history and examination area.

As an example, newborn records may include under history of the present illness (HPI) the details of the mother's pregnancy and the infant's status at birth; social history will focus on family structure; and family history will focus on congenital anomalies and hereditary disorders in the family. In addition, the content of a pediatric examination will vary with the age and development of the child. Although not specifically defined in these documentation guidelines, these patient group variations on history and examination are appropriate.

A. Documentation of History

The levels of E/M services are based on four types of history (Problem Focused, Expanded Problem Focused, Detailed, and Comprehensive). Each type of history includes some or all of the following elements:

- Chief complaint (CC)
- History of present illness (HPI)
- Review of systems (ROS)
- Past, family, and/or social history (PFSH)

The extent of history of present illness, review of systems, and past, family, and/or social history that is obtained and documented is dependent upon clinical judgment and the nature of the presenting problem.

The chart below shows the progression of the elements required for each type of history. To qualify for a given type of history all three elements in the table must be met. (A chief complaint is indicated at all levels.)

- DG: The CC, ROS, and PFSH may be listed as separate elements of history or they may be included in the description of the history of present illness

- DG: A ROS and/or a PFSH obtained during an earlier encounter does not need to be re-recorded if there is evidence that the physician reviewed and updated the previous information. This may occur when a physician updates his/her own record or in an institutional setting or group practice where many physicians use a common record. The review and update may be documented by:
  – Describing any new ROS and/or PFSH information or noting there has been no change in the information
  – Noting the date and location of the earlier ROS and/or PFSH

- DG: The ROS and/or PFSH may be recorded by ancillary staff or on a form completed by the patient. To document that the physician reviewed the information, there must be a notation supplementing or confirming the information recorded by others

- DG: If the physician is unable to obtain a history from the patient or other source, the record should describe the patient's condition or other circumstance that precludes obtaining a history

Definitions and specific documentation guidelines for each of the elements of history are listed below.

Chief Complaint (CC)
The CC is a concise statement describing the symptom, problem, condition, diagnosis, physician recommended return, or other factor that is the reason for the encounter, usually stated in the patient's words.

- DG: The medical record should clearly reflect the chief complaint

History of Present Illness (HPI)
The HPI is a chronological description of the development of the patient's present illness from the first sign and/or symptom or from the previous encounter to the present. It includes the following elements:

- Location
- Quality
- Severity
- Duration
- Timing
- Context
- Modifying factors
- Associated signs and symptoms

History of Present Illness	Review of systems (ROS)	PFSH	Type of History
Brief	N/A	N/A	Problem-focused
Brief	Problem Pertinent	N/A	Expanded Problem-Focused
Extended	Extended	Pertinent	Detailed
Extended	Complete	Complete	Comprehensive

Brief and extended HPIs are distinguished by the amount of detail needed to accurately characterize the clinical problem.

A brief HPI consists of one to three elements of the HPI.

- DG: The medical record should describe one to three elements of the present illness (HPI)

An extended HPI consists of at least four elements of the HPI or the status of at least three chronic or inactive conditions.

- DG: The medical record should describe at least four elements of the present illness (HPI) or for 1997 only the status of at least three chronic or inactive conditions

Review of Systems (ROS)

A ROS is an inventory of body systems obtained through a series of questions seeking to identify signs and/or symptoms that the patient may be experiencing or has experienced. For purposes of ROS, the following systems are recognized:

- Constitutional symptoms (e.g., fever, weight loss)
- Eyes
- Ears, nose, mouth, throat
- Cardiovascular
- Respiratory
- Gastrointestinal
- Genitourinary
- Musculoskeletal
- Integumentary (skin and/or breast)
- Neurological
- Psychiatric
- Endocrine
- Hematologic/lymphatic
- Allergic/immunologic

A problem pertinent ROS inquires about the system directly related to the problem identified in the HPI.

- DG: The patient's positive responses and pertinent negatives for the system related to the problem should be documented

An extended ROS inquires about the system directly related to the problem identified in the HPI and a limited number of additional systems.

- DG: The patient's positive responses and pertinent negatives for two to nine systems should be documented

A complete ROS inquires about the system directly related to the problem identified in the HPI plus all additional body systems.

- DG: At least 10 organ systems must be reviewed. Those systems with positive or pertinent negative responses must be individually documented. For the remaining systems, a notation indicating all other systems are negative is permissible. In the absence of such a notation, at least 10 systems must be individually documented

Past, Family, and/or Social History (PFSH)

The PFSH consists of a review of three areas:

- Past history (the patient's past experiences with illnesses, operations, injuries, and treatment)
- Family history (a review of medical events in the patient's family, including diseases that may be hereditary or place the patient at risk)
- Social history (an age appropriate review of past and current activities)

For certain categories of E/M services that include only an interval history, it is not necessary to record information about the PFSH. Those categories are subsequent hospital care, follow-up inpatient consultations, and subsequent nursing facility care.

A pertinent PFSH is a review of the history area directly related to the problem identified in the HPI.

- DG: At least one specific item from any of the three history areas must be documented for a pertinent PFSH

A complete PFSH is a review of two or all three of the PFSH history areas, depending on the category of the E/M service. A review of all three history areas is required for services that by their nature include a comprehensive assessment or reassessment of the patient. A review of two of the three history areas is sufficient for other services.

- DG: A least one specific item from two of the three history areas must be documented for a complete PFSH for the following categories of E/M services: office or other outpatient services, established patient; emergency department; domiciliary care, established patient; and home care, established patient

- DG: At least one specific item from each of the three history areas must be documented for a complete PFSH for the following categories of E/M services: office or other outpatient services, new patient; hospital observation services; hospital inpatient services, initial care; consultations; comprehensive nursing facility assessments; domiciliary care, new patient; and home care, new patient

B. Documentation of Examination 1997 Guidelines

The levels of E/M services are based on four types of examination:

- Problem Focused: A limited examination of the affected body area or organ system
- Expanded Problem Focused: A limited examination of the affected body area or organ system and any other symptomatic or related body area or organ system
- Detailed: An extended examination of the affected body area or organ system and any other symptomatic or related body area or organ system
- Comprehensive: A general multi-system examination or complete examination of a single organ system and other symptomatic or related body area or organ system

These types of examinations have been defined for general multi-system and the following single organ systems:

- Cardiovascular
- Ears, nose, mouth, and throat
- Eyes
- Genitourinary (Female)
- Genitourinary (Male)
- Hematologic/lymphatic/immunologic
- Musculoskeletal
- Neurological
- Psychiatric
- Respiratory
- Skin
- Gastrointestinal

Any physician regardless of specialty may perform a general multi-system examination or any of the single organ system examinations. The type (general multi-system or single organ system) and content of examination are selected by the examining physician and are based upon clinical judgment, the patient's history, and the nature of the presenting problem.

The content and documentation requirements for each type and level of examination are summarized below and described in detail in a table found later on in this document. In the table, organ systems and body areas recognized by CPT for purposes of describing examinations are shown in the left column. The content, or individual elements, of the examination pertaining to that body area or organ system are identified by bullets (•) in the right column.

Parenthetical examples "(e.g., ...)," have been used for clarification and to provide guidance regarding documentation. Documentation for each element must satisfy any numeric requirements (such as "Measurement of any three of the following seven...") included in the description of the element. Elements with multiple components but with no specific numeric requirement (such as "Examination of liver and spleen") require documentation of at least one component. It is possible for a given examination to be expanded beyond what is defined here. When that occurs, findings related to the additional systems and/or areas should be documented.

- DG: Specific abnormal and relevant negative findings from the examination of the affected or symptomatic body area or organ system should be documented. A notation of "abnormal" without elaboration is insufficient

- DG: Abnormal or unexpected findings from the examination of any asymptomatic body area or organ system should be described

- DG: A brief statement or notation indicating "negative" or "normal" is sufficient to document normal findings related to an unaffected areas or asymptomatic organ system

General Multi-System Examinations

General multi-system examinations are described in detail later in this document. To qualify for a given level of multi-system examination, the following content and documentation requirements should be met:

- Problem Focused Examination: It should include performance and documentation of one to five elements identified by a bullet (•) in one or more organ systems or body areas

- Expanded Problem Focused Examination: It should include performance and documentation of at least six elements identified by a bullet (•) in one or more organ systems or body areas

- Detailed Examination: It should include at least six organ systems or body areas. For each system/area selected, performance and documentation of at least two elements identified by a bullet (•) is expected. Alternatively, a detailed examination may include performance and documentation of at least 12 elements identified by a bullet (•) in two or more organ systems or body areas

- Comprehensive Examination: It should include at least nine organ systems or body areas. For each system/area selected, all elements of the examination identified by a bullet (•) should be performed, unless specific directions limit the content of the examination. For each area/system, documentation of at least two elements identified by a bullet (•) is expected

Single Organ System Examinations

The single organ system examinations recognized by CMS include eyes; ears, nose, and throat; cardiovascular; respiratory; gastrointestinal; genitourinary (male and female); musculoskeletal; neurologic; hematologic, lymphatic, and immunologic; skin; and psychiatric. Note that for each specific single organ examination type, the performance and documentation of the stated number of elements, identified by a bullet (•) should be included, whether in a box with a shaded or unshaded border. The following content and documentation requirements must be met to qualify for a given level:

- Problem Focused Examination: one to five elements

- Expanded Problem Focused Examination: at least six elements

- Detailed Examination: at least 12 elements (other than eye and psychiatric examinations)

- Comprehensive Examination: all elements (Documentation of every element in a box with a shaded border and at least one element in a box with an unshaded border is expected)

Content and Documentation Requirements

General Multisystem Examination 1997

System/Body Area	Elements of Examination
Constitutional	■ Measurement of any three of the following seven vital signs: 1) sitting or standing blood pressure, 2) supine blood pressure, 3) pulse rate and regularity, 4) respiration, 5) temperature, 6) height, 7) weight (May be measured and recorded by ancillary staff). ■ General appearance of patient (e.g., development, nutrition, body habitus, deformities attention to grooming)
Eyes	■ Inspection of conjunctivae and lids ■ Examination of pupils and irises (e.g., reaction to light and accommodation, size and symmetry) ■ Ophthalmoscopic examination of optic discs (e.g., size, C/D ratio, appearance) and posterior segments (e.g., vessel changes, exudates, hemorrhages)
Ears, nose, mouth, and throat	■ External inspection of ears and nose (e.g., overall appearance, scars, lesions, masses) ■ Otoscopic examination of external auditory canals and tympanic membranes ■ Assessment of hearing (e.g., whispered voice, finger rub, tuning fork) ■ Inspection of nasal mucosa, septum and turbinates ■ Inspection of lips, teeth and gums ■ Examination of oropharynx: oral mucosa, salivary glands, hard and soft palates, tongue, tonsils and posterior pharynx
Neck	■ Examination of neck (e.g., masses, overall appearance, symmetry, tracheal position, crepitus) ■ Examination of thyroid (e.g., enlargement, tenderness, mass)
Respiratory	■ Assessment of respiratory effort (e.g., intercostal retractions, use of accessory muscles, diaphragmatic movement) ■ Percussion of chest (e.g., dullness, flatness, hyperresonance) ■ Palpation of chest (e.g., tactile fremitus) ■ Auscultation of lungs (e.g., breath sounds, adventitious sounds, rubs)
Cardiovascular	■ Palpation of heart (e.g., location, size, thrills) ■ Auscultation of heart with notation of abnormal sounds and murmurs ■ Examination of: — carotid arteries (e.g., pulse amplitude, bruits) — abdominal aorta (e.g., size, bruits) — femoral arteries (e.g., pulse amplitude, bruits) — pedal pulses (e.g., pulse amplitude) — extremities for edema and/or varicosities
Chest (Breasts)	■ Inspection of breasts (e.g., symmetry, nipple discharge) ■ Palpation of breasts and axillae (e.g., masses or lumps, tenderness)
Gastrointestinal (Abdomen)	■ Examination of abdomen with notation of presence of masses or tenderness ■ Examination of liver and spleen ■ Examination for presence or absence of hernia ■ Examination (when indicated) of anus, perineum and rectum, including sphincter tone, presence of hemorrhoids, rectal masses ■ Obtain stool sample for occult blood test when indicated
Genitourinary	Male: ■ Examination of the scrotal contents (e.g., hydrocele, spermatocele, tenderness of cord, testicular mass) ■ Examination of the penis ■ Digital rectal examination of prostate gland (e.g., size, symmetry, nodularity tenderness) Female: ■ Pelvic examination (with or without specimen collection for smears and cultures), including: — examination of external genitalia (e.g., general appearance, hair distribution, lesions) and vagina (e.g., general appearance, estrogen effect, discharge, lesions, pelvic support, cystocele, rectocele) — examination of urethra (e.g., masses, tenderness, scarring) — examination of bladder (e.g., fullness, masses, tenderness) ■ Cervix (e.g., general appearance, lesions, discharge) ■ Uterus (e.g., size, contour, position, mobility, tenderness, consistency, descent or support) ■ Adnexa/parametria (e.g., masses, tenderness)
Lymphatic	Palpation of lymph nodes in **two or more** areas: ■ Neck Axillae ■ Groin Other

System/Body Area	Elements of Examination
Musculoskeletal	■ Examination of gait and station *(if circled, add to total at bottom of column to the left) ■ Inspection and/or palpation of digits and nails (e.g., clubbing, cyanosis, inflammatory conditions, petechiae, ischemia, infections, nodes) *(if circled, add to total at bottom of column to the left) Examination of joints, bones and muscles of **one or more of the following six** areas: 1) head and neck; 2) spine, ribs, and pelvis; 3) right upper extremity; 4) left upper extremity; 5) right lower extremity; and 6) left lower extremity. The examination of a given area includes: ■ Inspection and/or palpation with notation of presence of any misalignment, asymmetry, crepitation, defects, tenderness, masses, effusions ■ Assessment of range of motion with notation of any pain, crepitation or contracture ■ Assessment of stability with notation of any dislocation (luxation), subluxation, or laxity ■ Assessment of muscle strength and tone (e.g., flaccid, cog wheel, spastic) with notation of any atrophy or abnormal movements
Skin	■ Inspection of skin and subcutaneous tissue (e.g., rashes, lesions, ulcers) ■ Palpation of skin and subcutaneous tissue (e.g., induration, subcutaneous nodules, tightening)
Neurologic	■ Test cranial nerves with notation of any deficits ■ Examination of deep tendon reflexes with notation of pathological reflexes (e.g., Babinski) ■ Examination of sensation (e.g., by touch, pin, vibration, proprioception)
Psychiatric	■ Brief assessment of mental status including: — Orientation to time, place and person — Recent and remote memory — Mood and affect (e.g., depression, anxiety, agitation)

Content and Documentation Requirements

Level of exam	Perform and document
Problem focused	**One to five** elements identified by a bullet.
Expanded problem focused	**At least six** elements identified by a bullet.
Detailed	**At least 12** elements identified by a bullet, whether in a box with a shaded or unshaded border
Comprehensive	Performance of **all** elements identified by a bullet; whether in a box or with a shaded or unshaded box. Documentation of every element in each with a shaded border and at least one element in a box with un shaded border is expected

X. Documentation of the Complexity of Medical Decision Making 1995 and 1997

The levels of E/M services recognize four types of medical decision-making (straightforward, low complexity, moderate complexity, and high complexity). Medical decision-making refers to the complexity of establishing a diagnosis and/or selecting a management option as measured by:

- The number of possible diagnoses and/or the number of management options that must be considered

- The amount and/or complexity of medical records, diagnostic tests, and/or other information that must be obtained, reviewed, and analyzed

- The risk of significant complications, morbidity, and/or mortality, as well as comorbidities, associated with the patient's presenting problem, the diagnostic procedure, and/or the possible management options

The following chart shows the progression of the elements required for each level of medical decision-making. To qualify for a given type of decision-making, two of the three elements in the table must be either met or exceeded.

Number of Diagnoses or Management Options	Amount and/or Complexity of Data to be Reviewed	Risk of Complications and/or Morbidity or Mortality	Type of Decision Making
Minimal	Minimal or None	Minimal	Straightforward
Limited	Limited	Low	Low Complexity
Multiple	Moderate	Moderate	Moderate Complexity
Extensive	Extensive	High	High Complexity

Each of the elements of medical decision-making is described below.

Number of Diagnoses or Management Options

The number of possible diagnoses and/or the number of management options that must be considered is based on the number and types of problems addressed during the encounter, the complexity of establishing a diagnosis, and the management decisions that are made by the physician.

Generally, decision making with respect to a diagnosed problem is easier than that for an identified but undiagnosed problem. The number and type of diagnostic tests employed may be an indicator of the number of possible diagnoses. Problems that are improving or resolving are less complex than those that are worsening or failing to change as expected. The need to seek advice from others is another indicator of complexity of diagnostic or management problems.

- DG: For each encounter, an assessment, clinical impression, or diagnosis should be documented. It may be explicitly stated or implied in documented decisions regarding management plans and/or further evaluation

For a presenting problem with an established diagnosis, the record should reflect whether the problem is: a) improved, well controlled, resolving, or resolved; or b) inadequately controlled, worsening, or failing to change as expected

For a presenting problem without an established diagnosis, the assessment or clinical impression may be stated in the form of a differential diagnosis or as a "possible," "probable," or "rule-out" (R/O) diagnosis

- DG: The initiation of, or changes in, treatment should be documented. Treatment includes a wide range of management options including patient instructions, nursing instructions, therapies, and medications

- DG: If referrals are made, consultations requested, or advice sought, the record should indicate to whom or where the referral or consultation is made or from whom the advice is requested

Amount and/or Complexity of Data to be Reviewed

The amount and complexity of data to be reviewed is based on the types of diagnostic testing ordered or reviewed. A decision to obtain and review old medical records and/or obtain history from sources other than the patient increases the amount and complexity of data to be reviewed.

Discussion of contradictory or unexpected test results with the physician who performed or interpreted the test is an indication of the complexity of data being reviewed. On occasion, the physician who ordered a test may personally review the image, tracing, or specimen to supplement information from the physician who prepared the test report or interpretation; this is another indication of the complexity of data being reviewed.

- DG: If a diagnostic service (test or procedure) is ordered, planned, scheduled, or performed at the time of the E/M encounter, the type of service (e.g., lab or x-ray) should be documented

- DG: The review of lab, radiology, and/or other diagnostic tests should be documented. A simple notation such as WBC elevated" or "chest x-ray unremarkable" is acceptable. Alternatively, the review may be documented by initialing and dating the report containing the test results

- DG: A decision to obtain old records or a decision to obtain additional history from the family, caretaker, or other source to supplement that obtained from the patient should be documented

- DG: Relevant findings from the review of old records and/or the receipt of additional history from the family, caretaker, or other source to supplement that obtained from the patient should be documented. If there is no relevant information beyond that already obtained, that fact should be documented. A notation of "old records reviewed" or "additional history obtained from family" without elaboration is insufficient

- DG: The results of discussion of laboratory, radiology, or other diagnostic tests with the physician who performed or interpreted the study should be documented

- DG: The direct visualization and independent interpretation of an image, tracing, or specimen previously or subsequently interpreted by another physician should be documented

Risk of Significant Complications, Morbidity, and/or Mortality

The risk of significant complications, morbidity, and/or mortality is based on the risks associated with the presenting problem, the diagnostic procedure, and the possible management options.

- DG: Comorbidities/underlying disease or other factors that increase the complexity of medical decision making by increasing the risk of complications, morbidity, and/or mortality should be documented

- DG: If a surgical or invasive diagnostic procedure is ordered, planned, or scheduled at the time of the E/M encounter, the type of procedure (e.g., laparoscopy) should be documented

- **DG:** If a surgical or invasive diagnostic procedure is performed at the time of the E/M encounter, the specific procedure should be documented

- **DG:** The referral for or decision to perform a surgical or invasive diagnostic procedure on an urgent basis should be documented or implied

The following Table of Risk may be used to help determine whether the risk of significant complications, morbidity, and/or mortality is minimal, low, moderate, or high. Because the determination of risk is complex and not readily quantifiable, the table includes common clinical examples rather than absolute measures of risk. The assessment of risk of the presenting problem is based on the risk related to the disease process anticipated between the present encounter and the next one. The assessment of risk of selecting diagnostic procedures and management options is based on the risk during and immediately following any procedures or treatment. The highest level of risk in any one category (presenting problem, diagnostic procedure, or management options) determines the overall risk.

Table of Risk.

Level of Risk	Presenting Problem(s)	Diagnostic Procedure(s) Ordered	Management Options Selected
Minimal	One self-limited or minor problem (e.g., common cold, insect bite, tinea corporis)	Laboratory test requiring veinpuncture Chest x-rays EKG/EEG Urinalysis Ultrasound (e.g., echocardiography) KOH prep	Rest Gargles Elastic bandages Superficial dressings
Low	Two or more self-limited or minor problems One stable chronic illness (e.g., well controlled hypertension, non-insulin dependent diabetes, cataract, BPH) Acute, uncomplicated illness or injury (e.g., cystitis, allergic rhinitis, simple sprain)	Physiologic tests not under stress (e.g., pulmonary function tests) Non-cardiovascular imaging studies with contrast (e.g., barium enema) Superficial needle biopsies Clinical laboratory tests requiring arterial puncture Skin biopsies	Over-the-counter drugs Minor surgery with no identified risk factors Physical therapy Occupational therapy IV fluids without additives
Moderate	One or more chronic illnesses with mild exacerbation, progression or side effects of treatment Two or more stable chronic illnesses Undiagnosed new problem with uncertain prognosis (e.g., lump in breast) Acute illness with systemic symptoms (e.g., pyelonephritis, pneumonitis, colitis) Acute complicated injury (e.g., head injury with brief loss of consciousness)	Physiologic tests not under stress (e.g., cardiac stress test, fetal contraction stress test) Diagnostic endoscopies with no identified risk factors Deep needle or incisional biopsy Cardiovascular imaging studies with contrast and no identified risk factors (e.g., arteriogram, cardiac catheterization) Obtain fluid from body cavity (e.g., lumbar puncture, thoracentesis, culdocentesis)	Minor surgery with identified risk factors Effective major surgery (open, percutaneous or endoscopic) with no identified risk factors Prescription drug management Therapeutic nuclear medicine IV fluids with additives Closed treatment of fracture or dislocation without manipulation
High	One or more chronic illnesses with severe exacerbation, progression or side effects of treatment Acute chronic illnesses that may pose a threat to life or bodily function (e.g., multiple trauma, acute MI, pulmonary embolus, severe respiratory distress, progressive severe rheumatoid arthritis, psychiatric illness with potential threat to self or others, peritonitis, acute renal failure An abrupt change in neurologic status (e.g., seizure, TIA, weakness or sensory loss)	Cardiovascular imaging studies with contrast with identified risk factors Cardiac electrophysiological tests Diagnostic endoscopies with identified risk factors Discography	Elective major surgery (open, percutaneous or endoscopic) with identified risk factors Emergency major surgery (open, percutaneous or endoscopic) Parenteral controlled substances Drug therapy requiring intensive monitoring for toxicity Decision not to resuscitate or to de-escalate care because of poor prognosis

D. Documentation of an Encounter Dominated by Counseling or Coordination of Care

In the case where counseling and/or coordination of care dominates (more than 50 percent) the physician/patient and/or family encounter (face-to-face time in the office or other outpatient setting or floor-unit time in the hospital or nursing facility), time is considered the key or controlling factor to qualify for a particular level of E/M service.

- DG: If the physician elects to report the level of service based on counseling and/or coordination of care, the total length of time of the encounter (face-to-face or floor time, as appropriate) should be documented and the record should describe the counseling and/or activities to coordinate care

Orthopedic and Orthopedic Surgery Specifics

Each provider specialty has differences that typically lie in the approach and are likely to revolve around the physical exam.

There are 11 types of exams specified in the 1997 guidelines. Some of these exams will work better for some specialties than others. Not all specialists will find that the organ-system exam related to their specialty is the most practical. Find below suggestions related to the most problematic E/M audit areas: history and exam.

Many suggestions may pertain to the higher levels of service, new patient or consult levels four and five, or level four and five established patients. This is not an effort to steer a provider toward the use of those codes, but rather recognition that this is where the more demanding documentation elements reside.

Hospital admissions require comprehensive histories and exams at the two higher levels of admits. This is where documentation deficiencies most often occur. All admits for levels two and three require a complete (10) ROS. This area probably yields more deficiencies than any other. Hospitals generally require a complete "H & P." Under current guidelines, the history element can be met by indicating "all other ROS negative" after reviewing problem–pertinent systems.

For subsequent hospital visits, the exam is often not very substantial (the patient just having had a complete H & P on admission). It is best to use the general system-level approach.

Physical Exam Section

For orthopedics in general, the 1995 multi-system exam guidelines are much more friendly for follow-up patients.

The 1997 comprehensive single system exam requires that 28 or more individual elements be addressed to qualify for the highest level of exam. There is also a note under muskuloskeletal and skin sections that emphasizes that at least four major body areas must be examined in detail for the comprehensive level exams. For new patients and consults the 1997 approach may work well. Orthopods may wish to review the muskuloskeletal single system exam in case it in fact approximates key exam elements in certain situations. This is one of the more demanding single-system exams. The breadth of this exam poses a clear problem for an orthopod using this documentation approach when dealing with a severe problem limited to a single area (i.e., a severe disc problem). The overall code level would appear to be quite high, but under the documentation requirements for the higher level services it would be difficult to meet the exam requirements. An orthopedic template could be rather easily constructed and may be of benefit for ease of documentation.

See the 1997 single system muskuloskeletal exam on the following page.

Remember that you can always use the 1995 general multi-system approach, it tends to be much simpler.

Musculoskeletal Examination

System/Body Area	Elements of Examination
Constitutional	■ Measurement of **any three of the following seven** vital signs: 1) sitting or standing blood pressure, 2) supine blood pressure, 3) pulse rate and regularity, 4) respiration, 5) temperature, 6) height, 7) weight (May be measured and recorded by ancillary staff). ■ General appearance of patient (e.g., development, nutrition, body habitus, deformities, attention to grooming)
Head and face	
Eyes	
Ears, nose, mouth and throat	
Neck	
Respiratory	
Cardiovascular	■ Examination of peripheral vascular system by observation (e.g., swelling, varicosities) and palpation (e.g., pulses, temperature, edema, tenderness)
Chest (Breasts)	
Gastrointestinal (Abdomen)	
Genitourinary	
Lymphatic	■ Palpation of lymph nodes in neck, axillae, groin, and/or other location
Musculoskeletal	■ Examination of gait and station ■ Examination of joint(s), bone(s) and muscle(s) tendon(s) of **four of the following six areas:** 1) head and neck; 2) spine, ribs and pelvis; 3) right upper extremity; 4) left upper extremity; 5) right lower extremity; and 6) left lower extremity. The examination of a given area includes: ■ Inspection, percussion and/or palpation with notation of any misalignment, asymmetry, crepitation, defects, tenderness, masses or effusions ■ Assessment of range of motion with notation of any pain (e.g., straight leg raising), crepitation or contracture ■ Assessment of stability with notation of any dislocation (luxation), subluxation or laxity ■ Assessment of muscle strength and tone (e.g., flaccid, cog wheel, spastic) with notation of any atrophy or abnormal movements Note: For the comprehensive level of examination, all four of the elements identified by a bullet must be performed and documented for each of four anatomic areas. For the three lower levels of examination, each element is counted separately for each body area. For example, assessing range of motion in two extremities constitutes two elements.
Extremities	[See Musculoskeletal and Skin]
Skin	■ Inspection and/or palpation of skin and subcutaneous tissue (e.g., scars, rashes, lesions, cafe-au-lait spots, ulcers) in **four of the following six** areas: 1) head and neck; 2) trunk; 3) right upper extremity; 4) left upper extremity; 5) right lower extremity; and 6) left lower extremity. Note: For the comprehensive level, the examination of all four anatomic areas must be performed and documented. For the three lower levels of examination, each body area is counted separately. For example, inspection and/or palpation of the skin and subcutaneous tissue of two extremities constitutes two elements.
Neurological/ Psychiatric	■ Test coordination (e.g., finger/nose, heel/knee/shin, rapid alternating movements in the upper and lower extremities, evaluation of fine motor coordination in young children) ■ Examination of deep tendon reflexes and/or nerve stretch test with notation of pathological reflexes (e.g., Babinski) ■ Examination of sensation (e.g., by touch, pin, vibration, proprioception) ■ Brief assessment of mental status including: — orientation to time, place and person — mood and affect (e.g., depression, anxiety, agitation)

Content and Documentation Requirements

Level of exam	Perform and document
Problem focused	**One to five** elements identified by a bullet.
Expanded problem focused	**At least six** elements identified by a bullet.
Detailed	**At least 12** elements identified by a bullet, whether in a box with a shaded or unshaded border
Comprehensive	Performance of **all** elements identified by a bullet; whether in a box or with a shaded or unshaded box. Documentation of every element in each with a shaded border and at least one element in a box with un shaded border is expected

Index

A

Ablation
  Bone Tumor, 20982
  CT Scan Guidance, 77013
  Parenchymal Tissue
    CT Scan Guidance, 77013
Abscess
  Arm, Lower, 25028
    Excision, 25145
    Incision and Drainage, 25035
  Arm, Upper
    Incision and Drainage, 23930-23935
  Carpals
    Incision, Deep, 25035
  Clavicle
    Sequestrectomy, 23170
  Elbow
    Incision and Drainage, 23930-23935
  Excision
    Olecranon Process, 24138
    Radius, 24136
    Ulna, 24138
  Finger, 26010-26011
    Incision and Drainage, 26010-26011, 26034
  Hand
    Incision and Drainage, 26034
  Humeral Head, 23174
  Humerus
    Excision, 24134
    Incision and Drainage, 23935
  Posterior Spine, 22010-22015
  Radius
    Incision, Deep, 25035
  Scapula
    Sequestrectomy, 23172
  Shoulder
    Incision and Drainage, 23030
  Soft Tissue
    Incision, 20005
  Spine
    Incision and Drainage, 22010-22015
  Ulna
    Incision, Deep, 25035
  Wrist
    Excision, 25145
    Incision and Drainage, 25028, 25035
Absolute Neutrophil Count (ANC), 85048
Absorptiometry
  Dual Energy
    Bone
      Appendicular, 77079
      Axial Skeleton, 77078
      Vertebral, 77080-77082
  Dual Photon
    Bone, 78351
  Radiographic
    Photodensity, 77083
  Single Photon
    Bone, 78350
Absorption Spectrophotometry, 82190
  Atomic, 82190
Accessory Nerve
  Incision, 63191
  Section, 63191
ACD, 63075-63076
Acid
  Amino
    Blood or Urine, 82127-82131, 82136-82139
  Fast Bacilli (AFB)
    Culture, 87116

Acid—continued
  Fast Stain, 88312
  Guanylic, 83008
  Lactic, 83605
  Phosphatase, 84060
  Uric
    Blood, 84550
    Other Source, 84560
    Urine, 84560
Acidity/Alkalinity
  Blood Gases, 82800-82805
ACP, 84060
Acromioclavicular Joint
  Arthrocentesis, 20605
  Arthrotomy, 23044
    with Biopsy, 23101
  Dislocation, 23540-23552
    Open Treatment, 23550-23552
  X-ray, 73050
Acromion
  Excision
    Shoulder, 23130
Acromionectomy
  Partial, 23130
Acromioplasty, 23415-23420
  Partial, 23130
Activated Partial Thromboplastin Time, 85730-85732
Activities of Daily Living (ADL), 97535
  Training, 97535-97537
Acupuncture
  One or More Needles
    with Electrical Stimulation, 97813-97814
    without Electrical Stimulation, 97810-97811
Addam Operation, 26040-26045
Adhesion, Adhesions
  Epidural, 62263-62264
Adjustment
  External Fixation, 20693, 20696
ADL
  Activities of Daily Living, 97535-97537
Administration
  Injection
    Intramuscular Antibiotic, 96372
    Therapeutic, Diagnostic, Prophylactic
      Intra-arterial, 96373
      Intramuscular, 96372
      Intravenous, 96374-96376
      Subcutaneous, 96372
Adson Test, 95870
Advancement Flap
  Skin, Adjacent Tissue Transfer, 14000-14041, 14301-14350
After Hours Medical Services, 99051-99053, 99060
Aggregation
  Platelet, 85576
Alanine Amino (ALT), 84460
Albumin
  Serum, 82040
  Urine, 82042
Aldolase
  Blood, 82085
ALIF (Anterior Lumbar Interbody Fusion), 22558-22585
Alkaline Phosphatase, 84075-84080
  Leukocyte, 85540
  WBC, 85540
Allograft
  Bone, Structural, 20931
  Spine Surgery
    Morselized, 20930
    Osteopromotive Material, 20930

Allograft—continued
  Spine Surgery—continued
    Structural, 20931
Alloplastic Dressing
  Burns, 15002, 15004-15005
Amikacin
  Assay, 80150
Amino Acids
  Blood or Urine, 82127-82131, 82136-82139
Aminotransferase
  Alanine (SGPT), 84460
  Aspartate (SGOT), 84450
Ammonia
  Blood, 82140
  Urine, 82140
Amputation
  Arm and Shoulder, 23900-23921
  Arm, Lower, 25900-25905, 25915
    Revision, 25907-25909
    with Implant, 24931-24935
  Arm, Upper, 24900-24920
    and Shoulder, 23900-23921
    Revision, 24925-24930
    with Implant, 24931-24935
  Finger, 26910-26952
  Hand
    at Metacarpals, 25927
    at Wrist, 25920
      Revision, 25922
    Revision, 25924, 25929-25931
  Interthoracoscapular, 23900
  Metacarpal, 26910
  Thumb, 26910-26952
  Tuft of Distal Phalanx, 11752
Analysis
  Electronic
    Pulse Generator, 95970-95971
  Spectrum, 82190
Anesthesia
  Dressing Change, 15852
  External Fixation System
    Adjustment/Revision, 20693
    Removal, 20694
  Manipulation
    Spine, 22505
  Shoulder
    Dislocation
      Closed Treatment, 23655
  Suture Removal, 15850-15851
  Vertebral Process
    Fracture/Dislocation
      Closed Treatment, 22315
Angiography
  Arm Artery, 73206
  Extremity, Upper, 73225
  Neck, 70498, 70547-70549
Angiotensin I, 84244
Annuloplasty
  Percutaneous, Intradiscal, 22526-22527
Anti–Phosphatidylserine (Phospholipid) Antibody, 86148
Antibiotic Administration
  Injection, 96372
Antibiotic Sensitivity, 87181-87184, 87188
Antibodies, Thyroid–Stimulating, 84445
Antibody
  Anti–Phosphatidylserine (Phospholipid), 86148
  Cyclic Citrullinated Peptide (CCP), 86200
  Growth Hormone, 86277
Antidiuretic Hormone, 84588
Apoaminotransferase, Aspartate, 84550

Application
  Bone Fixation Device
    Multiplane, 20692
    Uniplane, 20690
  Caliper, 20660
  Cranial Tongs, 20660
  Fixation Device
    Shoulder, 23700
  Halo
    Cranial, 20661
      Thin Skull Osteology, 20664
  Intervertebral Device, 22851
  Stereotactic Frame, 20660
Aquatic Therapy
  with Exercises, 97113
Arm
  Excision
    Bone, 25145
  Removal
    Foreign Body
      Forearm or Wrist, 25248
  Repair
    Muscle, 24341
    Tendon, 24341
  Skin Graft
    Full Thickness, 15220-15221
    Muscle, Myocutaneous, or Fasciocutaneous Flaps, 15736
    Split, 15100-15101
  Tendon
    Excision, 25109
    Tissue Transfer, Adjacent, 14020-14021
Arm, Lower
  Abscess, 25028
    Excision, 25145
    Incision and Drainage Bone, 25035
  Amputation, 24900-24920, 25900-25905, 25915
    Revision, 25907-25909
  Angiography, 73206
  Biopsy, 25065-25066
  Bursa
    Incision and Drainage, 25031
  Cast, 29075
  CT Scan, 73200-73206
  Decompression, 25020-25025
  Fasciotomy, 24495, 25020-25025
  Hematoma, 25028
  Incision and Drainage, 23930
  Lesion, Tendon Sheath
    Excision, 25110
  Magnetic Resonance Imaging (MRI), 73218-73220, 73223
  Reconstruction
    Ulna, 25337
  Removal
    Foreign Body, 25248
  Repair
    Decompression, 24495
    Muscle, 25260-25263, 25270
    Secondary, 25265
  Secondary
    Muscle or Tendon, 25272-25274
    Tendon, 25260-25274, 25280-25295, 25310-25316
    Secondary, 25265
    Tendon Sheath, 25275
  Replantation, 20805
  Splint, 29125-29126
  Tenotomy, 25290
  Tumor, 25071-25073, 25078, 25120-25126
  Ultrasound, 76881-76882

Arm, Lower—continued
  X-ray, 73090
    with Upper Arm, 73092
Arm, Upper
  Abscess
    Incision and Drainage, 23930
  Amputation, 23900-23921,
    24900-24920
    Revision, 24925-24930
    with Implant, 24931-24935
  Angiography, 73206
  Biopsy, 24065-24066
  Cast, 29065
  CT Scan, 73200-73206
  Hematoma
    Incision and Drainage, 23930
  Magnetic Resonance Imaging (MRI),
    73218-73220, 73223
  Muscle Revision, 24330-24331
  Removal
    Cast, 29705
    Foreign Body, 24200-24201
  Repair
    Muscle Revision, 24301, 24320
    Muscle Transfer, 24301, 24320
    Tendon, 24332
    Tendon Lengthening, 24305
    Tendon Revision, 24320
    Tendon Transfer, 24301
    Tenotomy, 24310
  Replantation, 20802
  Splint, 29105
  Tumor, 24071-24073, 24079
  Ultrasound, 76881-76882
  Wound Exploration, 20103
    Penetrating, 20103
  X-ray, 73060
  X-ray with Lower Arm
    Infant, 73092
Arrest, Epiphyseal
  Radius, 25450-25455
  Ulna, 25450-25455
Artery
  Brachial
    Exploration, 24495
  Extremities
    Vascular Studies, 93922-93923
  Vascular Study
    Extremities, 93922-93923
Arthrectomy
  Elbow, 24155
Arthrocentesis
  Intermediate Joint, 20605
  Large Joint, 20610
  Small Joint, 20600
Arthrodesis
  Carpometacarpal Joint
    Hand, 26843-26844
    Thumb, 26841-26842
  Cervical Anterior
    with Discectomy, 22551-22554
  Elbow, 24800-24802
  Finger Joint, 26850-26863
    Interphalangeal, 26860-26863
    Metacarpophalangeal, 26850
  Hand Joint, 26843-26844
  Intercarpal Joint, 25820
    with Autograft, 25825
  Interphalangeal Joint, 26860-26863
  Metacarpophalangeal Joint,
    26850-26852
  Pre-Sacral Interbody, 0195T-0196T
  Radioulnar Joint, Distal, 25830
    with Resection of Ulna, 25830
  Shoulder Joint, 23800
    with Autogenous Graft, 23802
  Thumb Joint, 26841-26842
  Vertebra
    Additional Interspace
      Anterior/Anterolateral
        Approach, 22585
      Lateral Extracavitary, 22534
      Posterior/Posterolateral
        and/or Lateral Trans-
        verse Process, 22632
    Cervical
      Anterior/Anterolateral
        Approach, 22548

Arthrodesis—continued
  Vertebra—continued
    Cervical—continued
      Posterior/Posterolateral
        and/or Lateral Trans-
        verse Process,
        22590-22600
    Lumbar
      Anterior/Anterolateral
        Approach, 22558
      Lateral Extracavitary, 22533
      Posterior/Interbody, 22630
      Posterior/Posterolateral
        and/or Lateral Trans-
        verse Process, 22612,
        22630
      Presacral Interbody Tech-
        nique, 0195T-0196T
    Spinal Deformity
      Anterior Approach,
        22808-22812
      Posterior Approach,
        22800-22804
    Spinal Fusion
      Exploration, 22830
    Thoracic
      Anterior/Anterolateral
        Approach, 22556
      Lateral Extracavitary, 22532
      Posterior/Posterolateral
        and/or Lateral Traverse
        Process, 22610
    Vertebrae
      Posterior, 22614
  Wrist, 25800
    Radioulnar Joint, Distal, 25830
    with Graft, 25810
    with Sliding Graft, 25805
Arthrography
  Elbow, 73085
    Injection, 24220
  Shoulder, 73040
    Injection, 23350
  Wrist, 73115
    Injection, 25246
Arthroplasty
  Bower's, 25332
  Cervical, 0092T, 22856
  Elbow, 24360
    Total Replacement, 24363
    with Implant, 24361-24362
  Interphalangeal Joint, 26535-26536
  Lumbar, 0092T, 22857
  Metacarpophalangeal Joint,
    26530-26531
  Radius, 24365
  Removal
    Cervical, 22864
    Each Additional Interspace,
      0095T
    Lumbar, 22865
  Revision
    Cervical, 22861
    Each Additional Interspace,
      0098T
    Lumbar, 22862
  Shoulder Joint
    with Implant, 23470-23472
  Spine
    Cervical, 22856
    Each Additional Interspace,
      0092T
    Lumbar, 22857
    Vertebral, 0201T-0202T
  Wrist, 25332, 25441-25447
    Carpal, 25443
    Lunate, 25444
    Navicular, 25443
    Pseudarthrosis Type, 25332
    Radius, 25441
    Revision, 25449
    Total Replacement, 25446
    Trapezium, 25445
    Ulna, 25442
    with Implant, 25441-25445

Arthroscopy
  Diagnostic
    Elbow, 29830
    Metacarpophalangeal Joint,
      29900
    Shoulder, 29805
    Wrist, 29840
  Surgical
    Elbow, 29834-29838
    Metacarpophalangeal Joint,
      29901-29902
    Shoulder, 29806-29828
      Biceps Tenodesis, 29828
    Wrist, 29843-29848
Arthrotomy
  Acromioclavicular Joint, 23044,
    23101
  Carpometacarpal Joint, 26070,
    26100
    with Synovial Biopsy, 26100
  Elbow, 24000
    Capsular Release, 24006
    with Joint Exploration, 24101
    with Synovectomy, 24102
    with Synovial Biopsy, 24100
  Finger Joint, 26075
    Interphalangeal with Synovial
      Biopsy, 26110
    Metacarpophalangeal with
      Biopsy, Synovium, 26105
  Glenohumeral Joint, 23040
  Interphalangeal Joint, 26080, 26110
  Metacarpophalangeal Joint, 26075,
    26105
  Shoulder, 23044, 23105-23107
  Shoulder Joint, 23100-23101
    Exploration and/or Removal of
      Loose Foreign Body, 23107
  Sternoclavicular Joint, 23044,
    23101
  with Biopsy
    Acromioclavicular Joint, 23101
    Glenohumeral Joint, 23100
    Sternoclavicular Joint, 23101
  with Synovectomy
    Glenohumeral Joint, 23105
    Sternoclavicular Joint, 23106
  Wrist, 25040, 25100-25107
ASAT, 84450
Aspartate Aminotransferase, 84450
Aspiration
  Bone Marrow, 38220
  Bursa, 20600-20610
  Cyst
    Bone, 20615
    Ganglion Cyst, 20612
  Joint, 20600-20610
  Nucleus of Disc
    Diagnostic, 62267
Atomic Absorption Spectroscopy,
  82190
Augmentation
  Percutaneous
    Spine, 0200T-0201T,
      22523-22525
    Sacral, 0200T-0201T
    Spine, 22523-22525
    Vertebral, 22523-22525
Autograft
  Bone
    Local, 20936
    Morselized, 20937
    Structural, 20938
  Spine Surgery
    Local, 20936
    Morselized, 20937
    Structural, 20938
Avulsion
  Nails, 11730-11732
  Nerves, 64772
Axilla
  Skin Graft
    Full Thickness, 15240-15241
    Tissue Transfer, Adjacent,
      14040-14041

B

Back/Flank
  Biopsy, 21920-21925
  Tumor, 21931-21933, 21936
  Wound Exploration
    Penetrating, 20102
**Backbench Reconstruction Prior to
  Implant**
  Wound Exploration, Penetrating,
    20102
Bacteria Culture
  Additional Methods, 87077
  Aerobic, 87040, 87070-87071
  Anaerobic, 87073-87076
  Blood, 87040
  Other Source, 87070-87075
  Screening, 87081
Bankart Procedure, 23455
Barsky's Procedures, 26580
Bed Sores, 15931-15937
Benedict Test for Urea, 81005
Bennett Fracture
  Other Than Thumb
    Closed Treatment, 26670-26675
    Open Treatment, 26685-26686
    Percutaneous Treatment, 26676
  Thumb Fracture
    Open Treatment, 26665
    with Dislocation, 26645-26650
Bicarbonate, 82374
Biceps Tendon
  Insertion, 24342
  Tenodesis, 23430, 29828
Biopsy
  Arm, Lower, 25065-25066
  Arm, Upper, 24065-24066
  Back/Flank, 21920-21925
  Bone, 20220-20245
  Bone Marrow, 38221
  Carpometacarpal Joint
    Synovium, 26100
  Elbow, 24065-24066, 24101
    Synovium, 24100
  Forearm, Soft Tissue, 25065-25066
  Hand Joint
    Synovium, 26100
  Interphalangeal Joint
    Finger, 26110
    Finger Synovium, 26110
  Lymph Nodes, 38500-38505
    Needle, 38505
    Open, 38500
      Superficial, 38500
  Metacarpophalangeal Joint, 26105
  Muscle, 20200-20206
  Nail, 11755
  Neck, 21550
  Nerve, 64795
  Shoulder
    Deep, 23066
    Joint, 23100-23101
    Soft Tissue, 23065
  Thorax, 21550
  Vertebral Body, 20250-20251
  with Arthrotomy
    Acromioclavicular Joint, 23101
    Glenohumeral Joint, 23100
    Sternoclavicular Joint, 23101
  Wrist, 25065-25066, 25100-25101
Bischof Procedure
  Laminectomy, Surgical,
    63170-63172
Blatt Capsulodesis, 25320
Bleeding Time, 85002
Blood
  Bleeding Time, 85002
  Blood Clot
    Coagulation Time, 85345
  Hemoglobin Concentration, 85046
  Osmolality, 83930
  Patch, 62273
  Platelet
    Aggregation, 85576
    Count, 85008
  Reticulocyte, 85046

Blood Cell Count
  Blood Smear, 85007-85008
  Differential WBC Count, 85007, 85009
  Hematocrit, 85014
  Hemoglobin, 85018
  Hemogram
    Added Indices, 85025-85027
    Automated, 85025-85027
  Microhematocrit, 85013
  Red Blood Cell, 85041
  Red Blood Cells, 85041
  Reticulocyte, 85044-85046
  White Blood Cell, 85048
Blood Clot
  Coagulation Time, 85345
Blood Coagulation
  Factor III, 85730-85732
  Factor IV, 82310
Blood Flow Check, Graft, 15860
Blood Patch, 62273
Blood Smear, 85060
Blood Test(s)
  Panels
    Electrolyte, 80051
    General Health Panel, 80050
    Hepatic Function, 80076
    Lipid Panel, 80061
    Metabolic Panel, Basic
      Basic, 80048
      Comprehensive, 80053
      Ionized Calcium, 80047
      Total Calcium, 80048
Blood Urea Nitrogen, 84520-84525
Body Cast
  Halo, 29000
  Removal, 29700, 29710-29715
  Repair, 29720
  Risser Jacket, 29010-29015
  Turnbuckle Jacket, 29020-29025
  Upper Body and One Leg, 29044
  Upper Body Only, 29035
  Upper Body with Head, 29040
  Upper Body with Legs, 29046
Body Fluid
  Crystal Identification, 89060
Bone
  Ablation
    Tumor, 20982
  Biopsy, 20220-20245
  CT Scan
    Density Study, 77078-77079
  Cyst
    Drainage, 20615
    Injection, 20615
  Dual Energy X-ray
    Absorptiometry, 77080-77081
  Fixation
    Caliper, 20660
    Cranial Tong, 20660
    External, 20690
    Halo, 20661
    Multiplane, 20692
    Pin
      Wire, 20650
    Skeletal
      Humeral Epicondyle
        Percutaneous, 24566
    Stereotactic Frame, 20660
    Uniplane, 20690
  Nuclear Medicine
    Density Study, 78350-78351
    Imaging, 78300-78320
    SPECT, 78320
  Protein, 83937
  Removal
    Fixation Device, 20670-20680
  X-ray
    Dual Energy Absorptiometry, 77080-77081
    Osseous Survey, 77075-77077
Bone Density Study
  Appendicular Skeleton, 77079, 77081
  Axial Skeleton, 77078, 77080
  Ultrasound, 76977
  Vertebral Fracture Assessment, 77082

Bone Graft
  Allograft
    Morselized, 20930
    Structural, 20931
  Any Donor Area, 20900-20902
  Autograft, 20936
    Morselized, 20937
    Structural, 20938
  Harvesting, 20900-20902
  Spine Surgery
    Allograft
      Morselized, 20930
      Structural, 20931
    Autograft
      Local, 20936
      Morselized, 20937
      Structural, 20938
  Vascular Pedicle, 25430
Bone Healing
  Electrical Stimulation
    Invasive, 20975
    Noninvasive, 20974
  Ultrasound Stimulation, 20979
Bone Marrow
  Aspiration, 38220
  Needle Biopsy, 38221
  Smear, 85097
  Trocar Biopsy, 38221
Bone Osseous Survey, 77075
Bost Fusion
  Arthrodesis, Wrist, 25800-25810
Bosworth Operation, 23550-23552
Boutonniere Deformity, 26426-26428
Bower's Arthroplasty, 25332
Boxer's Fracture Treatment, 26600-26615
Brachial Plexus
  Decompression, 64713
  Neuroplasty, 64713
  Release, 64713
Bradykinin
  Blood or Urine, 82286
Braun Procedure, 23405-23406
Brisement Injection, 20550-20551
Bristow Procedure, 23450-23462
  Capsulorrhaphy, Anterior, 23450-23462
BUN, 84520-84545
Bunnell Procedure, 24301
Burns
  Debridement, 15002-15005
  Excision, 15002, 15004-15005
  Tissue Culture Skin Grafts, 15100-15101, 15120-15121
  Xenograft, 15400-15401
Burrow's Operation, 14000-14041, 14301-14350
Bursa
  Arm, Lower, 25031
  Elbow
    Excision, 24105
    Incision and Drainage, 23931
    Injection, 20600-20610
  Joint
    Aspiration, 20600-20610
    Drainage, 20600-20610
    Injection, 20600-20610
  Palm
    Incision and Drainage, 26025-26030
  Shoulder
    Drainage, 23031
  Wrist, 25031
    Excision, 25115-25116
    Incision and Drainage, 25020
    Infected Bursa, 25031

C

CA, 82310-82340
Calcareous Deposits
  Subdeltoid
    Removal, 23000
Calcitonin
  Blood or Urine, 82308

Calcium
  Blood
    Infusion Test, 82331
  Ionized, 82330
  Panel, 80047
  Total, 82310
    Panel, 80048
  Urine, 82340
Caliper
  Application
    Removal, 20660
Capsule
  Elbow
    Arthrotomy, 24006
    Excision, 24006
  Interphalangeal Joint
    Excision, 26525
    Incision, 26525
  Metacarpophalangeal Joint
    Excision, 26520
    Incision, 26520
  Shoulder, Incision, 23020
  Wrist
    Excision, 25320
Capsulodesis
  Blatt, 25320
  Metacarpophalangeal Joint, 26516-26518
Capsulorrhaphy
  Anterior, 23450-23462
  Multi-Directional Instability, 23466
  Posterior, 23465
  Wrist, 25320
Capsulotomy
  Metacarpophalangeal Joint, 26520
  Wrist, 25085
Carbon Dioxide
  Blood or Urine, 82374
Carpal Bone
  Arthroplasty
    with Implant, 25443
  Cyst
    Excision, 25130-25136
  Dislocation
    Closed Treatment, 25690
    Open Treatment, 25695
  Excision, 25210-25215
    Partial, 25145
  Fracture, 25622-25628
    Closed Treatment, 25622, 25630
    Open Treatment, 25628, 25645
    with Manipulation, 25624, 25635
    without Manipulation, 25630
  Incision and Drainage, 26034
  Insertion
    Vascular Pedicle, 25430
    Osteoplasty, 25394
  Repair, 25431-25440
  Sequestrectomy, 25145
  Tumor
    Excision, 25130-25136
Carpal Tunnel
  Injection
    Therapeutic, 20526
Carpal Tunnel Syndrome
  Decompression, 64721
  Arthroscopy, 29848
  Injection, 20526
Carpals
  Incision and Drainage, 25035
Carpectomy, 25210-25215
Carpometacarpal Joint
  Arthrodesis
    Hand, 26843-26844
    Thumb, 26841-26842
  Arthrotomy, 26070, 26100
  Biopsy
    Synovium, 26100
  Dislocation
    Closed Treatment, 26670
      with Manipulation, 26675-26676
    Open Treatment, 26685-26686
  Exploration, 26070
  Fusion
    Hand, 26843-26844
    Thumb, 26841-26842

Carpometacarpal Joint—*continued*
  Removal
    Foreign Body, 26070
  Repair, 25447
  Synovectomy, 26130
Cartilage Graft
  Harvesting, 20910
Cast
  Body
    Halo, 29000
    Risser Jacket, 29010-29015
    Turnbuckle Jacket, 29020-29025
    Upper Body and Head, 29040
    Upper Body and Legs, 29046
    Upper Body and One Leg, 29044
    Upper Body Only, 29035
  Finger, 29086
  Hand, 29085
  Long Arm, 29065
  Removal, 29700-29715
  Repair, 29720
  Short Arm, 29075
  Shoulder, 29049-29058
  Wedging, 29740
  Windowing, 29730
  Wrist, 29085
Cauda Equina
  Decompression, 63005-63011, 63017, 63047-63048, 63055
  Exploration, 63005-63011, 63017
Cauterization
  Skin Lesion
    Malignant, 17260-17276
CBC (Complete Blood Count), 85025-85027
Cerebrospinal Fluid, 86325
Chemiluminescent Assay, 82397
Chemistry Tests
  Organ or Disease Oriented Panel
    Electrolyte, 80051
    General Health Panel, 80050
    Hepatic Function Panel, 80076
    Lipid Panel, 80061
    Metabolic
      Basic, 80047-80048
      Calcium
        Ionized, 80047
        Total, 80048
      Comprehensive, 80053
Chemodenervation
  Extremity Muscle, 64614
  Trunk Muscle, 64614
Chemosurgery
  Skin Lesion, 17270
Chloramphenicol, 82415
Chlorhydrocarbon, 82441
Chloride
  Blood, 82435
  Urine, 82436
Chlorinated Hydrocarbons, 82441
Chlorohydrocarbon, 82441
Cholesterol
  Measurement, 83721
  Serum, 82465
  Testing, 83718-83719
Chromium, 82495
Cl, 82435-82436
Clavicle
  Craterization, 23180
  Cyst
    Excision, 23140
      with Allograft, 23146
      with Autograft, 23145
  Diaphysectomy, 23180
  Dislocation
    Acromioclavicular Joint
      Closed Treatment, 23540-23545
      Open Treatment, 23550-23552
    Sternoclavicular Joint
      Closed Treatment, 23520-23525
      Open Treatment, 23530-23532
      without Manipulation, 23540

Clavicle—continued
　Excision, 23170
　　Partial, 23120, 23180
　　Total, 23125
　Fracture
　　Closed Treatment
　　　with Manipulation, 23505
　　　without Manipulation, 23500
　　Open Treatment, 23515
　Osteotomy, 23480-23485
　Pinning, Wiring, Etc., 23490
　Prophylactic Treatment, 23490
　Repair Osteotomy, 23480-23485
　Saucerization, 23180
　Sequestrectomy, 23170
　Tumor
　　Excision, 23140, 23146, 23200
　　　with Allograft, 23146
　　　with Autograft, 23145
　　Radical Resection, 23200
　X-ray, 73000
Claviculectomy
　Partial, 23120
　Total, 23125
Claw Finger Repair, 26499
Cleft Hand
　Repair, 26580
Closure, 12001-12007, 12020-12047, 13120-13133, 13160
　Skin
　　Arm, Arms
　　　Complex, 13120-13122
　　　Intermediate, 12031-12037
　　　Layered, 12031-12037
　　　Simple, 12001-12007
　　　Superficial, 12001-12007
　　Axilla, Axillae
　　　Complex, 13131-13133
　　　Intermediate, 12031-12037
　　　Layered, 12031-12037
　　　Simple, 12001-12007
　　　Superficial, 12001-12007
　　Back
　　　Intermediate, 12031-12037
　　　Layered, 12031-12037
　　　Simple, 12001-12007
　　　Superficial, 12001-12007
　　Chest
　　　Intermediate, 12031-12037
　　　Layered, 12031-12037
　　　Simple, 12001-12007
　　　Superficial, 12001-12007
　　Extremity, Extremities
　　　Intermediate, 12031-12037
　　　Layered, 12031-12037
　　　Simple, 12001-12007
　　　Superficial, 12001-12007
　　Finger, Fingers
　　　Complex, 13131-13133
　　　Intermediate, 12041-12047
　　　Layered, 12041-12047
　　　Simple, 12001-12007
　　　Superficial, 12001-12007
　　Forearm, Forearms
　　　Complex, 13120-13122
　　　Intermediate, 12031-12037
　　　Layered, 12031-12037
　　　Simple, 12001-12007
　　　Superficial, 12001-12007
　　Hand, Hands
　　　Complex, 13131-13133
　　　Intermediate, 12041-12047
　　　Layered, 12041-12047
　　　Simple, 12001-12007
　　　Superficial, 12001-12007
　　Lower
　　　Arm, Arms
　　　　Complex, 13120-13122
　　　　Intermediate, 12031-12037
　　　　Layered, 12031-12037
　　　　Simple, 12001-12007
　　　　Superficial, 12001-12007
　　Neck
　　　Complex, 13131-13133
　　　Intermediate, 12041-12047
　　　Layered, 12041-12047
　　　Simple, 12001-12007
　　　Superficial, 12001-12007

Closure—continued
　Skin—continued
　　Palm, Palms
　　　Complex, 13131-13133
　　　Intermediate, 12041-12047
　　　Layered, 12041-12047
　　　Simple, 12001-12007
　　　Superficial, 12001-12007
　　Trunk
　　　Intermediate, 12031-12037
　　　Layered, 12031-12037
　　　Simple, 12001-12007
　　　Superficial, 12001-12007
　　Upper
　　　Arm, Arms
　　　　Complex, 13120-13122
　　　　Intermediate, 12031-12037
　　　　Layered, 12031-12037
　　　　Simple, 12001-12007
　　　　Superficial, 12001-12007
　　Extremity
　　　Intermediate, 12031-12037
　　　Layered, 12031-12037
　　　Simple, 12001-12007
　　　Superficial, 12001-12007
　Sternotomy, 21750
Coagulation
　Factor III, 85730-85732
　Factor IV, 82310
　Time, 85345
Coagulation Factor
　Factor III, 85730-85732
　Factor IV, 82310-82331
Coagulation Time, 85345
Coccyx
　X-ray, 72220
Cold Pack Treatment, 97010
Collagen Cross Links, 82523
Collar Bone
　Craterization, 23180
　Cyst
　　Excision, 23140
　　　with
　　　　Allograft, 23146
　　　　Autograft, 23145
　Diaphysectomy, 23180
　Dislocation
　　Acromioclavicular Joint
　　　Closed Treatment, 23540-23545
　　　Open Treatment, 23550-23552
　　Sternoclavicular Joint
　　　Closed Treatment, 23520-23525
　　　Open Treatment, 23530-23532
　　　with Manipulation, 23540
　Excision
　　Partial, 23120, 23180
　　Total, 23125
　Fracture
　　Closed Treatment
　　　with Manipulation, 23505
　　　without Manipulation, 23500
　　Open Treatment, 23515
　Osteotomy, 23480-23485
　Pinning, Wiring, Etc., 23490
　Prophylactic Treatment, 23490
　Repair Osteotomy, 23480-23485
　Saucerization, 23180
　Sequestrectomy, 23170
　Tumor
　　Excision, 23140
　　　with Allograft, 23146
　　　with Autograft, 23145
　　Radical Resection, 23200
　X-ray, 73000
Collateral Ligament
　Interphalangeal Joint, 26545
　Metacarpophalangeal Joint Repair, 26540-26542
Colles Fracture, 25600-25609
Common Sensory Nerve
　Repair, Suture, 64834
Community/Work Reintegration
　Training, 97537
Complete Blood Count, 85025-85027

Composite Graft, 15770
Computed Tomography (CT Scan)
　Bone
　　Density Study, 77078-77083
　　Follow-up Study, 76380
　Guidance
　　Cyst Aspiration, 77012
　　Localization, 77011
　　Needle Biopsy, 77012
　with Contrast
　　Arm, 73201, 73206
　　Head, 70496
　　Neck, 70491, 70498
　　Spine
　　　Cervical, 72126
　　　Lumbar, 72132
　　　Thoracic, 72129
　without Contrast
　　Arm, 73200
　　Neck, 70490
　　Spine, Cervical, 72125
　　Spine, Lumbar, 72131
　　Spine, Thoracic, 72128
　without Contrast, followed by Contrast
　　Arm, 73202
　　Neck, 70492
　　Spine
　　　Cervical, 72127
　　　Lumbar, 72133
　　　Thoracic, 72130
Computer Assisted Navigation
　Orthopedic Surgery, 20985
Computer-Assisted Navigation, 0054T-0055T, 20985
Computer-Assisted Surgical Navigation
　Imageless, 20985
　　Image Guidance
　　　Intraoperative, 20985
　　with Image Guidance, 0054T-0055T
Concentration of Specimen, 87015
Condyle
　Humerus
　　Fracture
　　　Closed Treatment, 24576-24577
　　　Open Treatment, 24579
　　　Percutaneous, 24582
Construction
　Finger
　　Toe to Hand Transfer, 26551-26556
Contracture
　Elbow
　　Release with Radical Resection of Capsule, 24149
　Palm
　　Release, 26121-26125
　Thumb
　　Release, 26508
Contrast Bath Therapy, 97034
Coracoacromial Ligament Release, 23415
Coracoid Process Transfer, 23462
Cordotomy, 63194-63199
Corpectomy, 63101-63103
Correction of Syndactyly, 26560-26562
Corticosterone
　Blood or Urine, 82528
Cortisol, 82530
　Total, 82533
Costotransversectomy, 21610
Cranial Bone
　Halo
　　for Thin Skull Osteology, 20664
Cranial Halo, 20661
Cranial Tongs
　Application
　　Removal, 20660
　Removal, 20665
Craterization
　Clavicle, 23180
　Humerus, 23184, 24140
　Metacarpal, 26230
　Olecranon Process, 24147

Craterization—continued
　Phalanges
　　Finger, 26235-26236
　　Radius, 24145, 25151
　　Scapula, 23182
　　Ulna, 24147, 25150
Creatine
　Blood or Urine, 82540
Creation
　Recipient Site, 15002-15005
Cryofibrinogen, 82585
Cryoglobulin, 82595
Cryosurgery, 17260-17276
　Lesion
　　Skin
　　　Malignant, 17260-17276
Crystal Identification
　Any Body Fluid, 89060
CSF, 86325, 89050-89051
CT Scan
　Bone
　　Density Study, 77078-77083
　　Follow-up Study, 76380
　Guidance
　　Localization, 77011
　　Needle Biopsy, 77012
　　Tissue Ablation, 77013
　　Vertebroplasty, 72292
　with Contrast
　　Arm, 73201, 73206
　　Brain, 70496
　　Head, 70496
　　Neck, 70491
　　Spine
　　　Cervical, 72126
　　　Lumbar, 72132
　　　Thoracic, 72129
　without Contrast
　　Arm, 73200
　　Neck, 70490
　　Spine
　　　Cervical, 72125
　　　Lumbar, 72131
　　　Thoracic, 72128
　without Contrast, followed by Contrast
　　Arm, 73202, 73220, 73223
　　Neck, 70492
　　Spine
　　　Cervical, 72127
　　　Lumbar, 72133
　　　Thoracic, 72130
CTS, 29848, 64721
Culture
　Acid Fast Bacilli, 87116
　Bacteria
　　Additional Methods, 87077
　　Aerobic, 87040, 87070
　　Anaerobic, 87073-87076
　　Blood, 87040
　　Other, 87070-87073
　　Screening, 87081
　Fungus
　　Identification, 87106
　　Nail, 87101
　　Other, 87102
　　Skin, 87101
　Mycobacteria, 87116
　Pathogen
　　by Kit, 87084
　Tubercle Bacilli, 87116
Curettement
　Skin Lesion, 17270
Cyclic Citrullinated Peptide (CCP), Antibody, 86200
Cyclic GMP, 83008
Cyst
　Bone
　　Drainage, 20615
　　Injection, 20615
　Carpal, 25130-25136
　Clavicle
　　Excision, 23140-23146
　Excision
　　Clavicle, 23140
　　　with Allograft, 23146
　　　with Autograft, 23145

Cyst—continued
  Excision—continued
    Humerus
      with Allograft, 23156
      with Autograft, 23155
    Olecranon Process
      with Allograft, 24126
      with Autograft, 24125
    Radius
      with Allograft, 24126
      with Autograft, 24125
    Scapula, 23140
      with Allograft, 23146
      with Autograft, 23145
    Ulna
      with Allograft, 24126
      with Autograft, 24125
  Ganglion
    Aspiration/Injection, 20612
  Humerus
    Excision, 23150-23156, 24110
      with Allograft, 24116
      with Autograft, 24115
  Metacarpal, 26200-26205
  Olecranon, 24120
  Phalanges
    Finger, 26210-26215
  Radius
    Excision, 24120, 25120-25126
  Scapula
    Excision, 23140-23146
  Spinal Cord
    Incision and Drainage,
      63172-63173
  Ulna, 24120, 25120-25126
  Wrist, 25130-25136
    Excision, 25111-25112
Cystine
  Urine, 82615

D

Dana Operation, 63185-63190
  Rhizotomy, 63185-63190
Darrach Procedure, 25240
Debridement
  Bone, 11044
  Muscle, 11046
  Nails, 11720-11721
  Skin
    Subcutaneous Tissue,
      11042-11047
    with Open Fracture and/or Dislocation, 11010-11012
  Sternum, 21627
  Subcutaneous, 11042-11043,
    11045-11047
  Wound
    Non-Selective, 97602
    Selective, 97597-97598
Decompression
  Arm, Lower, 24495, 25020-25025
  Carpal Tunnel, 64721
  Cauda Equina, 63011, 63017,
    63047-63048, 63056-63057,
    63087-63091
  Finger, 26035
  Gill Type procedure, 63012
  Hand, 26035-26037
  Nerve, 64702-64708, 64713,
    64718-64721, 64727
  Root, 63020-63048,
    63055-63103
  Nucleus of Disc
    Lumbar, 62287
  Spinal Cord, 63001-63017,
    63045-63103
    Anterolateral Approach,
      63075-63091
    Posterior Approach, 63001-63048
      Cauda Equina, 63001-63017
      Cervical, 63001, 63015,
        63020, 63035, 63045,
        63048
      Gill Type Procedure, 63012

Decompression—continued
  Spinal Cord—continued
    Posterior Approach—continued
      Lumbar, 63005, 63017,
        63030, 63042,
        63047-63048
      Sacral, 63011
      Thoracic, 63003, 63016,
        63046, 63048
      Transpedicular or Costovertebral
        Approach, 63055-63066
  Wrist, 25020-25025
Dehiscence
  Suture
    Skin and Subcutaneous Tissue
      Simple, 12020
        with Packing, 12021
      Superficial, 12020
        with Packing, 12021
  Wound
    Skin and Subcutaneous Tissue
      Simple, 12020
        with Packing, 12021
      Superficial, 12020
        with Packing, 12021
DeQuervain's Disease Treatment,
  25000
Derma-Fat-Fascia Graft, 15770
Destruction
  Lesion
    Skin
      Malignant, 17260-17276
  Muscle Endplate
    Extremity, 64614
    Trunk, 64614
  Nerve, 64614, 64622-64627, 64640
  Skin Lesion
    Malignant, 17260-17276
Diaphysectomy
  Clavicle, 23180
  Humerus, 23184, 24140
  Metacarpal, 26230
  Olecranon Process, 24147
  Phalanges
    Finger, 26235-26236
  Radius, 24145, 25151
  Scapula, 23182
  Ulna, 24147, 25150
Diathermy, 97024
Differential Count
  White Blood Cell Count, 85007,
    85009, 85540
Digit(s)
  Pinch Graft, 15050
  Replantation, 20816-20822
  Skin Graft
    Split, 15120-15121
Disarticulation
  Shoulder, 23920-23921
  Wrist, 25920, 25924
    Revision, 25922
Discectomy
  Anterior with Decompression
    Cervical Interspace, 63075
      Each Additional, 63076
    Thoracic Interspace, 63077
      Each Additional, 63078
  Arthrodesis
    Additional Interspace, 22534,
      22585
    Lumbar, 22533, 22558, 22630
    Thoracic, 22532, 22556
    Vertebra
      Cervical, 22554
  Cervical, 22220
  Lumbar, 22224, 22630
  Thoracic, 22222
    Additional Segment, 22226
Discography
  Cervical Disc, 72285
  Injection, 62290-62291
  Lumbar Disc, 72295
  Thoracic, 72285
Dislocation
  Acromioclavicular Joint
    Open Treatment, 23550-23552

Dislocation—continued
  Carpal, 25690
    Closed Treatment, 25690
    Open Treatment, 25695
  Carpometacarpal Joint
    Closed Treatment, 26641-26645,
      26670
      with Anesthesia, 26675
    Open Treatment, 26665,
      26685-26686
    Percutaneous Fixation, 26676
  Clavicle
    Closed Treatment, 23540-23545
    Open Treatment, 23550-23552
      with Manipulation, 23545
      without Manipulation, 23540
  Elbow
    Closed Treatment, 24600-24605,
      24640
    Open Treatment, 24586, 24615
      with Manipulation, 24620, 24640
  Interphalangeal Joint
    Finger(s)/Hand
      Closed Treatment,
        26770-26775
      Open Treatment, 26785
      Percutaneous Fixation, 26776
  Lunate, 25690-25695
    Closed Treatment, 25690
    Open Treatment, 25695
      with Manipulation, 25690,
        26670-26676,
        26700-26706
  Metacarpophalangeal Joint
    Closed Treatment, 26700-26706
    Open Treatment, 26715
  Percutaneous Fixation
    Metacarpophalangeal, 26705
  Radiocarpal Joint, 25660
  Radioulnar Joint
    Closed Treatment, 25675
      with Radial Fracture, 25520
    Open Treatment, 25676
      with Radial Fracture,
        25525-25526
  Radius
    Closed Treatment, 24640
      with Fracture, 24620-24635
      Closed Treatment, 24620
    Open Treatment, 24635
  Shoulder
    Closed Treatment
      with Manipulation,
        23650-23655
      with Fracture of Greater
        Humeral Tuberosity,
        23665
      Open Treatment, 23670
      with Surgical or Anatomical
        Neck Fracture,
        23675
      Open Treatment, 25680
    Open Treatment, 23660
    Recurrent, 23450-23466
  Sternoclavicular Joint
    Closed Treatment
      with Manipulation, 23525
      without Manipulation, 23520
    Open Treatment, 23530-23532
  Thumb
    Closed Treatment, 26641-26645
    Open Treatment, 26665
    Percutaneous Fixation, 26650
    with Fracture, 26645
      Open Treatment, 26665
      Percutaneous Fixation,
        26650-26655
      with Manipulation, 26641-26650
  Vertebrae
    Additional Segment, Any Level
      Open Treatment, 22328
    Cervical
      Open Treatment, 22326
    Closed Treatment
      with Manipulation, Casting
        and/or Bracing, 22315
      without Manipulation, 22310

Dislocation—continued
  Vertebrae—continued
    Lumbar
      Open Treatment, 22325
    Thoracic
      Open Treatment, 22327
  Wrist
    Intercarpal
      Closed Treatment, 25660
      Open Treatment, 25670
    Percutaneous, 25671
    Radiocarpal
      Closed Treatment, 25660
      Open Treatment, 25670
    Radioulnar
      Closed Treatment, 25675
      Open Treatment, 25676
      Percutaneous Fixation, 25671
    with Fracture
      Closed Treatment, 25680
      Open Treatment, 25685
Doppler Scan
  Arterial Studies, Extremities,
    93922-93923
  Extremities, 93965
Drainage
  Abscess
    Arm, Lower, 25028
      Incision and Drainage, 25035
    Arm, Upper
      Incision and Drainage,
        23930-23935
    Carpals
      Incision, Deep, 25035
    Clavicle
      Sequestrectomy, 23170
    Elbow
      Incision and Drainage,
        23930-23935
    Finger
      Incision and Drainage,
        26010-26011, 26034
    Ganglion Cyst, 20600-20605
    Hand
      Incision and Drainage, 26034
    Humeral Head, 23174
    Humerus
      Incision and Drainage, 23935
    Radius
      Incision, Deep, 25035
    Scapula
      Sequestrectomy, 23172
    Shoulder
      Incision and Drainage, 23030
    Soft Tissue
      Incision, 20005
    Ulna
      Incision, Deep, 25035
    Wrist
      Incision and Drainage, 25028,
        25035
  Bursa, 20600-20610
  Cyst
    Bone, 20615
    Ganglion, 20612
    Ganglion Cyst, 20612
  Hematoma
    Subungual, 11740
  Joint, 20600-20610
Dressings
  Change under Anesthesia, 15852
DREZ Procedure, 63170
Drug Assay
  Amikacin, 80150
  Gentamicin, 80170
  Gold, 80172
  Salicylate, 80196
  Tobramycin, 80200
  Vancomycin, 80202
Drug Delivery Implant
  Maintenance
    Epidural, 95990-95991
    Intrathecal, 95990-95991
    Intraventricular, 95990-95991
Dual X-ray Absorptiometry (DXA)
  Appendicular, 77081
  Axial Skeleton, 77080
  Vertebral Fracture, 77082

Duplex Scan
　Arterial Studies
　　Upper Extremity, 93930-93931
　Venous Studies
　　Extremity, 93970-93971
Dupuytren's Contracture,
　26040-26045
DXA (Dual Energy X-ray Absorptiometry), 77080-77082

E

Echography
　Arm, 76881-76882
　Intraoperative, 76998
　Leg, 76881-76882
Elbow
　Abscess
　　Incision and Drainage, 23930, 23935
　Arthrectomy, 24155
　Arthrocentesis, 20605
　Arthrodesis, 24800-24802
　Arthroplasty, 24360
　　Total Replacement, 24363
　　with Implant, 24361-24362
　Arthroscopy
　　Diagnostic, 29830
　　Surgical, 29834-29838
　Arthrotomy, 24000
　　Capsular Release, 24006
　　with Joint Exploration, 24101
　　with Synovectomy, 24102
　　with Synovial Biopsy, 24101
　Biopsy, 24065-24066, 24101
　Bursa
　　Incision and Drainage, 23931
　Dislocation
　　Closed Treatment, 24600-24605, 24640
　　Open Treatment, 24615
　　Partial, 24640
　　Subluxate, 24640
　Excision, 24155
　　Bursa, 24105
　　Synovium, 24102
　　Tumor, 24071-24073, 24079, 24120-24126, 24152
　Exploration, 24000-24101
　Fracture
　　Monteggia, 24620-24635
　　Open Treatment, 24586-24587
　Hematoma
　　Incision and Drainage, 23930
　Implant
　　Removal, 24164
　Incision and Drainage, 24000
　Injection
　　Arthrography (Radiologic), 24220
　Magnetic Resonance Imaging (MRI), 73221
　Manipulation, 24300
　Radical Resection
　　Capsule, Soft Tissue and Bone with Contracture Release, 24149
　Removal
　　Foreign Body, 24000, 24101, 24200-24201
　　Implant, 24160
　　Loose Body, 24101
　Repair
　　Epicondylitis, 24357-24359
　　Fasciotomy, 24357-24359
　　Flexorplasty, 24330
　　Hemiephyseal Arrest, 24470
　　Ligament, 24343-24346
　　Muscle, 24341
　　Muscle Transfer, 24301
　　Tendon, 24340-24342
　　　Lengthening, 24305
　　　Transfer, 24301
　　Tennis Elbow, 24357-24359
　Steindler Advancement, 24330
　Strapping, 29260
　Tenotomy, 24357-24359

Elbow—continued
　X-ray, 73070-73080
　　with Contrast, 73085
Elbow, Golfer, 24357-24359
Elbow, Tennis, 24357-24359
Electrical Stimulation
　Bone Healing
　　Invasive, 20975
　　Noninvasive, 20974
　Physical Therapy
　　Attended, Manual, 97032
　　Unattended, 97014
Electrocautery, 17260-17276
Electrodesiccation, 17260-17276
Electromyography
　Fine Wire
　　Dynamic, 96004
　Needle
　　Extremities, 95861-95864
　　Extremity, 95860
　　Other than Paraspinal, 95870
　　Single Fiber Electrode, 95872
　　Thoracic Paraspinal Muscles, 95869
　Surface
　　Dynamic, 96002-96004
Electronic Analysis
　Neurostimulator Pulse Generator, 95970-95973
　Pulse Generator, 95970-95971
Electrophoresis
　Immuno-, 86320-86327
　Immunofixation, 86334-86335
　Protein, 84165
Electrosurgery
　Skin Lesion, 17260-17276
EMG (Electromyography, Needle),
　95860-95864, 95869-95872
Enzyme Activity, 82657
　Radioactive Substrate, 82658
Epicondylitis, 24357-24359
Epidural
　Injection, 0228T-0231T
　Lysis, 62263-62264
Epiphyseal Arrest
　Radius, 25450-25455
　Ulna, 25450-25455
Epiphyseal Separation
　Radius
　　Closed Treatment, 25600
　　Open Treatment, 25607-25609
EPIS, 95925-95927
Equina, Cauda
　Decompression, 63005-63011, 63017, 63047-63048, 63055
　Exploration, 63005-63011, 63017
ESR, 85651-85652
Evacuation
　Hematoma
　　Subungual, 11740
Evaluation
　Occupation Therapy
　　Re-evaluation, 97004
　Physical Therapy
　　Re-evaluation, 97002
Evaluation and Management
　Athletic Training
　　Evaluation, 97005
　　Re-evaluation, 97006
　Occupation Therapy Evaluation, 97003
　　Re-evaluation, 97004
　Physical Therapy Evaluation, 97001
　　Re-evaluation, 97002
Evocative/Suppression Test,
　80428-80430, 80435
Evoked Potential
　Somatosensory Testing, 95925-95927
Exchange
　External Fixation, 20697
Excision
　Abscess
　　Olecranon Process, 24138
　　Radius, 24136
　　Ulna, 24138
　Acromion, 23130
　　Shoulder, 23130

Excision—continued
　Burns, 15002-15005
　Bursa
　　Elbow, 24105
　　Wrist, 25115-25116
　Carpal, 25145, 25210-25215
　Cartilage
　　Shoulder Joint, 23101
　　Wrist, 25107
　Clavicle
　　Partial, 23120, 23180
　　Sequestrectomy, 23170
　　Total, 23125
　　Tumor
　　　Radical Resection, 23200
　Constricting Ring
　　Finger, 26596
　Cyst
　　Carpal, 25130-25136
　　Clavicle, 23140
　　　with Allograft, 23146
　　　with Autograft, 23145
　　Finger, 26034, 26160
　　Hand, 26160
　　Humerus, 23150, 24110
　　　with Allograft, 23156, 24116
　　　with Autograft, 23155, 24115
　　Metacarpal, 26200-26205
　　Olecranon (Process), 24120
　　　with Allograft, 24126
　　　with Autograft, 24125
　　Phalanges
　　　Finger, 26210-26215
　　Radius, 24120, 25120-25126
　　　with Allograft, 24126
　　　with Autograft, 24125
　　Scapula, 23140
　　　with Allograft, 23146
　　　with Autograft, 23145
　　Ulna, 24120, 25120-25126
　　　with Allograft, 24126
　　　with Autograft, 24125
　Elbow Joint, 24155
　Ganglion Cyst
　　Wrist, 25111-25112
　Hemangioma, 11400-11426
　Humeral Head
　　Resection, 23195
　　Sequestrectomy, 23174
　Humerus, 23184, 23220, 24134, 24140, 24150
　Intervertebral Disc
　　Decompression, 63075-63078
　　Hemilaminectomy, 63040, 63043-63044
　　Herniated, 63020-63044, 63055-63066
　Lesion
　　Arm, Lower, 25110
　　Finger, 26160
　　Hand, 26160
　Lesion, Tendon Sheath
　　Arm, Lower, 25110
　　Hand/Finger, 26160
　Lymph Nodes, 38500
　　Superficial
　　　Needle, 38505
　　　Open, 38500
　Metacarpal, 26230
　Nail Fold, 11765
　Nails, 11750-11752
　Neurofibroma, 64788-64790
　Neurolemmoma, 64788-64792
　Neuroma, 64774-64786
　Odontoid Process, 22548
　Olecranon, 24147
　Phalanges
　　Finger, 26235-26236
　Pressure Ulcers, 15931-15937
　　Sacral, 15931-15936
　Radical Synovium
　　Wrist, 25115-25116
　Radius, 24130, 24136, 24145, 24152, 25145
　　Styloid Process, 25230
　Ribs, 21600-21616

Excision—continued
　Scapula
　　Ostectomy, 23190
　　Partial, 23182
　　Sequestrectomy, 23172
　　Tumor
　　　Radical Resection, 23210
　Skin, 11400-11426, 11600-11626
　　Lesion
　　　Benign, 11400-11426
　　　Malignant, 11600-11626
　Skin Graft
　　Preparation of Site, 15002-15005
　Spinal Cord, 63300-63308
　Sternum, 21620, 21630-21632
　Synovium
　　Carpometacarpal Joint, 26130
　　Elbow, 24102
　　Interphalangeal Joint, Finger, 26140
　　Metacarpophalangeal Joint, 26135
　　Shoulder, 23105-23106
　　Wrist, 25105, 25115-25119
　Tendon
　　Finger, 26180, 26390, 26415
　　Hand, 26390, 26415
　　Palm, 26170
　Tendon Sheath
　　Finger, 26145
　　Forearm, 25110
　　Palm, 26145
　　Wrist, 25115-25116
　Tumor
　　Arm, Lower, 25071-25078, 25120-25126, 25170
　　Arm, Upper, 23220, 24071-24079, 24110-24126, 24150-24152
　　Back
　　　Flank, 21930, 21935
　　Carpal, 25071-25078, 25130-25136
　　Clavicle, 23071-23078, 23140, 23200
　　Elbow, 24071-24079, 24120-24126, 24152
　　Finger, 26111-26118, 26210-26215, 26260-26262
　　Hand, 26111-26118, 26200-26205, 26250
　　Humerus, 23150, 23220, 24071-24079, 24110-24115, 24150
　　Metacarpal, 26111-26118, 26200-26205
　　Neck, 21552-21558
　　Olecranon Process, 24071-24079, 24120
　　Phalanges
　　　Finger, 26111-26118, 26210-26215, 26260-26262
　　Radius, 24152
　　Scapula, 23140
　　　with Allograft, 23146
　　　with Autograft, 23145
　　Shoulder, 23071-23078
　　Sternum, 21630
　　Thorax, 21552-21558
　　Ulna, 25071-25078
　　Vertebra
　　　Lumbar, 22102
　　　Thoracic, 22101
　　Wrist, 25071-25078, 25120-25126
　Ulna, 24147, 25145
　　Complete, 25240
　　Partial, 24147, 25150, 25240
　　Radical, 25170
　Vascular Malformation
　　Finger, 26115
　　Hand, 26115
　Vertebra
　　Additional Segment, 22103, 22116

Excision—continued
　Vertebra—continued
　　Cervical, 22110
　　　for Tumor, 22100, 22110
　　Lumbar, 22102
　　　for Tumor, 22114
　　Thoracic, 22112
　　　for Tumor, 22101
　Vertebral Body
　　Decompression, 63081-63091
　　Lesion, 63300-63308
　Wrist Tendon, 25110
Exercise Test
　Ischemic Limb, 95875
Exercise Therapy, 97110-97113
Exploration
　Abdomen
　　Penetrating Wound, 20102
　Arm, Lower, 25248
　Artery
　　Brachial, 24495
　Back, Penetrating Wound, 20102
　Cauda Equina, 63005-63011, 63017
　Elbow, 24000-24101
　Extremity
　　Penetrating Wound, 20103
　Finger Joint, 26075-26080
　Flank
　　Penetrating Wound, 20102
　Hand Joint, 26070
　Shoulder Joint, 23040-23044, 23107
　Spinal Cord, 63001-63011, 63015-63017, 63040-63044
　　Facetectomy, Foraminotomy
　　　Partial Cervical, 63045
　　　　Additional Segments, 63048
　　　Partial Lumbar, 63047
　　　　Additional Segments, 63048
　　　Partial Thoracic, 63046
　　　　Additional Segments, 63048
　　Fusion, 22830
　　Hemilaminectomy (including partial Facetectomy, Foraminotomy)
　　　Cervical, 63045
　　　　Additional Segments, 63048
　　　Lumbar, 63047
　　　　Additional Segments, 63048
　　　Thoracic, 63046
　　　　Additional Segments, 63048
　　Laminectomy
　　　Cervical, 63001, 63015
　　　Lumbar, 63005, 63017
　　　Thoracic, 63003, 63016
　　Laminotomy
　　　Initial
　　　　Cervical, 63020
　　　　　Each Additional Space, 63035
　　　　Lumbar, 63030
　　　Reexploration
　　　　Cervical, 63040
　　　　　Each Additional Space, 63043
　　　　Lumbar, 63042
　　　　　Each Additional Interspace, 63044
　Wrist, 25101, 25248
　Joint, 25040
External Fixation (System)
　Adjustment/Revision, 20693
　Application, 20690-20692
　Removal, 20694
Extracorporeal Shock Wave Therapy
　Lateral Humeral Epicondyle, 0102T
　Musculoskeletal, 0019T, 0101T
Extremity
　Penetrating Wound, 20103
Extremity Testing
　Physical Therapy, 97750

F

Factor
　III, 85730-85732
　IV, 82310
Fascia Graft
　Free Microvascular Anastomosis, 15758
　Harvesting, 20920-20922
　Open Treatment, Sternoclavicular Dislocation, 23532
Fascia Lata Graft
　Harvesting, 20920-20922
Fascial Graft
　Free
　　Microvascular Anastomosis, 15758
　Open Treatment
　　Sternoclavicular Dislocation, 23532
Fasciectomy
　Palm, 26121-26125
Fasciocutaneous Flap, 15732-15736
　Head and Neck, 15732
　Trunk, 15734
　Upper Extremity, 15736
Fasciotomy
　Arm, Lower, 24495, 25020-25025
　Elbow, 24357-24359
　Hand, Decompression, 26037
　Palm, 26040-26045
　Wrist, 25020-25025
Fern Test
　Smear and Stain, Wet Mount, 87210
Ferric Chloride
　Urine, 81005
Figure of Eight Cast, 29049
Finger
　Abscess
　　Bone
　　　Incision and Drainage, 26034
　　Incision and Drainage, 26010-26011
　Amputation, 26951
　　with Exploration or Removal, 26910
　Arthrocentesis, 20600
　Arthrodesis
　　Interphalangeal Joint, 26860-26863
　　Metacarpophalangeal Joint, 26850-26852
　Bone
　　Incision and Drainage, 26034
　Cast, 29086
　Decompression, 26035
　Excision, 26235-26236
　　Constricting Ring, 26596
　　Tendon, 26180, 26390, 26415
　Insertion
　　Tendon Graft, 26392
　Magnetic Resonance Imaging (MRI), 73221
　Reconstruction
　　Extra Digit, 26587
　　Toe to Hand Transfer, 26551-26554, 26556
　Removal
　　Implantation, 26320
　　Tube, 26392, 26416
　Repair
　　Claw Finger, 26499
　　Extra Digit, 26587
　　Macrodactylia, 26590
　　Tendon
　　　Dorsum, 26418-26420
　　　Extensor, 26415-26434, 26445-26449, 26460
　　　　Central Slip, 26426-26428
　　　　Distal Insertion, 26432-26433
　　　　Excision with Implantation, 26415
　　　　Hand, 26410
　　　　　with Graft, 26412
　　　　Realignment, Hand, 26437
　　　Flexor, 26356-26358, 26440-26442, 26455

Finger—continued
　Repair—continued
　　Tendon—continued
　　　Flexor Excision with Implantation, 26390
　　　Lengthening, 26476, 26478
　　　Opponensplasty, 26490-26496
　　　Profundus, 26370-26373
　　　Removal Tube or Rod
　　　　Extensor, 26416
　　　　Flexor, 26392
　　　Shortening, 26477, 26479
　　　Tenodesis, 26471-26474
　　　Tenolysis, 26440-26449
　　　Tenotomy, 26450-26460
　　　Transfer or Transplant, 26485-26489, 26497-26498
　　　Volar Plate, 26548
　　　Web Finger, 26560-26562
　Replantation, 20816-20822
　Reposition, 26555
　Sesamoidectomy, 26185
　Splint, 29130-29131
　Strapping, 29280
　Tendon Sheath
　　Excision, 26145
　　Incision, 26055
　　Incision and Drainage, 26020
　Tenotomy, 26060, 26460
　　Flexor, 26455
　Tumor, 25120, 26111-26113, 26118, 26260-26952
　X-ray, 73140
Finger Flap
　Tissue Transfer, 14350
Fixation (Device)
　Application, External, 20690-20697
　Insertion, 20690-20697, 22841-22844
　　Prosthetic, 22851
　　Reinsertion, 22849
　Pelvic
　　Insertion, 22848
　Removal
　　External, 20694
　　Internal, 20670-20680
　　Shoulder, 23700
　Skeletal
　　Humeral Epicondyle
　　　Percutaneous, 24566
　Spinal
　　Insertion, 22841-22847
　　Prosthetic, 22851
　　Reinsertion, 22849
Flap
　Grafts
　　Composite
　　　Derma-Fat-Fascia, 15770
　　Island Pedicle, 15740
　　Neurovascular Pedicle, 15750
Fluorescein
　Intravenous Injection
　　Vascular Flow Check, Graft, 15860
Fluoroscopy
　Hourly, 76000-76001
　Needle Biopsy, 77002
　Spine/Paraspinous
　　Guide Catheter
　　　Needle, 77003
　Vertebra
　　Osteoplasty, 72291-72292
Foreign Body
　Removal
　　Arm
　　　Lower, 25248
　　　Upper, 24200-24201
　　Elbow, 24000, 24101, 24200-24201
　　Finger, 26075-26080
　　Hand, 26070
　　Muscle, 20520-20525
　　Shoulder, 23040-23044
　　　Complicated, 23332
　　　Deep, 23331
　　　Subcutaneous, 23330

Foreign Body—continued
　Removal—continued
　　Skin
　　　with Debridement, 11010-11012
　　Subcutaneous
　　　with Debridement, 11010-11012
　　Tendon Sheath, 20520-20525
　　Wrist, 25040, 25101, 25248
Fracture, Treatment
　Boxer's, 26600-26615
　Carpal, 25622-25628
　　Closed Treatment
　　　with Manipulation, 25624, 25635
　　　without Manipulation, 25622, 25630
　　Open Treatment, 25628, 25645
　Carpal Scaphoid
　　Closed Treatment, 25622
　Carpometacarpal
　　Closed Treatment, 26645
　　Open Treatment, 26665
　　Percutaneous Fixation, 26650
　Clavicle
　　Closed Treatment, 23500-23505
　　　with Manipulation, 23505
　　　without Manipulation, 23500
　　Open Treatment, 23515
　Debridement
　　with Open Fracture, 11010-11012
　Elbow
　　Closed Treatment, 24620, 24640
　　Open Treatment, 24586-24587, 24635
　Humerus
　　Closed Treatment, 24500-24505
　　　with Manipulation, 23605
　　　without Manipulation, 23600
　　Condyle, 24582
　　　Closed Treatment, 24576-24577
　　　Open Treatment, 24579
　　　Percutaneous, 24582
　　Epicondyle
　　　Closed Treatment, 24560-24565
　　　Open Treatment, 24575
　　　Percutaneous Fixation, 24566
　　Greater Tuberosity Fracture
　　　Closed Treatment with Manipulation, 23625
　　　Closed Treatment without Manipulation, 23620
　　　Open Treatment, 23630
　　Open Treatment, 23615-23616
　　Shaft, 24500
　　　Open Treatment, 24515-24516
　　Supracondylar
　　　Closed Treatment, 24530-24535
　　　Open Treatment, 24545-24546
　　　Percutaneous Fixation, 24538
　　Transcondylar
　　　Closed Treatment, 24530-24535
　　　Open Treatment, 24545-24546
　　　Percutaneous Fixation, 24538
　　with Dislocation
　　　Closed Treatment, 23665
　　　Open Treatment, 23670
　　with Shoulder Dislocation
　　　Closed Treatment, 23675
　　　Open Treatment, 23680
　Metacarpal
　　Closed Treatment, 26600-26605
　　　with Fixation, 26607
　　Open Treatment, 26615
　　Percutaneous Fixation, 26608
　　with Manipulation, 26605-26607
　　without Manipulation, 26600

Fracture, Treatment—continued
  Navicular
    Closed Treatment, 25622
    Open Treatment, 25628
    with Manipulation, 25624
  Odontoid
    Open Treatment
      with Graft, 22319
      without Graft, 22318
  Phalanges
    Finger(s)
      Articular
        Closed Treatment, 26740
        Open Treatment, 26746
        with Manipulation, 26742
      Closed Treatment
        with Manipulation, 26725, 26742, 26755
        without Manipulation, 26720, 26740, 26750
      Distal, 26755-26756
        Closed Treatment, 26750
        Open Treatment, 26765
        Percutaneous Fixation, 26756
    Finger/Thumb
      Bennett Fracture, 26650-26665
      Closed Treatment, 26720-26725
      Percutaneous Fixation, 26650, 26727, 26756
      Shaft, 26720-26727
      with Manipulation, 26725-26727
      Open Treatment, 26735, 26746
      Distal, 26765
    Shaft
      Closed Treatment, 26725
      Open Treatment, 26735
      Percutaneous Fixation, 26727
  Radius
    Closed Treatment, 24650-24655, 25500-25505, 25520, 25560-25565, 25600-25605
    Colles, 25600-25605
    Distal, 25600-25609
      Open Treatment, 25607-25609
      Smith, 25600-25607, 25609
    Head/Neck
      Closed Treatment, 24650-24655
      Open Treatment, 24665-24666
    Open Treatment, 25515, 25607-25609
    Percutaneous Fixation, 25606
    Shaft, 25500, 25525-25526
      Closed Treatment, 25500-25505, 25520
      Open Treatment, 25515, 25525-25526, 25574
      with Manipulation, 25565, 25605
      with Ulna, 25560-25565
      Open Treatment, 25575
      without Manipulation, 25560, 25600
  Rib
    Closed Treatment, 21800
    External Fixation, 21810
    Open Treatment, 0245T-0248T, 21805
  Scaphoid
    Closed Treatment, 25622
    Open Treatment, 25628
    with Dislocation
      Closed Treatment, 25680
      Open Treatment, 25685
      with Manipulation, 25624
  Scapula
    Closed Treatment
      with Manipulation, 23575
      without Manipulation, 23570
    Open Treatment, 23585

Fracture, Treatment—continued
  Shoulder
    Closed Treatment
      with Greater Tuberosity Fracture, 23620, 23655
      with Surgical or Anatomical Neck Fracture, 23600, 23675
    Open Treatment, 23630, 23680
  Sternum
    Closed Treatment, 21820
    Open Treatment, 21825
  Thumb
    Closed Treatment, 26645-26650
    Percutaneous Fixation, 26650
    with Dislocation, 26645-26650
    Open Treatment, 26665
  Ulna
    Closed Treatment, 25560-25565
      Monteggia type, 24620
      of Shaft, 25530-25535
      and Radial, 25560
        with Manipulation, 25565
        with Manipulation, 25535
      Proximal end, 24670
        with Manipulation, 24675
      Ulnar Styloid, 25650
    Olecranon
      Closed Treatment, 24670-24675
        with Manipulation, 24675
      Open Treatment, 24685
    Open Treatment, 25574-25575
      Proximal End, 24685
      Radial AND Ulnar Shaft, 25574-25575
      Shaft, 25545
    Shaft
      Closed Treatment, 25530-25535
      Open Treatment, 25545, 25574
    Styloid Process
      Closed Treatment, 25650
      Open Treatment, 25652
      Percutaneous Fixation, 25651
    with Dislocation, 24620-24635
      Closed Treatment, 24620
      Monteggia, 24620-24635
      Open Treatment, 24635
    with Manipulation, 25535, 25565
    with Radius, 25560-25565
      Open Treatment, 25575
    without Manipulation, 25530, 25560
  Vertebra
    Additional Segment
      Open Treatment, 22328
    Cervical
      Open Treatment, 22326
    Closed Treatment
      with Manipulation, Casting and/or Bracing, 22315
      without Manipulation, 22310
    Lumbar
      Open Treatment, 22325
    Posterior
      Open Treatment, 22325-22327
    Thoracic
      Open Treatment, 22327
  Vertebral Process
    Closed Treatment, 22305
  Wrist
    with Dislocation, 25680-25685
      Closed Treatment, 25680
      Open Treatment, 25685
FT-4, 84439
FTG, 15220-15241
FTSG, 15220-15241
Full Thickness Graft, 15220-15241
Fungus
  Culture
    Hair, 87101
    Identification, 87106
    Nail, 87101
    Other, 87102

Fungus—continued
  Culture—continued
    Skin, 87101
Fusion
  Thumb
    in Opposition, 26820

G

Galeazzi Dislocation
  Fracture
    Closed Treatment, 25520
    Open Treatment, 25525-25526
Ganglion
  Cyst
    Aspiration/Injection, 20612
    Drainage, 20612
  Wrist
    Excision, 25111-25112
Gentamicin, 80170
  Assay, 80170
GH, 83003
Gill Operation, 63012
Glenohumeral Joint
  Arthrotomy, 23040
    with Biopsy, 23100
    with Synovectomy, 23105
  Exploration, 23107
  Removal
    Foreign or Loose Body, 23107
Globulin, Thyroxine-Binding, 84442
Glutamate Pyruvate Transaminase, 84460
Glutamic Alanine Transaminase, 84460
Glutamic Aspartic Transaminase, 84450
Glutamine, 82975
GMP (Guanosine Monophosphate), 83008
Gold
  Assay, 80172
  Blood, 80172
Golfer's Elbow, 24357-24359
Graft
  Bone
    Harvesting, 20900-20902
    Vascular Pedicle, 25430
  Cartilage
    Harvesting, 20910
  Dura
    Spinal Cord, 63710
  Fascia Lata
    Harvesting, 20920-20922
  Nail Bed Reconstruction, 11762
  Nerve, 64890-64907
  Skin
    Blood Flow Check, Graft, 15860
    Composite, 15770
    Free Flap, 15757
    Full Thickness, Free
      Axillae, 15240-15241
      Extremities (Excluding Hands/Feet), 15240-15241
      Feet, Hands, 15240-15241
      Mouth, Neck, 15240-15241
    Pinch Graft, 15050
    Preparation Recipient Site, 15002, 15004-15005
    Split Graft, 15100-15101, 15120-15121
    Vascular Flow Check, Graft, 15860
    Xenograft, 15400-15401
  Tendon
    Finger, 26392
    Hand, 26392
    Harvesting, 20924
  Tissue
    Harvesting, 20926
Greater Tuberosity Fracture
  with Shoulder Dislocation
    Closed Treatment, 23665
    Open Treatment, 23670
Gridley Stain, 88312

Growth Hormone, 83003
  Human, 80428-80430, 86277
  with Arginine Tolerance Test, 80428
Guanosine Monophosphate, 83008
Guard Stain, 88313

H

H-Reflex Study, 95934-95936
Halo
  Body Cast, 29000
  Cranial, 20661
    for Thin Skull Osteology, 20664
  Removal, 20665
Hand
  Amputation
    at Metacarpal, 25927
    at Wrist, 25920
      Revision, 25922
    Revision, 25924, 25929-25931
  Arthrodesis
    Carpometacarpal Joint, 26843-26844
    Intercarpal Joint, 25820-25825
  Bone
    Incision and Drainage, 26034
  Cast, 29085
  Decompression, 26035-26037
  Fracture
    Metacarpal, 26600
  Implantation
    Removal, 26320
    Tube/Rod, 26392, 26416
    Tube/Rod, 26390
  Insertion
    Tendon Graft, 26392
  Magnetic Resonance Imaging (MRI), 73218-73223
  Reconstruction
    Tendon Pulley, 26500-26502
  Repair
    Cleft Hand, 26580
    Muscle, 26591-26593
      Release, 26593
    Tendon
      Extensor, 26410-26416, 26426-26428, 26433-26437
      Flexor, 26350-26358, 26440
      Profundus, 26370-26373
  Replantation, 20808
  Skin Graft
    Full Thickness, 15240-15241
    Split, 15100-15101
  Strapping, 29280
  Tendon
    Excision, 26390
    Extensor, 26415
    Tenotomy, 26450, 26460
  Tissue Transfer, Adjacent, 14040-14041
  Tumor, 26111-26113, 26118, 26200-26205
  X-ray, 73120-73130
Harrington Rod
  Insertion, 22840
  Removal, 22850
Harvesting
  Bone Graft, 20900-20902
  Cartilage, 20910
  Fascia Lata Graft, 20920-20922
  Tendon Graft, 20924
  Tissue Grafts, 20926
Hct, 85013-85014
Headbrace
  Application
    Removal, 20661
Hematoma
  Arm, Lower, 25028
  Arm, Upper
    Incision and Drainage, 23930
  Elbow
    Incision and Drainage, 23930
  Shoulder
    Drainage, 23030

Hematoma—continued
  Subungual
    Evacuation, 11740
  Wrist, 25028
Hemiephyseal Arrest
  Elbow, 24470
Hemilaminectomy, 63020-63044
Hemoglobin
  Analysis
    O2 Affinity, 82820
Hemogram
  Added Indices, 85025-85027
  Automated, 85025-85027
  Manual, 85014-85018
Heparin, 85520
  Neutralization, 85525
  Protamine Tolerance Test, 85530
Heterograft
  Skin, 15400-15401
Hgb, 85018
HGH (Human Growth Hormone),
  80428-80430, 83003, 86277
Hibb Operation, 22841
Hicks–Pitney Test
  Thromboplastin, Partial Time,
    85730-85732
High Density Lipoprotein, 83718
Hoffman Apparatus, 20690
Home Services
  Home Infusion Procedures,
    99601-99602
  Intramuscular Injections, 99506
Homocystine
  Urine, 82615
Horii Procedure (Carpal Bone), 25430
Hormone Assay
  Corticosterone, 82528
  Cortisol
    Total, 82533
  Growth Hormone, 83003
    Suppression Panel, 80430
  Somatotropin, 80430, 83003
  Vasopressin, 84588
Hot Pack Treatment, 97010
Hubbard Tank Therapy, 97036
  with Exercises, 97036, 97113
Human
  Growth Hormone, 80428-80430
Humerus
  Abscess
    Incision and Drainage, 23935
  Craterization, 23184, 24140
  Cyst
    Excision, 23150, 24110
      with Allograft, 23156, 24116
      with Autograft, 23155, 24115
  Diaphysectomy, 23184, 24140
  Excision, 23174, 23184, 23195,
    23220, 24077-24079,
    24110-24116, 24134, 24140,
    24150
  Fracture
    Closed Treatment, 24500-24505
      with Manipulation, 23605
      without Manipulation, 23600
    Condyle
      Closed Treatment,
        24576-24577
      Open Treatment, 24579
      Percutaneous Fixation, 24582
    Epicondyle
      Closed Treatment,
        24560-24565
      Open Treatment, 24575
      Percutaneous Fixation, 24566
    Greater Tuberosity Fracture
      Closed Treatment with Manip-
        ulation, 23625
      Closed Treatment without
        Manipulation, 23620
      Open Treatment, 23630
      Open Treatment, 23615-23616
    Shaft
      Closed Treatment,
        24500-24505, 24516
      Open Treatment, 24515

Humerus—continued
  Fracture—continued
    Supracondylar
      Closed Treatment,
        24530-24535
      Open Treatment,
        24545-24546
      Percutaneous Fixation, 24538
    Transcondylar
      Closed Treatment,
        24530-24535
      Open Treatment,
        24545-24546
      Percutaneous Fixation, 24538
    with Dislocation, 23665-23670
  Osteomyelitis, 24134
  Pinning, Wiring, 23491, 24498
  Prophylactic Treatment, 23491,
    24498
  Radical Resection, 23220,
    24077-24079
  Repair, 24430
    Nonunion, Malunion,
      24430-24435
    Osteoplasty, 24420
    Osteotomy, 24400-24410
      with Graft, 24435
  Resection Head, 23195
  Saucerization, 23184, 24140
  Sequestrectomy, 23174, 24134
  Tumor
    Excision, 23150, 23220,
      24071-24079, 24110
  X-ray, 73060
Hydrotherapy (Hubbard Tank), 97036
  with Exercises, 97036, 97113

I

Ilizarov Procedure
  Application, Bone Fixation Device,
    20690-20692
  Monticelli Type, 20692
IM Injection
  Diagnostic, Prophylactic, Therapeu-
    tic, 96372
Immunoassay
  Analyte, 83518-83520
  Infectious Agent, 86317-86318
  Nonantibody, 83516-83519
Immunoblotting, Western
  Protein, 84181-84182
Immunoelectrophoresis,
  86320-86327, 86334-86335
Immunofixation Electrophoresis,
  86334-86335
Immunoglobulin
  Thyroid Stimulating, 84445
Implantation
  Nerve
    into Bone, 64787
    into Muscle, 64787
  Removal, 20670-20680
    Anesthesia, External Fixation,
      20694
    Elbow, 24164
    Radius, 24164
    Wire, Pin, Rod, 20670
    Wire, Pin, Rod/Deep, 20680
Incision
  Abscess
    Soft Tissue, 20005
  Accessory Nerve, 63191
  Dentate Ligament, 63180-63182
  Elbow, 24000
  Finger
    Decompression, 26035
    Tendon, 26060, 26455-26460
    Tendon Sheath, 26055-26060,
      26455-26460
  Hand Decompression, 26035-26037
    Tendon, 26450, 26460
  Hyoid, Muscle, 21685
  Intercarpal Joint
    Dislocation, 25670
  Interphalangeal Joint
    Capsule, 26525

Incision—continued
  Metacarpophalangeal Joint
    Capsule, 26520
  Nerve, 64702-64708, 64713,
    64718-64721, 64727, 64772
  Root, 63185-63190
  Palm
    Fasciotomy, 26040-26045
  Shoulder
    Bone, 23035
    Capsule Contracture Release,
      23020
    Removal
      Calcareous Deposits, 23000
    Tenomyotomy, 23405-23406
    Shoulder Joint, 23040-23044
  Spinal Cord
    Tract, 63170, 63194-63199
  Synovectomy, 26140
  Tendon
    Arm, Upper, 24310
    Wrist, 25100-25105
    Capsule, 25085
    Decompression, 25020-25025
    Tendon Sheath, 25000-25001
Incision and Drainage
  Abscess
    Arm, Lower, 25028, 25035
    Arm, Upper, 23930-23931
    Elbow, 23930
    Finger, 26010-26011
    Shoulder, 23030
    Spine, 22010-22015
    Wrist, 25028, 25040
  Bursa
    Arm, Lower, 25031
    Elbow, 23931
    Palm, 26025-26030
    Wrist, 25031
  Carpals, 25035, 26034
  Cyst
    Spinal Cord, 63172-63173
  Elbow
    Abscess, 23935
    Arthrotomy, 24000
  Hematoma
    Arm, Lower, 25028
    Arm, Upper, 23930
    Elbow, 23930
    Shoulder, 23030
    Wrist, 25028
  Humerus
    Abscess, 23935
  Phalanges
    Finger, 26034
  Radius, 25035
  Shoulder
    Abscess, 23030
    Arthrotomy
      Acromioclavicular Joint,
        23044
      Glenohumeral Joint, 23040
      Sternoclavicular Joint, 23044
    Bursa, 23031
    Hematoma, 23030
  Shoulder Joint
    Arthrotomy, Glenohumeral Joint,
      23040
  Tendon Sheath
    Finger, 26020
    Palm, 26020
  Ulna, 25035
  Wrist, 25028, 25040
Inclusion Bodies
  Smear, 87207, 87210
Infection
  Immunoassay, 86317-86318
Infectious Agent Detection
  Concentration, 87015
  Detection
    by Immunoassay
      Streptococcus, Group B,
        87802
      with Direct Optical Observa-
        tion, 87802
Infrared Light Treatment, 97026

Infusion
  Intra-Arterial
    Diagnostic, Prophylactic, Diag-
      nostic, 96373
  IV
    Diagnostic, Prophylactic, Thera-
      peutic, 96365-96368
Infusion Pump
  Maintenance, 95990-95991
Infusion Therapy
  Chemotherapy, 96450
  Home Infusion Procedures,
    99601-99602
  Intravenous, 96365-96368
Injection
  Aponeurosis, 20550
  Brisement, 20550-20551
  Bursa, 20600-20610
  Carpal Tunnel
    Therapeutic, 20526
  Chemotherapy, 96450
  Cyst
    Bone, 20615
  Elbow
    Arthrography, Radiologic, 24220
  Epidural, 0228T-0231T
  Ganglion Cyst, 20612
  Intervertebral Disc
    Radiological, 62290-62291
  Intra-arterial, 96373
  Intramuscular, 96372, 99506
  Intravenous, 96365-96368
    Diagnostic, 96365-96368
    Vascular Flow Check, Graft,
      15860
  Joint, 20600-20610
  Ligament, 20550
  Muscle Endplate
    Extremity, 64614
    Trunk, 64614
  Nerve
    Anesthetic, 64449
    Neurolytic Agent, 64614,
      64622-64627, 64640
  Paravertebral Facet Joint,
    0213T-0218T
  Platelet Rich Plasma, 0232T
  Shoulder
    Arthrography, Radiologic, 23350
  Spinal Cord
    Blood, 62273
    Radiologic, 62284
  Steroids
    Paravertebral Facet Joint,
      0213T-0218T
  Tendon Origin, Insertion, 20551
  Tendon Sheath, 20550
  Trigger Point(s)
    One or Two Muscle Groups,
      20552
    Three or More Muscle Groups,
      20553
  Wrist
    Carpal Tunnel
      Therapeutic, 20526
    Radiologic, 25246
  Zygaspophyseal, 0213T-0218T
Insertion
  Pin
    Skeletal Traction, 20650
  Posterior Spinous Process Distrac-
    tion Devices, 0171T-0172T
  Spinal Instrument, 22849
    Spinous Process, 0171T-0172T,
      22841
  Spinal Instrumentation
    Anterior, 22845-22847
    Internal Spinal Fixation, 22841
    Pelvic Fixation, 22848
    Posterior Non–segmental
      Harrington Rod Technique,
        22840
    Posterior Segmental,
      22842-22844
    Prosthetic Device, 22851
  Tendon Graft
    Finger, 26392
    Hand, 26392

Insertion—continued
  Vascular Pedicle
    Carpal Bone, 25430
  Wire
    Skeletal Traction, 20650
Instrumentation
  Spinal
    Insertion, 22840-22848, 22851
    Reinsertion, 22849
    Removal, 22850, 22852-22855
Insulin, 80435
Integumentary System
  Burns, 15002-15003, 15005,
    15100-15101, 15120-15121,
    15400-15401
  Debridement, 11010-11046
  Destruction
    Malignant Lesion, 17260-17276
  Excision
    Benign Lesion, 11400-11426
    Debridement, 11010-11046
    Malignant Lesion, 11600-11626
  Graft
    Autograft, 15050-15101,
      15120-15121
    Surgical Preparation,
      15002-15005
    Xenograft, 15400-15401
  Nails, 11719-11765
  Pressure Ulcers, 15931-15937
  Repair
    Adjacent Tissue Transfer
      Rearrangement, 14000-14041,
      14301-14350
    Complex, 13120-13133, 13160
    Flaps
      Other, 15740-15758, 15770
    Free Skin Grafts, 15002-15005,
      15050-15101,
      15120-15121,
      15220-15241
    Intermediate, 12031-12047
    Other Procedures, 15850-15860
    Simple, 12001-12007,
      12020-12021
    Skin and/or Deep Tissue,
      15732-15736
Intercarpal Joint
  Arthrodesis, 25820-25825
  Dislocation
    Closed Treatment, 25660
  Repair, 25447
Interphalangeal Joint
  Arthrodesis, 26860-26863
  Arthroplasty, 26535-26536
  Arthrotomy, 26080
  Biopsy
    Synovium, 26110
  Capsule
    Excision, 26525
    Incision, 26525
  Dislocation
    Closed Treatment, 26770
    Fingers/Hand
      Closed Treatment,
        26770-26775
      Open Treatment, 26785
      Percutaneous Fixation, 26776
      with Manipulation, 26340
    Open Treatment, 26785
    Percutaneous Fixation, 26776
    with Manipulation, 26340
  Exploration, 26080
  Fracture
    Closed Treatment, 26740
    Open Treatment, 26746
    with Manipulation, 26742
  Fusion, 26860-26863
  Removal
    Foreign Body, 26080
  Repair
    Collateral Ligament, 26545
    Volar Plate, 26548
  Synovectomy, 26140
Interstitial Cell Stimulating Hormone
  Fluid Pressure
    Monitoring, 20950

Intervertebral Disc
  Annuloplasty, 22526-22527
  Arthroplasty
    Cervical Interspace, 22856
    Each Additional Interspace,
      0092T
    Lumbar Interspace, 0163T,
      22857-22865
    Removal, 0095T, 0164T
      Removal, 0095T
    Revision, 0098T, 0165T
  Discography
    Cervical, 72285
    Lumbar, 72295
    Thoracic, 72285
  Excision
    Decompression, 63075-63078
    Herniated, 63020-63044,
      63055-63066
  Injection
    X-ray, 62290-62291
    X-ray with Contrast
      Cervical, 72285
      Lumbar, 72295
**Intradiscal Electrothermal Therapy
  (IDET),** 22526-22527
Intravenous Therapy, 96365-96368,
  96374-96376
Iontophoresis, 97033
Iron Hematoxylin Stain, 88312
Iron Stain, 88313
Island Pedicle Flaps, 15740
IV, 96365-96368, 96374-96376
IV Infusion Therapy, 96365-96368
IV Injection, 96374-96376
Ivy Bleeding Time, 85002

J

Joint
  Arthrocentesis, 20600-20610
  Aspiration, 20600-20610
  Drainage, 20600-20610
  Injection, 20600-20610
  Mobilization, 97140
  Nuclear Medicine
    Imaging, 78300-78315
  Radiology
    Stress Views, 77071
  Survey, 77077

K

K+, 84132
Keen Operation, 63198
Kinetic Therapy, 97530
Kloramfenikol, 82415
Kocher Operation, 23650-23680
Krukenberg Procedure, 25915
Kyphectomy
  More than Two Segments, 22819
  Up to Two Segments, 22818
Kyphoplasty, 22523-22525

L

Lactate, 83605
Lactic Acid, 83605
Lactic Dehydrogenase, 83615-83625
Laminectomy, 63001, 63005-63011,
  63015-63044, 63180-63199
  Decompression
    Cervical, 63001, 63015
      with Facetectomy and Foraminotomy, 63045, 63048
    Laminotomy
      Initial
        Cervical, 63020
        Each Additional Space,
          63035
        Lumbar, 63030
      Reexploration
        Cervical, 63040
        Each Additional Interspace, 63043

Laminectomy—continued
  Decompression—continued
    Laminotomy—continued
      Reexploration—continued
        Lumbar, 63042
        Each Additional Interspace, 63044
      Lumbar, 63005, 63017
        with Facetectomy and Foraminotomy, 63046, 63048
      Sacral, 63011
      Thoracic, 63003, 63016
        with Facetectomy and Foraminotomy, 63047-63048
    Lumbar, 22630, 63012
    Surgical, 63170-63199
      with Facetectomy, 63045-63048
Laminoplasty
  Cervical, 63050-63051
Laminotomy
  Cervical, 63042
  Cervical, One Interspace, 63020
  Lumbar, 63042
    One Interspace, 63030
    Each Additional, 63035
  Re-exploration, Cervical, 63040
Laser Surgery
  Lesion
    Skin, 17260-17276
  Spine
    Diskectomy, 62287
Laser Treatment, 17260-17276
LD (Lactic Dehydrogenase), 83615
LDH, 83615-83625
LDL, 83721
Lead, 83655
Lee and White Test, 85345
Lengthening
  Radius and Ulna, 25391, 25393
  Tendons
    Upper Extremities, 24305, 25280,
      26476, 26478
Lesion
  Arm, Lower
    Tendon Sheath Excision, 25110
  Finger
    Tendon Sheath, 26160
  Hand
    Tendon Sheath, 26160
  Nerve
    Excision, 64774-64792
    Sciatic Nerve
      Excision, 64786
  Skin
    Destruction
      Malignant, 17260-17276
    Excision
      Benign, 11400-11426
      Malignant, 11600-11626
  Wrist Tendon
    Excision, 25110
Leukocyte
  Alkaline Phosphatase, 85540
Leukocyte Count, 85048
Ligament
  Dentate
    Incision, 63180-63182
    Section, 63180-63182
  Injection, 20550
  Release
    Coracoacromial, 23415
    Transverse Carpal, 29848
  Repair
    Elbow, 24343-24346
Lipoprotein
  Blood, 83718-83721
  LDL, 83721
Living Activities, Daily, 97535-97537
Loose Body
  Removal
    Carpometacarpal, 26070
    Elbow, 24101
    Wrist, 25101
LP, 62270
Lumbar Plexus
  Injection, Anesthetic, 64449
Lunate
  Arthroplasty
    with Implant, 25444

Lunate—continued
  Dislocation
    Closed Treatment, 25690
    Open Treatment, 25695
Lymph Node(s)
  Biopsy, 38500
    Needle, 38505
  Excision, 38500
Lymphadenectomy
  Mediastinal, 21632
Lysis
  Adhesions
    Epidural, 62263-62264

M

MacLean–De Wesselow Test
  Clearance, Urea Nitrogen,
    84540-84545
Macrodactylia
  Repair, 26590
Magnesium, 83735
**Magnetic Resonance Angiography
  (MRA)**
  Arm, 73225
  Neck, 70547-70549
Magnetoencephalography (MEG),
  95965-95967
Magnuson Procedure, 23450
Malaria Smear, 87207
Mallet Finger Repair, 26432
Manipulation
  Dislocation and/or Fracture
    Acromioclavicular, 23545
    Carpometacarpal, 26670-26676
    Clavicle, 23505
    Elbow, 24300, 24640
    Epicondyle, 24565
    Finger, 26725-26727, 26742,
      26755
    Greater Tuberosity
      Humeral, 23625
    Hand, 26670-26676
    Humeral, 23605, 24505, 24535,
      24577
      Epicondyle, 24565
    Intercarpal, 25660
    Interphalangeal Joint, 26340,
      26770-26776
    Lunate, 25690
    Metacarpal, 26605-26607
    Metacarpophalangeal,
      26700-26706, 26742
    Metacarpophalangeal Joint,
      26340
    Phalangeal Shaft, 26727
      Distal, Finger or Thumb,
        26755
      Phalanges, Finger/Thumb,
        26725
    Phalanges
      Finger, 26742, 26755,
        26770-26776
      Finger/Thumb, 26727
    Radial, 24655, 25565
    Radial Shaft, 25505
    Radiocarpal, 25660
    Radioulnar, 25675
    Scapula, 23575
    Shoulder, 23650-23655
      with Greater Tuberosity,
        23665
      with Surgical or Anatomical
        Neck, 23675
    Sternoclavicular, 23525
      with Surgical or Anatomical
        Neck, 23675
    Thumb, 26641-26650
    Trans–Scaphoperilunar, 25680
    Ulnar, 24675, 25535, 25565
    Vertebral, 22315
    Wrist, 25259, 25624, 25635,
      25660, 25675, 25680,
      25690
  Interphalangeal Joint, Proximal,
    26742
  Osteopathic, 98925-98929

Manipulation—continued
  Physical Therapy, 97140
  Shoulder
    Application of Fixation Apparatus, 23700
  Spine
    Anesthesia, 22505
Manual Therapy, 97140
Marrow, Bone
  Aspiration, 38220
  Needle Biopsy, 38221
  Smear, 85097
Mass Spectrometry and Tandem Mass Spectrometry
  Analyte
    Qualitative, 83788
    Quantitative, 83789
Massage
  Therapy, 97124
MBC, 87181-87188
Median Nerve
  Decompression, 64721
  Neuroplasty, 64721
  Release, 64721
  Repair
    Suture
      Motor, 64835
  Transposition, 64721
Median Nerve Compression
  Decompression, 64721
  Endoscopy, 29848
  Injection, 20526
MEG (Magnetoencephalography), 95965-95967
Mercury, 83825
Metabolic Panel
  Calcium Ionized, 80047
  Calcium Total, 80048
  Comprehensive, 80053
Metacarpal
  Amputation, 26910
  Craterization, 26230
  Cyst
    Excision, 26200-26205
  Diaphysectomy, 26230
  Excision, 26230
    Radical for Tumor, 26250
  Fracture
    Closed Treatment, 26605
      with Fixation, 26607
    Open Treatment, 26615
    Percutaneous Fixation, 26608
    with Manipulation, 26605-26607
    without Manipulation, 26600
  Ostectomy
    Radical
      for Tumor, 26250
  Repair
    Lengthening, 26568
    Nonunion, 26546
    Osteotomy, 26565
  Saucerization, 26230
  Tumor
    Excision, 26200-26205
Metacarpophalangeal Joint
  Arthrodesis, 26850-26852
  Arthroplasty, 26530-26531
  Arthroscopy
    Diagnostic, 29900
    Surgical, 29901-29902
  Arthrotomy, 26075
  Biopsy
    Synovium, 26105
  Capsule
    Excision, 26520
    Incision, 26520
  Capsulodesis, 26516-26518
  Dislocation
    Closed Treatment, 26700
    Open Treatment, 26715
    Percutaneous Fixation, 26705-26706
    with Manipulation, 26340
  Exploration, 26075
  Fracture
    Closed Treatment, 26740
    Open Treatment, 26746
    with Manipulation, 26742

Metacarpophalangeal Joint—continued
  Fusion, 26516-26518, 26850-26852
  Removal of Foreign Body, 26075
  Repair
    Collateral Ligament, 26540-26542
  Synovectomy, 26135
Metadrenaline, 83835
Metanephrine, 83835
Methenamine Silver Stain, 88312
Methsuximide, 83858
Mg, 83735
Microbiology, 87015-87040, 87070-87084, 87101-87102, 87106, 87116, 87181-87188, 87205-87207, 87210, 87802
Microdissection, 88380
Microsurgery
  Operating Microscope, 69990
Microvascular Anastomosis
  Muscle Flap, Free, 15756
  Skin Flap, Free, 15757
Microvite A, 84590
Microwave Therapy, 97024
Midcarpal Mediocciptal Joint
  Arthrotomy, 25040
Minerva Cast, 29040
  Removal, 29710
Minimum Inhibitory Concentration, 87186
Molecular Oxygen Saturation, 82805-82810
Monitoring
  Interstitial Fluid Pressure, 20950
Monophosphate, Guanosine, 83008
Monophosphate, Guanosine Cyclic, 83008
Monteggia Fracture, 24620-24635
Monticelli Procedure, 20690-20692
Mosenthal Test, 81002
Motion Analysis
  by Video and 3-D Kinematics, 96004
  Computer-based, 96004
Motor and/or Sensory Nerve Conduction, 95900-95905
Move
  Finger, 26555
  Toe Joint, 26556
  Toe to Hand, 26551-26554
MRA (Magnetic Resonance Angiography), 73225
MRI (Magnetic Resonance Imaging)
  Arm, 73218-73220, 73223
  Elbow, 73221
  Finger Joint, 73221
  Guidance
    Needle Placement, 77021
  Hand, 73218-73220, 73223
  Joint
    Upper Extremity, 73221-73223
  Neck, 70540-70543
  Orbit, 70540-70543
  Spine
    Cervical, 72141-72142, 72156-72158
    Lumbar, 72148-72158
    Thoracic, 72146-72147, 72156-72158
  Wrist, 73221
Mucin
  Synovial Fluid, 83872
Mucous Cyst
  Antibody
    Hand or Finger, 26160
Mumford Operation, 29824
Mumford Procedure, 23120, 29824
Muscle
  Biopsy, 20200-20206
  Removal
    Foreign Body, 20520-20525
  Repair
    Forearm, 25260-25274
    Wrist, 25260-25274
  Revision
    Arm, Upper, 24330-24331
    Elbow, 24301

Muscle—continued
  Transfer
    Arm, Upper, 24301, 24320
    Elbow, 24301
    Shoulder, 23395-23397, 24301, 24320
Muscle Compartment Syndrome
  Detection, 20950
Muscle Division
  Scalenus Anticus, 21700-21705
  Sternocleidomastoid, 21720-21725
Muscle Flaps, 15732-15736
  Free, 15756
Muscle Testing
  Manual, 95831-95834
Musculoskeletal System
  Computer Assisted Surgical Navigational Procedure, 0054T-0055T, 20985
Musculotendinous (Rotator) Cuff
  Repair, 23410-23412
Mycobacteria
  Culture, 87116
Myelin Basic Protein
  Cerebrospinal Fluid, 83873
Myelography
  Brain, 70010
  Spine
    Cervical, 72240
    Lumbosacral, 72265
    Thoracic, 72255
    Total, 72270
Myelotomy, 63170
Myocutaneous Flaps, 15732-15736, 15756
Myofascial Release, 97140
Myoglobin, 83874
Myotomy
  Hyoid, 21685
Myxoid Cyst
  Aspiration/Injection, 20612
  Drainage, 20610
  Wrist
    Excision, 25111-25112

N

Na, 84295
Nail Bed
  Reconstruction, 11762
  Repair, 11760
Nail Fold
  Excision
    Wedge, 11765
Nails
  Avulsion, 11730-11732
  Biopsy, 11755
  Debridement, 11720-11721
  Evacuation
    Hematoma, Subungual, 11740
  Excision, 11750-11752
  Removal, 11730-11732, 11750-11752
  Trimming, 11719
Navicular
  Arthroplasty
    with Implant, 25443
  Fracture
    Closed Treatment, 25622
    Open Treatment, 25628
    with Manipulation, 25624
  Repair, 25440
Navigation
  Computer Assisted, 20985
NCS (Nerve Conduction Study), 95900-95904
Neck
  Angiography, 70498, 70547-70549
  Biopsy, 21550
  CT Scan, 70490-70492, 70498
  Magnetic Resonance Angiography (MRA), 70547-70549
  Magnetic Resonance Imaging (MRI), 70540-70543
  Skin Graft
    Full Thickness, 15240-15241
    Split, 15120-15121

Neck—continued
  Tissue Transfer, Adjacent, 14040-14041
  Tumor, 21552-21554, 21558
  Wound Exploration
  X-ray, 70360
Neck Muscle
  Division, Scalenus Anticus, 21700-21705
    Sternocleidomastoid, 21720-21725
Neck, Humerus
  Fracture
    with Shoulder Dislocation
      Closed Treatment, 23680
      Open Treatment, 23675
Needle Biopsy
  Bone, 20220-20225
  Bone Marrow, 38221
  CT Scan Guidance, 77012
  Fluoroscopic Guidance, 77002
  Lymph Node, 38505
  Muscle, 20206
Needle Localization
  Magnetic Resonance Guidance, 77021
Needle Manometer Technique, 20950
Neer Procedure, 23470
Negative Pressure Wound Therapy (NPWT), 97605-97606
Nephelometry, 83883
Nerve Conduction
  Motor and/or Sensory, 95905
  Motor Nerve, 95900-95903
  Sensory Nerve, 95904
Nerve Root
  Decompression, 63020-63048, 63055-63103
  Incision, 63185-63190
  Section, 63185-63190
Nerve Teasing, 88362
Nerves
  Avulsion, 64772
  Biopsy, 64795
  Decompression, 64702-64708, 64713, 64718-64721, 64727
  Destruction, 64614, 64622-64627, 64640
  Graft, 64890-64907
  Implantation
    to Bone, 64787
    to Muscle, 64787
  Incision, 64772
  Injection
    Anesthetic, 64449
    Neurolytic Agent, 64614, 64622-64627, 64640
  Lesion
    Excision, 64774-64792
  Neurofibroma
    Excision, 64788-64792
  Neurolemmoma
    Excision, 64788-64792
  Neurolytic
    Internal, 64727
  Neuroma
    Excision, 64774-64786
  Neuroplasty, 64702-64708, 64713, 64718-64721
  Repair
    Graft, 64890-64911
    Microdissection
      with Surgical Microscope, 69990
    Suture, 64831-64837, 64856-64857, 64859, 64872-64876
  Spinal Accessory
    Incision, 63191
    Section, 63191
  Suture, 64831-64837, 64856-64857, 64859, 64872-64876
  Transection, 64772
  Transposition, 64718-64721
Neurofibroma
  Cutaneous Nerve
    Excision, 64788

Neurofibroma—continued
    Extensive
        Excision, 64792
    Peripheral Nerve
        Excision, 64790
Neurolemmoma
    Cutaneous Nerve
        Excision, 64788
    Extensive
        Excision, 64792
    Peripheral Nerve
        Excision, 64790
Neurology
    Central Motor
        Electromyography
            Fine Wire
                Dynamic, 96004
            Ischemic Limb Exercise Test, 95875
            Needle, 95860-95864, 95869-95872
            Surface
                Dynamic, 96002-96004
        Magnetoencephalography (MEG), 95965-95967
        Motion Analysis
            by Video and 3-D Kinematics, 96004
            Computer-based, 96004
        Muscle Testing
            Manual, 95831-95834
        Nerve Conduction
            Motor Nerve, 95900-95903
            Sensory Nerve, 95904
        Neuromuscular Junction Tests, 95937
        Neurophysiological Testing
            Intraoperative, 95920
        Plantar Pressure Measurements
            Dynamic, 96004
        Range of Motion Test, 95851-95852
        Reflex
            H-Reflex, 95934
        Somatosensory Testing, 95925-95927
Neurolysis
    Nerve, 64704-64708
    Internal, 64727
Neuroma
    Cutaneous Nerve
        Excision, 64774
    Digital Nerve
        Excision, 64776-64778
    Excision, 64774
    Foot Nerve
        Excision, 64782-64783
    Hand Nerve
        Excision, 64782-64783
    Peripheral Nerve
        Excision, 64784
    Sciatic Nerve
        Excision, 64786
Neuromuscular Junction Tests, 95937
Neuromuscular Reeducation, 97112
    Intraoperative, Per Hour, 95920
Neurophysiologic Testing
    Intraoperative, Per Hour, 95920
Neuroplasty
    Digital Nerve, 64702-64704
    Peripheral Nerve, 64708, 64713, 64718-64721
Neurorrhaphy, 64831-64837,
    64856-64857, 64859,
    64872-64876
    Peripheral Nerve
        Conduit, 64910-64911
        with Graft, 64890-64907
Neurostimulator
    Analysis, 95970-95973
Neurovascular Pedicle Flaps, 15750
Nitrate Reduction Test
    Urinalysis, 81000-81025
No Man's Land
    Tendon Repair, 26356-26358
Non-Office Medical Services
    Emergency Care, 99060

NPWT (Negative Pressure Wound Therapy), 97605-97606
Nuclear Medicine
    Bone
        Density Study, 78350-78351
        Imaging, 78300-78320
        SPECT, 78320
        Ultrasound, 76977
Nucleotidase, 83915
Nursemaid Elbow, 24640

O

O2 Saturation, 82805-82810
Occupational Therapy
    Evaluation, 97003-97004
Odontoid Dislocation
    Open Treatment
        Reduction, 22318
        with Grafting, 22319
Odontoid Fracture
    Open Treatment
        Reduction, 22318
        With Grafting, 22319
Odontoid Process
    Excisions, 22548
Office Medical Services
    Extended Hours, 99051
Olecranon
    Bone Cyst
        Excision, 24120-24126
    Bursa
        Arthrocentesis, 20605
        Excision, 24105
    Tumor, Benign, 25120-25126
        Cyst, 24120
        Excision, 24125-24126
Olecranon Process
    Craterization, 24147
    Diaphysectomy, 24147
    Excision
        Cyst/Tumor, 24120-24126
        Partial, 24147
    Fracture
        Closed Treatment, 24670-24675
        Open Treatment, 24685
    Osteomyelitis, 24138, 24147
    Saucerization, 24147
    Sequestrectomy, 24138
Oligoclonal Immunoglobulin
    Cerebrospinal Fluid, 83916
OMT, 98925-98929
Onychectomy, 11750-11752
Onychoplasty, 11760-11762
Operating Microscope, 69990
Operation/Procedure
    Dana, 63185
    Green, 23400
    Mumford, 23120, 29824
Orbit
    Magnetic Resonance Imaging (MRI), 70540-70543
Orbits
    Skin Graft
        Split, 15120-15121
Organ or Disease Oriented Panel
    Electrolyte, 80051
    General Health Panel, 80050
    Hepatic Function Panel, 80076
    Lipid Panel, 80061
    Metabolic
        Basic
            Calcium Ionized, 80047
            Calcium Total, 80048
        Comprehensive, 80053
ORIF
    Dislocation
        Bennett, 26685-26686
        Bennett Thumb, 26665
        Carpometacarpal, 26685-26686
            Thumb, 26665
        Elbow, 24635
            Monteggia, 24635
            Galeazzi, 25525-25526

ORIF—continued
    Dislocation—continued
        Galeazzi—continued
            with—continued
                Repair—continued
                    Triangular Cartilage, 25526
        Interphalangeal
            Hand, 26785
        Lunate, 25695
        Metacarpophalangeal, 26715
        Monteggia, 24635
        Odontoid, 22318-22319
        Radioulnar
            Distal, 25676
        Shoulder
            with
                Fracture
                    Humeral, Humerus
                        Anatomical Neck, 23680
                        Surgical Neck, 23680
                        Tuberosity, 23670
        Trans-Scaphoperilunar, 25685
    Fracture
        Capitate, 25645
        Carpal (Other), 25645
            Navicular, 25628
            Scaphoid, 25628
        Clavicle, 23515
        Clavicular, 23515
        Colles, 25607-25609
        Elbow
            Monteggia, 24635
            Periarticular, 24586-24587
            Galeazzi, 25525-25526
                with
                    Fracture
                        Radial Shaft, 25525-25526
                    Repair
                        Triangular Cartilage, 25526
        Hamate, 25645
        Humeral, Humerus
            Anatomical Neck, 23615-23616
            Condylar
                Lateral, 24579
                Medial, 24579
            Epicondylar
                Lateral, 24575
                Medial, 24575
            Proximal, 23615-23616
            Shaft, 24515-24516
            Supracondylar, 24545-24546
                with
                    Intercondylar Extension, 24546
            Surgical Neck, 23615-23616
            Transcondylar, 24545-24546
                with
                    Intercondylar Extension, 24546
            Tuberosity, 23630
        Interphalangeal, 26746
        Lunate, 25645
        Metacarpal, 26615
        Metacarpophalangeal, 26715
        Monteggia, 24635
        Navicular
            Hand, 25628
        Odontoid, 22318-22319
        Olecranon process, 24685
        Phalange, Phalangeal
            Hand, 26735
            Distal, 26765
        Pisiform, 25645
        Radial, Radius
            and
                Ulnar, Ulna, 25575
            Distal, 25606-25609
            Head, 24665-24666
            Neck, 24665-24666
            or
                Ulnar, Ulna, 25574

ORIF—continued
    Fracture—continued
        Radial, Radius—continued
            Shaft
                with Dislocation
                    Distal
                        Radio-Ulnar Joint, 25525-25526
                    with Repair
                        Triangular Cartilage, 25526
        Rib, 21810
        Scaphoid, 25628
        Scapula, Scapular, 23585
        Smith, 25607-25609
        Sternum, 21825
        Thumb, 26665
        Trapezium, 25645
        Trapezoid, 25645
        Triquetral, 25645
        Ulna, Ulnar
            and Radial, Radius, 25575
            Monteggia, 24635
            Proximal, 24635, 24685
            Shaft, 25545
            or Radial, Radius, 25574
        Vertebral, 22325-22328
Orthopedic Surgery
    Computer Assisted Navigation, 20985
    Stereotaxis
        Computer Assisted, 20985
Orthosis/Orthotics
    Check-Out, 97762
    Management/Training, 97760
Osmolality
    Blood, 83930
    Urine, 83935
Osseous Survey, 77075-77076
Ostectomy
    Carpal, 25215
    Metacarpal, 26250
    Phalanges
        Fingers, 26260-26262
    Pressure Ulcer
        Sacral, 15933, 15935, 15937
    Scapula, 23190
    Sternum, 21620
Osteocalcin, 83937
Osteomyelitis
    Excision
        Clavicle, 23180
        Humerus, 24140
            Proximal, 23184
        Metacarpal, 26230
        Olecranon Process, 24147
        Phalanx (Finger)
            Distal, 26236
            Proximal or Middle, 26235
        Radial Head/Neck, 24145
        Scapula, 23182
        Ulna, 25150
    Incision
        Elbow, 23935
        Forearm, 25035
        Hand/Finger, 26034
        Humerus, 23935
        Shoulder, 23035
        Wrist, 25035
    Sequestrectomy
        Clavicle, 23170
        Forearm, 25145
        Humeral Head, 23174
        Humerus, Shaft or Distal, 24134
        Olecranon Process, 24138
        Radial Head/Neck, 24136
        Scapula, 23172
        Wrist, 25145
Osteopathic Manipulation, 98925-98929
Osteophytectomy, 63075-63078
Osteoplasty
    Carpal Bone, 25394
    Humerus, 24420
    Metacarpal, 26568
    Phalanges
        Finger, 26568
    Radius, 25390-25393

Osteoplasty—continued
  Ulna, 25390-25393
  Vertebra, 72291-72292
    Lumbar, 22521-22522
    Thoracic, 22520, 22522

Osteotomy
  Clavicle, 23480-23485
  Humerus, 24400-24410
  Metacarpal, 26565
  Phalanges
    Finger, 26567
  Radius
    and Ulna, 25365, 25375
    Distal Third, 25350
    Middle or Proximal Third, 25355
    Multiple, 25370
  Spine
    Anterior, 22220-22226
    Posterior/Posterolateral, 22210-22214
      Cervical, 22210
      Each Additional Vertebral Segment, 22208, 22216
      Lumbar, 22207, 22214
      Thoracic, 22206, 22212
      Three-Column, 22206-22208
  Ulna, 25360
    and Radius, 25365, 25375
    Multiple, 25370
  Vertebra
    Additional Segment
      Anterior Approach, 22226
      Posterior/Posterolateral Approach, 22208, 22216
    Cervical
      Anterior Approach, 22220
      Posterior/Posterolateral Approach, 22210
    Lumbar
      Anterior Approach, 22224
      Posterior/Posterolateral Approach, 22214
    Thoracic
      Anterior Approach, 22222
      Posterior/Posterolateral Approach, 22212

Oxidoreductase, Alcohol–Nad+, 84588
Oxygen Saturation, 82805-82810

P

Pain Management
  Epidural, 99601-99602
  Intrathecal, 99601-99602
  Intravenous Therapy, 96365-96368, 96374-96376

Palm
  Bursa
    Incision and Drainage, 26025-26030
  Fasciectomy, 26121-26125
  Fasciotomy, 26040-26045
  Tendon
    Excision, 26170
  Tendon Sheath
    Excision, 26145
    Incision and Drainage, 26020

Paraffin Bath Therapy, 97018
Parasites
  Blood, 87206-87207
  Concentration, 87015

Paravertebral Nerve
  Destruction, 64622-64627
  Injection
    Neurolytic, 64622-64627

Partial Claviculectomy, 23120, 23180
Partial Thromboplastin Time, 85730-85732
Patterson's Test
  Blood Urea Nitrogen, 84520-84525
Pedicle Fixation, 22842-22844
Pedicle Flap
  Island, 15740
  Neurovascular, 15750
Pelvic Fixation
  Insertion, 22848

Percutaneous Discectomies, 62287
Percutaneous Lumbar Discectomy, 62287
Percutaneous Lysis, 62263-62264
Percutaneous Vertebroplasty, 22520-22522
Performance Test
  Performance Test Physical Therapy, 97750
Peripheral Nerve
  Repair/Suture
    Major, 64856, 64859
pH
  Blood Gases, 82800-82805
Phalanges (Hand)
  Incision, Bone Cortex, 26034
Phalanx, Finger
  Craterization, 26235-26236
  Cyst
    Excision, 26210-26215
  Diaphysectomy, 26235-26236
  Excision, 26235-26236
    Radical
      for Tumor, 26260-26262
  Fracture
    Articular
      Closed Treatment, 26740
      Open Treatment, 26746
      with Manipulation, 26742
    Distal, 26755-26756
      Closed Treatment, 26750
      Open Treatment, 26765
      Percutaneous, 26756
    Open Treatment, 26735
      Distal, 26765
    Percutaneous Fixation, 26756
    Shaft, 26720-26727
      Open Treatment, 26735
  Incision and Drainage, 26034
  Ostectomy
    Radical
      for Tumor, 26260-26262
  Repair
    Lengthening, 26568
    Nonunion, 26546
    Osteotomy, 26567
  Saucerization, 26235-26236
  Thumb
    Fracture
      Shaft, 26720-26727
  Tumor, 26111-26118, 26260-26262
Phleborheography, 93965
Phosphatase
  Alkaline, 84075, 84080
  Blood, 84078
Phosphatase, Acid, 84060
Phosphohydrolases
  Alkaline, 84075-84080
Phospholipid, 86148
  Antibody, 86148
  Neutralization, 85598
Phosphomonoesterase, 84075-84080
Phosphoric Monoester Hydrolases, 84075-84080
Phosphorous, 84100
  Urine, 84105
Photodensity
  Radiographic Absorptiometry, 77083
Physical Medicine/Therapy/ Occupational Therapy
  Activities of Daily Living, 97535
  Aquatic Therapy
    with Exercises, 97113
  Athletic Training
    Evaluation, 97005
    Re-evaluation, 97006
  Check-Out
    Orthotics/Prosthetics
      ADL, 97762
  Community/Work Reintegration, 97537
  Evaluation, 97001-97002
  Hydrotherapy
    Hubbard Tank, 97036
    Pool with Exercises, 97036, 97113
  Joint Mobilization, 97140
  Kinetic Therapy, 97530

Physical Medicine/Therapy/ Occupational Therapy—continued
  Manipulation, 97140
  Manual Therapy, 97140
  Modalities
    Contrast Baths, 97034
    Diathermy Treatment, 97024
    Electric Stimulation
      Attended, Manual, 97032
      Unattended, 97014
    Hot or Cold Pack, 97010
    Hydrotherapy (Hubbard Tank), 97036
    Infrared Light Treatment, 97026
    Iontophoresis, 97033
    Microwave Therapy, 97024
    Paraffin Bath, 97018
    Traction, 97012
    Ultrasound, 97035
    Ultraviolet Light, 97028
    Vasopneumatic Device, 97016
    Whirlpool Therapy, 97022
  Orthotics Training, 97760
  Osteopathic Manipulation, 98925-98929
  Procedures
    Aquatic Therapy, 97113
    Direct, 97032
    Group Therapeutic, 97150
    Massage Therapy, 97124
    Neuromuscular Reeducation, 97112
    Physical Performance Test, 97750
    Supervised, 97010-97028
    Therapeutic Exercises, 97110
    Work Hardening, 97545-97546
  Prosthetic Training, 97761
  Sensory Integration, 97533
  Therapeutic Activities, 97530
  Wheelchair Management, 97542
  Work Reintegration, 97537
Pin
  Insertion
    Removal
      Skeletal Traction, 20650
  Prophylactic Treatment
    Humerus, 24498
    Shoulder, 23490-23491
Pinch Graft, 15050
Placement
  Intrafacet Implant(s), 0219T-0222T
  Stereotactic Frame, 20660
Plasma
  Injection, 0232T
Platelet
  Aggregation, 85576
  Blood, 85025
  Neutralization, 85597
Plethysmography
  Extremities, 93922-93923
  Veins, 93965
PLIF (Posterior Lumbar Interbody Fusion), 22630
Pollicization
  Digit, 26550
Polydactylism, 26587
Polydactylous Digit
  Reconstruction, 26587
  Repair, 26587
Pool Therapy with Exercises, 97036, 97113
Porphobilinogen
  Urine, 84106-84110
Porter–Silber Test
  Corticosteroid, Blood, 82528
Potassium
  Serum, 84132
  Urine, 84133
Pressure Ulcer (Decubitus)
  Excision, 15931-15937
  Sacral, 15931-15937
PROM, 95851-95852, 97110, 97530
Prophylactic Treatment
  Clavicle, 23490
  Humerus, 23491
    Pinning, Wiring, 24498

Prophylactic Treatment—continued
  Radius, 25490, 25492
    Nailing, 25490, 25492
    Pinning, 25490, 25492
    Plating, 25490, 25492
    Wiring, 25490, 25492
  Shoulder
    Clavicle, 23490
    Humerus, 23491
  Ulna, 25491-25492
    Nailing, 25491-25492
    Pinning, 25491-25492
    Plating, 25491-25492
    Wiring, 25491-25492
Prosthesis
  Check-Out, 97762
  Orthotic
    Check-Out, 97762
    Training, 97761
  Spinal
    Insertion, 22851
  Training, 97761
  Wrist
    Removal, 25250-25251
Protein
  Electrophoresis, 84165
  Myelin Basic, 83873
  Osteocalcin, 83937
  Serum, 84155, 84165
  Total, 84155, 84160
  Urine
    by Dipstick, 81000-81003
  Western Blot, 84181-84182
Protein Blotting, 84181-84182
Prothrombin Time, 85610-85611
Prothrombinase
  Partial Time, 85730-85732
Protime, 85610-85611
Provitamin A, 84590
PT, 85610-85611, 97001-97036, 97110-97530, 97533-97750
PTT, 85730-85732
Pulled Elbow, 24640
Pulmonology
  Diagnostic
    Hemoglobin Oxygen Affinity, 82820
Pulse Generator
  Electronic Analysis, 95970-95971
Puncture
  Lumbar, 62270
  Spinal Cord
    Diagnostic, 62270
    Lumbar, 62270
Putti–Platt Procedure, 23450
PVA (Percutaneous Vertebral Augmentation), 22523-22525
Pyruvate, 84210

Q

Quinine, 84228

R

RA Factor
  Qualitative, 86430
  Quantitative, 86431
Rachicentesis, 62270
Radial Head, Subluxation, 24640
Radiocarpal Joint
  Arthrotomy, 25040
  Dislocation
    Closed Treatment, 25660
Radiology
  Examination
    Stress Views, 77071
  Joint Survey, 77077
Radionuclide Tomography, Single-Photon Emission–Computed
  Bone, 78320
  Joint, 78320
Radioulnar Joint
  Arthrodesis
    with Ulnar Resection, 25830

Radioulnar Joint—continued
  Dislocation
    Closed Treatment, 25525, 25675
    Open Treatment, 25676
    Percutaneous Fixation, 25671

Radius
  Arthroplasty, 24365
    with Implant, 25441
  Craterization, 24145, 25151
  Cyst
    Excision, 24125-24126, 25120-25126
  Diaphysectomy, 24145, 25151
  Dislocation
    Partial, 24640
    Subluxate, 24640
    with Fracture
      Closed Treatment, 24620
      Open Treatment, 24635
  Excision, 24130, 24136, 24145, 24152
    Partial, 25145
    Styloid Process, 25230
  Fracture, 25605
    Closed Treatment, 25500-25505, 25520, 25600-25605
      with Manipulation, 25605
      without Manipulation, 25600
    Colles, 25600-25605
    Distal, 25600-25609
      Closed Treatment, 25600-25605
      Open Treatment, 25607-25609
    Head/Neck
      Closed Treatment, 24650-24655
      Open Treatment, 24665-24666
    Open Treatment, 25515, 25525-25526, 25574
    Percutaneous Fixation, 25606
    Shaft, 25500-25526
      Open Treatment, 25515, 25574-25575
    with Ulna, 25560-25565
    Open Treatment, 25575
  Implant
    Removal, 24164
  Incision and Drainage, 25035
  Osteomyelitis, 24136, 24145
  Osteoplasty, 25390-25393
  Prophylactic Treatment, 25490, 25492
  Repair
    Epiphyseal Arrest, 25450-25455
    Epiphyseal Separation
      Closed, 25600
      Closed with Manipulation, 25605
      Open Treatment, 25607-25609
      Percutaneous Fixation, 25606
    Malunion or Nonunion, 25400, 25415
    Osteotomy, 25350-25355, 25370-25375
      and Ulna, 25365
      with Graft, 25405, 25420-25426
  Saucerization, 24145, 25151
  Sequestrectomy, 24136, 25145
  Subluxation, 24640
  Tumor
    Cyst, 24120
    Excision, 24125-24126, 25120-25126, 25170

Range of Motion Test
  Extremities, 95851
  Hand, 95852
  Trunk, 97530

RBC, 85007, 85014, 85041, 85651-85652

Realignment
  Tendon, Extensor, 26437

Reconstruction
  Carpal, 25443
  Carpal Bone, 25394, 25430

Reconstruction—continued
  Elbow, 24360
    Total Replacement, 24363
    with Implant, 24361-24362
  Finger
    Polydactylous, 26587
  Hand
    Tendon Pulley, 26500-26502
    Toe to Finger Transfer, 26551-26556
  Interphalangeal Joint, 26535-26536
    Collateral Ligament, 26545
  Lunate, 25444
  Metacarpophalangeal Joint, 26530-26531
  Nail Bed, 11762
  Navicular, 25443
  Radius, 24365, 25390-25393, 25441
  Shoulder Joint
    with Implant, 23470-23472
  Thumb
    from Finger, 26550
    Opponensplasty, 26490-26496
  Toe
    Polydactylous, 26587
  Trapezium, 25445
  Ulna, 25390-25393, 25442
    Radioulnar, 25337
  Wound Repair, 13120-13133, 13160
  Wrist, 25332
    Capsulectomy, 25320
    Capsulorrhaphy, 25320
    Realign, 25335

Red Blood Cell (RBC)
  Count, 85041
  Hematocrit, 85014
  Morphology, 85007
  Platelet Estimation, 85007
  Sedimentation Rate
    Automated, 85652
    Manual, 85651

Reductase, Lactic Cytochrome, 83615-83625

Reduction
  Dislocation
    Acromioclavicular
      Closed Treatment, 23545
      Open Treatment, 23550-23552
    Bennet's
      Closed Treatment, 26670-26675
      Open Treatment, 26665, 26685-26686
      Percutaneous Fixation, 26650, 26676
    Carpometacarpal
      Closed Treatment, 26641-26645, 26670-26675
      Open Treatment, 26665, 26685-26686
      Percutaneous Fixation, 26650, 26676
    Clavicle
      Closed Treatment, 23540-23545
      Open Treatment, 23550-23552
    Elbow
      Closed Treatment, 24600-24605, 24620, 24640
      Monteggia, 24620
      Open Treatment
        Acute, 24615
        Chronic, 24615
        Monteggia, 24635
        Periarticular, 24586-24587
    Galeazzi
      Closed Treatment, 25520
      Open Treatment, 25525-25526
      with Fracture
        Radial Shaft, 25525-25526

Reduction—continued
  Dislocation—continued
    Galeazzi—continued
      Open Treatment—continued
        with Repair
          Triangular Cartilage, 25526
    Intercarpal
      Closed Treatment, 25660
      Open Treatment, 25670
    Interphalangeal Joint
      Hand/Finger
        Closed Treatment, 26770-26775
        Open Treatment, 26785
        Percutaneous Fixation, 26776
    Lunate
      Closed Treatment, 25690
      Open Treatment, 25695
    Metacarpophalangeal Joint
      Closed Treatment, 26700-26706
      Open Treatment, 26715
    Monteggia, 24635
    Odontoid
      Open Treatment, 22318-22319
    Radio-ulnar Joint
      Closed Treatment, 25675
        with Radial Fracture, 25520
      Open Treatment, 25676
        with Radial Fracture, 25525-25526
    Radiocarpal
      Closed Treatment, 25660
      Open Treatment, 25670
    Radius
      Closed Treatment, 24640
      with Fracture
        Closed Treatment, 24620
        Open Treatment, 24635
    Shoulder
      Closed Treatment with Manipulation, 23650-23655
        with Fracture of Greater Humeral Tuberosity, 23665
        with Surgical or Anatomical Neck Fracture, 23675
      Open Treatment, 23660
      Recurrent, 23450-23466
    Sternoclavicular
      Closed Treatment, 23525
      Open Treatment, 23530-23532
    Vertebral
      Closed Treatment, 22315
      Open Treatment, 22325-22328
  Fracture
    Bennett
      Closed Treatment, 26670-26675
      Open Treatment, 26665, 26685-26686
      Percutaneous Fixation, 26650, 26676
    Carpal Bone(s)
      Closed Treatment, 25624, 25635
        Capitate, 25635
        Hamate, 25635
        Lunate, 25635
        Navicular, 25624
        Pisiform, 25635
        Scaphoid, 25624
        Trapezium, 25635
        Trapezoid, 25635
        Triquetral, 25635
      Open Treatment, 25628, 25645
        Capitate, 25645
        Hamate, 25645
        Lunate, 25645
        Navicular, 25628

Reduction—continued
  Fracture—continued
    Carpal Bone(s)—continued
      Open Treatment—continued
        Pisiform, 25645
        Scaphoid, 25628
        Trapezium, 25645
        Trapezoid, 25645
        Triquetral, 25645
    Carpometacarpal
      Closed Treatment, 26645
      Open Treatment, 26665
      Percutaneous Fixation, 26650
    Clavicle
      Closed Treatment, 23505
      Open Treatment, 23515
    Colles
      Closed Treatment, 25605
      Open Treatment, 25607-25609
      Percutaneous Fixation, 25606
    Elbow
      Closed Treatment, 24620
      Open Treatment, 24586-24587
    Humeral, Humerus
      Anatomical neck
        Closed Treatment, 23605
        Open Treatment, 23615-23616
      Condylar
        Lateral
          Closed Treatment, 24577
          Open Treatment, 24579
          Percutaneous Fixation, 24582
        Medial
          Closed Treatment, 24577
          Open Treatment, 24579
          Percutaneous Fixation, 24566
      Epicondylar
        Lateral
          Closed Treatment, 24565
          Open Treatment, 24575
          Percutaneous Fixation, 24566
        Medial
          Closed Treatment, 24565
          Open, 24575
          Percutaneous Fixation, 24566
      Proximal
        Closed Treatment, 23605
        Open Treatment, 23615-23616
      Shaft
        Closed Treatment, 24505
        Open Treatment, 24515-24516
      Supracondylar
        Closed Treatment, 24535
        Open Treatment, 24545-24546
        with Intercondylar Extension, 24546
      Surgical Neck
        Closed Treatment, 23605
        Open Treatment, 23615-23616
      Transcondylar
        Closed Treatment, 24535
        Open Treatment, 24545-24546
        with Intercondylar Extension, 24546
      Tuberosity
        Closed Treatment, 23625
        Open Treatment, 23630
    Interphalangeal
      Closed Treatment
        Articular, 26742
      Open Treatment
        Articular, 26746

Reduction—*continued*
  Fracture—*continued*
    Lunate
      Closed Treatment, 25635
      Open Treatment, 25645
    Metacarpal
      Closed Treatment,
        26605-26607
      Open Treatment, 26615
      Percutaneous Fixation, 26608
    Metacarpophalangeal
      Closed
        Articular, 26742
      Open
        Articular, 26746
    Monteggia, 24635
    Navicular
      Hand
        Closed Treatment, 25624
        Open Treatment, 25628
    Odontoid
      Open Treatment,
        22318-22319
    Olecranon process
      Closed Treatment, 24675
      Open Treatment, 24685
    Phalange, Phalanges, Phalangeal
      Hand
        Closed Treatment, 26725
          Distal, 26755
        Open Treatment, 26735
          Distal, 26765
        Percutaneous Fixation,
          26727, 26756
    Pisiform
      Closed Treatment, 25635
      Open Treatment, 25645
    Radial, Radius
      Colles
        Closed Treatment, 25605
        Open Treatment,
          25607-25609
        Percutaneous Fixation,
          25606
      Distal
        Closed Treatment, 25605
          with Fracture
            Ulnar Styloid,
              25600-25605
        Open Treatment,
          25607-25609
      Head
        Closed Treatment, 24655
        Open Treatment,
          24665-24666
      Neck
        Closed Treatment, 24655
        Open Treatment,
          24665-24666
      Shaft
        Closed Treatment, 25505
          with Dislocation
            Radio-Ulnar Joint,
              Distal, 25520
        Open Treatment, 25515
          with Dislocation
            Radio-Ulnar Joint,
              Distal,
                25525-25526
            Repair, Triangular
              Cartilage,
                25526
      Smith
        Closed Treatment, 25605
        Open Treatment,
          25607-25609
        Percutaneous Fixation,
          25606
    Rib
      Open Treatment,
        21805-21810
    Scaphoid
      Closed Treatment, 25624
      Open Treatment, 25628
    Scapula, Scapular
      Closed Treatment, 23575
      Open Treatment, 23585

Reduction—*continued*
  Fracture—*continued*
    Sternum
      Open Treatment, 21825
    Thumb
      Bennett, 26645
        Closed Treatment, 26645
        Open Treatment, 26665
        Percutaneous Fixation, 26650
      Trans-Scaphoperilunar
        Closed Treatment, 25680
        Open Treatment, 25685
    Trapezium
      Closed Treatment, 25635
      Open Treatment, 25645
    Trapezoid
      Closed Treatment, 25635
      Open Treatment, 25645
    Triquetral
      Closed Treatment, 25635
      Open Treatment, 25645
    Ulna, Ulnar
      Proximal
        Closed Treatment, 24675
        Open Treatment, 24685
          Monteggia, 24635
          with Dislocation
            Radial Head, 24635
      Shaft
        Closed Treatment, 25535
        And
          Radial, Radius,
            25565
        Open Treatment, 25545
        and
          Radial, Radius,
            25574-25575
      Styloid, 25650
    Vertebral
      Closed Treatment, 22315
      Open Treatment,
        22325-22328,
        63081-63091
  Subluxation
    Radial, 24640
      Head, 24640
    Neck, 24640
Reflex Test
  H Reflex, 95934-95936
Reinsertion
  Spinal Fixation Device, 22849
Relative Density
  Body Fluid, 84315
Release
  Carpal Tunnel, 64721
  Elbow Contracture
    with Radical Release of Capsule,
      24149
  Muscle
    Thumb Contracture, 26508
  Nerve, 64702-64708, 64713,
    64718-64721
    Carpal Tunnel, 64721
    Neurolytic, 64727
  Tendon, 24332, 25295
  Thumb Contracture, 26508
Removal
  Artificial Disc, 0095T, 0164T,
    22864-22865
  Artificial Intervertebral Disc
    Cervical Interspace, 0095T,
      22864
    Lumbar Interspace, 0164T,
      22865
  Calcaneous Deposits
    Subdeltoid, 23000
  Cast, 29700-29715
  Cranial Tongs, 20665
  External Fixation System, 20694,
    20697
  Fixation Device, 20670-20680
  Foreign Bodies
    Arm
      Lower, 25248
      Upper, 24200-24201
    Elbow, 24000, 24101,
      24200-24201
    Finger, 26075-26080

Removal—*continued*
  Foreign Bodies—*continued*
    Hand, 26070
    Muscle, 20520-20525
    Shoulder, 23040-23044
      Complicated, 23332
      Deep, 23331
      Subcutaneous, 23330
    Skin
      with Debridement,
        11010-11012
    Subcutaneous
      with Debridement,
        11010-11012
    Tendon Sheath, 20520-20525
    Wrist, 25040, 25101, 25248
  Halo, 20665
  Harrington Rod, 22850
  Implant, 20670-20680
    Disc, 0164T, 22865
    Elbow, 24160
    Finger, 26320
    Hand, 26320
    Pin, 20670-20680
    Radius, 24164
    Rod, 20670-20680
    Screw, 20670-20680
    Wrist, 25449
  Loose Body
    Carpometacarpal Joint, 26070
    Elbow, 24101
    Wrist, 25101
  Nail, 11730-11732, 11750-11752
  Prosthesis
    Wrist, 25250-25251
  Shoulder Joint
    Foreign or Loose Body, 23107
  Spinal Instrumentation
    Anterior, 22855
    Posterior Nonsegmental
      Harrington Rod, 22850
    Posterior Segmental, 22852
  Suture
    Anesthesia, 15850-15851
  Tube
    Finger, 26392, 26416
    Hand, 26392, 26416
Renin, 84244
Repair
  Arm
    Lower, 25260-25263, 25270
      Fasciotomy, 24495
      Secondary, 25265,
        25272-25274
      Tendon, 25290
      Tendon Sheath, 25275
      Muscle, 24341
      Tendon, 24332, 24341, 25280,
        25295, 25310-25316
    Upper
      Muscle Revision, 24330-24331
      Muscle Transfer, 24301,
        24320
      Tendon Lengthening, 24305
      Tendon Revision, 24320
      Tendon Transfer, 24301
      Tenotomy, 24310
  Body Cast, 29720
  Carpal, 25440
  Carpal Bone, 25431
  Cast
    Spica, body, or jacket, 29720
  Clavicle
    Osteotomy, 23480-23485
  Cleft
    Hand, 26580
  Defect
    Radius, 25425-25426
    Ulna, 25425-25426
  Elbow
    Fasciotomy, 24357-24359
    Hemiepiphyseal Arrest, 24470
    Ligament, 24343-24346
    Muscle, 24341
    Muscle Transfer, 24301
    Tendon, 24340-24342
      Each, 24341
    Tendon Lengthening, 24305

Repair—*continued*
  Elbow—*continued*
    Tendon Transfer, 24301
    Tennis Elbow, 24357-24359
  Finger
    Claw Finger, 26499
    Macrodactyly, 26590
    Polydactylous, 26587
    Syndactyly, 26560-26562
    Tendon
      Extensor, 26415-26434,
        26445-26449, 26455
      Flexor, 26356-26358,
        26440-26442
      Joint Stabilization, 26474
      PIP Joint, 26471
    Toe Transfer, 26551-26556
    Trigger, 26055
    Volar Plate, 26548
    Web Finger, 26560
  Fracture
    Radius, 25526
  Hand
    Cleft Hand, 26580
    Muscles, 26591-26593
    Tendon
      Extensor, 26410-26416,
        26426-26428,
        26433-26437
      Flexor, 26350-26358, 26440
      Profundus, 26370-26373
    Humerus, 24420-24430
    Osteotomy, 24400-24410
      with Graft, 24435
  Interphalangeal Joint
    Volar Plate, 26548
  Laceration, Skin
    Abdomen
      Intermediate, 12031-12037
      Layered, 12031-12037
      Simple, 12001-12007
      Superficial, 12001-12007
    Arm, Arms
      Complex, 13120-13122
      Intermediate, 12031-12037
      Layered, 12031-12037
      Simple, 12001-12007
      Superficial, 12001-12007
    Axilla, Axillae
      Complex, 13131-13133
      Intermediate, 12031-12037
      Layered, 12031-12037
      Simple, 12001-12007
      Superficial, 12001-12007
    Back
      Intermediate, 12031-12037
      Layered, 12031-12037
      Simple, 12001-12007
      Superficial, 12001-12007
    Chest
      Intermediate, 12031-12037
      Layered, 12031-12037
      Simple, 12001-12007
      Superficial, 12001-12007
    Extremity, Extremities
      Complex/Intermediate,
        12031-12037
      Layered, 12031-12037
      Simple, 12001-12007
      Superficial, 12001-12007
    Finger, Fingers
      Complex, 13131-13133
      Intermediate, 12041-12047
      Layered, 12041-12047
      Simple, 12001-12007
      Superficial, 12001-12007
    Forearm, Forearms
      Complex, 13120-13122
      Intermediate, 12031-12037
      Layered, 12031-12037
      Simple, 12001-12007
      Superficial, 12001-12007
    Hand, Hands
      Complex, 13131-13133
      Intermediate, 12041-12047
      Layered, 12041-12047
      Simple, 12001-12007
      Superficial, 12001-12007

Repair—continued
  Laceration, Skin—continued
    Lower
      Arm, Arms
        Complex, 13120-13122
        Intermediate, 12031-12037
        Layered, 12031-12037
        Simple, 12001-12007
        Superficial, 12001-12007
      Neck
        Complex, 13131-13133
        Intermediate, 12041-12047
        Layered, 12041-12047
        Simple, 12001-12007
        Superficial, 12001-12007
      Palm, Palms
        Complex, 13131-13133
        Intermediate, 12041-12047
        Layered, 12041-12047
        Layered Simple, 12001-12007
        Superficial, 12001-12007
      Trunk
        Intermediate, 12031-12037
        Layered, 12031-12037
        Simple, 12001-12007
        Superficial, 12001-12007
      Upper
        Arm, Arms
          Complex, 13120-13122
          Intermediate, 12031-12037
          Layered, 12031-12037
          Simple, 12001-12007
          Superficial, 12001-12007
        Extremity
          Complex, 13120-13122
          Intermediate, 12031-12037
          Layered, 12031-12037
          Simple, 12001-12007
          Superficial, 12001-12007
  Ligament
    Collateral
      Elbow, 24343, 24345
      Metacarpophalangeal or interphalangeal joint, 26540
  Macrodactylia, 26590
  Malunion
    Humerus, 24430
    Radius, 25400-25420
    Ulna, 25400-25420
  Metacarpal
    Lengthen, 26568
    Nonunion, 26546
    Osteotomy, 26565
  Metacarpophalangeal Joint
    Capsulodesis, 26516-26518
    Collateral Ligament, 26540-26542
    Fusion, 26516-26518
  Microsurgery, 69990
  Muscle
    Hand, 26591
    Upper Arm or Elbow, 24341
  Musculotendinous Cuff, 23410-23412
  Nail Bed, 11760
  Navicular, 25440
  Neck Muscles
    Scalenus Anticus, 21700-21705
    Sternocleidomastoid, 21720-21725
  Nerve, 64876
    Graft, 64890-64907
    Microrepair
      with Surgical Microscope, 69990
    Suture, 64831-64837, 64856-64857, 64859, 64872-64876
  Nonunion
    Carpal Bone, 25431
    Humerus, 24430
    Metacarpal, 26546
    Navicular, 25440
    Phalanx, 26546
    Radius, 25400-25420
    Scaphoid, 25440
    Ulna, 25400-25420

Repair—continued
  Osteotomy
    Radius and Ulna, 25365
    Ulna and Radius, 25365
    Vertebra
      Additional Segment, 22216, 22226
      Cervical, 22210, 22220
      Lumbar, 22214, 22224
      Thoracic, 22212, 22222
  Phalanges
    Finger
      Lengthening, 26568
      Osteotomy, 26567
      Nonunion, 26546
  Radius
    Epiphyseal, 25450-25455
    Malunion or Nonunion, 25400-25420
    Osteotomy, 25350-25355, 25370-25375
    with Graft, 25405, 25420-25426
  Rotator Cuff, 23410-23412, 23420, 29827
  Scalenus Anticus, 21700-21705
  Scapula
    Fixation, 23400
    Scapulopexy, 23400
  Shoulder
    Capsule, 23450-23466
    Cuff, 23410-23412
    Ligament Release, 23415
    Muscle Transfer, 23395-23397
    Musculotendinous (Rotator) Cuff, 23410-23412
    Rotator Cuff, 23415-23420
    Tendon, 23410-23412, 23430-23440
    Tenomyotomy, 23405-23406
  Simple, Integumentary System, 12001-12007, 12020-12021
  Skin
    Wound
      Complex, 13120-13133, 13160
      Intermediate, 12031-12047
      Simple, 12020-12021
  SLAP Lesion, 29807
  Spica Cast, 29720
  Spine
    Lumbar Vertebra, 22521-22522, 22524-22525
    Osteotomy, 22210-22226
    Thoracic Vertebra, 22520, 22522-22523, 22525
  Sternocleidomastoid, 21720-21725
  Syndactyly, 26560-26562
  Tendon
    Extensor, 26410-26412, 26418-26428, 26433-26434
    Flexor, 26350-26358
    Profundus, 26370-26373
    Upper Arm or Elbow, 24341
  Thumb
    Muscle, 26508
    Tendon, 26510
  Triangular Fibrocartilage, 29846
  Trigger Finger, 26055
  Ulna
    Epiphyseal, 25450-25455
    Malunion or Nonunion, 25400-25415
    Osteotomy, 25360, 25370-25375, 25425-25426
    with Graft, 25405, 25420
  Wound
    Complex, 13120-13133, 13160
    Intermediate, 12031-12047
    Simple, 12001-12007, 12020-12021
  Wound Dehiscence
    Skin and Subcutaneous Tissue
      Complex, 13160
      Simple, 12020-12021

Repair—continued
  Wrist, 25260-25263, 25270, 25447
    Bones, 25440
    Carpal Bone, 25431
    Cartilage, 25107
    Muscles, 25260-25274
    Removal
      Implant, 25449
    Secondary, 25265, 25272-25274
    Tendon, 25280-25316
    Sheath, 25275
    Total Replacement, 25446
Replacement
  Arthroplasty
    Spine, 22856-22862
  Elbow
    Total, 24363
  External Fixation, 20697
  Intervertebral Disc
    Cervical Interspace, 0092T, 22856
    Lumbar Interspace, 0163T, 22862
  Strut, 20697
Replantation, Reimplantation
  Arm, Upper, 20802
  Digit, 20816-20822
  Forearm, 20805
  Hand, 20808
  Thumb, 20824-20827
Reposition
  Toe to Hand, 26551-26556
Reptilase
  Test, 85635
Resection
  Humeral Head, 23195
  Radical
    Arm, Lower, 24152, 25077-25078, 25170
    Arm, Upper, 23220, 24077-24079, 24150
    Back, 21935-21936
    Elbow, 24077-24079, 24152
      Capsule Soft Tissue, 24149
    Finger, 26117-26118, 26260-26262
    Flank, 21935-21936
    Forearm, 25077-25078, 25170
    Hand, 26117-26118, 26250
    Humerus, 23220, 24077-24079
    Metacarpal, 26117-26118, 26250
    Neck, 21557-21558
    Phalanges
      Fingers, 26117-26118, 26260-26262
    Radius, 24152, 25077-25078, 25170
    Scapula, 23077-23078, 23210
    Shoulder, 23077-23078, 23220
    Sternum, 21557-21558, 21630-21632
    Thorax, 21557-21558
    Ulna, 25077-25078, 25170
    Wrist, 25077-25078, 25115-25116, 25170
  Ulna
    Arthrodesis
      Radioulnar Joint, 25830
Reticulocyte
  Count, 85044-85045
Revascularization
  Other Tissue Grafts, 20926
Revision
  Arthroplasty
    Spine, 22861-22862
  External Fixation System, 20693
Rheumatoid Factor, 86430-86431
Rhizotomy, 63185-63190
Rib
  Excision, 21600-21616
  Fracture
    Closed Treatment, 21800
    External Fixation, 21810
    Open Treatment, 0245T-0248T, 21805
Risser Jacket, 29010-29015
  Removal, 29710
ROM, 95851-95852, 97110, 97530

Ropes Test, 83872
Rotation Flap, 14000-14041, 14301-14350
Rotator Cuff
  Repair, 23410-23420

S

Sacroplasty, 0200T-0201T
Sacrum
  augmentation, 0200T-0201T
  Pressure Ulcer, 15931-15937
  X-ray, 72220
Salicylate
  Assay, 80196
SALT, 84460
SAST, 84450
Saucerization
  Clavicle, 23180
  Humerus, 23184, 24140
  Metacarpal, 26230
  Olecranon Process, 24147
  Phalanges
    Finger, 26235-26236
  Radius, 24145, 25151
  Scapula, 23182
  Ulna, 24147, 25150
Sauve-Kapandji Procedure
  Arthrodesis, Distal Radioulnar Joint, 25830
Scalenotomy, 21700-21705
Scalenus Anticus
  Division, 21700-21705
Scaphoid
  Fracture
    Closed Treatment, 25622
    Open Treatment, 25628
    with Manipulation, 25624
Scapula
  Craterization, 23182
  Cyst
    Excision, 23140
      with Allograft, 23146
      with Autograft, 23145
  Diaphysectomy, 23182
  Excision, 23172, 23190
    Partial, 23182
  Fracture
    Closed Treatment
      with Manipulation, 23575
      without Manipulation, 23570
    Open Treatment, 23585
  Ostectomy, 23190
  Repair
    Fixation, 23400
    Scapulopexy, 23400
  Saucerization, 23182
  Sequestrectomy, 23172
  Tumor
    Excision, 23140, 23210
      with Allograft, 23146
      with Autograft, 23145
    Radical Resection, 23210
  X-ray, 73010
Scapulopexy, 23400
Sciatic Nerve
  Lesion
    Excision, 64786
  Neuroma
    Excision, 64786
Section
  Cranial Nerve
    Spinal Access, 63191
    Dentate Ligament, 63180-63182
    Nerve Root, 63185-63190
    Spinal Accessory Nerve, 63191
    Spinal Cord Tract, 63194-63199
Seddon-Brookes Procedure, 24320
Sedimentation Rate
  Automated, 85652
  Manual, 85651
Self Care
  Training, 97535
Semiquantitative, 81005

Sensitivity Study
  Antibiotic
    Agar, 87181
    Disc, 87184
    Enzyme Detection, 87185
    Macrobroth, 87188
    MIC, 87186
    Microtiter, 87186
    MLC, 87187
Sensory Nerve
  Common
    Repair/Suture, 64834
SEP (Somatosensory Evoked Potentials), 95925-95927
Sequestrectomy
  Carpal, 25145
  Clavicle, 23170
  Forearm, 25145
  Humeral Head, 23174
  Humerus, 24134
  Olecranon Process, 24138
  Radius, 24136, 25145
  Scapula, 23172
  Ulna, 24138, 25145
  Wrist, 25145
Serum
  Albumin, 82040
Sesamoid Bone
  Finger
    Excision, 26185
  Thumb
    Excision, 26185
Sever Procedure, 23020
SG, 84315
SGOT, 84450
SGPT, 84460
Shock Wave (Extracorporeal) Therapy, 0019T, 0101T-0102T
Shoulder
  Abscess
    Drainage, 23030
  Amputation, 23900-23921
  Arthrocentesis, 20610
  Arthrodesis, 23800
    with Autogenous Graft, 23802
  Arthrography
    Injection
      Radiologic, 23350
  Arthroplasty
    with Implant, 23470-23472
  Arthroscopy
    Diagnostic, 29805
    Surgical, 29806-29828
  Arthrotomy
    with Removal Loose or Foreign Body, 23107
  Biopsy
    Deep, 23066
    Soft Tissue, 23065
  Bone
    Excision
      Acromion, 23130
      Clavicle, 23120-23125
      Clavicle Tumor, 23140-23146
    Incision, 23035
    Tumor
      Excision, 23140-23146
  Bursa
    Drainage, 23031
  Capsular Contracture Release, 23020
  Cast
    Figure Eight, 29049
    Removal, 29710
    Spica, 29055
    Velpeau, 29058
  Disarticulation, 23920-23921
  Dislocation
    Closed Treatment
      with Manipulation, 23650-23655
    Open Treatment, 23660
    with Greater Tuberosity Fracture
      Closed Treatment, 23665
      Open Treatment, 23670

Shoulder—continued
  Dislocation—continued
    with Surgical or Anatomical Neck Fracture
      Closed Treatment with Manipulation, 23675
      Open Treatment, 23680
    Excision
      Acromion, 23130
      Torn Cartilage, 23101
    Exploration, 23107
    Hematoma
      Drainage, 23030
    Incision and Drainage, 23040-23044
    Joint
      X-ray, 73050
    Manipulation
      Application of Fixation Apparatus, 23700
    Prophylactic Treatment, 23490-23491
    Radical Resection, 23077
    Removal
      Calcareous Deposits, 23000
      Cast, 29710
      Foreign Body, 23040-23044
        Complicated, 23332
        Deep, 23331
        Subcutaneous, 23330
      Foreign or Loose Body, 23107
    Repair
      Capsule, 23450-23466
      Ligament Release, 23415
      Muscle Transfer, 23395-23397
      Rotator Cuff, 23410-23420
      Tendon, 23410-23412, 23430-23440
      Tenomyotomy, 23405-23406
    Strapping, 29240
    Tumor, 23071-23073, 23078
    X-ray, 73020-73030
      with Contrast, 73040
Shoulder Bone
  Excision
    Acromion, 23130
    Clavicle, 23120-23125
  Tumor
    Excision, 23140-23146
Shoulder Joint
  Arthroplasty
    with Implant, 23470-23472
  Arthrotomy
    with Biopsy, 23100-23101
    with Synovectomy, 23105-23106
  Dislocation
    Open Treatment, 23660
    with Greater Tuberosity Fracture
      Closed Treatment, 23665
      Open Treatment, 23670
    with Surgical or Anatomical Neck Fracture
      Closed Treatment with Manipulation, 23675
      Open Treatment, 23680
  Excision
    Torn Cartilage, 23101
  Exploration, 23040-23044, 23107
  Foreign Body Removal, 23040-23044
  Incision and Drainage, 23040-23044
  X-ray, 73050
Siderophilin, 84466
Single Photon Absorptiometry
  Bone Density, 78350
Skeletal Fixation
  Humeral Epicondyle
    Percutaneous, 24566
Skeletal Traction
  Insertion/Removal, 20650
  Pin/Wire, 20650
Skin
  Adjacent Tissue Transfer, 14000-14041, 14301-14350
  Debridement, 11010-11047
    Subcutaneous Tissue, 11042-11046
    with Open Fracture and/or Dislocation, 11010-11012

Skin—continued
  Decubitus Ulcer(s)
    Excision, 15931-15937
  Destruction
    Malignant Lesion, 17260-17276
  Excision
    Debridement, 11010-11046
    Hemangioma, 11400-11426
  Lesion
    Benign, 11400-11426
    Malignant, 11600-11626
  Fasciocutaneous Flaps, 15732-15736
  Grafts
    Free, 15220-15241
  Muscle Flaps, 15732-15736
  Myocutaneous Flap, 15732-15736
  Wound Repair
    Arm, Arms
      Complex, 13120-13122
      Intermediate, 12031-12037
      Layered, 12031-12037
      Simple, 12001-12007
      Superficial, 12001-12007
    Axilla, Axillae
      Complex, 13131-13133
      Intermediate, 12031-12037
      Layered, 12031-12037
      Simple, 12001-12007
      Superficial, 12001-12007
    Back
      Intermediate, 12031-12037
      Layered, 12031-12037
      Simple, 12001-12007
      Superficial, 12001-12007
    Chest
      Intermediate, 12031-12037
      Layered, 12031-12037
      Simple, 12001-12007
      Superficial, 12001-12007
    Extremity, Extremities
      Complex/Intermediate, 12031-12037
      Layered, 12031-12037
      Simple, 12001-12007
      Superficial, 12001-12007
    Finger, Fingers
      Complex, 13131-13133
      Intermediate, 12041-12047
      Layered, 12041-12047
      Simple, 12001-12007
      Superficial, 12001-12007
    Forearm, Forearms
      Complex, 13120-13122
      Intermediate, 12031-12037
      Layered, 12031-12037
      Simple, 12001-12007
      Superficial, 12001-12007
    Hand, Hands
      Complex, 13131-13133
      Intermediate, 12041-12047
      Layered, 12041-12047
      Simple, 12001-12007
      Superficial, 12001-12007
    Lower
      Arm, Arms
        Complex, 13120-13122
        Intermediate, 12031-12037
        Layered, 12031-12037
        Simple, 12001-12007
        Superficial, 12001-12007
    Neck
      Complex, 13131-13133
      Intermediate, 12041-12047
      Layered, 12041-12047
      Simple, 12001-12007
      Superficial, 12001-12007
    Palm, Palms
      Complex, 13131-13133
      Intermediate, 12041-12047
      Layered, 12041-12047
      Simple, 12001-12007
      Superficial, 12001-12007
    Trunk
      Intermediate, 12031-12037
      Layered, 12031-12037
      Simple, 12001-12007
      Superficial, 12001-12007

Skin—continued
  Wound Repair—continued
    Upper
      Arm, Arms
        Complex, 13120-13122
        Intermediate, 12031-12037
        Layered, 12031-12037
        Simple, 12001-12007
        Superficial, 12001-12007
      Extremity
        Complex, 13120-13122
        Intermediate, 12031-12037
        Layered, 12031-12037
        Simple, 12001-12007
        Superficial, 12001-12007
Skin Graft and Flap
  Autograft
    Split-Thickness, 15100-15101, 15120-15121
  Composite Graft, 15770
  Derma-Fat-Fascia Graft, 15770
  Fascial
    Free, 15758
  Fasciocutaneous Flap, 15732-15736
  Free
    Microvascular Anastomosis, 15756-15758
  Free Skin Graft
    Full Thickness, 15220-15241
  Island Pedicle Flap, 15740
  Muscle, 15732-15736
    Free, 15756
  Myocutaneous, 15732-15736, 15756
  Pedicle Flap
    Island, 15740
    Neurovascular, 15750
  Pinch Graft, 15050
  Recipient Site Preparation, 15002-15005
  Skin
    Free, 15757
  Split Graft, 15100-15101, 15120-15121
  Tissue Transfer, 14000-14041, 14301-14350
  Vascular Flow Check, 15860
  Xenograft, 15400-15401
Smear and Stain
  Fluorescent, 87206
  Gram or Giesma, 87205
  Intracellular Parasites, 87207
  Parasites, 87206-87207
  Wet Mount, 87210
Smith Fracture, 25600-25605, 25607-25609
Smith-Robinson Operation
  Arthrodesis, Vertebra, 22614
Sodium, 84295
  Urine, 84300
Sofield Procedure, 24410
Soft Tissue
  Abscess, 20005
Solitary Cyst, Bone
  Drainage, 20615
  Injection, 20615
Somatomedin, 84305
Somatosensory Testing
  Trunk or Head, 95927
  Upper Limbs, 95925
Somatotropin, 83003
Somatropin, 80428-80430, 86277
Sore, Bed
  Excision, 15931-15937
Special Services
  Emergency Care in Office
    Out of Office, 99060
  Extended Hours, 99051-99053
Specific Gravity
  Body Fluid, 84315
  with Urinalysis, 81000-81003
Specimen Concentration, 87015
SPECT
  Bone, 78320
Spectometry
  Mass
    Analyte
      Qualitative, 83788
      Quantitative, 83789

Spectrophotometry, 84311
  Atomic Absorption, 82190
Spectroscopy
  Atomic Absorption, 82190
Spectrum Analyses, 84311
Spica Cast
  Repair, 29720
  Shoulder, 29055
Spinal Accessory Nerve
  Incision, 63191
  Section, 63191
Spinal Cord
  Cyst
    Incision and Drainage, 63172-63173
  Decompression, 63001-63103
    with Cervical Laminoplasty, 63050-63051
  Exploration, 63001-63044
  Graft
    Dura, 63710
  Incision
    Dentate Ligament, 63180-63182
    Nerve Root, 63185-63190
    Tract, 63170, 63194-63199
  Injection
    Blood, 62273
    CT Scan, 62284
    X-ray, 62284
  Lesion
    Excision, 63300-63308
  Puncture (Tap)
    Diagnostic, 62270
    Lumbar, 62270
  Reconstruction
    Dorsal Spine Elements, 63295
  Section
    Dentate Ligament, 63180-63182
    Nerve Root, 63185-63190
    Tract, 63194-63199
Spinal Fluid
  Immunoelectrophoresis, 86325
Spinal Instrumentation
  Anterior, 22845-22847
  Removal, 22855
  Internal Fixation, 22841
  Pelvic Fixation, 22848
  Posterior Nonsegmental
    Harrington Rod Technique, 22840
    Harrington Rod Technique Removal, 22850
  Posterior Segmental, 22842-22844
  Posterior Segmental Removal, 22852
  Prosthetic Device, 22851
  Reinsertion of Spinal Fixation Device, 22849
Spinal Nerve
  Avulsion, 64772
  Transection, 64772
Spinal Tap
  Lumbar, 62270
Spine
  Allograft
    Morselized, 20930
    Structural, 20931
  Arthroplasty
    Cervical, 0098T, 22861
    Lumbar, 0163T-0165T, 22857-22865
  Augmentation
    Lumbar Vertebra, 22524-22525
    Thoracic Vertebra, 22523, 22525
  Autograft
    Local, 20936
    Morselized, 20937
    Structural, 20938
  Biopsy, 20250-20251
  CT Scan
    Cervical, 72125-72127
    Lumbar, 72131-72133
    Thoracic, 72128-72130
  Fixation, 22842
  Fusion
    Anterior, 22808-22812
    Anterior Approach, 22548-22585, 22812
    Exploration, 22830

Spine—*continued*
  Fusion—*continued*
    Lateral Extracavitary, 22532-22534
    Posterior Approach, 22590-22802
  Incision and Drainage
    Abscess, 22010-22015
  Insertion
    Instrumentation, 22840-22848, 22851
  Kyphectomy, 22818-22819
  Magnetic Resonance Imaging
    Cervical, 72141-72142, 72156-72158
    Lumbar, 72148-72158
    Thoracic, 72146-72147, 72156-72158
  Manipulation
    Anesthesia, 22505
  Myelography
    Cervical, 72240
    Lumbosacral, 72265
    Thoracic, 72255
    Total, 72270
  Reconstruction
    Dorsal Spine Elements, 63295
  Reinsertion Instrumentation, 22849
  Removal Instrumentation, 22850, 22852-22855
  Repair, Osteotomy
    Anterior, 22220-22226
    Posterior, 22210-22214
      Cervical Laminoplasty, 63050-63051
      Posterolateral, 22216
  Standing X-ray, 72069
  X-Ray, 72020, 72090
    Absorptiometry, 77080, 77082
    Cervical, 72040-72052
    Lumbosacral, 72100-72120
    Standing, 72069
    Thoracic, 72070-72074
    Thoracolumbar, 72080
    Total, 72010
    with Contrast
      Cervical, 72240
      Lumbosacral, 72265
      Thoracic, 72255
      Total, 72270
Spine Chemotherapy
  Administration, 96450
Splint
  Arm
    Long, 29105
    Short, 29125-29126
  Finger, 29130-29131
Split Grafts, 15100-15101, 15120-15121
SPR (Selective Posterior Rhizotomy), 63185-63190
Sprengel's Deformity, 23400
SQ, 96372
Standing X-ray, 72069
Steindler Type Advancement, 24330
Stereotactic Frame
  Application
    Removal, 20660
Stereotaxis
  Computer-Assisted
    Orthopedic Surgery, 20985
Sterile Coverings
  Change
    under Anesthesia, 15852
Sternal Fracture
  Closed Treatment, 21820
  Open Treatment, 21825
Sternoclavicular Joint
  Arthrotomy, 23044
    with Biopsy, 23101
    with Synovectomy, 23106
  Dislocation
    Closed Treatment
      with Manipulation, 23525
      without Manipulation, 23520
    Open Treatment, 23530-23532
      with Fascial Graft, 23532
Sternocleidomastoid
  Division, 21720-21725

Sternotomy
  Closure, 21750
Sternum
  Debridement, 21627
  Excision, 21620, 21630-21632
  Fracture
    Closed Treatment, 21820
    Open Treatment, 21825
  Ostectomy, 21620
  Radical Resection, 21630-21632
  Reconstruction, 21750
STG, 15100-15101, 15120-15121
STH, 83003
Stimson's Method Reduction, 23650-23655
Stimulating Antibody, Thyroid, 84445
Stoffel Operation
  Rhizotomy, 63185-63190
Strapping
  Elbow, 29260
  Finger, 29280
  Hand, 29280
  Shoulder, 29240
  Wrist, 29260
Streptococcus, Group B
  by Immunoassay
    with Direct Optical Observation, 87802
STSG, 15100-15101, 15120-15121
Styloid Process
  Fracture, 25645-25650
  Radial
    Excision, 25230
Styloidectomy
  Radial, 25230
Subacromial Bursa
  Arthrocentesis, 20610
Subcutaneous
  Injecton, 96372
Subcutaneous Tissue
  Repair
    Complex, 13120-13133, 13160
    Intermediate, 12031-12047
    Simple, 12020-12021
Subluxation
  Elbow, 24640
Sulfation Factor, 84305
Supernumerary Digit
  Reconstruction, 26587
  Repair, 26587
Suppression/Testing, 80428-80430, 80435
Surgeries
  Laser
    Lesion
      Skin, 17260-17276
      Spine, 62287
Surgical
  Avulsion
    Nails, 11730-11732
    Nerve, 64772
  Diathermy
    Lesions
      Malignant, 17260-17276
  Microscopes, 69990
Suspension
  Hyoid, 21685
Suture
  Nerve, 64831-64837, 64856-64857, 64859, 64872-64876
  Removal
    Anesthesia, 15850-15851
  Wound
    Skin
      Complex, 13120-13133, 13160
      Intermediate, 12031-12047
      Simple, 12020-12021
Sweat Test
  Chloride, Blood, 82435
Sympathectomy
  with Rib Excision, 21616
Syndactyly
  Repair, 26560-26562
Syndesmotomy
  Coracoacromial
    Arthroscopic, 29826
    Open, 23130, 23415

Syndesmotomy—*continued*
  Transverse Carpal, 29848
Syndrome
  Carpal Tunnel
    Decompression, 64721
Synovectomy
  Arthrotomy with
    Glenohumeral Joint, 23105
    Sternoclavicular Joint, 23106
  Elbow, 24102
  Excision
    Carpometacarpal Joint, 26130
    Finger Joint, 26135-26140
    Interphalangeal Joint, 26140
    Metacarpophalangeal Joint, 26135
    Palm, 26145
    Wrist, 25105, 25115-25119
    Radical, 25115-25116
Synovial
  Bursa
    Joint Aspiration, 20600-20610
  Cyst
    Aspiration, 20612
Synovium
  Biopsy
    Carpometacarpal Joint, 26100
    Interphalangeal Joint, 26110
    Metacarpophalangeal Joint
      with Synovial Biopsy, 26105
  Excision
    Carpometacarpal Joint, 26130
    Finger Joint, 26135-26140
    Interphalangeal Joint, 26140
System
  Hemic/Lymphatic, 38220-38221, 38500-38505
  Integumentary, 11010-11047, 11400-11426, 11600-11626, 11719-11765, 12001-12007, 12020-12047, 13120-13133, 13160-14041, 14301-15005, 15050-15101, 15120-15121, 15220-15241, 15400-15401, 15732-15736, 15740-15758, 15770, 15850-15860, 15931-15937, 17260-17276
  Musculoskeletal, 20005, 20102-20103, 20200-20251, 20520-20553, 20600-20661, 20664-20827, 20900-20910, 20920-20950, 20974-20985, 21550-21725, 21750-21825, 21920-22865, 23000-23921, 23930-24365, 24400-24935, 25000-25931, 26010-26952, 29000-29131, 29240-29280, 29700-29740, 29805-29848, 29900-29902
  Nervous, 62263-62267, 62270, 62273, 62284-62291, 63001-63199, 63295-63308, 63710, 64449, 64614, 64622-64627, 64640, 64702-64708, 64713, 64718-64721, 64727, 64772-64795, 64831-64837, 64856-64857, 64859, 64872-64876, 64890-64911

T

T-4
  Thyroxine, 84436-84439
T-7 Index
  Thyroxine, Total, 84436
T4 Total, 84436
Tap
  Lumbar Diagnostic, 62270
TBG, 84442
Temporomandibular Joint (TMJ)
  Arthrocentesis, 20605
Tendon
  Arm, Upper
    Revision, 24320
  Finger
    Excision, 26180

Tendon—continued
  Forearm
    Repair, 25260-25274
  Graft
    Harvesting, 20924
  Insertion
    Biceps Tendon, 24342
  Lengthening
    Arm, Lower, 25280
    Arm, Upper, 24305
    Elbow, 24305
    Finger, 26476, 26478
    Forearm, 25280
    Hand, 26476, 26478
    Wrist, 25280
  Palm
    Excision, 26170
  Release
    Arm, Lower, 25295
    Arm, Upper, 24332
    Wrist, 25295
  Shortening
    Finger, 26477, 26479
    Hand, 26477, 26479
  Transfer
    Arm, Lower, 25310-25312, 25316
    Arm, Upper, 24301
    Elbow, 24301
    Finger, 26497-26498
    Hand, 26480-26489
    Thumb, 26490-26492, 26510
    Wrist, 25310-25312,
      25316-25320
  Wrist
    Repair, 25260-25274
Tendon Origin
  Insertion
    Injection, 20551
Tendon Pulley Reconstruction of Hand, 26500-26502
Tendon Sheath
  Arm
    Lower
      Repair, 25275
  Finger
    Incision, 26055
    Incision and Drainage, 26020
    Lesion, 26160
  Hand
    Lesion, 26160
    Injection, 20550
  Palm
    Incision and Drainage, 26020
  Removal
    Foreign Body, 20520-20525
  Wrist
    Excision, 25115-25116
    Incision, 25000-25001
    Repair, 25275
Tenectomy, Tendon Sheath
  Forearm/Wrist, 25110
  Hand/Finger, 26160
Tennis Elbow
  Repair, 24357-24359
Tenodesis
  Biceps Tendon
    at Elbow, 24340
    at Shoulder, 23430, 29828
  Finger, 26471-26474
  Wrist, 25300-25301
Tenolysis
  Arm, Lower, 25295
  Arm, Upper, 24332
  Finger
    Extensor, 26445-26449
    Flexor, 26440-26442
  Hand
    Extensor, 26445-26449
    Flexor, 26440-26442
  Wrist, 25295
Tenomyotomy, 23405-23406
Tenosuspension
  at Wrist, 25300-25301
  Biceps, 29828
    at Elbow, 24340
    Long Tendon, 23430
  Interphalangeal Joint, 26471-26474
Tenosynovectomy, 26145

Tenotomy
  Arm, Lower, 25290
  Arm, Upper, 24310
  Elbow, 24357
  Finger, 26060, 26455-26460
  Hand, 26450, 26460
  Wrist, 25290
TENS, 97014, 97032
Testing
  Neuropsychological
    Intraoperative, 95920
  Range of Motion
    Extremities, 95851
    Hand, 95852
    Trunk, 97530
THBR, 84479
Therapeutic Activities
  Music
    Per 15 Minutes, 97530
Therapies
  Exercise, 97110-97113
  Occupational
    Evaluation, 97003-97004
Thermocoagulation, 17260-17276
Thiersch Operation
  Pinch Graft, 15050
Thompson Test
  Smear and Stain, Routine, 87205
  Urinalysis, Glass Test, 81020
Thoracic
  Vertebra
    Corpectomy, 63085-63101,
      63103
    Intraspinal Lesion,
      63301-63302,
      63305-63306, 63308
    Decompression, 63055,
      63057-63066
    Discectomy, 63077-63078
    Excision for Lesion, 22101,
      22112
    Injection Procedure
      for Discography, 62291
    Laminectomy, 63003, 63016,
      63046, 63048
Thorax
  Biopsy, 21550
  Tumor, 21552-21554, 21558
Thrombocyte (Platelet)
  Aggregation, 85576
  Count, 85008
Thromboplastin
  Partial Time, 85730-85732
Thumb
  Amputation, 26910-26952
  Arthrodesis
    Carpometacarpal Joint,
      26841-26842
  Dislocation
    with Fracture, 26645-26650
    Open Treatment, 26665
    with Manipulation, 26641
  Fracture
    with Dislocation, 26645-26650
    Open Treatment, 26665
  Fusion
    in Opposition, 26820
  Reconstruction
    from Finger, 26550
    Opponensplasty, 26490-26496
  Repair
    Muscle, 26508
    Muscle Transfer, 26494
    Tendon Transfer, 26510
  Replantation, 20824-20827
  Sesamoidectomy, 26185
Thyrocalcitonin, 82308
Thyroid Hormone Binding Ratio, 84479
Thyroid Hormone Uptake, 84479
Thyroid Stimulating Hormone (TSH), 84443
Thyroid Stimulating Immune Globulins (TSI), 84445
Thyrotropin Stimulating Immunoglobulins, 84445

Thyroxine
  Free, 84439
  Neonatal, 84437
  Total, 84436
  True, 84436
Thyroxine Binding Globulin, 84442
Time
  Bleeding, 85002
  Prothrombin, 85610-85611
Tissue
  Closure
    Arm, Arms
      Complex, 13120-13122
      Intermediate, 12031-12037
      Layered, 12031-12037
      Simple, 12001-12007
      Superficial, 12001-12007
    Axilla, Axillae
      Complex, 13131-13133
      Intermediate, 12031-12037
      Layered, 12031-12037
      Simple, 12001-12007
      Superficial, 12001-12007
    Back
      Intermediate, 12031-12037
      Layered, 12031-12037
      Simple, 12001-12007
      Superficial, 12001-12007
    Chest
      Intermediate, 12031-12037
      Layered, 12031-12037
      Simple, 12001-12007
      Superficial, 12001-12007
    Extremity, Extremities
      Complex/Intermediate,
        12031-12037
      Layered, 12031-12037
      Simple, 12001-12007
      Superficial, 12001-12007
    Finger, Fingers
      Complex, 13131-13133
      Intermediate, 12041-12047
      Layered, 12041-12047
      Simple, 12001-12007
      Superficial, 12001-12007
    Forearm, Forearms
      Complex, 13120-13122
      Intermediate, 12031-12037
      Layered, 12031-12037
      Simple, 12001-12007
      Superficial, 12001-12007
    Hand, Hands
      Complex, 13131-13133
      Intermediate, 12041-12047
      Layered, 12041-12047
      Simple, 12001-12007
      Superficial, 12001-12007
    Lower
      Arm, Arms
        Complex, 13120-13122
        Intermediate, 12031-12037
        Layered, 12031-12037
        Simple, 12001-12007
        Superficial, 12001-12007
    Neck
      Complex, 13131-13133
      Intermediate, 12041-12047
      Layered, 12041-12047
      Simple, 12001-12007
      Superficial, 12001-12007
    Palm, Palms
      Complex, 13131-13133
      Intermediate, 12041-12047
      Layered, 12041-12047
      Simple, 12001-12007
      Superficial, 12001-12007
    Trunk
      Intermediate, 12031-12037
      Layered, 12031-12037
      Simple, 12001-12007
      Superficial, 12001-12007
    Upper
      Arm, Arms
        Complex, 13120-13122
        Intermediate, 12031-12037
        Layered, 12031-12037
        Simple, 12001-12007
        Superficial, 12001-12007

Tissue—continued
  Closure—continued
    Upper—continued
      Extremity
        Complex, 13120-13122
        Intermediate, 12031-12037
        Layered, 12031-12037
        Simple, 12001-12007
        Superficial, 12001-12007
  Culture
    Skin Grafts, 15050-15101,
      15120-15121
  Enzyme Activity, 82657
  Grafts
    Harvesting, 20926
  Soft
    Abscess, 20005
  Subcutaneous Tissue
    Arm, Arms
      Complex, 13120-13122
      Intermediate, 12031-12037
      Layered, 12031-12037
      Simple, 12001-12007
      Superficial, 12001-12007
    Axilla, Axillae
      Complex, 13131-13133
      Intermediate, 12031-12037
      Layered, 12031-12037
      Simple, 12001-12007
      Superficial, 12001-12007
    Back
      Intermediate, 12031-12037
      Layered, 12031-12037
      Simple, 12001-12007
      Superficial, 12001-12007
    Chest
      Intermediate, 12031-12037
      Layered, 12031-12037
      Simple, 12001-12007
      Superficial, 12001-12007
    Extremity, Extremities
      Complex/Intermediate,
        12031-12037
      Layered, 12031-12037
      Simple, 12001-12007
      Superficial, 12001-12007
    Finger, Fingers
      Complex, 13131-13133
      Intermediate, 12041-12047
      Layered, 12041-12047
      Simple, 12001-12007
      Superficial, 12001-12007
    Forearm, Forearms
      Complex, 13120-13122
      Intermediate, 12031-12037
      Layered, 12031-12037
      Simple, 12001-12007
      Superficial, 12001-12007
    Hand, Hands
      Complex, 13131-13133
      Intermediate, 12041-12047
      Layered, 12041-12047
      Simple, 12001-12007
      Superficial, 12001-12007
    Lower
      Arm, Arms
        Complex, 13120-13122
        Intermediate, 12031-12037
        Layered, 12031-12037
        Simple, 12001-12007
        Superficial, 12001-12007
    Neck
      Complex, 13131-13133
      Intermediate, 12041-12047
      Layered, 12041-12047
      Simple, 12001-12007
      Superficial, 12001-12007
    Palm, Palms
      Complex, 13131-13133
      Intermediate, 12041-12047
      Layered, 12041-12047
      Simple, 12001-12007
      Superficial, 12001-12007
    Trunk
      Intermediate, 12031-12037
      Layered, 12031-12037
      Simple, 12001-12007
      Superficial, 12001-12007

Tissue—continued
  Subcutaneous Tissue—continued
    Upper
      Arm, Arms
        Complex, 13120-13122
        Intermediate, 12031-12037
        Layered, 12031-12037
        Simple, 12001-12007
        Superficial, 12001-12007
      Extremity
        Complex, 13120-13122
        Intermediate, 12031-12037
        Layered, 12031-12037
        Simple, 12001-12007
        Superficial, 12001-12007
  Transfer
    Adjacent
      Skin, 14000-14041, 14301-14350
    Finger Flap, 14350
    Toe Flap, 14350
Tissue Factor
  Partial Time, 85730-85732
Tissue Transfer
  Adjacent
    Arms, 14020-14021
    Axillae, 14040-14041
    Finger, 14350
    Hand, 14040-14041
    Limbs, 14020-14021
    Neck, 14040-14041
    Skin, 14000-14041, 14301-14350
    Trunk, 14000-14001
  Finger Flap, 14350
  Toe Flap, 14350
TMJ
  Arthrocentesis, 20605
TNA (Total Nail Avulsion), 11730-11732
Tobramycin, 80200
  Assay, 80200
Tolerance Test(s)
  Glucagon, 82946
  Heparin–Protamine, 85530
  Insulin, 80435
Tomography, Computed
  Head, 70496
Total
  Elbow Replacement, 24363
Toxin, Botulinum
  Chemodenervation
    Extremity Muscle, 64614
    Trunk Muscle, 64614
Traction Therapy
  Manual, 97140
  Mechanical, 97012
Training
  Activities of Daily Living, 97535
  Community
    Work Reintegration, 97537
  Home Management, 97535
  Management
    Propulsion, 97542
  Orthotics, 97760
  Prosthetics, 97761
  Self Care, 97535
  Sensory Integration, 97533
  Wheelchair Management
    Propulsion, 97542
Trans–Scaphoperilunar
  Fracture
    Dislocation, 25680-25685
      Closed Treatment, 25680
      Open Treatment, 25685
Transaminase
  Glutamic Oxaloacetic, 84450
  Glutamic Pyruvic, 84460
Transection
  Nerve, 64772
Transfer
  Adjacent Tissue, 14000-14041, 14301-14350
  Finger Position, 26555
  Toe Joint, 26556
  Toe to Hand, 26551-26554, 26556

Transferase
  Aspartate Amino, 84450
  Glutamic Oxaloacetic, 84450
Transferrin, 84466
Transplant
  Bone
    Allograft, Spine, 20930-20931
    Autograft, Spine, 20936-20938
Transplantation
  Heterologous
    Skin, 15400-15401
  Muscle, 15732-15736, 15756
  Tissue, Harvesting, 20926
Transposition
  Nerve, 64718-64721
  Peripheral Nerve
    Major, 64856
Trapezium
  Arthroplasty
    with Implant, 25445
Triacylglycerol, 84478
Triangular Cartilage
  Repair with Fracture
    Radial shaft, 25526
Triangular Fibrocartilage
  Excision, 29846
Trichrome Stain, 88313
Trigger Finger Repair, 26055
Trigger Point
  Injection
    One or Two Muscle Groups, 20552
    Two or More Muscle Groups, 20553
Triglycerides, 84478
Triiodothyronine
  Resin Uptake, 84479
Trioxopurine, 84550-84560
Trocar Biopsy
  Bone Marrow, 38221
Trunk
  Skin Graft
    Muscle, Myocutaneous, or Fasciocutaneous Flaps, 15734
    Split, 15100-15101
  Tissue Transfer, Adjacent, 14000
Tsalicylate Intoxication, 80196
TSH, 84443
TSI, 84445
TT-4, 84436
Tubercle Bacilli
  Culture, 87116
Tuberculosis
  Culture, 87116
Tumor
  Arm, Lower, 24152, 25071-25078
  Arm, Upper, 23220, 24071-24079, 24110-24126, 24150
  Back, 21931-21933, 21936
  Carpal, 25130-25136
  Clavicle
    Excision, 23140, 23200
      with Allograft, 23146
      with Autograft, 23145
  Elbow, 24071-24073, 24079, 24110-24126, 24152
  Finger
    Excision, 26111-26117
  Flank, 21930-21936
  Forearm
    Radical Resection, 25077
  Hand, 26111-26117
  Humerus, 24150
  Metacarpal, 26200-26205, 26250
  Neck, 21552-21554, 21558
  Olecranon Process, 24071-24077
  Phalanges
    Finger, 26210-26215, 26260-26262
  Radius, 25120-25126, 25170
    Excision, 24120
      with Allograft, 24126
      with Autograft, 24125
  Scapula, 23140
    Excision, 23140, 23210
      with Allograft, 23146
      with Autograft, 23145
  Shoulder, 23071-23073, 23078

Tumor—continued
  Soft Tissue
    Elbow
      Excision, 24075
    Finger
      Excision, 26115
    Forearm
      Radical Resection, 25077
    Hand
      Excision, 26115
  Thorax, 21552-21554, 21558
  Ulna, 25120-25126, 25170
    Excision, 24120
      with Allograft
        Excision, 24126
      with Autograft
        Excision, 24125
  Vertebra
    Additional Segment
      Excision, 22103, 22116
    Cervical
      Excision, 22100
    Lumbar, 22102
    Thoracic
      Excision, 22101
  Wrist, 25071-25078
Turnbuckle Jacket, 29020-29025
  Removal, 29715

U

Ulcer
  Pinch Graft, 15050
  Pressure, 15931-15937
Ulna
  Arthrodesis
    Radioulnar Joint
      with Resection, 25830
  Arthroplasty
    with Implant, 25442
  Centralization of Wrist, 25335
  Craterization, 24147, 25150
  Cyst
    Excision, 24125-24126, 25120-25126
  Diaphysectomy, 24147, 25150-25151
  Excision, 24147
    Abscess, 24138
    Complete, 25240
    Partial, 25145-25151, 25240
  Fracture, 25605
    Closed Treatment, 25530-25535
    Olecranon, 24670-24675
    Open Treatment, 24685
    Open Treatment, 25545
    Shaft, 25530-25545
      Open Treatment, 25574
    Styloid Process
      Closed Treatment, 25650
      Open Treatment, 25652
      Percutaneous Fixation, 25651
    with Dislocation
      Closed Treatment, 24620
      Open Treatment, 24635
    with Manipulation, 25535
    with Radius, 25560-25565
      Open Treatment, 25575
    without Manipulation, 25530
  Incision and Drainage, 25035
  Osteoplasty, 25390-25393
  Prophylactic Treatment, 25491-25492
  Reconstruction
    Radioulnar, 25337
  Repair, 25400, 25415
    Epiphyseal Arrest, 25450-25455
    Osteotomy, 25360, 25370-25375
      and Radius, 25365
    with Graft, 25405, 25420-25426
    Malunion or Nonunion, 25400, 25415
  Saucerization, 24147, 25150, 25151
  Sequestrectomy, 24138, 25145
  Tumor
    Cyst, 24120

Ulna—continued
  Tumor—continued
    Excision, 24125-24126, 25120-25126, 25170
Ulnar Nerve
  Decompression, 64718
  Neuroplasty, 64718-64719
  Reconstruction, 64718-64719
  Release, 64718-64719
  Repair
    Suture
      Motor, 64836
  Transposition, 64718-64719
Ultrasound
  Arm, 76881-76882
  Bone Density Study, 76977
  Computer Aided Surgical Navigation
    Intraoperative, 0054T-0055T
  Extremity, 76881-76882
  for Physical Therapy, 97035
  Guidance
    Injection Facet Joint, 0213T-0218T
    Needle Biopsy, 76942
    Thoracentesis, 76942
  Intraoperative, 76998
  Leg, 76881-76882
  Physical Therapy, 97035
  Stimulation to Aid Bone Healing, 20979
Ultraviolet Light Therapy
  for Physical Medicine, 97028
Unlisted Services or Procedures
  Physical Therapy, 97139
Unna Paste Boot
  Removal, 29700
Urea Nitrogen, 84525
  Blood, 84520-84525
  Clearance, 84545
  Quantitative, 84520
  Semiquantitative, 84525
  Urine, 84540
Uric Acid
  Blood, 84550
  Other Source, 84560
  Urine, 84560
Urinalysis, 81000-81025
Urine
  Albumin, 82042
  Blood, 81000-81005
  Tests, 81000-81025
Urine Sensitivity Test, 87181-87188
Urothromboplastin
  Partial Time, 85730-85732

V

V-Y Plasty
  Skin, Adjacent Tissue Transfer, 14000-14041, 14301-14350
Valentine's Test
  Urinalysis, Glass Test, 81020
Vancomycin
  Assay, 80202
Vascular Flow Check, Graft, 15860
Vascular Malformation
  Finger
    Excision, 26115
  Hand
    Excision, 26115
Vascular Studies
  Artery Studies
    Extremities, 93922-93923
    Lower Extremity, 93922-93923
    Upper Extremity, 93930-93931
  Venous Studies
    Extremities, 93965-93971
Vasopneumatic Device Therapy, 97016
Vasopressin, 84588
Vein
  Extremity
    Non-Invasive Studies, 93965-93971
Velpeau Cast, 29058
Venography
  Thoracic, 22520-22522

Vertebra
  Additional Segment
    Excision, 22103, 22116
  Arthrodesis
    Anterior, 22548-22585
    Exploration, 22830
    Lateral Extracavitary,
      22532-22534
    Posterior, 22590-22802
    Spinal Deformity
      Anterior Approach,
        22808-22812
      Posterior Approach,
        22800-22804
  Arthroplasty, 0202T
  Cervical
    Artificial Disc, 22864
    Excision for Tumor, 22100,
      22110
    Fracture, 23675-23680
  Fracture
    Dislocation
      Additional Segment
        Open Treatment, 22328
      Cervical
        Open Treatment, 22326
      Lumbar
        Open Treatment, 22325
      Thoracic
        Open Treatment, 22327
  Kyphectomy, 22818-22819
  Lumbar
    Artificial Disc, 22865
    Distraction Device, 0171T-0172T
    Excision for Tumor, 22102,
      22114
  Osteoplasty
    CT Scan, 72292
    Fluoroscopy, 72291
    Lumbar, 22521-22522
    Thoracic, 22520-22522
  Osteotomy
    Additional Segment
      Anterior Approach, 22226
      Posterior/Posterolateral
        Approach, 22216
    Cervical
      Anterior Approach, 22220
      Posterior/Posterolateral
        Approach, 22210
    Lumbar
      Anterior Approach, 22224
      Posterior/Posterolateral
        Approach, 22214
    Thoracic
      Anterior Approach, 22222
      Posterior/Posterolateral
        Approach, 22212
  Thoracic
    Excision for Tumor, 22101,
      22112

Vertebrae
  Arthrodesis
    Anterior, 22548-22585
    Lateral Extracavitary,
      22532-22534
  Spinal Deformity, 22818-22819

Vertebral Body
  Biopsy, 20250-20251
  Excision
    Decompression, 63081-63091
    Lesion, 63300-63308
  Fracture
    Dislocation
      Closed Treatment, 22305
        without Manipulation,
          22310
  Kyphectomy, 22818-22819

Vertebral Corpectomy, 63081-63199,
  63295-63308

Vertebral Fracture
  Closed Treatment
    with Manipulation, Casting,
      and/or Bracing, 22315
    without Manipulation, 22310
  Open Treatment
    Additional Segment, 22328
    Cervical, 22326

Vertebral Fracture—continued
  Open Treatment—continued
    Lumbar, 22325
    Posterior, 22325-22327
    Thoracic, 22327

Vertebral Process
  Fracture
    Closed Treatment, 22305

Very Low Density Lipoprotein, 83719

Vitamin
  A, 84590
  D, 82306, 82652
  K, 84597
  Dependent Bone Protein, 83937

VLDL, 83719

Volkman Contracture, 25315-25316

W

W-Plasty
  Skin Surgery, Adjacent Tissue
    Transfer, 14000-14041,
    14301-14350

WBC, 85007, 85009, 85025, 85048,
  85540

Westergren Test
  Sedimentation Rate, Blood Cell,
    85651-85652

Western Blot
  Protein, 84181-84182

Wheelchair Management
  Propulsion
    Training, 97542

Whirlpool Therapy, 97022

White Blood Cell
  Alkaline Phosphatase, 85540
  Count, 85048
  Differential, 85007, 85009

Wick Catheter Technique, 20950

Wintrobe Test
  Sedimentation Rate, Blood Cell,
    85651-85652

Wire
  Insertion
    Removal
      Skeletal Traction, 20650

Wiring
  Prophylactic Treatment
    Humerus, 24498

Work Hardening, 97545-97546

Work Reintegration, 97545-97546

Wound
  Debridement
    Non–Selective, 97602
    Selective, 97597-97598
  Dehiscence
    Repair
      Secondary
        Skin and subcutaneous tis-
          sue
          Complex, 13160
          Complicated, 13160
          Extensive, 13160
        Skin and subcutaneous tissue
          Simple, 12020
            with packing, 12021
          Superficial, 12020
            with packing, 12021
    Suture
      Secondary
        Skin and subcutaneous tis-
          sue
          Complex, 13160
          Complicated, 13160
          Extensive, 13160
        Skin and subcutaneous tissue
          Simple, 12020
            with packing, 12021
          Superficial, 12020
            with packing, 12021
  Exploration
    Penetrating
      Abdomen/Flank/Back, 20102
      Extremity, 20103

Wound—continued
  Exploration—continued
    Penetrating Trauma,
      20102-20103
  Negative Pressure Therapy,
    97605-97606
  Repair
    Skin
      Complex, 13120-13133,
        13160
      Intermediate, 12031-12047
      Simple, 12001-12007,
        12020-12021
  Secondary
    Skin and subcutaneous tissue
      Complex, 13160
      Complicated, 13160
      Extensive, 13160
      Simple, 12020
      Simple with packing, 12021
      Superficial, 12020
        with packing, 12021

Wrist
  Abscess, 25028
  Arthrocentesis, 20605
  Arthrodesis, 25800
    with Graft, 25810
    with Sliding Graft, 25805
  Arthrography, 73115
  Arthroplasty, 25332, 25443, 25447
    Revision, 25449
    Total Replacement, 25446
      with Implant, 25441-25442,
        25444-25445
  Arthroscopy
    Diagnostic, 29840
    Surgical, 29843-29848
  Arthrotomy, 25040, 25100-25105
    for Repair, 25107
  Biopsy, 25065-25066, 25100-25101
  Bursa
    Excision, 25115-25116
    Incision and Drainage, 25031
  Capsule
    Incision, 25085
  Cast, 29085
  Cyst, 25130-25136
  Decompression, 25020-25023
  Disarticulation, 25920
    Reamputation, 25924
    Revision, 25922
  Dislocation
    Closed Treatment, 25660
    Intercarpal, 25660
      Open Treatment, 25670
    Open Treatment, 25660-25670,
      25676
    Percutaneous Fixation, 25671
    Radiocarpal, 25660
      Open Treatment, 25670
    Radioulnar
      Closed Treatment, 25675
      Percutaneous Fixation, 25671
    with Fracture
      Closed Treatment, 25680
      Open Treatment, 25685
    with Manipulation, 25259,
      25660, 25675
  Excision
    Carpal, 25210-25215
    Cartilage, 25107
    Tendon Sheath, 25115-25116
    Tumor, 25071-25078
  Exploration, 25040, 25101
  Fasciotomy, 25020-25025
  Fracture, 25645
    Closed Treatment, 25622, 25630
    Open Treatment, 25628
    with Dislocation, 25680-25685
    with Manipulation, 25259,
      25624, 25635
  Ganglion Cyst
    Excision, 25111-25112
  Hematoma, 25028
  Incision, 25040, 25100-25105
    Tendon Sheath, 25000-25001

Wrist—continued
  Injection
    Carpal Tunnel
      Therapeutic, 20526
    X–ray, 25246
  Lesion
    Excision, 25110
    Tendon Sheath, 25000
  Magnetic Resonance Imaging, 73221
  Reconstruction
    Capsulectomy, 25320
    Capsulorrhaphy, 25320
    Carpal Bone, 25394, 25430
    Realign, 25335
  Removal
    Foreign Body, 25040, 25101,
      25248
    Implant, 25449
    Loose Body, 25101
    Prosthesis, 25250-25251
  Repair, 25447
    Bone, 25440
    Carpal Bone, 25431
    Muscle, 25260, 25270
      Secondary, 25263-25265,
        25272-25274
    Tendon, 25260, 25270,
      25280-25316
      Secondary, 25263-25265,
        25272-25274
    Tendon Sheath, 25275
  Strapping, 29260
  Synovium
    Excision, 25105, 25115-25119
  Tendon
    Excision, 25109
  Tendon Sheath
    Excision, 25115-25116
  Tenodesis, 25300-25301
  Tenotomy, 25290
  X-ray, 73100-73110
    with Contrast, 73115

X

X-ray
  Acromioclavicular Joint, 73050
  Arm, Lower, 73090
  Arm, Upper, 73092
  Bone
    Dual Energy Absorptiometry,
      77080-77082
    Osseous Survey, 77075-77076
      Complete, 77075
      Infant, 77076
    Ultrasound, 76977
  Clavicle, 73000
  Coccyx, 72220
  Elbow, 73070-73080
  Fingers, 73140
  Hand, 73120-73130
  Humerus, 73060
  Joint
    Stress Views, 77071
  Neck, 70360
  Sacrum, 72220
  Scapula, 73010
  Shoulder, 73020-73030, 73050
  Spine, 72020, 72090
    Cervical, 72040-72052
    Lumbosacral, 72100-72120
    Thoracic, 72070-72074
    Thoracolumbar, 72080
    Total, 72010
  Standing
    Spine, 72069
  with Contrast
    Brain, 70010
    Elbow, 73085
    Intervertebral Disc
      Cervical, 72285
      Lumbar, 72295
      Thoracic, 72285
    Joint
      Stress Views, 77071
    Shoulder, 73040

X-ray—*continued*
  with Contrast—*continued*
    Spine
      Cervical, 72240
      Lumbosacral, 72265
      Thoracic, 72255
      Total, 72270
    Wrist, 73115
  Wrist, 73100-73110

Xenograft, 15400-15401
Xenotransplantation
  Skin, 15400-15401

Z

Z-Plasty, 26121-26125
Zinc, 84630